D1275269

# Handbook of Psychooncology

# Handbook of Psychooncology

---

## PSYCHOLOGICAL CARE OF
## THE PATIENT WITH CANCER

Edited by

### Jimmie C. Holland, M. D.

*Chief, Psychiatry Service*
*Memorial Sloan-Kettering Cancer Center*
*and*
*Professor, Department of Psychiatry*
*Cornell University Medical College*

### Julia H. Rowland, Ph.D.

*Clinical Assistant Psychologist*
*Psychiatry Service*
*Memorial Sloan-Kettering Cancer Center*
*and*
*Instructor of Psychology in Psychiatry*
*Department of Psychiatry*
*Cornell University Medical College*

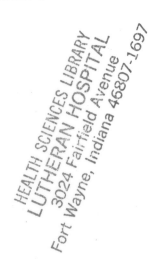
New York    Oxford
OXFORD UNIVERSITY PRESS
1989

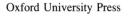
Oxford University Press

Oxford   New York   Toronto
Delhi   Bombay   Calcutta   Madras   Karachi
Petaling Jaya   Singapore   Hong Kong   Tokyo
Nairobi   Dar es Salaam   Cape Town
Melbourne   Auckland

and associated companies in
Berlin   Ibadan

Published by Oxford University Press, Inc.,
200 Madison Avenue, New York, New York 10016

Oxford is a registered trademark of Oxford University Press

Library of Congress Cataloging-in-Publication Data
Handbook of psychooncology : psychological care of the patient with
cancer / edited by Jimmie C. Holland and Julia H. Rowland.
p. cm.   Includes bibliographies and index.
ISBN 0-19-504308-1
1. Cancer—Psychological aspects.
2. Cancer—Patients—Mental health.
I. Holland, Jimmie C.   II. Rowland, Julia Howe.
[DNLM: 1. Neoplasms—psychology.   QZ 200 H235]
RC262.H285   1989
616.99′4′0019—dc20
DNLM/DLC   for Library of Congress   89-8603   CIP

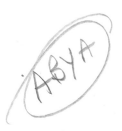

2 4 6 8 9 7 5 3 1

Printed in the United States of America
on acid-free paper

# Foreword

Thanks to a wide range of technical advances achieved over the past 30 years in surgery, radiation biology, and chemotherapy, the treatment of cancer has been substantially transformed in many different types of neoplasia. Of course, these new technologies are most effective in patients whose cancers are detected early on, and spectacularly effective in the neoplasms of early childhood. The more common solid tumors of later life, for example those affecting the lung, breast, colon, and prostate, are considerably less vulnerable to the new technologies, but even here there are enough examples of cure or prolonged survival to warrant the most intensive therapeutic efforts, whatever the side effects.

As a regrettable but seemingly unavoidable result, the treatment of cancer has come to be an extremely technical undertaking, based almost entirely within the busiest and most active wards of the hospital, and involving the strenuous efforts of highly specialized professionals, each taking his or her responsibility for a share of the patient's problem, but sometimes working at a rather impersonal distance from the patient as an individual. To many patients, stunned by the diagnosis, suffering numerous losses and discomforts, moved from place to place for one procedure after another, the experience is bewildering and frightening; at worst, it is like being trapped in the workings of a huge piece of complicated machinery.

It is only in quite recent years that oncologists in general have begun to confront squarely the emotional impact of these ordeals and the fact that emotional states play a large role in the tolerability of treatment and, perhaps, in the outcome as well.

Within less than a decade, the term psychooncology, viewed at first with deep suspicion by most oncologists, has at last emerged as a respectable field for both application and research. In my own view,

having passed through both stages as a skeptical clinician and administrator, the appearance on the scene of psychiatrists and experimental psychologists has so vastly improved the lot of cancer patients as to make these new professionals indispensable.

There could not be a better time than now for the presentation of a volume with the scope and depth of this one. The clinical oncologists of all stripes have, for too long, overlooked or ignored the psychological factors that may, for all we know at present, play a surprisingly large role in individual susceptibility to neoplasia. They are certainly influential in affecting the course of treatment, the adaptation to the illness, and hence, in some ways, not all of which are yet understood, affect the outcome of treatment. These matters are dealt with in various chapters of the book, with abundant citations and illustrations taken from clinical experience, and with balance and skepticism wherever needed (which, as in any new young field, is often). In addition, the entire spectrum of psychological factors involved in cancer risk, treatment, and survival is addressed in this book, providing both practical detail and theory.

The chapter on psychoneuroimmunology was of special interest to me. When I first encountered the term some years back, I was appalled until confronted by the impressive data from the animal research laboratories of Ader, Bovbjerg, and others that underpinned the term. The linkage between the central nervous system and the immunologic apparatus has now assumed the status of a complex, conjoined information system, feedback loops and all, and nothing could be more exciting than pursuing these concepts for their future implications.

But now the hazard is for overextension of the data at hand, overapplication of conceivable uses of the new information, and even the introduction of pure magic. One has only to glance at the paperback stands in airports to see the books claiming knowledge of do-it-yourself techniques for instructing your lymphocytes to prevent or cure cancer, crowding the earlier books on curing by strange diets or by changing one's personality overnight off the shelves. It is, therefore, a great satisfaction to see this new field of proper science handled, as in this book, with such care for the available facts of the matter and, at the same time, with such high, but restrained hopes for the scientific future.

Lewis Thomas, M.D.
*Scholar-in-Residence*
*Cornell University Medical College*
*President Emeritus*
*Memorial Sloan-Kettering Cancer Center*

# Preface

The idea of this book grew out of the awareness of the need for a better answer to the frequent query: "Where can I learn about the psychological problems of cancer patients and how to treat them?" This was asked often of us in the early years of the Psychiatric Service, which was established in 1977, at Memorial Sloan-Kettering Cancer Center. There were many books and journals that an interested reader could turn to, but no summary of the broad range of issues that one needed to know to be informed was available. We began to conceive of a small book that would serve as an introduction to this emerging area of oncology. Using a developmental model, we sought to understand and to describe the patients' life stage, the disruptions caused by cancer at that stage, and the interventions needed to promote adaptation. During the early 1980s, family obligations for us both led to procrastination. Meanwhile, an explosion of information and research made it clear that the simple answer we hoped to provide was not so simple after all. In fact, by the mid-1980s, psychooncology had become a respectable subspecialty of oncology and psychiatry with its own body of information.

It was at this point that we began to conceive of an edited book with the major contributors from our own group that, by then, was nearing a decade of experience. We decided to provide a far broader book where both oncologic and mental health professionals, or students in either field, could find information about the range of psychiatric and psychological issues in oncology. The handbook that resulted attempts to put in context the cultural, psychological, and medical aspects that contribute to adaptation, the special problems posed by childhood or older age, by treatment modality, and special problems, such as pain and central nervous system complications. In addition, it reviews the problems of families, home care, staff, ethical, and research problems, and offers treatment principles to be used in providing psychotherapy and behavioral and pharmacologic interventions.

We also became aware that, by 1985, we had learned most from our patients with cancer at Memorial Sloan-Kettering, the *true* experts, who were willing to share their feelings and reactions with us. Robert Fisher, founding Patient Volunteer Counselor of the Patient Volunteer Program, was critically important to our work. Bob inspired us through his courage, his dedication to helping others, and his extraordinary insights into coping with leukemia.

Several members of the Psychiatric Service also became experts in specific areas, such as psychotherapy, family issues, sex counseling, and problems of patients with specific tumors. Expertise of other staff and a few individuals outside the institution were added to provide a comprehensive overview of psychooncology.

We wish to particularly recognize Robert Fisher, who inspired and helped us; the members of the Psychiatric Service, who toiled long and hard to offer critiques of the effort and to provide state-of-the-art overviews of areas, some of which required extensive effort; to members of the Neurology Department, Pain Service, Social Work Department, and Chaplaincy Service, who provided special areas of information; to the individuals outside Memorial Sloan-Kettering who participated; and especially to our families who tolerated the stresses.

We are particularly grateful to Dr. Lewis Thomas in his role 12 years ago as President of the Memorial Sloan-Kettering Cancer Center, who was instrumental in establishing the Psychiatry Service at Memorial Sloan-Kettering, and without whom the psychiatric activities on which this book is based would not have happened.

*New York*　　　　　　　　　　　　　　　　　　J.C.H.
*March 1989*　　　　　　　　　　　　　　　　　J.H.R.

# Contents

# Contributors

**Margaret Adams-Greenly, A.C.S.W.**
Assistant Director, Department of Social Work, Memorial Sloan-Kettering Cancer Center, New York, New York

**Sarah Auchincloss, M.D.**
Clinical Assistant Attending Psychiatrist, Psychiatry Service, Department of Neurology, Memorial Sloan-Kettering Cancer Center; Assistant Professor, Department of Psychiatry, Cornell University Medical College, New York, New York

**Lucanne Bailey, C.M.T.**
Music Therapist (Private Practice), Woodstock, New York

**Dana Bovbjerg, Ph.D.**
Assistant Professor, Department of Medicine, Cornell University Medical College, New York, New York

**William Breitbart, M.D.**
Assistant Attending Psychiatrist, Psychiatry Service, Department of Neurology, Memorial Sloan-Kettering Cancer Center; Assistant Professor, Department of Psychiatry, Cornell University Medical College, New York, New York

**David Cella, Ph.D.**
Assistant Professor, Department of Psychology and Social Sciences and Department of Internal Medicine, Rush Medical College; Director of Psychological Services and Research, Rush Cancer Center, Rush-Presbyterian-St. Luke's Medical Center, Chicago, Illinois

**Harvey Chochinov, M.D.**
Assistant Professor of Psychiatry, Department of Psychiatry, University of Manitoba, Winnipeg, Canada; Psychiatric Consultant, Manitoba Cancer Treatment and Research Foundation, Winnipeg, Canada

**Grace Christ, M.A., A.C.S.W.**
Director, Department of Social Work, Memorial Sloan-Kettering Cancer Center, New York, New York

**Kenneth H. Cohn, M.D.**
Assistant Professor, Department of Surgery, State University of New York Health Science Center at Brooklyn, Brooklyn, New York

**Nessa Coyle, R.N., M.S.**
Director, Supportive Care Program, Pain Service, Department of Neurology, Memorial Sloan-Kettering Cancer Center, New York, New York

**Carol Farkas, R.N., M.P.H.**
Director, Home Care Program, Psychiatry Service, Department of Neurology, Memorial Sloan-Kettering Cancer Center, New York, New York

**Stewart B. Fleishman, M.D.**
Attending Psychiatrist, Division of Psychiatric Oncology, Long Island Jewish Medical Center; Assistant Professor of Psychiatry, City University of New York Medical School, New York, New York

**Kathleen Foley, M.D.**
Chief, Pain Service, Attending Neurologist, Department of Neurology, Memorial Sloan-Kettering Cancer Center; Associate Professor, Department of Neurology, Cornell University Medical College, New York, New York

**Alice Furman, B.A.**
Medical Student, Mount Sinai School of Medicine, New York, New York

**Natalie Geary, B.A.**
Medical Student, Johns Hopkins School of Medicine, Baltimore, Maryland

**Reverend George Handzo**
Chaplain, Chaplaincy Service, Memorial Sloan-Kettering Cancer Center, New York, New York

**Phyllis Hansell, Ed.D., R.N.**
Professor and Director of Nursing Research, Department of Nursing, Seton Hall University, South Orange, New Jersey

**Eric Heiligenstein, M.D.**
Assistant Attending Psychiatrist, Psychiatry Service, Department of Neurology and Department of Pediatrics, Memorial Sloan-Kettering Cancer Center; Assistant Professor, Department of Psychiatry, Cornell University Medical College, New York, New York

**Jimmie C. Holland, M.D.**
Chief and Attending Psychiatrist, Psychiatry Service, Department of Neurology, Memorial Sloan-Kettering Cancer Center; Professor, Department of Psychiatry, Cornell University Medical Center, New York, New York

**Paul Jacobsen, Ph.D.**
Assistant Attending Psychologist, Psychiatry Service, Department of Neurology, Memorial Sloan-Kettering Cancer Center; Assistant Professor, Department of Psychiatry, Cornell University Medical College, New York, New York

**Kathryn M. Kash, R.N., Ph.D.**
Clinical Assistant Psychologist, Psychiatry Service, Department of Neurology, Memorial Sloan-Kettering Cancer Center, New York, New York

**Marguerite S. Lederberg, M.D.**
Associate Attending Psychiatrist, Psychiatry Service, Department of Neurology, Memorial Sloan-Kettering Cancer Center; Clinical Associate Professor of Psychiatry, Cornell University Medical College, New York, New York; Associate Attending Psychiatrist, The New York Hospital, New York, New York

**Lynna M. Lesko, M.D., Ph.D.**
Assistant Attending Psychiatrist, Psychiatry Service, Department of Neurology, Memorial Sloan-Kettering Cancer Center; Assistant Professor, Department of Psychiatry, Cornell University Medical College, New York, New York

**Matthew Loscalzo, A.C.S.W.**
Assistant Director, Department of Social Work, Memorial Sloan-Kettering Cancer Center, New York, New York

**Mary Jane Massie, M.D.**
Associate Attending Psychiatrist, Psychiatry Service, Department of Neurology, Memorial Sloan-Kettering Cancer Center; Associate Clinical Professor, Cornell University Medical College, New York, New York

**Rene Mastrovito, M.D.**
Attending Psychiatrist, Psychiatry Service, Department of Neurology, Memorial Sloan-Kettering Cancer Center; Clinical Professor of Psychiatry, Cornell University Medical College, New York, New York

**Sr. Rosemary T. Moynihan, A.C.S.W.**
Assistant Director, Department of Social Work, Memorial Sloan-Kettering Cancer Center, New York, New York

**Lisa Parsonnet, M.S., A.C.S.W.**
Administrative Supervisor, Department of Social Work, Memorial Sloan-Kettering Cancer Center, New York, New York

**Roy A. Patchell, M.D.**
Assistant Professor, Departments of Neurology and Neurosurgery, University of Kentucky College of Medicine, Lexington, Kentucky

**Betty Pfefferbaum, M.D.**
Associate Professor, Department of Psychiatry and Behavioral Sciences and Department of Pediatrics, University of Texas Medical School; Adjunct Associate Professor, Department of Pediatrics (Psychiatry), University of Texas, M.D. Anderson Cancer Center, Houston, Texas

**Russell Portenoy, M.D.**
Assistant Attending Neurologist, Pain Service, Department of Neurology, Memorial Sloan-Kettering Cancer Center; Assistant Professor, Department of Neurology, Cornell University Medical College, New York, New York

**Jerome B. Posner, M.D.**
Chairman and Attending Neurologist, Department of Neurology, Memorial Sloan-Kettering Cancer Center; Professor and Vice-Chairman, Department of Neurology, Cornell University Medical College, New York, New York

**Douglas Rait, Ph.D.**
Director, Family Therapy Program, Department of Psychiatry, Beth Israel Medical Center, New York, New York; Instructor, Department of Psychiatry, Mount Sinai School of Medicine, New York, New York

**William H. Redd, M.D.**
Associate Attending Psychologist, Psychiatry Service, Department of Neurology, Memorial Sloan-Kettering Cancer Center; Associate Professor, Department of Psychiatry, Cornell University Medical College, New York, New York

**Julia H. Rowland, Ph.D.**
Clinical Assistant Attending Psychologist, Psychiatry Service, Department of Neurology, Memorial Sloan-Kettering Cancer Center; Instructor of Psychology in Psychiatry, Department of Psychiatry, Cornell University Medical College, New York, New York

**Norman Straker, M.D.**
Adjunct Attending Psychiatrist, Psychiatry Service, Department of Neurology, Memorial Sloan-Kettering Cancer Center; Clinical Associate Professor, Department of Psychiatry, Cornell University Medical College, New York, New York

**Susan Tross, Ph.D.**
Clinical Assistant Attending Psychologist, Psychiatry Service, Department of Neurology, Memorial Sloan-Kettering Cancer Center; Assistant Professor, Department of Psychiatry, Cornell University Medical College, New York, New York

**Marianne Zimberg, R.N., M.A.**
Psychiatric Nurse Clinician, Department of Nursing, Memorial Sloan-Kettering Cancer Center, New York, New York

# PART I

## Social Factors and Adaptation

# 1

# Historical Overview

Jimmie C. Holland

## A HISTORICAL PERSPECTIVE

Several broad changes in society and medicine have heightened interest in the psychological aspects of cancer (Table 1-1). These include attitudes toward cancer reflecting greater optimism about its treatment; concerns about patients' autonomy in decision making and the human aspects of medical care; advances permitting earlier diagnosis of cancers that can be treated by more effective combinations of surgery, radiation, and chemotherapy; the recognition of psychological and behavioral factors associated with cancer risk, detection, and prevention; the emergence of consultation–liaison psychiatry with its focus on the psychological problems of the medically ill. These changes in society, medicine, and psychiatry have also interacted with each other. Table 1-2 outlines some key events in medicine over the past 200 years including advances in the treatment of cancer and the practice of psychiatry, and suggests how these may have influenced attitudes toward disease, doctors, and death. This chapter reviews the early interface of cancer and social attitudes, the later growth and development of oncology, and finally the maturing relationship between oncology and the social sciences in recent years.

## Early Attitudes of Society Toward Cancer

In the 1800s a definitive diagnosis of cancer was often hard to make. Even when the disease was correctly identified, little treatment was available except for supportive care. Surgical extirpation as a curative treatment became possible only after general anesthesia came into use at midcentury. Even then, cure was rare; death was the expected outcome for most cancer patients. Adequate methods to control the pain and distressing symptoms associated with advanced disease were also few. Little was known about the causes

of either cancer or most of the infectious diseases that took the lives of children and young adults. Thus, an aura of fear and dread surrounded cancer as it did some of the other fatal diseases common at the time (Patterson, 1987).

By the early part of the twentieth century, three major diseases predominated in the Western world: heart disease, tuberculosis, and cancer. Heart disease never aroused the same abhorrence and fear as tuberculosis and cancer. A diagnosis of either of the other two diseases was a death sentence and caused the person to be stigmatized, isolated, and humiliated, a fate similar to that of persons with leprosy and syphilis. The information that someone had cancer was whispered among family members and often witheld from children in the family. Reluctantly shared with friends, the diagnosis was rarely publicly stated. Obituaries never gave cancer as a cause of death; instead, a euphemism such as "a lingering illness"—which was known to mean cancer—was employed.

The word cancer carried such dread that the doctor revealed the diagnosis only to the family and never to the patient. In *The Death of Ivan Ilyich,* Tolstoy (1886) provided a poignant literary example of how a patient in the nineteenth century felt when his physician and family refused to acknowledge that he was dying of cancer. He recognized his serious condition, yet all those around him maintained a pretense that he was scarcely ill. He was grateful to his servant who alone acknowledged his condition.

There were other special problems associated with cancer: pain, disfiguring tumors with foul-smelling secretions, concerns about contagion and communicability, loss of attractiveness and self-image, and loss of sexual function. All of these contributed to the special revulsion associated with the diagnosis of a malignant tumor. The visibility of cancer of the breast and genital organs, and the resemblance of these inoperable le-

**Table 1-1** Factors contributing to greater emphasis on psychological aspects of cancer

---

- Societal changes in attitudes toward cancer with shift toward less pessimism
- Increased concern for patient autonomy and human aspects of care
- Earlier diagnosis of cancer by improved methods with treatment by more effective combinations of surgery, chemotherapy, and in radiation
- Recognition of psychological and behavioral influences in cancer risk, early detection, and prevention
- Emergence of consultation–liaison psychiatry with its emphasis on psychological care of medically ill

---

sions to the gummas of syphilis, frequently led to the erroneous assumption of sexual transmission, adding further to the patient's shame, stigma, and guilt. Sontag traced the social symbols used by society in relation to cancer. She powerfully argues in *Illness as Metaphor* that the anguish of having cancer is compounded by the social stigma:

Illness is the night-side of life, a more onerous citizenship. Everyone who is born holds a dual citizenship, in the kingdom of the well and the sick. Although we all prefer to use only the good passport, sooner or later, each of us is obligated, at least for a spell, to identify ourselves as citizens of that other place. . . . it is hardly possible to take up one's residence in the kingdom of the ill unprejudiced by the lurid metaphors with which it has been landscaped. (Sontag, 1977, p. 3)

Cancer is often the metaphor chosen for any social state or condition that slowly but inexorably destroys or erodes. Such expressions as "the cancer of our society," the "growing cancer of the political system," convey its sinister meaning and contribute to the stigmatization of the person who has cancer.

Early in this century surgery began to offer a possible cure for cancer when the tumor could be removed before it had spread, but success depended on "getting it all out." For the first time educating the public about the possibility of cure associated with early diagnosis became important. Educational programs encouraging people to seek treatment early began and represented the first step in altering the negative attitudes toward cancer.

The first pioneering effort in public cancer education began in Europe in the 1890s when Winter, a gynecologist in East Prussia, urged women to be better informed on the danger signals of cancer. A newspaper campaign in East and West Prussia in 1903 publicized the early warning signs of cancer. Childe began a similar campaign in England to educate the public that cancer, when diagnosed early, was not a death warrant; early cancer could be cured by surgery. Childe

also advocated the establishment of cancer control societies worldwide to create a more informed public (Fact Book, American Cancer Society, 1980).

The American Society for Control of Cancer was formed in 1913. The mandate of this organization, later renamed the American Cancer Society (ACS), was to "disseminate knowledge concerning the symptoms, treatment and prevention of cancer." To counter the ignorance and fears, warning signals of cancer were publicized; emphasis was placed on information as a way to combat fear by such slogans as "Fight cancer with knowledge." Physicians also needed education to counter their pessimism about treatment (Wainwright, 1911).

As part of the American Cancer Society's efforts, a special Women's Field Army was developed to teach women about the early symptoms of breast and uterine cancer and reduce the reluctance to consult a physician for gynecological problems. In this regard, the first consumer awareness article to appear in the popular press was published in 1912 in the *Ladies' Home Journal*. It said, in part:

Be careful of persistent sores and irritations, external and internal. Be watchful of yourself, without undue worry. At the first suspicious symptoms go to a good physician and demand the truth . . . . The risk is not in *surgery*, but in *delayed* surgery. (Fact Book, American Cancer Society, 1980).

Early surgical efforts were directed toward developing radical and extensive procedures to attempt cure. Although the efforts increasingly offered cure to some, attitudes toward cancer reflected the awareness that the prognosis continued to be dire for tumors that were not surgically resectable. In cases not curable by surgery, the doctor's role was one of offering comfort and "laying on of hands" when no more could be done. The view was common that life was "in God's hands."

In the nineteenth century, psychiatrists were known as *alienists* whose major role was to remove the mentally ill from society, placing them in mental hospitals. By 1850, however, there was keen interest in teaching psychological medicine to medical students and physicians who cared for medical patients in general hospitals (Lipowski, 1981). In 1902 a psychiatric ward was placed in a general hospital in Albany, New York, representing the first effort to bring psychiatry into the general medical care setting. The psychobiological concepts of Adolph Meyer had an impact on psychiatric thought, which was felt in the first quarter of the century; the psychophysiological experiments of Walter Cannon furthered interest in what later became psychosomatic medicine. Typically, however, psychiatrists had no role in the understanding or care of cancer patients until they began to participate in debates about

**Table 1-2** Events and attitudes influencing perception of and response to cancer

| Decade | Medicine and cancer | Society | | Psychiatry and psychology |
|--------|---------------------|---------|---|---------------------------|
| | | Attitudes toward disease and doctors | Attitudes toward death | |
| 1800s | Mortality highest from infectious diseases, tuberculosis common<br>Syphilis and cancer have similar lesions<br>Effective cancer treatment unknown<br>Introduction of anesthesia and antisepsis, opening way for surgical excision of cancer (1847) | Expectation of high mortality among infants and children<br>Stigma, shame, guilt associated with having tuberculosis, cancer, and syphilis<br>Fears of transmission of infectious diseases and cancer | Patient is "in God's hands"<br>Physician's role seen to comfort<br>*"Death is part of life,"* person died at home, simple "pine box" burial | Concern with major mental illness—"Alienists"<br>Psychiatric hospitals largely removed from general hospitals, but movement began after 1850 to bring psychological medicine into medical education and general hospitals |
| 1900–1920s | Successful surgical removal of some cancers<br>Radiation used for palliative cancer treatment<br>American Cancer Society (ACS) started (1913) | In 1890s efforts began in Europe to inform public of warning signs of cancer; first focus on public education about cancer in United States<br>Fear of going to doctors and hospitals, fear of diagnosis of cancer, patients generally never told cancer diagnosis diagnosis | Doctors assumed authoritarian and paternalistic role, did not reveal diagnosis or medications, "trust me and don't worry" philosophy | Psychopathic ward in a general hospital in Albany, N.Y. (1902)<br>Psychobiological approach of Adolph Meyer<br>Psychophysiologic approach to disease by Cannon |
| 1930s | National Cancer Institute and International Union against Cancer formed (1937) | Visitor–volunteer programs for cancer patients by ACS | Deaths in hospitals; embalming, elaborate funerals; person "only sleeping" as euphemism for death | Consultation and general psychatric hospital units flourished<br>Psychosomatic movement begun<br>Dunbar's landmark review of psychosomatic disorders |
| 1940s | Nitrogen mustards, developed in World War II, found to have antitumor action<br>First remission of acute leukemia by use of drug | Pervasive pessimism about outcome of cancer treatment by surgery and irradiation<br>Cancer diagnosis given to family, never patient | "Cancer = death"; expression of grief encouraged; education of caregivers about therapeutic value of expressing grief<br>Concern for cost of funerals; increased use of cremation | Psychodynamic approach to psychosomatic medicine by Alexander; search for a cancer personality and life events as stimulus for cancer growth<br>First systematic study of acute grief |
| 1950s | Beginning of cancer chemotherapy; first cure of choriocarcinoma by drugs alone (1951); increasing medical technology and life-sustaining supports for critical illness<br>Psychiatric clinical and research group established at Memorial Sloan-Kettering Cancer Center (1950) under A. M. Sutherland | Debates about the practice of not revealing cancer diagnosis reach the public, who are becoming better informed about issues in medicine | Fatal outcome of cancer revealed to family but not to patient | First papers on psychological reactions to cancer (1951–1952)<br>Beginning of community psychiatry; education of "gatekeepers" and primary caregivers in crisis theory and intervention<br>Psychiatrists strongly favor revealing cancer diagnosis, and debates with cancer physicians ensue |

*(continued)*

**Table 1-2**  *(Continued)*

| Decade | Medicine and cancer | Society | | Psychiatry and psychology |
| | | Attitudes toward disease and doctors | Attitudes toward death | |
| --- | --- | --- | --- | --- |
| 1960s | Combined-modality treatment of cancer; successful treatment of Hodgkin's disease | Cancer more openly discussed, less taboo | More open discussion of death; concern for death and dignity; criticism of conspiracy of silence | Beginning of thanatology movement in United States; influence of Kubler-Ross in psychological management. Hospice movement begun in England by Saunders reaches United States; increased concern about care for terminally ill |
| 1970s | Increasing development of life-sustaining technology; new chemotherapy drugs | Statement of Patient's Rights; development of federal guidelines for patients' participation in investigational protocols | First formal hospice unit in United States (1974), although religious groups long had a tradition of care of the terminally ill. Legal and ethical discussion of right to die; first hospital guidelines for care of hopelessly ill (1976). Legal decisions about definition of death, right to stop life-sustaining efforts | Resurgence of general hospital psychiatry as consultation–liaison psychiatry, first in ICUs, recovery rooms, later in cancer units; development of health psychology and behavioral medicine; biopsychosocial concept of disease by Engel. Support for psychological studies in cancer rehabilitation from National Cancer Institute |
| 1980s | Number of survivors increase: childhood leukemia, Hodgkin's disease, and testicular cancer | Consumer movement; concerns about human aspects of patient care, adequate symptom control (particularly pain), and "quality of life" of patients during active and palliative treatment | Legal right of "natural death". "Do not resuscitate" guidelines in several teaching hospitals; guidelines for termination of life-sustaining measures beginning to be developed. Impact of President's Commission for the Study of Ethical Problems in Medicine and Biomedical and Behavioral Research | Studies of ethical, legal, and emotional issues around informed consent, resuscitation, and stopping of life-sustaining supports. First major studies of cancer survivors. Studies of psychological behavioral, and pharmacological management of stress with cancer. ACS support for fellowships in psychiatric oncology and for psychosocial research studies |

whether a cancer diagnosis should be withheld from a patient.

## Cancer Treatment Advances and Early Psychosocial Efforts

In the 1920s radium provided the second treatment modality for cancer. The development of radiotherapy was a big step forward, although it mainly offered only palliation after surgical failure (Shimkin, 1977). Indeed, referral for radiation was commonly recognized by the patient and family as evidence of incurable disease. Clearly, investigation of new treatments was required and became a major focus of biomedical research. The International Union Against Cancer and the National Cancer Institute (NCI) were both established in 1937 and provided new resources to support research. Over the past 40 years, the NCI has provided the most successful model for federally supported biomedical cancer research and has been emulated throughout the world.

Consonant with the greater research effort in the 1940s, new support for cancer patients was initiated through the American Cancer Society's field and service programs. These programs provided patients with supplies such as bandages and transportation. Trained volunteers provided information and counseling specifically designed for and directed to the patient with cancer. It soon became apparent that the best providers of information about a specific cancer and support were other patients and their families. Surgeons began to ask patients who had had a laryngectomy or colostomy to speak with patients anticipating similar surgery. This was often a critical intervention in encouraging a person to consent to such radical procedures leading to the loss of voice or normal bowel function. Laryngectomy and ostomy clubs developed as the first cancer self-help groups. By the 1950s, the first self-help group for the increasing numbers of cured patients was developed. The Cured Cancer Club was formed to offer assistance to those patients who faced the severe stigma and prejudices at that time against one who had had cancer.

Psychological support for women following mastectomy by those who had themselves had a mastectomy was started by Teresa Lasser and Fannie Rosenau in New York in the late 1940s. Both of these women had undergone a mastectomy and perceived the great sense of isolation and alienation women felt because they could not discuss their experience with others. The impact of their efforts was particularly significant, occurring as it did at a time when mention of either cancer or the sexual organs was taboo in polite society and in the news media. In the 1950s the integration by the ACS of their postmastectomy support program, Reach-to-Recovery, led to the program's worldwide expansion as a highly successful self-help resource for mastectomy patients.

Despite widespread endorsement by patients, these organizations had an uphill battle to gain acceptance in the medical community. Except in special situations, physicians were slow to acknowledge that there was a unique and useful role for patients to support and encourage others with the same diagnosis and treatment. Such efforts were viewed by many as an intrusion into the doctor–patient relationship, even though few adverse effects have ever been reported (see Chapter 41 on self-help support).

The development in the late 1940s of the first anticancer agent initiated chemotherapy in cancer treatment, which today has more than 60 active agents against cancer. The first responses of acute leukemia to nitrogen mustard, a drug that was developed from World War II research on war gases, were seen in the early 1950s. The first cure of a cancer, choriocarcinoma, by a single chemotherapeutic agent, methotrexate, was achieved in the early 1950s. Growth of this field soon led to the creation of the subspecialty of medical oncology, with its own professional standards and certification within the field of internal medicine. The rapid increase in the number of medical oncologists quickly provided a group of physicians who were trained in administering chemotherapy and who provided continuity of care throughout the course of the illness. This had been difficult to achieve when surgeons and radiotherapists were responsible primarily for administering their specific treatments to cancer patients during palliative treatment and advanced disease. They, and their pediatric oncological counterparts, spearheaded many efforts to improve supportive care, which included psychological support.

The advent of chemotherapy in the treatment of cancer dramatically altered the prognosis for several previously fatal tumors of children and young adults. Figure 1-1 shows for the years from 1940 to 1980 the dramatic, steady increase in survival for eight childhood cancers treated with multimodal therapies. For example, Hodgkin's disease, previously largely incurable, is now over 90% curable (Hammond, 1981). Figure 1-2 shows the same trend in survival for children with acute lymphocytic leukemia treated by the Cancer and Leukemia group B from 1956 to 1980. In 1956 all children with this disease died in a little over a year; however, today, 60 to 80% of all newly diagnosed children can expect to be cured. Figure 1-3 shows overall cancer mortality trends from 1954 to 1976 (DeVita et al., 1979). The remarkably improved survival of cancer patients under 30 is shown, the same but less dramatic change for patients under 45, and a leveling off in cancer deaths for those under 60.

The psychosocial issues in cancer have dramatically changed as treatments have become more successful. Initially, when childhood tumors and many adult cancers were uniformly fatal, efforts were directed toward assisting the patient and family to adapt to the inevitable outcome. It was considered more humane to shield the patient from the frightening word equated with death. Doctors, who saw their role as protectors, chose to withhold the news for as long as possible. The primary psychological issue was dealing with death, because the numbers of survivors were few and their coping problems were largely kept secret because of the attitude that "one should be thankful to be alive." However, as more patients survived, concerns broadened to include those associated with cancer as a chronic disease and even one from which patients were cured. The psychosocial issues of cancer reflect sub-

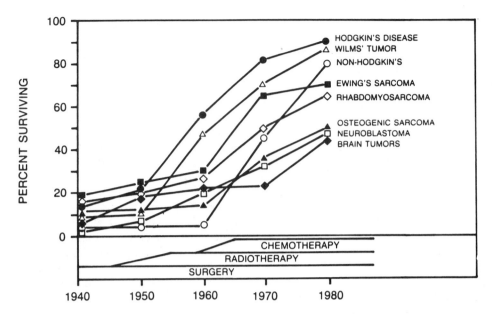

**Figure 1-1.** Progressive improvement in survival of children with solid tumors, 1940–1980. Proportion surviving 2 years from diagnosis. Data from multiple sources are shown relative to the chronology of the general application of the three principal therapeutic modalities to the tumors of children. *Source:* Reproduced by permission from D. Hammond (1981). Progress in the study, treatment, and cure of the cancers of children. In J.H. Burchenal and H.F. Oettgen (eds.), *Cancer: Achievements, Challenges, and Prospects for the 1980s,* Vol. 2. New York: Grune & Stratton.

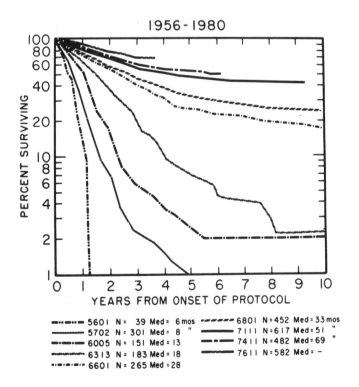

**Figure 1-2.** Cancer and Leukemia Group B, acute lymphocytic leukemia survival in children under 20 years of age, 1956–1980. *Source:* Reprinted with permission of J.F. Holland, CALGB 1956–1983.

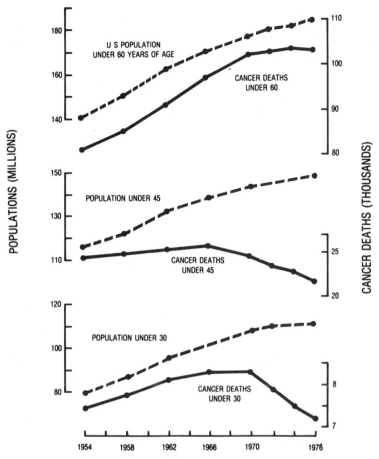

**Figure 1-3.** Cancer mortality and U.S. population trends, 1954–1976. *Source:* Reproduced from V.T. De Vita, V.T. Oliverio, F.M. Muggia, P.W. Wiernik, J. Ziegler, A. Goldin, D. Rudin, J. Henney, and S. Schepartz (1979). The drug development and clinical trials programs of the Division of Cancer Treatment, National Cancer Institute. *Cancer Clin. Trials* 2:195–216.

stantially both the medical reality of likely survival and the societal attitudes at any given time, changing rapidly over the past 20 years with the sharp increase in predicted survival from cancer.

## A Growing Interface Between the Social Sciences and Oncology

Between the 1930s and 1950s, increasing numbers of psychiatric consultation services and psychiatric units in general hospitals resulted in rising concern with the psychological care of medically ill patients (Lipowski, 1981). The first two studies of psychological adaptation to cancer came from the psychiatric group at the Massachusetts General Hospital. They reported that patterns of communication changed with the stage of cancer. The tendency in advanced stages for communication to become more limited, and for guilt—a prominent psychological response—to increase, was

noted (Shands et al., 1951; Abrams and Finesinger, 1953). Social workers and nurses contributed to early observations of the psychosocial aspects of care and played a crucial role in understanding the cancer patients' emotional problems.

Early papers about psychological adaptation dealt also with how patients responded to radical surgery as the primary treatment for cancer. Major physical and functional deficits were often necessary to obtain a possible cure. In 1950 Sutherland established the first psychiatric group in the United States, which was devoted to study of the psychosocial consequences of cancer and surgical treatment. The group carried out several seminal studies at Memorial Sloan-Kettering Cancer Center, describing responses to colostomy and radical mastectomy (Sutherland et al., 1952; Bard and Sutherland, 1955).

Following World War II, cancer patients were studied for psychosomatic links between personality and disease, similar to studies in hypertension, rheumatoid arthritis, and asthma. These studies were usually anecdotal accounts of patients with cancer, which attempted retrospectively to deduce a premorbid personality pattern that might have predisposed the individual to develop cancer. Most of them had no control groups, studied small samples, and failed to take into account the difficulty of assuming the premorbid personality of a patient after diagnosis of cancer. These studies focused primarily on the etiological question, failing to focus on the psychological impact of cancer on the patient, and to explore the role of psychiatrists in the active care of cancer patients. Important insights, however, into the psychological issues faced by the patient and physician during dying were provided, particularly by Eissler and Norton, whose psychiatric clinical case studies included terminally ill cancer patients (Eissler, 1955; Norton, 1963).

At about the same time that Sutherland's group was exploring the impact of radical surgery, and psychiatrists were researching personality traits in physical diseases, the first debates began to arise about the wisdom of never revealing the diagnosis of cancer. A group of oncologists and psychiatrists suggested to the "never tellers," who constituted more than 90% of physicians polled in a survey by Oken in 1961, that more harm was being done by telling a lie, with the loss of trust in the physician, than would be the case if patients were informed of the actual diagnosis (Oken, 1961). Doctors working with cancer began to change their practice in this regard and found that both they and the patient were more comfortable when false pretenses were dropped, which resulted in greater understanding between them. Over the next 25 years, the public's sophistication about diseases, the development of informed-consent guidelines, and the increasingly successful treatment of cancer have contributed to a far more open discussion of cancer diagnosis, treatment, and prognosis.

The same questions were used in a survey in 1977 that showed that 97% of the doctors studied generally told patients their cancer diagnosis (Novack et al., 1979). It should be noted that the candor of American doctors in revealing cancer is not matched in most other countries. The custom of "not telling" continues in most. However, the general trend is moving gradually toward fuller disclosure. Even so, the American practice of informing the patient is sharply criticized by those physicians in other countries who are still accustomed to concealing cancer diagnosis.

The wide publicity given to the work of Elisabeth Kubler-Ross (1969) sharply focused medical and public attention on the psychological dimension of patients dying with cancer. Kubler-Ross' seminal work on open communication with the dying cancer patient heralded the beginning of the thanatology movement in this country and brought American attitudes toward death under scrutiny. Her work underscored the tendency of doctors and staff to avoid the discussion of death as they had avoided that of the diagnosis of cancer. She observed that death had become a taboo subject that was spurned by the healthy as well. The thanatology movement encouraged exploration of social attitudes about death. It particularly fostered better communication with cancer patients during the terminal stages of disease.

Because Kubler-Ross' work focused on cancer patients reactions to the anticipation of death, it had a profound impact on professionals, especially the nurses who were working with cancer patients. For a time this perspective overshadowed psychological studies on rehabilitation and cure. Dr. Kubler-Ross spoke at all major cancer centers and recounted, with a remarkably charismatic delivery, her experiences with dying patients. For some years attention was directed toward her "stages of dying," assuming that the course of cancer was a predictable and inexorable downhill path from diagnosis to death, with equally predictable psychological stages. Overzealous application of her principles led to attempts by staff to categorize patients into these psychological stages. Health professionals were encouraged to approach patients with questions concerning their thoughts about death and sometimes failed to be sensitive to the needs of the individual and to recognize that many patients preferred not to discuss feelings that they considered intimate. The work of Weisman (1972) and his coworkers, as well as others, countered this trend by emphasizing the need for a healthy respect for the complexity of the psychological issues of the individual patient.

## Recent Interface of Psychiatry and Oncology

In the past 15 years converging trends within society, oncology, and psychiatry have led to the thoughtful study of the psychological responses of patients with cancer. A body of knowledge regarding the psychological aspects of cancer treatment and care have led to an emerging subspecialty within oncology devoted to psychosocial issues. The public's increased knowledge of health care and disease has forced a dialogue with physicians about diagnosis, and the risks and benefits of treatment options. Increasing numbers of cured patients have led to studies of the delayed effects of cancer treatment on both physical and psychological functions (Koocher and O'Malley, 1981).

Concern about the ethics of clinical investigation

has led to the establishment of federal guidelines requiring disclosure of all relevant facts about participation in research studies. The consumer-oriented philosophy, combined with a more critical view of physicians and medicine, has led to communication between doctor and patient with respect not only to the physical aspects of the disease, but also to the impact the disease and treatments have on personal goals and quality of life (American Cancer Society Conference, 1982). The need for a multidisciplinary team to address the diverse needs of cancer patients has become apparent.

The growth of consultation–liaison psychiatry since the early 1970s has had a significant impact on cancer patient care. Psychiatrists trained in consultation–liaison have influenced primary care physicians in the psychological management of patients. Clinical investigations examining the psychological responses of patients, in intensive care units (ICUs), recovery rooms, and coronary care units were undertaken and had an immediate impact on patient care. By the mid-1970s, oncologists, especially those specializing in pediatrics, began to invite psychiatrists to their units as consultants, and cancer centers began to appoint psychiatric consultants to examine the problems of patients, families, and staff. The clinical consultations provided by psychiatrists to oncological units quickly expanded to include a liaison role, conducting multidisciplinary teaching rounds and groups that focused on psychological and behavioral problems, ethical dilemmas, conflicts between patient and staff, and staff members with each other (Artiss & Levine, 1973).

Psychological issues related to prevention, early detection, and compliance with cancer treatment became apparent as epidemiologists became aware of the importance of habits that resulted in exposure to environmental carcinogens (Doll and Peto, 1981; Doll, 1983). The evidence that lung cancer was associated with cigarette smoking, an acquired habit, focused on the need for psychological studies to promote abstinence and cessation.

Psychological variables also loomed large in determining the best approaches to encouraging individuals to pursue early detection of cancer. Individual willingness to change behavior and to practice self-examination emerged as key health-related behaviors that required study (Roberts, 1967; Rosenstock, 1963). At the same time, while cancer therapy became effective, it also became more lengthy and arduous, demanding a high level of commitment from the patient to comply with treatment and tolerate side effects. Thus, several issues emerged in oncology that highlighted a need for more psychological and social research.

Very little support for psychosocial research in cancer existed before 1970. However, with the advent of the National Cancer Plan in 1972 and the establishment of the Division of Cancer Control and Rehabilitation, demonstration projects (but not research studies) to improve rehabilitation became possible (Burke, 1981). The first conference that brought together the handful of psychosocial researchers was held in San Antonio in 1975 (Cullen et al., 1976). The Psychosocial Collaborative Oncology Group, chaired by Arthur Schmale, carried out several multiinstitutional studies addressing psychosocial problems and research methods (see Part XII, ''Research Methods in Psychooncology''). The American Cancer Society became concerned that psychosocial and behavioral issues receive additional support. They sponsored two workshops that were also benchmarks. The first reviewed the state of the art and goals in educational and research efforts in psychological, social, and psychiatric aspects of cancer (ACS Conference, 1982). The second workshop, which focused on the status of research methods in psychosocial and behavioral aspects of cancer, provided recommendations for future directions and ways to improve the quality of research efforts (ACS Conference, 1984). The result was the development of national advisory committees on psychosocial education and research for adult and childhood cancer, and the formation of a peer review committee to review behavioral and psychosocial research proposals. Psychosocial studies had been previously reviewed largely by basic scientists and clinicians not versed in methods of social science research. By the end of 1986, the American Cancer Society had supported over 25 research studies, which received more than $2.5 million in funding.

## The Emergence of Psychooncology

The total care of cancer patients today incorporates psychological management as one of its key elements. Research on prevention and detection depends on the social sciences for tackling some of the basic questions in behavior modification. Theory and practice in both the impact of cancer and its prevention rely heavily on clinical investigations that are identified as an emerging subspecialty called psychosocial oncology or, simply *psychooncology*. This subspecialty of oncology seeks to study the two psychological dimensions of cancer: (1) the impact of cancer on the psychological function of the patient, the patient's family, and staff; and (2) the role that psychological and behavioral variables may have in cancer risk and survival. The latter area is also considered by some as behavioral medicine in cancer; certain aspects represent the new field of psychoneuroimmunology, addressing the impact of emotions on the immune and endocrine systems that may contribute to cancer risk. The next decade will likely see a major expansion of work in these areas by investigators from both the social and physical sciences.

# REFERENCES

Abrams, R.D. and J.E. Finesinger (1953). Guilt reactions in patients with cancer. *Cancer* 6:474–82.

American Cancer Society. (1980). *Fact Book for the Medical and Related Professionals*. New York: Author.

American Cancer Society Working Conference (1982). The psychological, social, and behavioral medicine aspects of cancer: Research and professional education needs and directions for the 1980s. *Cancer* 50 (Suppl.):1919–78.

American Cancer Society Workshop Conference (1984). Methodology in behavioral and psychosocial cancer research. *Cancer* 53 (Suppl.):2217–2384.

Artiss, L.K. and A.S. Levine (1973). Doctor–patient relation in severe illness: A seminar for oncology Fellows. *N. Engl. J. Med.* 288:1210–14.

Bard, M. and A.M. Sutherland (1955). Psychological impact of cancer and its treatment. IV. Adaptation to radical mastectomy. *Cancer* 8:656–72.

Burke, L.D. (1981). A national planning program for cancer rehabilitation. In J. Burchenal and H.F. Oettgen (eds.). *Cancer: Achievements, Challenges, and Prospects for the 1980s,* Vol. 2. New York: Grune & Stratton, pp. 771–91.

Cullen, J.W., B.H. Fox, and R.N. Isom (eds.). (1976). *Cancer: The Behavioral Dimensions*. DHEW Publ. No. (NIH) 76-1074. Washington, D.C.: National Cancer Institute.

DeVita, V.T., V.T. Oliverio, F.M. Muggia, P.W. Wiernik, J. Ziegler, A. Goldin, D. Rubin, J. Henney, and S. Schepartz (1979). The drug development and clinical trials programs of the Division of Cancer Treatment, National Cancer Institute. *Cancer Clin. Trials* 2:195–216.

Doll, R. (1983). Prospects for the prevention of cancer. *Clin. Radiol.* 34:609–23.

Doll, R. and R. Peto (1981). *The Causes of Cancer. Quantitative Estimates of Avoidable Risks of Cancer in the United States Today*. Oxford: Oxford University Press.

Eissler, K.R. (1955). *The Psychiatrist and the Dying Patient*. New York: International Universities Press.

Hammond, D. (1981). Progress in the study, treatment, and cure of the cancers of children. In J.H. Burchenal and H.F. Oettgen (eds.), *Cancer: Achievements, Challenges, and Prospects for the 1980s*, Vol. 2. New York: Grune & Stratton, pp. 171–90.

Holland, J.C. (1982). Psychologic aspects of cancer. In J.F. Holland and E. Frei III (eds.), *Cancer Medicine,* 2nd ed. Philadelphia: Lea & Febiger, pp. 1175–1203, 2325–31.

Koocher, G. and J. O'Malley (1981). *The Damocles Syndrome*. New York: McGraw-Hill.

Kubler-Ross, E. (1969). *On Death and Dying.* New York: Macmillan.

Lipowski, Z.J. (1981). Holistic-medical foundations of American psychiatry: a bicentennial. *Am. J. Psychiatry* 138:888–95.

Norton, J. (1963). Treatment of a dying patient. *Psychoanl. Study Child* 18:541–60.

Novack, D.H., R. Plumer, R.L., Smith, H. Ochitill, G.R. Morrow, and J.M. Bennet (1979). Changes in physicians' attitudes toward telling the cancer patient. *J.A.M.A.* 241:897–900.

Oken, D. (1961). What to tell cancer patients: A study of medical attitudes. *J.A.M.A.* 175:1120–28.

Patterson, J.J. (1987). *The Dread Disease: Cancer and Modern American Culture*. Cambridge, MA: Harvard University Press.

Roberts, B. (1967). Factors and forces influencing decision-making related to health behavior. In *Health Education in Cancer Control. Proc. Semin. Health Educ. Uterine Cancer Programs*. Ann Arbor, Mich.: University of Michigan School of Public Health, pp. 75–86.

Rosenstock, I.M. (1963). Public response to cancer screening and detection programs: Determinants of health behavior. *J. Chron. Dis.* 16:407–18.

Shands, H.C., J.E. Finesinger, S. Cobb, and R.D. Abrams (1951). Psychological mechanisms in patients with cancer. *Cancer* 4:1159–70.

Shimkin, M. (1977). *Contrary to Nature*. National Institutes of Health Publ. No. 76-7291977. Washington, D.C.: U.S. Department of Health and Human Services, Public Health Service.

Sontag, S. (1977). *Illness as Metaphor*. New York: Farrar, Straus & Giroux.

Sutherland, A.M., C.E. Orbach, R.B. Dyk, and M. Bard (1952). The psychological impact of cancer and cancer surgery: I. Adaptation to the dry colostomy; Preliminary report and summary of findings. *Cancer* 5:857–72.

Tolstoy, L. (1967). The death of Ivan Ilyich. In L. Maude and A. Maude (trans.). *Great Short Works of Leo Tolstoy*. New York: Harper & Row (original work published 1886).

Wainwright, J.M. (1911). The reduction of cancer mortality. *N.Y. Med. J.* 94:1165–68.

Weisman, A.D. (1972). *On Dying and Denying: A Psychiatric Study of Terminality*. New York: Behavioral Publications.

# 2

# Fears and Abnormal Reactions to Cancer in Physically Healthy Individuals

Jimmie C. Holland

The fear of cancer has stigmatized patients with the disease for centuries. Although it is far more treatable and can be more openly discussed today, the fear persists and has an impact on current attitudes toward cancer.

Over the past two decades, extensive media coverage of cancer has exacerbated this fear. At times it has reached the proportions of hysteria with the publication of sensational reports on environmental carcinogens, as with Love Canal. For the public it is difficult to weigh the importance of information about new "cancer-causing agents" and distinguish between real and hypothetical risks.

Ingelfinger identified cancerophobia in American society as a serious problem in 1975:

American cancerophobia, in brief, is a disease as serious to society as cancer is to the individual—and morally more devastating. For this state of affairs, many are to blame—not only high-pressure advertisers foment and exploit our cancerophobia, but also the well-meaning but yet baneful practices of other groups: activist consumer organizations, politicians, and even the American Cancer Society, which points direly accusatory fingers at you if you do not give money to "cure cancer." Among the guilty are the media. Because of our society's disease, any news about cancer, no matter how trivial, is ipso facto sensational. Whether it is the latest tentative suggestion that some agent or condition is oncogenic, or the most recent molecular definition of the cancer cell's wall, the media treat the tentative indictment as if it were an actual catastrophe, and the minor laboratory discovery is heralded as another "breakthrough" in our "war" against cancer. So the vicious circle spirals upward and outward: cancerophobia elicits sensationalist reporting, which in turn fosters the demonology of cancer.

Bianchi (1971) noted that specific phobias of disease, nosophobias, usually parallel the medical preoccupations of the times. Syphilophobia and fears of infections dominated earlier periods; they have been replaced by phobias about cancer and most recently AIDS (Brandt, 1985). A nosophobia usually focuses on a serious disease about which the person may have only fragmentary knowledge but experiences excessive fears by virtue of some prior association. Given that one in four families experiences cancer, and the high visibility of cancer in the media, it is not surprising that cancerophobia has been so common. Plays, television dramas, and movies based on both true and fictional stories of patients with cancer, mostly with a fatal outcome, have appeared more frequently in recent years. Despite the flood of dramatic cancer information, most psychologically healthy individuals maintain an equilibrium with respect to their own and their family's risk of disease. For these individuals, the fear of cancer is not overriding. When this balance is upset, however, this fear can become a preoccupation. This abnormal reaction to cancer in a physically healthy individual, which interferes with function, constitutes cancerophobia. It is associated with underlying emotional problems which range from mild to severe.

Cancerophobia is a symptom of psychological distress that requires careful evaluation to determine its etiology and to assess the proper treatment. Few psychiatric studies have examined specific phobias of cancer (Ryle, 1948; Branch, 1952; Garner, 1964; Bianchi, 1971; Sanborn and Seibert, 1975, 1976). These early papers described differences between transient cancerophobia related to anxiety and a fixed cancerophobia related to a more pervasive underlying psychiatric disorder. These two forms of cancerophobia must be distinguished from a morbid preoccupation that represents a delusion of having cancer and occasionally involves factitious symptoms of the disease (Table 2-1).

**Table 2-1**  Abnormal reactions to cancer
in physically healthy individuals

| Abnormal reaction | Examples |
| --- | --- |
| Cancerophobia: a type of nosophobia | Transient (anxiety-related) <br> • Related to new dramatic disclosures in mass media (exposures in food, environment) <br> • During a life crisis <br> • Following personal contact with cancer through illness or death of someone close <br> • Health professionals and students who work with cancer patients for the first time <br> Fixed, chronic <br> • Siblings of a child who dies of cancer (often, history of chronic cancerophobia) <br> • Individuals at known enhanced risk of cancer (familial polyposis, breast cancer) <br> • Hypochondriacal conviction of cancer, fearful preoccupation with body symptoms; persistent visits to doctors <br> • Somatization in briquet's syndrome, hysterical conversions, anxiety disorders, depression, borderline personality, schizophrenia |
| Delusion of having cancer | • Schizophrenia <br> • Major depression with psychotic features <br> • Schizoaffective |
| Factitious symptoms of cancer | • Malingering <br> • Munchausen's syndrome—factitious symptoms to attain patient status; prior association with cancer and knowledge of symptoms (e.g., leukemia and bleeding) |

## Transient Cancerophobia

Anxiety about cancer can produce transient cancerophobia in psychologically healthy individuals. Several situations predispose individuals to this response: major coverage in the media of some new cancer risk, an anxiety-producing life crisis, coming into close personal contact with cancer through the illness or death of a close friend or relative, and encountering cancer as a health professional or student in the clinical setting for the first time. In these stressful situations a symptom that would ordinarily be ignored becomes a source of anxiety. The following case is an example of cancerophobia developing during an anxiety-provoking life crisis.

### CASE REPORT

A young doctor was experiencing marital stress at a transitional point in his career when he wished to pursue an academic goal not shared by his wife. She resented his career and its confining goals. After accepting a position he did not want, he became concerned about some small shotty nodes in his neck, night sweats, and tachycardia. He became convinced that he had Hodgkin's disease which he recognized would preclude his beginning the position and thus fulfill his unspoken wish to escape his situation. Several psychotherapeutic visits and a workup for Hodgkin's which proved negative allowed him to cope more realistically with his marital and career conflicts without further physical illness.

Occasionally a healthy individual who is experiencing grief after death of a loved one from cancer, develops a symptom that the deceased had during the terminal phase of the illness. This leads the grieved survivor to seek medical advice for a symptom feared to be cancer. When a careful medical history, thorough physical examination, and laboratory data reveal no sign of cancer, the person is reassured and the symptom disappears. It is important to explain to the individual that increased anxiety about developing cancer is not uncommon in these situations. Questions the patient has about contagion, hereditary predisposition, and risk factors should be answered frankly. Reassurance that a symptom does not indicate emotional instability is important, because most people are embarrassed about the possibility of having developed an imaginary symptom.

Fears of cancer can also become heightened when a member of the staff rotates for the first time on to an oncology unit or begins to work in a cancer setting. For medical students, nurses and house staff, this may be the first time they have cared for cancer patients. Taking medical histories of these very ill hospitalized patients is frightening because a minor symptom such as a bruise or headache, is often described as the onset of leukemia or brain tumor. When a similar minor symptom occurs in the individual, or a family member, acute anxiety is provoked about its cause. Embarrassment about entertaining these fears often results in an anxious silence, which adds to the normal stress health professionals experience in the early months of working with cancer patients. Orientation for new staff should include discussions of these feelings as common and normal. Encouraging new staff to discuss these feelings is important and can make the transition to work in a cancer unit emotionally easier. Sometimes negative laboratory results and reassurance by a physician are necessary to convince a staff member of good health.

## Fixed Cancerophobia

A persistent, fixed cancerophobia that is not responsive to reassurance occurs in individuals with either an unusual association with cancer in the past or those who have an underlying psychiatric disorder. In one of the few studies of phobias of cancer, Ryle (1948) reported the frequency of death from cancer in the family of patients with cancerophobia to be 39%. Sanborn and Seibert (1975, 1976) found that 78% of cancerophobics who committed suicide had a history of cancer in the family, an increased incidence confirmed in a controlled study that compared them to other suicides. Thus, family history is an important consideration in the workup of such cancerophobic patients, which may provide added weight to the likelihood of the diagnosis.

Several studies have noted the powerful impact that death of a sibling from cancer has in provoking death and disease phobias in the survivors (Cain, 1964; Binger et al., 1969). Binger observed that the healthy siblings of childhood leukemia patients were more apt to fear developing leukemia themselves when their parents were overprotective and hypervigilant for signs of disease. Although more research is needed in this area, it is reasonable to expect that the contact of the family with doctors and hospitals during the illness of a child with leukemia, which is then followed by excessive disease concerns, creates a setting that may encourage the development of hypochondriasis and cancerophobia in surviving siblings.

Another group in whom cancerophobia can be difficult to assess is that of individuals at high risk for developing cancer of a particular site. Because they do require careful monitoring and their cooperation in regular checkups is important, vigilance about symptoms is both appropriate and vital. Some individuals, however, become so obsessed by their fear of cancer that they become dysfunctional; this sometimes occurs in families with a high genetic risk for specific tumors, as in cases of familial polyposis. Another example of such a fear is the woman who has had frequent biopsies for fibrocystic breast disease or the woman at high genetic risk of breast cancer because a mother or sisters have died of it. Some request a bilateral mastectomy to deal with the fear. Such women who prefer to "get it over" rather than tolerate the anxiety require careful psychological evaluation in reaching a decision about prophylactic procedures, such as mastectomy, that are occasionally indicated and helpful (see Chapter 14).

In the individual with a chronic cancerophobia, it is critical to rule out presence of an occult neoplasm by doing a careful medical workup. When this has been done to the physician's satisfaction, and there is a suggestive history of underlying hypochondriacal preoccupations or somatization, the patient should be referred to the psychiatric consultant. The psychiatric disturbance may be related to hypochondriasis in which there is a conviction of cancer or preoccupation with minor symptoms that might be cancer. Barsky and Klerman (1983) have conceptualized hypochondriasis as a somatic style that amplifies body sensations. This perspective is useful in considering individuals who constantly monitor their body for signs of cancer, indict trivial symptoms as evidence of cancer, and frequently become panic-stricken and seek immediate and usually repeated examinations by the primary physician or multiple specialists. The reassurance these patients gain by a visit to the doctor is usually short-lived, and they must constantly repeat the cycle.

The individual who has had hypochondriacal concerns about cancer and who then actually develops a neoplasm poses a difficult psychiatric problem in the posttreatment period. During this time, they have similar preoccupations about recurrence, and usually require psychotherapy and medication.

In somatization seen in Briquet's syndrome, hysterical conversions, anxiety disorders, depression, borderline states, and schizophrenia, the focus may be on cancer, and a thorough psychiatric evaluation will be required to determine both etiology and therapeutic approach.

## Delusion of Cancer

Cancerophobia that assumes delusional and psychotic proportions is likely associated with a borderline state, major depression, or schizophrenia with a strong depressive component. The delusion is usually one of having a fatal form of cancer, such as acute leukemia or stomach cancer; it is especially common in psychotic depressive states. The delusion of cancer may be accompanied by bizarre sensations such as "I feel it eating my stomach and killing me." These patients often say, "I deserve to die" or "I'm being punished." Suicidal thoughts and serious suicide attempts are not uncommon. They should be observed carefully, preferably in a psychiatric hospital, to monitor the suicidal risk. Some patients maintain the delusion over many years as a chronic, but less disabling mental symptom. In these cases, the patient's symptoms become well known to the responsible psychiatrist and physician, but both must continue to monitor the patient carefully.

CASE REPORT

A 25-year-old college student was admitted to a psychiatric unit with recent onset of disorganized thought, poor school performance, and increasingly withdrawn behavior. She experienced fears that she had acute leukemia, although no evidence of physical illness was present. She had delusions about her body function and was preoccupied with having a fatal illness. Before workup could be completed, she made a serious suicide attempt by multiple cuts on her arms. Subsequent diagnosis was that of a schizoaffective disorder. She responded to medication, a protected environment, and psychotherapy.

## Factitious Symptoms

Some patients who de elop factitious symptoms initially show simulated symptoms of a neoplasm or a hematological malignancy. They fall within one of two groups: those with malingering or those with Munchausen's syndrome. In the first group are individuals for whom a secondary gain is associated with the development of symptoms of a neoplasm. The other group is of individuals who have a pathological need to be a patient and who show no evidence of attaining a secondary gain. They usually have a prior association with cancer and often appear to have a masochistic need to undergo painful diagnostic procedures and treatment. The latter group fits the criteria for Munchausen's syndrome. These individuals tend to go from one cancer center to another, presenting plausible and convincing symptoms to obtain admission. Factitious fever or self-induced bleeding are often accompanied by a bizarre, vague, or inconsistent history of leukemia or a neoplasm. Often, these individuals have had repeated admissions and workups in well-known cancer centers until they become "notorious." A telephone call often reveals numerous prior workups, which leads the house staff to become frustrated, resentful, and unsympathetic to the deceptive patient who is physically healthy but psychiatrically ill. Confrontation with the truth and referral to psychiatry usually are sufficient to cause them to sign out against advice. Psychiatric treatment or follow-up is rare, resulting in a paucity of information about the actual psychodynamics of these individuals.

Personal history of the patient usually reveals some prior association with cancer: they are usually familiar with medical terms and hospital routine, and they know the symptoms and treatment for cancer of a particular site. These patients have a severe underlying psychiatric disorder. Borderline personality or an actual thought disorder characteristic of schizophrenia may be present. The several cases we have seen have also generally involved one or more relatives who also accepted the factitious disease as fact. The Munchausen's syndrome by proxy seen in pediatric settings may also appear in pediatric oncology clinics, where a disturbed parent forces repeated examinations for factitious or induced symptoms resembling cancer in the child.

### CASE REPORTS

A 25-year-old man saw several different individual physicians and appeared in the diagnostic clinic in a cancer center with complaints that could be consistent with hematological disease, lymphoma, or head and neck cancer. He described severe pain in his neck with ostensibly enlarged hard nodes, and made it clear that admission to the hospital was necessary. He was found to have had extensive evaluations in two other cancer centers, where calls to the physicians found that none of the diagnoses could be confirmed. Psychiatric evaluation in one center suggested a likely diagnosis of chronic undifferentiated schizophrenia with paranoid features and a belief that he had cancer and required treatment. This impression was supported by the interview in which the patient gave little information to the psychiatric consultant. His mother shared the delusion; she refused to accept the psychiatric diagnosis or recommendation for psychiatric treatment. She continued to attempt to have him admitted to cancer facilities in several different cities.

A 20-year-old man who claimed to be a medical student with history of homosexual contacts was seen at the hospital with a history that he had a diagnosis of AIDS and lymphoma made a year earlier at another institution. No laboratory data confirmed AIDS or lymphoma, and a call to the institution revealed he had told the physician there that the diagnosis of AIDS and lymphoma of the brain had been made at this institution. He had shaved his head to simulate alopecia from chemotherapy and had deceived his family and support services organized in his behalf, both of whom he accused of refusing to help him. When confronted with the facts, he rejected psychiatric treatment and did not return.

These patients raise difficult treatment and ethical issues in regard to their management. Because they are exploitative and manipulative of staff, the relationship of trust is breached (Kass, 1985). Guidelines for physicians' behavior must consider the patient's right to confidentiality, which is sometimes outweighed by the potential injury to the person of multiple diagnostic procedures by virtue of the absence of the history of factitious illness. Information about the patient's behavioral history can ethically be disclosed to others, although the patient should be so informed when possible.

## EARLY CANCER SYMPTOMS

Between the healthy individual with cancer phobias and the person who receives a diagnosis of cancer is that gray zone in which a person recognizes a symptom that might or might not be cancer. How rapidly or slowly the person responds to warning symptoms of cancer has a profound impact on disease outcome. Who will seek early detection and diagnosis by virtue of being well informed? Who will delay, and why? These questions are central in attaining higher survival from cancer. Every person has a response pattern to a physical discomfort or malfunction. Some people become fearful and respond to "false alarms" (hypochondriasis), whereas others experience significant discomfort and even pain, recognize the suspicious symptom, but still fail to seek help. This section examines delay and its counterpart—early cancer detection.

**Table 2-2**  Summary of nine studies of patient delay

| Authors | Study population | Percent of patients who delayed >3 months |
|---|---|---|
| Antonovsky and Hartman (1974) | Review of 22 studies, 1938–1969 | 44 (range:23–76%) |
| Worden and Weisman (1975) | 125 Consecutive cancer patients | 34 |
| E. R. Fisher et al. (1977) | 1539 Stages I and II breast cancer patients | 34 |
| Macadam (1979) | 150 Gastrointestinal cancer patients | Mean delay 9 weeks (range:1 week to >2 years) |
| Post and Belis (1980) | 50 Men with intrascrotal mass | 48 |
| Fruchter et al. (1980) | 80 Invasive cervical cancer patients | 38 |
| DiClemente et al. (1982) | 98 Malignant melanoma patients | 45 |
| Nemoto et al. (1982) | 7397 (Self-detected) breast cancer patients | 29 |
| Feldman et al. (1983) | 395 Breast cancer patients breast lump— only symptom | 40 |
|  | 227 Breast cancer patients no breast lump—other symptoms | 51 |

*Source*: Published with permission of D.M. Eddy and J.F. Eddy (1984). Delay factors in the detection of cancer. *Proc. Am. Cancer Soc. Fourth Ntl. Conf. on Human Values and Cancer*, New York, March 15–17. New York: American Cancer Society, pp. 32–40.

## Psychological Influences in Delay

The first study of delay by Pack and Gallo (1938) defined it as a lapse of more than 3 months between appearance of a definite symptom and seeking consultation. Their definition continued to be widely used, despite the suggestion of use of the less perjorative term of "lagtime" and a clearly delineated time frame (Worden and Weisman, 1975). Several studies of delay were done in the 1950s and 1960s when education about the seven warning symptoms of cancer were being widely promulgated (Cobb et al., 1954; S. Fisher, 1967; Kegeles, 1974; E.R. Fisher et al., 1977; 1967). Kalmer and others reexamined the problem in the 1970s (Kalmer, 1974; DiClemente et al., 1982; Macadam, 1979; Fruchter et al., 1980; Feldman et al., 1983). These showed that three-fourths of those studied delayed at least 1 month after the recognition of a symptom of cancer; 35 to 50% delayed over 3 months (Kalmer, 1974). In 25% of the cases, a month or more elapsed between the initial visit to the doctor and the beginning of treatment. In 1973 a survey of delay was done of 583 cancer patients treated at the Massachusetts General Hospital. Surprisingly, no appreciable decrease in the proportion of patients who delayed was seen when the numbers were compared to a study done 30 years earlier at the same hospital, (Hackett et al., 1973). Because knowledge of cancer and suspicious symptoms had improved, psychological reasons contributing to delay, despite education, were likely responsible.

Eddy and Eddy (1984) reviewed studies of delay and its effect on survival (Table 2-2). Their summary of nine studies, using 3 months or more as defining delay, showed that, although the studies suffered from biases and methodological flaws, one-fourth to three-fourths of the cancer patients examined had delayed more than 3 months, and their chances of long-term survival had been reduced by 10 to 20%. Perception of the risk of disease, the potential for likely benefit from treatment, the "hassle" obtaining a workup, the presence of symptoms, and the need for reassurance were reasons that affected delay. Recommendations were to diminish immobilizing fear and the tendency to deny by reducing the "hassles" of evaluation, providing more public information about cancer symptoms, and, at the same time, emphasizing the benefits of early detection.

Principal reasons associated with delay are outlined in Table 2-3 (Antonovsky and Hartman, 1974; Green and Roberts, 1974; Green et al., 1981). Sociodemographic variables may limit access to adequate health care and are important. Limited or inaccurate knowledge of cancer symptoms may cause delay, as will prior association with cancer, excessive fear, attitudes of guilt, and fatalism. Preexisting personality problems or actual psychiatric illness may result in delay. The absence of easily accessible health care is particularly apparent for older individuals who may have difficulty with an unfamiliar, complex and expensive medical system. The patient who can call a physician without fear of ridicule for undue alarm, and receive an early appointment and examination, has confidence in moving rapidly. A call or visit to an unknown physician, clinic or emergency room is far more apt to be postponed, especially by the elderly.

**Table 2-3** Factors associated with delay in seeking care for cancer symptoms

| Factors | Specific aspects |
| --- | --- |
| Sociodemographic variables | Older age<br>Lower educational level<br>Lower socioeconomic class |
| Knowledge, attitudes, and beliefs about cancer | Poor knowledge of cancer symptoms<br>Previous association with cancer<br>Excessive fears of cancer<br>Emotional meaning, attitudes, and beliefs about cancer (guilt, shame, pessimism, fatalism) |
| Personality and coping styles | Preexisting emotional difficulties or psychiatric illness<br>Tendency to deny or repress disturbing information<br>Rejection of dependent role, with secure feeling of body integrity |
| Poor or absent doctor–patient relationship | |

Individuals whose coping style relies heavily on avoidance, suppression, repression, and denial of threatening or distressing information may ignore obvious cancer risks. When there is also a strong sense of invulnerability to illness and a dislike for yielding control to another, risk of delay is high.

There is evidence that a medical education may affect negatively the reaction time to a cancer symptom. In a study of 569 patients with breast cancer treated at a community hospital, the 7 of 27 who were health professionals reported delays of more than 6 months between finding a mass and reporting it to a physician. Their lesions were somewhat larger than the other women (Buttlar and Templeton, 1983). Pack and Gallo in their 1938 study noted that physicians responded to potential problems no sooner than anyone else. The impact of education and daily work in a medical setting may be an additional largely unrecognized reason for delay.

## Extended Delay

Special attention has been devoted to individuals who tolerate extensive symptoms for extended periods of time. The two primary contributing reasons are psychiatric disorder or illness and site of cancer (Lynch et al., 1966; Lynch and Krush, 1969). Chronically hospitalized schizophrenics have been observed at annual physical examinations to have large, fungating cancerous lesions that they have not reported or complained of pain. Yet the patients had seemingly ignored or been unaware of the discomfort. The reason for this

is not understood. Studies by Talbot and Linn (1978) suggested that this apparent disregard had either a psychological basis of profound mental preoccupation or a possible biochemical basis, involving the perturbation of neurotransmitters that control response to pain. Further studies would be of great interest.

The site of the tumor results in long delays in some individuals, especially penile and testicular neoplasms in men (Post and Belis, 1980) and breast neoplasms in women. The following two cases give examples of unusual reactions of delay and suicide. When the cancer site carries a stigma and compromises the physical self-image, some personality types may be unable to consider or tolerate the diagnosis of cancer. These individuals are at risk of long delay or suicide. There may be attempts to hide evidence of the tumor from others, maintaining the ''secret'' and bearing the burden alone. Also, these patients may be cognizant that they have lost the chance of cure by having permitted extensive tumor growth and when the symptoms can no longer be contained, they may commit suicide. The following case reports the psychological response of two women who demonstrated this uncommon type of extended delay.

### CASE REPORTS

A 50-year-old married mother of four children was an attractive, avid athlete who valued her appearance and her active social and family life. She developed a breast mass and did not reveal its presence to her husband, children, or physician, managing to hide its presence until it began to ulcerate, requiring dressings. She managed, however, to maintain her usual activities, did not show evidence of distress, and hid the breast even from her husband. She was found dead in bed at home, having taken a drug overdose. Autopsy revealed an extensive breast cancer.

A 38-year-old housewife, mother of two children, was admitted to the hospital following a massive hemorrhage from a fungating lesion of the right breast. She had been aware of the lump growing in her breast for over a year. Anxious about it, she told herself that it couldn't be cancer. She began to drink alcohol excessively to relieve her anxiety, causing her family grave concern as she became alcoholic. She was able to hide the breast from her husband. Nevertheless, as the lesion grew larger, she became depressed and ashamed to consult her physician. She then began to develop a fatalistic outlook that she described as, ''I know it's cancer, and I'm going to die anyway; what difference does it make now?'' This alternation of denial and fatalism served effectively to immobilize her until it was too late.

## Physician and Delay

Physicians can also contribute to the delay between the patient's workup of a symptom and the beginning of definitive treatment. Inappropriate reassurance or misdiagnosis by the doctor ordinarily reinforces the pa-

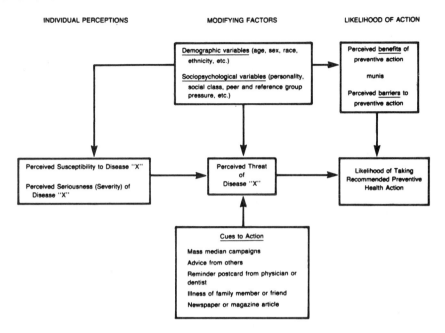

**Figure 2-1.** The "health belief model" as predictor of preventive health behavior. *Source:* Reprinted with permission from M.H. Becker and B.A. Maiman (1975). Sociobehavioral determinants of compliance with health and medical care recommendations. *Med. Care* 13:10–24.

tient's wishful thinking and provides false relief. Patients with advanced or recurrent disease often think back with anger, regret, and depression that, had the physician been more attentive to an early symptom, the course of their disease might have been different.

Physicians contribute to delay in treatment because of inadequate physical examination, too little suspicion of the potential seriousness of a problem and too ready assurance to the patient that a symptom can safely be ignored or watched. Some sites of cancer, because of their psychological meaning are more apt to lead to the physician's decision to procrastinate, such as a testicular lesion where surgical excision has great psychological impact on the patient. Reassurance without sound proof that delay is appropriate is extremely hazardous. The importance of scheduling follow-up appointments to assure that a suspicious lesion or symptom will be monitored, and that the individual recognizes the need for continued vigilance, cannot be overestimated.

The major impetus for early detection comes from well-trained physicians who see their responsibility as extending to include patient teaching and even serving as a role model of good health practices. Teaching breast self-examination to women for their own monthly practice contributes to earlier recognition of breast cancer (Nemoto et al., 1982).

## Early Detection

The means for assuring early detection are based today on a more sophisticated knowledge of the best approach to the public. The health belief model, widely applied today as an explanation of individual health behavior, is derived from psychological and behavioral theory associated with decision making under circumstances of uncertainty and has helped to conceptualize approaches to early cancer detection (see Fig. 2-1) (Leventhal, 1965; Becker and Maiman, 1975). Negative attitudes often center on a perceived lack of probable benefit from the proposed preventive action. The remedial action is most effective when it is paired with an opportunity for immediate action (Kirscht et al., 1966). Fear is an additional influence on the effectiveness of education about cancer (Leventhal, 1965). Similar to the work of Rosenstock, Leventhal found that creating a level of fear is an effective motivator *if* it is coupled with ready access to a simple preventive action. If no action can be taken immediately, fear dissipates and the person may not be aroused by the message when heard a second time. Effective cancer prevention and detection programs must draw upon epidemiology and the behavioral and social sciences (see Part XII, "Research Methods in Psychooncology") (Green et al., 1981; Greenwald et al., 1978).

## SUMMARY

Attitudes about cancer have changed as medicine has learned more about the causes and has applied more effective treatments by combining surgery, radiation, and chemotherapy. Psychiatry (through consultation–liaison, health psychology, and behavioral medicine) has responded to the increased interest in the humanistic and supportive aspects of care, as well as the research initiative in cancer prevention, to provide a new focus in oncology, called psychooncology. The emotional problems embedded in delay in seeking consultation for cancer symptoms, the fears and phobias of cancer seen in healthy individuals, and the attitudes that assure early detection and preventive behaviors, fall within the purview of this newly emerging area.

## REFERENCES

Antonovsky, A. and H. Hartman (1974). Delay in the detection of cancer: A review of the literature. *Health Educ. Monogr.* 2:98–128.

Barsky, A.J. and G.L. Klerman (1983). Overview: Hypochondriasis, bodily complaints and somatic styles. *Am. J. Psychiatry* 14:272–83.

Becker, M.H. and L.A. Maiman (1975). Sociobehavioral determinants of compliance with health and medical care recommendations. *Med. Care* 13:10–21.

Bianchi, G.N. (1971). Origins of disease phobia. *Aust. N.Z. J. Psychiatry* 5:241–57.

Binger, C.M., A.R. Ablin, R.C. Feuerstein, J.H. Kushner, S. Aoger, and C. Mikkelsen (1969). Childhood leukemia. *N. Engl. J. Med.* 280:414–18.

Branch, C.H. (1952). The psychiatric approach to patients with malignant disease. *Rocky Mt. Med. J.* 49:749–53.

Brandt, A. (1985). *No Magic Bullet: A Social History of Venereal Disease in the United States since 1880.* New York: Oxford University Press.

Buttlar, C.A. and A.C. Templeton (1983). The size of breast masses at presentation: The impact of prior medical training. *Cancer* 51:1750–3.

Cain, A.C., I. Fast, and M.E. Erickson (1964). Children's disturbed reactions to the death of a sibling. *Am. J. Orthopsychiatry* 34:741–52.

Cobb, B., R.L. Clark, C. McGuire, and C.D. Howe (1954). Patient-responsible delay of treatment in cancer. *Cancer* 7:920–26.

Di Clemente, R.J. L. Temoshok, L.W. Pickle, A.R. Barrow, and G. Ehlke (1982). Patient delay in the diagnosis of cancer, emphasizing malignant melanoma of the skin. *Prog. Clin. Biol. Res.* 83:185–94.

Eddy, D.M. and J.F. Eddy (1984). Delay factors in the detection of cancer. *Proc. Am. Cancer Soc. Fourth Ntl. Conf. on Human Values and Cancer,* New York, March 15–17. New York: American Cancer Society, pp. 32–40.

Feldman, J.G., M. Saunders, A.C. Carter, and B. Gardner (1983). The effects of patient delay and symptoms other than a lump on survival in breast cancer. *Cancer* 51:1226–29.

Fisher, E.R., C. Redmond, and B. Fisher (1977). A perspective concerning the relation of duration of symptoms to treatment failure in patients with breast cancer. *Cancer* 40:3160–67.

Fisher, S. (1967). Motivation for patient delay. *Arch. Gen. Psychiatry* 16:676–78.

Fruchter, R.G., J. Boyce, M. Hunt, F. Sillman, and I. Medhat (1980). Invasive cancer of the cervix: Failure in prevention II. Delays in diagnosis. *N.Y. State J. Med.* 80:913–17.

Garner, H.H. (1964). Management of the patient with cancerophobia and cancer. *Psychosomatics* 5:147–56.

Green, L.W. and B.J. Roberts (1974). The research literature on why women delay in seeking medical care for breast symptoms. *Health Educ. Monogr.* 2(2):129–77.

Green, L.W., E.T. Rimer, and J.M. Elwood (1981). Behavioral approaches to cancer prevention and detection. In S. Weiss, A. Herd, and B. Fox (eds.), *Perspectives on Behavioral Medicine.* New York: Academic Press, pp. 215–34.

Greenwald, H.P., S. Becker, and M. Nevitt (1978). Delay and noncompliance in cancer detection. *Milbank Mem. Fund Q.* 56:212–30.

Hackett, T.P., N.H. Cassem, and J.W. Rake (1973). Patient delay in cancer. *N. Engl. J. Med.* 289:14–20.

Ingelfinger, F.J. (1975). Cancer! Alarm! Cancer! (Editorial). *N. Engl. J. Med.* 293(25):1319–20.

Kalmer, H. (ed.). (1974). Reviews of research and studies related to delay in seeking diagnosis of cancer. *Health Educ. Monogr.* 2 (2).

Kass, F.C. (1985). Identification of persons with Munchausen's syndrome: Ethical problems. *Gen. Hosp. Psychiatry* 7:195–200.

Kegeles, S. (1967). Attitudes and behavior of the public regarding cervical cytology: Current findings and new directions for research. *J. Chron. Dis.* 20:911–22.

Kirscht, J.P., D.P. Haefner, S.S. Kegeles, and I.M. Rosenstock (1966). A national study of health beliefs. *J. Health Hum. Behav.* 7:248–54.

Leventhal, H. (1965). Fear communications in the acceptance of preventive health practices. *Bull. N.Y. Acad. Med.* 41;1144–68.

Lynch, H.T. and A.J. Krush (1969). Breast carcinoma and delay in treatment surgery. *Gynecol. Obstet. Invest.* 128:1027–32.

Lynch, H.T., T.P. Krush, and A. Krush (1966). Psychodynamics in cancer detection: A patient with advanced cancer of the lip. *Psychosomatics* 7:152–57.

Macadam, D.B. (1979). A study in general practice of the symptoms and delay patterns in the diagnosis of gastrointestinal cancer. *J. R. Coll. Gen. Pract.* 29:723–29.

Nemoto, T., N. Natarajan, C.R. Smart, C. Mettlin, and G.P. Murphy (1982). Patterns of breast cancer detection in the United States. *J. Surg. Oncol.* 21:183–88.

Pack, G.T. and S.J. Gallo (1938)., The culpability for delay in the treatment of cancer. *Am. J. Cancer* 33:443–62.

Post, G.J., J.A. Belis, (1980). Delayed presentation of testicular tumors. *South. Med. J.* 73:33–35.

Ryle, J.A. (1948). The Twenty-First Maudsley Lecture: Nosophobia. *J. Ment. Sci.* 94:1–17.

Sanborn, D. and D. Seibert (1975). The relationship of cancer to suicide. In B. Comstock and R. Maris (ed.). *Proc. Eighth Annu. Mtg. Am. Assoc. Suicidol.* Denver: American Association of Suicidology, pp. 111–18.

Sanborn, D. and D. Seibert (1976). Cancerophobic suicides and history of cancer. *Psychol. Rep.* 38:602.

Talbot, J.A. and L. Linn (1978). Reactions of schizophrenics to life-threatening disease. *Psychiatric Q.* 50:218–27.

Worden, J.W. and A.D. Weisman (1975). Psychosocial components of lagtime in cancer diagnosis. *J. Psychosom. Res.* 19:69–79.

# PART II

## Psychological Factors and Adaptation

# 3

# Developmental Stage and Adaptation: Adult Model

Julia H. Rowland

## BACKGROUND

Three broad variables influence the psychological adjustment of patients to cancer. The first is the sociocultural context in which the cancer occurs (see Part I). Social attitudes and cultural beliefs about cancer can affect not only how we treat patients and their families, but also how patients view themselves, their illness, and future. The medical context of a given patient is another crucial consideration. "Medical context" refers to the stage of disease being treated, the type of treatment being used, and the particular site or sites affected (see Part III). Finally, the individual psychological context within which cancer occurs constitutes a third set of variables and is the focus of this section.

As with overall adjustment, three sets of individual or patient-related variables affect psychological adaptation to cancer. The *developmental stage* is where the person is with respect to life cycle-related biological, personal, and social life goals and tasks when cancer develops. The *intrapersonal style* is what the person brings to the illness by way of previous cancer or medical experience, personality, coping style, and defenses. The *interpersonal resources* are what family, friends, groups of people and other social support structures contribute to the person's environment. Because a patient's status with respect to each of these conditions can materially influence psychological adjustment, medical staff must assess each of these as separate variables to identify sources of strength and weakness. This knowledge can be used to develop a plan for individualized interventions that promote optimal psychological adaptation and psychosocial function during, as well as after, treatment. The chapters in Part II address the specific influences encompassed in these three conditions, review the literature relevant to their meaning in cancer patients, and outline methods for assessing a patient's status with respect to each.

Whereas it is generally acknowledged that one of the fundamental goals of medical education is the acquisition of a global understanding of the patient in both sickness and health (a tradition well described by Peabody in 1929), the multidimensional approach often receives short shrift in medical school teaching and in clinical settings (Schildkraut, 1980; Silverman et al., 1983). Engel has been one of the most vocal proponents of the importance of the biopsychosocial model in clinical medicine as a move away from the predominantly biomedical modes promulgated in Western medical practice (Engel, 1962, 1977; Kimball, 1981; Reiser and Rosen, 1984). The limitations of this latter approach and its contrast to the biopsychosocial perspective are well summarized by Silverman and colleagues (1983):

Derived from molecular biology, the biomedical model assumes that all disease can ultimately be explained in terms of deviations from norms of measurable biological processes. Such a model at once removes disease from its psychological and social contexts and explains all physical and behavioral abnormality as the result of disordered biochemical or neurophysiological events. In so doing, the biomedical, in distinction to the bio-psychosocial, model fails to consider the "crucial stabilizing and destabilizing potential" of intrapsychic, interpersonal, familial, cultural, and societal phenomena in the development, expression, natural history, and outcome of the patient's disease . . . . In addition to placing limitations on the physician's understanding of the cause, course, and treatment of disease, the biomedical model may also serve to depersonalize the practice of medicine and encourage the doctor to neglect the patient's subjective experience of his or her illness as a critical source of data. This in turn may lead the physician to place undue emphasis on more impersonal technical diagnostic procedures and on laboratory measurements. (p. 1154)

In this chapter and those that follow, an effort has been made to illustrate not only the relevance of eliciting personal, familial, and social information from patients, but also the benefits of incorporating this material in plans for management to minimize fragmentation and improve the quality of cancer patient care. Although the chapters address specifically the psychological care of the cancer patient and family, many of the principles covered apply to all patients with life-threatening disease.

In evaluating the psychological context within which treatment occurs, the first consideration is the developmental stage of the patient. How does the use of a developmental model apply to the care of patients with cancer? Cancer, or any other life-threatening disease, naturally has a profound impact on how patients perceive themselves and their environment, whenever it occurs. The main utility of applying a developmental perspective is to draw on the general observations of large populations as they are examined or are obliged to defer or forego major "life tasks," and to relate these insights to the person confronted with cancer. Information about the time at which cancer occurs in the life cycle, and what tasks are threatened or interrupted as a consequence, provides insight into the psychological problems likely to result from the diagnosis and to arise during the treatment and course of the illness.

Like all life-threatening illnesses, cancer poses a real or potential threat to an individual's immediate and future goals. These goals arise from biological, developmental, social, and personal time clocks, that may be explicit or implicit. For example, the young dancer must be helped to aspire to a new career when osteogenic sarcoma causes the loss of a leg. In some cases the natural stresses of a period of life are compounded by an illness. For example, the recently retired couple who have carefully planned and budgeted for their retirement worry when cancer strikes one of them and the escalating medical costs deplete their financial reserves. Diagnosis of cancer may precipitate bitterness in a couple who have worked hard to raise and educate a family, and who then find that the long-denied pleasures of life are precluded. Recognition of where the cancer patient is in life physically, socially, and psychologically is especially useful in interpreting the emotional impact of a particular cancer on the patient; it is even more helpful in anticipating problem areas and planning for appropriate interventions (Eisenberg et al., 1984).

Health professionals working in oncology cannot be expected to assimilate all the information about biological and psychosocial development for all ages. Indeed, even developmental psychologists who have set out to broaden the perspectives of medical professionals must recognize the problems raised by specialization within their own discipline. Most of them generally specialize in a narrow range of age groups (e.g., Bowlby's work in neonatal development and attachment, Offer's research on adolescence, or Neugarten's studies among the aging adult population). In response to this specialization, we have devised a chart that attempts to summarize the major biological, social, and psychological tasks associated with each life stage that are generally regarded as part of normal development; contrasted with this is a body of illness-related material. In its totality, this material is designed to highlight the potential disruptions to an individual's "developmental agenda" when illness is experienced at a given stage of life. It also serves to draw attention to the differences in individuals' responses to cancer that are in part a function of the specific goals, responsibilities, and resources associated with a given life stage. The chart is summarized in Appendices A–H.

However, there is a general pattern that reflects universal areas of disruption. In reviewing the impact of cancer at all life stages, we found that the common disruptions of illness could be divided into five categories that denote major themes of stress: *altered interpersonal relationships, dependence–independence, achievement disruption, body–sexual image and integrity,* and *existential issues*. These are not ordered in terms of their importance. Indeed, the importance of a specific disruption may vary by stage as well as by individual. To make them easier to remember, these disruptions have been simplified to "the five D's": distance, dependence, disability, disfigurement, and death. Looking at the chart by age group, it can be seen that although the themes remain constant, the specific context or meaning of each varies greatly.

By identifying areas likely to cause special stress, and understanding the source of life task disruptions, we can hypothesize and devise appropriate psychosocial interventions. As noted earlier, this information is outlined in a format designed to provide the clinician with a quick overview of life cycle stages, expected milestones, common sites of tumors, likely psychosocial disruptions, and suggested interventions. However, as with any highly generalized scheme of information, several caveats to its use are in order.

First, this sort of approach is intended only as a starting point. Clinicians can use the chart as a quick reference or, by checking the source materials summarized, can pursue in greater depth an area of special interest. Although it would be possible to refer only to the illness-related aspects of the chart, the developmental sections provide information useful to understanding the origins or dynamics of particular psychological problems typical of a specific age group. The information in the chart provides general guidelines meant to be interpreted, elaborated, and applied by readers in conjunction with their prior clinical training and experience.

As a corollary to this point, it should be noted that the content of the chart reflects current societal mores and expectations of individuals at each life stage. Obviously, as social demands related to age change, modifications in the time schema or tasks outlined in the chart must be adjusted accordingly. Similarly, available psychosocial interventions vary by geographic area and type of facility. Clinicians should take into account the kind of resources available to the hospital and patient or family when using the chart as a guideline for planning.

Second, although the biological norms described in the chart are widely applicable, the developmental norms have been generated from largely middle-class and in some cases, predominantly Caucasian, samples. Norms may vary by ethnicity, social class, and sex. For example, children of a lower-class background are more often exposed to death caused by violence than are children from families of the middle and upper classes, who tend to experience death as a consequence of illness and old age (Nagy, 1948). Neugarten (1968a) has reported that individuals in lower social classes have a different sense of the timing of major life events (e.g., marriage, age at first job, grandparenthood), and experience them as occurring earlier than more affluent groups. With regard to changes related to sex, we have seen a recent increase in the numbers of women working and on the importance placed by society on women's career potentials.

Third, although we have assigned age ranges to identify each of the eight labeled stage periods, these should not be viewed as absolute. Patients may exhibit developmental attributes characteristic of individuals in a stage that, by age alone, would classify them above or below their designated level. For example, the 24-year-old Hodgkin's patient who has two aging parents to support may face many of the problems that the "mature adult" confronts, in addition to those of his or her own age group. Moreover, as stage transition is not viewed as an all-inclusive process, a person may exhibit behaviors or responses typical of more than one stage. For example, a child may be socially very competent and mature but have a concept of death more similar to that of a younger child. For these reasons one must take into account those characteristics that might make either side of the given age group within which a patient falls more appropriate than the one usually assigned.

Fourth, and of special importance for *prospective* counseling, the practitioner must have a general knowledge of developmental tasks the individual is likely to confront over his or her entire life span. This is particularly critical in interventions developed during primary treatment, which have implications for later developmental stages in patients with good prognosis for cure and a normal life span. A 24-year-old young man with Hodgkin's disease should be informed of the risk of chemotherapy-related sterility and offered sperm banking prior to initial treatment. Knowing what future tasks may be affected by current treatment facilitates effective rehabilitation efforts.

Fifth, though separated here for purposes of simplification, the life cycle models for the child, adolescent, and the adult obviously form a continuum. A working familiarity with the whole life cycle is essential for all oncological staff members, irrespective of primary responsibility in adult or childhood cancer. Cancer in one family member affects all other members as well, disrupting certain of their life cycle goals. Children with cancer must be considered in conjunction with their parents; children often become psychologically vulnerable when their parents have cancer. In particular, an appreciation of the changes that occur over time in the concept of death is helpful in caring for the affected relatives. Thus, the use of the chart should not be restricted to an understanding of a patient's emotional response. Families follow their own developmental patterns, which are described more fully in Chapter 47. For organizational reasons the chart emphasizes individuals, but the family context is a highly important variable.

Finally, staff reaction to work in the oncology setting, where they deal often with sadness and loss, has developmental overtones. Awareness of these is helpful in understanding and interpreting strong identification with certain patients and unusual grief reactions, such as those illustrated in Chapter 51.

The primary purpose of the chart is to provide a framework for looking at individuals under stress of cancer; by referring to the chart, caregivers can look at the person and affected family from the perspective of their normal life course, in which cancer is an unwelcome intruder requiring major accommodation and adaptation. How this is done, the courage with which individuals, families, and professionals face these problems, is as personal as any autobiography. The developmental approach, however, can offer a context and general guidelines from which to view and care for the individual.

The remainder of this chapter describes in detail the four outlined adult developmental stages. The major psychological themes for each stage are reviewed, with examples of problems and interventions. Information on the four childhood stages are detailed in Chapter 43 as part of the introduction to the childhood cancer section, Part VIII.

## ADULT DEVELOPMENTAL MODEL

The use of a life cycle model in assessing adult populations is a relatively new development. Although those working with psychological and physical problems of children and adolescents have long been trained to evaluate their patients by age and developmental milestones, differences in the responses of adults by age and life cycle stage have been poorly recognized and are thus often neglected. The notion that adults no less than children undergo continuing developmental stages with similar opportunities for emotional growth is a relatively recent analytical concept.

Early childhood development is marked by a fairly predictable progression of physical changes that can be used as milestones and studied in terms of related social and emotional growth. Childhood lends itself well to a developmental model, because signs of growth are easily defined, are sometimes dramatic, and follow a generally uniform course (regardless of culture or social experience). In the early adult years there is a decreased primacy of the biological clock and an increased emphasis on the social clock, until midlife and the older adult years when the biological clock reasserts itself.

Entry into adulthood is typically characterized by a slowing or stabilization of physical and physiological changes, and an increasing complexity of socioemotional growth. Because social development is more variable in terms of its definition, direction, and the timing of changes, creation of a coherent and universally applicable model of development is difficult. Previously, most studies focused on discrete periods of adult development in which a physical or major social change was primary. The impact of pregnancy and menopause in women, retirement in men, and aging in both sexes served as common topics. More recently, however, researchers have systematically studied cohorts of adults to obtain information about a spectrum of life tasks (cf. Vaillant and Milofsky, 1980; Vaillant, 1977; Lowenthal et al., 1975; Levinson et al., 1978). As a consequence, although there is not yet a universal model of adult life cycle milestones, there are a number of theoretical overviews developed by such researchers as Eric Erikson, Bernice Neugarten, Daniel Levinson, and George Vaillant, which, though probably culture-specific, provide a framework within which to appreciate biological and social tasks, thereby highlighting those areas most likely to be affected by a disease such as cancer.

The differences between child and adult developmental models when viewed from a historical perspective serve to illustrate the different forces in these two life periods. The models of Freud and Piaget are directly tied to the evolving biological organism: Freud to the unfolding psychosexual being and Piaget to the developing cognitive structure and capacity (Freud, 1952, 1962; Piaget, 1952; Ginsburg and Opper, 1969). In contrast, Erikson's developmental life span model and the work of Neugarten, Levinson, and Vaillant emphasize the influence of societal forces, and are less driven by biology and focus on the changing psychosocial self (Erikson, 1958, 1963; Neugarten, 1968a,b; Levinson, 1978, 1986; Levinson et al., 1978; Levinson and Gooden, 1985; Vaillant, 1977; Mages and Mendelsohn, 1980). The adult-stage theorists also differ in that, in addition to delineating tasks of each period, they afford perhaps even greater attention to the consequences to the individual of a crisis or life task not well navigated. Rather than chronicling the stages and tasks themselves and the negative consequences of failure to progress, the adult theorists emphasize the requisites of mastery. This is particularly so in Erikson's research, but is also true of Levinson. Taking this emphasis one step further, Vaillant's work attempts to evaluate which ego-adaptive coping mechanisms characteristic of young adulthood are predictive of an older adult who is healthy, well adjusted, and happy. Like child developmental theorists, adult-stage theorists see a cyclic pattern in growth over the life span with periods of stability alternating with periods of change (Vaillant and Milofsky, 1980; Levinson, 1986).

Despite wide individual variability, the greater predictability of biological (e.g., walking, talking, sexual maturation) and social (e.g., entry and progression through school, adolescence) stages during childhood facilitates the assignment of relative age ranges. This is not the case once one enters adulthood. In the first place, the rationale for dividing adulthood into four eras appears at times to be merely pragmatic.

In their provocative essay reflecting on the changes of age, the Neugartens speak of "the fluid life cycle," in which there is a blurring of the distinctions between life periods (Neugarten and Neugarten, 1987). That increasing numbers of women are having their first child before age 15 or after 35, and that more adults, particularly women, exit and reenter school and the work force (and undertake serial careers) is taken as evidence that the very rhythm and timing of life events is changing. The median age at first marriage for both men and women is rising. In global terms, the rapidly changing social realities have softened the sharp distinctions between events occurring too late or too early. To the cancer patient whose development may be delayed during illness or need to be later restructured, this may be a boon. Living at home or alone longer, a delay in starting a family or the decision not to have one, or entering school or a career later are more common, resulting in less stigma for individuals who follow these paths as a consequence of illness. Charting the expected tasks and responsibilities of adulthood for purposes of planning interventions has thus become more complex.

Erikson saw adult development as having only three stages (Erikson, 1963). However, the increasing emphasis on the period called "youth," the time after adolescence but before the assumption of full adult responsibilities, has made important the inclusion of four periods—at least in samples from the middle and upper class (Keniston, 1975; Erikson, 1968).

If segmenting and assigning prescribed tasks to different periods of life has become increasingly complex, then with adulthood the finding of age markers with which to label each era is even more difficult. There are some who would argue that this attempt should be abandoned entirely (Gould, 1978; Butler, 1963a). Though not entirely arbitrary, the age brackets assigned must be interpreted with flexibility. As the baby boom generation ages, we are likely to see the retirement age being pushed past 65, even though there is still a psychological aura associated with this age for many. This is also true for ages 30 and 45, which serve as the upper boundaries for the earlier periods of life. In the case of these latter ages, however, there is also research to suggest that transitions do occur around these periods and that they thus serve as appropriate demarcations of developmental change (Neugarten, 1968c, 1979; Levinson, 1977). What becomes apparent in reading through the adult sections of this chart is the enormous overlap in demands from one period to the next. In childhood, as a rule, developmental tasks are more clearly (or with greater frequency) relegated to one period or another (e.g., walking 9–18 months, puberty, 10–14 years). In adulthood they may span all four eras (e.g., marriage for both sexes, getting a first job for women, having children for men). In addition, age is becoming an increasingly poor indicator of health status (Birren and Schaie, 1977; Neugarten, 1974). Thus, although general characteristics of an era are important, it is equally important to look ahead and back at tasks that may be more common at earlier and later periods to understand what hurdles a patient and family face.

In the text that follows, information for each of the four adult periods defined is covered in a format that closely follows the way it is presented in the chart. Material is grouped within each period under four sections. The *Developmental Tasks* section summarizes the details of the relevant physical, cognitive, linguistic, affective, social, and psychosexual tasks. This section also elaborates on the life cycle model theories, as well as the life–death concepts germain to the period though not shown in the chart. The *Common Tumors* (not included in the chart) are listed for each period,

and the more salient characteristics of the impact of these on stage-specific functions are highlighted. Under *Disruptions of Illness*, the concerns most typical of the period are addressed in the order that they are covered in the chart: (1) *altered relationships*, (2) *dependence–independence issues*, (3) *achievement disruptions*, (4) *impact on body–sexual image and integrity*, and (5) *existential issues*. Finally the specific *Interventions* derived from this knowledge and that serve to guide patient management are detailed for each period.

## THE YOUNG ADULT (19–30 YEARS)

### Developmental Tasks

The individual's transition from adolescence to young adulthood, usually assumed to occur by age 20, is typically marked by maturity both physically and psychologically. Intellectually the young adult tends to be egocentric about the origin of ideas, believing at times that he or she is the first to experience profound feelings or to see the world in all its complexity. One of the tasks of this period is to put progressively this egocentric tendency into perspective. Writing and speaking skills also improve and peak by the end of the period. Most individuals complete their formal education, including—for some—advanced technical or professional degrees. Jobs consonant with career goals are undertaken, and plans for advancement in a specific area are mapped out.

In the affective and social area, autonomy from the family of origin is usually achieved, as personal values and goals are formulated. The key life cycle task of the young adult is centered on the achievement of intimacy and closeness to others, particularly sexual. Sexual identity is established, with a satisfactory relationship with a sexual partner as a goal. Commitment to another (usually with marriage and acceptance of a parental role), a more mature perspective about one's own parents, and the identification of long-term career plans are significant milestone achievements associated with this period. A reconciliation of sexual identity that is consonant with work, career, parental, and nurturing roles must be achieved. Concepts of death for the young adult are essentially the same as in adolescence, except that there is greater clarity about the universality of death, especially as personal contact with death in the extended family is experienced (e.g., grandparents, and accidental death or fatal illness among peers).

Because much of what occurs in the early part of this period may reflect late adolescent changes, it is helpful to review the developmental changes expected in these years as detailed in Chapter 43. Erikson (1963) has defined the early-adult period as one characterized by *intimacy versus isolation*. A mature sexual relationship is an important dimension to the normal development of close and intimate ties. Inability to achieve this aim results in isolation and poses a threat to the person's ability to reach the usual developmental milestones of the period. Vaillant (1977), extending Erikson's model, saw as a substage of this period the need to balance *career consolidation versus self-absorption*.

Both Neugarten (1968a) and Levinson (1978) describe the period as one in which the individual strives to find a comfortable fit between self and society, and explores the adult role to find an acceptable and stable life structure that permits individuation while enabling investment in another. Levinson (1978) sees this period as one in which individuals enter the adult world and create and explore their own first adult life structure. The end of the period is heralded by incipient efforts at changing this structure, a point referred to in Levinson's model as the "age 30 transition," seen as spanning the years from 28 to 33. At this point, life goals and structure become more reality oriented. This is a time when energies are directed toward recognizing and working with the flaws and limitations of the first adult structure and thus creating the basis for a more satisfactory structure, one that can carry the individual through the next era of development.

In Levinson's broader model, the years from age 17 to 45 are defined as the era of early adulthood. He notes that, although this is the era of greatest energy and abundance, it can also be one of crushing stresses. "Early adulthood is the era in which we are most buffeted by our own passions and ambitions from within and by the demands of family, community, and society from without" (Levinson, 1986, p. 5).

## Common Tumors

The common hematological malignancies of young adulthood are acute leukemia, Hodgkin's disease, and lymphoma. Testicular cancer in men, breast cancer in women, and osteogenic sarcoma and brain tumors in both sexes are the most common solid tumors. The impact of a given tumor necessarily varies by site involved, the clinical course of the cancer, and the treatment required. These medical and related considerations in adaptation are covered in the chapters of Part III. However, each of these tumors, irrespective of the specific effects, has a dramatic impact on the young adult's ability to develop or sustain close relationships, to commit to another, to achieve work goals, and to maintain independence. Physical appearance and often fertility may be compromised as well. As survival has become more common, attention to the delayed or long-term psychological sequelae has also increased in importance.

## Disruptions of Illness

### ALTERED RELATIONSHIPS

The young man or woman who is diagnosed as having cancer questions developing a close bond with another. Similarly, the physically healthy partner may seriously question commitment to a person with cancer. Even a close, established relationship is strained because of fear and guilt about the potential consequences of the illness (fatality, disability, and dysfunction). The individual may opt to remain emotionally isolated rather than deal with the real or perceived demands of maintaining old or beginning new relationships. The stigma of cancer is often keenly felt in this population, and the person may actually be shunned by healthy peers who "can't handle it." This is particularly true for those with Hodgkin's disease, which evokes public and private concerns about contagion and potential transmissibility to others. The demands of personal life, domestic routines, and concerns for the future, particularly when children are involved, are exaggerated. Fears of death in the young parent focus on leaving a young child or children. The single parent must deal realistically with guardianship, sometimes with settlement of a divorce. The couple must address how the single parent will manage alone. Aging parents' care is a concern as well.

### DEPENDENCE–INDEPENDENCE

Cancer usually makes it necessary to depend on others. Inability to carry out usual family roles, which must then be assumed by another, has a deleterious effect on self-esteem. Reliance on another for personal hygiene is difficult to accept. The need for the patient to assume a submissive, dependent role in relation to the oncologist who outlines a treatment, coexists with demands for a high level of participation and cooperation if the full therapeutic effects of the treatment are to be achieved. Finding a balance between these two seemingly conflicting roles requires effort. For many, this period in their life may be one in which there are few ties to a health care system; sudden dependence on one for survival can thus produce anger and resentment. Rebellious feelings, though more frequently associated with adolescence, are also common in this age group. Demonstrations of anger are manifested by refusal of or poor compliance with treatment. The family may attempt to overprotect the patient and yield poorly to demands for independence after treatment. Similarly, excessive dependence may be difficult to give up for some individuals with emotional problems and may result in their achieving less than expected rehabilitation goals.

## ACHIEVEMENT DISRUPTIONS

Uncertainty associated with cancer is felt no more poignantly than in relation to meeting aspirations and expectations about career. The young adult is pursuing advanced educational goals or beginning in a trade or professional apprenticeship that in every sense is geared toward ''moving up'' and ahead. The diagnosis of cancer places a cloud over these expectations and is associated with realistic anxieties that the future may be substantially altered by virtue of treatment sequelae. The disruption in the ability to meet expectations of a job and fears that cancer affects an employer's decisions about advancement, are major concerns, even in those long cured of cancer. This is reviewed in detail by Tross in Chapter 7. The milestones by which one normally measures career success or failure at a given point may be delayed during illness or subsequently unachieved as a result of illness and treatment. A reassessment of goals is often needed, but not easy to accomplish. Disappointment and despair are not uncommon.

## BODY IMAGE AND INTEGRITY

Cancer causes a major psychological disruption by its feared or actual association with diminished attractiveness, effect on the patient's ability to elicit affection from others, and the effect on the ability to establish or maintain a sexual relationship. In general, treatment of the common tumors in the young-adult age group have significant side effects: alopecia, nausea and vomiting, anorexia, weight loss, fatigue, weakness, and lowered libido—all symptoms that can lead the patient to be or feel less attractive as a potential or actual sexual partner or spouse.

Uncertainty about whether reduced fertility or sterility will result from a chemotherapy regimen that is cytotoxic to germ cells in both sexes, or from radiation to pelvic areas, raises real issues about the ability to have children. When the libido is diminished by the effects and treatment of illness, and the threat of infertility is high, these combined influences may cause profound disruption to the sexual and marital role of the patient. Significant anxiety and depression may occur, resulting in both a psychological and a physical basis for sexual dysfunction.

## EXISTENTIAL ISSUES

The fear that cancer will recur and cause death is a constant worry with any new, even minor, symptom after a cancer diagnosis. The acknowledged finality of death represents a threat to the individual's personal identity and to his or her sense of continuity with subsequent generations. This latter issue has particular impact on individuals who are the only children or who are childless.

### Interventions

The central theme for interventions with young adults is counseling with emphasis on restoring and buttressing interpersonal relations. Toward this end, frequent visits by friends and family while the patient is in the hospital are important. At home, usual role functions should be encouraged and maintained, even if this is at times limited to decision making alone. Visits from friends and colleagues from the work place, aside from providing an important source of social support, serve to keep contact with roles outside the family.

Although these visits are important to maintaining the individual's interpersonal relations and minimizing a sense of isolation, they can also be stressful. Patients often need guidance in how much information about their illness should be given to their children, family, employer, and friends. Group discussions with other patients who have the same disease or who received the same treatment can be useful. (See also Chapter 41 on self-help groups.) Such meetings enable patients to express and explore their fears, expectations, and concerns. The new relationships formed in peer group meetings are also important in themselves, because they are active proof that social life need not end or atrophy with cancer. Recognizing and helping patients express and manage the conflicts that arise between dependencies imposed by illness and the desire for self-sufficiency can also minimize the likelihood that a patient will seek to assert control counterproductively through noncompliance.

The patient's core relationships with intimate friends and relations require special attention. What are the attitudes, beliefs, and feelings about cancer held by the patient and this intimate circle? Is counseling required to correct misperceptions? For young adult patients with young children, planning for financial security is an important task, including the drawing up of wills and arranging for additional help at home and the substitute caregivers for young children. Clarification of health and life insurance benefits, job security, and related benefits, as well as a review and restructuring of financial liabilities and obligations are a necessary part of this process.

Because of the intense interpersonal and social demands of this developmental period, it is important to assess the individual's potential for recovery early, and to reassess it frequently. Information, including uncertainties, should be shared openly with patient and spouse or relevant family members. Clarification of the level of rehabilitation possible and early identification of problems in achieving this can prevent the development of maladaptive responses such as overdependency on family, friends, or hospital staff, and poor motivation (giving up or hopelessness), or the opposite emotions of anger and frustration arising out of overly ambitious or unrealistic expectations and efforts.

Work, career, family, and interpersonal goals may all need to be reassessed and reformulated with the onset of cancer. Managing the unavoidable changes in the least disruptive way can help the individual maintain self-esteem and keep his or her relative accomplishments in view. Planning chemotherapy to cause minimal work disruption is helpful. If home life is significantly disrupted, the availability of support homemaker services may be important, especially for the children. Often neglected, it is of extreme importance to monitor the adaptation of children and other family members at home for the effects of parental illness. (See also Chapter 47 on family.)

As with adolescents, discussions with young adult patients about the meaning of the illness to their sense of self-worth and future are essential. Attention should be given to special problems of altered appearance. Normal appearance, as nearly as possible, should be encouraged. Psychological preparation for possible alopecia should be initiated and if necessary the purchase of a wig. If necessary a prosthesis should be encouraged with training for its use begun as early as possible.

Issues concerning sexual function are likely to be particularly sensitive and may be difficult for the patient to discuss without encouragement. It is all the more important, therefore, for the doctor to address these questions frankly and promptly. Referral of both the patient and partner for sexual counseling may be suggested. Tangible measures such as sperm banking may be appropriate before undertaking chemotherapy.

Counseling offered in the course of routine treatment by the doctor, nurse, or social worker often covers many of the salient issues outlined earlier. One should not, however, overlook the importance of religion. Pastoral counseling can be a valuable source of psychological support, providing an opportunity for the patient and family to explore and come to terms with existential issues and the meaning of life.

## THE MATURE ADULT (31–45 YEARS)

### Developmental Tasks

This period in development is characterized by personal growth and consolidation of career and social goals.

It is, perhaps, in general terms the most stable period in the life course. In their research with a sample of men initially seen as Harvard freshmen, Vaillant and his colleagues (1977) reported that those considered to be doing best in their late forties "regarded the period from 35 to 49 as the happiest in their lives, and the seemingly calmer period from 21–35 as the unhappiest." Although subtle signs of aging begin to appear (e.g., decreased bone density, mild decrements in functional capacity of major organs, tendency to put on and keep extra weight, appearance of facial wrinkles, changes in vision), physical capacity remains constant. In terms of cognition, many feel this season in the life span encompasses the peak period of intellectual ability. Social and emotional tasks center on childrearing or, increasingly, establishing a family for the first time and nurturing of a younger generation in their social and work contexts. Personal identity stabilizes and solidifies.

As the adult matures, so too does the family, requiring the adjustment and redefinition of ties to growing children and aging parents. Anticipation of illness and preparation for parental death occurs. Roles become more closely defined, both at home and at work. Special efforts are required to maintain a satisfactory home environment on the one hand, and achieve entrepreneurial success, job recognition, and upward mobility on the other. For many individuals this period is also associated with their optimal sexual life. As desired family size is achieved and the associated pressures to produce or perform are relieved, sexual activity can assume a new level of intimacy and provide a more relaxed and recreational outlet. Gould (1972) found a growing satisfaction with marriage and friends in the period from ages 44 to 50.

For Erikson (1963) the central task of this developmental period (commencing around age 40) is the resolution of the conflict between *generativity versus stagnation*. The individual needs to be engaged in establishing and guiding the next generation. For this reason the period can be typified as one of productivity and caring. Failure to achieve a productive and creative sense can lead to personal impoverishment, pseudointimacy, excessive dependency, or premature disengagement from society. Vaillant (1977) added a stage to Erikson's model. He saw as stage 7a the individual's need to adopt the role as "keeper of the meaning" of life, hopes, and goals for the next generation, thereby avoiding the risk of becoming rigid, unable to grow further or share.

Levinson (1978) describes the years from 33 to 40 as a "settling-down" period, a time during which the individual establishes a niche in society, works at "making it," "becoming one's own person," and adjusts to what Levinson calls the "second adult life structure." This is the outgrowth and resolution of the age 30 transition tasks described in the preceding developmental section. Indeed, in Levinson's model (1977), what are referred to here as the mature-adult years are seen as bounded on either side by periods of transition; the age 30 transition on one side and the midlife transition, occurring some time between the ages of 40 and 45, as the other. In this latter stage, every aspect of life is questioned; there is a search for an optimum balance among a variety of choices: expression of desires, aspirations, talents, values, and previously neglected parts of the self. Satisfactory resolution of these "intentionality" questions for each individual is a necessary and important task of this developmental stage. "To the extent that this occurs, we can become more compassionate, more reflective and judicious, less tyrannized by inner conflicts and external demands, and more genuinely loving of ourselves and others. Without it, our lives become increasingly trivial or stagnant" (Levinson, 1986, p. 5).

That the time around age 40 is stressful for many, both in marriage and personally, is echoed by other adult development researchers (Vaillant, 1977; Gould, 1972, 1978). Gould (1978) emphasizes the importance of the individual's ability to change early expectations. "Childhood delivers most people into adulthood with a view of adults that few could ever live up to." Work by Vaillant (1977) and his team suggests that those who embrace this period of change adapt best while those who may seek to retreat to earlier (calmer, less painful) periods adapt more poorly. Jacques (1965) suggests that fundamental to the midlife crisis is confrontation with mortality.

## Common Tumors

Cancers of the lung, breast, colon and rectum, uterus, ovary, pancreas, brain, and nervous system are the common solid tumors. Leukemia and lymphoma are the common hematological malignancies. The treatment for most cancers in these sites is aggressive, involving surgery, often combined with radiation and multidrug chemotherapy.

## Disruptions of Illness

Because many of the tasks of this period grow out of those of the preceding stage, similar disruptions are faced by patients with cancer in both of these life cycle stages. For this reason, it is useful to review the disruptions noted in the preceding section, as well as this one to gain a full appreciation of the issues patients may confront.

## ALTERED RELATIONSHIPS

As in the preceding period, diagnosis and treatment may separate patient from family. Fears of being abandoned are experienced by both patient and partner. Patients and family members alike may feel further isolated by real or perceived social stigmatization. While good relationships may become even stronger in such crises, the stresses of illness can further strain already faltering relations. The family may become preoccupied by what to tell aging parents or young children. The threat to life precipitates regrets about leaving a partner, children, and other family, and concern for the social, financial, and educational well-being of these individuals—feelings that may alternate at times with a sense of anger and despair that they and not he or she will be survivors.

## DEPENDENCE–INDEPENDENCE

Responsibilities ordinarily carried by the patient may have to be assumed by a partner; the active partner may need to be more passive. Such role reversals create an additional burden on families. The assumption of the more dependent role may be particularly stressful for men. Such a situation can also result in overdependency and a yielding to illness, or the opposite of overcompensation that is exhibited in a premature return to physical activity and excessive effort in work.

## ACHIEVEMENT DISRUPTIONS

A premature return to work may be fueled by anxieties about one's employment status. Both illness-related job disruptions and the high cost of medical care may also threaten long-term personal and familial financial commitments (e.g., children's education, business obligations, mortgages, and loans). Depending on the course of the illness and treatment, certain life goals may have to be altered or abandoned.

## BODY IMAGE AND INTEGRITY

In addition to the considerable costs in time, money, and emotional energies, cancer and cancer therapy often impose enormous physical burdens. Combination treatment may result in hair loss, fatigue, nausea and vomiting, and anorexia, as well as sterility, infertility, impotence or frigidity, and disfigurement. Any existing sexual problems are frequently exacerbated by the effects of illness. Associated changes in body image, physical or cognitive disability, or reproductive capacity serve to accentuate the sense of physical vulnerability experienced normally with aging. In the same vein, for patients who have no evidence of disease and are in remission or actually cured, minor physical symptoms of aging (e.g., arthritic pain or change in vision) may be interpreted as signs of a return or progression of disease.

## EXISTENTIAL ISSUES

Because it has an impact on all aspects of a person's life, present and future, illness represents a major threat to the individual's identity. Individuals who have drawn on their religious beliefs for strength may feel that illness threatens even this source of personal support. A questioning of cosmic purpose, of long-held spiritual value, and religious beliefs may be interpreted by the patient and family as an indication of faltering faith. For others, cancer can restore and re-affirm beliefs that were held more strongly at an earlier age, and serve as a comfort and source of strength.

### Interventions

The mature adult surrounds himself or herself with family members, close friends, and possibly work associates. Maintaining and fostering optimal interpersonal relations within this support group should be the central theme for interventions. Several approaches can be appropriate. Daily routines should remain as normal as possible. Family, friends, and peers should be encouraged to visit during periods of hospitalization or confinement. The counselor can contribute by identifying areas of stress and seeking to manage them. Patient and family groups can be useful vehicles for sharing feelings, correcting misinformation (e.g., communicability of disease), and combatting despondency. Counseling can also address practical questions such as financial planning (including insurance coverage, decreased income, alternate income sources, and debt refinancing) and the need for live-in or paid help at home. The counselor can encourage families to communicate openly with children about the parent's illness. Their responses to the illness of a mother or father, and the changes in their routine it necessitates, should also be monitored by the oncologist as a routine part of a clinic visit. Older children, especially adolescents, may develop deviant or hostile behavior that, in turn, is poorly understood or tolerated by the parents under stress. Parent and child alike are uncomfortable with parental vulnerability, but the children should not be "protected," even though both may instinctively favor such an approach.

The most successful interventions are those that minimize social isolation and loss of home and work routines, and that preserve to the extent possible the patient's sense of vitality and ability to contribute. Assumption of maximal self-care with realistic rehabilitation goals supports this approach. If work roles and patterns are irretrievably altered, consider vocational counseling and retraining.

Scheduling radiotherapy and chemotherapy treatments and follow-up visits to cause minimal home and work disruption, though not always easy, has dramatic positive effects. Relaxation techniques and other psychotherapeutic approaches can mitigate the stress and disruption of radiotherapy and chemotherapy (see Chapters 35, 38, 40). While helping to ease the discomfort associated with treatment, they also provide the patient with an element of control and allow the feeling of active participation in the treatment plan.

For many patients, the opportunity to speak to a veteran patient, someone who has faced and dealt with similar disease, treatment, and life issues can represent a unique source of support (see Chapter 41). These individuals not only provide emotional support to the patient, but are also frequently a special resource for dealing with concrete problems of illness, such as finding a good place to buy wigs or breast prostheses, learning how to manage colostomy care or master esophageal speech, or adjusting to alterations in sexual activities necessitated by pelvic, urological, and gynecological, cancer surgery. Patient counselors are an invaluable asset to the overall rehabilitative effort toward supporting normal appearance and function.

An opportunity to discuss any changes in sexual function should be provided to all patients, with referral for sexual counseling as needed. These sessions, generally conducted by specially trained individuals, include review of past and present psychosexual functioning, with special attention given to specific problems resulting from disease or treatment (e.g., need for sperm banking, penile prostheses, and advice about adoption). (See Chapter 33 for a general elaboration of sexual therapy for cancer patients.) Minor physical symptoms continue to elicit anxiety about recurrence even years after a cure has been achieved. A thorough physical examination is warranted, accompanied by a discussion geared toward helping the patient reformulate an appropriate level of body monitoring. If reassurance from a normal examination by the oncologist is inadequate, referral to a psychiatrist would be helpful.

Like physical concerns, a patient's existential concerns also produce fears about the future. The patient may need guidance in the search for meaning to the past as well as the rest of life and ultimately death. Pastoral, lay, and group counseling each provide a forum for reviewing these issues and should be available to all.

## THE OLDER ADULT (46–65 YEARS)

As the average life expectancy increases, the period referred to as "middle age" has been shifting to a later time in the life span. For most contemporary Americans, it probably occurs somewhere between the end of the preceding period (e.g., age 40–45) and extends into the older adult period. The life review and reflection associated with this time are a forerunner to and, in a sense, set the stage for adjustments in later years. Whereas the earlier period only alerted the individual to tasks or approaching changes, the older adult actually sees the realization of many of those anticipated alterations.

Despite enormous individual variability, most adults between the ages of 45 and 65 experience and adapt to a range of physical, emotional, and social changes. A number of physical changes associated with this period include the redistribution of fatty deposits, skin changes, the incipient loss of musculoskeletal integrity, decrements in bone density and mass (osteoporosis in women), a trend toward increased weight despite a decrease in body mass, and gradual vertebral compression. Women must adjust to menopausal hormonal changes that serve as biological reminders of the aging process. Toward the end of this period, signs of a slow decrease in intellectual acumen may be noted. The changes are more pronounced on tasks involving sensorimotor and visuoperceptual skills as a result of the compromising of the physical determinants of these functions by aging (e.g., poorer eyesight and slower reaction time). Such changes contribute to the sense of physical vulnerability and result in a focus on body monitoring.

Physical changes are also accompanied by modifications in the individual's psychosexual identity. Following the male climacteric, men generally assume a more passive mode of mastery, both sexually and socially, and become more nurturing. The role reversal (or reclaiming of submerged aspects of personality—cf. Jung, 1933) at this stage is prompted by social as well as hormonal alterations. Women, generally more involved in early child care, often adapt to children leaving home by becoming active in work, in late-career development, or in altruistic volunteering of time outside the home (Notman, 1979). As increasing numbers of women join the work force, the phenomenon of "the empty-nest syndrome" and its associated stresses have become less common. Rather, in some cases, stress may be felt by families experiencing the "return to the nest" or "failure to leave the nest" of adult children.

New family roles must be established between parents and adult child or children, and also between spouses. A reclaimed intimacy between partners can be a special outcome, bringing with it a sense of freedom to focus on more personal issues that were postponed by prior responsibilities. The assumption of the role as nurturer to grandchildren evolves and heightens the introspection and reflection appropriate to this era.

Careers or business success usually peak during the early years of this stage. Career goals have been reached by the end of the period, or more often, the person has been progressively adjusting the goals to conform to realistic expectations. Few adults would honestly claim that all their youthful goals had been fulfilled. There is a natural inclination toward stock taking and a growing awareness during these years of being on the upper half of the age curve. Change in attitude is reflected by a gradual reformulation of time perspective from "years since birth" to "years left" (Neugarten, 1968c). There begins to be mental rehearsal of death with a new personal meaning associated with it. Writing of wills, financial planning for survivors, and passing on of family sentimental treasures begins more seriously.

For Levinson (1986), the years from 40 to 65 encompass the era of middle adulthood, the period of the second adult life structure. Commencing some time between ages 40 and 45, or the midlife transition, this period is one marked by changes in crucial aspects of the individual's life. These may be dramatic (e.g., divorce or a change in profession) or subtle (e.g., increase or decrease in satisfaction and creativity). Also typical of the period is a shift from outer to inner-world orientation, an emphasis on "interiority." An important point of middle adulthood is seen in the age 50 transition (ages 50–55), during which time these authors feel the individual adjusts the second or begins to build a new life structure with revised goals and purpose.

Levinson is careful to note that a normal personal development does not always occur in middle adulthood. Indeed, he observes that decline is "*statistically* normal in the sense that it occurs frequently. It is not, however, *developmentally* normal. Drastic decline occurs only when development has been impaired by adverse psychological, social, and biological circumstances" (Levinson, 1978, p. 41).

The eighth and final of Erikson's life stages (1963), and that which influences the course of this last life structure, is the resolution of the conflict between *ego integrity versus despair*. This begins in older adulthood (around age 60) and carries over into the person's remaining decades. This stage is characterized by one who "has taken care of things and people and has adapted himself to the triumphs and disappointments inherent to being the originator of others or the generator of products and ideas.'' Inadequate resolution of this conflict can result in despair about one's accomplishments and meaningfulness, leading to difficulty in facing death or (at the opposite extreme) a despairing embrace of death.

## Common Tumors

The common tumors of this era are the solid tumors of the lung, breast, colon and rectum, prostate, pancreas, ovary, uterus, stomach, and brain. These are the less curable cancers today; several, such as pancreatic cancer, have a particularly poor prognosis. Threat to life is undeniable, as is the knowledge that treatment is arduous and not always successful. The acute concerns for survival are accompanied by additional worries about the extent to which treatment side effects will affect attractiveness, sexuality, and ability to work and socialize.

## Disruptions of Illness

The very nature of the tasks and adjustments that are the hallmarks of this period in the life span make the associated disruptions of illness particularly keenly felt.

## ALTERED RELATIONSHIPS

In the interpersonal domain, responsibilities to the patient's parents and children are altered by cancer. Whereas financial obligations may be less significant than in the preceding period, concern for the social, financial, and educational well-being of survivors is an important issue. People who start families later, or have a second family following remarriage, may still have major responsibilities. Adults who have responsibility for the care of an aging parent or parents worry about who will assume responsibility for their welfare. Patients with grandchildren fear the possible loss of opportunity to know and nurture them.

For patient and spouse, cancer may make it difficult to maintain prior social ties. This may be a particularly difficult disruption for the healthy spouse and other family members who need socially supportive relationships not only to provide substantial physical help, but also psychological help in caring for an ill partner or relative.

In a similar vein, illness may accelerate or intensify the confrontation with a chronically unhappy marriage or social life. Disability in one partner can also spark conflicts about the changing nature of a couple's interactions; a husband may resent being moved into a passive role because of physical limitations. The wife, especially one whose husband has a brain tumor, may resent the suddenly enforced role of both caretaker and decision maker. A wife may also resist returning to a more passive role, particularly if she has had her own career or has just had a taste of being more assertive and career oriented after many years devoted primarily to bringing up her family.

## DEPENDENCE–INDEPENDENCE

For both patient and caretaker, there may be bad feelings about having to be ''cared for'' and ''caring for.'' The patient fears becoming an invalid, dependent on others for physical care, especially on the older children. Resentment and guilt can build on both sides.

The financial costs of cancer also threaten an individual or couple's ability to be independent. Conflicts about not wishing to be a burden on others yet worrying about the ability to meet treatment costs on a fixed income can be a particular problem for a retired couple, or the widowed or single person. Living arrangements may require giving up independence and living with others, including placement in a residence for older individuals.

## ACHIEVEMENT DISRUPTIONS

Anger and frustration arise when cancer poses a possible enforced early retirement. For individuals in an earlier point in this period, illness may cause disappointment about any necessary curtailment of potential achievements. This is especially true in cases in which the individual has embarked on a second career. There may be concern about the loss of ability to manage an emotionally significant enterprise such as a business or home. For individuals approaching retirement or who have already retired, there is a sense of being cheated out of a much anticipated healthy retirement. A couple or individual may see years of planning and dreams dissolve as cancer progresses, and hard-earned savings disappear as months of treatment pass. Suicidal ideation is often expressed by the patient as being a preferable option to financial ruin for the surviving spouse and children.

## BODY IMAGE AND INTEGRITY

A similar sense of premature acceleration of changes may be experienced in the physical realm as a consequence of cancer diagnosis. The patient may experience a speeding up of the aging process because of the effects of disease or treatment. Weakness, weight loss, and older appearance are alterations that occur with cancer, but represent aging as well. They pose a threat to the individual's sense of physical invulnerability and to the ability to cope. Individuals who have used denial as a defense against the fear of aging and who have placed great emphasis on youthful appearance and perfection of body integrity and function have special difficulty in adjusting to the changes of cancer and treatment. Some of these patients are at risk for serious psychological difficulties, which include depression and suicide (see Chapters 23 and 24).

Concerns typical of this period about a changing sexual image may be exacerbated by the side effects of treatment. Acute embarrassment and demoralization may accompany alopecia, especially in women, but also in men for whom wigs are a greater problem. Distress may also be caused by the feminizing effects of female hormones in men (e.g., the association of prostate cancer therapy with the development of female habitus, loss of libido, and breast enlargement), and masculinizing effects of hormonal therapy in women (e.g., the association of breast cancer treatment with a hirsute face, deepening voice, and altered libido).

## EXISTENTIAL ISSUES

Finally, with respect to existential issues, there may be a marked increase in depression associated with less denial of death as a possible outcome. In addition, a heightening of the introspection and reflection characteristic of this period of life review may lead to potential despair about unattained accomplishments and the meaningfulness of one's life. Overemphasis on an introspective orientation can put the individual at risk for closing out others or giving up prematurely.

### Interventions

Many of the adjustments (and potential sources of disruption) of this period resonate with earlier periods, particularly adolescence: the coming to terms with the self, important physical changes, alterations in the social relations of home and work. For this reason and because of the many transitions that are hallmarks of this stage, the theme for interventions is often the maintenance of personal integrity.

The impact of illness on interpersonal relationships is usefully monitored by a social work consultation. The focus of this contact should be to assess the welfare (social, psychological, physical, and financial) of the family and patient, to evaluate the adequacy of available social support systems, and to assist in the development of resources where they are lacking. Consideration of referral for conjoint or personal therapy to deal with conflicts arising in the context of disease and possible death may be appropriate.

Rehabilitative measures following major treatments that produce functional deficits should be quickly and effectively instituted to prevent problems of dependency. Mechanical aids should be provided as needed to facilitate activities of daily living. Patients, however, should be helped to tolerate dependence on others for specific needs, a task facilitated by pointing out or reinforcing independence in other areas. Nursing care needs should be carefully explored, especially when they are apt to be prolonged at home. Decisions must take into account available insurance, public, private, and personal resources, often discreetly examined by a social worker.

Disruptions in lifetime achievement associated with cancer may lead to personal crisis. Counseling should focus on fears and concerns about the possible loss of targeted life-style and goals, taking into account medical data about prognosis. Sessions should cover realistic issues of financial planning, treatment costs, and family needs.

The adverse impact of changes in body image and sexuality can be tempered by counseling on these issues, which incorporates information about the practical management of alterations in appearance (e.g., facial prostheses) and body functions (e.g., colostomy). Nurses can best provide explanations before therapy about the nature of side effects and about personal hygiene during treatment. The more sophisticated, information-oriented approaches used in contemporary patient education are helpful in preparing the patient and responsible relative for anticipated changes and facilitating the development of adequate concrete (e.g., deciding on the response to "embarrassing" questions) as well as intellectual coping mechanisms. Patients who receive hormonal treatment need particular preparation for any associated sexual changes and reassurance about their transient nature.

Most important, the older adult may need counseling to maintain self-esteem. Life review of meaningful accomplishments, achievements, and relationships should be supported and patients encouraged to regard these in light of their importance and contribution to individuals, to the overall good, and to a sense of the meaning of a life well lived. Adaptive coping mechanisms and behaviors need to be reinforced and the philosophical and religious meaning of life and death explored.

## THE AGING ADULT (66 YEARS AND OVER)

### Developmental Tasks

Although individuals in each period of life vary in character, circumstances, and relative position vis-à-vis life tasks, the potential for disparity between representative members is perhaps no more dramatic than toward the end of the life span. At this developmental period, knowing an individual's age is probably the least helpful piece of information, especially for those older than age 70, in constructing a picture of that person's strengths or stresses. For example, learning that someone is 80 may conjure up an image of a person with substantial memory loss, who is frail and living in a nursing home; or, the picture of this same person may be of a spry and wiry individual who is actively engaged in gardening and volunteer work, and is valued as a senior consultant and public speaker. Because of the growing disparity between functional and physical age, some members of this group are now referred to as the "young old" (Neugarten, 1974). Bearing in mind the physical manifestations of the latter end of the life span that may be widely disparate, there are nevertheless features commonly expected of this population.

Although there is variability in the magnitude and the rapidity with which they occur, a number of changes are common in the physical ability and performance of the aging adult that have impact for psychological, social, and physical functioning (Storandt, 1986). These are related to "primary aging" or the built-in clock that begins early in life and affects all body systems. These effects include a decline in the functional capacity of key organ systems, in basal metabolic rate, cardiac output, respiratory capacity, and renal filtration rate. One by-product is less energy reserve, resulting in both a decline in physical work capacity and a decrease in physical activity. Although perhaps not as readily apparent (or acknowledged) earlier, there are naturally going to be limitations (sometimes sharp, usually gradual) on activities that at prior times were easy. A tennis or golf game may fall off, long periods of standing or bending become difficult, walking distances or climbing stairs produces fatigue, reflexes are slower. This period is also associated with a sharp increase in the prevalence of chronic diseases (e.g., diabetes, emphysema, and heart disease) and metabolic dysfunction. Homeostatic systems that continue to function well at rest may become unable to react rapidly to stress or perturbation, leading to progressive impairment. As a group, older persons are characteristically less effective than the young in adapting to environmental challenges and take longer to readjust their internal environment after displacements occur. Though becoming less common with the more widespread use in younger generations of dental prophylaxis, a frequently overlooked expression of physical aging that can demand significant adaptation is change in teeth and gums. Major dental or oral problems can at times necessitate major modification of diet and, in cases where dentures are ill-fitting or absent, lead to restriction of social intercourse because of

discomfort or embarrassment. We are beginning to learn how much of this process or its impact is under individual control. Some researchers feel that many of the problems associated with old age are the result of "secondary aging," the product of diseases, abuse, and disuse, often under the individual's control. As older people engage in more physical exercise, eat better, and remain involved socially, the deleterious effects of natural aging appear to be less. Improved financial well-being in this group has also led to better mental health.

As people approach the end of their lives, increasingly overt evidence of intellectual as well as physical senescence becomes more common. This may include an acceleration in the decrease of intellectual acumen that began at the end of the preceding life phase, in particular with respect to sensorimotor and visuoperceptual skills. Occasionally there is progressive memory loss and difficulty remembering common words or referents. Recent research among aging samples leads us to caution the assumption that these latter changes are limited to or even typical of aging adults (Schaie and Gribben, 1975; Birren and Schaie, 1985; Botwinick, 1984). Forgetting is an experience at all age groups; the difference is that when it occurs in the 19-year-old we are far more likely to attribute it to youthful absentmindedness or "being in love," whereas in the 75-year-old it is not uncommonly interpreted as a symptom of senility. In addition, studies with groups of healthy aging populations indicate that memory loss is not a sine qua non of normal aging (Kra, 1986). Public consciousness has also been raised with respect to what actually constitutes senility. Most cases of severe memory loss, which were once considered to be senility, are now known as Alzheimer's disease, a specific form of organic brain dysfunction. Rather than being endemic to the aging process, such severe alterations represent a very unusual and infrequent course. Primary degenerative dementia occurs in only 2–4% of the population over 65, although the prevalence increases with advancing age, particularly after age 75, and is more common in women than men, presumably because women outnumber men in the older population and not because of any, as yet, identified genetic predisposition (Smith and Bierman, 1973; Finch and Hayflick, 1977). Changes in personality, social or occupational functioning, and general intellectual ability are not an expected consequence of aging, and when they occur they should be evaluated to rule out a possible underlying organic etiology. (See also Chapter 30, "Delirium and Dementia.") It is important to note that depression following the loss of a spouse or problems with medication for hypertension can produce disorientation and symptoms that resemble Alzheimer's. At times progressive hearing loss can cause an older adult to become socially withdrawn and to appear paranoid and suspicious. (See review by Corso in Birren and Schaie, 1977).

If the individual is to weather these later years successfully, gracefully, and fully, he or she must adapt to the changes associated with normal aging, regardless of their nature or magnitude. The individual must understand and deal with the implications of the changes and the accompanying fears of physical and mental deterioration leading to dependency. A balance in these concerns must be achieved to avoid preoccupation or even obsession about such issues. The older person who is repeatedly apologetic for being in the way shows such a problem.

There are also a number of adaptational changes and adjustments that must be made in the social and affective sphere. Chief among these is retirement, typically at age 65 or 70 in our society. The individual must deal with the issues surrounding the yielding of authority and status and the review of life success and failure inherent in such a change. There is a focus on plans associated with creating a legacy for colleagues and family alike. Traditionally this step has been considered more stressful for men than women. Perhaps this is because women have traditionally always been more involved in, and received socially sanctioned support for, extraprofessional concerns (e.g., homemaking and volunteer work). Because these can continue after retirement and indeed may increase (e.g., grandparenting), women may not experience as abrupt a transition in status when a career ends. Fox (1977), however, suggests this picture may be misleading and notes the paucity of research on women's adjustment to retirement.

Looking at retirement from the point of view of a spouse or partner, even this can be equally stressful, if in a different way, for each. The person whose life partner retires may find adjusting to his or her being home all day a strain. Part of the task of adapting to retirement is working out new schedules that provide enough interaction for the member accustomed to a work setting while still preserving the valued hours of privacy of the member accustomed to the empty house, learning to share projects and interests, and learning to enjoy time together. At times, these adjustment periods may mean having to come to grips with previously ignored differences.

Over time there are generally increasing limitations on physical abilities, income, and mobility. These alterations lead to a restriction of usual social contacts. They may, at the extreme, erode the sense of purpose in living, a circumstance to which women who outlive their mates may be especially vulnerable (Levy, 1981). The individual's social milieu becomes further restricted as he or she accommodates to the frequent personal losses of later life: death of spouse, siblings, and friends of many years. There is a shift from a sense of controlling, to yielding to the environment's demands, thereby submitting to external control. Some older people exhibit an ''adaptational paranoia'' and adopt a combative stance, a quality that once would have been labeled maladaptive but which if not excessive can serve as a survival asset in these later years. In contrast is the attitude of pessimism and hopelessness, despair about one's accomplishments, or lack of meaningfulness that can lead to a fear of death. The key word for this delicate balance is ''wisdom,'' a sense of knowledge, understanding, and appreciation of one's life. This may be reflected in an emotional integration as well as a new and different love of parents and children.

Although there may be some other later stage (or stages), the last period in the life cycle model is the *late adult transition,* marking entry into the era of late adulthood (i.e., age 60 and older) (Levinson et al., 1978; Levinson, 1986). Levinson and colleagues feel that this period is between ages 60 and 65, although it may be earlier in persons of lower socioeconomic status and in individuals with chronic illness, or later as mandatory retirement is being abandoned and people are working longer. Emphasis on this transition should be technically related to the preceding developmental section, but its thrust seems more appropriate here and underscores the weakness of an age-delimited model. Characteristic of this period as Levinson and colleagues define it is the preparation for the next life era, or putting the store of memories in order. Some memories are dramatized while in others there may be a search for consistency. There is a reworking of the past (Butler, 1963b). Levinson notes that the developmental task of this period is to ''overcome the splitting of youth and age, and find in each season an appropriate balance of the two'' (Levinson et al., 1978, p. 46). Everyone is likely to feel despair at one point or another during this late transition. Though less well elaborated than other periods in his model, the tasks of late adulthood for Levinson are finding a balance in the degree of societal and self-involvement, making peace with inner and external enemies, and finally, making peace with dying.

## Common Tumors

The leading cancer sites among women in this age group are colon and rectum, breast, lung, pancreas, uterus, and ovary. For men, the common cancers include lung, prostate, colon and rectum, pancreas, bladder, and stomach. Cancer is second only to heart disease as a cause of death in persons of either sex over age 55. In the case of many of these tumors (stomach, pancreas, ovary, and lung), the disease is often already widely spread at time of diagnosis. In addition, the adult over age 70 may have other diseases that compromise the ability to undergo definitive surgery or a potentially curative course of radiation or chemotherapy.

## Disruptions of Illness

While the diagnosis of a serious, life-threatening illness like cancer in an aging adult is more common, individuals in this life era are perhaps the least prepared to handle the attendant complications and demands of treatment and care. Coming as it does in the context of multiple personal losses, the added loss of health by cancer and restricted physical, financial, and social resources, places the aging adult at particular risk for major psychosocial disruptions (see also Chapter 37).

### ALTERED RELATIONSHIPS

The aging adult is already experiencing a sense of isolation and loss through death or distance, both social and geographic, from family members. Cancer, by imposing further limitations on activity, may contribute to an even greater isolation. As a group, aging adults are less adaptable to the stresses of unfamiliar environments and treatments. Suspiciousness about treatment and staff, and fear of abandonment by staff, healthy spouse, family, and friends are not uncommon reactions. So, too, are fears of being an invalid and a burden to others, particularly to children.

### DEPENDENCE–INDEPENDENCE

There may be a deep sense of shame about having to ask for help, especially with regard to personal hygiene or incontinence. For the older adult who has been able to live and function independently, the sudden need to be cared for by others is particularly stressful. Questions about the well-being and future of a beloved pet can also arise and become a major concern when a move to a relative's home or special care setting requires giving up a companion of many years. The opposite, however, may also occur and the patient may "give up" upon diagnosis, becoming inappropriately dependent.

### ACHIEVEMENT DISRUPTIONS

Additional financial strain put on an income already reduced by retirement can lead to anxiety about the dissolution of planned financial security for oneself and the survivors. As noted in the preceding develop-

mental period, illness may precipitate anger about having been cheated out of a "healthy" retirement, mourning for the loss of expected enjoyment in later life (the pursuit of avocations, relaxing, and traveling), and despair in individuals who view their lives as unsatisfying, and create great distress.

## BODY IMAGE AND INTEGRITY

Treatment may lead to an inability to carry out adequate personal hygiene, making interaction uncomfortable for patient, family, and staff alike. The masculinizing in women or feminizing in men from the effects of hormonal therapy can be acutely upsetting. Alopecia is also a major cause of demoralization. Cancer also tends to compound the diseases of aging (e.g., organ failure, deafness, failing eyesight, and heart disease). In addition, older bodies are more susceptible to the complications of illness; there is lower tolerance for treatment side effects and greater risk for the development of delirium in the hospitalized aged patient (see Chapter 30). Finally, there is at times greater difficulty for the elderly adult in perceiving and assimilating complex information (e.g., pill schedules).

## EXISTENTIAL ISSUES

Cancer has a cumulative effect on the multiple life losses of the aging adult, leading at times to bereavement overload and a depressive response to illness. There is often an accelerated need for a life review, which, if it falls short, can lead to remorse, a sense of inability to contribute, and despair. An accompanying urgency to settle one's spiritual affairs or religious beliefs may also be seen. The assault of illness and treatment on the already vulnerable physical and social being can deprive the aging adult of personal dignity, a quality needed for self-respect and self-esteem. Finally, the existential concern for *"How* I will die" takes on new meaning when cancer occurs, usually with fears of a prolonged period of dying with progressive disability and pain.

## Interventions

The aging adult population is already at great risk for isolation, a situation accentuated by cancer and its attendant fears. Their heightened needs for additional practical, financial, and the important social resources make it appropriate to center interventions around providing and maintaining social supports and resources. To help with the daily physical as well as emotional needs of the patient, support sources need to be identified. Those in place should be maintained. New ones may need to be established or developed.

This may mean tightening bonds to the immediate family or reengaging a distant family member who was previously involved, or creating or reestablishing appropriate religious or social group connections. Shared activities and affectional ties need to be supported.

In caring for the patient, emphasis should be given to providing detailed information about diagnosis and all treatments to be undertaken. When a complex drug regimen is involved, careful monitoring by others may be required to prevent poor compliance or inadvertent overdose. Hospital routines such as meal and care schedules and use of call bells should be clearly described. Continuity of care by trusted and familiar staff is important to foster a sense of security. The patients' family physician should stay involved during care in a treatment center. Ideally, treatment in a hospital, when needed, should be near the home. One physician should coordinate care and answer the patient's questions. The nursing staff must judge the patient's level of self-care ability and strive for the proper level of care that does not exceed need.

Where the patient is best treated after primary treatment is ended is an important issue; home or alternative care options should be explored. With the growth of home health agencies, and home and hospice care programs, home care is an increasingly viable and, for some families, a desirable alternative option to hospital or institutional care. (See also Chapters 48 and 49 on home and terminal care.) A nursing home setting allows elderly patients to bring their own furniture and in some cases to keep a special pet; such considerations may be important in placement. Counseling should address feelings about dependency, hopelessness, and the grief associated with illness and loss. Appointment of a conservator of resources, when the patient is unable to manage them, should be made. Best use of available financial assets, health insurance, community financial resources, and Medicare should be considered. Continued involvement in meaningful hobbies and recreation should be explored and supported to the extent possible.

Physical disruptions can be minimized by a variety of approaches: planning daily routine so that part-time homemaker help is available (especially for bathing and the use of the bathroom), obtaining aids to counter sensory losses (hearing aids, glasses, large-print newspapers and talking books), and supporting awareness of environment (use of large clocks, calendars, and nightlights). Regular oncologist or physician visits to monitor for medical problems should also include assessment of mental function and mood.

Finally, some individuals want to plan their funeral and make burial arrangements; others do not want to be reminded of this eventuality. A sensitive ear is needed to meet these needs. The cleric who is a friend and religious counselor is best suited for this, if not a family member. A positive review of past life and achievements with an opportunity to recall the "good days," good memories, and an existential perspective of life and death provides a helpful forum for this discussion. This is an opportunity for venting feelings and for engaging in life review that builds self-esteem and reinforces personal dignity.

## SUMMARY

As can be seen from the preceding sections, cancer, especially when treatments are arduous and lengthy, constitutes a major stress that is added to the normal stresses of adaptation to the age-appropriate tasks across the life cycle. This chapter is intended to provide a rational basis for generating psychosocial interventions in cancer, derived from a logical understanding of the individual's background and by having a general appreciation of the problems related to age or place in the life cycle. Such an approach is based on the premise that the psychological toll exacted by cancer is experienced emotionally as a threat or inability to carry out life tasks expected at a given stage of life. Therefore, knowledge of these enables the oncological staff to anticipate potential problem areas. General awareness of life cycle norms also provides a broad yardstick against which to measure a person's maturity and developmental milestones, not only as they existed prior to the diagnosis but also the extent to which they may have deviated from the norms as a result of the illness. By applying such a framework, health professionals are in a better position to respond to common and predictable psychosocial responses and to recognize those that are uncommon or maladaptive.

This review in no way attempts to offer cookbook solutions to an individual patient's needs. These are in each case unique and require great sensitivity to assure that the individual's concerns are met. Like all good reviews, it should change as new information accumulates about the cancer patient and as new sources of help for cancer patients and their families evolve. Nevertheless, it is important to move away from a position in which interventions are planned on a totally individual basis, without reference to a framework or contextual model, toward one in which guidelines are based on and developed out of a model that recognizes common stress-producing issues as a function of the person's overall developmental growth and adaptation.

Engel (1977, p. 129) defines neatly the purpose of applying a biopsychosocial model as follows:

to identify and emphasize the mental health needs of medically ill patients and their families during the stress of severe illness, when significant post-illness psychological morbidity may be prevented with appropriate anticipatory education and crisis-intervention oriented techniques.

To be successful, however, the efforts at troubleshooting must be moved to the front-line staff, those individuals who are in a better position to assess patient adaptation and who can learn to make efficient and appropriate referrals. Much of the kind of information needed to determine where a patient is in developmental terms is covered in good history taking, at times supplemented by careful nursing or social work notes. Special or specific relevant issues with respect to a patient's status vis-à-vis life cycle tasks should be touched on during initial evaluation. One useful way to accomplish this is to keep in mind the five potential areas of disruption when assessing the patient's needs and then reviewing how the treatment will compromise adjustment in each area. Attention to these areas offers a guide whereby appropriate developmentally relevant psychological support is provided, thus serving as a preventive measure against psychosocial dysfunction.

## REFERENCES

Birren, J.E. and K.W. Schaie (eds.). (1977). *The Handbook of the Psychology of Aging*. New York: Van Nostrand Reinhold.

Birren, J.E. and K.W. Schaie (eds.). (1985). *The Handbook of the Psychology of Aging,* 2nd ed. New York: Van Nostrand Reinhold.

Botwinick, J. (1984). *Aging and Behavior,* 3rd ed. New York: Springer.

Butler, R. (1963a). The facade of chronological age. *Am. J. Psychiatry* 119:722–28.

Butler, R.N. (1963b). The life review: An interpretation of reminiscence in the aged. *Psychiatry* 26:65–76.

Eisenberg, M.G., L.C., Sutkin, and M.A. Jansen (ed.). (1984). *Chronic Illness and Disability through the Life Span: Effects on Self and Family.* New York: Springer.

Engel, G.L. (1962). *Psychological Development in Health and Disease.* Philadelphia: W.B. Saunders.

Engel, G.L. (1977). The need for a new medical model: A challenge for biomedicine. *Science* 196:129–36.

Erikson, E.H. (1958). *Young Man Luther.* New York: Norton.

Erikson, E.H. (1963). *Childhood and Society,* 2nd ed. New York: Norton.

Erikson, E. (1968). *Identity: Youth and Crisis.* New York: Norton.

Finch, C.E. and L. Hayflick (1977). *The Handbook of the Biology of Aging.* New York: Van Nostrand Reinhold.

Fox, J. (1977). Effects of retirement and former work life on women's adaptation in old age. *J. Gerontol.* 32:196–202.

Freud, S. (1952). *A General Introduction to Psychoanalysis.* New York: Garden City Books.

Freud, S. (1962). *The Ego and the Id.* New York: Norton.

Ginsburg, H. and S. Opper (1969). *Piaget's Theory of Intellectual Development: An Introduction.* Englewood Cliffs, N.J.: Prentice-Hall.

Gould, R.L. (1972). The phases of adult life. A study of developmental psychology. *Am. J. Psychiatry* 129:521–31.

Gould, R.L. (1979). *Transformations: Growth and Change in Adult Life.* New York: Simon & Schuster.

Jacques, E. (1965). Death and the mid-life crisis. *Int. J. Psychoanal.* 46:502–14.

Jung, C. (1933). *Modern Man in Search of a Soul.* New York: Harcourt.

Kastenbaum, R. (1977). Death and development through the lifespan. In H. Feifel (ed.), *New Meanings of Death.* New York: McGraw-Hill, pp. 18–45.

Keith, P.M. (1979). Life changes and perceptions of life and death among older men and women. *J. Gerontol.* 34:870–78.

Keniston, K. (1975). Youth as a stage of life. In W.C. Sze (ed.), *Human Life Cycle.* New York: Jason Aronson, pp. 331–49.

Kimball, C. (1981). *The Biopsychosocial Approach to the Patient.* Baltimore: Williams & Wilkins.

Kra, S. (1986). *Aging Myths: Reversible Causes of Mind and Memory Loss.* New York: McGraw-Hill.

Levinson, D.J. (1977). The mid-life transition. *Psychiatry* 40:99–112.

Levinson, D.J. (1978). Eras: The anatomy of the life cycle. *Psychiatric Opinion* 15:10–11, 39–48.

Levinson, D.J. (1986). A conception of adult development. *Am. Psychol.* 41:3–13.

Levinson, D.J. and W.E. Gooden (1985). The life cycle. In H.I. Kaplan and B.J. Sadock (eds.), *Comprehensive Textbook of Psychiatry,* 4th ed. Baltimore: Williams & Wilkins, pp. 1–13.

Levinson, D.J., with C.N. Darrow, E.B. Klein, M.H. Levinson, and B. McKee (1978). *The Seasons of a Man's Life.* New York: Alfred A. Knopf.

Levy, S. (1981). The aging woman: developmental issues and mental health needs. *Professional Psychology* 12:92–102.

Lowenthal, M.F., M. Thurnher, and D. Chiriboga (1975). *Four Stages of Life: A Comparative Study of Women and Men Facing Transitions.* San Francisco: Jossey-Bass.

Mages, N.L. and G.A. Mendelsohn (1980). Effects of cancer on patients' lives: A personalogical approach. In G.C. Stone, F. Cohen, and N.E. Adler (eds.), *Health Psychology.* San Francisco: Jossey-Bass, pp. 255–84.

Nagy, M. (1948). The child's theories concerning death. *J. Genet. Psychol.* 73:3–27.

Neugarten, B.L. (1968a). Adult personality: Toward a psychology of the life cycle. In B.L. Neugarten (ed.), *Middle Age and Aging: Reader in Social Psychology* Chicago: University of Chicago Press, pp. 137–47.

Neugarten, B.L. (1968b). *Middle Age and Aging: Reader in Social Psychology.* Chicago: University of Chicago Press.

Neugarten, B.L. (1968c). The awareness of middle age. In B.L. Neugarten (ed.), *Middle Age and Aging: Reader in Social Psychology* Chicago: University of Chicago Press, pp. 93–98.

Neugarten, B.L. (1974). Age groups in American society

and the rise of the young-old. *Ann. Am. Acad. Polit. Soc. Sci.* 415:187–98.

Neugarten, B.L. (1979). Time, age, and the life cycle. *Am. J. Psychiatry* 136:887–94.

Neugarten, B.L. and D.A. Neugarten (1987). The changing meanings of age. *Psychology Today* 21:29–33.

Notman, M. (1979). Midlife concerns of women: Implications of the menopause. *Am. J. Psychiatry* 136:1270–74.

Piaget, J. (1952). *The Origins of Intelligence in Children.* New York: International Universities Press.

Reiser, D.E. and D.H. Rosen (1984). *Medicine as a Human Experience.* Baltimore: University Park Press.

Schaie, K. and K. Gribbin (1975). Adult development and aging. *Ann. Rev. Psychol.* 26:65–96.

Schildkraut, E. (1980). Medical residents' difficulty in learning and utilizing a psychosocial perspective. *J. Med. Educ.* 55:962–64.

Silverman, D., N. Gartrell, M. Aronson, M. Steer, and S. Edbril (1983). In search of the biopsychosocial perspective: An experiment with beginning medical students. *Am. J. Psychiatry* 140:1154–59.

Smith, D.W. and E.L. Bierman (1973). *The Biologic Ages of Man: From Conception through Old Age.* London: W.B. Saunders.

Storandt, M. (1986). Psychological aspects of aging. In I. Rossman (ed.), *Clinical Geriatrics.* Philadelphia: Lippincott, pp. 606–17.

Vaillant, G.E. (1977). *Adaptation to Life.* Boston: Little, Brown & Co.

Vaillant, G.E. and E. Milofsky (1980). Natural history of male psychological health: IX. Empirical evidence for Erikson's model of the life cycle. *Am. J. Psychiatry* 137:1348–59.

# 4

# Intrapersonal Resources: Coping

## Julia H. Rowland

The second set of patient-related variables contributing to psychosocial adjustment in illness, along with developmental stage and social support, encompasses the intrapsychic or intrapersonal issues (see Table 6-1). This describes what the individual brings to the illness by way of personality, coping style, and defenses. The past two decades have seen an intensification of interest in human responses to stress. This reflects in part a growing awareness of the multiple demands made on people in our increasingly complex and pressured world, and concern about the potentially negative effects. (For summaries of the literature and controversies in this area, see Monat and Lazarus, 1977; Goldberger and Breznitz, 1982; Jemott and Locke, 1984.) It also reflects a growing appreciation of human adaptability and its impact on stress management (Coelho et al., 1974; Meichenbaum et al., 1975; Antonovsky, 1979; Moos, 1977, 1984; Burish and Bradley, 1983). Although theorists and researchers frequently argue about the nature and definition of stress, many have adopted the definition proposed by Caplan (1981, p. 414), who defines as stressful those situations "in which there is a marked discrepancy between the demands made on an organism and the organisms's capability to respond." Within this framework, illness, particularly cancer, is unquestionably a major life stress.

Increased attention to quality-of-life issues has led to interest in how normal people cope with stress and how to enhance these skills. "Coping" is an expression widely used by the public; it is also a term echoed in the name of many of the self-help programs that have formed over the last several years (e.g., "I can Cope," "Coping with Cancer," and "Hope and Cope") and reflects the efforts of these grassroots movements to promote self-efficacy in dealing with cancer. For these reasons it is important that the clinician have some understanding of how coping is de-

fined, what its determinants are, how to evaluate its effectiveness, and what impact it has in cancer. Each of these issues is discussed in the sections that follow.

## DEFINING COPING

Although cancer is emotionally experienced differently by each individual, it constitutes a threat to life and integrity that must be faced by every patient. This threat requires that the ill person devote his or her cognitive and physical activities to preserving physical and psychic integrity. Early studies of individuals' responses to life-threatening illness emphasized adverse impact, distress, and incapacity, resulting in the clinical literature being "long on stress (and defense) and short on coping" (Hamburg, 1974). Today, research has shifted away from a model that looks for the psychopathological correlates or sequelae of illness, to one that emphasizes the adaptational aspects in human responses to stressful life events. As a consequence, although there are many different perspectives on what constitutes coping (See Table 4-1), there has been over time a general shift away from a view of human beings as being under siege (cf. early view of Lazarus), to an adaptational view of human beings, in which life's stresses are seen as challenges or tasks to be mastered through thoughtful use of available social and psychological resources (cf. Mechanic, 1968; Caplan, 1981). White (1974) sees the definition and domain of coping as being quite specific. According to his approach, the central issue in any definition is "adaptation." Under the general rubric of adaptation are subsumed three characteristics, each closely defined:

*Defense*—concerned with the reflexive responses associated with danger and safety
*Mastery*—having to do with successful performance in meeting task requirements

**Table 4-1** Definitions of coping

| Reference | Definitions |
| --- | --- |
| Lazarus (1966) | When we use the term "coping" we are referring to strategies for dealing with threat. |
| Mechanic (1968) | . . . instrumental behavior and problem-solving capacities of persons in meeting life demands and goals. It involves the application of skills, techniques, and knowledge that a person has acquired. |
| Lipowski (1970) | . . . all cognitive and motor activities which a sick person employs to preserve his bodily and psychic integrity, to recover reversibly impaired function and compensate to the limit for any irreversible impairment. |
| White (1974) | Coping is adaptation under very difficult conditions. |
| Weisman and Worden (1976–1977) | Coping is what one does about a perceived problem in order to bring about relief, reward, quiescence, or equilibrium. |
| Pearlin and Schooler (1978) | . . . any response to external life strains that serves to prevent, avoid, or control emotional distress. |
| Caplan (1981) | . . . behavior by the individual that (1) results in reducing to tolerable limits physiological and psychological manifestations of emotional arousal during and shortly after the stressful event and also (2) mobilizes the individual's internal and external resources and develops new capabilities in him that lead to his changing his environment or his relation to it, so that he reduces the threat or finds alternate sources of satisfaction for what is lost. |
| Lazarus and Folkman (1984) | We define coping as constantly changing cognitive and behavioral efforts to manage specific external and/or internal demands that are appraised as taxing or exceeding the resources of the person. |

*Coping*—deals with the difficult and unusual in situations for which the development of new strategic maneuvers and instrumental behaviors is required

This nomenclature is useful in distinguishing between coping (e.g., reflective) and defensive (e.g., reflexive and routine) responses. Serious illness calls on both; the threat to life makes defense a primary concern, but the need for new strategies to meet the unusual demands of cancer also places a premium on coping capacity (Lipowski, 1970). White's nomenclature is also helpful in that it emphasizes the concept that defense and coping are separate and independent

of outcome. Each, in his view, is dependent on the *nature* of the stress and either may be used to achieve mastery. Thus, neither is inherently better or worse than the other. The importance of distinguishing coping from degree of success of outcome is a theme echoed by others (Folkman and Lazarus, 1980). Weisman and Worden (1976–1977) would add one further refinement to the distinction between coping and defending. Because the nature of the stress eliciting these two categories of response is different, so, too, is the goal of the process employed to manage it. As they point out, coping seeks resolution of a declared problem, while defense seeks relief through avoidance and disavowal.

Having defined coping, we should distinguish other commonly used terms. Coping style refers to the relatively enduring and characteristic ways in which an individual responds to stressful situations such as illness (Lipowski, 1970). Coping strategies are the patterns that emerge as a result of the person's coping style and represent behaviors, cognitions, and perceptions employed to maintain equilibrium in the face of illness. The purpose served by a given coping strategy is designated a coping function. Within the model advanced by Pearlin and Schooler (1978), coping is seen as having three main (protective) functions: management of the problem causing the distress through elimination or modification of the conditions giving rise to it, alteration of (perceptually controlling) the meaning of the experience so as to neutralize its problematic character, and regulation of the emotional distress produced by the problem. These functions have been supported in their own research and are widely recognized by others (Mechanic, 1977; Kahn et al., 1964; Folkman and Lazarus, 1980). The three coping functions are also referred to, respectively, by the terms problem-focused or instrumental coping, appraisal-focused coping, and emotion-focused or palliative coping (Moos and Schaeffer, 1984; Folkman and Lazarus, 1980). The latter two functions are sometimes paired and referred to as palliative functions (versus active and problem-solving). Which function predominates is based on the individual's assessment of the situation. Problem-focused forms of coping are more apt to be employed when circumstances are viewed as changeable, whereas appraisal-focused and emotion-focused coping occur more often in the context of situations deemed uncontrollable, as is frequently the case in adapting to cancer (Folkman, 1984).

Research on coping falls generally into two areas. One set of studies focuses on coping style (e.g., Ilfeld, 1980a,b; McCrae and Costa, 1986). A second set of studies examines active coping strategies, particularly as they are used in a given situation (e.g., Weisman,

1979). Interest in the latter area has been increasing rapidly in the last decade for a number of reasons. First, some studies have revealed that knowledge of the individual's "characteristic" coping style is *not* always useful in predicting how he or she will respond in a novel situation (F. Cohen and R. Lazarus, 1973; Silver and Wortman, 1980). Second, researchers have also found that any given coping strategy or those characteristics of a person's coping style can have both positive and negative, as well as short-term and long-term consequences (Monat and Lazarus, 1977). Thus, labeling an individual's style as uniformly maladaptive or ineffectual may not be appropriate or accurate. Third, it may be easier to alter characteristics of a person's coping repertoire than to change the person's response style. Furthermore, achieving a clearer understanding of the "adaptive" value of various coping processes or strategies may lead to the design of more effective interventions. From a pragmatic standpoint and that of the oncology staff, this latter point is probably the most compelling rationale for emphasizing a situational (state) rather than a personality (trait) orientation to understanding and facilitating coping. It is not surprising, therefore, that much of the literature on coping with cancer has embraced just such an approach.

## DETERMINANTS OF COPING

Three broad influences determine patients' coping with cancer (see Table 4-2). Of prime importance is the nature of the stress: cancer, and the disease-related variables (e.g., site of disease, stage, treatment, and course). Next come the individual variables, such as when in the life course cancer occurs and what emotional and social resources are available. Finally, the sociocultural climate within which the diagnosis and treatment of cancer occur also contributes to coping (Lipowski, 1969).

The stresses engendered by the disease and its treatment are discussed in Chapter 6, with emphasis placed on those points during the course of treatment that place maximal demands on the individual's ability to adjust. In considering the impact of the nature of the stress, Lazarus and co-workers (Lazarus, 1966; Lazarus, et al., 1974) differentiate between coping or problem-solving behavior in low-stakes versus high-stakes situations. Low-stakes situations (e.g., having dental work) permit flexible, deliberate, reality-oriented, rational efforts at mastery. High-stakes situations, by contrast, are those that occur in the context of a demanding environment and high drive and emotion. In high-stakes situations, such as facing cancer, there is a shift to more primitive, rigid, reflexive (versus reflective), and less realistic efforts at mastery, paral-

**Table 4-2**  Determinants of coping

| Type of determinant | Examples |
|---|---|
| Disease-related | Nature of illness, symptoms |
| | Site |
| | Stage |
| | Type of treatment |
| | Course of treatment |
| | Rehabilitation options |
| Individual | Developmental stage (includes issues of age cognition, skills) |
| | Values and beliefs (includes previous illness and cancer experience, internalized cultural mores, religious beliefs) |
| | Social support |
| Sociocultural | Community attitudes |
| | Resources available |

leling White's description of defenses and Freud's concept of ego defenses (cf. Haan, 1977). Thus, the nature of the stressor, cancer, is key in examining and interpreting coping responses.

However, beyond this broadly stated classification, there are gradations in response to the crisis of cancer reflective of the stress associated with a particular diagnosis and treatment. For example, the woman who is told that she has an in situ lesion of the cervix faces a very different set of adaptational demands than the woman who is told she has an invasive tumor of the cervix with likely metastatic involvement. Although both hear a diagnosis of cervical cancer, the treatment course and prognosis for the two women is vastly different and will demand different coping skills. As highlighted in Chapters 6-21, the course of illness, treatment, site, and rehabilitative measures available, by dictating the nature and degree of adaptation required, influence coping.

The point in an individual's life at which cancer occurs is also considered a major determinant of coping in the present model. Even in the absence of illness there are, over the course of an individual's life, tasks that he or she must accomplish (e.g., learning to walk, getting a job). The nature of these varies over time, as detailed in Chapter 3 for adults and Chapter 43 for children and adolescents. To what extent specific tasks are disrupted by illness affects the ability to cope. Again using the example of cervical cancer, it is apparent that a diagnosis of this type of tumor has a different impact depending on the age of the woman. Prospects for marriage and childbearing will be an issue for the young woman; management of a family in her absence may worry the middle-aged woman, whereas concern for financial burden and social support during convalescence or prolonged illness are more apt to be problems for the older, widowed woman.

In addition, the sophistication of personal skills and cognitive capacity at the outset and over the course of illness affect coping capacity (D.A. Hamburg and B. Hamburg, 1981). The impact of age is especially significant. First, children have a more limited repertoire of coping skills and strategies available to them than adults. Second, children are also exquisitely vulnerable to the reactions and behaviors of the adults responsible for their care, in ways that have an enduring impact on future coping, both during the index illness and in all later episodes. As Lipowski (1970) points out, the quality of initial experiences with illness takes on added importance; the strategies established or learned early in life are more likely to be used first in future illness situations.

Values and beliefs also affect coping. The importance of previous illness experience is not just an issue in childhood. Indeed, everyone's prior illness experience has important repercussions for coping in subsequent times of sickness. Lipowski (1970) in particular has stressed the importance of the personal meaning of, and attitudes toward, sickness, injury, and dysfunction in determining an individual's coping. The individual's idiosyncratic perception of the illness is what dictates the selection of particular coping strategies. The most typical meanings of illness are as challenge, enemy, punishment, weakness, relief, irreparable loss or danger, and finally, even positive value (Lipowski, 1970). Certainly, cancer is often perceived as a challenge to be met; the disease is the ''enemy'' and treatment ''the battlefield.'' Though more often associated with childhood, the perception of illness as punishment or relief from tasks is also very common in adults, but less openly acknowledged. Many cured patients will say that, as bad as it was, their illness and treatment had positive aspects (Taylor, 1983; Taylor et al., 1983; Pearlin and Schooler, 1978).

Previous personal experiences with cancer also dramatically influence coping strategies, and hence are determinants of the individual's formulation of his or her concept of cancer. For example, the individual who has lost several relatives to cancer (particularly of the same site) will fear the disease more, be more likely to delay seeking treatment, or may adopt a futile, hopeless stance in the face of a diagnosis of cancer than the person whose experience has been with cancer cures. Bard and Sutherland (1955) and Jamison and co-workers (1978) found that knowledge of someone who did well and confidence in the therapy, both aid in patient recovery from breast cancer. Individuals who firmly expect to be successfully treated will probably battle their disease more actively. Indeed, some feel this issue is critical; individuals must *believe* that they can

succeed in an endeavor in order to attempt to master it. Central to Erikson's theory (1963) of human development is the importance of self-efficacy in adaptation, which is also stressed by Moos and Schaefer (1984) with respect to adjustment to physical illness. In addition, several studies suggest that sense of control relates to type of coping activity employed. Those individuals who have an internal locus of control are more likely to use problem-focused coping (Strickland, 1978; Anderson, 1977). Thus, understanding people's beliefs about their illness is an important dimension of understanding how they cope.

Religious values and beliefs similarly affect coping. Although there is strong anecdotal support for the positive impact of religious attitudes and activities on individuals' responses to serious illness, this relationship has not been well studied. Research by Blazer and Palmore (1976) and Comstock and Partridge (1972) suggests that religious convictions and beliefs are associated with higher levels of self-reported well-being. In a study by Yates and colleagues (1981), religious patients with advanced cancer reported significantly lower levels of pain. A strong positive correlation was also seen between religious beliefs and life satisfaction, as well as between religious activity and connections, and both happiness and life satisfaction. Although the research by Yates and colleagues emphasized the importance of religion as a source of social support, the role of religion in coping is much more complex, as touched on by Rev. Handzo in Chapter 57. Kaplan and Blazer (1989) provide an elegant theoretical framework within which to conceptualize and research the role of religion in the stress, coping, support, and adaptation model. Though difficult at present to evaluate, the role of spirituality in adaptation to cancer needs to be acknowledged and its potential impact appreciated (Vastyan, 1986).

The role of social support and coping is an area gaining increasing attention. A number of studies have shown that social support can reduce or buffer the negative impact of illness (S. Cohen and T.A. Wills, 1985; S. Cohen and S.L. Syme, 1985; Wortman, 1984). Thoits (1986) goes so far as to argue that social support be reconceptualized as coping assistance. She and others (Lieberman, 1982; House, 1981) delineate a number of ways in which social support affects coping. Social resources can (1) intervene directly and alter the likelihood of the occurrence of a stressful event (e.g., by providing a loan, taking over child care, and providing information on a strategy to avoid a problem), (2) reinterpret the meaning of the situation so it seems less threatening (e.g., help an individual solve specific problematic issues so adjustment is not viewed as overwhelming, or provide reminders that being upset is normal and that nothing more serious is indicated), (3) influence use of a coping strategy (e.g., provide distraction and encourage humor), (4) help persons alter their physiological state (e.g., providing food, drink, or relaxation coaching), and (5) modify and bolster self-esteem often eroded by stressful events. (See Chapter 5 for a detailed review of the use and assessment of social support in cancer.)

Finally, as already noted, the sociocultural context within which cancer occurs, the nature of public response to and support for resources to patients with cancer, all influence coping. The extent to which the patient feels stigmatized by having cancer or penalized financially or socially, contributes to the degree of burden with which he or she must cope. Social attitudes and cultural beliefs about cancer can profoundly affect not only how patients view themselves, their illness, and the future, but also how the oncology staff treat patients and their families. A positive approach to the treatment and care of the patient communicates hopefulness and also assures the patient that supports are available. Thus, it is important to appreciate society's view of cancer and to be sensitive to one's own or the prevailing cultural biases about cancer causes and cures when evaluating patient coping.

## EVALUATING THE EFFICACY OF COPING

In order to define what constitutes successful coping, it is necessary first to establish the goals of a coping response. In the most general terms, the goals of coping can be said to be to reduce physiological and psychological arousal to a tolerable level, and to adapt to the realities of the stressful situation (Caplan, 1981). On a more theoretical level, Taylor (1983) sees three themes in the coping, or readjustment, process: "a search for meaning in the experience, an attempt to gain mastery over the event in particular and over one's life more generally, and an effort to enhance one's self-esteem—to feel good about oneself again despite the personal setback" (p. 1161). In their research, D.A. Hamburg and J.E. Adams (1967) distinguished five goals of effective coping behavior in serious illness (see Table 4-3). These goals reflect the basic areas threatened by serious illness: psychological organization, self-esteem, affiliations, body functions, and assumptions about the future. Applying their criteria, successful coping would be defined as that which keeps stress within manageable limits, maintains self-esteem, maintains or restores relations with significant other people, enhances prospects for the recovery of body functions, and increases the likelihood of working out a personally valued and socially acceptable situation after maximal physical recovery, which may include modification of the ego ideal. To this list should be added: maximizes the individual's ability to

**Table 4-3**　Goals of effective coping behavior in serious illness

To keep distress within manageable limits
To maintain a sense of personal worth
To restore relations with significant other people
To enhance prospects for recovery of physical functions
To increase the likelihood of working out a personally valued and socially acceptable situation after maximum physical recovery has been attained

*Source*: Adapted from Hamburg, D.A. and J.E. Adams (1967). A perspective on coping behavior: Seeking and utilizing information in major transitions. *Arch. Gen. Psychiatry* 17:277–284, pp. 278.

meet the requirements of the stressful task (e.g., treatment and care), and enables the individual to benefit from opportunities provided (such as information concerning treatment options or availability of social support).

The extent to which individual coping is successful in meeting a specified goal or goals is one measure of its efficacy. As a consequence, the stated or perceived goals to be achieved themselves influence coping efficacy. Goals must often be reformulated to reflect changes in the problems to be managed (e.g., as a consequence of changes in disease status). They can also shift in response to changes in the way the patient or staff define the existing problems. Thus, what was adaptive initially can become maladaptive over time. For example, although increased dependency on parents is expected as a means of coping with hospitalization during adolescence, such behavior would be considered maladaptive if it continued at the same level after the youth was well enough to return to school.

In a similar vein, under the stress of illness, it is frequently observed that a variety of behaviors may fall within the range of "normal" (appropriate and adaptive) that at other times of less stress would be considered grossly abnormal (immature and maladaptive). The use of denial is a prime example. In Vaillant's hierarchy and other psychoanalytically derived classifications (cf. Haan, 1977), denial is considered a more primitive or immature coping response. If employed to an excessive degree, denial may result in the person's failing to request medical consultation or follow-up for even an acute symptom. However, denial is commonly encountered in medically ill patients at a level that serves an important protective function in the initial phase of adaptation to life-threatening illness. Its use allows the individual time to "regroup" and face the challenges imposed more gradually (Hamburg and Adams, 1967; Hackett and Weisman, 1969. See also Janoff-Bulman, and Timko, 1986, for a discussion). Some researchers have suggested that what patients exhibit may in fact be "suppression" of information rather than denial of illness, a nomenclature that may make the protective function more acceptable.

Clearly, the level of a patient's denial cannot be assessed without the oncologist or staff member having an accurate picture of the medical facts. Even then it is a subjective assessment on the part of a healthy individual of the "appropriateness" of denial in another who is ill. It is hard for any person to live daily with hopelessness about cancer, and most individuals use denial as a way to make reality more tolerable. Only when it interferes with treatment or family decisions does it become necessary to discourage or confront it. These points further serve to highlight the issue that there are important subjective as well as objective criteria that enter into any evaluation of the success of coping.

The effectiveness of coping is also strongly influenced by the duration and intensity of the stress. Cancer illness, when it extends over long periods of time, can deplete psychic and social resources needed to cope effectively. Similarly, as noted earlier, the acute, life-threatening nature of cancer elicits different coping responses than non-life-threatening events or chronic problems.

Singer (1984) notes two additional features about coping that have an impact on its efficacy and management. First, coping is "costly" in terms of the emotional, physical, and interpersonal energy and resources required. As he points out, "most patients have pressures not to overexpend resources in coping. Some of the pressures are self-imposed; others are imposed from those around them. Each patient must decide on not only the appropriate level of these costs to be expended, but upon their distribution as well" (Singer, 1984, p. 2307). Second, effective coping may necessitate a variety of strategies and behaviors that are at times in conflict with each other, and require that patients and their environment disregard occasional inconsistencies in the greater interest of permitting effective functioning. An example is the case of the highly independent individual who, when faced by the burdens of serious illness, must accept the dependency of the patient role. Such an action is inconsistent with self-image and a restriction of a primary source of satisfaction, that of doing and accomplishing for oneself and others. Thus, the patient has to suppress the sense of dissonance associated with accepting support without providing it, and his or her family has to be understanding of the change in role and behavior necessary for such a strategy to succeed.

In broad terms, the degree of success achieved depends on the nature of the stress, the goals dictated, the type of coping responses prompted by the situation, and most importantly, the suitability of the strategies chosen to meet the tasks with minimal cost to the pa-

**Table 4-4** Vaillant's theoretical hierarchy of adaptive ego mechanisms

| Level | Mechanisms |
|---|---|
| IV. Mature | Altruism |
| | Humor |
| | Suppression |
| | Anticipation |
| | Sublimation |
| III. Neurotic | Intellectualization–rationalization |
| | Repression |
| | Displacement |
| | Reaction formation |
| | Dissociation |
| II. Immature | Projection |
| | Schizoid fantasy |
| | Hypochondriasis |
| | Passive-aggressive behavior |
| | Acting out |
| I. Narcissistic | Delusional projection |
| | Denial (psychotic) |
| | Distortion |

*Source*: Vaillant, G.E. (1971) Theoretical hierarchy of adaptive ego mechanisms. *Arch. Gen. Psychiatry* 24:107–117. pp. 111.

tient. Because this process is dynamic, success in prior coping itself serves to inspire more rigorous and persistent efforts in subsequent coping.

As with general coping studies, the research on coping with illness has proceeded largely on two main lines. The first develops theoretical constructs to explain coping behavior, explores strategies to facilitate categorization of people according to the constructs, and then correlates these with health outcomes. Vaillant's work (1971, 1977) is an example of such an approach. In his longitudinal study of a group of "healthy" men, he and his colleagues used a developmental and psychoanalytically derived hierarchy of defense mechanisms, arranged along a continuum of maturity to evaluate the subsequent adaptation and functioning mechanisms of his subjects in daily and major life crisis (Vaillant, 1977). His categorizations are presented in Table 4-4. In general, patients with cancer reflect psychologically healthy individuals under stress, and the use of humor, suppression, anticipation, and sublimation (level IV mechanisms) are commonly seen. Vaillant's level III mechanisms, though called neurotic, are also effective and adaptive, when not used to a pathological degree. With the exception of denial, the mechanisms of levels II and I are not often seen in cancer patients and serve as an indicator for early psychiatric consultation. The second type of study focuses on a particular illness and seeks to evaluate individuals with respect to the types of coping associated with successful adaptation to that illness. The series of studies by Weisman and Worden (1976–1977) on coping in cancer is an example of this approach and will be discussed later in more detail.

Both approaches have their strengths and weaknesses. The former approach leads to more generalizable results. However, its usefulness is often restricted by a tendency to focus on improving the theoretical model while neglecting practical application of the principles (toward mediating the stress of illness). The latter approach, though less generalizable across different illness settings (Moos and Tsu, 1977), can yield information of importance to the development of specific interventions.

## MODELS FOR COPING IN CANCER

Considerable information from other illnesses can be used to help in understanding the coping process in cancer. Many of the illness and treatment issues faced by patients with other serious, life-threatening medical conditions parallel those that confront the cancer patient, such as the disfigurement and pain experienced with burns (D.A. Hamburg et al., 1953; Andreason and Norris, 1972), the emotional and physical disability associated with traumatic amputations (Parkes, 1972), the problems with central nervous system complications associated with poliomyelitis (Visotsky et al., 1961), the issues of chronic medication and slow deterioration attached to diabetes (B.A. Hamburg et al., 1980), and the silent nature of the illness and uncertainty and fear of the future attached to the diagnosis of heart disease (Hackett and Weisman, 1969). Cancer patients have recently come under closer scrutiny in order to determine patterns of coping that are specific to cancer. A summary of the findings of a representative sample of these studies across site and stage is shown in Table 4-5. (For reviews see also Penman, 1980; Stewart, 1982.)

In their seminal work, Weisman and Worden (1976–1977) evaluated the use of 15 commonly observed coping strategies in a sample of cancer patients during the first 3 months following diagnosis. The list of strategies was based on an outline by Sidle and colleagues (1969) and included both defensive and adaptive behaviors. The relative effectiveness of each in bringing about relief and resolution to predominant concerns was then assessed. (See Table 4-6 for a list of strategies used.) Weisman and Worden concluded that the most effective strategies reflected open acceptance of the cancer (without, however, preoccupation with illness, as "accept, but find something favorable"), followed by responses designed to deal with the illness and current problems according to realistic considerations (e.g., "take firm action based on understanding," "seek direction from an authority and comply"). Least effective strategies were those that emphasized retreat, avoidance, passivity, yielding, blaming, acting out, and apathy (e.g., "try to forget; put it out of mind," "submit to and accept the inevitable," "withdraw socially into isolation"). Weisman and Worden also found a number of characteristics associated with high and low emotional distress and vulnerability. These are listed in Table 4-7.

Penman (1980, 1982), in a similar study among 27 postmastectomy patients, identified those coping strategies associated with adaptive or maladaptive coping at 1 week and at 4 months following surgery. In the coping strategies inventory developed for the study, 45 behaviors were grouped into five broad strategies: tackling, rationalizing, avoiding, capitulating, and tension-relieving. In her research, Penman found that women judged to be coping best after surgery used a greater range of tackling behaviors, exhibiting active engagement with issues raised by diagnosis and surgery. At 4 months, better copers showed more rationalizing behaviors than poorer copers and were less distressed. In contrast, poorer copers were characterized by greater use of avoiding and capitulating behaviors, demonstrating more evasion of illness-related issues and a more passive, fatalistic outlook with respect to illness and treatment. Tension-relieving behaviors were used by both groups. Penman interpreted the wider use of rationalizing behaviors by the better coping group in the first assessment period, as suggestive of persistence of and growing emphasis over time on cognitive defense maneuvers in the maintenance of postcrisis adjustment.

Feifel and co-workers (1987) evaluated the use and efficacy of three major coping strategies (confrontation, avoidance, and acceptance–resignation) among patients. They looked at three groups of male patients. Two consisted of men with life-threatening illness: cancer and heart disease. The third sample involved men with non-life-threatening conditions (e.g., orthopedic disability, rheumatoid arthritis, or a dermatological ailment). In their study, use of confrontation was found to be significantly correlated with treatment for a life-threatening illness. In addition, use of confrontation as a coping strategy was greatest among those who were more extroverted and who perceived their illness as being serious. In contrast, use of avoidance was more prevalent among those of the lower socioeconomic classes, who were less self-directed, and who had a more negative self-perception. Acceptance–resignation as a coping strategy was most often used by patients exhibiting little expectation of recovery and lacking hope. With regard to coping efficacy, it was found that cancer patients who estimated themselves to be coping poorly were more willing to use avoidance and acceptance–resignation as coping modes.

Despite variations in populations, disease sites and

**Table 4-5** Selected studies of coping and adaptation to cancer illness

| Author(s) | Sample | Coping assessment | Outcome variable(s) | Findings |
|---|---|---|---|---|
| Schoenfield (1972) | 42 Cancer patients with good prognosis | Coping per se not assessed; rather, psychological adaptation measured by (1) three MMPI subscales—morale loss, health concern, sense of well-being (a factor of Barron's ego strength scale); (2) Cattell's self-analysis form (to assess manifest anxiety); (3) Holtzman ink-blot test | Return to previous life-style and full-time employment | Those who returned to work ($n = 33$) had significantly lower morale loss scores, higher well-being scores, and less covert anxiety than those who did not ($n = 9$). |
| Weisman and Worden (1976–1977); Weisman (1976) | 120 Newly diagnosed patients | Clinical interview and self-report ratings of adjustment to "plight" of cancer | Multiple outcome measures: coping resolution (COPE scale), predominant concerns, vulnerability, and total mood disturbance (POMS) | Patients who were good copers (e.g., high resolution, low vulnerability, low-mood disturbance) used confrontation, redefinition, and compliance with authority; poor copers employed suppression–passivity and stoic acceptance. Regrets about the past, pessimism, multiple family problems, and little expectation of support were associated with high vulnerability. |
| Sanders and Kardinal (1977) | 6 Adult patients with acute leukemia in remission | Detailed interviews over 6-month period assessing present perception of condition, life-style changes, coping patterns used in past, expectations for future | Derived adaptational "pattern" used to adjust to illness and remission, reduce fear and anxiety, permit return to as normal as possible functioning | Three adaptive coping behaviors were identified: denial of being sick, identification with fellow patients to form "hospital family," anticipatory grieving. |
| O'Malley et al. (1979) | 115 Survivors of pediatric cancer | Interview eliciting information on various coping mechanisms used in adjusting to illness | Standardized psychiatric interview and adjustment ratings, mental status exam, and measures of self-esteem, social adjustment, anxiety, depression, and death anxiety | Effective use of denial facilitates adjustment; group rated as "well" on interview and self-report worried least about recurrence, and looked forward to and actively planned for the future. |
| Penman (1982) | 27 Postmastectomy patients | Coping strategies and their adequacy rated on semi-structured interview using specially developed instruments | Coping adequacy and mood state (POMS) | Tackling and mastering behaviors, combined with rationalizing and reinterpretive strategies (versus avoiding–capitulating), were predictive of better later adjustment as manifested in higher coping adequacy and less distressed mood. |
| Felton and Revenson (1984) | 151 Adult patients with chronic illnesses: rheumatoid arthritis, cancer, hypertension, and diabetes | Assessed use of two strategies: information seeking and wish-fulfilling fantasy (from Folkman and Lazarus Ways of Coping Scale) | Ratings on Acceptance of Illness Scale (eight items from Sickness Impact Scales), and five-item positive and negative affect subscales of Bradburn Affect Balance Scale | Information seeking was linked to decreased negative affect and better acceptance of illness regardless of "controllability" of disease. (Effects of coping on adjustment to illness, however, were modest.) |

*(continued)*

**Table 4-5** *(Continued)*

| Author(s) | Sample | Coping assessment | Outcome variable(s) | Findings |
|---|---|---|---|---|
| Taylor et al. (1984) | 78 Breast cancer patients | Coping indirectly assessed with respect to patient's sense of control over illness | Questionnaire rating of belief in illness controllability and multiple measure-derived adjustment scale | Belief in one's own control over the cancer and belief that others (e.g., physician) could now control the disease were significantly associated with good adjustment. Blaming another person was associated with poorer adjustment. |

**Table 4-6** Models for coping in illness

| Moos and Schaefer (1984) | Weisman and Worden (1976–1977) | Lipowski (1970) | Penman (1980) |
|---|---|---|---|
| *Appraisal-focused coping* | | | |
| Logical analysis | — | Minimization<br>Denial | Rationalizing, reinterpreting (e.g., minimizes; emphasizes self-sufficiency; puts in "perspective") |
| Cognitive redefinition | Accept, but find something favorable (redefinition). | Rationalization | |
| Cognitive avoidance | Try to forget; put it out of mind (suppression). | Selective misinterpretation/interpretation | |
| | Do other things to distract self (displacement). | Avoiding<br>Avoidance | Avoiding (e.g., withdraws, avoids, seeks distraction) |
| | Blame someone or something (disown responsibility). | Denial | |
| *Problem-focused coping* | | | |
| Seek information or advice | Seek more information about the situation (rational-intellectual). | Vigilant focusing<br>Seek as much information as possible | Tackling and mastering (e.g., seeks information, fights disability, works at problem solving) |
| | Seek direction from an authority and comply (compliance). | | |
| Take problem-solving action | Take firm action based on present understanding (confrontation). | Tackling<br>Confronting<br>Actively dealing with illness | |
| Develop alternative rewards | Negotiate feasible alternatives (if *x*, then *y*). | | |
| *Emotion-focused coping* | | | |
| Affective regulation | Laugh it off; make light; of situation (reversal of affect). | | |
| Resigned acceptance | Withdraw socially into isolation (stimulus reduction). | Capitulating<br>Adapting a passive dependent stance<br>Withdrawal | Capitulating (e.g., accepts stoically; complies passively; expresses futility) |
| | Submit to and accept the inevitable (fatalism). | | |
| | Blame yourself, sacrifice or atone (self-pity). | | |
| Emotional discharge | Reduce tension by drinking, overeating, drugs (tension reduction). | | Tension-relieving (e.g., expresses and shares feelings; uses humor; blames others) |
| | Talk with others to relieve distress (shared concern). | | |
| | Do something, anything, however reckless, impractical (act out). | | |

**Table 4-7** Characteristics associated with high and low emotional distress*

| High distress | Low distress |
| --- | --- |
| Pessimistic | Optimistic, including outcome, regardless of time required |
| Many regrets about past life | Fewer regrets and marital problems |
| Marital problems | |
| History of psychiatric treatment or suicidal ideation | |
| High anxiety; lower ego strength (MMPI) | Low anxiety; higher ego strength |
| More recent life changes (Holmes and Rahe) | Fewer recent life changes (Holmes and Rahe) |
| More physical symptoms | Fewer physical symptoms |
| Higher IPC scores | Lower IPC scores |
| Less effective RES | Better problem resolution (RES scores higher) |
| Expects little support from family | Expects full support or adequate support from family and doctor |
| Doctor is seen as less helpful | Doctor is helpful enough for present needs |
| Foresees more interference by illness on family, work, and personal life | Foresees little interference by illness on family, work, and personal life |
| Feels isolated or given up, and feels like giving up | Feels not at all ignored or victimized; encouraged about future adjustment |
| Tendency to submit passively, or blame others for their plight | Active desire to live with the problems that turn up |

*IPC, Inventory of Personal Concerns; RES, resolution or outcome of strategies used.
*Source*: Reprinted with permission from Weisman, A.D. and J.W. Worden (1976–1977). The existential plight of cancer: Significance of the first 100 days. *Int. J. Psychiatry Med.* 7:1–15, pp 9.

stages, methods and time frames of evaluation, several common themes emerge from the body of coping research and adaptation to cancer. First, strategies or styles that promote an active (versus passive and helpless) response to problem-solving and coping behavior are consistently found to be the most effective. Second, coping with illness is a dynamic process, changing as a function of the circumstances and of the individual's continuing appraisal of its meaning with respect to his or her survival, future, relationships, self-esteem, and achievement of goals. Third, individuals who exhibit flexibility in their efforts are better able to cope. This can be seen as a corollary to the second point; because adaptation to illness is necessarily a dynamic process, the person who can more readily respond to changing demands by developing new strategies will cope more effectively. Fourth, the nature and amount of social support available to the individual strongly influences capacity to cope. Though often not directly assessed, presence or absence of supportive others is cited in many of the studies as a powerful determinant of successful outcome.

Review of the studies in coping with cancer, as well as those in other serious illnesses, does indicate that there are characteristics that, if present in a given patient, may put him or her at increased risk for problems in coping. These are shown in Table 4-8. Although an attempt was made to arrange the characteristics on the list in order of potential seriousness, this was based on the prevalence with which a given attribute was cited as a poor prognosticator and its potential for mediation (viability as a point of interventions), rather than on an empirical assessment of rank order of impact on coping. Poor prognosticators for coping may occur singly, but more often occur in multiple combinations. Presence of any one, however, should alert staff that additional assessment is warranted. Social support (reviewed extensively in Chapter 5 that follows) is probably the most manageable risk variable for poor coping, and one well worth addressing because absence of a functioning support system can have a dramatic negative impact on the patient's ability to cope, by depriving him or her of a buffer against the stress of illness, of needed feedback on alternative coping strategies, and of additional coping resources. The changing nature of illness demands, and the dynamic interaction between stress and coping virtually assure, that the rigid patient incapable of altering coping strategies is at high risk. So, too, is the individual who faces his or her situation with a grim outlook. Pessimism precludes the opportunity to explore alternative action-oriented options and may encourage the patient to adopt a passive stance toward illness, a coping style shown to be less effective. In both cases, discussion of the usefulness of strategies used or the implications of the style adopted is helpful in reorienting a patient's coping efforts. Though often considered characterological, these patterns have been found to be amenable to change (Weisman and Sobel, 1979). When there are multiple external obligations, competing demands on emotional and physical resources may leave the patient with little energy to deal with illness. Identification of these obligations and help in minimizing them by allocating resources and delegating responsibility to oth-

**Table 4-8** Predictors of poor coping with cancer

Social isolation (perceived or actual)
Low socioeconomic status
Alcohol or drug abuse
Previous psychiatric history
History of recent losses
Inflexibility and rigidity of coping
Pessimistic philosophy of life
Multiple obligations

ers may be necessary to free the patient sufficiently to manage his or her own personal problems in adjusting to illness. Similarly with low socioeconomic status, the increasing demands in the face of reduced or limited resources results in poor coping capacity. The limitations on cognitive capacity imposed as a consequence of extreme youth or age may limit the coping strategies available and their efficacy. Alcohol and drug abuse seriously compromise patients' cognitive abilities and hence limit their intellectual coping skills. Because these problems often arise in the context of a long history of difficulty managing day-to-day stress, substance abuse and prior psychiatric history put the patient at high risk of difficulty in coping with life-threatening illness and call for early consultation. Finally, multiple losses that deprive the individual of a needed social network, strain self-esteem, optimism, and general coping resources, and result in multiple bereavement, may lead to inadequate reserve when he or she is faced by the demands of illness. Although the tangible consequences can sometimes be mitigated (e.g., supplying a new social network), the psychological devastation resulting from a loss of social supports may prevent a patient from coping effectively or even attempting to undertake coping efforts.

There is some evidence to suggest that "good" coping strategies as defined earlier are likely to be concomitants of "good" ego strength (Worden and Sobel, 1973; Vaillant, 1977). Using the Barrons Scale of Ego Strength from the Minnesota Multiphasic Personality Inventory (MMPI), Worden and Sobel (1973) found that cancer patients who showed good (high) ego strength also chose more effective coping strategies and made a better adjustment to their illness. Thus, in very broad terms, it is likely that whatever means we use to identify the more emotionally "healthy" individual will also select the one more likely to make a positive adjustment to illness.

## INTERVENTIONS TO ENHANCE COPING WITH CANCER

In relation to the amount and complexity of literature on coping and stress, there have been fewer studies to test interventions designed to maximize coping efforts. However, most of the psychosocial intervention studies in cancer have had this as a goal. (See Chapter 38 for a review of these.) Also, a number of studies that were designed with specific interventions to improve cancer coping have reported improvement in patient adjustment and functioning (Gordon et al., 1980; Worden, 1982; Telch and Telch, 1986).

Clinical observation and systematic research among cancer patients reveals a remarkable resilience of these individuals and their families in adapting to adversity.

It is clear, however, that a person's ability to cope with the many stresses of illness is multidetermined. Understanding all the determinants that contribute, though desirable, is probably not feasible in caring for the patient; however, an understanding of the nature and effectiveness of the individual patient's coping ability is vital.

How a patient responds to the crisis brought about by cancer can in extreme situations spell the difference between optimum recovery and psychological invalidism. Lipowski (1970) emphasizes that physical illness constitutes a psychological stress that results in adaptational tasks, challenges, and goals to be mastered. If effective, the effort to meet the challenges can result in emotional growth, but if ineffective, it may lead to psychic distress or regression. When either the stress is too great or the adaptive capacity too limited, then actual psychiatric syndromes may occur that require diagnosis and intervention (see also chapters in Part IV).

Researchers have begun recently to explore the question of whether the use of different coping strategies affects survival in cancer. The theoretical and clinical issues involved in coping in relation to cancer survival are discussed in detail in Chapters 60 and 61 (see also Temoshok, 1987). It is noteworthy that among studies showing a positive impact of coping on survival, many have identified a pattern of active, "fighting spirit," responses similar to those found in studies of adaptation that are associated with good general adjustment (Greer et al., 1979; Derogatis et al., 1979; Pettingale et al., 1985). Similarly, other studies have indicated that responses characterized by emotional inhibition, stoicism, and hopelessness are associated with higher rates of mortality (Stavraky et al., 1968; Rogentine et al., 1979; DiClemente and Temoshok, 1985; Goodkin et al., 1986). However, other researchers, using more sophisticated models and controlling for confounding medical variables, have seen no impact on coping and outcome of disease (Cassileth et al., 1985, 1987; Holland et al., 1986; R.N. Jamison et al., 1987). As research in this area continues, it will have an impact both on how we interpret coping responses and the direction of interventions to promote optimal coping both in the immediate and long-term adaptational process.

## SUMMARY

It is important that staff caring for the patient recognize the modes of coping being used and help the patient employ the most adaptive and effective strategies possible. In order to do this, it is necessary to understand the tasks demanded of the patient and the resources available to meet these challenges physically, socially, and emotionally. Facilitating a patient's active participation in managing illness appears to have a dramatic impact not only on day-to-day activities and adjustment, but also possibly on long-term survival.

## REFERENCES

Anderson, C.R. (1977). Locus of control, coping behaviors and performance in a stress setting: A longitudinal study. *J. Appl. Psychiatry* 62:446–51.

Andreason, N.J.C. and A.S. Norris (1972). Long-term adjustment and adaptation mechanisms in severely burned adults. *J. Nerv. Ment. Dis.* 154:352–62.

Antonovsky, A. (1979). *Health, Stress and Coping*. San Francisco: Jossey-Bass.

Bard, M. and A. Sutherland (1955). Psychological impact of cancer and its treatment. IV. Adaptation to radical mastectomy. *Cancer* 8:656–72.

Blazer, D. and E. Palmore (1976). Religion and aging in a longitudinal panel. *Gerontologist* 16:82–85.

Burish, T.G. and L.A. Bradley (eds.). (1983). *Coping with Chronic Disease: Research Applications*. New York: Academic Press.

Caplan, G. (1981). Mastery of stress. *Am. J. Psychiatry* 138:413–20.

Cassileth, B.R., E.J. Lusk, D.S. Miller, L.L. Brown, and C. Miller (1985). Psychosocial correlates of survival in advanced malignant disease? *N. Engl. J. Med.* 312:1551–55.

Cassileth, B.R., E. Lusk, W. Walsh, H. Altman, and M. Pisano (1987). Psychosocial correlates of unusually good outcome 3 years after diagnosis (Abstract). *Proc. Am. Soc. Clin. Oncol.* 6:253.

Coelho, G.V., D.A. Hamburg, and J.E. Adams (eds.). (1974). *Coping and Adaptation*. New York: Basic Book.

Cohen, F. and R. Lazarus (1973). Active coping processes, coping dispositions, and recovery from surgery. *Psychosom. Med.* 35:375–89.

Cohen, S. and S.L. Syme (eds.). (1985). *Social Support and Health*. New York: Academic Press.

Cohen, S. and T.A. Wills (1985). Stress, social support, and the buffering hypothesis. *Psychol. Bull.* 98:310–57.

Comstock, G.W. and J.D. Partridge (1972). Church attendance and health. *J. Chron. Dis.* 25:665–72.

Derogatis, L.R., M.D. Abeloff, and N. Melisaratos (1979). Psychological coping mechanisms and survival time in metastatic breast cancer. *J.A.M.A.* 242:1504–8.

DiClemente, R.J. and L. Temoshok (1985). Psychological adjustment to having cutaneous malignant melanoma as a predictor of follow-up clinical status. *Psychosom. Med.* 47:81 (Abstract).

Erikson, E.H. (1963). *Childhood and Society*, 2nd ed. New York: Norton.

Feifel, H., S. Strack, and V.T. Nagy (1987). Coping strategies and associated features of medically ill patients. *Psychosom. Med.* 49:616–25.

Felton, B.J. and T.A. Revenson (1984). Coping with chronic illness: A study of illness controlability and the influence of coping strategies on psychological adjustment. *J. Consult. Clin. Psychol.* 52:343–53.

Finlayson, A. (1976). Social networks as coping resources. *Soc. Sci. Med.* 10:97–103.

Folkman, S. (1984). Personal control and stress and coping processes: A theoretical analysis. *J. Pers. Soc. Psychol.* 46:839–52.

Folkman, S. and R.S. Lazarus, (1980). An analysis of coping in a middle-aged community sample. *J. Health Soc. Behav.* 21:219–39.

Goldberger, L. and S. Breznitz (eds.). (1982). *Handbook of Stress*. New York: The Free Press.

Goodkin, K., M.H. Antoni, and P.H. Blaney (1986). Stress and hopelessness in the promotion of cervical intraepithelial neoplasia to invasive squamous cell carcinoma of the cervix. *J. Psychosom. Res.* 30:67–76.

Gordon, W.A., I. Freidenbergs, L. Diller, M. Hibbard, C. Wolfe, L. Levine, R. Lipkins, O. Ezrachi, and D. Lucido (1980). Efficacy of psychosocial intervention with cancer patients. *J. Consult. Clin. Psychol.* 48:743–59.

Greer, S., T. Morris, and K.W. Pettingale (1979). Psychological response to breast cancer: Effect on outcome. *Lancet* 2:785–87.

Haan, N. (1977). *Coping and Defending. Processes of Self-Environment Organization*. New York: Academic Press.

Hackett, T.P. and A.D. Weisman (1969). Denial as a factor in patients with heart disease and cancer. *Ann. N.Y. Acad. Sci.* 164:802–11.

Hamburg, B.A., L.F. Lipsett, G.E. Inoff, and A.L. Drash (eds.). (1980). *Behavioral and Psychosocial Issues in Diabetes*. NIH Publ. No. 80-1993. Washington, D.C.: U.S. Govt. Printing Office.

Hamburg, D.A. (1974). Coping behavior in life-threatening circumstances. *Psychother. Psychosom.* 23:13–25.

Hamburg, D.A. and J.E. Adams (1967). A perspective on coping behavior: Seeking and utilizing information in major transitions. *Arch. Gen. Psychiatry* 17:277–84.

Hamburg, D.A., G.V. Coelho, and J.E. Adams (1974). Coping and adaptation: Steps towards a synthesis of biological and social perspectives. In G.V. Coelho, D.A. Hamburg, and J.E. Adams (eds.), *Coping and Adaptation*. New York: Basic Books, pp. 403–40.

Hamburg, D.A., B. Hamburg, and S. deGoza (1953). Adaptive problems and mechanisms in severely burned patients. *Psychiatry* 16:1–20.

Hamburg, B.A., and D. Hamburg, (1981). Adaptation and health: a life span perspective. In B. Kaplan and M. Ibrahim (eds.), *Family Medicine and Supportive Interventions: An Epidemiological Approach*, Chapel Hill, NC: University of North Carolina Press, Institute for Research in Social Sciences, pp. 41–54.

Holland, J.C., A.H. Korzun, S. Tross, D.F. Cella, L. Norton, and W. Wood (1986). Psychosocial factors and disease-free survival in Stage II breast cancer (Abstract). *Proc. Am. Soc. Clin. Oncol.* 5:237.

House, J.S. (1981). *Work Stress and Social Support*. Reading, Mass.: Addison-Wesley.

Ilfeld, F.W. (1980a). Coping styles among Chicago adults: Description. *J. Human Stress* 6:2–10.

Ilfeld, F.W. (1980b). Coping styles of Chicago adults: Effectiveness. *Arch. Gen. Psychiatry* 37:1239–43.

Jamison, K.R., D.K. Wellisch, and R.O. Pasnau (1978).

Psychosocial aspects of mastectomy. I. The woman's perspective. *Am. J. Psychiatry* 135:432–36.

Jamison, R.N., T.G. Burish, and K.A. Wallston (1987). Psychogenic factors in predicting survival of breast cancer patients. *J. Clin. Oncol.* 5:768–72.

Janoff-Bulman, R. and C. Timko (1986). Coping with traumatic life events: The role of denial in light of people's assumptive worlds. In C.R. Snyder and C. Ford (eds.), *Coping with Negative Life Events: Clinical and Social Psychological Perspectives.* New York: Plenum.

Jemott, J.B. III and S.E. Locke (1984). Psychosocial factors, immunologic mediation, and human susceptibility to infectious diseases: How much do we know? *Psychol. Bull.* 95:78–108.

Kaplan, B.H. and D.G. Blazer (1989). Religion in the stress and adaptation paradigm. In P. Barchas (ed.), *Sociophysiology.* New York: Oxford University Press.

Kahn, R., D.M. Wolfe, R.P. Quinn, and J.D. Snoek (1964). *Organizational Stress: Studies in Role Conflict and Ambiguity.* New York: Wiley.

Lazarus, R.S. (1966). *Psychological Stress and the Coping Process.* New York: McGraw-Hill.

Lazarus, R.S. (1974). Psychological stress and coping in adaptation and illness. *Int. J. Psychiatry Med.* 5:321–33.

Lazarus, R.S. and S. Folkman, (1984). *Stress Appraisal and Coping.* New York: Springer.

Lazarus, R.S., J. Averill, and E. Opton (1974). The psychology of coping: Issues of research and assessment. In G. Coelho, D. Hamburg, and J. Adams (eds.), *Coping and Adaptation.* New York: Basic Books, pp. 249–315.

Levy, S.M. and B.H. Fox (1987). Psychological risk factors and mechanisms in cancer prognosis. Unpublished manuscript.

Lieberman, M.A. (1982). The effects of social support on responses to stress. In L. Goldberger and S. Breznitz (eds.), *Handbook of Stress: Theoretical and Clinical Aspects.* New York: The Free Press, pp. 764–83.

Lipowski, Z.J. (1969). Psychosocial aspects of disease. *Ann. Intern. Med.* 71:1197–1206.

Lipowski, Z.J. (1970). Physical illness, the individual and the coping processes. *Psychiatry Med.* 1:91–102.

McCrae, R.R. and P.T. Costa (1986). Personality, coping, and coping effectiveness in an adult sample. *J. Pers. Soc. Psychol.* 54:385–405.

Mechanic, D. (1968). *Medical Sociology.* New York: The Free Press.

Mechanic, D. (1977). Illness behavior, social adaptation, and the management of illness. *J. Nerv. Mental Dis.* 165:79–87.

Meichenbaum, D., D. Turk, and S. Burstein, (1975). The nature of coping with stress. In I.G. Sarason and C.D. Spielberger (eds.), *Stress and Anxiety,* Vol. 2. New York: Wiley, pp. 337–60.

Monat, A. and R.S. Lazarus (eds.). (1977). *Stress and Coping: An Anthology.* New York: Columbia University Press.

Moos, R.H. (ed.). (1977). *Coping with Physical Illness,* Vol. 1. New York: Plenum.

Moos, R.H. (ed.). (1984). *Coping with Physical Illness.* Vol. 2, *New Perspectives.* New York: Plenum.

Moos, R.H. and J.A. Schaefer (1984). The crisis of physical illness: An overview and conceptual approach. In R.H. Moos (ed.), *Coping with Physical Illness.* Vol. 2, New Perspectives New York: Plenum, pp. 3–25.

Moos, R.H. and V.D. Tsu (1977). The crisis of physical illness: An overview. In R.H. Moos (ed.), *Coping with Physical Illness,* Vol. 1. New York: Plenum, pp. 3–21.

O'Malley, J.E., G. Koocher, D. Foster, and L. Slavin (1979). Psychiatric sequelae of surviving childhood cancer. *Am. J. Orthopsychiatry* 49:608–16.

Parkes, C.M. (1972). Components of the reaction to loss of a limb, spouse or home. *J. Psychosom. Res.* 16:343–49.

Pearlin, L.I. and C. Schooler (1978). The structure of coping. *J. Health Soc. Behav.* 19:2–21.

Penman, D.T. (1980). Coping strategies in adaptation to mastectomy. *Diss. Abstr. Int.* 40(12):5825-B.

Penman, D.T. (1982). Coping strategies in adaptation to mastectomy. *Psychosom. Med.* 44:117 (Abstract).

Pettingale, K.W., T. Moris, S. Greer, and J.L. Haybittle (1985). Mental attitudes to cancer: An additional prognostic factor. *Lancet* 1:750.

Rogentine, G.N., D.P. van Kammen, B.H. Fox, J.P. Dockerty, J.E. Rosenblatt, S.C. Boyd, and W.E. Bunney (1979). Psychological factors in the prognosis of malignant melanoma: A prospective study. *Psychosom. Med.* 41:647–55.

Sanders, J.B. and C.G. Kardinal (1977). Adaptive coping mechanisms in adult acute leukemia patients in remission. *J.A.M.A.* 238:952–54.

Schonfield, J. (1972). Psychological factors related to delayed return to an earlier life-style in successfully treated cancer patients. *J. Psychosom. Res.* 16:41–46.

Sidle, A., R. Moos, J. Adams, and P. Cady (1969). Development of a coping scale. *Arch. Gen. Psychiatry* 20:226–32.

Silver, R.L. and C.B. Wortman (1980). Coping with undesirable life events. In J. Garber and M.E. Seligman (eds.), *Human Helplessness.* New York: Academic Press, pp. 279–345.

Singer, J.E. (1984). Some issues in the study of coping. *Cancer* 53:2303–13.

Stavraky, K., C. Buck, J. Lott, and J.M. Wanklin (1968). Psychological factors in the outcome of human cancer. *J. Psychosom. Res.* 12:251–59.

Stewart, A.L. (1982). *Measuring Coping with Serious Illness.* Unpublished doctoral dissertation. University of California, Los Angeles.

Strickland, B.R. (1978). Internal–external experiences and health-related behaviors. *J. Consult. Clin. Psychol.* 46:1192–1211.

Taylor, S.E. (1983). Adjustment to threatening events. A theory of cognitive adaptation. *Am. Psychol.* 38:1161–73.

Taylor, S.E., R.R. Lichtman, and J.V. Wood (1984). Attributions, beliefs about control, and adjustment to breast cancer. *J. Pers. Soc. Psychol.* 46:489–502.

Taylor, S.E., J.V. Wood, and R.R. Lichtman (1983). It could be worse: Selective evaluation as a response to victimization. *J. Soc. Issues* 39:19–40.

Telch, C.F. and M.J. Telch (1986). Group coping skills instruction and supportive group therapy for cancer patients: A comparison of strategies. *J. Consult. Clin. Psychol.* 54:802–8.

Temoshok, L. (1987). Personality, coping style, emotion and cancer: Towards an integrative model. *Cancer Surveys* 6:545–567.

Thoits, P.A. (1986). Social support as coping assistance. *J. Consult. Clin. Psychol.* 54:416–23.

Vaillant, G.E. (1971). Theoretical hierarchy of adaptive ego mechanisms. *Arch. Gen. Psychiatry* 24:107–17.

Vaillant, G.E. (1977). *Adaptation to Life.* Boston: Little, Brown & Co.

Vastyan, E.A. (1986). Spiritual aspects of the care of cancer patients. *CA* 36:110–14.

Visotsky, H., D. Hamburg, M.E. Goss, and B.Z. Lebovits (1961). Coping behavior under extreme stress: Observation of patients with severe poliomyelitis. *Arch. Gen. Psychiatry* 5:423–48.

Weisman, A.D. (1976). Early diagnosis of vulnerability in cancer patients. *Am. J. Med. Sci.* 271:187–96.

Weisman, A.D. (1979). *Coping with Cancer,* New York: McGraw-Hill.

Weisman, A.D. and H.J. Sobel (1979). Coping with cancer through self instruction: A hypothesis. *J. Human Stress* 5:3–8.

Weisman, A.D. and J.W. Worden (1975). Psychosocial analysis of cancer deaths. *Omega* 6:61–75.

Weisman, A.D. and J.W. Worden (1976–1977). The existential plight of cancer: Significance of the first 100 days. *Int. J. Psychiatry Med.* 7:1–15.

White, R.W. (1974). Strategies of adaptation: An attempt at systematic description. In G.V. Coelho, D.A. Hamburg, and J.E. Adams (eds.), *Coping and Adaptation.* New York: Basic Books, pp. 47–48.

Worden, J.W. (1982). Psychosocial screening and intervention with newly diagnosed cancer patients. *Proc. Internationale Union Contre le Cancer,* p. 158, No. 885.

Worden, J.W. and H.J. Sobel (1973). Ego strength and psychosocial adaptation to cancer. *Psychosom. Med.* 40:585–92.

Wortman, C.B. (1984). Social support and the cancer patient. Conceptual and methodologic issues. *Cancer* 53:2339–60.

Yates, J.W., B.J. Chalmer, Rev. P. St. James, Rev. M. Follansbee, and F.P. McKegney (1981). Religion in patients with advanced cancer. *Med. Pediatr. Oncol.* 9:121–28.

# 5

# Interpersonal Resources: Social Support

Julia H. Rowland

It is proposed that there are three variables that affect adaptation to illness. The first two variables involve the life stage at which illness occurs and the individual's interpersonal style or coping capacity. The third context within which the individual's psychological adaptation must be considered is that of interpersonal resources, or namely, what other people or social support structures contribute to his or her adjustment to illness. Although given its own chapter, the issue of interpersonal resources necessarily enters into discussions in all the chapters within Part II. Its importance has already been highlighted in Chapter 3 as a necessary feature of normal development (cf. Erikson's stage of intimacy versus isolation), as a major focus of illness-related disruptions (e.g., impact on interpersonal relations), and as an important characteristic of developmentally generated interventions at *all* levels (in particular with respect to the older adult), and in Chapter 4 as a powerful modifier of capacity for coping. Similar to the area of stress and coping, research into the impact of social support and health has blossomed in the last 10 to 15 years as evidenced by the number of articles (Berkman and Syme, 1979; Bloom, 1982b; Cobb, 1976; Greenblatt et al., 1982; Jemott and Locke, 1984; Kaplan et al., 1977; Mitchell et al., 1982; Murawski et al., 1978; Schaefer et al., 1981; Thoits, 1982; Wortman and Conway, 1985) and books (Caplan, 1974; Cohen and Syme, 1985; H.S. Friedman and M.R. DiMatteo, 1982; Gottlieb, 1981; House, 1981; Kaplan and Cassel, 1975; Sarason and Sarason, 1985) published in this area. Indeed, the parallel growth of interest in the two areas may well reflect a common source of increased public awareness of and research concern with determinants that mediate stress and illness. From a practical standpoint, the relative benefits to improved mental and physical health by modifying social support suggest that social support represents an area in which it may be easiest, most effective, and most economical to intervene.

That a positive relationship exists between social support and health or illness outcomes is a consistent finding (for reviews see Broadhead et al., 1983; Wallston et al., 1983; DiMatteo and Hayes, 1981). Determining precisely what is meant or encompassed by the term "social support" and explaining how it works, however, is more problematic. Camille Wortman's scholarly review, published in 1984, provided the first major critique of research on social support and cancer. Although the main thrust of Wortman's article is the elaboration of research design issues in the study of social support in a cancer setting, it highlights points critical to the clinician's understanding of the meaning and impact of a person's social supports, and which have a direct bearing on clinicians' ability to facilitate optimal communication with and support of their patients. The outline that follows is similar to that of Wortman, but gives special attention to application of the information to clinical care.

This chapter addresses the nature of social support and the criteria used to assess support status. Particular attention is given to those variables that influence successful use of social support systems. Research on the effects on well-being from social support in cancer is reviewed and guidelines provided concerning the evaluation and management of social support in the cancer setting.

## NATURE OF SOCIAL SUPPORT

One of the primary issues in the study of social support is how to define the term. Authors vary in the emphasis and specificity of content that they feel falls under the aegis of "social support" (see Table 5-1). For the researcher, how the term is defined provides essential

**Table 5-1** Definitions of social support

| Reference | Definitions |
|---|---|
| Caplan (1974) | . . . others who (1) help people mobilize their psychological resources in order to deal with emotional problems; (2) share people's tasks; (3) provide individuals with money, materials, tools, skills, information, and advice in order to help them deal with the particular stressful situation to which they are exposed. |
| Cobb (1976) | . . . information leading the subject to believe that he or she is cared for and loved, esteemed and valued, and a member of a network of communication and mutual obligations. |
| Kaplan et al. (1977) | . . . the degree to which a person's basic needs are gratified through interaction with others. |
| Lin et al. (1979) | . . . support accessible to an individual through social ties to other individuals, groups, and the larger community. |
| Wallston et al. (1983) | . . . social support describes the comfort, assistance, and/or information one receives through formal or informal contacts with individuals or groups. |

guidelines for how it will be employed or studied and evaluated. For example, in evaluating support resources, does one count numbers of relatives available or only those to whom the individual speaks once a week (a more realistic ''support'')? But such a definition is also important for the clinician. From a clinical care standpoint, it is probably more useful to have a knowledge of the concrete characteristics of social support (the operational definition) than a general definition or vague concept of what is meant by the term. Toward this end, it is helpful to follow the outline a researcher might use to ''operationalize'' the concept of social support.

There are five criteria for assessing social support: the type of support being provided or needed, the source of support (providers), the quantity and availability of support, the quality and content of support given, and the perceived need by the recipient for support. Aspects of each have special ramifications on the usefulness and impact of the interpersonal domain on the patient's well-being. The definition of the term social support also dictates what information regarding a patient's social support is elicited (or omitted).

## TYPE OF SUPPORT

Even a cursory review of the literature reveals that there are a variety of taxonomies or lists of what constitutes social support (Cobb, 1976; Weiss, 1974; House, 1981). Principal areas of support provided include informational, emotional-affectional, tangible (e.g., financial, physical—sometimes referred to as instrumental), affirmational (providing a sense that one's feelings are understood), affiliational (providing a sense of belonging or maintenance of social identity), and appraisal (support that gives feedback to the patient). There is a tendency in evaluating support to overemphasize one aspect or another, specifically emotional support. Research carried out by Dunkel-Schetter (1984) provides empirical evidence that emotional support may in fact be the most helpful kind of support for cancer patients. In her study, 81% of 79 breast and colon cancer patients interviewed mentioned emotional support as one of the most helpful behaviors, and 41% indicated informational support as most helpful.

However, the relative importance of the various kinds of support may vary with the individual, as well as over time. For example, the 24-year-old Hodgkin's patient who is single may especially depend on the emotional support provided by her or his parents and peers to cope during the stress of active treatment. In contrast, the 24-year-old Hodgkin's patient who is married with a small child at home may rely more on (hence value more greatly) the baby-sitting and cooking, or the instrumental support, provided by neighbors during the same period. However, as treatment terminates, both patients may feel a great need for informational support from their physician, desiring reassurance that they will still be monitored and cared for, although visits will become less frequent. (For an elaboration of how a specific type of support might be used to manage particular problems in cancer, such as depression or grief, see also Peteet, 1982).

Because it is not always feasible for a clinician to assess all of the types of support needs and resources of each patient as well as their importance during various treatments, a simpler approach must be adopted. One useful approach to this task is suggested by Cohen and McKay (1984). They emphasize the importance of achieving a match between the coping requirements of a task and the support given.

## SOURCE OF SUPPORT

Who provides the support is another important consideration in assessing social support. Most studies indicate that it is the ill person's spouse or parent (if the

**Table 5-2**  Sources of support

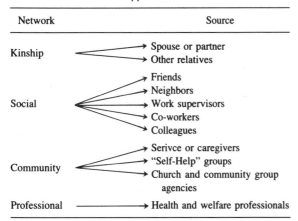

| Network | Source |
|---------|--------|
| Kinship | Spouse or partner<br>Other relatives |
| Social | Friends<br>Neighbors<br>Work supervisors<br>Co-workers<br>Colleagues |
| Community | Serivce or caregivers<br>"Self-Help" groups<br>Church and community group agencies |
| Professional | Health and welfare professionals |

*Source*: Modified from J.S. House (1981). *Work Stress and Social Support.* Reading, Mass.: Addison-Wesley, p. 23.

patient is a child) who is the central support figure, but it may at times be a child (if the patient is older and alone), or an extended family member, friend, or even staffperson. In her study, Dunkel-Schetter (1984) found that physicians and other medical care providers were mentioned about as frequently as family members (30% versus 34%) as sources of the greatest help, a result consistent with that reported earlier by Bloom (1981).

As seen in Table 5-2, the primary social support provider may come from a wide range of sources. Two points need to be made about the variety within a patient's sources of support. First, it is important to recognize that different sources of support often provide different types of support. For example, a spouse may provide vital affectional needs, while a friend may help with more tangible support, such as doing errands or looking after children. Even when the same type of support is given, it may be received differently by the patient depending on who provides it, which is the second feature to note about multiple sources. For example, patients may feel greatly reassured when their physician assures them that they are doing well, yet find themselves anxious or resentful when a spouse provides the same reassurance. A more classic, and likely familiar, example is the case of the person who hears the words "I understand how you feel." When uttered by someone who has experienced the same situation (a fellow cancer patient), such words may be deeply reassuring; however, when spoken by a solicitous friend or even staff member they can elicit anger and disgust. Far from being supportive, some statements made by healthy friends may be perceived by patients, parents of ill children, and bereaved individuals as trivializing a serious problem (Wortman and Lehman, 1985; Lehman et al., 1986).

A study by Lieberman (1982) found that spouses served as the most effective source of help for psychological problems. Friends were the second most helpful, followed by professionals and self-help groups. Relatives proved to be the least helpful for managing such problems. In another study, Bozeman and colleagues (1955) reported that, for parents whose child was being treated for leukemia, other parents with leukemic children "were regarded by most mothers as the most important source of emotional support" (p. 15). Dunkel-Schetter (1984) reported that health care professionals who provided a combination of direct assistance information and emotional support are seen as most effective. This was in contrast to the specialization found in support from family and friends. Thus, although maximizing the use of support services available is often a helpful overall goal when evaluating social support, it is also necessary to ensure that particular individuals (e.g., spouse and attending physician) or groups of individuals (family and medical care team) are called on to provide specific types of support. Stated somewhat differently, the provider needs to be appropriately matched to the task.

## QUANTITY AND AVAILABILITY OF SUPPORT

There are a variety of different ways in which the quantity and availability of social support to the patient can be determined. The most general, and probably most commonly used, is the structural approach. This entails a review of marital or partner status, membership in social and professional groups, involvement in social activities, amount of social contacts, and so on. This kind of information is often easy to obtain and constitutes a relatively objective and generally stable indicator of the person's level of social activity and "connectedness." It can serve as a simple screening approach to identify the patient who has a history of being isolated, or alternately of being bound by multiple obligations (overextended or overcommitted), and is hence at risk for increased stress when illness is diagnosed.

Wortman covers two other techniques that can also be used to assess social support. One is relatively quick but may be more stressful for the patient. The second, mentioned here only because there have been some interesting dynamic ramifications of information collected in this way, is principally a research-analytical, approach. The first approach entails having the individual indicate whether particular sources or types of support are available. In such cases the patient is asked if there are supportive family members, friends, staff, and others on whom he or she can depend or can turn to for support. As Wortman notes (1984, p. 2344), it may be particularly helpful to assess the emotional and physical availability of "key members" of each group, in particular the spouse, the physician, and peer patients. If, as is usually the case, the interviewer is unable to obtain information about all these sources, a simpler approach might be adopted. One such method is to adopt the phrasing proposed by Abbey and co-workers (1981), in which the emphasis is on determining if there is "some one person" who makes you feel loved and needed, depends on you, listens to what you have to say. This approach has several advantages. It enables the person doing the evaluation to determine if the patient has within his or her network some source for each of the various types of support. If one type of support is missing, then information about the specific need enables the evaluator to plan out the means of filling those special needs, particularly if this is an area in which the patient has always had support. Such an approach is also quick, less directed than queries regarding "the person closest to you," yet more specific than wording emphasizing "the people in your life." Finally, Abbey and co-workers (1981) found that the phrasing "some one person" yielded the strongest and most consistent relationships between social support and emotional well-being.

The second and more empirically oriented approach to exploring a person's social support is to conduct what is referred to as a network analysis. This involves examining a number of properties related to the social network, namely, the size (or number of direct contacts), density (or frequency of contacts), stability, accessibility, and reciprocity. Network analysis has been used in the context of research in mental health and is detailed elsewhere (Fischer, 1982; McCallister and Fischer, 1978; House and Kahn, 1985). Although the technique has not been applied specifically in research with cancer patients, as Wortman (1984, p. 2349) points out, the results of related studies among stressed and critically ill samples are provocative. For example, though generally considered the most supportive in periods of crisis, the small and intense networks can also lead the individual to feel entrapped under other circumstances (Caplan, 1974). Such situations may be more common for patients and families from different ethnic or cultural backgrounds who travel to a major cancer treatment center for care. Language or social barriers may prevent the foreign patient from obtaining help beyond the small social network of members traveling with him or her who themselves may have limited resources, knowledge, or skills. Additionally, when the crisis situation makes obtaining new information a premium, it may be that a loosely connected (low-density) network is an asset because where close friends may hear the same news at the same time, weaker ties are more frequently the source of novel news (Hirsch, 1981; Thomas and Weiner,

1974). For example, the breast cancer patient who has in her support network friends from diverse backgrounds, who are also geographically dispersed, may learn of a variety of self-help groups and rehabilitative options following her mastectomy because of the variety of experience and knowledge available to her diverse friends. Such information may not be as readily available to the woman whose support network depends on a close group of friends who all grew up together and live in close proximity.

The quantity and availability, both physical and emotional, of supports is itself dependent on a number of variables. The most obvious of these is the individual's prior resources. It is unlikely that the isolated individual will be able to mobilize a social network any more readily once he or she becomes ill than previously. However, it is not advisable to assume a previously well-supported patient's needs will be adequately met. The person who comes from a close family and who was socially active may find that supports fall away during illness. The disappointment in withdrawal of friends is particularly painful for these individuals, even when they can recognize the reasons for the response. The stresses of illness on both recipient patient and support provider often precipitates a realignment of ties and interactions. A consistent theme voiced by cancer patients is a sense of surprise at the unexpected sources of support that emerge during a crisis; a casual friend may at times emerge to provide the more intense and personal support expected only from closer family. Thus, while the individual with poor or few social support should always be evaluated for additional supportive intervention, the well-supported patient should also be periodically monitored for disruptions or gaps in support areas.

Availability of social supports is also dependent on the impact of disease. Greater restriction in access to supports is to be expected when disease or treatment cause significant physical impairment or disruption of daily routine.

Finally, availability of social supports may vary as a function of the individual's ability to utilize the resources offered. This statement is in part a corollary to the preceding one, as ability to utilize supports is related to disease limitations. For example, the housebound patient who is unable to travel to the homes of others or to entertain guests at home, loses access to a vital source of ongoing social intercourse. Bloom and Spiegel (1984) have shown that disease-related restrictions on social exchange have a negative impact on outlook on life as well as social functioning. However, a recipient's personality also affects capacity to elicit and utilize support.

Some research has shown that easygoing, self-confident, "hardy" individuals are best able to use social supports in times of crisis (Holahan and Moos, 1986). In contrast, there is evidence that people who externalize the source of health outcome, who take less responsibility for their illness and recovery, or use avoidance as a means of coping, may be less likely or able to mobilize social resources (Eckenrode, 1983; Billings and Moos, 1981). On the basis of their research, Sarason and co-workers maintain that social support should be viewed as an individual difference variable and reflects a stable personality trait (Sarason et al., 1986).

Emotions of the patient can also affect the utilization of the support network. Family members, friends, and staff alike may find that their genuine offers of support are rejected by a patient who may feel embarrassed, angered, or confused about accepting help. Reaction to illness often affects use of support. Work by Coyne (1978) has shown that depressed patients tend to alienate themselves from people close to them at the times they need their family's help the most.

The ability to utilize support may demand not only a willingness to call on one's support network, but also a flexibility to develop or use alternate means of obtaining specific types of support. Using the example cited earlier of the housebound patient, adaptive responses might include arranging to have friends come for short visits or bring their own food (or order out) if a meal is to be shared, or to visit by phone.

## QUALITY OF SUPPORT

A fourth issue in assessing social support is gauging the quality of support given. Two aspects are important to assessment here: whom you ask and when you ask. Although it is desirable to ask the patient directly about social resources, it is equally important to ask the primary providers about how things are going as well. This is especially true if the patient is critical of the support received. The relationship between poor mental health and lack of perceived support is well documented. Without assessing supportgivers separately, it would not be possible in cases of social support failure to determine if the structures and/or individuals required to fill the patients' needs were lacking or the patient was simply unable or unwilling to utilize them. Discrepancies between provider–recipient responses can also help highlight sources of distress. For example, the wife of the patient who claims that she is abandoning him may tell the interviewer that she has terminated her visits specifically at his request, stating that he asks repeatedly that she not visit so often because he worries about her traveling so far. Hearing both sides of the problem alerts the interviewer to possible communication difficulties with this couple.

The quality of social support available may also vary

over time. Over the course of illness there will be peak demand periods for additional social support or for specific types of support. There will likely also be times when the system is overextended and/or the patient is more needy or less effective at utilizing available resources. Just as the patient's needs and demands may vary over time, so also do those of his or her support network. It may be that onset of illness or an illness-related crisis occurs at a time when the patients' usual source of support is already under pressure to assume additional responsibilities. The wife who is having trouble managing two teenage children at home may find it more difficult to find time to prepare all the special foods for or to spend the extra time chatting with her hospitalized husband, activities that both used to enjoy in an earlier period. Other situations that point up the importance of monitoring periodically levels of social support include an abrupt change in the patient's emotional or physical status (e.g., depression, relapse, and acute treatment-related side effects), or a transition in treatment (e.g., termination of therapy, admission for bone marrow transplant) or in treatment staff (e.g., change in or absence of primary physician or nurse).

## PERCEIVED NEED FOR SUPPORT

The last issue in the evaluation of social support is the determination of the patient's perceived need for intervention. When it becomes apparent to the interviewer that there are specific deficits in a patient's support system, the final aspect of assessment is first to find out from the patient whether these are recognized, and second, if their absence is viewed by the patient as stressful. In her research, Dunkel-Schetter (1984) found that 95% of interviewed cancer patients reported receiving as much love, advice, approval, assistance, information, and understanding from the important people in their lives as needed. Attempts to institute support interventions for patients who do not perceive or who deny their isolation is distressing and is doomed to failure. For example, the schizoid person will experience attempts at close social interaction as an additional stress. Similarly, the young adult who acknowledges that his or her family does not visit often may also state with further questioning that the patient has asked the family to limit their visits in an effort to gain a sense of autonomy and independence. Attempts on the part of staff to reverse such a situation, undertaken without an appreciation for the patient's reasons for limiting visits, may be met by the patient with anger and a sense of defeat. In cases in which patients acknowledge a deficit in their support system yet claim that it is of little consequence, the nature of the reasons must be carefully explored by the clinician. At times, a patient may see a need yet be unable or unwilling to ask for more support for fear of being a burden, an issue discussed in greater detail under special problems later.

## SOCIAL SUPPORT IN CANCER

Considerable research exists to substantiate the observation that the interpersonal environment of the person with cancer is of paramount importance in adaptation (Bloom, 1982a, 1982b; Dunkel-Schetter, 1984; Dunkel-Schetter and Wortman, 1982; Lindsey et al., 1981; Peteet, 1982; Peters-Golden, 1982; Wortman and Dunkel-Schetter, 1979). The next of kin or closest person to the patient is frequently cited as a critical figure in adjustment. Serious illness of any kind makes the ill person need increased closeness to other important people to counteract the feelings of insecurity and vulnerability (Leiber et al., 1976; Weisman and Worden, 1976–1977; Bloom, 1982b; Thomas and Weiner, 1974). If anything, this need for support, love, and affiliation increases over time, reflecting in part the patient's reactions to the effects of the disease and treatment and—a principal concern for many patients—the fear that they will no longer be loved or cared for. There are, however, special considerations to issues of social support in the cancer patient that need to be addressed briefly.

The diagnosis of cancer elicits adaptational demands that, though perhaps not unique to cancer patients, may make the cancer patient especially dependent on social supports. Fears of abandonment and rejection, experienced by other critically ill patients, may be keenly felt by the cancer patient in the context of gaps in communication with both families (Dunkel-Schetter and Wortman, 1982) and the public (*National Survey on Breast Cancer,* 1980), regarding the causes and cure of cancer (see also Chapter 1). At the same time, during illness people tend to feel less in control, less powerful, more inferior, especially when they cannot help themselves and must rely on others. It has been found that in these circumstances social support can actually decrease self-esteem, because it emphasizes the recipient's vulnerability. Indeed, the whole area of the recipient's reactions to aid is of growing interest (Fisher et al., 1982; Coates et al., 1983; Rook, 1984).

Misunderstanding by members of a support network about the illness or the patient's needs seem to be more common among cancer patients than other populations of patients. One of the questions friends and family most frequently ask staff members is "how" they should offer help. Because of either their own fears and/or what are perceived to be explicit or implied messages given by the patient, friends and family are also more likely to adopt an overly optimistic de-

meanor in dealing with the cancer patient, a stance that often makes the patient feel isolated and resentful. In one study, 66% of healthy individuals surveyed said they would "go out of their way" to cheer up a patient with cancer (Peters-Golden, 1982). This same report also indicated that 60% of the cancer patients sampled stated that they felt separated by what they considered "unrelenting optimism that seemed unauthentic." Work among parents of children with cancer reveals they too feel the victims of unwanted, or misdirected sympathy (S.B. Friedman et al., 1963).

Finally, the manner in which support is assessed in the cancer patient may need to be modified if accuracy is to be achieved. With respect to help offered by the social support system, most studies indicate that the "perceived" level of social support is a sufficient indicator of a patient's status with respect to this health dimension (Lieberman, 1982; Wethington and Kessler, 1986); however, as Wortman notes (1984, p. 2348), for cancer patients the *actual* support may be more critical to well-being. Because patients' support needs are frequently intense, concrete evidence of help offered and received is probably a more accurate means of assessing social support in cancer. This may be particularly the case for patients who have access to a large number of supports but who may be reluctant to ask for specific assistance. Guilt about being a burden, though not unique to this group of patients, is a common issue in cancer.

Table 5-3 summarizes a number of studies of cancer patients that incorporated as the basis or as part of the study design the evaluation of the impact of social support on outcome or adaptation (for reviews, see also Lindsey et al., 1981; DiMatteo and Hayes, 1981). Although there are specific aspects of support that proved more helpful than others, the overall finding is that the degree of social support is positively associated with both better adjustment and longer survival.

In addition to the correlational evidence of a positive link between social support and adaptation in cancer, there is a small but growing body of research providing empirical validation of these findings. In a study by Bloom and co-workers (1978), 21 women who had had mastectomies were provided with a comprehensive supportive intervention consisting of information, opportunities for expression of feelings, and support from a team of medical and mental health professionals. Women who received this intervention had higher self-esteem and self-efficacy scores 2 months after the mastectomy than a comparison group of 18 women who did not receive the treatment. In a similar study by Maguire and colleagues (1983), 152 women were randomly assigned to receive either supportive counseling by a specially trained nurse clinician following mastectomy ($n = 75$) or standard care ($n = 77$).

**Table 5-3** Selected studies examining the relationship of social support to adjustment and survival in cancer

| Author(s) | Sample | Method/type support assessed | Outcome |
|---|---|---|---|
| *Impact on Adjustment* | | | |
| Jamison et al. (1978) | 41 Mastectomy patients | Self-report questionnaire items examined aspects of mastectomy procedure, perceptions of effects of surgery on relationships with spouses, and attitudes toward health care staff. | Women who reported better emotional adjustment also perceived their spouses, children, physicians, and nurses as more supportive than those with lower self-reported adjustment. |
| Morrow et al. (1981) | 107 Parents of pediatric cancer patients | Subjects rated 11 sources of potential psychosocial support on "how helpful and supportive each source has been to you during your illness" (1 = very, to 5 = not at all); psychosocial adjustment rated using the Psychosocial Adjustment to Illness Scale (PAIS). | Perceived support from spouse, relatives, friends, and primary physician, and average amount of support correlated significantly with overall adjustment to child's illness. Psychosocial adjustment of parents with a child in treatment correlated more frequently with perceived social support than that for those whose child was off therapy or had died. |
| Koocher and O'Malley (1981) | 15 Long-term survivors of pediatric cancers | Detailed patient and family interviews assessed changes in family interactions, social relations and supports. | Maintenance of social contacts at time of diagnosis and good communication (information) within family was associated with better long-term adjustment. |
| Bloom (1982a) | 130 Mastectomy patients | Employed four measures of social support: (1) perception of family cohesiveness; (2) perception of social contact; (3) perception of leisure activity; (4) social identity feedback (having a confidant). | Perception of family cohesiveness and amount of social contact directly influence coping and indirectly affect adjustment as reflected in improved self-concept, increased sense of power, and diminished psychological distress. |
| Funch and Mettlin (1982) | 151 Breast cancer patients (3–12 months after surgery) | Assessed extent of three forms of social, support: social, professional, financial. | Social and professional support were positively related to psychological adjustment. Financial support was positively related to physical recovery. |
| Taylor et al. (1983) | 78 Breast cancer patients | Included multiple interview and questionnaire variables such as marital adjustment, family support, social involvement. | Satisfaction with her relationship with and ability to share concerns with a significant other, perceived support from family members, perceived support from friends, and close and highly interactive family status all were associated with good adjustment. Overall social support was a strong predictor of adjustment, as hypothesized. |
| *Relation to Disease Status* | | | |
| Peters-Golden (1982) | 100 Breast cancer patients | Conducted interviews of 30–40 minutes covering perceived social support and attitudes. | Patients reporting good support also expressed less difficulty in adjusting to their illness. Patients with recurrent disease reported less satisfaction with support, and those undergoing chemotherapy experienced the least adequate levels of support. |

**Table 5-3** (*Continued*)

| Author(s) | Sample | Method/type support assessed | Outcome |
|---|---|---|---|
| Dunkel-Schetter (1984) | 59 Breast and 20 colorectal patients (7–20 months postdiagnosis) | Multidimensional analysis was used to generate three measures of support: (1) quantity of support, (2) satisfaction with support from spouse or significant other, (3) interviewer-rated strength of support. | Support was significantly associated with adjustment, but outcome differed by prognosis: more support in good-prognosis group was associated with more positive affect and higher self-esteem but not in poor-prognosis group. Also, patients with poor physical condition were rated as having stronger social support (perhaps because it was needed). Patients with more advanced disease experienced more problems in social relationships and support. |
| *Impact on Survival* | | | |
| Weisman and Worden (1975) | 35 Patients, multiple sites | Cases were reviewed postmortem, and assessment was based on open-ended interviews, social service contacts, nursing reports, and psychological testing documented in the premorbid period. | Longer survival was associated with presence of good relationships with others and tendency to maintain cooperative and mutually responsive relationships until the very last. |
| Funch and Marshall (1983) | 208 Women treated for breast cancer (20-year follow-up) | Social involvement was assessed as the sum of standardized scores on self-report variables measuring (1) total number of acquaintances and relatives, (2) number of religious and nonreligious meetings attended, and (3) marital status as measured around the time of diagnosis and treatment. | For women younger than 46, those with the least social involvement had the poorest average survival length; for older groups, social support appeared to have no impact on survival. |

In addition to reviewing proper physical care, arm mobility exercises, and information about how to obtain a well-fitting prosthesis, the nurse encouraged the woman to view the scar and discuss her feelings about the surgery. She also emphasized the need for the woman to be open with her spouse about her response to having breast cancer and supported the woman's efforts to return as quickly as possible to work and prior social activities. After 12 to 18 months, those helped by the nurse showed greater social recovery, return to work, adaptation to breast loss, and satisfaction with their breast prostheses than women in the standard care group.

The majority of published intervention studies have been conducted among breast cancer populations. However, work carried out by Gordon and co-workers (1980) indicates that such psychological and social support programs benefit most cancer patients. Also using a team model, Gordon and his colleagues investigated the efficacy of providing three types of support interventions: educational (informational), counseling (emotional and affiliational appraisal), and environmental (instrumental) to 157 breast, lung, and melanoma patients. Both immediate (at discharge) and long-term (6 months postdischarge) effects were associated with intervention, as evidenced by more rapid decline in anxiety and hostility, a more realistic outlook on life, and an activity pattern suggestive of more active time usage in intervention versus control ($n = 151$) patients.

As noted at the beginning of this chapter, it is unclear *how* social support works. A number of possible mechanisms of action are outlined in Table 5-4. Although its influence is frequently manifest as an indi-

**Table 5-4**  Ways in which social support may buffer the deleterious effects of stress

Social resources can decrease the likelihood of the occurrence of stressful events.

If the event occurs, interaction with significant others can modify or alter the individual's perception of the particular event and hence mitigate the stress potential

Stress levels are partially contingent on the degree to which a potentially stressful event alters role functioning. Social resources can alter the relationship between role strain and the stress-inducing event.

Social resources can influence coping strategies and in this way modify the linkage between stress event and effect.

To the degree that stressful events erode self-esteem and feelings of personal mastery, social resources can modify such effects.

There may be a direct influence of social resources on adaptation level.

*Source*: From M.A. Lieberman (1982). The effects of social supports on responses to stress. In L. Goldberger and S. Breznitz (eds.), *Handbook of Stress*. New York: The Free Press, p. 778.

rect or buffering effect on well-being (Cohen and Wills, 1985; Dean and Lin, 1977), social support may also have a direct impact. A review by Levy (1983) provides provocative evidence that compliance with medical treatment may be closely tied to degree of social support. Thoits (1986) has conceptualized social support as coping assistance and used this model to develop new support strategies to promote adaptation. It is probable that the impact of social support exerts its influence in all the ways listed in Table 5-4, with different mechanisms being more or less important at different times. For example, during diagnosis and the early treatment period, social supports may provide important reassurance that the person is still needed, loved, and esteemed, thus buffering the impact of illness on sense of self. Later in the course of therapy, provision of social resources (e.g., financial aid and role assistance) may be more salient in enhancing a sense of well-being and may facilitate adaptation by minimizing environmental stressors.

## SPECIAL PROBLEMS IN EVALUATING AND MANAGING SOCIAL SUPPORT

For the health professional managing a cancer patient's care, some additional issues enter into both evaluation of the need for and effective management of social support interventions. Though already noted as an influence on the quality of social support, the question of whom you ask has important clinical implications. Reliance solely on patient report of actual or perceived levels of social support puts the evaluator at risk of (most commonly) *over*estimating availability of interpersonal resources. Although there is evidence that

psychiatric impairment is strongly correlated with expressed lack of social support, there is no clear association between dysphoric responses in the cancer patient and perceived failure in the support system. Cancer patients may feel more commonly that they are failing the support system, in particular spouse or family, rather than the expected opposite.

Another broad area of problems may be in the content of the supportive interactions provided, or more specifically, *how* the support is provided. Antonucci (1984) defines a supportive transaction as one that encompasses the intent of a person to be supportive, behavior that expresses that intent, and an effect such that the other person feels supported. However, in any social relationship there are both positive and negative elements, and when the patient is asked about how things are going vis-à-vis a specific social interaction (e.g., marriage and patient–doctor relationship) the response generally represents a summary of the good and bad areas of that relationship. Fiori and co-workers (1983), as well as Rook (1984), found that unpleasant social relationships—those characterized by tension, discord, and negative affect—are associated with greater psychiatric morbidity. As Wortman (1984, p. 2346) emphasized, the diagnosis of cancer is unique in its ability to elicit negative feelings in others. The cancer patient is particularly vulnerable to feelings of being misunderstood, avoided, and feared. Going back to an illustration provided earlier, the loving spouse who presents a cheerful, optimistic attitude may not realize that such a stance could have a negative impact on the patient. Research by Dunkel-Schetter and Wortman (1982) suggested that family members, friends, and staff frequently exhibit negative as well as positive behaviors as a reflection of conflicting feelings about cancer. They noted that these individuals may outwardly voice reassurance but manifest negative nonverbal behaviors as well as inconsistencies in behavior over time. The dependent position of the patient and the stresses of illness make it hard to change negative relationships. Patients may feel that they cannot help themselves and often have little energy to terminate an unpleasant interaction or develop new, more supportive ones. It is not safe to assume that the support provided will always be valued by the recipient. When supportive interventions are deemed by the patient to be unhelpful or result in negative consequences, the clinician may need to reexamine how the support is being delivered. This brings us to the last point, which deals with problems in giving and receiving support (see Table 5-5).

Failure of a social network to provide adequate social support may be a result of a mismatch between patient needs and the type of support given, its source, and/or the timing of supportive efforts; that is, the

**Table 5-5** Problem sources in obtaining and maintaining adequate social support in illness

| Types of issues | Problem areas |
|---|---|
| Provider | Availability |
| |   Physical |
| |   Emotional |
| | Awareness of need |
| | Appropriateness (goodness of provider–task match) |
| | Ability to initiate supportive efforts |
| |   Knowledge of what is helpful |
| |   Skills and experience |
| |   Flexibility |
| | Adequacy of backup (relief or alternate supportgivers) |
| Receiver | Prior support network status |
| | Ability to ask for help |
| | Current physical and emotional state (limitations on ability to accept help; change in support needs) |
| | Perceived need for support |

wrong person may offer inappropriate help at the worst possible time. On a more fundamental level, problems in providing support can also arise from the inability of the providers to offer the support needed either because of personal limitations, fears, and concerns, or out of a lack of understanding of the "how to" of helping. Silver and Wortman (1980) have noted that, although we are all essentially able to approach a sick or needy person, our response is to avoid them. In interviews with 100 healthy men and women, Peters-Golden (1982) found that 61% "said they would avoid a person with cancer (56%), or might (5%) avoid contact with someone they knew who had cancer" (p. 484). Of the respondents, 94% said they would feel sorry for anyone with cancer. Of the patients with cancer, 52% in her study felt they *were* avoided or feared.

Intellectual as well as motivational reasons may lead members of a social network to avoid, blame, and reject the family member, friend, or patient with cancer. (See also Chapters 1 and 2, and Peters-Golden, 1982, for a discussion of the derivation of social roles and social stigma surrounding cancer.) People feel vulnerable themselves to becoming ill and therefore feel uncomfortable around the sick person. This point is well illustrated in the research by Lichtman and colleagues among the daughters of mothers with breast cancer (Lichtman et al., 1984). To be effective, support providers need, at times, to be sensitive to the negative ramifications of the diagnosis or impact of cancer in a loved one, friend, or patient has on them. Toward this end, it is important that support providers be encouraged to take care of themselves; this includes being able to air grievances and concerns, and to mobilize extra resources for the patient and themselves

when appropriate. Support groups for spouses, family, and staff provide important forums for dealing with these issues (see Taylor et al., 1986, as well as Chapters 38 and 51 in this volume). Discussion of problems in fulfilling social support roles is helpful in identifying sources of conflict, encouraging continued support of the patient, and, when necessary, "permitting" a support source to limit his or her care to those areas in which he or she can be most comfortable and effective.

## CASE REPORTS

A 36-year-old man hospitalized for treatment of a lymphosarcoma made repeated requests of various staff members for information about his treatment and when he would be going home, and received various responses. Formerly cheerful and cooperative, he was observed by the staff to be becoming more irritable and withdrawn. At a staff meeting it was decided that the attending physician be designated as the sole information source concerning this patient's medical status; nursing and house staff would provide only emotional and physical care. The patient was also encouraged to ask his doctor about specific treatment-related questions. The patient reported feeling much less confused, angry, and frustrated after this system was instituted, and his mood improved.

A young single mother whose 4-year-old son was placed in a special isolation unit preparatory to undergoing bone marrow transplant for leukemia had practically "moved into" the transplant unit. She was constantly at her child's side, at times interfering with nursing care, and refused to take a break from her caretaking duties despite her apparent fatigue. The staff noticed that she was beginning to lose patience with her son, who in turn became more whining and tearful.

At a staff meeting it was proposed that a steady team of "substitutes" be arranged to stay with the child for a period each day and every third or fourth evening in order to enable the mother to have some time to herself. This was discussed with the mother and, after initial reluctance, agreed upon.

At the end of 2 weeks on this system, the mother looked rested and more relaxed. She acknowledged how hard it had been for her to leave her only child and how grateful she was to get some relief, knowing he was well cared for. Her son's behavior improved dramatically as the mother's mood, energy, and spirits lifted.

A common problem for members of the extended social network (e.g., relatives outside the immediate family, friends, and associates) is knowing "how to" provide support. There are always fears one will make the patient feel worse, embarrassed, or offended. These concerns are heightened by media reports indicating that emotional support can backfire (Goleman, 1985). Jimmie Holland, Memorial Sloan-Kettering Cancer Center social workers, chaplains, and patient representatives outline several useful guidelines for those visiting patients in the hospital (see Table 5-6). In many cases these points are also applicable to visits made with patients recuperating at home. In this context it is

**Table 5-6** Guidelines for structuring patient visits

- Ask before going. Surprise visits are not always welcome. Calling ahead gives the patient a chance to look and feel his or her best and to schedule visits so they won't interfere with medical care or result in a "crowd" of well-wishers.
- When arriving, knock and wait for a greeting before entering.
- When you see the patient, do not be alarmed if he or she is surrounded by equipment, tubes, and bottles. These are *not* necessarily indicative of the patient's condition.
- Greet the patient as you normally would (e.g., shake hands, or give the person a kiss).
- Find a chair and sit down near the patient. Proximity and eye contact help make the patient feel comfortable. Do *not*, however, hover.
- Do not compare the patient's present condition to previous states of health. Instead of asking "how are you?" ask "How are you feeling today?" or "How is your day going?" Inquire about their experience in the hospital. "How is the food?" or "How is the service?"
- Let the patient take the lead in conversation. Be a good listener, and don't be unnerved by lulls in the conversation. You need not feel you have to say something. If the patient confides in you, listen and communicate openly.
- Remember that patients do not want to think about their illness all the time. It is human to want to laugh and ignore the most serious realities for brief periods. Sports, politics, fashion, music, or news about mutual friends are often good topics offering the opportunity for mutual exchange.
- Focus the visit on the patient. Ask: "What can I get you?" or "How can I help?"
- If the patient can walk or sit in a wheelchair, suggest a trip around the floor, to a lounge, a gift shop, or a recreation area.
- Give the patient realistic support and reassurance. For help in talking about concerns, you can urge the patient to utilize the hospital social workers, support services, or the chaplains.
- Visits need not take up long blocks of time. Indeed, it may help if you plan some breaks. Go get something to eat or drink, make a phone call, check the parking meter, or run an errand for the patient.
- Knowing when to leave is important. For some patients 10 minutes is a long time, for others an hour is too short. Simply say, "I think I've been here long enough." If the patient replies, "No" or "please stay," you can stay a while longer. If the patient agrees with you, it is certainly time to leave.

*Source*: Modified from J.E. Mullane (1981). Visiting a friend with cancer. *Cancer Center (Memorial Sloan-Kettering Cancer Center)* 3(3):17.

important to note a common misconception highlighted by Wortman and Dunkel-Schetter (1979). In their research, they found that others believe that those patients who make few or no references to their disease are the "healthiest." As Holland notes, "it is important to neither ignore nor overemphasize the patient's disease." Since improved survival time is possible with many types of cancer, social interactions often return to, if not their pre-illness status, at least a "normal" level, with both patient and friends usually welcoming the new, less stressed interchange.

Having addressed issues of giving support, we turn now to a final area of problems, those concerned with receiving adequate support. Problems receiving support may be seen as consequent to lack of availability of support, changing patterns of communication and coping, and discrepancies in perceived need for support. Lack of availability of support can be due to emotional or physical reasons. The emotional reasons and their remedy were covered earlier and arise principally from fear of illness or misunderstanding of the appropriate response. In some cases, however, a patient may be physically cut off from social resources because of hospitalization (distance from home), degree of illness, or previous social isolation. This problem is more common in the older patient or the patient with a psychiatric history. In these instances it is important to create new or revitalize old social networks through family, social, or community resources. Availability of social support is also mediated by life stage. The relationship between social support and life course is a relatively new area of study (for reviews see Schulz and Rau, 1985; Kahn and Antonucci, 1980; Lieberman, 1982). Although aspects of the relationship of support at given life intervals affect both provider and receiver, it is mentioned here as an issue in obtaining adequate support. First, there may be periods in the individual's life when support is naturally more readily available (e.g., school years) or less available (e.g., in late retirement years). Second, the timing and nature of illness may evoke different support responses at different life stages. Schulz and Rau (1985) have put forth a model for viewing life course events in the context of their temporal and statistical normality. For example, marriage in one's twenties and thirties is both statistically and temporally normative; however, becoming widowed at a young age is statistically normative but not temporally normative. Illness in old age is normal—almost *too well* accepted! Schulz and Rau make a strong case for evaluating the support available to persons on the basis of how an event is so categorized. In such a model, pediatric cancer is both statistically and temporally nonnormative, and may be viewed as eliciting less support because fewer people have experienced it and it evokes more feelings of vulnerability and helplessness in caregivers. (For a thoughtful review of issues related to providing support during pediatric illness see Chesler and Barbarin, 1984.) Even if a social support structure is present and active, the patient may feel unsupported because he or she is unable to ask for additional or different kinds of help as his or her needs change. The individual may be concerned about what others will think of him or her if demands are made for more or even less involvement. There may be cultural taboos or stigma associated with asking for help. Issues of disclosure can also be a concern. Patients having sexual problems following abdominal surgery may feel too embarrassed to seek information from their physician. Others may drop out of social activities because they are afraid that their friends will "treat them differently" if their friends find out that they had cancer. Periodic monitoring of patients over the course of illness and follow-up is important to detect difficulties in social functioning and support.

Finally, a support network may be present and active but the patient may feel the attention is inappropriate or unwanted. As noted earlier, the oversolicitous family member or friend may make the patient feel dependent and helpless. Members of a support system need to recognize signals about what is not as well as what is helpful, and to recognize that needs change over time. In addition, patients may need help accepting certain types of support (e.g., emotional and financial) without feeling guilty, losing self-esteem, or becoming passive. At times it is important for the provider to persevere even when a recipient is reluctant to accept the support given. For example, patients may want the staff to tell them only good news about their illness despite potential maladaptive consequences. In this difficult situation, although even gently given "honest feedback" may be seen as unhelpful, it may be critical to optimal recovery in the long run (Visotsky et al., 1961).

## SUMMARY

A consistent finding in research among cancer patients is that illness is frequently associated with considerable difficulty in interpersonal relationships. A second finding, which can be viewed perhaps as a corollary to the first, is that one of the most important "buffers" against the harmful effects of the stress of illness is the presence or availability of persons in the patient's environment with whom the experience can be shared. This role is usually filled by a member (or members) of the nuclear family (spouse, child, or parent), but may be an extended family member or friend(s). Research indicates that the presence of positive social support not only diminishes the psychic distress of cancer, but may be also important in modulating survival as well. Conversely, absence of social support, or loss of a significant person who withdraws during the patient's illness, becomes an additional stressor that may be more painful than the illness itself.

In order to maximize the beneficial impact of social support, attention must be paid not only to those features constituting support (i.e., type, source, availability, quality, and perceived use for), but also to those characteristics of the provider as well as recipient that influence the adequacy of support both given and re-

ceived. There is no question that early identification of and intervention with patients with few social supports and extensive needs, or with those who perceive their social supports to be inadequate, is important in comprehensive care. As a general form of intervention, modification of the patient's social support system is appealing because it is generally not time-consuming, is inexpensive, and has few negative consequences. In the future, a major task for researchers and clinicians will be to refine our knowledge about "how, when and for whom supportive social relationships are beneficial" (House, 1981), particularly in adapting to the special stresses of cancer.

## REFERENCES

Abbey, A., D. Abramis, and R. Caplan (1981). *Measuring Social Support: The Effects of Frame of Reference on the Relationship between Social Support and Strain*. Paper presented at the American Psychological Association conference, Los Angeles, 1981.

Antonucci, T. (1984). Personal characteristics, social support and social behavior. In E. Shanas and B.H. Binstock (eds.), *Handbook of Aging and the Social Sciences*, 2nd ed. New York: Van Nostrand Reinhold, pp. 94–128.

Berkman, L.F. and S.L. Syme (1979). Social networks, host resistance, and mortality: A nine-year follow-up study of Alameda County residents. *Am. J. Epidemiol.* 109:186–204.

Billings, A.G. and R.H. Moos (1981). The role of coping resources in attenuating the stress of life events. *J. Behav. Med.* 4:139–57.

Bloom, J. (1981). Cancer-care providers and the medical care system: Facilitators or inhibitors of patient coping responses. In P. Ahmed (ed.), *Coping with Medical Issues.* Vol. 3, *Living and Dying with Cancer.* New York: Elsevier, pp. 253–72.

Bloom, J.R. (1982a). Social support, accommodation to stress and adjustment to breast cancer. *Soc. Sci. Med.* 16:1329–38.

Bloom, J.R. (1982b). Social support systems and cancer: A conceptual view. In J. Cohen, J.W. Cullen, and L.R. Martin (eds.), *Psychosocial Aspects of Cancer.* New York: Raven Press, pp. 129–49.

Bloom, J.R. and D. Spiegel (1984). The relationship of two dimensions of social support to the psychosocial well-being and social functioning of women with advanced breast cancer. *Soc. Sci. Med.* 19:831–37.

Bloom, J.R., R. Ross, and G.M. Burnell (1978). The effect of social support on patient adjustment after breast surgery. *Patient Counseling Health Educ.* 1:50–59.

Bozeman, M.F., C.E. Orbach, and A.M. Sutherland (1955). Psychological impact of cancer and its treatment: The adaptation of mothers to the threatened loss of their children through leukemia. *Cancer* 8:1–33.

Broadhead, W.E., B.H. Kaplan, S.A. James, E.H. Wagner, V.J. Schoenbach, R. Grimson, S. Heyden, G. Tiblin, and S.H. Gehlbach (1983). The epidemiologic evidence for a relationship between social support and health. *Am. J. Epidemiol.* 117:521–37.

Caplan, G. (1974). *Social Support Systems and Community Mental Health.* New York: Behavioral Publications.

Chesler, M.A. and O.A. Barbarin (1984). Difficulties of providing help in a crisis: Relationships between parents of children with cancer and their friends. *J. Soc. Issues* 40:113–34.

Coates, D., G.J. Renzaglia, and M.C. Embree (1983). When helping backfires: Help and helplessness. In J.D. Fisher and A. Nadler (eds.), *New Directions in Helping. Vol. 1, Recipient Reactions to Aid.* New York: Academic Press, pp. 251–79.

Cobb, S. (1976). Social support as a moderator of life stress. *Psychosom. Med.* 38:300–314.

Cohen, S. and G. McKay (1984). Social support, stress and the buffering hypothesis: A theoretical analysis. In A. Baum, J.E. Singer, and S.E. Taylor (eds.), *Handbook of Psychology and Health,* Vol. 4. Hillsdale, N.J.: Erlbaum, pp.253–67.

Cohen, S. and S.L. Syme (eds.). (1985). *Social Support and Health.* New York: Academic Press.

Cohen, S. and T.A. Wills (1985). Stress, social support, and the buffering hypothesis. *Psychol. Bull.* 98:310–57.

Coyne, J.C. (1978). Depression and responses of others. *J. Abnorm. Psychol.* 85:186–93.

Dean, A. and N. Lin (1977). The stress buffering role of social support. *J. Nerv. Ment. Dis.* 165:403–17.

DiMatteo, M.R. and R. Hayes, (1981). Social support and serious illness. In B.H. Gottlieb (ed.), *Social Networks and Social Support.* London: Sage Publications, pp. 117–48.

Dunkel-Schetter, C. (1984). Social support and cancer: Findings based on patient interviews and their implications. *J. Soc. Issues* 40:77–98.

Dunkel-Schetter, C. and C. Wortman (1982). The interpersonal dynamics of cancer: Problems in social relationships and their impact on the patient. In H.S. Friedman and M.R. DiMatteo (eds.), *Interpersonal Issues in Health Care.* New York: Academic Press, pp. 69–100.

Eckenrode, J. (1983). The mobilization of social supports: Some individual constraints. *Am. J. Community Psychol.* 2:509–28.

Fiori, J., J. Becker, and B. Coppel (1983). Social network interactions: A buffer or a stress? *Am. J. Community Psychol.* 11:423–39.

Fischer, C.S. (1982). *To Dwell among Friends: Personal Networks in Town and City.* Chicago: University of Chicago Press.

Fisher, J.D., A. Nadler, and S. Whitcher-Alagna (1982). Recipient reactions to aid. *Psychol. Bull.* 91:27–54.

Friedman, H.S. and M.R. DiMatteo (eds.). (1982). *Interpersonal Issues in Health Care.* New York: Academic Press.

Friedman, S.B., P. Chodoff, J.W. Mason, and D.A. Hamburg (1963). Behavioral observations on parents anticipating the death of a child. *Pediatrics* 32:610–25.

Funch, D.P. and J. Marshall (1983). The role of stress, social support and age in survival from breast cancer. *J. Psychosom. Res.* 27:77–83.

Funch, D.P., and C. Mettlin (1982). The role of support in relation to recovery from breast surgery. *Soc. Sci. Med.* 16:91–98.

Goleman, D. (1985). Emotional support has its destructive side. *The New York Times,* August 27, pp. C1, C3.

Gordon, W., I. Friedenbergs, L. Diller, M. Hibbard, C. Wolf, L. Levine, R. Lipkins, O. Ezrachi, and D. Lucido (1980). Efficacy of psychosocial interventions with cancer patients. *J. Consult. Clin. Psychol.* 48:743–59.

Gottlieb, B.H. (eds.). (1981). *Social Networks and Social Support.* Beverly Hills, Calif.: Sage Publications.

Greenblatt, M., R.M. Becerra, and E.A. Serafetinides (1982). Social networks and mental health: An overview. *Am. J. Psychiatry* 139:977–84.

Hirsch, B. (1981). Social networks and the coping process: Creating personal communities. In B. Gottlieb (ed.), *Social Networks and Social Support.* Beverly Hills, Calif.: Sage Publications, pp. 149–70.

Holahan, C. and R. Moos (1986). Personality, coping and family resources in stress resistance: A longitudinal analysis. *J. Pers. Soc. Psychol.* 51:381–95.

House, J.S. (1981). *Work Stress and Social Support.* Reading, Mass.: Addison-Wesley.

House, J.S. and R. Kahn (1985). Measures and concepts of social support. In S. Cohen and L. Syme (eds.), *Social Support and Health.* New York: Academic Press, pp. 83–108.

Jamison, K.R., D.K. Wellisch, and R.O. Pasnau (1978). Psychosocial aspects of mastectomy: I. The woman's perspective. *Am. J. Psychiatry* 135:432–36.

Jemott, J.B. III and S.E. Locke (1984). Psychosocial factors, immunologic mediation, and human susceptibility to infectious diseases: How much do we know. *Psychol. Bull.* 95:78–108.

Kahn, R.L. and T. Antonucci (1980). Convoys over the life course: Attachment, roles, and social support. In P.B. Baltes and O.G. Brim, Jr. (eds.), *Life-span Development and Behavior,* Vol. 3. New York: Academic Press, pp. 253–86.

Kaplan, B.H. and J.C. Cassel (eds.). (1975). *Family and Health: An Epidemiological Approach.* Chapel Hill: University of North Carolina Press.

Kaplan, B.H., J.C. Cassel, and S. Gore (1977). Social support and health. *Med. Care* 15:47–58.

Koocher, G. and J. O'Malley (1981). *The Damocles Syndrome: Psychological Consequences of Surviving Childhood Cancer.* New York: McGraw-Hill.

Lehman, D.R., J.H. Ellard, and C.B. Wortman (1986). Social support for the bereaved: Recipients' and providers' perspectives on what is helpful. *J. Consult. Clin. Psychol.* 54:438–46.

Leiber, L., M. Plumb, M.L. Gerstenzang, and J. Holland (1976). The communication of affection between cancer patients and their spouses. *Psychosom. Med.* 38:379–89.

Levy, R.L. (1983). Social support and compliance: A selective review and critique of treatment integrity and outcome measurement. *Soc. Sci. Med.* 17:1329–38.

Lichtman, R.R., S.E. Taylor, J.V. Wood, A.Z. Bluming, G.M. Dosik, and R.L. Leibowitz (1984). Relations with children after breast cancer: The mother–daughter relationship at risk. *J. Psychosoc. Oncol.* 2:1–19.

Lieberman, M.A. (1982). The effects of social supports on responses to stress. In L. Goldberger and S. Breznitz (eds.), *Handbook of Stress*. New York: The Free Press, pp. 764–83.

Lin, N.R., S. Simeone, W.M. Ensel, and W. Kwo (1979). Social support, stressful life events, and illness: A model and an empirical test. *J. Health Soc. Behav.* 20:108–19.

Lindsey, A.M., J.S. Norbeck, V.L. Carrieri, and E. Perry (1981). Social support and health outcomes in postmastectomy women: A review. *Cancer Nurs.* 4(5):377–84.

Maguire, P., M. Brooke, C. Thomas, and R. Sellwood (1983). The effect of counselling on physical disability and social recovery after mastectomy. *Clin. Oncol.* 9:319–24.

McCallister, L. and C.S. Fischer (1978). A procedure for surveying personal networks. *Sociol. Methods Res.* 7:131–48.

Mitchell, R.E., A.G. Billings, and R.H. Moos (1982). Social support and well-being: Implications for prevention programs. *J. Primary Prevention* 3:77–98.

Morrow, G.R., A. Hoagland, and C.L.M. Carnrike, Jr. (1981). Social support and parental adjustment to pediatric cancer. *J. Consult. Clin. Psychol.* 49:763–65.

Murawski, B.J., D. Penman, and M. Schmitt, (1978). Social support in health and illness: The concept and its measurement. *Cancer Nurs.* 1(5):365–71.

*National Survey on Breast Cancer: A Measure of Progress in Public Understanding.* (1980). Washington, D.C.: National Cancer Institute, Department of Health and Human Services.

Peteet, J.R. (1982). A closer look at the concept of support: Some applications to the care of patients with cancer. *Gen. Hosp. Psychiatry* 4:19–23.

Peters-Golden, H. (1982). Breast cancer: Varied perceptions of social support in the illness experience. *Soc. Sci. Med.* 16:483–91.

Rook, K. (1948). The negative side of social interaction: Impact on psychological well-being. *J. Pers. Soc. Psychol.* 46:1097–1108.

Sarason, I.G. and B. Sarason (eds.). (1985). *Social Support: Theory, Research and Applications*. The Hague, The Netherlands: Martinus Nijhof.

Sarason, I.G., B.R. Sarason, and E.N. Shearin (1986). Social support as an individual difference variable: Its stability, origins, and relational aspects. *J. Pers. Soc. Psychol.* 50:845–55.

Schaefer, C., J.C. Coyne, and R.S. Lazarus (1981). The health-related functions of social support. *J. Behav. Med.* 4:381–406.

Schulz, R. and M.T. Rau (1985). Social support through the life course. In S. Cohen and S.L. Syme (eds.), *Social Support and Health*. New York: Academic Press, pp. 129–49.

Silver, R.L. and C.B. Wortman (1980). Coping with undesirable life events. In J. Garber and M.E. Seligman (eds.), *Human Helplessness*. New York: Academic Press, pp. 279–345.

Taylor, S.E., R.L., Falke, S.J. Shoptaw, and R.R. Lichtman (1986). Social support, support groups, and the cancer patient. *J. Consult. Clin. Psychol.* 54:608–15.

Taylor, S.E., R.R. Lichtman, and J.V. Wood (1983). *Adjustment to Breast Cancer: Physical, Sociodemographic, and Psychological Predictors*. Paper presented at the American Psychological Association meetings, Anaheim, Calif., August 1983.

Thoits, P.A. (1982). Conceptual, methodological, and theoretical problems in studying social support as a buffer against life stress. *J. Health Soc. Behav.* 23:145–59.

Thoits, P.A. (1986). Social support as coping assistance. *J. Consult. Clin. Psychol.* 54:416–23.

Thomas, J. and E.A. Weiner (1974). Psychological differences among groups of critically ill hospitalized patients, noncritically ill hospitalized patients, and well controls. *J. Clin. Psychol.* 42:274–79.

Visotsky, H.M., D.A. Hamburg, M.E. Gross, and B.Z. Lebovits (1961). Coping behavior under extreme stress. *Arch. Gen. Psychiatry* 5:423–48.

Wallston, B.S., S.W. Alagna, B.M. DeVellis, and R.F. DeVellis, (1983). Social support and physical health. *Health Psychol.* 2:367–91.

Weisman, A.D. and J.W. Worden (1975). Psychosocial analysis of cancer deaths. *Omega* 6:61–75.

Weisman, A.D. and J.W. Worden (1976–1977). The existential plight in cancer: Significance of the first 100 days. *Int. J. Psychiatry Med.* 7:1–15.

Weiss, R. (1974). The provisions of social relationships. In S. Rubin (ed.), *Doing unto Others*. Englewood Cliffs, N.J.: Prentice-Hall, pp. 17–26.

Wethington, E., and R.C. Kessler (1986). Perceived support, received support, and adjustment to stressful life events. *J. Health Soc. Behav.* 27:78–89.

Wortman, C.B. (1984). Social support, and the cancer patient. Conceptual and methodologic issues. *Cancer* 53:2339–60.

Wortman, C.B. and T.L. Conway (1985). The role of social support in adaptation and recovery from physical illness. In S. Cohen and S.L. Syme (eds.), *Social Support and Health*. New York: Academic Press, pp. 281–302.

Wortman, C.B. and C. Dunkel-Schetter (1979). Interpersonal relationships and cancer: A theoretical analysis. *J. Soc. Issues* 35:120–55.

Wortman, C.B. and D.R. Lehman (1985). Reactions to victims of life crisis: Support attempts that fail. In I.G. Sarason and B.R. Sarason (eds.), *Social Support: Theory, Research, and Application*. The Hague, The Netherlands: Martinus Nijhof. pp. 463–89.

# PART III

# Medical Factors and Adaptation

# 6

## Clinical Course of Cancer

Jimmie C. Holland

Parts I and II have reviewed two of the three major determinants of psychological adjustment to cancer: the sociocultural attitudes of society about cancer (Part I), and the patient-related intrapsychic and interpersonal contributions (Part II). Part III adds the third parameter: the medically related determinants of disease stages and clinical course (Chapters 6 and 7), the treatment variables (Chapters 8–12), and those problems related to specific sites of cancer (Chapters 13–21). Table 6-1 outlines these determinants and their primary characteristics.

The medical facts to which the patient must adjust include the diagnosis, prognosis, treatment, and the events that will likely follow in the clinical course. With cancer, this may be total cure, a long disease-free state followed by recurrence, a chronic illness state with rehabilitation to counter dysfunction, or illness leading to death. In a sense, the modulating determinants that have an impact on these medical situations are the patient's own psychological strength (predicted in part from prior behavior under stress), developmental level, and available social supports (family, friends, physician, and the health care team). Societal attitude modifies potential social support by influencing disclosure of the diagnosis and by affecting the responses of others to the individual with cancer (see Part I). The clinical course, site of tumor, treatment, and personal variables must all be considered in determining the psychological management.

A patient's quality of life and adaptation at a given point in illness represents the balance between the medical facts and the mitigating effects of psychological state and social supports. This balance is a delicate, dynamically changing one that can be tipped toward better or poorer quality of life by changes in the medi-

cal condition or alteration of psychological state or key supports. A schema graphically shows the interaction of these determinants (Fig. 6-1). Patients who are psychologically stable with a good support network and minimal illness have few serious psychological difficulties; consequently they cope well. Conversely, the person with poor psychological, personal, and social resources may have difficulties and need help, even if the disease severity is not great and the disability is minimal. Furthermore, in the presence of severe illness, even the individual with good psychological resources may naturally find it hard to cope and hence may need help. When an individual with poor resources develops a severe illness, the likelihood of significant psychological disturbance is very high and is likely to require psychosocial intervention. Such patients need to be identified early and provided with support to reduce the risk of psychological decompensation.

In all situations, the psychological management of the patient by the health care team is central to the quality of life of all patients at all stages of disease. Integration of good psychological care within the context of total care can make the difference in both the subjective experience of the patient and cooperation with treatment. Optimal comprehensive care recognizes that emotional distress is a part of the illness of cancer, and includes attention to this normal level of distress in every patient. Therefore, the basic level of psychosocial care (Table 6-2) addresses the normal emotional distress and is given as a part of the routine care in the hospital and the office. The physician has the key role, followed by the nurse, other specialists, and support staff in the particular treatment setting. In basic or level 1 care, the physician, on whose decisions

**Table 6-1**  Primary issues in psychological adjustment
to cancer

| Determinants | Characteristics |
|---|---|
| Sociocultural | Social attitudes about cancer and the stigma and meaning attached |
| Patient-related | Intrapersonal |
| |   Age-specific developmental life tasks that are threatened or disrupted by cancer |
| |   Personality, prior capability to cope with major life stresses |
| | Interpersonal |
| |   Nature and availability of social supports: family, friends, affiliated groups |
| Medical-related | Clinical facts |
| |   Stage and clinical course |
| |   Site of cancer |
| |   Nature of dysfunction and symptoms produced |
| | Treatment required |
| |   Surgery |
| |   Chemotherapy |
| |   Radiotherapy |
| |   Combined modalities |
| |   Protected environment with BMT |
| |   Immunotherapy |
| | Rehabilitative options |
| | Psychological management by the health care team |

*Source*: Holland and Rowland (1987).

and actions the patient feels survival depends, is the primary support. The physician with primary responsibility for a given patient should, as part of total care,

1. Provide adequate explanation and information about illness to the patient and relative (usually together).
2. Develop an alliance with the patient about the treatment plan.
3. Listen to concerns; support and reassure as appropriate.
4. Monitor for signs of psychological problems.
5. Refer the patient for psychiatric consultation when appropriate.
6. Be aware of resources for psychosocial support, their function and appropriateness for the individual patient (e.g., psychiatrist, social worker, clergy, self-help groups).

The nurse often clarifies information given by the physician to the patient and provides education about details of the treatment and procedures, particularly in regard to chemotherapy. Because of her frequent contact and work with a patient, the nurse often serves as an extremely sensitive observer of a patient's level of distress.

It is crucial that support staff with whom patients come into contact recognize the importance of their role (see Chapters 51–53). The pleasant secre-

**Figure 6-1.**  Interaction of medical and patient-related variables in prediction of psychological adjustment to cancer diagnosis.

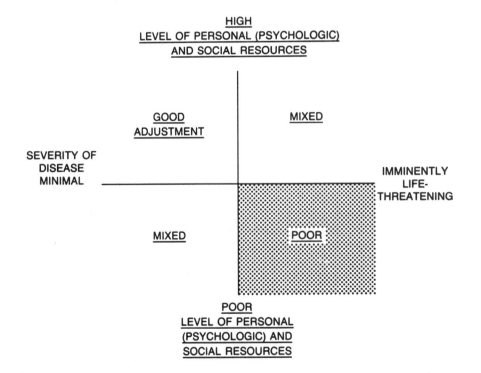

**Table 6-2** Psychosupportive aspects of routine patient care

| Support person | Function | Support person | Function |
|---|---|---|---|
| *Level 1. Basic psychosocial support* | | | May suggest referral |
| Physician | Provides information about diagnosis and treatment | | Knows psychosocial resources |
| | Forms therapeutic alliance | Clergy | Available on patient request |
| | Listens to concerns; gives support | | Provides spiritual perspective and support, religious counseling |
| | Monitors for signs of greater than normal distress | Veteran patient, self-help | Available to patient experiencing same disease and treatment |
| | Refers for consultation | | Gives own "expertise" about coping and practical problems |
| | Knows psychosocial resources | | |
| Nurse | Provides detailed education about treatment to patient and relative; may counsel | *Level 3. Referral for special problems* | |
| | Monitors; may suggest referral | Psychiatrist | Makes differential diagnosis of mental symptoms |
| Office, clinic, floor staff | Provide pleasant environment | | Decides appropriate treatment |
| | Encourage patient | | Implements psychotherapeutic/pharmacological management |
| | Monitor patient's mood | Psychologist, mental health professionals | Provide psychotherapeutic, behavioral, psychosocial support |
| *Level 2. Available support* | | Physiatrist | Aids in special rehabilitative problems; interacts with psychosocial supports |
| Social worker | Available on request to manage practical problems associated with illness | | |
| | Monitors; counsels | | |

tary/receptionist who is concerned and empathic can "make the day" for the patient who feels despondent upon arrival at the door for a visit or treatment. The sour, unconcerned receptionist can have an equally powerful negative effect on the emotionally vulnerable patient. In the hospital, the aides and housekeeping staff who enter the room to carry out specific tasks add to the perceived ambiance as supportive or hostile. Attention paid to interpersonal skills of these staff members through support and education is well rewarded. However, the staff sometimes become demoralized by a perceived lack of appreciation of their responsibilities and support for their effort. At Memorial Sloan-Kettering, courses are given by the personnel department and patient representatives using videotapes to model constructive interactions with patients (Chapter 51 on staff support).

Level 2 of routine psychological care (Table 6-2) should ideally include the availability of a social worker who can provide, on request, management of practical problems arising from illness for patient and fami-

ly. A medical setting in which the social worker can see all patients is helpful, but it is often not available. The social worker monitors for abnormal distress, counsels as a part of total management, and refers to other available resources as required.

The clergy provide an important level 2 resource, available on request or offered regularly, for patients in their own faith. Patients whose primary way of coping with illness is from a spiritual perspective find the support of a religious counselor critical to their successful adaptation. (See also Chapter 57 by Handzo on role of the clergy.)

Level 2 psychological support also includes veteran patients who are available through physicians, institutions, and a range of independent sources (e.g., Reach to Recovery, Can Surmount, Make Today Count) (see Chapter 41). These veteran patients provide a view of illness and treatment that has credibility as a result of their own personal experiences, offering a kind of intimate knowledge of illness that the medical staff cannot provide.

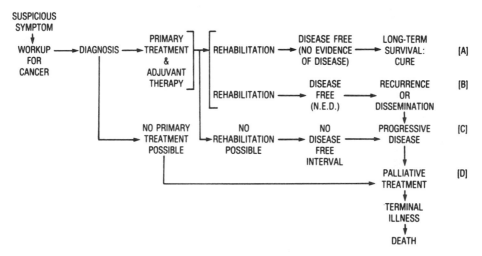

**Figure 6-2.** Clinical course and outcome of cancer.

Level 3 (Table 6-2) represents the psychosocial level which provides mental health referral that may be necessary for the patient who has significant mental symptoms or psychological distress, which require differential diagnosis, especially in distinguishing between a psychological and medical etiology. Patients for whom this level is appropriate may have problems requiring decisions about psychotherapeutic and psychopharmacological management. There is overlap with level 2 resources because, in the last several years, more patients themselves request a psychiatric consultation, particularly because of the emphasis given to this area. At this level of care, psychologists and other mental health professionals also provide psychotherapeutic management. Many who are skilled in behavioral interventions provide a range of these techniques for control of pain and anxiety (see Chapter 40). Consultation with a physiatrist, if a rehabilitation medicine division is available, will ensure integration of physical and emotional rehabilitation.

The severity of problems encountered will dictate the necessary level of care beyond level 1. Over time, the level of need varies for each patient, particularly as different problems arise from the changing course of the illness. Section 1, which includes this chapter and Chapter 7 on survivors outlines the psychological problems as they relate to the stages of disease.

The clinical course of a specific cancer follows one of three possible outcomes: complete cure; a long disease-free interval followed by recurrence and usually progressive disease (despite treatment); or no disease-free interval followed by progressive disease leading to death (Fig. 6-2). The psychological issues for a patient with cancer must be considered in relation to the medical situation at the particular time, because it dictates the immediate problems and symptoms to which the patient must adapt. However, that day-to-day adjustment is markedly colored by the realistic expectations about the future. Thus, one can better understand a patient's psychological adaptation at a given point by understanding the common psychological issues at that stage of disease, while recognizing that the issues will not be static any more than the illness itself. Problems are outlined below as they may be expected, based on the clinical course, recognizing that periods of emotional crisis are usually associated with major transitional points in the illness course or treatment.

One of the cardinal issues that confronts every cancer patient is the constant uncertainty about the future. The single most salient psychological issue for every cancer patient is that prediction of outcome is difficult and uncertainty about the future is a pervasive concern. Even when the survival statistics for a given tumor at a given stage are outlined, they offer a poor substitute for the desired 100% assurance, and do not address the uncertainty reflected in the query, "Into which percentage do *I* fall?" Patients without evidence of disease ask, "*Did* I have cancer, or *do* I have cancer?" Patients weighing the odds and dealing with their emotions must also manage the social pressures. Although optimism grows about cancer, there is still a strong societal message that, "Once you have cancer, you always have it." These concerns about the clinical course are present in patients from the outset, even before the diagnosis is confirmed (see Part I).

The schema in Fig. 6-2 shows the possible clinical courses cancer can take. By looking at this clinical "map" of cancer, one can consider the general issues for a patient at a specific point: suspicious symptom, workup, diagnosis, primary treatment, rehabilitation, long survival, cure, and progressive and terminal disease (Holland, 1982). The trajectory of each course presents vastly different psychological problems; thus each must be considered separately:

1. Course A, long survival and cure
2. Course B, survival with no evidence of disease, followed by recurrence
3. Course C, no response to primary treatment
4. Course D, no primary treatment possible

The patient responses in Courses A–D, at each point along the trajectory, correspond closely to the psychosocial staging proposed by Weisman (1976–77). The four trajectories represent the "roller coaster rides" of cancer, with the many ups and downs and unpredictable turns along the way. Specific symptoms, especially pain, affect behavior and mood; and they vary by site. Side effects of treatment can be life-threatening and often place different demands on the individual in terms of return to prior levels of activity and function. It is these stages, treatment, and site-related variables that constitute the medical determinants. Common to all four courses, however, are the initial phases and crises associated with discovery of a symptom, diagnostic workup, and primary treatment planning, which are associated with unique psychological reactions and problems.

## DIAGNOSIS

### The Workup for Cancer

The schema outlining stage-specific psychological issues (Fig. 6-2) begins with the person's reaction to finding a suspicious sign of cancer. Workup by a physician follows after a longer or shorter period. (See Chapter 2 for a discussion of reasons for delay.) The doctor may have to tell the patient that he or she has cancer. When and how the physician does this, and how the treatment plan is presented, are critical to the patient's well-being and willingness to accept and adhere to the treatment offered. This doctor–patient interaction has been the object of considerable study and is discussed more fully later.

Most people recognize when they have a suspicious symptom of cancer. They also recognize when the physician is considering cancer among the possible diagnoses by the tests that are ordered, such as a computerized tomography (CT) scan, biopsy, or bone marrow aspiration. This is an emotionally difficult period during which the person may not want to alarm family members, and may choose to carry the burden of knowledge and fear alone. The question, "What if it *is* cancer?" is central. Thoughts often alternate between "It's nothing" and "I know it is the worst." The fears are greater in individuals who have had a close family member or friend experience cancer. These individuals may remember an earlier death when treatment and comfort were limited. Anxiety is high when symptoms suggest a cancer for which an increased hereditary risk is known to be present. Women from families with a high frequency of breast cancer who find a breast lump have great anxiety as they await biopsy. Similarly, patients with AIDS-related complex (ARC), or lesions suspicious of Kaposi's sarcoma, many of whom have seen friends die of AIDS, go through panic and sometimes experience suicidal thoughts in anticipation of what they might do if a diagnosis of AIDS were confirmed (see Tross, Chapter 21).

During workup for cancer, the thoughtful clinician is assessing the patient psychologically in the course of taking the medical and family history. Psychological stability is tapped by questions about how prior experiences with personal illness or loss of family members were handled. The mood, attitude, and demeanor of the patient during the medical history and physical examination provide important cues for psychological management (see Chapter 22).

After completion of the initial history and physical examination, the doctor should outline his or her thinking and discuss the tests required to make a definitive diagnosis. The word cancer should be used when it is being considered among the differential diagnoses and presented in a forthright manner such as, "We must be thorough and consider all the possibilities, including, of course, cancer." The patient is warned in this way of the serious nature of the workup, the necessity to complete it, and the possibility of cancer. For most patients, this level of frankness is appreciated and their cooperation is assured. Others, however, especially those who have strong fears of cancer, may refuse to continue the diagnostic tests, responding, "If it *is* cancer, I don't want to know." The physician must be supportive but firm about the necessity of carrying out the diagnostic tests, using a family member to support the effort if needed. The psychological management at this time may be critical to enlist cooperation. Sometimes, a minor tranquilizer (diazepam, lorazepam, or alprazolam) may be helpful, if some of the diagnostic procedures are anxiously anticipated and sleeplessness is a problem.

Sensitive psychological care during this period includes thoughtful attention not only to how to convey the findings, but also to assuring that the patient and family are given the information in a timely fashion, recognizing the distress they are going through. The physician must avoid allowing an unnecessary time lag between doing the biopsy and other key tests, and reporting it to the patient. Many personal decisions are suspended as all await the "news." For many patients, this period of "not knowing" is recalled as one of the worst times.

## Psychiatric Intervention During Workup

Psychological support is provided essentially by the primary physician and the specialist who is doing the workup. Some physicians have highly skilled nurses who offer psychological support informally. The medical community's concern that misinformation might be given from a source other than the physician at this juncture is understandable. Nevertheless, the high anxiety of patients during this period makes it clear that professional or veteran patient counseling would be helpful for some to supplement the information provided by the physicians. The diagnostic period, by virtue of its ambiguity, discourages other psychosocial interventions, yet it is a time of major emotional upheaval. The few formal prediagnosis support programs that have arisen were largely developed for women with breast cancer, at a time when the one-stage procedure, combining biopsy and mastectomy in one surgical procedure, predominated. These programs utilized nurse counselors, informational records, and cassettes for women during the preoperative period (Weider et al., 1978). For patients anticipating laryngectomy or colostomy, veteran patient counseling is particularly helpful when patients have difficulty agreeing to a surgical procedure which produces a major functional deficit.

Psychiatric consultation, infrequently requested during workup, is primarily needed in situations in which anxiety is extremely high, when there is ambivalence and indecision about medical treatment, or when the patient's ability to understand the nature of the procedures is in question. Presence of mental retardation, major mental illness, or dementia brings up the question of capacity to make judgments. Consent of a family member or appointment of a guardian may be necessary. The presence of severe anxiety requires a psychiatric evaluation to determine the cause (e.g., prior association with cancer, preexisting anxiety disorder, or phobia of disease or hospitals) and to plan for treatment involving psychological assistance to tolerate the diagnostic procedures. Especially frightening are total-body scans or scans of the head, which involve lengthy periods of being alone and immobilized in a small enclosed space. The magnetic resonance imaging (MRI) procedure is frightening to a significant percentage of patients (as high as 10–15%), some of whom cannot go through the procedure (Brennan et al., 1988). Special management, including the use of

medication, may be required to assist these patients (see Chapter 39 on psychopharmacology). For the very fearful patient, or one who has a preexisting anxiety disorder with panic attacks or phobias (particularly of enclosed spaces, illness, doctors, needles, and/or hospitals), some of the diagnostic tests pose major hurdles to overcome before treatment can be determined.

The following case illustrates some of these problems.

### CASE REPORT

A 35-year-old married mother of one small child required diagnostic staging for Hodgkin's disease. A long-standing history of generalized anxiety disorder and fears of needles, illness, and doctors made it difficult for her to agree to a bone marrow aspiration and lymphangiogram. The initial lymphangiogram attempted could not be completed because of her anxiety and inability to remain still. Arrangements were made by the consulting psychiatrist to reschedule the procedure with the presence of a familiar staff member, and careful advance planning with nursing staff who were prepared for her high level of distress. Sedation before the procedure followed by an intravenous, short-acting anesthetic during the procedure were used to permit the lymphangiogram to be completed.

## Telling The Diagnosis of Cancer

Since the 1950s, the norm in U.S. clinical practice has progressively changed from telling almost no cancer patient his or her diagnosis of cancer (revealing it only to the family), to the current policy of informing most patients of the name and nature of their illness (Oken, 1961; Novack et al., 1979; Morrow and Hoagland, 1981). Morrow and Hoagland, in a review of practice in the United States, charted the changes in practice over time, using data from four studies (Fig. 6-3). The drastic change from nearly 90% never revealing the diagnosis in 1961, to less than 10% in 1977 stating this policy, shows how rapidly the change occurred. Debated began in the 1960s when psychiatrists, on the basis of their knowledge of responses to stressful information, encouraged more open disclosure. Doctors who began to work exclusively with cancer found that more open communication enhanced the sense of trust between them and their patients. Lies or euphemisms were no longer necessary, and the facts could more often be safely revealed to the patient, as well as to the family member. The conspiracy of silence, a common consequence of the prior practice of not telling the diagnosis, was avoided.

Other social changes occurring in the United States contributed to the change in attitudes toward disclosure. These included increasing medical information and sophistication among laypersons about all diseases, the knowledge that some forms of cancer are

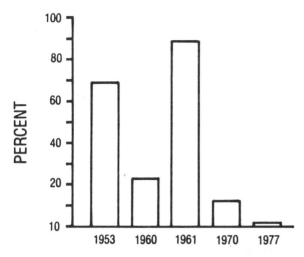

**Figure 6-3.** Percentage of physicians whose policy was not to inform cancer patients of their diagnosis. *Source:* Reprinted with permission from G.R. Morrow and A.C. Hoagland (1981). Physician–patient communications in cancer treatment. *Proc. Am. Cancer Soc. Third Ntl. Conf. on Human Values and Cancer.* Washington, D.C., April 23–25, pp. 27–37.

treatable and curable, the social trend toward viewing patients as consumers of health care as a product, a diminished trust in doctors and the medical system in general, and the emergence of concern about the moral and legal rights of the patient to autonomy expressed in the doctrine of "informed consent." Guidelines promulgated by federal regulations for research in humans mandated full disclosure of disease, as well as the risks and benefits associated with each treatment option.

It should be noted that how revealing the diagnosis of cancer is handled is greatly influenced by the social attitudes in a particular society. In most of Europe, the Soviet Union, and Asia, the diagnosis of cancer is still not commonly told to the patient. There is evidence, however, from a study done through the International Psycho-Oncology Society, that this pattern is changing worldwide. There is a trend toward more open discussion of the diagnosis. Numbers of physicians appear to be increasing who feel that the benefits of better coping and cooperation with treatment outweigh the risk of distress associated with learning the cancer diagnosis (Holland et al., 1986).

In the United States today, the word cancer is, with rare exception, used in discussions of diagnosis that include site of cancer, extent, and often prognosis, depending on the patient's request for information. Open communication of the diagnosis eliminates the duplicity of a "secret" shared by the physician with the relative in which the patient is excluded. Withholding the information today can be counterproductive because the patient may discover the diagnosis inadvertently, either by hearing it discussed or by reading a consent form for a diagnostic procedure or treatment. It is far more desirable that the patient hear the information from the trusted physician who can couple the word *cancer* with a proposed treatment plan. In this context the word cancer becomes less frightening. In fact, the U.S. physician's concern over whether to utter the word cancer is no longer as critical an issue as the way in which the diagnosis is given; how and when the physician reveals it becomes the central issue.

*Who* tells the diagnosis is equally important from a psychological perspective. It should not be the specialist who may have made the definitive diagnosis if he or she has not known the patient before and is a poor judge of the "how" to tell. Instead, the physician who knows the patient and the family best, and who in turn is trusted by them, is preferably the one to carry out the discussion of the diagnosis. The family or primary doctor usually knows the patient, is trusted by him, and is in the best position to decide how, when and what should be told. The place for such a discussion is in a quiet, private place where emotions can be expressed without embarrassment and interruptions. Individuals given news of such importance over the telephone never forget the implicit lack of consideration and sensitivity that is suggested by an offhanded means of presentation. Language and, as appropriate, drawings should be used that the patient can understand. Medical jargon should be avoided. Anxiety is usually very high, and for this reason, the "telling process" may need to be spread over several interviews, starting with less frightening terms such as "tumor," "blood disease," or "growth," and following this with more definitive terms as the person adapts to the idea of a neoplasm or hematological disorder. Some physicians find it helpful to audiotape the initial discussion of the diagnosis and treatment, and give the cassette to the patient to carry home (Rosenbaum et al., 1981). They can then listen in the quiet atmosphere of their own home with a relative, when anxiety is lower and questions can be formulated. The result is a far better informed patient who has appropriate questions at the next visit.

The honesty associated with revealing the diagnosis must be tempered with sensitivity by the physician. Though not telling lies, the physician must also avoid giving the unvarnished truth without any hope. Patients have sometimes been told, "You have cancer that has spread and there is nothing I can do for you"; or, "You have 6 months to live and there is no treatment for your problem." The patient's psychological reaction to these remarks is a feeling of hopelessness, anger, and abandonment. Giving an estimated survival time is particularly damaging because it is often experienced as a "death sentence." Such an approach can result in a search for alternative methods that *do* offer hope. The physician can give hope in the context of the reality of the illness: hope to attain short-term desired goals; by pointing out recognition that today not all cancer patients die, because many are cured, some have long periods of clinical remission, and new therapies are constantly being developed. It is equally important that the doctor convey a sense of commitment to the patient and to ongoing care, irrespective of the stage of disease or nature of the treatment. Honesty, realistic hope, and awareness of the physician's commitment to excellence in his or her care provide a climate for the patient to sense the physician's full psychological support and for participation to the fullest in his or her own care (Holland, 1982).

One response to the sweep of the pendulum toward a "harsh facts without hope" approach has been put forward by Spingarn (1982), an articulate cancer survivor. She reminds us that patients still must have the right *not* to know if they so choose. She is critical of the practice of some physicians who not only tell the diagnosis but also rob patients of hope for cure or arrest at a time when hope is crucial. This is especially important to keep in mind with certain groups of patients, for example, some older individuals whose experiences with cancer span the "never tell" days, and for whom the word *cancer* remains devastating. Such persons, especially those who insist that they do not want to know all the facts, should not be forced to receive more details than are needed to inform them. The important issue is to couple the diagnostic discussion with a treatment plan, offered with optimism and a sense of commitment to the best possible outcome.

The withholding of depressing facts has support from many who advocate alternative treatment methods. They feel that eliminating hope has an impact on treatment outcome and may be biologically deleterious. Although there are no data to support a biological response to diagnosis, there are clearly negative psychological consequences when facts are presented insensitively. Certainly, the change in practice to open disclosure of medical information has had a positive effect on patient participation in care. However, the burden on the doctor to reveal the diagnosis and still maintain hope is greater than ever.

## FAMILY REFUSAL TO REVEAL THE DIAGNOSIS

The family that insists, "He can't take it," and stipulates that the diagnosis, if it is cancer, not be revealed to the patient, is a troubling problem for the physician. When this occurs, the emotional problem usually lies with the relative rather than the patient. Often the patient knows or suspects the cancer diagnosis and is in turn seeking to protect the family, sensing that "*they* can't take it.*" Insistence from the onset on one set of facts stated to patient and family together, avoids many problems later. By insisting on discussing the diagnosis and treatment only when both the patient and the family are present, the charade of presenting one set of facts to the patient at the bedside and another to the family outside the patient's room, is eliminated. Although it is difficult at the outset to convince some families of the importance of this approach, such a discussion often serves an educational purpose that hastens the family's more realistic acceptance of the situation.

The most common rationale previously employed by physicians for not telling the diagnosis, and one that is still put forth by relatives who do not wish the patient to be told, is the argument that "he will commit suicide." The risk appears far less than is often assumed. It is even less likely today, as cancer is more openly discussed and is known to be more treatable (Oken, 1961). However, the issue of suicide in cancer is important and is discussed in Chapter 24.

## Reactions To The Diagnosis

The initial period following the diagnosis of cancer has been the most widely studied with respect to the range of coping strategies used and the means by which the stress of cancer diagnosis may be modulated. The earliest studies (see Part I) during the 1950s were based on clinical interviews and, using psychodynamic insights, provided our first psychosocial data. An early paper by Shands and co-workers (1951) corrected a widely held view at that time that there was an encompassing psychological response to cancer diagnosis, and pointed out the range of responses that are related to specific medical and personal circumstances.

The question we wished in the study to answer is: What is the emotional reaction exhibited by a patient with cancer? The first answer that has emerged is that it is a poor and even unanswerable question. We have had to replace it with some such questions as: How does this person, of such an age, background, habit of life and so son, react at this time to this aspect of the malignant lesion in this organ? Reactions vary from patient to patient, and, even in the same individuals, there is a constantly shifting reaction pattern depending upon a great variety of essential and accidental variables encountered by the patient. A given individual does, however, tend to exhibit consistent trends of reaction even though the details differ from time to time. The same general tendencies are present in everyone, but the specific form and intensity vary according to heredity, environment, and circumstance. (p. 1159)

They made other observations of the period following diagnosis, noting the violently disruptive effect on personality as the individual seeks to integrate the idea of cancer, using defense mechanisms to avoid being overwhelmed. The need to assign a cause (sometimes perceived as retribution for prior behavior), to process the information, and to deal with the impact on relationships was well described:

The occurrence of a serious illness disrupts the entire system of relationships: (1) the outcome of the illness is unknown and consequently, the individual is faced with the problem of alternative readjustment to several possibilities; (2) he is forced to attempt to adjust at a time when his "adaptational energies" are occupied with the illness; and (3) he has to integrate into his context a central relationship with a stranger or a series of strangers [who] holds the patient's life in his hands. The patient then is forced into a sudden, decisive dependent relationship, the extent of which is proportional to the severity of the symptoms or to the patient's understanding of the severity of illness. (Shands et al., 1951, p. 1164)

The seminal decade-long work of Project Omega at the Massachusetts General Hospital made extensive observations on patients with cancer in the period following diagnosis (Weisman and Worden, 1976; Weisman, 1979a,b). Their series of observations led to a concept that cancer is experienced as a series of expectable psychosocial crises, or phases that occur in relation to the existential concerns associated with different periods following diagnosis. They identified several correlations with the presence of high or low distress during the period after diagnosis. This Index of Vulnerability provides key indicators of risk for distress that are helpful to keep in mind in evaluating a patient (see Table 6-3). In addition to psychological influences (e.g., prior psychiatric history, pessimism, high anxiety), status and social risk factors (e.g., lower socioeconomic status, prior marital problems), they also found that seriousness or degree of illness, symptoms, or perception of lack of support from physicians were correlated with high distress.

One of the early research concerns in psycho-oncology has been the search for ways to rapidly, at an early point in illness, identify the patient vulnerable to poor adjustment and high distress. Data from a Psychosocial Collaborative Oncology Group (PSYCOG) study showed a high correlation between presence of a psychiatric disorder and elevated scores on the Hopkins Symptom Checklist (SCL-90), a brief screening inventory. Other research by this multicenter group indicated that oncology staff can be trained to use several brief simple measures to obtain a reliable assessment of patient distress or vulnerability such as the Global Adjustment to Illness Scale (Morrow et al., 1981).

The period that coincides with reaction to diagnosis in our own schema coincides with phase 1 of the four psychosocial phases of cancer identified by Weisman

**Table 6-3** Indicators associated with vulnerability to poor psychosocial adjustment

| Adjustment areas | Indicators |
|---|---|
| Medical | More physical symptoms |
| | More advanced cancer at diagnosis |
| | Doctor perceived as less helpful |
| | Dubious about effect of treatment |
| | Short time perspective about survival |
| Social | Lower socioeconomic status |
| | More marital problems |
| | More background problems |
| | Expects and/or gets little support from others |
| | Little or no church attendance |
| Psychological and psychiatric | History of psychiatric problems |
| | High anxiety |
| | Low ego strength |
| | More suppression |
| | More concerns of all kinds |
| | Feels like giving up |
| | Alcohol abuse |
| | Coping less effective |

*Source*: Adapted from Weisman (1979).

(1979b). It is characterized by acute distress reflecting the impact of diagnosis that subsides as the person returns to normal activity. Both Shands and co-workers (1951) and Weisman described the distress of this period as being like a fever or "psychic inflammation"; it is a transient response that leaves no aftermath (similar to a febrile response) in psychologically healthy individuals. This response is called the "existential plight" by Weisman and represents a period during which the person has cure as an aim, is optimistic, experiences transient functional impairment, uses denial as a temporary mechanism, and copes actively with the stress. The transient nature of response to the crises was demonstrated by McCorkle and Quint-Benoliel (1983), who showed that although existential concerns were greater in patients following diagnosis of cancer, as compared to patients with their first myocardial infarction, distress had significantly subsided after 2 months in both groups. Penman (1980) found better coping with breast cancer at 3 months in women who "tackled" the problem as compared to those who coped by avoiding confrontation with the problem.

Caplan (1981) also described stress in terms relevant to cancer. The diagnosis of cancer, in his conceptual model, is a time when emotional demands on the individual exceed the ability to respond, resulting in psychological and physiological arousal. Mastery of the stress results in reduction of the arousal (symptoms) to tolerable limits. (See Chapter 4 on coping and Chapter 22 on normal responses.)

Taylor (1982), in studying responses to threatening events, notes that the search for meaning is also important. A sense of mastery is enhanced by assigning cause. Believing one has control over threatening events and attributing personal benefit from the experience are constructive in promoting behavior to regain control. Though lacking factual basis, these beliefs simultaneously protect and prompt constructive thought and action.

Clinical observations and data from studies support the assumption that a highly adaptive response can be expected in most patients at the time of the initial diagnosis of cancer. (Chapter 22 describes these normal responses.) Shock, numbness, and denial constitute a frequent initial response. At times the response may be an immediate sense of despair and hopelessness. Minimizing the frightening nature of the facts, if it does not interfere with treatment, may be a transiently helpful mechanism protecting against overwhelming anxiety and allowing the person to ''hear'' the news more gradually. Dysphoria and anxiety, depression, anger, and difficulty with concentration and maintenance of daily function and activities may be part of the clinical picture. Anger may predominate: ''I just got my life together. Why did it have to happen now?'' The distress dissipates over 7 to 14 days, and the adaptation to the bad news is seen with its incorporation into a constructive plan of action. Longer term adaptation of course goes on over months. A good therapeutic alliance with the doctor makes the adaptation easier. A prolonged or overly intense response, which may be due to any number of causes, can become sufficient to be recognizable as a psychiatric disorder (Part IV). Most often the disorder is reactive anxiety, combined with depressive symptoms, that fits the diagnosis of an adjustment reaction with depressed, anxious, or mixed mood disturbance (Chapter 22).

Persons who have been deeply religious before receiving news of a cancer diagnosis usually find great solace in placing the outcome ''in God's hands,'' using their religion and beliefs to face the crises. People who have strong spiritual beliefs often reveal a calmer, more accepting attitude toward disease and possible death, relying on both the comfort of their belief system and the support of their religious community. It is important that this spiritual support be available in the hospital. (Chapter 57 describes the role of the clergy.) However, people who have not had a religious orientation usually rely on their own personal philosophical approach to life and death. They may especially benefit from discussions with members of the health care team that enable them to explore their thoughts about existential issues as they seek a perspective from which to view this threat to life and possible death.

Coming to terms with the diagnosis is coupled with obtaining information about treatment options and making a decision about the best plan to be followed. Primary treatment, irrespective of type, carries with it the next set of stresses.

## PRIMARY TREATMENT

The primary treatment for cancer today is usually multimodal, consisting of surgery, radiation, chemotherapy, and to a lesser extent, immunotherapy. The specific psychological issues associated with the major treatment modalities are discussed in Chapters 8–12. For most patients, the goal of the initial treatment is cure. In aiming for this outcome, the individual is optimistic and willing to tolerate whatever is necessary to attain that goal. Psychological support is needed largely to assist the person in dealing with treatment side effects, maintaining high morale, and cooperating in such a way that a full treatment course can be given. Studies show that nonadherence to a chemotherapy regimen results in poorer survival for several tumor sites (see Chapter 10). This can become a central issue, particularly with teenagers.

Although psychological problems of therapy vary by modality, one issue is a consistent concern with all treatments: informed consent. It is important in all medical settings in this country, but it is especially important with cancer when conventional therapies fail and treatments under clinical investigation must be considered. Both the definition of informed consent, and the elements which are necessary to assure it, become important issues with which the oncology staff should be familiar.

## INFORMED CONSENT

During the era when the medical diagnosis was withheld to protect the patient from distress, decisions about treatment were made by the physician in conjunction with family consultation. At that time, the approach was both justified and was considered to be morally defensible. The view of the physician was that of an authority figure who protected patients from emotional distress and chose appropriate treatment for their illness, providing it in a humane way. Such a position is now viewed by society as having been inappropriately paternalistic and overprotective (Herbert, 1980). Far greater emphasis has been placed on patients' autonomy and their rights to be informed and to chart their own destiny in terms of treatment decisions. The ethical issues associated with informed consent have, at a practical level, become complicated by legal ones in the past decade. There is, at times, overlap of ethical, legal, and psychological issues that complicates the interface between the three fields, especially in relation to cancer (Chapter 59).

Rules governing consent for investigational treatment require lengthy written consent forms, which contain detailed exposition of risks and benefits. Despite this, a study by Penman and colleagues (1984), showed that the sense of trust the patient had in the doctor was still a major reason for the patient's decision to accept treatment by investigational chemotherapy. In this study, trust in the doctor, belief that the treatment would help, and fear that their condition would worsen otherwise were the three main reasons cited by patients for accepting investigational treatment. Although Cassileth and co-workers (1980) found that younger patients desired more participation in decisions than older patients, those who did participate, irrespective of age, were more hopeful and preferred the greater communication and maximal information.

An additional problem in obtaining truly informed consent is that the discussion in which consent is given is held in the period following diagnosis when the ability to concentrate is transiently impaired. In a study conducted by a surgeon who tape-recorded his preoperative discussion of risks and benefits for a thoracic operation, the majority of patients did not recall having been told of the possible undesirable outcomes even after listening to the tapes, when interviewed several months after the operation (Robinson and Merav, 1976). Scott (1983) has shown that women anticipating biopsy of a lump with suspicion of breast cancer actually had difficulty in processing information. Those with highest anxiety had the most difficulty in concentrating and reasoning, suggesting it to be a period in which decision making may be particularly difficult. Those who had negative biopsy results had normal mental function 6 weeks later (Chapter 14 on breast cancer).

The study of Penman and colleagues (1984) found that recall of possible side effects was low, even when they were described in the informed-consent document and presented verbally by the doctor for consent to treatment by an investigational protocol. The informed-consent document, a central part of clinical research, is a written outline of the key aspects of informed consent. It should ideally be used only to complement the discussion with the doctor. The consent form should (in understandable nontechnical language) outline the treatment, its proposed risks and benefits, other treatment options, and the person's rights to confidentiality of information and to optimal care whether accepting the treatment or not. The person must also know that he or she is free to withdraw from the treatment without compromise of care. Many early forms were written in legal terms that led some

patients to perceive them as documents more for the legal protection of the doctor than for assistance in giving information to the patient, their primary purpose. They were also written in medically technical terms that reduced possible comprehension. When several were subjected to a commonly used readability scale, they were found to be at comprehension level almost equivalent to that required for reading medical journals (Fig. 6-4; Morrow, 1980). A major effort by Institutional Review Boards (IRB), set up to protect patients' rights, has begun to correct this problem, and consent forms are carefully reviewed to assure that they can be understood by patients and families.

There are inherent problems for both patient and physician in obtaining truly informed consent, even when both are seeking rational decision making and self-determination. Considerations on both sides make it difficult (Penman et al., 1984). Anxiety, maximal at the time when a patient with cancer must make the choice about treatment is heightened by conflicting second opinions and media coverage. On the other side, treating physicians who are also clinical investigators must present the proposed treatment in a way to encourage the patients to make their own decision. Yet in cancer treatment, there may be few options available except supportive care. The physician, who feels the treatment may offer at least a hope of response, even if partial or temporary, may find it difficult to be completely neutral. Penman and colleagues (1984) noted:

The patient depends on the physician for information about treatment, but may reject some of this information, particularly the negative, selecting the more positively therapeutic aspects. Also reliant on the physician for guidance, patients eager to follow physicians' recommendations may also eagerly relegate the decision to the physician unless deliberation is fostered. This underscores the strong obligation that rests on the physician to encourage the patients' autonomy in making their decision, while still conveying the mandated information.

Investigative protocols that offer patients the current best treatment available versus one that has promise of being better—but which can only be proven in a double-blind randomized clinical trial—places both the doctor and patient in the ambiguous position of choice based on random selection. Yet the improvement of survival rates, still low for many common tumor sites, depends on participation in such clinical trials. Clinical investigational protocols have been brought to community hospitals to assure access to more patients through the Cancer Community Oncology Program of the National Cancer Institute (NCI). This has assured more patients the opportunity to receive drugs that were previously available only at approved cancer centers.

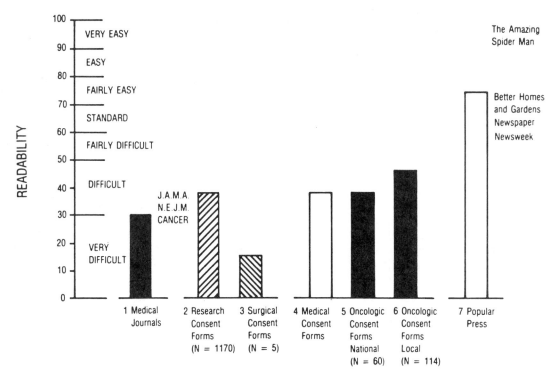

**Figure 6-4.** Readability of medical journals, informed-consent forms, and popular press, studied by readability scales. *Source:* Reprinted with permission from G.R. Morrow and A.C. Hoagland (1981). Physician–patient communications in cancer treatment. *Proc. Am. Cancer Soc. Third Ntl. Conf. on Human Values and Cancer.* Washington, D.C., April 23–25, pp. 27–37.

## ELEMENTS OF INFORMED CONSENT

The ethical principles of informed consent that protect the autonomy of patients participating in clinical investigations also protect professionals and benefit society by allaying public fears, encouraging self-scrutiny of the medical profession, and maintaining relations of trust (Beauchamp and Childress, 1983). The elements of consent that protect patient autonomy are important bioethical issues for oncology staff, because they are applied in clinical situations to evaluate whether informed consent has been established. To assume informed consent there have to be competency of the person, adequate disclosure of information, comprehension of the information by the patient, and evidence of a voluntary decision without coercion. A person is viewed as having capacity to decide if he or she can make a decision based on rational reasons; that is, the person must be able to understand a proposed treatment, weigh its risks and benefits, and make a decision in light of such knowledge, even choosing not to utilize the information. The psychiatrist is often asked to determine the degree to which the patient understands the proposed treatment and its risks and benefits. This is a clinical judgment and is not the same as a legal test of "competency" (Schwartz and Blank, 1986). For example, at times, even in the presence of a mild transient impairment of mental function, it may be determined that the person does understand the nature and quality of the procedure proposed and can give consent. In such cases, it may be useful to have a relative consent as well, but it does not warrant a legal judgment. However, if understanding is impaired such that the person does not understand the need for or outcome of a proposed elective procedure, a relative should be legally appointed to assume responsibility as guardian for the patient who has been legally declared incompetent. If an emergency exists, then a decision may have to be made to proceed with the relatives' consent and patient's assent.

The second element, that of adequate disclosure of information, is judged by the "reasonable person" standard. It is required that the patient be provided with information that a "reasonable person," in the patient's circumstances, would find relevant and would be able to assimilate. In the current climate of full disclosure, the person who expresses a wish to receive less information than the "reasonable person" standard requires, poses a difficult problem (Spingarn, 1982). The young physician who has been trained in the period in which patient autonomy has been emphasized may find it hard to accept. However, forcing a patient to face information also violates the principle of autonomy. The shift in favor of greater patient autonomy is recent and may be distressing to some. Many patients, particularly older ones, prefer not to make decisions or to be fully informed.

Each institution in which clinical investigations are conducted has a federally mandated Institutional Review Board (IRB), consisting of a multidisciplinary panel with representatives from law, the community, the clergy, the social sciences, as well as biomedical sciences. A study, to be approved, must ask valid questions, indicate protection of patients' rights, and show that all elements of informed consent have been met. The IRBs are supplemented today by Institutional Ethics Committees (IECs), which provide advice on ethical issues that relate to the interface of research, institutional policies, and patient care.

## AWAITING TREATMENT

Patients and their relatives experience high anxiety while awaiting the initiation of primary treatment, whether it is surgery, chemotherapy, radiation, or some combination of these modalities. It is a period when memories of a close relative or friend who died with cancer may become vivid. Horror stories about the side effects of cancer treatments are repeated, often based on the realities of treatment in an earlier period. Radiation and chemotherapy especially carry fears of side effects. (See Chapters 9 and 10 on problems associated with each therapy.) The very anxious patient will need special attention to reduce the fears during this time. Description of the procedure using drawings or videotapes help. Actual rehearsal of the events and sensations to be expected contribute to a sense of control when the treatment or procedure begins. Training in relaxation, or an antianxiety drug such as benzodiazepine (for either daytime or bedtime sedation, or both) will reduce anxious anticipation.

The different clinical courses that may follow primary treatment (Fig. 6-1), each associated with predictable crises, are outlined in the following paragraphs.

### Clinical Course A: Treatment Followed by Rehabilitation, Long-Term Survival, and Cure

In clinical course A, primary treatments—surgery, chemotherapy, and radiotherapy—are followed by rehabilitation that has physical and psychological components. Participation in rehabilitation procedures to achieve the maximal functional outcome is important at this time. Many problems arise: return home to responsibilities, adaptation to side effects or sequelae of treatment, return to job, and resumption of normal family role and function. There is often an assumption that getting discharged from the hospital will be followed by a sense of "it's all over." It is a disappointment to discover that there are still intermittent periods of anxiety and reactive depression. This early posttreatment period is characterized by a central emotion: uncertainty about the future. Optimism about having achieved a cure is high. But with the end of active treatment, the fear that "perhaps they didn't get it all," and "perhaps it will start to grow now that the treatment is over" are major emotional hazards. The need for reassurance from the doctor may require extra visits and telephone calls. The person may even joke about how any ache or pain triggers a feeling of panic that the cancer is returning in that place, even if it is the earlobe or the big toe. Fears of recurrence are highest at this point, and for some, create a dysfunctional state requiring intervention. As time goes by, confidence builds and the person returns to previous levels of functioning and coping. The problems of the cured patients—the survivors—are a subject of great interest as more patients join this group (Chapter 7).

### Clinical Course B: Disease-Free Interval Followed by Recurrence

In clinical course B, a patient may enjoy the elation of a positive response to the curative treatment attempt, experience a short to lengthy disease-free interval (as seen in course A), only to have the hope for cure suddenly shattered by the discovery of a metastasis, extension, recurrence or relapse of disease. Despite the fears of recurrence that may have characterized the prior months or years, the actual diagnosis of recurrence is sometimes experienced as "the other shoe finally dropped." As distressing as the news may be, it ends the painful uncertainty. Tross and co-workers (1986) have found a similar response in HIV positive patients with Aids Related Complex who, after many months of fearing progression to an AIDS diagnosis, actually feel relieved that it has finally happened (see Chapter 21 on AIDS).

Weisman and Worden (1986) studied 102 patients at time of recurrence. They found a correlation between the degree of distress experienced at time of recurrence and the degree of expectation of recurrence. Those who were surprised about recurrence had the highest distress; those who had never believed themselves to be cured, including all with remissions under a year, experienced least distress. They found adaptation to recurrence better than expected by the nature of the information.

The information from the doctor that the illness has

entered a new phase, however, requires a major re-orientation similar to that seen at the time of diagnosis (Schmale, 1976). A new level of adaptation is required to deal with the idea that the treatment that offered the greatest hope for cure has failed. The threat to life cannot be denied; second-line therapies must be considered, and sometimes, participation in an investigational treatment.

When the patient is told about recurrence, the acute emotional turmoil is similar to that experienced at the time of diagnosis, with intensified existential concerns, sadness, and depression. Insomnia, restlessness, anxiety, depressive symptoms, and poor concentration may again temporarily disrupt daily activities, as at the time of diagnosis. As the information is assimilated, mastery of the new situation is slowly established. There is a tendency again to search for a cause of the catastrophe. Some patients blame themselves. Others blame the doctor who delayed the initial diagnosis or treatment, or failed to detect the recurrence at the earliest possible time. Anger may be the primary emotion, masking the depression. However, usually depression is the predominant emotion, colored by anxiety. The patient must struggle to control emotions while attempting to find the best treatment plan in the context of a reality in which treatments are directed toward disease control, not cure. Coming to grips more directly with death leads to fears of dying, which exceed those of death itself. Fear of a painful death causes the greatest distress. Suicidal thoughts and plans are common, usually planned for a time in the future "when it gets bad enough." The plans, which may include lethal doses of drugs kept in a special place, seem to serve as a comfort to ensure that there is a means of asserting ultimate control by suicide if the illness becomes intolerable. Most patients never act out these plans. Rational suicide, though widely publicized when it occurs, is quite uncommon (see Chapter 24). However, risk of rational suicide poses ethical and clinical dilemmas for all concerned. Evaluation of such individuals requires an attempt to detect any underlying psychiatric or neurological disturbance. At times, however, in the face of advanced or terminal illness, the patient's thoughts seem truly rational and management centers around encouraging family, friends, and staff to create maximal emotional support.

Severe, even psychotic reactions do sometimes occur at the time of diagnosis of recurrence, especially among persons with prior significant psychiatric problems. The following two brief case histories illustrate two extreme responses.

## CASE REPORTS

A 51-year-old married mother of three adult children who had had a 3-year remission from lymphoma noted a mass in her neck that she suspected to be a recurrence. A call to her physician confirmed the necessity for him to evaluate the new symptoms by an office visit. She became depressed, agitated, and preoccupied with the thought that she would require chemotherapy again, which had been difficult for her the first time. She became sure that treatment would fail anyway. At home alone, she took 2 mg diazepam to sleep and to "try to forget"; she then swallowed the remaining 60 pills in the bottle. She required care in an intensive care unit initially, followed by admission for psychiatric hospitalization. Treatment with antidepressants and psychotherapy led to prompt recovery. She returned to her home and family, and her physician reinstituted chemotherapy with good results.

A 35-year-old married father of two young children had appeared to be cured by surgery for lung cancer, but evidence of extensive metastases to the liver appeared 2 years later. Long noted to be suspicious and contentious, and an avid hunter, he became acutely paranoid toward his family and physician over several days after receiving confirmation of the recurrence. He attempted to find his guns and threatened the lives of his wife and children, to be followed by suicide. Hospitalized in a psychiatric unit, he had no signs of brain metastases. He developed florid paranoid and persecutory delusions that responded poorly to antipsychotic medication and psychotherapy up to the time of his death.

In discussing the recurrence, the physician must explain the ramifications of the new development and outline a revised treatment plan. The physician should convey his or her continuing commitment to the patient's care, explaining that although a cure is not possible, control of disease is. Statements, such as "We have treatments that are directed toward control of your disease, and if the first treatment doesn't work, there are others that we will use," are important. Hope, optimism, and assurance that the doctor will continue treatment are crucial. Fear of abandonment by the doctor and family is great at this time. Assurance that pain can be controlled is critical, because that is a central fear. Opportunity to ask exploring questions, including those concerning the possibility of a fatal outcome, is important. The treatment options should be discussed honestly, setting the stage for a close doctor–patient relationship that will be a source of strength later, especially when this relationship is characterized by trust and open communication.

A serious mistake is made by the doctor who says "There is nothing more I can do for you." This conveys a hopeless situation, and an attitude that is perceived by the patient as rejection. The NCI-funded study of laetrile showed that patients who participated had most often been told "nothing could be done" and sought alternative methods because "medicine had failed them" (Redding et al., 1981). The physician must present a treatment plan that conveys an equal commitment to the patient, irrespective of the goal of the treatment. Conveying that there will be an aggressive approach to the control of cancer and distressing symptoms is critical for the patient. During the new treatment phase, only the goal of treatment has changed. Usually, once a strategy has been outlined, most patients begin to cope effectively with the new reality and cooperate with the doctor in the effort to obtain maximum benefit from a revised treatment plan.

## Clinical Course C: Primary Treatment Failure with Progressive Disease

An attempt at curative treatment may be planned and carried out with enthusiasm, only to have no significant effect on disease progression. The patient whose cancer fails to respond to initial therapy may receive second-line treatments or participate in investigative protocols. Although transient responses occur with an equally transient sense of optimism and elation, disease progression continues, bringing sadness and despair. Investigational protocols are often proposed at these stages, bringing up again the choice between supportive care at home or in a hospice, or participation in an experimental study of an investigative therapy.

## Clinical Course D: When No Primary Treatment Is Possible

Some patients at the time of diagnosis are found to have a cancer for which no curative effort is possible. Under these conditions the oncologist must convey not only the diagnosis of cancer, but also that treatment to be undertaken, similar to the situation for patients in course C, is aimed at control and palliation. Therapy may arrest and control tumor growth for some time, but no hope of cure is possible. Adjusting to this news requires great courage from patient and family, who suffer equally in absorbing the information. Optimism that there will be a period of time with maximal quality of life—however long or short—provides the opportunity to make plans for the ensuing period, and to decide about investigative treatments versus supportive or hospice care. It can be pointed out to patients that many others have experienced lengthy periods in which they enjoyed a reasonable quality of life. Indeed, the course of some incurable tumors can be quite protracted, extending over months to years, during which time the quality of life is good. Unexplainable prolonged remissions also occur.

In some patients the time from diagnosis to death is precipitously short. Adults with acute leukemia are most representative of this group, in which the illness onset is acute and the course is fulminating. The rapid onset of illness, arising as a sudden deviation from usual health and requiring immediate hospitalization and aggressive induction treatment, is emotionally overwhelming (see Hematological Malignancies, Chapter 16). In certain diseases, like leukemia, talking with someone who has survived the initial stages of the same illness and who understands the feelings of panic as no one else can, can be extremely reassuring (see Self-Help, Chapter 41).

## Day-To-Day Adjustment

After recurrent disease becomes a day-to-day reality, adjustment depends to a large measure on the severity of symptoms, particularly pain and discomfort. Optimism and more enjoyment of surroundings is seen on days when the physical state is good, however, the converse is equally readily apparent. Pessimism, depressed mood, and poor physical status go hand in hand. Awareness of the fatal nature of the illness is always present, but a variable conscious awareness is related to level of denial, a helpful mental mechanism that will vary from being totally absent on some days to totally active on other days. The presence of denial does not mean that a full awareness of reality does not still exist, but that the person temporarily modifies that reality. Patients with cancer, as do physically healthy persons, transiently change the meaning of reality to make it acceptable. Henry (1971) called this "as-if-ness"; we behave as if certain facts were true, knowing they may not be. Hope, "as-if-ness," and denial have a similar implication, that of altering the person's perception of reality in a more acceptable way at this stage. Weisman (1975) has described the simultaneous existence of denial, awareness, and acceptance of death. The delicate balance that determines which coping mechanism is most apparent at a given time is tipped by circumstances and these, in turn, alter perception of illness. For example, good news of a response to a new treatment may encourage plans for the "last trip to—," which previously seemed too much to undertake.

Increasing dependence on others, inability to work and to maintain the role in the family as the breadwinner or homemaker, are painful adjustments to increasing severity of illness. Physical dependency, characterized by the inability to walk, to feed oneself, or to meet personal needs unaided, cause additional psychological burdens. The unaccustomed helplessness and relentless progression of advancing cancer require enormous adjustment. Most patients, however, manage these difficulties with remarkable courage and strength. Studies by Casselith and colleagues (1984), using a Mental Health Index, found patients with several different chronic illnesses, including cancer, were quite similar in their level of mental health and well-being. However, with advanced stages of each disease (renal, diabetes, arthritis, and cancer), well-being was more impaired with poorer mental health. Patients with cancer, however, showed no higher levels of distress than equally ill patients with the other chronic diseases.

Increased emotional attachments to and dependence on others is also a consequence of severe illness (Lieber et al., 1976). Patients with advanced cancer and their spouses, when asked how their relationship had changed with illness, both noted the increased need for verbal and physical expressions of affection, with greater need for physical closeness and touching, although sexual relations were less frequent because of illness.

Response of family members to a relative's advanced stage of cancer was examined by Plumb and Holland (1977). The level of depression in patients with advanced disease and their next of kin (spouse or child) were remarkably similar on the Beck Depression Inventory. The assumption is usually made that the family member is not as distressed. Staff may underestimate the distress the next of kin is experiencing in terms of depression. When patients in this study were asked to rank their concerns in order of priority, the first three were "my spouse," "my children," and "God." Next appeared "my future" and "my illness"; death was near the end of a lengthy list. These findings are supported by those of Gotay (1984), who found that concern for the spouse was central for advanced-cancer patients and their mates.

Interpersonal relationships with medical personnel also take on increased meaning at this stage of disease for the patient. Medical staff should be aware of the importance to the patient of even casual interactions. This explains, in part, the highly compliant and uncomplaining manner of many patients with advanced cancer, who fear that expression of anger might alienate those persons they most need. A change of doctors, because new specialists may be required for treatment, is particularly distressing and frightening at this point. Patients' dependency on the physician for their treatment equips them poorly to express their discontent or fear of change. Thoughtful preparation for each change of staff allows for anticipation and adjustment. Assurance that the present and proposed specialist will coordinate efforts promotes a sense of security that there will be continuity of care.

## The Search For Alternative Treatments

The need to explore alternative unproven remedies is apt to be considered when it is discovered that the disease is unresponsive to traditional treatment (Schmale, 1976). Awareness that traditional medicine has failed, coupled with the fears of advancing disease, the sense of helplessness, and the need to reestablish mastery of their situation, contribute to the interest in alternative treatments (see Chapter 42). Well-meaning colleagues, friends, and relatives feel responsible for telling the patient about all extant cancer "cures" and their anecdotal successes. Today, these remedies tend to be naturalistic, purporting to support the body's own defenses, and thus aiding the fight against cancer. Nutritional approaches with the use of vitamins, vaccines that build the immune system, and psychological techniques to stop tumor growth by visual imagery all reflect our culture's contention that one can control disease by means of mind–body links. This distraught patient and family cannot separate the valid from the invalid approaches, especially in the psychological area, because they are torn between what they perceive as the inevitability of the cancer's course and the need to feel they have done or tried everything to save themselves or a family member.

Physicians who treat cancer patients should understand the compelling emotional need of patients to pursue such remedies. They should encourage discussion of the facts about treatments of interest without being judgmental or punitive (Holland, 1981). This should include pointing out alternative opportunities to participate in the trials of new and promising treatments under investigation, in which ethical guidelines provided by federal and institutional regulations are carefully followed to protect the patients' rights. No treatment is assumed to be efficacious without some evidence from research laboratories; no claims are made that cannot be substantiated. These basic tenets, required of new traditional therapies, are not held by those who support alternative therapies. Many patients are comforted by the thought of helping future patients, if not clearly themselves. This altruism is apparent in many patients.

## Psychological Exhaustion of Protracted, Severe Illness

Treatment of the life-threatening complications of cancer is common, even when effective control of the tumor is not possible. Bleeding, infection, and organ failure occur and are often treated successfully with the outstanding supportive care available in many hospitals and cancer centers. A patient may appear preterminal, only to have a complication successfully treated and return to the prior level of illness. The treatment may entail periods in an intensive care unit, on dialysis, or receiving courses of antibiotics or transfusions of platelets, leukocytes, or whole blood. Such events are becoming an expected part of treatment, with increasing numbers of patients living over protracted periods with more severe levels of illness. Many patients begin to show demoralization and emotional exhaustion with protracted illness of this kind. Withdrawal and apathy are common.

In the context of the physical symptoms of fatigue and weakness, depression is common, varying from mild to severe. The data of Bukberg and colleagues (1984), showed that severe depressive symptoms were more apt to appear in the advanced stages of illness. The prevalence, diagnosis, and management of depression in cancer patients is reviewed in Chapter 23.

When patients require treatment in the Intensive Care Unit, families undergo great stress; despite their concern, they are excluded from the bedside and isolated from the patient who may be comatose or intermittently awake. They struggle with the dilemma of whether to prepare for the patient's death, recovery, or improvement with permanently altered physical or mental function. They live in a state of limbo and uncertainty that may be drawn out over days or even weeks. Staff members' communications take on enormous meaning as families anxiously await each minute-to-minute report. Information received from several individuals can lead to needless "yo-yo-ing" of their emotions, because the families are oversensitive to nuances of tones of voice and expressions of face in relation to their relative's condition. Limiting the number of staff who give reports provides greater stability for families.

## TERMINAL ILLNESS AND DEATH

The factors that influence a patient's response to terminal illness and death are the same as those that prevailed earlier in the illness, except that there is an escalation in the intensity of both the psychological and the medical problems. Weisman (1975) has pointed out that the concerns of the dying are the same as those of the living, except that the dying must bear the added strains, both physical and mental, of being "sick unto death." The psychological issues are complex. At times, a psychiatric consultant can be helpful in clarifying issues. A legal and bioethical consultant is also most apt to be needed at this stage. The opportunity to request review by an Ethics Committee can be helpful when conflict arises.

The issues now have the same relevance as those of the earlier illness: ability to cope with stress, the unique perception and meaning of death to the individual, presence of a close tie to another person(s), and availability of physical care that can be given by family are all important. At this point, value judgments of the patients, family, and physician, as well as the medical reality, begin to play a role in decisions about care.

How aggressively treatment will be pursued, how long life supports will be continued, and where the person will be best treated require these judgments.

## RESPONSES TO TERMINAL ILLNESS

People's philosophy about death reflect their longstanding approach to both living and dying. The philosophy is usually abiding, evident far earlier in life, and may explain the homily that "people die as they have lived." Those who have depended on religion will likely depend even more on it at this stage. Those who have other value systems that give meaning to life and death will reexamine them, as the existential issues are put into bold relief. The period is one in which profound emotions are evoked. Although responses to dying may include acceptance in some and decathexis in others, there is no single pattern of response nor should it be anticipated or encouraged to occur in any particular form.

The prior partial denial continues, with acknowledgments made at one moment or another to a selected person, that death is anticipated. Such statements may be followed by a discussion with someone else of plans for a possible long-anticipated trip or an event spoken of with pleasure in hope that it might occur, suggesting that dual levels of knowledge are present. Yates et al. (1981) found a sustained sense of optimism among patients who maintained a positive outlook (despite advancing illness) during their last 3 months of life, suggesting that denial is often maintained and that hope often coexists, even within the recognition of a painful reality of advancing illness.

## PERCEPTION OF DEATH: PATIENT VERSUS PHYSICIAN

It is important to remember that the patient's perceptions of death are related closely to life cycle stage (see Chapter 3, adult, and Chapter 43, child). So are the perceptions of death by the physician, nurse, and health professional who are of young, middle, or older age which impact on the care of the patient. Indeed, Feifel (1959) showed that individuals who choose to go into medicine have greater fears of death than those who choose other professions. The young physician caring for an adolescent or young adult is more likely to share similar feelings of anger and outrage toward the prematurity of death. The closer in age and, more important, in developmental stage, that the physician is to the dying patient, the greater the possibility for his or her identification with the patient. The terminal stage of illness of a young patient may threaten the younger doctor's sense of invulnerability. The meaning is clear: "This could happen to me too." Guilt about inability to cure may lead to inappropriate use of heroic measures and life supports, and to refusal to give up when, in the view of others, the time to allow the patient to die has clearly been reached (Spikes and Holland, 1975).

The same young physician may be singularly less interested and able to mount a vigorous effort to treat the critically ill older patient. The young person sees death as appropriately coming to the older and elderly. When this perception is combined with culturally sanctioned negative views of the elderly, a callous manner may result, leading an older patient to perceive that he or she is less compassionately treated.

In another context, the middle-aged and older physician who takes care of the young patient may appear to the young person as not sharing in the "fighting spirit of never giving up." The sensitive physician must be attentive to that need among his or her young patients. The older mature physician will share with his or her older patient a similar orientation toward death, contributed to by having shared the same historical period, and sharing views toward death that make the relationship comfortable in dealing with terminal care issues.

The reactions to patient care of physician and staff and their management are discussed more extensively in Chapter 51.

## COMMUNICATION ABOUT TERMINAL ILLNESS

One of the important aspects of the art of medicine is management of terminal illness: How and when should patients be informed? The family? What and how and when? No pat answer exists for these questions. A thoughtful approach to each patient and his or her unique needs and situation is needed. Myers (1979), a physician respected for his compassionate management of this stage of illness, suggests that several questions will assure the thoughtful doctor that the humane issues have been addressed:

1. What does the patient know about his or her situation?
2. What is the patient's attitude regarding the prospect of death?
3. Does he or she have pain, and if so, is it relieved?
4. Is the patient being comforted physically, mentally, and spiritually?
5. Is the physician prepared to go "down to the wire" with the patient?
6. What is the attitude of the patient's family and how is it being dealt with?
7. Is the patient undergoing experimental study, and if so, are humanitarian principles being observed?

Guidelines for communication combine common sense, compassion, sensitivity, and knowing a patient's wishes. Cassem (1978) points out nine features of care of the dying patient that are based on observations of patients themselves: the need for competence, concern, comfort, communication, visits by children, support of family cohesion, cheerfulness, consistency, and equanimity. Latitude, however, in the management of the patient's knowledge and awareness of terminal illness has been sharply reduced in the wake of the societal attempts to develop legal guidelines for decisions. These changes are best reviewed in the context of the use since the 1950s of cardiopulmonary resuscitation and the writing of the "Do Not Resuscitate" (DNR) order.

## PSYCHOLOGICAL ISSUES AND THE "DO NOT RESUSCITATE" (DNR) ORDER

When seen from a historical perspective, the issue of DNR comes after generations of physicians who have traditionally had little to offer except to make the dying patient more comfortable. Few "heroic" measures were available for sustaining life until the 1950s when it became clear that in cases of cardiac arrest in an otherwise healthy individual, for example, after drowning or electrical shock, the heart could be restarted by external cardiac massage. Later, cardiopulmonary resuscitation (CPR) procedures were developed and the application of CPR spread to all patients in hospitals and those receiving emergency care (Table 6-4). Decisions about when to use CPR, and how aggressively to try to sustain life were viewed as the physician's responsibility, and it was regarded as unethical to place such a burden on the patient and family. The decisions were rarely discussed privately and never publicly. Over the past 25 years, the development of life-sustaining techniques has been so remarkable that fears have arisen that our technology has leaped ahead of our ability to handle the ethical and moral questions that arise from these advances. There has also been a significant change in the view of society about how these decisions should be made, brought about by the parallel development of increasing technology and societal demands for patient participation in treatment decisions, including decisions about terminal care and resuscitation.

In 1965 the first public decision about DNR was announced in England. It was decided not to resuscitate certain elderly patients if they had a cardiac arrest or stopped breathing, because of the medical costs, the age of the patients, and the stage of the disease. This led to an enormous public outcry against these "death squads." In the United States the issue was discussed, but the law and custom continued to forbid "predeter-

**Table 6-4**  "Do not resuscitate" (DNR) history

| Time period | Status |
| --- | --- |
| Before 1950s | Few "heroic" measures available |
| After 1960s | External cardiac massage, then cardiopulmonary resuscitation (CPR) |
| 1965 | In England, certain elderly identified not to be resuscitated |
| | In United States, custom forbade "predetermination" regarding CPR |
| | Surreptitious lists kept: no notes in chart |
| 1974 | AMA proposed that decisions not to resuscitate be placed in chart |
| 1976 | Karen Quinlan case decision |
| 1976 | Massachusetts general hospital and Beth Israel hospital developed DNR guidelines |
| 1982–1983 | Report of President's Commission on Ethical Problems in Medicine |

mination" of a decision about whether resuscitation would be performed for a particular patient. However, in order to communicate physicians' decisions to other staff members, surreptitious lists were kept indicating the level of care appropriate for different critically ill patients, including those who should not be resuscitated. These were usually entered on blackboards in nursing stations, or by a symbol on a chart and no entries about such decisions were written in the patient's chart. The responsible physician often did not discuss the decision with nurses or house staff.

In 1976 two hospitals in Boston, Beth Israel and Massachusetts General Hospital, in a single issue of the *New England Journal of Medicine,* described guidelines adopted by their physicians. In each case they determined that a DNR order must be written in the patient's chart (Rabkin et al., 1976; Pontoppidian, 1976). At Massachusetts General Hospital, decisions regarding terminal care were referred to an Optimum Care Committee for the Hopelessly Ill, which determined levels of care to be given and also intervened as advisers when disagreements occurred (Pontoppidian, 1976). The editorial that accompanied these two articles was entitled "Terminating Life Supports—Out of the Closet!" The article by Rabkin and colleagues noted that, although the policy had not been tested legally, it was their decision to require that the DNR order be written in the chart and in the order book after discussion with the patient and family. In the same year, there was wide publicity surrounding the Karen Quinlan case, in which the decision of the court was that the respirator could be unplugged and life support for this young woman terminated, following review by a panel of physicians who had agreed on prognosis.

The panel review method was the beginning of the institutional ethics committees. Since then, other states have developed "natural death" laws supporting this position. In 1983, the President's Commission on Ethical Problems in Medicine encouraged hospitals to make public their "no code policies." Since that time, many teaching hospitals have developed and implemented DNR guidelines.

In 1984 12 eminent physicians, whose clinical work included care of many fatally ill patients, defined the physician's responsibility toward hopelessly ill patients (Wanzer et al., 1984). They provided a clear review of the issues and problems involved in terminal care and put them forth in the context of both medical and social change. They highlighted three major issues of concern in the clinical setting of DNR: the patient's role in the decision making, the physician's role in the decision making, and the nature of the communication between doctor, patient, and family about the decisions.

## THE PATIENT'S ROLE IN DECISION MAKING

Legal decisions have supported the right of patients to make decisions about their own medical care and to refuse life-sustaining treatment. This right, however, is assumed to be exercised in the context of three conditions: first, that the diagnosis, treatment, and prognosis are firmly established; second, that the physician is sensitive and skilled; third, and most important, that the patient has mental capacity to make decisions. Unfortunately, these three conditions are often difficult to establish with certainty. It is helpful when the patient has prepared a "living will" so that his or her wishes are known as well as the person who is to act as a proxy on behalf of the patient has been identified. Although the legal status of such documents is still unclear, they are respected by most physicians.

Discussions with patients should occur as early as possible because, as they become more ill, ability to participate in decisions is likely to fluctuate markedly due to confusion related to drugs, organ failure, and central nervous system complications. There are several problems that may impair or suggest that the patient's ability to make a decision is impaired:

1. A delirium that alters judgment or results in inability to understand the facts of the situation
2. Presence of a depression severe enough that it may alter judgment
3. The patient's frequent self-contradiction in decision making, an excessive indecisiveness that suggests lack of competent judgment
4. Excessive fear of intubation, cardioresuscitation, or the intensive care unit, often as a consequence of

having seen other patients undergo these measures or having personally experienced them, and resulting in a judgment based on fear

5. Problems between the patient and the family about the DNR
6. Mild mental retardation
7. Long-standing psychiatric illness

A judgment of capacity (or lack of it) to participate in a decision must be entered in the chart. Guidelines today often require the judgment of two physicians, one of whom is a psychiatrist.

## PHYSICIAN'S ROLE IN DECISION MAKING

The physician, central to the decision making, must first of all be confident about the medical grounds for the decision not to resuscitate. Wanzer and colleagues (1984) agreed that a "decrease in aggressive treatment of the hopelessly ill patient is advisable when such treatment would only prolong a difficult and uncomfortable process of dying." The need for such a decision arises when one or more of the four following conditions is met: that further treatment is futile, that the patient wishes a DNR order, that the quality of life is unacceptable, or that the cost is too great. One of the problems, especially in a teaching hospital, is the subjective nature of these four points and that there may be conflict among staff members about the interpretation of medical data. However, when the physician feels secure about the decision, based on medical facts, he then has the obligation to present the issues to the patient in as kind and sensitive way as possible.

There are several problems that make it difficult for the physician to deal with both a decision concerning DNR and the discussion of DNR options with the patient.

1. Concerns about malpractice and legal issues can stand in the way of reaching what may be a clear medical decision.
2. Limited bed space in intensive care units leads to agonizing decisions about who can be transferred there after resuscitation.
3. There may be uncertainty and disagreement about prognosis and whether a further treatment is or is not entirely futile, underscoring the difficulty in making a clear decision.
4. Such decisions often seem contrary to medical training. Physicians are taught to be aggressive in their approach to care, and they often perceive the decision to institute comfort care as a decision to give up. In a sense, they must abandon the stance that they have been taught to take and which they contracted with the patient to assume. Some physi-

cians perceive the decision as a failure of medicine and of themselves.

5. Patients with cancer who come to major cancer centers for care have a strong determination to "fight to the end." They have already made the decision for aggressive, even experimental treatment by seeking such care, and inherent in that decision is a determination to fight to the end despite poor odds.

## COMMUNICATION BETWEEN DOCTOR AND PATIENT ABOUT DNR

Given a competent patient, and that a decision about DNR is appropriate, there are then issues about how information necessary for informed decision making is communicated to the patient. Questions concerning how much information a patient should have, when it should be given, and how to discuss it, are central. These questions are so profound that many physicians find reasons not to discuss the matter at all. In the Bedell and Delbanco (1984) study, carried out in the Beth Israel Hospital in Boston, where the first guidelines were promulgated in 1976, only 19% of patients who were successfully resuscitated and who were mentally competent stated that they had actually been asked about DNR, despite explicit guidelines set by the hospital requiring prior discussion of such action. A repeat of the survey done at the same hospital found that physicians frequently continued to delay the discussion until the patient was too ill to participate, with the result that patient participation in the decision continued to be low (Bedell et al., 1986).

The justification doctors give for not communicating about this issue included several common:

1. This patient really had "told me in other ways by nonverbal means, and therefore I didn't have to discuss it with him."
2. "I knew what the patient wanted."
3. "It was very hard to discuss the painful prospects with him."
4. "I wanted to protect the patient."
5. "I prefer to rely on the family who know the patient best."
6. "I felt the patient couldn't stand it; he would be too upset."
7. "I can never find the *right* time to do it."

Wanzer and colleagues (1984) concluded that both physicians and families avoid frank discussions with the patient, but that practically all patients, even disturbed ones, are better off knowing and having a frank discussion of the issue. The decision not to discuss DNR issues on emotional grounds should be extremely

**Table 6-5**  Communication with patient

Fear of emotionally harming patient is rarely justified.
Give only as much information as the patient wants.
Discuss use of life-prolonging treatment *early*, in ongoing
  physician–patient relationship.
Discussion conducted by person who knows patient best.
Continue the communication process while monitoring patient's
  reactions.
Do not destroy hope; listen to patient's doubts and fears.
Ascertain that conditions of informed consent have been met.

rare; it is usually harder for patients to anticipate the unknown than to have some clear idea of what is happening to them (Table 6-5). Efforts to protect the patient or family member have a tendency also to isolate them from the rest of the family and the doctor and reflect beliefs held in the earlier period when even the diagnosis of cancer was withheld.

Ideally it is desirable to have discussed these issues with the patient well before a critical episode of illness occurs. Some hospitals have materials available for patients and families about code versus no code to explain what it is and asks them to raise questions they may have about it. New York state, since April, 1988, has required hospitals to have booklets available. It will surely be easier for a physician to bring up if it appears that the patient already knows something about it. Initial discussion with a patient upon admission of the issue through statements such as, "and if treatments do not work, as happens sometimes, we will need to discuss how you feel about treatments aimed at just sustaining life." "Individuals vary in their philosophy about these issues. I need to know yours." Initiation of life support measures should be considered as any other procedure for which the patient has the right to understand and to give informed consent. In this context, one uses the guidelines to establish that the patient has the capacity to understand, and does understand the risks, benefits, prognosis, and alternatives, and can make the decision without coercion. Discussion about DNR options becomes easier.

The doctor's attitude is crucial to ensure that a discussion of DNR is not perceived by the patient as abandonment. In fact, the patient must be assured of continuing care, with discussion of the specific measures, beyond DNR, which will and will not be employed. This can vary from full efforts to comfort care only. The responsible physician must indicate a therapeutic plan to reduce ambiguity for nurses and house staff when he writes a DNR order which includes a description in the progress notes of which measures are to be continued and which withdrawn (e.g., antibiotics, nutrition, oxygen, blood products).

It is normal to feel self-conscious about giving such dire information. However, this should not interfere with a sense of sincere concern. Guilt at having failed the patient, fear that the patient will lose control, and concerns about what to say are all problems that can lead to less sensitive presentation of the issues. Nobody wants to give bad news.

In planning how best to carry out a discussion of life support options with the patient, there are several points to remember. First, it is important to sit down, appear unhurried, establish eye contact that shows concern and sensitivity, and allows one to observe how the patient is reacting as the discussion ensues. While the exact words used will be determined by each individual, the discussion must be conducted in such a way as not to destroy all hope. By the same token, it must also convey the situation accurately: "Although you are all right today, you may reach a point where certain treatments that have significant risks and side effects may be needed. I am reluctant to institute these without first discussing them with you. We want you to be comfortable. There is a question of whether or not you would want resuscitation should you require it. We are going to do all that we can, but we need to know your feelings about this."

The DNR Committee at Memorial Sloan-Kettering developed a film with the support of the American Cancer Society that shows a typical scenario in the hospital of a patient who appears unlikely to survive resuscitation with any acceptable quality of life. The doctor's and hospital staff's dilemma about the DNR discussion describe the ramifications of the issues. It finally demonstrates a sensitive and compassionate model of communication about the DNR order with the patient (Carle Medical Communications, 1987).

It is important to listen to questions and to be sensitive to the concerns voiced. The doctor should be ready to respond to the question, "What would you do, Doctor?" The physician can reassure the patient by saying, "While I will continue to make the medical judgments, I want input from you." After the discussion, it is important to return for frequent visits to ensure that they understand that no abandonment was implied and to determine how they responded to the impact of what was said.

Finally, the interview with the family should include a discussion of the patient's prognosis and the patient's wishes. Here again, it is important to listen to the concerns raised. Family members who feel guilty about prior problems and conflicts or who choose to deny the realities of the situation can be real problems in such dialogues. The conflict that is most often seen is between the family that wishes the doctor to do everything and the doctor who feels that the issue, based on medical data, should be resolved in favor of no resuscitation, especially when such efforts will only prolong the act of dying.

Two studies at the Beth Israel Hospital in Boston examined their cardioresuscitation experience in relation to the application of DNR guidelines. The first, carried out in 1983, looked at 294 patients who were resuscitated (Bedell et al., 1983). Only 14% of the total number were discharged. However, of those, 70% had an intact mental status. Although they were profoundly depressed at the time of discharge, these individuals had a normal mood and no psychiatric impairment at 6 months. The patients with the worst prognosis were those who at the time of resuscitation had pneumonia, hypotension, renal failure, cancer (only 7% survival), homebound life-style, intubation (91% mortality), or longer than 15 minutes arrest time (95% mortality).

The second study, reported in 1984, examined doctors' attitudes and philosophy. Results of this study noted that most interviewed physicians (91%) and house officers felt that patients should at least sometimes participate in decisions about CPR (Bedell and Delbanco, 1984). In actual practice, however, 49% of the doctors and 67% of the house officers had spoken to neither the patient nor the family prior to CPR. In the case of 24 mentally competent patients who were interviewed later, it was revealed that the doctors had correctly perceived those who wished CPR, but they had incorrectly perceived those 5 patients who stated that, had they been asked, they would have not wanted to be resuscitated.

DNR issues are of great concern in cancer centers where, increasingly, hospitalized patients are largely those who are seriously ill. In two surveys done at Memorial Sloan-Kettering, clinical judgment, based on chart review of 100 medical oncology patients, suggested that about 20% more patients should have had a DNR order than the 20% that was documented in the chart at two weeks after admission (T. Hakes, personal communication). The issue is being increasingly raised as to whether, in patients such as those with cancer, resuscitation should be offered when the physician considers it medially unfeasible but offers it because of the right of autonomy. Blackhall (1987), following review of studies of survival after resuscitation, found patients with underlying extensive cancer to have received virtually no survival advantage from CPR. There is need for discussion of the obligation to offer CPR when it has no chance of benefit in the physician's opinion.

Staff education is needed to ensure the successful and sensitive implementation of life support guidelines. Nurses are particularly vulnerable to distress when physicians procrastinate in making a judgment about DNR, leaving them from shift to shift without a clear management plan. The potential for conflict among nurse, house staff, and attending physician in a teaching hospital is great. Ethics committees at times play a mediating as well as consultative and educational role. Psychiatrists also play a consultative role, determining capacity and when, on those rare occasions, it would "do harm" to discuss DNR with a patient. DNR guidelines, as outlined by Younger (1987), should include the following: documentation with regular review, specification of the nature of the treatment to be withheld, patient and family participation, nurses and staff understanding of the decision and the plan of treatment, and that it not be equivalent of medical or psychological abandonment.

## PSYCHIATRIC CONSULTATION FOR THE TERMINALLY ILL

The most commonly cited reasons for requesting a psychiatric consultation for patients during terminal stages are the following (Massie et al., 1983).

### Competency Evaluation

A psychiatrist may be called in to determine the patient's capacity to consent to a procedure, including DNR. It is necessary that the patient have enough understanding of the nature of the proposed procedure and its consequences to be able to make an independent decision.

### Presence of Delirium

A psychiatric consultation is often required whenever there is agitated or disruptive behavior. A determination of the cause, if possible, is required, and a combined psychological intervention with the patient, family, and staff with, if needed, behavior management by the use of psychotropic drugs. Delirium is a common problem and reflects the frequency with which the CNS is impaired in terminal illness by hypoxia, metabolic derangement, infections, bleeding, and drug side effects (see Chapters 29 and 30 on delirium and dementia).

### Suicidal Risk

When patients experience severe discomfort or pain, expressions of "I'd rather be dead" or "If I could jump, I would" may be heard as expressions of frustration. Actual suicide attempts are unusual, but the risk must be evaluated. Patients at highest risk are those who are depressed, mildly confused, and agitated, in which normally controlled impulses may be acted out.

Feeble but, at time, serious attempts may be made. We have encountered suicide attempts in terminally ill patients in whom cerebral hypoxia and hypercalcemia have been causes of encephalopathy. Often, in terminal illness, the risk is discussed with family and physician and one-to-one nursing is employed, along with low-dose haloperidol for management of the confusional state. Suicide, when it does occur in terminal illness, is often not predicted and appears to be impulsively motivated (see Chapter 4 on suicide).

## Staff Conflict

When decisions about terminal care have not been fully shared with the individuals who must implement them, a conflict arises, usually between doctor and nurse. The nurse may be ordered to administer a medication that she or he feels will hasten dying, or to give a medication or procedure to prolong life when she or he sees no reason to do so. Similar conflicts occur between the house staff and the attending physician. Both situations may reflect less than adequate communication and result in difficulty in resolving differences about complex and uncertain situations. Judgments in terminal care are rarely clearly defined and absolute, and discussion of issues is important in maintaining good morale on units where death is frequent.

## Family Conflict

Decisions about "letting the patient go" or "fighting on" are painful judgments made daily in intensive care units. Family members are now drawn into the decisions more fully, leading at times to conflicts with staff when the family insist on a course the staff feel is not medically indicated. Family members may also be divided among themselves about the choice. They may become angry and blame one another.

## Multispecialty Problems

The patient's level and complexity of illness may require numerous specialists as consultants. Each specialist tends to see the problem in terms of the needed specialization. One consultant may blame another for missing a diagnosis or introducing treatment that causes a complication. Anger and blame can ensue, causing disruption for patient, family, and staff alike.

## Fluctuating Terminal Course

When a patient has been near death (sometimes more than once) and temporarily gets better, staff and family (having emotionally prepared for death) may seem to withdraw from the patient. Their emotions may seem to be "out of sync."

## Management of Pain and Sedation

Problems with pain are experienced by 60% of terminally ill patients with cancer. In addition to pain, the patient may have extreme fearfulness, anxiety, and distress related to shortness of breath, weakness, or awareness of deteriorating function. It may be necessary to introduce careful titration of drugs for sedation and analgesia. This must be planned with minimal compromise of vital functions and requires special attention to the interaction between specific psychotropic drugs and analgesics (see Psychopharmacology, Chapter 39).

## Management of Depression and Anxiety

These two emotions dominate the psychological picture during end-stage disease; each will need careful attention to determine psychological and medical state and the need for counseling and drug management.

## TALKING TO THE TERMINALLY ILL PATIENT

It is helpful for the person who attempts to counsel or offer support to a fatally ill person to keep several points in mind:

1. *Remember that the patient is the same person he or she was before the illness.* The primary concerns are the same as in earlier stages of the illness, only now they are intensified and tinged with the grief of anticipated loss and separation. Being a good listener and asking questions that allow the patient to tell you what he or she was like before the illness, as suggested by Weisman (1975), make the interviewer more comfortable and offer the staff a fresh view of the very ill person. The stigma assigned to the label of "dying" should not alter communication. Only the physical status, not the person, has changed. An observation about the person's courage in the face of a difficult situation conveys understanding and support.

2. *A quiet, unhurried manner is important, even though the visit may be short.* A 20-minute visit is often long for an ill patient. Shorter visits may be necessary if fatigue is evident. The conversation should also be sensitive to the person's mood, allowing for discussion of their concerns.

3. *Physical affections as communication is important.* Touching the person and showing feeling by a pat on the arm or by holding his or her hand often conveys an understanding that cannot be expressed in words.

4. *"Am I dying?"* and *"How long will I live?"* are

questions from the patient that cause anxiety in the staff, because they may not know how to respond. The result may be avoidance of the dying patient. It is helpful to recognize that a positive or negative answer or a definite time frame is not necessary and may not even be wanted. Asking the patient about their emotional state and identifying the patient's primary concerns are important. By no means do all patients want to discuss dying. From our experience many patients do not, or, if they do, they will select a family member who knows them well with whom to share their feelings. The popularity of books and discussions about death has led some young students to assume that they have not done an adequate job with a patient who is dying if they have not attempted to discuss death. Although the opportunity should be made available and the staff member must feel able to respond if the patient wants to talk, most patients will not wish to share such intimate feelings with a staff member unless they know the person well. They may choose a single individual with whom to speak about these issues, while maintaining denial of them with others. The chosen person may be a clergyman, a family member, or a member of the health care team. Respect for patients' need for privacy about their feelings concerning death is as important in care as open and full communication.

5. *For a person who visits a terminally ill patient, the proper demeanor is important.* A superficially cheery attitude, which appears to negate the seriousness of the situation, is not appropriate. The "gloom and doom" look, however, is also unwelcome. The approach to the patient should show respect and concern for the situation, and should reflect a willingness to speak of shared interests or other aspects of the patient's life without focus on illness.

6. *Unhurried companionship is the type of interaction needed.* Archbishop Coggan (1977), a noted theologian, put this into perspective when he wrote:

Death in the western world is more lonely than in eastern cultures where one dies surrounded by family. Death should not be lonely. . . . A man as he comes to die should have around him not only the apparatus of modern technical medicine designed to extend his life or to ease his physical suffering, but also the unhurried companionship of people who are not frightened by the fact of death and are prepared to go with the man concerned as far as they may to the point of his departure.

## SUMMARY

Each stage of cancer creates its own constellation of psychological problems that must be understood in order to be able to offer proper support and guidance through diagnosis and treatment. The advanced stages of disease, irrespective of site, are associated with a greater likelihood of pain, distressing symptoms, and existential concerns that must be addressed in management. Terminal illness care must consider the use of life-sustaining interventions and the patient and family's wishes vis-à-vis their use. Discussion of resuscitation with the patient and family requires great sensitivity, and review with nurses and staff is necessary to outline a treatment plan and to avoid any perception of abandonment.

## REFERENCES

Beauchamp, T.L. and J.F. Childress (1983). The principle of autonomy [I. Conceptual Foundations: A Informed Consent]. In N. Abrams and M.D. Buckner (eds.), *Medical Ethics: A Clinical Textbook and References for the Health Care Professions.* Cambridge, Mass.: MIT Press, pp. 3–12.

Bedell, S.E. and T.L. Delbanco (1984). Choices about cardiopulmonary resuscitation in the hospital: When do physicians talk with patients? *N. Engl. J. Med.* 310:1089–93.

Bedell, S.E., T.L. Delbanco, E.F. Cook, and F.H. Epstein (1983). Survival after cardiopulmonary resuscitation in the hospital. *N. Engl. J. Med.* 309:569–76.

Bedell, S.E., D. Pelle, P.L. Maher, and P.D. Cleary (1986). Do-not-resuscitate orders for critically ill patients in the hospital. How are they used and what is their impact? *J.A.M.A.* 256:233–37.

Blackhall, L.J. (1987). Must we always use CPR? N.E.J.M. 317:1281–1285.

Brennan, S., Redd, W.H., Jacobsen, P., Schorr, O., Heelan, R.T., Sze, G.K., Kroe, G., Peters, B.E., & Morrissey, J.K. (1988). Anxiety and panic during magnetic resonance scans. The Lancet, p. 512.

Bukburg, J., D. Penman, and J.C. Holland (1984). Depression in hospitalized cancer patients. *Psychosom. Med.* 46:199–212.

Caplan, G. (1981). Mastery of stress: Psychosocial aspects. *Am. J. Psychiatry* 138:413–20.

Carle Medical Communications (1987). The DNR Dilemma (Videotape). Urbana, IL.

Cassem, N.H. (1978). The dying patient. In T.P. Hackett and N.H. Cassem (eds.), *Massachusetts General Hospital: Handbook of General Hospital Psychiatry.* St. Louis: C.V. Mosby, pp. 300–318.

Cassileth, B.R., R.V. Zupkis, K. Sutton-Smith, and V. March (1980). Information and participation preferences among cancer patients. *Ann. Intern. Med.* 92:832–36.

Cassileth, B.R., E.J. Lusk, T.B. Strouse, D.S. Millay, L.L. Brown, P.A. Cross, and A.N. Tonaglia (1984). Psychosocial status in chronic illness: A comparative analysis of six diagnostic groups. *N. Engl. J. Med.* 311:506–11.

Coggan, D. (1977). On dying well: Moral and spiritual aspects. *Proc. R. Soc. Med.* 70:71–81.

Feifel, H.J. (ed.). (1959). *The Meaning of Death.* New York: McGraw-Hill.

Gotay, C.C. (1984). The experience of cancer during early and advanced stages: The views of patients and their mates. *Soc. Sci. Med.* 18:605–13.

Henry, J. (1971). *Pathways to Madness.* New York: Random House.

Herbert, V. (1980). Informed consent: A legal evaluation. *Cancer* 46:1042–44.

Holland, J.C. (1981). Why patients seek unproven cancer remedies: A psychological perspective. *CA* 30:10–14.

Holland, J.C.B. (1982). Psychological aspects of cancer. In J.F. Holland and E. Frei III (eds.), *Cancer Medicine,* 2nd ed. Philadelphia: Lea & Febiger, pp. 1175–1203.

Holland, J.C., A. Marchini, and S. Tross (1986). An international survey of physician practices in regard to revealing the diagnosis of cancer. *Fourteenth Int. Cancer Congr. Abstr. Lect. Symp. Free Commun.,* Vol. 3 Basel: Karger (Abstract No. 3964).

Leiber, L., M. Plumb, M. Gerstenzang, and J. Holland (1976). The communication of affection between cancer patients and their spouses. *Psychosom. Med.* 38: 379–89.

Massie, M.J., J.C. Holland, and E. Glass (1983). Delirium in terminally ill patients. *Am. J. Psychiatry* 140:1048–50.

McCorkle, R. and J. Quint-Benoliel (1983). Symptom distress, current concerns and mood disturbance after diagnosis of life-threatening disease. *Soc. Sci. Med.* 17:431–38.

Morrow, G.R. (1980). How readable are subject consent forms? *J.A.M.A.* 244:56–58.

Morrow, G.R. and A.C. Hoagland (1981). Physician–patient communications in cancer treatment. *Proc. Am. Cancer Soc. Third Natl. Conf. on Human Values and Cancer,* Washington, D.C., April 23–25, pp. 27–37.

Morrow, G.R., M. Feldstein, L.M. Adler, L.R. Derogatis, A.J. Enelow, C. Gates, J.C. Holland, N. Melesaratos, B.J. Murawski, D. Penman, A. Schmale, M. Schmitt, and I. Morse (1981). Development of brief measures of psychosocial adjustment to medical illness applied to cancer patients. *Gen. Hosp. Psychiatry* 3:79–88.

Myers, W.P.L. (1979). The care of the patient with terminal illness. In P.B. Beeson, W. McDermott, and J.B. Wyngaarden (eds.), *Cecil Textbook of Medicine,* 15th ed. Philadelphia: W.B. Saunders, pp. 1941–48.

Novack, D.H., R. Plumer, R.L. Smith, H. Ochtill, G.R. Morrow, and J.M. Bennett (1979). Changes in physicians' attitudes toward telling the cancer patient. *J.A.M.A.* 241:897–900.

Oken, D. (1961). What to tell cancer patients: A study of medical attitudes. *J.A.M.A.* 175:1120–28.

Penman, D.T. (1980). Coping strategies in adaptation to mastectomy. Doctoral dissertation, Yeshiva University, 1979. *Diss. Abstr. Int.* 40:5825 B.

Penman, D.T., J.C. Holland, G.F. Bahna, G.R. Morrow, A.H. Schmale, L.R. Derogatis, C.L. Carnrike, and R. Cherry (1984). Informed consent for investigational chemotherapy: Patients' and physicians' perceptions. *J. Clin. Oncol.* 2:849–55.

Plumb, M. and J. Holland (1977). Comparative studies of psychological function in patients with advanced cancer. 1. Self-reported depressive symptoms. *Psychosom. Med.* 39:264–76.

Pontoppidian, H. (1976). Optimum care for hopelessly ill patients: A report of the Clinical Care Committee of the Massachusetts General Hospital. *N. Engl. J. Med.* 295:362–64.

Rabkin, M.T., G. Gillerman, and N.R. Rice (1976). Orders not to resuscitate. *N. Engl. J. Med.* 295:364–66.

Redding, K., L. Beutler, S. Jones, F. Meyskens, and T. Moon (1981). Psychosocial attitudes of cancer patients treated with lactrile or other phase II agents [Abstract C-243]. *Proc. Seventy-Second Annu. Mtg. Am. Assoc. Cancer Res. and Seventeenth Annu. Mtg. Am. Soc. Clin. Oncol.* 22:394.

Robinson, G. and A. Merav (1976). Informed consent: Recall by patients tested postoperatively. *Ann. Thorac. Surg.* 22:209–12.

Rosenbaum, E.H., I.R. Rosenbaum, A. Sweet, and A. Mohr (1981). Audio aids in improving communications with patients. *Proc. Am. Cancer Soc. Third Natl. Conf. on Human Values and Cancer,* Washington, D.C., April 23–25, pp. 51–57.

Schmale, A. (1976). Psychological reactions to recurrent metastasis or dissemination cancer. *Int. J. Radiat. Oncol. Biol. Phys.* 1:515–20.

Scott, D.W. (1983). Anxiety, critical thinking and information processing during and after breast biopsy. *Nurs. Res.* 32:24–29.

Schwartz, H.I. and K. Blank (1986). Shifting competency during hospitalization: A model for informed consent decisions. *Hosp. Community Psychiatry* 37:1256–60.

Shands, H.C., J.E. Finesinger, S. Cobb, and R.D. Abrams (1951). Psychological mechanisms in patients with cancer. *Cancer* 4:1159–70.

Spikes, J. and J. Holland (1975). The physician's response to the dying patient. In J.J. Strain and S. Grossman (eds.), *Psychological Care of the Medically Ill.* New York: Appleton-Century-Crofts.

Spingarn, N.D. (1982). *Hanging in There, Living Well on Borrowed Time.* New York: Stein & Day.

Taylor, S.E. (1982). *Adjustment to Threatening Events: A Theory of Cognitive Adaptation.* Unpublished manuscript, Tenth Katz-Newcomb Lecture, University of Michigan, Ann Arbor.

Tross, S., J.C. Holland, D. Hirsch, M. Schiffman, J. Gold, B. Safai, and P. Myskowski (1986). *Psychological and Social Impact of AIDS Spectrum Disorders.* CDC Int. Conf. on AIDS, Atlanta, Ga.

U.S. President's Commission for the Study of Ethical Problems in Medicine and Biomedical and Behavioral Research (1983). *Deciding to Forego Life-Sustaining Treatment.* Washington, D.C.: U.S. Govt. Printing Office.

Wanzer, S.H., S.J. Adelstein, R.E. Cranford, D.D. Federman, E.D. Hook, C.G. Moertel, P. Safar, A. Stone, H.B. Taussig, and J. Van Eys (1984). The physician's responsibility toward hopelessly ill patients. *N. Engl. J. Med.* 310:955–59.

Weisman, A.D. (1975). The dying patient. In R.O. Pasnau (ed.), *Consultation–Liaison Psychiatry.* New York: Grune & Stratton, pp. 237–44.

Weisman, A.D. (1979a). *Coping with Cancer.* New York: McGraw-Hill.

Weisman, A.D. (1979b). A model for psychosocial phasing in cancer. *Gen. Hosp. Psychiatry* 3:187–95.

Weisman, A.D. and J.W. Worden (1976). The existential plight in cancer: Significance of the first 100 days. *Int. J. Psychiatry Med.* 7:1–15.

Weisman, A.D. and J.W. Worden (1986). The emotional impact of recurrent cancer. *J. Psychosoc. Ongol.* 3:5–16.

Wieder, S., J. Schwarzfeld, J. Fromewick, and J.C. Holland (1978). Team effort: Psychosocial support program for patients with breast cancer at Montefiore Hospital. *Q.R.B.* 4(1):10–13.

Yates, J.W., F.P. McKegney, and L.E. Kun (1981). A comparative study of home nursing care of patients with advanced cancer. *Proc. Am. Cancer Soc. Third Natl. Conf. on Human Values and Cancer,* pp. 207–18.

Younger, S.J. (1987). Do-not-resuscitate orders: No longer a secret, but still a problem. *Hastings Cent. Rep.* 17:24–33.

# 7

## Psychological Sequelae In Cancer Survivors

Susan Tross and Jimmie C. Holland

Advances in detection and treatment have transformed cancer from a nearly uniformly fatal disease to one that is often curable. The current 5-year survival rate for all sites of cancer combined is greater than 50% (National Cancer Institute, 1984); earlier in this century, it was only 10%. There are now over 3 million individuals in the United States who are 5-year cancer survivors; most of these former patients can consider themselves cured. For some neoplasms, especially Hodgkin's disease, testicular, endometrial, cervical, and several childhood malignancies (e.g., acute lymphocytic leukemia, Wilms' tumor, osteogenic sarcoma), the overwhelming majority of patients may look forward to cure.

This dramatic progress in cancer treatment has given the behavioral sciences one of its happiest tasks: the description and monitoring of the psychological sequelae among patients who have come so close to the prospect of death. The earliest research on survivors focused on the delayed effects of treatment that were of concern to medical oncology proper: second malignancies and organ system dysfunction or failure. The early psychological studies of survivors followed, with sharp differences between the psychiatric investigators who took a relatively alarmist view of the seriousness of psychological sequelae, and the epidemiologists who took a relatively "Pollyannaish" view that tended to minimize the psychological and social legacy of cancer diagnosis. The difference in findings in large part represented the difference in definition of outcome, and the way in which it was measured. The epidemiological research used survey techniques, large samples, and, in some instances, case–control comparison. They also mainly used gross social indicators (e.g., occupational or disability status, marital status, parenthood status, educational level, and socioeconomic status) to infer psychological quality of survival. The psychiatric investigators had rarely un-

dertaken systematic studies, however, their intensive case study approach did afford their work greater psychological depth. The question of whether delayed psychological effects—of cancer or its therapies—accompanied the patient into the cure period has remained debatable, although the answer is gradually emerging as more individuals survive cancer and are studied for both general psychosocial function and for more subtle forms of psychological impairment. A national conference sponsored by the American Cancer Society was devoted to review of the state-of-the art information available in 1987 on psychological, social and work problems in survivors. It provides a helpful bench mark for research in this emerging area (ACS, 1987).

In addition to scientific investigations, another source of information has come from survivors of cancer who have been increasingly willing to reveal their cancer diagnosis, to describe their personal responses to it, and to offer their own experience to help others (Spingarn, 1982; Bloch and Bloch, 1985; Mullan, 1985). Mullan described his psychological reactions to three periods after treatment that he called the "seasons of survival": acute survival immediately after completion of treatment, extended survival in which cure was hopeful but uncertain, and finally, permanent survival. Mullan felt that the increasing numbers of "extended and permanent" survivors needed a network to provide information and to serve as an advocacy group. The National Coalition of Cancer Survivors was formed in 1986. It has already brought increased public attention to the needs of cancer survivors.

Two institutions, St. Jude's Children's Cancer Research Center and Fox Chase Cancer Center, have also established an "alumni" program for their cured child and adult patients. Memorial Sloan-Kettering is the first cancer center to establish a special program in

1988 to meet the range of psychosocial, legal, and counseling needs of survivors in a special program. This clinical program is intimately associated with a research effort whose studies are aimed at the better understanding of the problems of survivors and their management.

Psychological sequelae arise in survivors from five major sources: the medical late or delayed effects of treatment, the sexual complications of treatment, the CNS complications of treatment resulting in neuropsychological late effects, the psychological responses to having had a life-threatening illness, and the practical and social complications of reentry into normal activities and work.

## MEDICAL LATE EFFECTS OF TREATMENT

Psychological sequelae results from concerns about adverse effects of treatment that do not appear until years later as well as about the chances of recurrence versus cure. Although multimodal therapy has improved survival rates, the prospect of mortality and morbidity in the 5-year period after treatment has also increased as a result of treatment-related late effects of second malignancy, organ dysfunction or failure, and infection due to immunosuppression. Table 7-1 summarizes the medical late effects reported in childhood cancer survivors, for whom the earliest cures were achieved. Survival rates of 20 years were found to be significantly lower for 5-year survivors of childhood cancer than for their peers in the general population (Li and Stone, 1976). In a pair of studies by Li (1977) and Li and co-workers (1978), risk of mortality from recurrence, second malignancy, organ failure, and infection increased between 5 and 9 years after the diagnosis, whereas risk of second malignancy peaked in the period between 15 and 19 years after the diagnosis. The incidence of developing a second malignancy by 20 years after treatment is 17%, or 20 times that of the general population (Byrd, 1983). Initial concerns about the progeny of long-term survivors in regard to cancer risk and birth defects related to teratogenicity of radiation and chemotherapy have not been borne out (Li and Jaffe, 1974). In a review of late effects in treatment of childhood cancer, Byrd (1983) noted the cardiovascular effects as among the most serious. Endocrine abnormalities that develop relate primarily to hypothalamic–pituitary axis damage, thyroid gland, and gonads (discussed later). Small stature is common with cranial irradiation of greater than 3000 rads for brain and head and neck tumors, and with CNS prophylaxis for acute leukemia as a result of failure of normal growth hormone production. Bushhouse and colleagues (1987) reported significant risk for children

**Table 7-1** Physical late effects of treatment in childhood cancer survivors

| Investigators | Tumor sites | Time from diagnosis (years) | Results |
|---|---|---|---|
| Li et al. (1975) | Mixed | 6–21 | Second malignancy in 28 of 410 survivors |
| Li (1977) | Mixed | 5–9 | Risk for mortality from recurrence, second malignancy, organ failure, or infection |
|  |  | 15–19 | Peak risk for second malignancy |
| Li et al. (1978) | Mixed | 20 | Projected survival rate for cancer survivors 78–83% (versus 97% rate for controls) |
| Li and Jaffe (1974) | Mixed | — | Normal rates of birth defects, morbidity, and mortality in offspring ($n = 92$) or pregnancies ($n = 107$) of 46 survivors |
| Thompson et al. (1987) | Mixed | >10 | 75% Normal or minor bone or soft-tissue changes from radiation |
|  |  |  | 1% Second malignancies |
|  |  |  | 6% Benign tumors |
|  |  |  | 5% Thyroid dysfunction |
|  |  |  | 12% Sterility |
|  |  |  | 2% Severe obesity |
|  |  |  | 3% Hepatic, cardiac, or pulmonary problems |
|  |  |  | 12% Lack of growth in irradiated areas |

who received body irradiation or single-dose lymphoid irradiation (750 cGy), or reduction in age-appropriate height 4 years later. Slightly greater impact was noted by the total-body irradiation. Both chemotherapy and irradiation cause interstitial pneumonitis and pulmonary fibrosis. Thompson and colleagues (1987) at St. Jude's studied 269 adolescents and young adults treated 10 years earlier for childhood tumors. Despite the risks already mentioned, 75% were normal or had only minor problems. Dobkin and Morrow (1985-1986) provided a review of the long term treatment effects which affect quality of life.

In both children and adults, irradiation or chemotherapy alone has carcinogenic effects that cause the appearance of second cancers years later. When chemotherapy and radiation are given together, the oncogenic effect appears greater than for either one alone. The most common types of radiation-induced malignancy are breast and thyroid tumors, osteogenic sarcoma, and leukemia. Alkylating agents are the cytotoxic chemotherapeutic agents that are most likely to cause second malignancies. Patients who receive both modalities, particularly survivors of Hodgkin's disease, may develop leukemia. According to a major study at Stanford University, survivors of non-Hodgkin's lymphoma and malignant melanoma were found to have a risk of second cancers of 9.9% at 10 years. Tucker and colleagues (1988) extended the follow-up to 15 years and found that there was a 17.6% cumulative risk (i.e., a sixfold excess risk) of second cancers over 15 years. Although leukemia prevalence did not rise after 10 years, occurrences of non-Hodgkin's lymphoma and solid tumors continued to increase with time, particularly lung cancer among survivors who were still smokers. These findings confirm the need for continued monitoring and counseling about smoking.

Another less dramatic but strong contributor to the quality of life in survivors is the persistence of low energy level and physical stamina in some patients. In one study, 37% of Hodgkin's disease survivors reported that they were not satisfied with their energy level at a median of 9 years after treatment (Fobair et al., 1986). Patients also appear to require long periods before stamina returns to normal after leukemia and lymphoma treatment (L.M. Lesko, personal communication).

Another persistent treatment effect was identified by Cella and co-workers (1986) in a study of Hodgkin's survivors treated by the MOPP regimen (mechlorethamine + vincristine + procarbazine + prednisone) and radiation. Among 60 patients studied 6 months to 12 years after completion of treatment, 80% reported developing a feeling of anxiety and nausea (but not vomiting) when they experienced a reminder of the prior chemotherapy treatments or the clinic. Smells (alcohol, cleaning solution, and perfume) were most apt to trigger the response, although visual and auditory cues also did (Table 7-2). This surprising persistence of a conditioned response years later suggests that the experience of cyclic chemotherapy leaves greater psychological residue than previously assumed.

Long-term cancer survivors are now followed indefinitely to monitor the development of delayed treatment effects and late recurrence of the primary tumor. Their awareness of their greater vulnerability to recurrence, a second cancer, or death is a major cause of psychological morbidity in survivors. Table 7-3 outlines the major areas from which psychological morbidity is derived: physical, psychological, and reentry problems regarding social and job concerns. Those concerns that relate to illness lie at the core of the

**Table 7-2**  Sensations eliciting nausea in Hodgkin's patients off treatment ($n = 60$ men)

| Sensation | Frequency |
|---|---|
| *Smells and tastes* | |
| Clinic/hospital smell | 19 |
| Rubbing alcohol | 16 |
| Commercial products (cleaning solutions) | 10 |
| Foods | 8 |
| Perfume | 6 |
| Other (house, New York City) | 3 |
| Total | 62 |
| *Sights, sounds, and thoughts* | |
| Clinic/hospital sight | 15 |
| Thoughts | 3 |
| Physician's voice | 1 |
| Total | 19 |

*Source*: Reprinted with permission from D.F. Cella, A. Pratt, and J.C. Holland (1986). Persistent anticipatory nausea, vomiting and anxiety in cured Hodgkin's patients after completion of chemotherapy. *Amer. J. Psychiatry* 143:641–43.

increased levels of psychological distress discussed later.

## SEXUAL COMPLICATIONS

The sexual problems of long-term cancer survivors are of two types: (1) those that alter sexual function directly by tissue changes or indirectly by hormonal changes resulting in altered physiological function and responsivity, and (2) those treatments that have a spe-

**Table 7-3**  Psychological morbidity in cancer survivors

| Concerns | Types of morbidity |
|---|---|
| Physical | Continued preoccupation with illness |
| | Fears of recurrence or relapse |
| | Increased fears of death |
| | Feelings of physical damage and infertility |
| | Concerns about sexuality and fertility |
| Psychological | Greater sense of vulnerability and uncertainty about the future (Damocles syndrome) |
| | Sense of personal inadequacy about "being on own" |
| | Fear of social rejection |
| | Diminished sense of control |
| | Anxiety and depression |
| Reentry, social and job | Transition from patient to healthy status (Lazarus syndrome) |
| | Regarded by others as "special": hero versus victim |
| | Job insecurity, discrimination: employer and peer attitudes |
| | Health and life insurance problems |

cific effect on *gonadal* function either directly by damaging the germ cells or indirectly by altering hormonal production resulting in infertility or sterility. Surgery, chemotherapy, and radiation can all produce these changes; the latter two can particularly affect fertility, while sexual function remains normal. Treatment, age, and sexual maturity must be considered as crucial in sexual adjustment. Chapter 33 reviews sexual dysfunction, evaluation, and management, by cancer site and treatment.

In studies of adolescents and young adults who had childhood cancer, emphasis has been primarily on assessing the impact of treatment on reproductive function. The earliest delayed effects of cancer treatment on sexual and reproductive function were reported in childhood tumors. More extensive psychosexual interviewing has examined the impact of gonadal dysfunction on sexual functioning and adjustment. Puberty is the time when impact of sexual problems are greatest because it is the time when the body itself changes and performance issues are critically important (Schain, 1980). Awareness of infertility for the first time, as revealed by parents or the physician, may be difficult. Cella and Smith (1987) also found a high number of adolescents who were not aware of their fertility status. Many also chose to deny the possibility of sterility. The adolescent boy survivors in their sample equated sterility with impotence.

The effect of chemotherapy on male gonadal function has been most widely investigated with Hodgkin's disease or leukemia treated with alkylating agents (Table 7-4). Sherins and DeVita (1973) reported azoospermia and germinal aplasia in 63% of 16 lymphoma patients studied, without any change in sexual function. However, adolescent boys treated by the MOPP regimen had oligospermia and azoospermia, elevated follicle-stimulating and luteinizing hormones (FSH and LH), and decreased testosterone. They also developed Leydig's cell failure accounting for gynecomastia (Blatt et al., 1985). Studies of prepubertal boys have also shown changes in the testis after chemotherapy and irradiation, suggesting it is vulnerable even when physiologically quiescent. Chapman and co-workers (1979a, 1981) found azoospermia and germinal aplasia with decreased libido, impotence, and psychological distress in over 90% of men (Table 7-4). The potential for reversibility of azoospermia is unclear, although it is not likely high.

In men there is a dose–response relationship between irradiation and damage to sperm count and recovery rate. Azoospermia is produced at doses of 140–300 rads. Lower dose results in oligospermia, which may be reversible. Irradiation doses of 400–700 rads produce ovarian failure in women 40 and older (Meadows and Silber, 1985).

**Table 7-4** Sexual morbidity in survivors of Hodgkin's disease and other lymphomas

| Study | Time from treatment | Results |
|---|---|---|
| *Males* | | |
| Sherins and Devita (1973) | From 6 months to 7 years | Azoospermia and germinal aplasia (63%; $n = 16$); no impotence or decreased libido |
| Chapman et al. (1979a) | Median of 27 months | Azoospermia and germinal aplasia (95%); decreased libido (50%); marked personality and mood change |
| Chapman et al. (1981) | ≤3 years | Azoospermia and germinal aplasia (90%); decreased libido (50%); marked personality and mood disturbance (50%) |
| *Females* | | |
| Chapman et al. (1979b) | Median of 36 months | Menstrual irregularity and decreased libido (73%); excessive separation/divorce rate (30%); marked mood change |

The alkylating agents, primarily cyclophosphamide, administered for at least 9 months in women, produce amenorrhea or menstrual irregularities, loss of libido, and menopausal symptoms. Chapman and colleagues (1979b) reported severe disruption in sexual function and secondary emotional distress based on ovulation failure, which was exacerbated by lack of psychological preparation (Table 7-4).

In girls and women, ovulation failure was reported in up to 60% of postpubertal females treated with cyclophosphamide (Andrieu and Ochoa-Molina, 1983). Younger women, however, had lower risk for gonadal failure, in fact prepubertal girls had no gonadal dysfunction with cyclophosphamide.

Lesko and colleagues (1987) examined sexual functioning and satisfaction in 126 young adult male survivors of Hodgkin's disease, leukemia, and testicular cancer and 35 age-matched comparison subjects. When these men, mean age 32, were divided by marital status, and by high risk of infertility (Hodgkin's and testicular) versus low risk (leukemics treated by chemotherapy and comparison subjects), the married men with high risk of infertility exhibited poorer body image, sexual satisfaction, and general satisfaction than any other subgroup. Thus, negative meaning and impact of infertility appeared to be enhanced by marriage, whereas it could be avoided in the single cancer survivors.

An examination of 71 acute leukemia male and female survivors (mean age 24 years old) treated by either chemotherapy or bone marrow transplant revealed similar levels of problems (Lesko et al., 1987). Women had significantly lower sexual drive than healthy normals. Both reported poorer body image than normals. Lower sexual drive was correlated with amount of time since the diagnosis, being more psychologically distressed, having more illness-related problems, and poorer body image and sexual satisfaction. These data suggest that, even in the absence of infertility, patients need evaluation for sexual problems.

In a major review article, Andersen (1985) argued for a broad conceptualization of the causes of sexual sequelae in cancer survivors, including affective (i.e., especially depressive and anxious) disturbance, concern with body function, and body image disturbance, as well as the actual physical changes caused by treatments. Existing sexual research is dominated by studies of the major cancer sites where direct impairment of sexual function occurs from the surgical procedure or the effects of irradiation: gynecological, genitourinary, and colorectal cancer. Pelvic tumors result in sexual dysfunction by virtue of the direct effect of surgical deficits and irradiation and indirectly by the gonadotoxic effects of chemotherapy. It is clear that severity of sequelae is directly related to extent and aggressiveness of treatment required for therapeutic benefit.

Among women, cervical cancer has been the most frequently studied site for psychological consequences. In the early stage of disease, radiation can cause dyspareunia, decreased vaginal sensitivity, and postcoital bleeding (Abitol and Davenport, 1974; Kaufman et al., 1961; Vasicka et al., 1958). Dysfunction was reported in 44–79% of the patients studied retrospectively (Abitol and Davenport, 1974; Seibel et al., 1980; Vasicka et al., 1958; Decker and Schwartzman, 1962; Bertelsen, 1983). Under more careful study, this percentage decreased by 29% (Vincent et al., 1975). Radical hysterectomy causes vaginal shortening and consequent coital pain (Abitol and Davenport, 1974; Seibel et al., 1980). Dysfunction was reported in 6–19% of patients studied retrospectively (Abitol and Davenport, 1974; Seibel et al., 1980; Vasicka et al., 1958; Decker and Schwartzman, 1962; Bertelsen, 1983). Under more careful study, this percentage increased to 33% (Vincent et al., 1975). In advanced cervical cancer, pelvic exenteration with the wide excision of the uterus, tubes, ovaries, bladder, rectum, and vagina, results in both loss of sexual function and

depression (Brown et al., 1972; Dempsey et al., 1975; Knorr, 1967; Vera, 1981). This is similar to the general sexual dysfunction associated with radical vulvectomy in vulvar cancer patients (Anderson and Hacker, 1983; Moth et al., 1983).

Bos-Branolte (1987) has studied more than 100 women survivors treated in Leiden, The Netherlands, for the range of gynecological malignancies. As discussed by Auchincloss (Chapter 33), she noted that sexual functioning becomes a major concern only after the existential crises of illness are over and treatment has been completed. Her study found severe to moderately severe dysfunction in a third of the women evaluated. Bos-Branolte has also examined the effect of psychotherapy on women's psychosocial function and rehabilitation. Psychotherapy was accepted by 30% of those to whom it was offered. After 9 months, women with severe problems who had had psychotherapy showed decreased anxiety and depression, and had a better body image and self-esteem. Bos-Branolte also studied patients' sexual partners, highlighting the negative impact of illness on the partner and the relationship, resulting from treatment-related sexual dysfunction and the negative impact on desire and arousal in both patients and partners.

Among men, prostatic cancer has been frequently studied for psychosexual dysfunction. Erectile dysfunction has been detected along the entire treatment spectrum—from open perineal biopsy (in 24%) (Dahlen and Goodwin, 1957; A.L. Finkle and T.G.M. Moyers, 1960a,b), to transurethral resection (in 32%) (A.L. Finkle and I.G. Moyers, 1960b; and Madorsky et al., 1976), to radical prostatectomy (in 90%) (Kopecky et al., 1970; Middleton, 1981; Walsh and Donker, 1982; Correa et al., 1977; J.E. Finkle and A.B. Taylor, 1975). Even when erectile and orgasmic function are intact, ejaculatory ability may often be impaired, resulting in diminished or dry ejaculation. When treatment also includes hormone therapy and/or bilateral orchiectomy, total erectile dysfunction and ejaculatory impairment are universal (Scott and Boyd, 1969; Veenema et al., 1977). (See Chapter 10 for consequences of hormonal therapy.) Radiation implantation therapy has been reported to spare the most severe aspects of sexual dysfunction (Fowler et al., 1979; Herr, 1979).

For both men and women, abdominoperineal rectal excision for colorectal cancer causes impairment of libido and performance. Among men the disturbance of libido has been reported in 32–59% (Aso and Yasutomi, 1974; Druss et al., 1969), and erectile disturbance in 28–76% of patients (Aso and Yasutomi, 1974; Bernstein and Berstein, 1966; Sutherland et al., 1952). However, the surgical procedure has been modified to spare some of the pelvic innervation, with a decrease in sexual dysfunction (see Chapters 15 and 33). Among women, disturbance of libido was reported in 28% and dyspareunia in 21% of patients (Druss et al., 1969). Those patients who require colostomy have particularly sensitive problems concerning sexual function, which are aided by veteran patient counseling and participation in an ostomy group.

In breast cancer patients, the acute effects of mastectomy on psychosocial adjustment, including sexual function, have been well documented (see Chapters 14 and 33). However, fewer studies have provided long-term follow-up of the sexual sequelae of breast cancer therapy. Both Morris et al. (1977) and Maguire et al. (1978) found impairment in sexual satisfaction or performance in approximately 30% of women after 2 years and 1 year, respectively. However, in the former, this rate did not exceed that obtained for benign comparison subjects, whereas in the latter it did.

Psychosexual research on testicular cancer offers a good model in which one can examine the sexual and reproductive sequelae in young adult men cured of cancer. Infertility due to retrograde or dry ejaculation is a well-documented consequence of surgical treatment, which includes retroperitoneal lymph node dissection. Little or no physiological effect on sexual function has been observed in men undergoing such treatment unless wider or bilateral dissection of the retroperitoneal node chain occurs. In the research of Thachil and colleagues (1981), neither infertility nor sexual dysfunction was associated with unilateral orchiectomy; however, psychological concerns about both were apparent. Infertility or associated sexual dysfunction on a psychological basis may be reason for counseling (Schover and von Eschenbach, 1984; Rieker et al., 1985). Although testicular patients had greater distress, and greater sexual concerns and dysfunction, than did a comparable group of patients who had had benign genitourinary disease, the level of disturbance was only mild and did not jeopardize function (Tross et al., 1984).

Testicular cancer is also a good current model for a solid tumor in which stage I and II nonseminomatous cancer is virtually uniformly cured by surgery and adjuvant chemotherapy containing cisplatin. Trials of surgery plus immediate adjuvant chemotherapy versus surgery with chemotherapy given only at time of relapse have resulted in comparable cure rates, thus preserving fertility and avoiding delayed side effects of unneeded adjuvant therapy. Vogelzang and colleagues (1987) have reported on a sample of men with stage I testicular cancer treated by orchiectomy alone and follow-up, in which infertility was a major issue: among these men 65% expressed concern about infertility and 71% had considered banking sperm at a mean follow-up of 14 months, but only 18% had done so.

Andersen (1985) warned that research on sexual dysfunction has probably underestimated the true incidence of sexual sequelae because of its emphasis on frequency of sexual activity. A broader definition of sexual dysfunction is needed that includes perceived desire and satisfaction. This need for more sensitive indicators of sexual dysfunction is apparent in more recent research, with a careful emphasis on sexual rehabilitation and counseling. In a study of 308 men and women evaluated for sexual rehabilitation, Schover and co-workers (1987) observed that decreased sexual desire was common in both men and women after cancer treatment; in the arousal phase, men showed erectile dysfunction and as many women had loss of lubrication and vaginal expansion; in the orgasm phase, both men and women recognized an increased difficulty in reaching orgasm.

Sexual counseling should include adequate preparation for immediate and delayed treatment effects on gonadal and sexual function, opportunity for sperm-banking for men, counseling and support during and following treatment, opportunity for penile prostheses for men with erectile dysfunction, and hormonal replacement when possible (von Eschenbach and Schover, 1984).

## NEUROPSYCHOLOGICAL LATE EFFECTS

Cancer treatment may have major physical late effects on the CNS and intellectual function. Children treated for brain tumors exhibit the most profound decline in intellectual ability, with greater loss in younger children. Neuropsychological late effects have also been observed in children with acute lymphocytic leukemia (ALL) who have undergone prophylaxis against CNS spread by treatment with cranial irradiation and intrathecal methotrexate. These sequelae have generally been characterized as deficits in attention and concentration and school achievement (McIntosh et al., 1976; Meadows and Evans, 1976; Eiser, 1978; Goff et al., 1980; Moss et al., 1981; Meadows et al., 1981; Pavlovsky et al., 1983). Only one study emphasized the presence of broad deficits in general intelligence, achievement, and fine-motor and tactile functioning (Rowland et al., 1984). However, reports in the literature vary regarding the presence of these deficits. Several studies reported no differences between patients treated with radiation and those not treated (Soni et al., 1975; Verzosa et al., 1976; Eiser and Landsdown, 1977; Obetz et al., 1979; Berg et al., 1983; Whitt et al., 1984). Some authors have argued additionally that ALL itself, or the neurotoxic chemotherapy alone (especially when delivered intrathecally), plays a role in the development of neuropsychological sequelae (Whitt et al., 1984). Others have described higher intelligence in ALL subjects, as compared to their healthy peers (Moss et al., 1981; Tamaroff et al., 1982; Rowland et al., 1984). There is general consensus that even when sequelae have been detected, they have been relatively mild, with scores rarely falling below normal limits (Goff et al., 1980; Rowland et al., 1984). However, the Rowland study showed a mean IQ drop of 10 points in children treated with cranial irradiation and intrathecal methotrexate, with greater impact in the younger children. Peckham and colleagues (1988) found that specific patterns of learning disabilities in children they studied responded positively to early educational intervention by tutoring, individualized instruction, and parental support. They found that early recognition and intervention allowed attention to poor concentration and specific losses, which prevented more significant academic achievement problems. These studies of the adverse effects of ALL treatment on intellectual function have led to the development of alternative forms of CNS prophylaxis in treatment of childhood ALL. A study from the Children's Cancer Study group by Browers and colleagues (1987) showed that children with ALL who were randomized to high-dose systemic methotrexate had an equal disease-free survival at almost 5 years with no adverse effect on mental function, as compared to children who were randomized to intrathecal methotrexate and cranial irradiation, who showed the mental acuity losses reported in other studies.

## PSYCHOLOGICAL RESPONSE TO LIFE-THREATENING ILLNESS

Some psychiatric investigators view the cancer survivor as heir to the same psychological problems that beset the patient at the time of the initial diagnosis or during active treatment. Psychological sequelae in the survivor are actually quite different and are produced by two complementary mechanisms associated with life-threatening illness: an anticipatory response to death and a residual response to diagnosis and treatment. On the one hand, psychological sequelae are an expected result of the anticipated threat of death, arising from personal confrontation with mortality. Even after cure has been achieved, the survivor may anticipate an only tenuous sense of longevity, producing anxiety, depressive mood, damaged body image, and fears of recurrence. This has been called the "Damocles syndrome" by Koocher and O'Malley (1981). It is similar in manifestations to the anticipatory grief reaction observed in the families of patients dying from prolonged illness (Futterman and Hoffman, 1973). On the other hand, the psychological sequelae can also be conceptualized as a form of residual stress syndrome

(Selye, 1956), grief reaction (Parkes, 1972), or traumatic disorder (Horowitz, 1970) following the catastrophic burden of initial diagnosis. This response has been designated as the "existential plight" belonging to the first 100 days of diagnosis, and is marked by preoccupation with mortality, sense of personal vulnerability, and heightened emotional distress (Weisman and Worden, 1976–1977). The most widely discussed psychological issues in the cancer survival literature are presented in Table 7-3.

The work of Koocher and O'Malley (1981) represents a prototype for the comprehensive evaluation of psychological sequelae of cancer survival. They conducted a controlled study of pediatric cancer survivors and chronically nonfatally ill children, using indices of both social and psychological adjustment. Children surviving cancer were found to have a high incidence (59%) of subtle, nonimpairing psychological disturbance in the areas of general adjustment, self-esteem, uncertainty about the future, anxiety, and depressive symptoms.

Studies of adult cancer survivors have been built on a design similar to the Koocher and O'Malley study. The early studies have focused on testicular cancer, Hodgkin's disease, and more recently, leukemia survivors. These malignancies are now associated with a high rate of cure and provide excellent settings for examining the impact of successful cancer treatment on young adults. They have a high incidence in late adolescence and early adulthood, when impact on active work, sexual, and social functioning is most visible, and may have the most profound long-term effects. Treated by multimodal therapy (surgery, chemotherapy, and radiotherapy), they are also comparable to other major cancer sites. Finally, the reproductive system is affected by the disease or treatment, permitting emphasis on a critical, but understudied, area of disturbance in cancer survivors. The early studies of psychological function are summarized in Table 7-5. In general, their results highlight the absence of clinical psychiatric disorders or discrete functional impairment. However, mild psychological concerns in survivors are evident, with a greater sense of vulnerability, higher levels of anxiety and depression, diminished sense of control, fear of social rejection, and sense of personal inadequacy (Table 7-3). The salience of illness- and treatment-specific sexual and physical problems are obvious in the survivors studied (Koocher and O'Malley, 1981; Tross et al., 1984; Cella, 1983; Rieker et al., 1985; Fobair et al., 1986). Studies have also identified determinants of this distress. Cella and Tross (1986) found patients treated for advanced disease were a high-risk subgroup for psychological distress. Rieker and colleagues (1985) emphasized the role of infertility and sexual dysfunc-

**Table 7-5**  Psychological sequelae of cancer survival

| Study | Site | Time from diagnosis (years) | Findings |
|---|---|---|---|
| Koocher and O'Malley (1981) | Mixed pediatric | ≥5 | Mild psychological distress without behavioral dysfunction |
| Tross et al. (1984) | Testicular | 2–4 | Mild clinical-rated distress related to anxiety and depression but no self-reported distress or behavioral dysfunction |
| Cella (1983) | Hodgkin's disease | 5–12 | Decreased intimacy, motivation, and increased appreciation of life |
| Rieker et al. (1985) | Testicular | 2–10 | Increased sexual (especially ejaculatory) dysfunction and infertility-related distress, but no general distress or behavioral dysfunction |
| Fobair et al. (1986) | Hodgkin's disease | 10–21 | Decreased energy (37%), decreased divorce (32%), increased fertility-related distress (18%), decreased libido (20%), increased work difficulty (42%), increased depression (18%) |
| Lesko et al. (1987) | Acute leukemia | 5–9 | Psychological distress level comparable to other cancer survivors; treatment-related maladjustment slightly lower; both genders with decreased body image; woman with decreased sex drive and satisfaction and increased psychological distress |

tion as causes of psychological distress. Mumma and co-workers (1988) have identified a subgroup of survivors whose general distress correlated with more intrusive illness-related concerns and distress. Cella and Tross (1987) found anxiety about death to be a separate concern but related to general anxiety, depression, and overall distress. Leukemics had more illness-specific concerns than Hodgkin's disease or testicular survivors (Tross et al., 1987), although their overall distress levels were not greater than others (Lesko et al., 1987).

In a review of psychosocial sequelae in children surviving childhood cancer, van Dongen-Melman and Sanders-Woutstra (1986) noted that the variables associated with optimal long-term psychosocial adjustment were a short treatment course, no relapse of disease, an early knowledge of the diagnosis, a supportive and openly communicating family, ability to use denial effectively, and onset of disease at a young age. This last point of younger age (Koocher et al., 1980) is of interest because a greater disturbance might have been expected later. Children appear to be more resilient and adaptable. However, such problems as a posttraumatic stress disorder and other responses to reminders of illness have been inadequately studied in children. As more children survive cancer, they may also experience less psychological distress because survival is an expected outcome.

Ongoing studies by the Memorial Sloan-Kettering group of adolescent survivors of hematological malignancies (Cella and Smith, 1987) have found teenagers as a group functioning well in school and social life; however, individual teenagers have significant problems with family and peer relations. Evaluation is needed at time of reentry to detect and prevent maladaptive patterns from developing.

## SOCIAL SEQUELAE

Investigations of social indicators by epidemiologists have generally found the life of the cancer survivor to be virtually identical to that of his or her healthy peers. The early studies, conducted to assess social sequelae in childhood cancer survivors, found no difference in rates of marriage, work function (i.e., levels of job turnover, absenteeism, and performance), and school achievement among cancer survivors as compared to healthy controls (Table 7-6) (Eisenberg and Goldenberg, 1966). In fact, Kennedy and co-workers (1976) identified normal work and social function with a dramatic elevation in optimism and appreciation of life as a psychological benefit of having survived the cancer experience. Other studies of breast cancer survivors supported the findings of few or no psychosocial sequelae of cancer cure (Schottenfeld and Robbins, 1970; Craig et al., 1974). Holmes and Holmes (1975) and Li and Stone (1976) studied children and found normal school, job, and marital status. It may be seen that the major area of liability for the adult cancer survivor in these studies was illness-related morbidity in the form of poorer health or physical disability, with fewer evidences of social dysfunction.

**Table 7-6** Social adjustment of cancer survival

| Study | Site | Time from diagnosis (years) | Findings |
|---|---|---|---|
| Eisenberg and Goldenberg (1966) | Breast | 1.5 | Increased positive attitude and physical recovery from diagnosis |
| Schottenfeld and Robbins (1970) | Breast | 5 10 15 | Recovery of physical function within median of 3 months after diagnosis; increased rate of recovery at 10 and increased at 15 years |
| Craig et al. (1974) | Breast | ≥5 | Normal work, marital, leisure, and psychological function and attitude toward life and future; increased physical disability and poor health |
| Holmes and Holmes (1975) | Mixed pediatric | Average 16.5 | Normal school achievement and job range |
| Li and Stone (1976) | Mixed pediatric | Median 15 | Normal school achievement, work, marriage; occasional job and/or insurance discrimination |
| Kennedy et al. (1976) | Mixed | ≤20 | Normal work and social function; increased optimism and life appreciation |

## REENTRY AND JOB–INSURANCE PROBLEMS

### Reentry

The survivor must also confront the problems of reentry into prior normal responsibilities, roles, and lifestyle. The psychological consequences arise from having been identified (by oneself and by others) as a cancer patient, which may confer a sense of personal vulnerability and may result in financial and job insecurity, and health–life insurance discrimination (Table 7-3). The transition from "patient" to "healthy" status may be psychologically problematic. Cured patients often experience a new sense of vulnerability about being "on their own" vis-à-vis the medical system. The fear of recurrence or relapse may escalate, especially in the early period after completion of treatment. Diminished stamina with which to meet standard, full-time work demands may pose a problem (Fobair et al., 1986). Interpersonal relationships may be complicated by a sense of physical (especially reproductive) damage, inferiority, social withdrawal, and rejection sensitivity. Financial insecurity, caused by cumulative medical expenses and job discrimination (i.e., in obtaining, being promoted, or changing jobs), may be increased. In the United States, it is common for patients to become locked into their jobs because of difficulty in acquiring health insurance coverage under other plans after cancer diagnosis. Sullivan et al. (1987) observed greater concerns about financial security among U.S. versus Swedish survivors, as well as greater reluctance to reveal the diagnosis to an employer.

### Job and Insurance Problems

Two major group of investigators have studied the employment and insurance problems of workers diagnosed with cancer: the management of companies who employ or insure workers and who share the cost of the medical bills, and the cancer service organizations who advocate for workers and lobby for their social and economic protection. Irrespective of survey data, the public is being repeatedly confronted with greater numbers of prominent individuals who are cancer survivors. The cancer diagnosis of President Reagan in 1985 and of Mrs. Reagan in 1987, followed by their rapid return to full work and great responsibility, has served in its own way to demonstrate that a cancer diagnosis is not incompatible with even the most important jobs in the country. The growing coalition of survivors, who advocate for others and use their influence to lobby for the rights of survivors, is having an impact on long-apparent employment problems, which were slow to surface because most cancer survivors preferred to keep their diagnosis a secret because of their negative experiences when they had revealed it.

The major industrial surveys were carried out by Wheatley and co-workers (1974) and Stone (1975) (Table 7-7). The former study analyzed employment records of 74 employees of the Metropolitan Life Insurance Company who had been diagnosed and treated for cancer between 1959 and 1971. They varied from 1 month to 25 years after the treatment at the time of the interview: Among these employees, 55% were working, and 75% of these were full-time. The turnover rate

**Table 7-7** Employability and insurability in cancer survivors

| Study | Type of cancer | Findings |
|---|---|---|
| Wheatley et al. (1974) | Mixed | 47% Medical acceptability rate (at ≥5 years off treatment)<br>55% Employment rate<br>3% Disability rate<br>42% (Voluntary) discontinuation rate<br>85% Satisfactory performance rating<br>51% <5 Days/year absenteeism |
| Stone (1975) | Mixed | 77% Employment rate; after mean absence of 106 days, 5.2% disability rate |
| Feldman (1976, 1978, 1980) | Mixed (white-collar employee) | 50% Experienced some form of job discrimination |
| | Mixed (blue-collar employee) | 84% Experienced job discrimination (more problems for less skilled workers) |
| | Adults with prior childhood tumors | 50% Experienced discrimination at time of first job application |
| Mashberg and Lesko (1987) | Acute leukemia | 55% Were employed<br>>80% Informed employers of illness status<br><22% Denied life insurance<br><10% Denied health insurance |

did not differ from that of other employees. Chiefly because of job dissatisfaction, 42% had left their jobs, and no patient had been fired. Only 2 patients had resigned for health reasons. Job performance was rated high and a modest rate of absenteeism was reported. On this basis, the investigators recommended that cancer survivors be "selectively hired," provided they had passed the 5-year survival point without evidence of disease; they estimated that 50% of all applicants with cancer history would meet this criterion. Stone (1975) analyzed employment trends for 1351 cancer patients from 800,000 employees of the Bell System Operating Telephone Companies for FY 1972. This study found a 77% employment rate with 5.2% disability. They identified the young cancer survivor–employee as a person who was less likely to have accumulated enough work years to be eligible for a pension if disability was necessary, and who also was at higher risk for exhausting illness benefits before being able to resume work.

Under the auspices of the California Division of the American Cancer Society, Feldman conducted studies with white-collar employees in 1976, with blue-collar employees in 1978, and with adults with prior childhood tumors in 1980. The first was a comprehensive prevalence study of the problems and service needs of 810 cancer patients and 142 of their families 30 months after diagnosis. The patients studied were predominantly married women, 46 years of age or older. At follow-up, 49% were employed as compared to 54% at diagnosis. In part, Feldman attributed this level of work stability to the continuation of these patients with their previous jobs, which assured benefits in the event of future disease. The majority of the patients had comprehensive insurance coverage for their past treatment, but 25% subsequently experienced negative adjustments in their health benefits, including loss of further coverage from cancer (5%) and reduction or cancellation of their insurance. Blue-collar workers studied by Feldman had experienced more job-related discriminatory problems, probably because their work depended on need for greater strength and stamina than that required of white-collar workers. Her third study (1980) showed that with young adults seeking their first job a diagnosis of childhood cancer as long as 15 years earlier was still problematic in half of those studied.

## LEGISLATION

The primary legislation that has been used to protect cancer patients from discrimination is the Rehabilitation Act of 1973 (Sec. 503 and 504), which offers general protection to handicapped individuals. It mandates that within any federal department or agency, which has entered into a contract in excess of $2500, affirmative action must be taken to employ, advance, or preserve the benefits of any "qualified handicapped" individuals. A violation may be filed as a grievance with the Department of Labor. It indirectly covers patients with cancer. In addition, more than 37 states have affirmative-action fair employment acts to prevent discrimination against the handicapped. This gives cancer patients protection as disabled individuals. However, coverage under this law is somewhat inappropriate for many cancer patients who are not disabled. Discrimination is often due to the stigma of the diagnosis in healthy recovered patients. However, it does give them a basis from which to seek recourse when they have experienced discrimination. The California Division of the American Cancer Society had documented 44 cases of employment discrimination by 1979, but cancer patients have constituted a very small percentage of the cases brought under the Rehabilitation Act of 1973 (Hoffman, 1986). A project between the Legal Aid Society of San Francisco and the American Cancer Society has resulted in a center that offers assistance and psychological support for patients who have experienced discrimination. A greater effort to inform patients of their rights is being actively encouraged by the American Cancer Society. The Memorial Sloan-Kettering survivor center also offers counseling about job discrimination in New York.

Cured cancer patients also experience discrimination when seeking new jobs. Certain government agencies, such as the armed forces and municipalities (including the police), knowingly discriminate against applicants with a cancer history. With adequate education in the public and private sectors this unequal treatment can be changed. Efforts have been made to develop legislation that specifically deals with the problems of the cancer patient and the person with a history of cancer by eliminating employment discrimination (Hoffman, 1986).

Feldman, in her three seminal studies, pointed out that negative attitudes on the part of the employer, co-workers, and the survivors' self–attitudes collude to make the workplace a difficult setting for reentry after cancer treatment. Table 7-8 presents some of the major employer, co-worker and survivor barriers to workplace reentry. The employer may fear low productivity, absenteeism, and higher costs, as well as be concerned about co-workers' morale. Co-workers may erroneously fear contagion of cancer and shun the cancer survivor. Returning cancer patients may have self-doubts about their ability to perform, the return of

cancer, social rejection by co-workers, concerns about job stability, and loss of health benefits. The result is often that the very place that is usually an important source of self-esteem becomes a source of stress.

One of the most widespread consequences of having had cancer is a tendency for survivors to lock themselves into existing jobs. The person becomes locked into a particular job because of the risk of changing jobs, and experiencing a period without insurance coverage is too great to tolerate. The careers of young people appear sometimes to plateau prematurely, in part because of their own fears of "taking a risk." This happens also with fathers who have a child with cancer. The Consolidated Omnibus Budget Reconciliation Act of 1986 (COBRA) law protects individuals for 18 months after leaving a job with assured coverage at the same rate by the group insurance policy of the prior job. This is an important cushion. Irrespective of legal protection, survivors are likely to be safer in changing jobs and obtaining a new one when the period of extended survival already suggests a likely cure.

## INTERVENTIONS TO PROMOTE HEALTHY SURVIVORSHIP

Thoughtful reports by cancer survivors themselves and the psychosocial studies have begun to provide us with guidelines for interventions. Mullan (1985) stressed the importance of education of the cancer patient on (1) reentry, to anticipate the fears of recurrence, (2) the adjustment to living with compromises entailed by treatment (e.g., mastectomy, ostomy), (3) the emotions of anger (about compromise), anxiety, and depression, (4) the need to self-monitor for physical symptoms (but not become preoccupied), (5) and the need to become part of a community of survivors (to offer a network, information, and support). The National Coalition of Cancer Survivors is such a group, started by him. Natalie Spingarn, another survivor who has devoted herself to writing and advocacy for cancer patients, gave the key note address at the group's meeting in 1987. She recounted the "anomic aspects" of recovering from cancer identified by sociologist, Maher (1982). Based on their work, Table 7-9 outlines interventions from the time of diagnosis to optimal rehabilitation. Diagnosis and possible treatment side effects must be fairly presented to prevent "surprises" later. Awareness of the option for sperm banking reduces concerns about infertility and inability to father a child. Psychological preparation prior to treatment for anticipated amenorrhea and menopausal symptoms in women is important. The point of completion of treatment, even when it has been arduous, is one that is best handled by awareness that the paradoxical anxiety about recurrence and a sense of

**Table 7-8** Workplace and cancer survivor issues

| Source of attitudes | Issues |
|---|---|
| Employer | Fear of low productivity, absenteeism, and work inability of survivor |
| | Fear of effect of cancer patient on morale of office personnel |
| | Fear that cancer survivor will increase costs of health benefits and insurance |
| Coworkers | Misconception that cancer is contagious |
| | Avoidance of survivor contact |
| | View of survivor as victim |
| Survivors | Uncertainty about ability to do job as well as before |
| | Uncertainty about future health and recurrence |
| | Fear of rejection by coworkers |
| | Fear of negative attitude of supervisors and management |
| | Fear of loss of health insurance through job termination |
| | Fear of inability to get another job with cancer diagnosis |

**Table 7-9**   Interventions to assist cancer survivors' adjustment

| Adjustment situation | Types of intervention |
|---|---|
| At time of diagnosis | Honesty about diagnosis and possible delayed treatment effects |
| | Opportunity for sperm banking prior to treatment when infertility is anticipated |
| | Sense of alliance with doctor about treatment |
| | Concept of full rehabilitation from the outset |
| On completion of treatment | Anticipation of increased anxiety in the immediate period after completion of treatment |
| | Anticipation of no longer being "a patient" and the reduction of special support and concern |
| | Adjustment to physical side effects of treatment |
| Reentry in early survival | Counseling about how to deal with expectations of others: family, friends, workplace |
| | Counseling to deal with personal feelings of increased anxiety about self-adequacy and future health |
| | Help for family to prevent overprotection |
| | Practical advice and support from veteran patient(s) with same illness |
| Extended and permanent survival | Monitoring of physical and mental state by same medical staff (checking developmental milestones in children) |
| | Early referral for evaluation for signs of psychological distress |
| | Becoming a veteran patient and helping others (promotes mastery) |

vulnerability and inadequacy is normal (see Chapters 9 and 10 on completion of chemotherapy and radiation). The emotional leap from "patient," with special status, to "healthy," with full expectations for meeting all roles and obligations, is great and may require psychological assistance, especially if treatment residuals remain. Preparation at reentry must deal with work stresses and with attitudes of employer, co-workers, and family, while also recognizing the potential for feelings of physical inferiority and inadequacy. Long-term survivors today must continue to have medical monitoring, preferably by the same trusted staff, for possible development of delayed treatment effects or recurrence of some tumors. Receiving information and

support from other veteran patients and then becoming one who helps others consolidates mastery of problems as well as enhancing the survivor network.

## SUMMARY

Early studies of cancer survivors were appropriately concerned with delayed physical effects of treatment. Initial studies of social adjustment used social indicators (e.g., occupational or disability status, marital status, parenthood, educational level, and socioeconomic status) that showed little adverse effect of having had cancer treatment. Only later with study of psychological parameters (especially affective symptoms, concerns about illness and death, and modes of coping) did the more subtle signs of emotional stress in cancer survivors begin to appear. As more attention is given to psychosocial, psychosexual, and job function, evidence of problems for survivors become more evident. Cancer survivors have become a potent force in making needs and problems known and suggesting interventions. Before treatment begins, counseling that informs the patient of possible long-term treatment effects offers preemptive protection against later distress. Special measures to offset the impact of the late effects of treatment, such as the use of sperm-banking in anticipation of possible infertility, must be initiated at this time. The end of the treatment is another critical juncture at which the problems of full reentry into work, social, and sexual life can be expected to surface. Finally, arriving at remission and facing the psychological challenge of putting the cancer experience in the past identifies another juncture at which counseling may be particularly helpful.

## REFERENCES

Abitol, M.M. and J.H. Davenport (1974). Sexual dysfunction after therapy for cervical carcinoma. *Am. J. Obstet. Gynecol.* 119:181–89.

American Cancer Society, Proceedings of the Fifth National Conference on Human Values in Cancer—1987. A Service and Rehabilitation Education Publication. Atlanta: Amer. Cancer Society, Inc.

Andersen, B.L. (1985). Sexual functioning morbidity among cancer survivors: Current status and future research directions. *Cancer* 55:1835–42.

Andersen, B.L. and N.F. Hacker (1983). Psychosexual adjustment after vulvar surgery. *Obstet. Gynecol.* 62:457–62.

Andrieu, J.M. and M.E. Ochoa-Molina (1983). Menstrual cycle pregnancies and offspring before and after MOPP therapy for Hodgkin's disease. *Cancer* 52:435–38.

Aso, R. and M. Yasutomi (1974). Urinary and sexual disturbances following radical surgery for rectal cancer, and pudendal nerveblock as a countermeasure for urinary disturbance. *Am. J. Proctol.* 32:60–70.

Berg, R.A., L.T. Ch'ien, W.P. Bowman, J. Ochs, W. Lancaster, J.R. Goff, and H.R. Anderson, Jr. (1983). The neuropsychological effects of acute lymphocytic leukemia and its treatment—A three-year report: Intellectual functioning and academic achievement. *Int. J. Clin. Neuropsychol.* 5:9–13.

Bernstein, W.C. and E.F. Bernstein (1966). Sexual dysfunction following radical surgery for cancer of the rectum. *Dis. Colon Rectum* 9:328–32.

Bertelsen, K. (1983). Sexual dysfunction after treatment of cervical cancer. *Dan. Med. Bull.* 30:31–34.

Blatt, J., R. Sherins, D. Niebrugge, W. Bleyer, and D. Poplack (1985). Leydig cell function in boys following treatment for testicular relapse of acute lymphoblastic leukemia. *J. Clin. Oncol.* 3:1227–31.

Bloch, R. and A. Bloch (1985). *Fighting Cancer.* Kansas City: The Cancer Connection.

Bos-Branolte, G. (1987). *Psychological Problems in Survivors of Gynaecologic Cancers: A Psychotherapeutic Approach.* Leiden, The Netherlands: DeKempenaer Oogstgeest.

Brouwers, P., H. Moss, G. Reaman, T. McGuire, E. Trupin, K. Libow, W. Tarnowski, J. Bleyer, J. Feusner, F. Ruymann, J. Miser, D. Hammond, and D. Poplack (1987). Central nervous system preventive therapy with systematic high dose methotrexate versus cranial radiation and intrathecal methotrexate. *Proc. Am. Soc. Clin. Oncol.* 6:158 (Abstract No. 622).

Brown, R.S., V. Haddox, A. Posada, and A. Rubio (1972). Social and psychological adjustment following pelvic exenteration. *Am. J. Obstet. Gynecol.* 114:162–71.

Bushhouse, S., N. Ramsey, O. Pescovitz, T. Kim, L. Robison (1987). Growth patterns following bone marrow transplantation (BMT) in pediatric patients (PTS). *Proc. Am. Soc. Clin. Oncol.* 6:159 (Abstract No. 627).

Byrd, B.L. (1983). Late effects of treatment of cancer in children. *Pediatr. Ann.* 12:450–60.

Cella, D.F. (1983). *Psychosocial Adjustment over Time to the Successful Treatment of Early versus Late Stage Hodgkin's Disease in Young Adult Men.* Doctoral thesis, Graduate School of Loyola University, Chicago.

Cella, D.F. and K. Smith (1987). Sexual and reproductive problems in cancer survivors: Males. *Proc. Workshop on Psychosexual and Reproductive Issues in Cancer Survivors,* American Cancer Society, San Antonio, Texas, January 13–17.

Cella, D.F. and S. Tross (1986). Psychological adjustment to survival from Hodgkin's disease. *J. Consult. Clin. Psychol.* 54:1–7.

Cella, D.F. and S. Tross (1987). Death anxiety in cancer survival: A preliminary cross-validation study. *J. Pers. Assess.* 51:451–61.

Cella, D.F., A. Pratt, and J.C. Holland (1986). Persistent anticipatory nausea, vomiting and anxiety in cured Hodgkin's disease patients after completion of chemotherapy. *Am. J. Psychiatry* 143:641–43.

Chapman, R.M., S.B. Sutcliffe, L.H. Rees, G.R. Edwards,

and J.S. Malpas (1979a). Cyclical combinations chemotherapy and gonadal function: Retrospective study in males. *Lancet* 1:285–89.

Chapman, R.M., S.B. Sutcliffe, and J.S. Malpas (1979b). Cytotoxic-induced ovarian failure in women with Hodgkin's disease: I. Hormone function. *J.A.M.A.* 242:1882–84.

Chapman, R., S. Sutcliffe, and J. Malpas (1981). Male gonadal dysfunction in Hodgkin's disease. *J.A.M.A.* 245:1323–28.

Correa, R.J., R.P. Gibbons, K.B. Cummings, and J.T. Mason (1977). Total prostatectomy for Stage B carcinoma of the prostate. *J. Urol.* 117:328–29.

Craig, T.J., G.W. Comstock, and P.B. Geiser (1974). The quality of survival in breast cancer: A case–control comparison. *Cancer* 33:1451–57.

Dahlen, C.D. and W.E. Goodwin (1957). Sexual potency after perineal biopsy. *J. Urol.* 77:660–69.

Decker, W.H. and E. Schwartzman (1962). Sexual function following treatment for carcinoma of the cervix. *Am. J. Obstet. Gynecol.* 83:401–5.

Dempsey, G.M., H.J. Buchsbaum, and J. Morrison (1975). Psychosocial adjustment to pelvic exenteration. *Gynecol. Oncol.* 3:325–34.

Dobkin, P.L. and G.R. Morrow (1985–1986). Long-term side effects in patients who have been treated successfully for cancer. *J. Psych. Oncol.* 3:23–51.

Druss, R.G., J.F. O'Connor, J.F. Prudden, and L.O. Stern (1969). Psychological response to colectomy II. *Arch. Gen. Psychiatry* 30:419–27.

Eisenberg, H.S. and I.S. Goldenberg (1966). A measurement of quality of survival of breast cancer patients. In J.L. Hayward and R.D. Bulbrook (eds.), *Clinical Evaluation in Breast Cancer: Symposium on Clinical Evaluation in Breast Cancer, London, 1965.* New York: Academic Press, pp. 93–108.

Eiser, C. (1978). Intellectual abilities among survivors of childhood leukemia as a function of CNS irradiation. *Arch. Dis. Child.* 53:391–95.

Eiser, C. and R. Landsdown (1977). Retrospective study of intellectual development in children with lymphoblastic leukemia. *Arch. Dis. Child.* 52:525–29.

Feldman, F.L. (1976). *Work and Cancer Health Histories: A Study of the Experiences of Recovered Patients.* Oakland, Calif.: American Cancer Society, California Division.

Feldman, F.L. (1978). *Work and Cancer Health Histories: A Study of the Experiences of Recovered Blue-Collar Workers.* Oakland, Calif.: American Cancer Society, California Division.

Feldman, F.L. (1980). *Work and Cancer Health Histories: Work Expectations and Experiences of Youth (Ages 13–23) with Cancer Histories.* Oakland, Calif.: American Cancer Society, California Division.

Finkle, A.L. and T.G. Moyers (1960a). Sexual potency in aging males: IV. Status of private patients before and after prostatectomy. *J. Urol.* 84:152–57.

Finkle, A.L. and T.G. Moyers, (1960b). Sexual potency in aging males: V. Coital ability following open perineal prostatic biopsy. *J. Urol.* 84:649–53.

Finkle, J.E. and A.B. Taylor (1975). Encouraging preservation of sexual function after prostatectomy. *Urology* 6:697–702.

Fobair, P., R.T. Hoppe, J. Bloom, R. Cox, A. Varghese, and D. Spiegel (1986). Psychosocial problems among survivors of Hodgkin's disease. *J. Clin. Oncol.* 4:805–14.

Fowler, J.E., Jr., W. Barzell, B.S. Hilaris, and W.F. Whitmore Jr. (1979). Complications of 125-iodine implantation and pelvic lymphadenectomy in the treatment of prostatic cancer. *J. Urol.* 121:447–51.

Futterman, E. and I. Hoffman (1978). Crisis and adaptation in the families of fatally ill children. In E.J. Anthony and C. Koupernik (eds.), *The Child in His Family: The Impact of Disease and Death.* New York: Wiley, pp. 127–44.

Goff, J.R., H.R. Anderson, and P.F. Cooper (1980). Distractibility and memory deficits in long-term survivors of acute lymphoblastic leukemia. *Dev. Behav. Pediatr.* 1:158–63.

Graham, S. and R.W. Gibson (1983). Social epidemiology of cancer of the testis. *Cancer* 51:211–15.

Herr, H.W. (1979). Preservation of sexual potency in prostatic cancer patients after pelvic lymphadenopathy and retropubic 125I implantation. *J. Urol.* 121:621–23.

Hoffman, B. (1986). Employment discrimination based on cancer history: The need for federal legislation. *Temple Law Q.* 59:1–34.

Holmes, H.A. and F.F. Holmes (1975). After ten years, what are the handicaps and life styles of children treated for cancer? *Clin. Pediatr.* 14:819–23.

Horowitz, M. (1976). *Stress response syndromes.* New York: Aronson.

Kaufman, R.H., N.J. Topek, and J.A. Wall (1961). Late irradiation changes in vaginal cytology. *Am. J. Obstet. gynecol.* 81:859–63.

Kennedy, B.J., A. Tellegen, S. Kennedy, and N. Havernick (1976). Psychological response of patients cured of advanced cancer. *Cancer* 38:2184–91.

Knorr, N.J. (1967). A depressive syndrome following pelvic exenteration and ileostomy. *Arch. Surg.* 94:258–60.

Koocher, G.P. and J.E. O'Malley (1981). *The Damocles Syndrome: Psychosocial Consequences of Surviving Childhood Cancer.* New York: McGraw-Hill.

Koocher, G.P., J.E. O'Malley, J.L. Gogan, and D.J. Foster (1980). Psychological adjustment among pediatric cancer survivors. *J. Child Psychol. Psychiatry* 21:163–73.

Kopecky, A.A., T.Z. Laskowski, and R. Scott (1970). Radial retropubic prostatectomy in the treatment of prostatic carcinoma. *J. Urol.* 103:641–44.

Lesko, L.M., D.F. Cella, S.E. Tross, C. Fredrick, and J.C. Holland (1987). Marital status and risk of infertility as predictors of sexual adjustment in cancer survivors. In *Program and Abstracts: Int. Conf. Reprod. Hum. Cancer,* Poster No. 18 (sponsored by the NCI and National Institute of Child Health and Human Development, Bethesda, Md.).

Lesko, L.M., G. Mumma, and D. Mashberg (1987). Psychosocial functioning of adult acute leukemia survivors treated with bone marrow transplantation (BMT) or standard chemotherapy (SC). *Proc. Am. Soc. Clin. Oncol.* 255 (Abstract No. 1002).

Li, F.P. (1977). Follow-up of survivors of childhood cancer. *Cancer* 39:1776–78.

Li, F.P. and N. Jaffe (1974). Progeny of childhood cancer survivors. *Lancet* 2:707–9.

Li, F.P. and R. Stone (1976). Survivors of cancer in childhood. *Ann. Intern. Med.* 84:551–53.

Li, F.P., J.P. Cassady, and N. Jaffe (1975). Risk of second tumors in survivors of childhood cancer. *Cancer* 35:1230–35.

Li, F.P., M.H. Myers, H.W. Heise, and N. Jaffe (1978). The course of five-year survivors of cancer in childhood. *J. Pediatr.* 93:185–87.

Madorsky, M.L., M.G. Ashamalla, I. Schussler, H.R. Lyons, and G.H. Miller, Jr. (1976). Post-prostatectomy impotence. *J. Urol.* 115:401–3.

Maguire, G.P., E.G. Lee, D.J. Bevington, C.S. Kuchemann, R.J. Crabtree, and C.E. Cornell (1978). Psychiatric problems in the first year after mastectomy. *Br. Med. J.* 1:963–65.

Maher, E. (1982). Anomic aspects of recovery from cancer. *Soc. Sci. Med.* 16:907–14.

Mashberg, D. and L. Lesko (1987). Insurance and employment status of adult leukemia survivors. In M.J.M. Massie and L.M. Lesko (eds.), *Current Concepts in Psycho-Oncology and AIDS* (Poster No. 13). Syllabus of the postgraduate course sponsored by the Memorial Sloan-Kettering Cancer Center, New York City, September 17–19, 1987. New York: Memorial Sloan-Kettering Cancer Center.

McIntosh, S., E.H. Klatskin, R.T. O'Brien, G.T. Aspnes, B.L. Kammerer, C. Snead, S.M. Kalavsky, and H.A. Pearson (1976). Chronic neurologic disturbance in childhood leukemia. *Cancer* 37:853–57.

Meadows, A.T., J. Gordon, D.J. Massari, P. Littman, J. Fergusson, and K. Moss (1981). Declines in IQ scores and cognitive dysfunctions in children with acute lymphocytic leukemia treated with cranial irradiation. *Lancet* 2:1015–18.

Middleton, T. (1981). Pelvic lymphadenectomy with modified radical retropubic prostatectomy as a single operation: Techniques used and results in 50 consecutive cases. *J. Urol.* 125:353–56.

Morris, T., H.S. Greer, and P. White (1977). Psychological and social adjustment to mastectomy: A two-year follow-up study. *Cancer* 40:2381–87.

Moss, H.A., E.D. Nannis, and D.G. Poplack (1981). The effects of prophylactic treatment of the central nervous system on the intellectual functioning of children with acute lymphocytic leukemia. *Am. J. Med.* 71:47–52.

Moth, I., B. Andreasson, S.B. Jensen, and J.E. Bock (1983). Sexual function and somatopsychic reactions after vulvectomy. *Dan. Med. Bull.* 30:27–30.

Mullan, F. (1985). Seasons of survival: Reflections of a physician with cancer. *N. Engl. J. Med.* 313:270–73.

Mulland, F. (1986). Re-entry: The educational needs of the cancer survivor. *Health Educ. Q.* 1:88–94.

Mumma, G., D. Cella, L. Lesko, and S. Tross (1988). *Subgroups of Psychologically Distressed Cancer Survivors* (Abstract). Submitted for presentation at the twenty-fourth annual meeting, Am. Soc. Clin. Oncol.

National Cancer Institute (1984). Surveillance, Epidemiology, and End Results Program (SEER) cancer patient survival statistics. *Update: Annu. Cancer Stat. Rev.*, Nov. 24, pp. 1–8.

Obetz, S.W., R.J. Ivnik, W.A. Smithson, et al. (1979). Neuropsychologic follow-up study of children with acute lymphocytic leukemia: A preliminary report. *Am. J. Pediatr. Hematol. Oncol.* 1:207–13.

Parkes, C.M. (1972). Components of the reaction to loss of a limb, spouse, or home. *J. Psychosom. Res.* 16:343–49.

Pavlovsky, S., N. Fisman, R. Arizaga, J. Castano, N. Chamoles, R. Leiguarda, and R. Moreno (1983). Neuropsychological study in patients with ALL: Two different CNS prevention therapies—Cranial irradiation plus IT methotrexate vs IT methotrexate alone. *Am. J. Pediatr. Hematol. Oncol.* 5:79–86.

Peckham, V.C., A.T. Meadows, N.S. Bartel, and O. Marrero (1988). Educational late effects in long-term survivors of childhood lymphocytic leukemia. *Pediatrics* 81:127–33.

Rieker, P., S.D. Edbril, and M.B. Garnick (1985). Curative testis cancer therapy: Psychosocial sequelae. *J. Clin. Oncol.* 3:1117–26.

Rowland, J.H., O. Glidewell, R. Sibley, J.C. Holland, R. Tull, A. Berman, M.L. Brecher, M. Harris, A.S. Glicksman, E. Forman, B. Jones, M.E. Cohen, P.K. Duffner, and A.I. Freeman (1984). Effects of different forms of central nervous system prophylaxis on neuropsychologic function in childhood leukemia. *J. Clin. Oncol.* 1:1327–35.

Schain, W. (1980). Sexual functioning self-esteem and cancer care. *Front. Radiat. Ther. Oncol.* 14:12–19.

Schottenfeld, D. and G.F. Robbins (1970). Quality of survival among patients who have had radical mastectomy. *Cancer* 26:650–54.

Schover, L.R. and A.C. von Eschenbach (1984). Sexual and marital counseling with men treated for testicular cancer. *J. Sex. Marital Ther.* 10:29–40.

Schover, L.R., R.B. Evans, and A.C. von Eschenbach (1987). Sexual rehabilitation in a cancer center: Diagnosis and outcome in 384 consultations. *Arch. Sex. Behav.* 16:445–61.

Scott, W.W. and H.L. Boyd (1969). Combined hormonal control therapy and radical prostatectomy in the treatment of selected cases of advanced carcinoma of the prostate: A retrospective study based upon 25 years of experience. *J. Urol.* 101:86–92.

Seibel, M.M., M.G. Freeman, and W.L. Graves (1980). Carcinoma of the cervix and sexual function. *Obstet. Gynecol.* 55:484–87.

Selye, H. (1956). *The Stress of Life.* New York: McGraw-Hill.

Sherins, R.J., and V.T. DeVita (1973). Effect of drug treatment for lymphoma on male reproductive capacity. *Ann. Intern. Med.* 79:216–20.

Soni, S., G. Marten, S. Pitner, D. Duenas, and M. Powaizk (1975). Effects of CNS irradiation on neuropsychologic function. *N. Engl. J. Med.* 293:113–18.

Spingarn, N. (1982). *Hanging in There: Living Well on Borrowed Time.* New York: Stein & Day.

Spingarn, N. (1987). *Hanging in There: New Challenges.* Keynote address delivered at the meeting of the National Coalition of Cancer Survivors, Albuquerque, N.M.

Stone, R.W. (1975). Employing the recovered cancer patient. *Cancer* 36:285–86.

Sullivan, M., J. Cohen, and I. Branehog (1987). Psychosocial responses to cancer in the U.S. and Sweden: A comparative patient and family study. *EECO-4: Fourth Eur. Conf. Clin. Oncol. Cancer Nurs.: Satellite Symp. Proc.*, p. 30.

Sutherland, A.M., C.F. Orbach, R.B. Dyk, and M. Bard (1952). The psychological impact of cancer and cancer surgery: I. Adaptation to the dry colostomy. *Cancer* 5:857–72.

Tamaroff, M., D.R. Miller, M.L. Murphy, R. Salwen, F. Ghavimi, and Y. Nir (1982). Immediate and long-term posttherapy neuropsychologic performance in children with acute lymphoblastic leukemia treated without central nervous system radiation. *J. Pediatr.* 101:524–29.

Thacil, J.V., M.A.S. Jewitt, and W.D. Rider (1981). The effects of cancer and cancer therapy on male fertility. *J. Urol.* 126:141–45.

Thompson, E., D. Fairclough, D. Crom, and J. Simone (1987). Normal physical and psychosocial function in the majority of childhood cancer patients surviving 10 years or more from diagnosis. *Proc. Am. Soc. Clin. Oncol.* 6:258 (Abstract No. 1013).

Tross, S., D. Cella, L. Lesko, and J.C. Holland (1987). General versus cancer-specific distress in cancer survivors. *Proc. Am. Soc. Clin. Oncol.* 6:258 (Abstract No. 1001).

Tross, S., J.C. Holland, G. Bosl, and N. Geller (1984). A controlled study of psychosocial sequelae in cured survivors of testicular cancer. *Proc. Am. Soc. Clin. Oncol.* 3:74 (Abstract No. C-287).

Tucker, M.A., C.N. Coleman, R.S. Cox, A. Varghese, and S.A. Rosenberg (1988). Risk of second cancers after treatment for Hodgkin's disease. *N. Engl. J. Med.* 318:76–81.

Van Dongen-Melman, J.E.W.M. and J.A.R. Sanders-Woutstra (1986). Psychosocial aspects of childhood cancer: A review of the literature. *J. Child. Psychol. Psychiatry* 27:145–80.

Vasicka, A., N.R. Popovich, and C.C. Brausch (1958). Post irradiation course of patients with cervical carcinoma. *Obstet. Gynecol.* 11:403–14.

Veenema, R.J., E.O. Gersel, and J.K. Lattimer (1977). Radical retropubic prostatectomy for cancer: A 20-year experience. *J. Urol.* 117:330–31.

Vera, M.I. (1981). Quality of life following pelvic exenteration. *Gynecol. Oncol.* 12:355–66.

Verzosa, M.S., R.J. Aur, J.V. Simone, H. Hustu, and D. Pinkel (1976). Five years after central nervous system irradiation of children with leukemia. *Int. J. Radiat. Oncol. Biol. Phys.* 1:209–315.

Vincent, C.E., B. Vincent, F.C. Greiss, and E.B. Linton (1975). Some marital–sexual concomitants of carcinoma of the cervix. *South. Med. J.* 68:552–58.

Vogelzang, N.J., D. Magid, M. Kozloff, and R. Desser (1987). Psychosocial function in clinical stage I germ cell testicular cancer. *Proc. Am. Soc. Clin. Oncol.* 6:260 (Abstract No. 1021).

Von Eschenbach, A.C. and L.R. Schover (1984). The role of sexual rehabilitation in the treatment of patients with cancer. *Cancer* 54:2662–67.

Walsh, P.C. and P.J. Donker (1982). Impotence following radical prostatectomy: Insight into etiology and prevention. *J. Urol.* 128:492–97.

Wasserman, A.L., E.I. Thompson, J.H. Williams, and D.L. Fairclough (1987). The psychological status of survivors of childhood/adolescent Hodgkin's disease. *Am. J. Dis. Child.* 141:626–31.

Weisman, A. and J.W. Worden (1976–1977). The existential plight in cancer: Significance of the first 100 days. *Int. J. Psychiatry Med.* 7(1):1–15.

Wheatley, G.M., W.W. Cunnick, B.P. Wright, and D. van Keuren (1974). The employment of persons with a history of treatment of cancer. *Cancer* 33:441–45.

Whitt, J.K., R.J. Wells, M. Lauria, C.L. Wihelm, and W. McMillan (1984). Cranial radiation in childhood acute lymphocytic leukemia: Neuropsychologic sequelae. *Am. J. Dis. Child.* 138:730–36.

# Section 2  Treatment-Specific Psychological Issues

# 8

## Psychological Reactions to Cancer Surgery

Paul Jacobsen and Jimmie C. Holland

## HISTORICAL PERSPECTIVE

Surgical removal is the oldest recorded form of treatment for solid tumors. Egyptian papyruses dating from 1600 B.C. show evidence of tumors being cut out (Shimkin, 1977). However, the modern history of cancer surgery began in the early nineteenth century (Rosenberg, 1985). In 1809, Ephraim MacDowell reported removing a 22-pound ovarian tumor; the patient survived for 30 years after the operation. More radical removal of tumors became possible after ether anesthesia was introduced by Warren in 1846. The introduction of antisepsis by Lister in 1867 reduced the high frequency of postoperative infections and deaths from this common complication. These events paved the way for the development of new procedures that allowed radical excision of several previously inoperable neoplasms: gastrectomy, laryngectomy, mastectomy, and hysterectomy (Rosenberg, 1985) (Table 8-1). Over the past few decades, primary surgical treatment has been followed, first by radiotherapy, and since the 1960s, by chemotherapy. The combined-modality approach came about as the result of better understanding of tumor biology, which made it clear that increasingly radical surgery could not deal with the micrometastases that were already present in 70% of solid tumors at the time of presentation (Fisher, 1983).

Current surgical interventions in cancer are not limited to tumor removal (Table 8-2). Far more accurate histological diagnosis can be obtained today through use of bronchoscopy, mediastinoscopy, and exploratory laparotomy for tissue biopsy. Debulking procedures help in the management of recurrent disease. Solitary

metastatic lesions in the liver, lungs, and brain are treated surgically with curative outcome. In cases of advanced disease, palliative surgical procedures are used to provide pain relief and symptom control. The increasingly sophisticated reconstructive procedures and application of prostheses have significantly reduced psychological distress resulting from procedures that alter appearance, such as facial and breast surgery.

Surgery also plays a role in prevention of cancer (Rosenberg, 1985) (Table 8-3). With certain familial conditions that are associated with a high incidence of subsequent cancer, prophylactic removal of the organ concerned can prevent the development of a predictable malignancy. Presurgical counseling is important in cases in which a preventive procedure (e.g., colectomy or mastectomy) has a significant impact on function and appearance.

It is of interest that the psychological responses of patients to radical surgical procedures done for cancer received little attention until the 1950s, more than half a century after several procedures had been developed and widely applied. During the 1950s Sutherland, a psychiatrist, and his group at Memorial Hospital in New York, where much early cancer surgery was developed, carried out the first studies of psychological adaptation to mastectomy and dry colostomy (Sutherland and Orbach, 1953; Bard and Sutherland, 1955). Their early observations remain classics in the field of psychooncology at a time when cancer diagnosis was not revealed and cancer was viewed solely as a surgical discipline. Psychological studies of response to treatment were barely accepted as a scientific discipline. Mastectomy and response to breast cancer were also

117

**Table 8-1**   Selected historical milestones
in surgical oncology

| Year | Surgeon | Event |
|------|---------|-------|
| 1809 | Ephraim McDowell | Elective abdominal surgery (excised ovarian tumor) |
| 1846 | John Collins Warren | Use of ether anesthesia (excised submaxillary gland) |
| 1867 | Joseph Lister | Introduction of antisepsis |
| 1850–1880 | Albert Theodore Billroth | First gastrectomy, laryngectomy, and esophagectomy |
| 1878 | Richard von Volkmann | Excision of cancerous rectum |
| 1880s | Theodore Kocher | Development of thyroid surgery |
| 1890 | William Stewart Halsted | Radical mastectomy |
| 1896 | G. T. Beatson | Oophorectomy for breast cancer |
| 1904 | Hugh H. Young | Radical prostatectomy |
| 1906 | Ernest Wertheim | Radical hysterectomy |
| 1908 | W. Ernest Miles | Abdominoperineal resection for cancer of the rectum |
| 1912 | E. Martin | Cordotomy for the treatment of pain |
| 1910–1930 | Harvey Cushing | Development of surgery for brain tumors |
| 1913 | Franz Torek | Successful resection of cancer of the thoracic esophagus |
| 1927 | G. Divis | Successful resection of pulmonary metastases |
| 1933 | Evarts Graham | Pneumonectomy |
| 1935 | A. O. Whipple | Pancreaticoduodenectomy |
| 1945 | Charles B. Huggins | Adrenalectomy for prostate cancer |

*Source*: Reprinted with permission from S.A. Rosenberg (1985). Principles of surgical oncology. In V.T. DeVita, Jr., S. Hellman, and S.A. Rosenberg (eds.), Philadelphia: Lippincott.

studied in this period by Renneker and Cutler (1952). Far more interest in the psychological issues of cancer surgery developed in the 1960s as the debate grew about whether patients should be told their diagnosis. This directly affected surgeons, who traditionally had obtained consent for surgery without revealing the likely or confirmed diagnosis. The common explanation was, "Your condition might run into cancer and therefore I must remove it." They also never revealed cancer as the diagnosis made at surgery, because it was viewed at that time as information too painful to be revealed to the patient. Surgeons began to write thoughtfully in the 1960s about the psychological man-

**Table 8-2**   Surgeon's role in the treatment of cancer patients

1. Definitive surgical treatment for primary cancer
    Selection of appropriate local therapy
    Integration of surgery with other adjuvant modalities
2. Surgery to reduce the bulk of residual disease
    (Examples: Burkitt's lymphoma, ovarian cancer)
3. Surgical resection of metastatic disease with curative intent
    (Examples: pulmonary metastatses in sarcoma patients, hepatic metastases from colorectal cancer)
4. Surgery for the treatment of oncologic emergencies
5. Surgery for palliation
6. Surgery for reconstruction and rehabilitation

*Source*: Reprinted with permission from S.A. Rosenberg (1985). Principles of surgical oncology. In V.T. DeVita, Jr., S. Hellman, S.A. Rosenberg (eds.). *Cancer: Principles and Practice of Oncology,* 2nd ed. Philadelphia: Lippincott.

agement of their curable and incurable patients (Pack, 1962; Stehlin and Beach, 1966). Stehlin and Beach (1966) provided an excellent outline of how to establish rapport in the preoperative period to allay the patient's fears, how to tell the patient that curable cancer was found at surgery, and how to establish close communication with the patient whose cancer was found to be incurable at surgery. In regard to the latter, they wrote:

If the doctor–patient relationship is one in which each feels free to communicate with the other, telling the patient that he is incurable, although never easy, is less painful. Here, again, if we listen to the patient he will let us know when he can be told and how much he can tolerate hearing. Once the essentials of truth are explained in the proper manner, the way becomes clear for the next phase . . . hope; . . . the words "incurable" and "hopeless" are not synonymous. To tell a patient that his condition is hopeless is both cruel and technically incorrect. Incurability is a state of mind, a giving up—a situation that must be avoided at all cost. A patient can tolerate knowing he is incurable; he cannot tolerate hopelessness. (p. 103)

**Table 8-3**   Surgery that can prevent cancer

| Underlying condition | Associated cancer | Prophylactic surgery |
|----------------------|-------------------|----------------------|
| Cryptorchidism | Testicular | Orchiopexy |
| Polyposis coli | Colon | Colectomy |
| Familial colon cancer | Colon | Colectomy |
| Ulcerative colitis | Colon | Colectomy |
| Multiple endocrine neoplasia, types II and III | Medullary cancer of the thyroid | Thyroidectomy |
| Familial breast cancer | Breast | Mastectomy |
| Familial ovarian cancer | Ovary | Oophorectomy |

*Source*: Reprinted with permission from S.A. Rosenberg (1985). Principles of surgical oncology. In V.T. DeVita, Jr., S. Hellman, S.A. Rosenberg (eds.), *Cancer: Principles and Practice of Oncology,* 2nd ed. Philadelphia: Lippincott.

Surgery today continues to play a central role in curative treatment of cancer. Yet it cannot be applied effectively without attention to possible psychological influences on the person's ability to understand the procedure proposed, recognize its necessity, and tolerate the stress and discomforts associated with the procedure in order to reap the benefit of improved survival. In most instances the surgeon, through interaction with the patient, is aware of the patient's psychological needs. Only when serious psychopathological conditions arise is collaboration between the surgeon and psychiatrist necessary to assure that patients can tolerate a needed procedure. Several common issues require immediate attention: a disturbed relationship to the surgeon or staff, inability to give consent, severe preoperative anxiety and refusal of surgery, exacerbation of a preexisting psychiatric disorder, postoperative psychiatric delirium or mental disorder, and poor compliance with rehabilitation. It is here that knowledge of the common types of psychiatric disturbance that occur in surgical cancer patients and their management becomes important.

This chapter describes the range of normal and abnormal psychological reactions that occur in the period surrounding surgery (the perioperative period): this includes (1) the preoperative period, which may be brief or may extend over weeks of tests and medical preparation for the procedure, (2) the intraoperative period in the operating room and the recovery room, and (3) the postoperative recovery period in the hospital and at home. Specific emotional problems that relate to procedures for particular neoplasms such as breast, head and neck, and colon are mentioned. Rehabilitation of patients after surgery, which depends heavily on the individual's psychological state, commitment, and perseverance, is also reviewed.

## THE PERIOPERATIVE PERIOD: NORMAL AND ABNORMAL REACTIONS

As with the determinants of psychological reactions to cancer generally (Chapter 3), there are two principal sets of determinants in the psychological adaptation of a patient to cancer surgery (Table 8-4). First is the combination of *medical* variables that includes site, stage, and curability of the tumor by surgery alone or with other treatment modalities, functional deficits resulting from surgery, rehabilitation available, and the surgeon's psychological management of the patient. Second is the constellation of patient-related issues represented by the meaning the person attaches to the cancer diagnosis or its possibility, the surgical procedure itself and its consequences, the psychological stability of the patient to tolerate a stressful event, and the relationship established with the surgeon. When

**Table 8-4** Psychological adaptation to cancer surgery

| Considerations | Examples |
| --- | --- |
| Medical | Site |
| | Stage |
| | Surgical resection: operable or inoperable |
| | Functional deficits resulting from surgery |
| | Rehabilitation available |
| | Surgeon's psychological management of the patient |
| Patient | Meaning the person attaches to possible (or actual) cancer diagnosis, anesthesia, the surgical procedure, and functional consequences |
| | Psychological stability: ability to cope with stress of surgery; absence of psychiatric disorder |
| | Relationship to surgeon |

these are considered carefully, the patient who is likely to have trouble adapting can usually be identified early. The discussion that follows reviews these considerations as they relate to the preoperative and postoperative periods; however, the division is arbitrary because psychological adaptation to the postoperative period is strongly influenced and can often be predicted by variables evident in the preoperative period, some of which are amenable to interventions that increase likelihood of a smoother postoperative course.

## Normal Preoperative Responses and Their Management

The universal reaction to an anticipated surgical procedure is fear and anxiety. These feelings take different forms depending on the patient's prior experiences, personality, and the nature of the procedure planned. Fears of anesthesia, pain, and death during the operation are common. Strain and Grossman (1977) outlined concerns evoked by impending surgery: the threat to the sense of personal invulnerability, the concern that one's life is being entrusted largely to strangers, separation from the familiar environment of home and family members, fears of transient loss of control or death while under anesthesia, fear of being partially awake during surgery, and fears of damage to body parts. These fears are greatest in individuals who have chronically high levels of anxiety or a past history of phobias, as discussed later. In addition to preoperative fear, many patients feel hopeless, helpless, and angry. Although these preoperative reactions occur in all patients, there is a significantly greater stress involved when cancer is the suspected diagnosis or the condition for which surgery is being performed (Gottesman and Lewis, 1982). These normal concerns, heightened in

**Table 8-5**  Preoperative sources for patients' psychological preparation

| Source | Type of preparation |
|---|---|
| Surgeon | Information and emotional support<br>Psychological management |
| Anesthesiologist | Information and support |
| Nurse | Preoperative education: orientation to procedures, operating room, care in recovery room, postoperative breathing and coughing |
| Veteran patient of same procedure | Experiential information and reassurance; good model of coping |
| Nurse–counselor | Communication between surgeon in the operating room and waiting family |
| Psychiatrist or psychologist | Supportive psychotherapy<br>Behavioral techniques (rehearsing, models, instructions, stress inoculation) |

cancer, are addressed by all members of the surgical team, but the surgeon who will perform the procedure is central (Table 8-5).

When one considers the stresses surgery presents, it is not surprising that the surgeon is invested with the strong emotions that come from entrusting one's life to another. By virtue of this fact, however, the surgeon may elicit reactions similar to those associated with authority figures in the individual's past (Small, 1976). This accounts for some of the special feelings of affection and admiration patients develop for the surgeon, as well as for some of the unwarranted hostile and angry responses. These transference reactions can complicate the relationship and impede good cooperation and optimal surgical outcome. Surgeons who are alert to such responses try to avoid a personal response, but at times the subtlety of the response, or its extreme nature, may require evaluation and intervention.

For many years surgeons have made use of the veteran patient in helping a patient make the difficult decision to consent to surgery that will produce a major functional deficit. Patients who have had a laryngectomy and those who have adapted to a colostomy are an extremely important resource for the anxious patient. They are credible models of how well another has adapted and, as such, are far more effective than anyone else in encouraging an optimistic approach to surgery.

Ideally, psychological management begins with the family doctor who refers the patient to the surgeon. The patient should arrive at the surgeon's office with some explanation of the reason for the consideration of an operation. This preparation provides a sense of security about the continuity of care. The preoperative consultation visit with the surgeon is a critically impor-

tant opportunity for the surgeon to assess the patient's emotional stability and to begin psychological preparation for the procedure. It is in this conversation that a sense of respect and trust develops and a positive doctor–patient relationship is established, which makes it easier for the patient to face the anticipated procedure. It is most important that the patient be given an adequate explanation of all aspects of the proposed procedure: the type of anesthesia to be administered, the nature of the surgical procedure itself, the expected length of time in the recovery room and in the hospital, the body part(s) that may be removed, the functions that may be temporarily or permanently lost, and the corrective and rehabilitative procedures that are available. It is very important that the surgeon develop a relationship with the patient, rather than with some self-designated relative spokesperson who has decided to protect the patient from any bad news, such as with the attitude expressed in ''We know she will give up if she knows she has cancer,'' or ''Don't tell her what's wrong, doctor.'' In addition to providing information, preoperative discussions should also be used to clarify misconceptions or unrealistic expectations. This point is particularly important with children, who are prone to misunderstand information about medical procedures and who therefore experience greater distress (Seeman and Rockoff, 1986). Because all patients are anxious, explanations must be given clearly, in nonmedical terms, and with adequate opportunity to ask questions. Drawings that depict the procedure may aid the patient in understanding what will be done. Having a relative present allows for later discussion at home. Tape-recording the interview allows the patient and relative to listen together at home when they are less stressed. Moreover, because the patient is anxious, the information the surgeon has conveyed may not be ''heard,'' and may need to be repeated at more than one visit. Patients will sometimes have no recall months later of the preoperative discussion for informed consent.

Finally, it is important that the surgeon in a tertiary center obtain the informed consent and request the patient's signature himself or herself, because the consent document reflects the contract between them. Also, a visit the evening before the surgery conveys a sense of personal concern and may enhance the patient's confidence for facing the procedure the following day. A note in the chart confirms the patient's consent and understanding of the procedure. The loss of personal identity inherent in accepting hospital attire, acquiring a number, giving up jewelry, and loss of personal dignity that accompanies preoperative shaving of an operative site or bowel preparation, make the personal relationship to the surgeon and not his or her surrogate all the more important. Another valuable reinforcement is a visit by the surgeon in the early morning to see the patient who may have to wait until 3 or 4 P.M. for an operation. A moment or two of reassurance is all that is required.

One of the most striking attempts to improve communication between the surgeon and waiting family once surgery has begun is the Surgical Nurse Counseling Program at the Memorial Sloan-Kettering Center in New York (Watson and Hickey, 1984). A major aim of the program, developed by two surgical nurses at the center, is to reassure the patient the evening before the surgery that the nurses will help the family through the waiting period. The nurse–counselors familiarize themselves daily with the operating room schedule and visit each patient the afternoon before surgery to ask if he or she wishes them to maintain contact with their closest relative before and during the procedure the following day. They are careful to respect the patient's wishes about the amount and nature of news to be told. Most patients welcome the opportunity for a link between the surgeon in the operating room and the waiting family. The nurses circulate through the several operating rooms and obtain firsthand information from the surgeon about the patient's condition, the progress of the surgery, and the information the surgeon wishes conveyed to the relatives. In addition to relieving anxiety in family members, the program has reduced the angry and disruptive inquiries made to operating room and floor staff by worried relatives. These calls had previously been handled by harried recovery room staff who were not given information with which to answer questions, and hence often inadvertently increased anxiety. This simple intervention by nurse–counselors who are knowledgeable about both surgery and counseling has been highly successful, inexpensive, and well received by the medical staff. The surgeons rapidly became accustomed to these surgical nurses' new role and saw the benefit of improved communication with relatives. The initially feared problems of inaccurate or inappropriate messages being conveyed never materialized, and the program is now an integral part of surgical management.

Today patient education is a far more important aspect of preoperative preparation. Nurses are responsible for much of this development. At our hospital, surgical patients see a film that orients them to procedures on the floors and prepares them for postoperative discomforts. Patients awaiting thoracic surgery learn the importance of coughing and deep breathing after surgery. Women undergoing breast surgery know that daily classes are held for women after surgery that instructs them in arm exercises and allow for discussion of emotional responses.

## Empirical Studies of Preoperative Interventions

Most work on preoperative anxiety and postoperative adjustment derives from the observations of Janis (1958). He found that patients who were moderately fearful before surgery were better adjusted and tolerated postoperative discomforts better than patients who had a high or low level of fear. Patients with low preoperative fear showed more anger, resentment, and less cooperation; those with high preoperative fear were less involved in their treatments and developed hypochondriacal concerns. Janis argued that moderate fear promoted the "work of worrying" by forcing the patient to rehearse mentally the procedure and obtain information to fill the gaps in understanding, thus resulting in more self-assurance and ability to cooperate. Low preoperative fear did not stimulate the work of worrying and high preoperative fear precluded the process from occurring.

Much subsequent research has not confirmed Janis' finding of a curvilinear relationship between the level of preoperative fear and postoperative emotional difficulties, although Auerbach (1973) and, more recently, Andersen and Tewfik (1985) confirmed the findings. The latter showed that the level of anxiety before receiving external beam radiation predicted adaptation. Those with high and low anxiety levels had more anger or hostility than those with moderate anxiety, suggesting that there is a desirable and constructive level of anxiety in anticipation of a threatening situation. (See Chapter 9 on response to radiotherapy.) Most research has demonstrated a linear relationship, with high fear causing the greatest postoperative emotional disturbance and low fear causing the least disturbance. These relationships, however, are altered by the presence of pain, in that more severe pain is associated with greater postoperative anxiety (Wolfer and Davis, 1970; Chapman and Cox, 1977).

Following Janis' work, studies began to be reported on psychological reactions to head and neck surgery (Adsett, 1963), and to psychological reactions to open-heart surgery (Kimball, 1969; Kornfeld et al., 1965). Hackett and Weisman (1960) described the common psychiatric operative syndromes and placed them in perspective by identifying them as disorders that "frequently trouble the surgeon, harass the nursing staff, impede the course of recovery, and may be fully as dangerous as the infections or embolic complications of surgery." These observations were followed by evidence of the effect of psychological decompensation on the hypothalamic–pituitary–adrenal axis prior to mastectomy by Katz and colleagues (1970). The studies that began to emphasize the importance of psychological responses of patients to surgery, for both benign and malignant conditions, resulted in a body of information on which we have drawn to understand reactions of patients currently undergoing cancer surgery.

Anesthesiologists are traditionally seen as technicians administering anesthesia and as having little interaction with patients. However, they always have a preoperative review of the patient's chart and visit the patient to explain the anesthesia, which is often the most frightening aspect of surgery. In 1964, Egbert and colleagues at the Massachusetts General Hospital randomized 97 patients undergoing intraabdominal procedures to a group who were told about postoperative pain by the anesthesiologist or a group who did not receive similar instructions. Neither patients nor staff were aware of the randomization, which preceded formal consent procedures for participation in clinical research. Of the 97 surgical procedures, 57 were gastrectomy, colectomy, and bowel resection; it is likely that these procedures were largely done for cancerous disease, although it is not reported. The anesthesiologist described during the preoperative visit the postoperative pain that patients would have, the medication they would receive, and that the painful muscle spasms could be diminished by deep breathing. The anesthesiologist continued to make daily visits after surgery, giving encouragement and reassurance. Results indicated that, compared to the control group, the intervention group used significantly fewer analgesics. They also went home an average of 3 days earlier. The study by Egbert and colleagues (1964), demonstrating that preoperative reassurance by the anesthesiologist reduced postoperative narcotics requirement of surgical patients was a landmark; unfortunately, it still has not led to change in clinical practice.

Other studies have confirmed that such interventions reduce hospital stay and the use of analgesics (Lindeman and Van Aernam, 1971; Schmitt and Wooldridge, 1973). However, the multifaceted nature of the interventions employed by Egbert and others prevented understanding of how psychological considerations affect recovery. Later, efforts have tried to isolate and examine the principal determinants: psychological support, provision of information, and skills training.

Several studies in the 1970s examined the psychological effects of providing patients with detailed information about the procedure(s) to be performed (Andrew, 1970; Chapman and Cox, 1977; Vernon and Bigelow, 1974). Anderson and Masur (1983), however, concluded that patients receiving such information scored only slightly better than controls on measures of postoperative adjustment and recovery. Several investigators have examined the efficacy of providing different types of information (Kendall et al., 1979; Johnson and Leventhal, 1974; Johnson, 1973; Wilson, 1981; Anderson, 1987). In these studies patients were provided with information about the visual, auditory, and kinesthetic sensations they would experience during an anticipated procedure. The addition of sensory information increased the beneficial effects, perhaps because sensory information permits more accurate expectations of postoperative sensations, including those that are uncomfortable.

Brief psychotherapy has also been used to prepare patients for surgery. In fact the intervention employed by Egbert and colleagues was called superficial psychotherapy. Few studies have systematically evaluated its effects on postoperative recovery. Two early studies suggested that a preoperative psychotherapy visit was associated with decreased incidence of postoperative psychiatric complications (Kornfeld et al., 1974; Layne and Yudofsky, 1971). However, results of other studies questioned the efficacy of brief psychotherapy (Dumas and Johnson, 1972; Streltzer and Leigh, 1978). It is a common assumption that allowing patients to express concerns and fears, and providing emotional support and reassurance are the major contributors to better postoperative adjustment (Anderson and Masur, 1983). However, an alternative explanation is that psychotherapy is helpful because it provides information. It is difficult to reassure without giving information, and more systematic psychotherapeutic research may be needed to tease out the components.

Several studies have examined the effects of behavioral interventions such as active and passive relaxation training, stress inoculation training, and modeling of postoperative recovery. The active form of relaxation training involves teaching patients to tense and relax muscle groups progressively as a means of inducing relaxation. The passive form of relaxation training is similar to self-hypnosis or meditation, and typically involves calming self-statements and the use of pleasant mental imagery (see Chapter 40, 46). In controlled studies, passive relaxation training reduced intraoperative and postoperative anxiety in ambulatory surgery patients (Domar et al., 1987). Active relaxation training reduced length of stay and the use of analgesics in abdominal surgery patients (Wilson, 1981). In both studies, patients received training in relaxation techniques by use of audiocassette tapes, an inexpensive simple intervention.

Another behavioral technique that was recently evaluated is stress inoculation training (Turk et al., 1983). Wells and colleagues (1986) developed a stress inoculation procedure for surgical patients that was administered during a 1-hour training session the day before surgery. During this session, patients received instruction in monitoring themselves for cognitive and physiological signs of stress, deep breathing, muscle relaxation, induction of pleasant imagery, and substitution of coping self-statements for negative self-statements. In addition to experiencing less preoperative anxiety, the patients who underwent stress inoculation training experienced less postoperative anxiety and pain than a control group of patients receiving standard hospital care. Moreover, patients who received training went home an average of 3.5 days earlier than their control group counterparts.

Modeling is a behavioral technique that has been used extensively with children undergoing surgery by having them view films showing another child going through the same procedure. In one study children viewed the film, "Ethan Has an Operation," a detailed realistic portrayal of the hospitalization, preparation, hernia surgery, and recovery of a 7-year-old boy (Melamed and Siegel, 1975). Results indicated that children who viewed the film before surgery were more cooperative with medical personnel, reported less anxiety, and had fewer medical concerns. In oncology, modeling has been used to reduce the distress of bone marrow aspiration, usually performed without anesthesia. Jay and colleagues have developed a group of behavioral therapy techniques to be used before aspiration procedures, which consist of breathing exercises, rewards, and the viewing of a film of a child undergoing the procedure. Children who had received the intervention showed less distress as evidenced by crying, and were less likely to require restraint during bone marrow aspiration (Jay et al., 1985).

There is considerable evidence that psychological preparation for surgery facilitates postoperative emotional adjustment and recovery in both adults and children. The research supports the early observations of Janis that the "work of worry" is an important part of the psychological preparation for a stressful event. The more the anxiety is constructively directed, by rehearsal of anticipated events or discussion of what is anticipated, the better the psychological outcome. Strain (1985) noted that "it is less important which caretaker performs this intervention—nurse, anesthesiologist, surgeon, primary physician, house staff, psychiatrist—than that it is done." Table 8-5 outlines the major preoperative interventions that support healthy psychological adaptation. Indeed, two metaanalyses of studies in this area concluded that brief psychological interventions were superior to standard hospital care in reducing postoperative pain and in increasing satisfaction with care and psychological well-being (Mumford et al., 1982; Devine and Cook, 1986). These analyses also indicated that psychological interventions possess cost-saving effects, because patients who received psychological preparation were discharged an average of 2 days sooner than patients who

received standard care. Gil (1984) has suggested that there are at least four ways in which psychological interventions may enhance patients' ability to cope with the physical and psychological demands of surgery: by directing the patient's attention to the demands of the situation, by clarifying the demands so that expectations more closely reflect the reality of the situation, by providing information that can make the consequences of the situation more predictable and thereby increase the patient's sense of personal control, and by directly promoting control over the demands of the situation through training in specific responses (e.g., with breathing and relaxation).

Normal postoperative psychological responses are varied and depend heavily on medical considerations that are highly variable. The acute postoperative pain can usually be controlled with narcotics given in adequate doses. Physicians unfamiliar with drug pharmacology, half-life, and excretion patterns may undertreat postoperative pain. Uncontrolled pain results in acute agitation and anxiety, which can be alleviated by adequate pain relief (Massie and Holland, 1987). High preoperative anxiety or depression also results in increased postoperative pain and need for analgesics and sedatives following abdominal surgery. All clinical experience points toward better control of pain postoperatively in the psychologically prepared patients, as shown by Egbert and colleagues. However, two empirical studies have given contradictory results (Scott et al., 1983; Sime, 1976). In general, given the absence of complications or unusually severe pain, anxiety rapidly returns to normal over several days.

Depressed mood often accompanies the early postoperative days. It may be much worse when bad news is reported about surgical findings and prognosis. Longitudinal studies of women undergoing mastectomy found that initial distress reduced rapidly over a year, reaching comparable levels to those of women who had had cholecystectomy (Penman et al., 1986). Women who had persistent distress at a year had received chemotherapy after surgery (see Chapter 14 on breast cancer). This study of over 1000 women suggests that women adapt to mastectomy better than previously assumed. However, predictors of poor adjustment were other concurrent illness or adverse life events, as well as stage II disease requiring chemotherapy.

## Common Psychiatric Operative Syndromes and Issues

Several psychiatric determinants can lead to distress that exceeds normal limits. These are reviewed in order of likely appearance, from the period before to that after the operation (see Table 8-6).

**Table 8-6**  Common psychiatric disorders and problems in surgical patients

---

- Perioperative management of patients receiving psychotropic drugs
- Inability to understand and give consent
- Preoperative panic and refusal of surgery
- Postoperative delirium
- Depression and suicidal risk
- Personality disorders

---

## PATIENTS RECEIVING PSYCHOTROPIC DRUGS

Patients who require psychotropic drugs pose a particularly difficult problem when they are awaiting surgery that raises the possibility of cancer. Their known vulnerability to the exacerbation of symptoms of schizophrenia, major depression, or manic-depressive illness in a stressful situation makes the psychiatrist reluctant to stop medication for a lengthy period in advance of major surgery. Although some psychiatrists and anesthesiologists suggest the conservative approach of suspending the use of all psychotropic drugs 2 weeks before surgery (DiGiacomo, 1985), our experience has not supported such a blanket guideline for management of this problem. In fact, in a survey of 50 patients with severe psychiatric illness who were studied for prevalence of psychiatric complications in their postoperative hospital course (Solomon et al., 1987), both chronic schizophrenics and chronic depressives tolerated surgery well without exacerbation of symptoms. Only those who had acute symptoms in the preoperative period tended to have significant postoperative psychiatric difficulties. Flexibility is possible when the psychiatrist and the anesthesiologist coordinate their care. The guidelines we suggest are as follows:

1. At the time that a patient who is receiving a tricyclic antidepressant, a monoamine oxidase inhibitor (MAOI), lithium, or a major tranquilizer is referred for surgery, a consultation between the anesthesiologist and the psychiatrist should take place in order to develop a coordinated plan based on the particular patient's needs and the drug involved.

2. The drug that is of most concern is the MAOI, because its metabolism alters the sympathetic amines, serotonin, norepinephrine, and dopamine. Narcotics interact with an MAOI to cause an exaggerated response to the usual dose, thus producing hypotension and apnea. The narcotic chosen is important. Meperidine is contraindicated because of its interaction with MAOIs to produce hyperpyrexia and hypertension. A hypertensive crisis, should it occur, is treated by an alpha adrenergic blocker such as chlorpromazine. The effect of succinylcholine may be exaggerated, and the dose will need to be adjusted. MAOI administration should be stopped well in advance of the anticipated surgery, by at least 1 week.

3. When the patient is receiving a tricyclic antidepressant, it can be continued until the day before surgery if the anesthesiologist is aware of the situation and can plan the anesthesia with that in mind. Scopolamine and other anticholinergic drugs will act synergistically with a tricyclic, raising the risk of postoperative anticholinergic delirium. Physostigmine is the drug of choice in treating delirium (see Chapter 30 for detailed discussion). The hypnotic effect of barbiturates is potentiated by tricyclic antidepressants, requiring lower doses of sedating drugs.

4. Major tranquilizers block the dopamine receptor, and the low-potency drugs (e.g., thioridazine and chlorpromazine) produce hypotension by central and peripheral anticholinergic action. They also increase the risk of postoperative delirium when other drugs (e.g., scopolamine) are used (DiGiacomo, 1985).

5. Lithium carbonate can be continued until the time of surgery and poses few difficulties that cannot be anticipated. Muscle relaxants such as succinylcholine may be potentiated by lithium, and this should be taken into account in the dosage.

6. All of the preceding medications can be resumed at the time that the patient resumes taking liquids orally. Starting the drug again must take into account the patient's needs for the drug and any possible contraindications that result from the surgery, as with bowel resection.

## INABILITY TO UNDERSTAND AND GIVE CONSENT

Some patients appear for surgery who are unable to understand the nature and consequences of the procedure proposed. When it is lifesaving and relatives are absent, the surgery may be performed with a note from the psychiatrist and agreement of the hospital to accept responsibility. If the surgery is elective and there is need for a guardian to be appointed for the individual, one is justified in requesting a legal test of competency and the appointment of a legal guardian. This procedure is usually followed for dementia and does not occur often in oncology situations. More common are cases that involve a patient with an alcoholic history who understands in part the need for a major resection of a head and neck tumor, but whose ability to cooperate after surgery is minimal. These cases require thoughtful evaluation.

CASE REPORT

A 62-year-old who had a concerned family had a long history of alcoholism despite many efforts by the family to obtain treatment for her. She had had two early lesions of the tongue excised, continued to drink, and came in for symptoms of a recurrence that required wide excision of tongue and jaw. A psychiatric consultation revealed that the patient had mild cognitive impairment and poor ability to understand the postoperative situation and need for self-care, suggesting inability to give fully informed consent. The concerned family met with the surgeon and psychiatrist and decided that palliative radiation was preferable to the excision of tongue and partial jaw resection, with which she would have trouble coping, and her inability to participate in self-care was likely to result in painful and troublesome complications.

## PREOPERATIVE PANIC AND REFUSAL OF SURGERY

Paralyzing anxiety or panic occurs most often in situations involving either a preexisting severe anxiety disorder (accompanied by a phobia of being alone in an unfamiliar environment, or a morbid fear of anesthesia, or fear of having an operation), or a special meaning of the surgery or some prior association with surgery or cancer. Data from our studies of psychiatric consultations with cancer patients and data from general surgical patients indicate that there is a low percentage of such cases, less than 5% (Massie and Holland, 1987; Strain, 1985). Nevertheless, these unusual cases present difficult management problems as surgical cases. The following cases illustrate the problems and their management.

CASE REPORT

A 57-year-old man with severe hypochondriacal concerns for many years and severe anxiety attacks was found to have an early resectable lung cancer. His chronic anxiety became worse and resulted in several severe anxiety attacks with chest pain requiring workup for heart attack; all were negative. The thoracic surgeon requested consultation and careful coordination of care with the psychiatrist, who met with the patient several times before admission and placed him on imipramine to control the attacks. With the anesthesiologist, they developed a plan in which he was admitted with a relative who was allowed to stay the night before surgery. The nursing staff were alerted to the unusual demands and problems in care that this patient might present. The surgeon put him first on the morning surgery schedule after preanesthesia had been started 24 hours earlier. The nurse–counselor accompanied him to the operating room. He managed the operation and became far more cooperative in the postoperative period when his fears were lessened.

Management of this type of patient led to the plan outlined in Table 8-7. It is implemented early when such cases are identified, resulting in their more effective management.

**Table 8-7** Guidelines for preoperative anxiety and/or panic

1. Refer to psychiatrist early (preferably prior to admission for surgery).
2. Provide psychiatric consultation.
   A. Evaluate symptoms.
   B. Call for anesthesiology consultation.
   C. Coordinate psychotropic medications 12–24 hours before surgery with anesthesia and surgery:
      • Benzodiazepines
      • Neuroleptics
      • Antidepressants
   D. Request surgical nurse-counselor for continuity from floor to operating room for patient.
   E. Advise floor staff of special needs of patient and need for presence of family.
3. Maximize "familiar" staff; minimize conflicting information.
4. Schedule as first case, when possible.

CASE REPORT

A 45-year-old married woman was admitted to the surgery floor for mastectomy. She appeared calm and composed, without evidence of any emotional distress or anxiety. She complied with all requests until, while waiting in the holding area for the operating room, she became panic-stricken, crying wildly and stating that she could not go through with the operation. She was returned to her room and her surgeon discharged her to allow the psychological problem to be explored. Psychiatric evaluation revealed a traumatic series of events in which her mother had died a year earlier from breast cancer and her sister had just been found to have metastatic breast disease. She viewed her own outlook as bleak and hopeless, although she had not expressed it to anyone. A conversation with another patient had suddenly led her to become overwhelmed by the meaning of her own operation. A chance to reassess the reality of the situation and remove the unrealistic meaning she had given to it allowed her to be able to be readmitted and have the surgery.

This case is similar to the one described by Abram and Gil (1961), in which identification with another patient who had died of breast cancer resulted in severe anxiety and depression.

CASE REPORT

A 55-year-old unmarried businesswoman came in for resection of a colon cancer that appeared to be fully resectable. She appeared calm and assured, but asked to see a psychiatrist. She stated that she felt embarrassed by her intense fear of surgery and her concern that she might not go through with it. She then recounted that she had had tonsillectomy at age 10. Her parents had not prepared her for the surgery. She had frightening memories of having a mask placed on her face and smelling the drip ether used at that time. She also had vague memories of not being asleep as the doctor began the procedure. These memories had resulted in nightmares for many years and great fear of how she would face surgery should it ever become necessary. This posttraumatic stress response was somewhat relieved by reliving the memories. She was given mild bedtime sedation for insomnia that had been present since the time was set for the surgery. A meeting with the anesthesiologist was planned in which the intravenous preanesthesia was described and she was reassured that intubation would occur only when she was well asleep. She was assured she would have no recall of the procedure and would awaken in the recovery room. The evening before the surgery, the surgeon and anesthesiologist again reassured her about the procedure. She tolerated the preoperative period well and did well postoperatively.

## POSTOPERATIVE DELIRIUM

The postoperative period is a time when acute postoperative confusional states (i.e., organic mental syndromes) occur. They usually appear within 3 to 4 days after surgery. The initial signs are often subtle, with slight loss of memory, changes in behavior, irritability, or misinterpretation of sights or sounds. Patients often develop delusions and fears of being harmed. Organic affective syndrome is common in response to analgesics. It is important that the mental change be recognized early and that a psychiatric consultation be called to assist in determining etiology and management. The delirium, when unrecognized, usually becomes worse with disruptive behavior (e.g., pulling out tubes) and fatigue resulting from agitation and lack of rest. (See Chapter 10 on delirium and dementia for signs, symptoms, diagnosis, and management.) In the early stages, a screening instrument (Cognitive Capacity Screening Examination—Jacobs et al., 1977; or the Mini Mental State Examination—Folstein et al., 1975) may be helpful for differentiating between a functional state and metabolic encephalopathy.

Most postoperative disorders relate to the procedure or a complication of it. Table 8-8 outlines the common causes of postoperative disorders: response to anesthesia or analgesics; anticholinergic syndrome based on the additive effects of several drugs with anticholinergic side effects; electrolyte, fluid, or metabolic imbalance; delirium tremens caused by alcohol withdrawal; CNS complications; and loss of circadian pattern and the stress of an unfamiliar environment (especially in the elderly). (Chapter 30 reviews the common causes and diagnostic characteristics of delirium.) Seymour and colleagues (1986) provide extensive reviews of these issues. Older individuals are at greater risk, as are those with any preexisting mild dementia, particularly alcohol-related.

The most common postoperative delirium seen in patients with head and neck cancer is in those who have an alcoholic history, transient hypoxia, and cerebral anoxia. They drink until admission, have the operation, and develop withdrawal with delirium tremens on

**Table 8-8** Common causes of postoperative delirium (mental organic syndromes)

Response to anesthesia or analgesia
Anticholinergic syndrome (due to additive effect of several anticholinergic drugs used during and after surgery)
Electrolyte, fluid, or metabolic imbalance
Delirium tremens
CNS complication (e.g., hypoxia, infection, bleeding, emboli)
Loss of circadian pattern and stress of unfamiliar environment (in elderly)

the second or third day. (See Chapter 17 on head and neck cancer for management of delirium tremens.) Management depends on determining the etiology and controlling behavior with one-to-one observation and low dose of a major tranquilizer, preferably haloperidol. At times, emotional influences complicate the delirium.

### CASE REPORTS

A 55-year-old attorney had a pneumonectomy followed by a reasonable postoperative course, despite a cardiac complication and a period of transient hypoxia and cerebral anoxia. He had been more fearful due to memories of his father dying of lung cancer. On the third day he was told gently by the surgeon that the diagnosis of cancer had been made at surgery. He became morose, then agitated, and for several hours he felt he was dying and visualized his funeral in which he saw himself in a casket. His confusion slowly cleared and 3 days later he had poor recall of the episode.

A 65-year-old man required an unusually high dose of narcotics following gastrectomy. On the fourth postoperative day he reported that he heard people talking about drugs being sold outside his room and that there was a plot to take his life. He was fearful, had illusions of frightening objects on the ceiling of his room related to the pattern of the tiles on the ceiling, and saw alterations of the figures in the picture in his room. The analgesic was changed and with one-to-one observation, his delirium cleared over 24 hours, and he recalled the events with curiosity.

## DEPRESSION AND SUICIDAL RISK

The presence of depressive symptoms, both before and after surgery, relate most often to presence of uncontrolled pain and appear usually with anxiety symptoms, resulting in a diagnosis of an adjustment disorder with mixed anxiety and depressive mood (Strain, 1985). Uncomplicated recovery from surgery for a benign condition is accompanied by decrease in depression by the third postoperative day (Chapman and Cox, 1977). This pattern, however, may not be the case when cancer is the diagnosis.

Depression—often major—most often occurs following surgery for cancer when the results are particularly ominous, for example, when a tumor was found unresectable and the prognosis is poor, when a limb or breast was amputated, or when gynecological or urological surgery is known to result in sterility or sexual dysfunction. The postoperative period then is one of recovery from the procedure but also confrontation with and adaptation to loss and possible death. This process resembles anticipatory grieving. The initial shock is usually followed by emotional turmoil, and resolution may be difficult. Suicidal ideation is not uncommon. "Why put my family through more?" "What do I have to live for?" "My life is over, I might as well end it." These patients require urgent attention because they sometimes attempt suicide, usually after discharge. Families need help in planning care at home, and referral for help from a mental health professional is important.

### CASE REPORT

A 61-year-old teacher had had a brief history of gastric distress that led to a diagnostic workup for suspected gastric cancer. On exploratory laparotomy, widespread disease was found; no resection was attempted. The patient was informed of the findings after she recovered from anesthesia and was able to talk with the surgeon. She had never permitted herself to be seen as ill by her family and vowed they would remember her as she was, not as she felt she would become over the next few months she had to live. She wanted no chemotherapy or radiation, and began serious plans for suicide at home. Psychiatric consultation with her and her family focused on the present and that her present quality of life was such that she could enjoy her family. Suicide, while always an option she wanted to consider, could be postponed. She accepted friends and family's solicitations and accepted some alternative therapies that had no adverse effect on her appearance. She met regularly with the psychiatrist about her fears, her concerns for an aged parent, and young children. She requested mild daytime and bedtime sedation. Over 2 months, she adjusted to the situation and was able to see the value of her husband and children of living out the time she had with them.

## PERSONALITY DISORDERS

Patients who cause the most distress to staff are those who have long-standing personality problems that are exacerbated by the stresses of surgery. They are reviewed in Chapter 26 in detail. Briefly, patients who are excessively meticulous and obsessive often are concerned about the details of care and the competence of the staff. Suspicious patients are constantly doubting and querulous about information given them. The histrionic patient often sets one staff member against another, and symptoms may be difficult to assess because of their dramatic description. Management of these problems largely depends on the staff to recog-

nize and handle difficult behavior, because the basic personality problems are too complex to address in any substantive way during hospitalization.

## PSYCHOLOGICAL REACTIONS RELATED TO SITE OF SURGERY

In addition to the common postoperative reactions already described, psychological reactions are largely related to the site of surgery and the functional loss sustained. Adverse emotional reactions correlate with the psychological significance of the loss, especially with the face, breast, genitals, or colon. Site-specific problems also arise when surgery results in a major loss of a particular function. Loss of normal bowel function following colostomy and loss of normal speech following laryngectomy are the two most notable examples. This section briefly reviews the site-specific problems that occur following mastectomy, colostomy, head and neck surgery, limb amputation, and genitourinary surgery. More detailed discussion can be found in the chapters on each site (breast cancer, Chapter 14; gastrointestinal cancer, Chapter 15; head and neck cancer, Chapter 17; malignant bone tumors, Chapter 20).

### Mastectomy

In the 1950s, Sutherland and colleagues at Memorial Hospital conducted one of the first studies of psychosocial reactions to radical mastectomy. A majority of the women studied were found to be experiencing significant postoperative depression, anxiety, and low self-esteem along with prolonged impairments in physical and sexual functioning. For many of the women, the loss of a breast signified the loss of an organ intimately associated with their sense of self-esteem, sexuality, and femininity. Among the variables that appear to determine the severity of the patient's reaction are the point in the life cycle during which breast surgery occurs and the social tasks that are threatened or interrupted. Threats to femininity and self-esteem occur in all women, but may be more pronounced in young women for whom attractiveness and fertility are major life issues. The meaning of the surgery may be quite different among older women for whom the risk to life may be the paramount concern. Also associated with more severe postmastectomy reactions are a history of psychiatric disorder, problems in body image, a history of unsatisfying or negative sexual experiences, and difficulty discussing personal, especially sexual, problems (Holland and Rowland, 1987). During the past decade, several important changes have occurred in the treatment of breast cancer. Today, most women undergo modified radical mastectomy or lumpectomy procedures that are less extensive than radical mastectomy and are associated with better postoperative physical functioning, less extensive chest deformity, and the opportunity for breast reconstruction. The switch to less radical surgery has had psychological benefits as well. Recent studies suggest that women who undergo breast-conserving cancer surgery are less self-conscious and experience greater satisfaction with sexual activity postoperatively.

## Colostomy

In oncology, the colostomy procedure is performed chiefly for colorectal cancer. This procedure results in the loss of normal bowel function, which is replaced by fecal elimination through a surgically constructed stoma. For some patients, the diversion of their fecal stream to an observable stoma violates their sense of cleanliness. In the first days following surgery it is not uncommon for patients to refuse to look at the stoma. Even thoughts about it evoke feelings of disgust, anger, embarrassment, and shame. When the colostomy starts to work, patients may be embarrassed by the gas and noise that cannot be controlled. In one of the first psychosocial studies of cancer patients who had undergone colostomy, Sutherland and colleagues surveyed patients who had survived disease-free for 5 or more years from rectal cancer. In general, these patients were significantly impaired in both their sexual and social functioning. Among patients who were employed prior to surgery, the majority had experienced decreases in their work status and earning capacity. Difficulties with practical management of the colostomy were common, as were depression, chronic anxiety, and a sense of social isolation. In the years since this study was completed, a number of changes have been made aimed at improving the adjustment of cancer patients undergoing colostomy. Perhaps the most important advance has been the development of improved equipment, which virtually eliminates problems with odor and spillage of feces. In addition, the location of the stoma site has been given more attention preoperatively to take into account skin folds, patient preference, and style of dress. Sexual difficulties in male patients have also been addressed with penile implant procedures that can successfully remedy erectile problems that are of physiological origin.

A recent study suggests that these improvements in patient care have resulted in less distress and better postoperative adjustment. Oberst and James (1985) followed 20 ostomy patients and their spouses until 6 months following hospital discharge. Results indicated that at hospital discharge, most patients anticipated having difficulties with stoma management. In many cases mastery of self-care tasks did not occur as quickly as patients would have liked and thus delayed a return to previous levels of activity. However, most patients reported that by 3 months their lives were returning to normal with the exception of sexual functioning. It is interesting to note that despite their difficulties in attaining control and regulation of the stoma, most patients did not view the ostomy as particularly stigmatizing. Their attitude could generally be described as, "If I have to live with it, everyone else can too" (Oberst and James, 1985, p. 54). The same group found that spouses continued to have distress after the patients improved, suggesting a need for their support.

## Head and Neck Surgery

Although all parts of the body have psychological significance, the head and neck area is central. Attractiveness, social interaction, and emotional expression all depend to a great extent on the integrity of facial features. For most persons, the disfigurement of the head and neck from cancer surgery is difficult to contemplate. Suicidal thoughts are not uncommon preoperatively, especially if the patient is to undergo extensive surgery. Following surgery many patients are concerned about the reactions of others and express fears of isolation and rejection. Unlike the mastectomy and colostomy patient, head and neck surgery cannot be hidden. It has a strong negative impact on self-esteem and self-confidence (Scott et al., 1980). In addition to the stress of an altered facial appearance, many patients must also cope with the loss or impairment of speech, sight, taste, or smell. The psychological impact of surgery appears to be directly related to the extent of disfigurement and sensory impairment. More severe structural and functional loss has been shown to be associated with a slower recovery, more prolonged social isolation, lower self-esteem, and more severe postoperative depression. Postoperative adjustment is also complicated by the association of malignancies in the head and neck region with previous histories of chronic, excessive use of alcohol and tobacco. Chronic alcoholism presents more serious problems from a psychiatric standpoint. Alcoholics who abruptly discontinue alcohol use are likely to experience symptoms of withdrawal (i.e., delirium tremens) in the days following surgery. Moreover, cognitive deficits and dementia related to chronic alcohol abuse may impair the ability of patients to cooperate with or become involved in postoperative self-care. A history of chronic alcohol abuse is also likely to have an adverse effect on the progress of postoperative rehabilitation. The common sequelae of chronic alcoholism (e.g., limited economic resources and family disruptions) and the possibility of a resumption of alcohol intake are among the contributors to noncompliance and poor outcome of rehabilitative efforts.

## Limb Amputation

Limb amputation is performed in oncology primarily for treatment of osteosarcoma, the most common form of bone tumor. Osteosarcoma typically presents in the long bones of the arms or legs in young people between 10 and 25. In recent years an alternative to amputation, known as limb salvage, has been developed for the treatment of osteosarcoma. The affected limb is spared; only malignant bone tissue is removed, being replaced with a specially constructed implant. These two procedures raise different psychological issues. Psychological recovery from amputation entails grieving for the lost limb, similar to the grief that occurs following the death of a loved one. The adolescent osteosarcoma patient also mourns the loss of athletic and social activities that required the use of the affected limb. Another commonly occurring postamputation reaction is phantom limb sensations, which usually abate within a few weeks after surgery. With limb salvage, other psychological issues arise. During the postoperative period, limb salvage patients are at risk for a number of complications, chiefly infection, which can lead to amputation. Many patients focus attention on the limb to "save" it. Comparisons of osteosarcoma patients who underwent amputation versus limb salvage do not indicate that one procedure is superior to the other in terms of either the physical or psychological adjustment patients achieve postoperatively (Sugarbaker et al., 1982; Weddington et al., 1985). Thus, the assumption that sparing a limb rather than amputating it would be associated with improved quality of life has, to date, not been supported by empirical research.

## Genitourinary Surgery

Malignant tumors of the genitourinary tract arise in men in the prostate, bladder, testes, and penis. In women, the uterus, cervix, bladder, and ovaries are the common sites of genitourinary neoplasms. This group of diseases share at least two major features. First, treatment typically involves surgery, either alone or in conjunction with chemotherapy and radiotherapy. Second, both the disease and the treatments result in disturbances in sexual functioning. The physiological effects of the disease and side effects of treatment often affect the patient's sexual desire and capacity for stimulation and orgasm. These same aspects of sexual functioning can also be disrupted by the patient's psy-

chological reactions to the disease and its treatment. The partner's usual sexual function may also be impaired by the psychological impact of the meaning of cancer in the genital organs, or fears aroused by its treatment. The reader is referred to Chapter 33 for a more detailed discussion of sexual problems and their management.

In men the most common site of genitourinary cancer is the prostate. It is also the second most common malignancy in American men. In cases where the tumor is localized, treatment generally involves radical prostatectomy (removal of the prostate gland). Most patients experience erectile dysfunction following this procedure. However, 10–15% of patients do eventually recover normal erectile function (Schover, 1987). This problem has been attributed to damage incurred during surgery to the autonomic nerve plexus that runs along the lateral surface of the prostate (von Eschenbach, 1980). A recently developed surgical technique spares these nerves and may yield significant reductions in the prevalence of postoperative impotence (Walsh and Lepar, 1987). For patients who do not recover erectile function postoperatively, implantation of a penile prosthesis is often a rehabilitative option. Another physiological effect of radical prostatectomy is dry ejaculation, a condition that may decrease the subjective intensity of the patient's orgasm. The nature and prevalence of psychologically based sexual dysfunctions associated with prostate cancer have been less well researched. Because these patients are generally older men, the lack of research data may be attributable to assumptions that sexual interest is low in this group or that patients would be unwilling to discuss their sexual functioning. When prostate cancer has metastasized, treatment involves hormonal therapy (daily estrogen), bilateral orchiectomy (removal of the testes), or a combination of the two. Many men are distressed by the prospect of being "castrated" or of receiving "female hormones," and often fear that they will become asexual or effeminate. Schover and colleagues (1984) have suggested that these fears can be addressed by emphasizing to the patient that masculinity is a function of the total person, not just the testicles, and that in the adult male the loss of testosterone should not have a major effect on personality. However, patients need to be informed that the administration of estrogen leads to a lessening of sexual desire.

Cancer of the bladder is the second most frequently occurring urological genitourinary cancer in American males. When bladder tumors are localized but have invaded surrounding muscle tissue, radical cystectomy combined with either radiation therapy or chemotherapy is the most common treatment. The impact of this surgical procedure on male sexual functioning is similar to that of radical prostatectomy: approximately 15% of patients retain or recover erectile function postoperatively (Schover et al., 1984). In addition to possible problems with erectile function, all radical cystectomy patients must contend with impact of the urostomy appliance on sexual activity. Urostomy patients often benefit from brief counseling on more comfortable positions for lovemaking and on ways of keeping the appliance as unobtrusive as possible (Schover, 1987).

Cancer of the testes accounts for only 2% of all male malignancies, but it is the second most common tumor in men between the ages of 20 and 34 (von Eschenbach, 1980). Treatment for localized disease involves only unilateral orchiectomy. The procedure does not produce impairment in fertility or in endocrine function; however, it can result in psychologically based sexual problems. Along with orchiectomy, many patients with testicular cancer undergo retroperitoneal lymph node dissection. This procedure produces dry ejaculation and associated infertility (see Chapter 7 on survivors; Chapter 33 on sexual dysfunction). Psychological preparation for this outcome by the surgeon is essential. The patient should also be offered the opportunity for sperm banking, which is also discussed in the chapters indicated.

Cancer of the penis is a relatively uncommon tumor in the United States and rarely occurs before the fifth decade of life. It is more prevalent among uncircumcised men from lower socioeconomic groups. Moreover, it is a form of cancer in which there are long delays between the appearance of symptoms and the patient's seeking of medical attention. Delays may be attributable to modesty about examination of the genitalia as well as to fears about surgery on the penis. Treatment usually requires either total or partial penectomy. However, most patients retain the capacity for sexual stimulation and ejaculations (Schover, 1987).

As stated previously, the major genitourinary cancers in women arise in the uterus, cervix, bladder, and ovaries. The impact of these malignancies on psychological and sexual functioning are reviewed in Chapter 33.

In any patient with genitourinary cancer it is important that the surgeon explain preoperatively to the patient and his or her partner the expected impact of surgery on sexual functioning. At the same time, the available rehabilitative options for the expected sexual dysfunction should also be discussed. This discussion by the surgeon serves to dispel common misconceptions and may thereby prevent the development of certain psychologically based postoperative sexual problems (e.g., avoidance of sexual activity for fear of transmitting cancer).

## REHABILITATION

Cancer rehabilitation is that part of treatment that assists patients in attaining maximal physical, social, psychological, and vocational functioning within the limits imposed by their disease and its treatment (Cromes, 1978). In order to provide comprehensive rehabilitation, professionals from many disciplines must collaborate in a team approach to patient care, including the psychological aspects. The role of the mental health professional in the interdisciplinary rehabilitation team is reviewed here.

The rehabilitation of the patient undergoing cancer surgery begins before the procedure is undertaken. Ideally, it begins at the first preoperative visit. It is important to review with the patient the plan for rehabilitation and to begin planning for rehabilitative procedures as soon as possible after surgery. From a psychological standpoint, there are at least two issues that should be addressed preoperatively. First, it is important to determine if any psychosocial determinants are present that could lead to a poor rehabilitation outcome. This task is accomplished by a brief preoperative interview. Compliance could be limited by a previous psychiatric disorder, alcoholism, a chaotic family situation, or circumstances that could limit access to treatment, such as limited finances and geographic distance. With the identification of potential problems preoperatively, it is possible to anticipate and prevent them rather than wait until they arise and impede rehabilitation. The second preoperative task is to discuss available rehabilitative options. This preoperative discussion reduces the patient's fears of surgery, and strengthens motivation to begin rehabilitation in the immediate postoperative period.

There is general agreement that the sooner rehabilitation is initiated after surgery, the more successful the outcome will be. However, the readiness to learn, the ability to work in physical therapy, and the willingness to make life-style changes are all dependent on the patient's psychological state. Patients who have not come to terms with the loss of body parts or functions may not be ready to begin rehabilitation. A number of psychological interventions can be employed in the immediate postoperative period to motivate the patient to engage in rehabilitation, such as individual counseling, couples counseling, and group meetings with other patients who have undergone similar procedures. Visits by previously rehabilitated patients are also very beneficial. This form of peer support is the basis of many self-help programs, such as the American Cancer Society's Reach to Recovery. An individual whose experience is close to that of the patient provides an effective role model for coping and is an important source of emotional support during the stressful postoperative period.

Following hospital discharge, most patients continue to recuperate from their cancer surgery at home. Given the trend toward shorter hospital stays, patients often require considerable physical care in the period immediately following discharge. Providing this level of care and mobilizing the patient to resume activities of daily living can place severe burdens on family members. Oberst and James (1985) have shown that spouses typically suffer an increase in somatic complaints and emotional problems after the cancer surgery patient comes home. The demands placed on the spouse frequently lead to physical complaints (e.g., diffuse aches and pains as well as upper respiratory infections) and emotional responses (e.g., irritability and dysphoria) associated with exhaustion. In a novel approach to this problem, Heinrich and Schag (1985) developed a stress and activity management group for ambulatory cancer patients and their spouses. Over a 6-week period, group members received information about coping with cancer, a relaxation and exercise program, and reviewed strategies for solving cancer-related problems. Participation in the group was found to increase the level of knowledge about cancer and coping for both the patient and the spouse. Moreover, spouses who completed the program had a more positive attitude toward the patient's health care team and felt better able to handle stressful situations. Almost all participants said that they would recommend the group to other patients and spouses.

## SUMMARY

The psychological problems associated with cancer surgery represent those of surgery in general, with the added meaning of cancer and its threat to life. Understanding patients' normal reactions to surgery and to rehabilitation will help the clinician recognize abnormal responses early. Adequate emotional support and information, especially in the preoperative period, have an impact on postoperative course and adjustment. Attention to these issues of surgical care enhances both the well-being of the patient and outcome of the surgery.

## REFERENCES

Abram, H.S. and B.F. Gill (1961). Predictions of postoperative psychiatric complications. *N. Engl. J. Med.* 265: 1123–28.

Adsett, C.A. (1963). Emotional reactions to disfigurement from cancer therapy. *Can. Med. Assoc. J.* 89:385–91.

Andersen, B.L. and H.H. Tewfik (1985). Psychological reactions to radiation therapy: Reconsideration of the adaptive aspects of anxiety. *J. Pers. Soc. Psychol.* 48:1024–32.

Anderson, E.A. (1987). Preoperative preparation for cardiac surgery facilitates recovery, reduces psychological distress, and reduces the incidence of acute postoperative hypertension. *J. Consul. Clin. Psychol.* 55:513–20.

Anderson, K.O. and F.T. Masur (1983). Psychological preparation for invasive medical and dental procedures. *J. Behav. Med.* 6:1–40.

Andrew, J.M. (1970). Recovery from surgery, with and without preparatory instruction, for three coping styles. *J. Pers. Soc. Psychol.* 15:223–26.

Auerbach, S.M. (1973). Trait-state anxiety and adjustment to surgery. *J. Consult. Clin. Psychol.* 40:264–71.

Bard, M. and A.M. Sutherland (1955). Psychological impact of cancer and its treatment: IV. Adaptation to radical mastectomy. *Cancer* 8:652–72.

Chapman, C.R. and G.B. Cox (1977). Anxiety, pain, and depression surrounding elective surgery: A multivariate comparison of abdominal surgery patients with kidney donors and recipients. *J. Psychosom. Res.* 21:1–15.

Cromes, G.F., Jr. (1978). Implementation of interdisciplinary cancer rehabilitation. *Rehab. Counsel. Bull.* 21:230–37.

Devine, E.C. and T.D. Cook (1986). Clinical and cost-saving effects of psychoeducational interventions with surgical patients: A meta-analysis. *Res. Nurs. Health* 9:89–105.

Domar, A.D., J.M. Noe, and H. Benson (1987). The preoperative use of the relaxation response with ambulatory surgery patients. *J. Human Stress* 13:101–07.

DiGiacomo, J.N. (1985). Preoperative considerations concerning psychotropic drugs. *Med. Psychiatry* 2:4–6.

Dumas, R.G., and B.A. Johnson (1972). Research in nursing practice: a review of five clinical experiments. *International J. Nurs. Stud.* 9:137–49.

Dyk, R.B. and A.M. Sutherland (1956). Adaptation of the spouse and other family members to the colostomy patient. *Cancer* 9:123–38.

Egbert, L.D., G.E. Battit, C.E. Welch, and M.K. Bartlett (1964). Reduction of postoperative pain by encouragement and instruction of patients. *N. Engl. J. Med.* 270(16):825–27.

Fisher, B. and P. Barboni (1982). Breast Cancer. J.F. Holland and E. Frei, III (eds.). In Cancer Medicine Philadelphia, Lea and Febiger (2nd ed.), 2025–56.

Folstein, M.F., S.E. Folstein and P.R.H. McHugh (1975). Mini-mental states. *J. Psychiatr. Res.* 2:189–98.

Gil, K.M. (1984). Coping effectively with invasive medical procedures: A descriptive model. *Clin. Psychol. Rev.* 4:339–62.

Gottesman, D. and M.S. Lewis (1982). Differences in crisis reactions among cancer and surgery patients. *J. Consult. Clin. Psychol.* 50:381–88.

Hackett, T.P. and A.D. Weisman (1960). Psychiatric management of operative syndromes: I. Therapeutic consultation and effect of noninterpretive intervention. *Psychosom. Med.* 22:267–82.

Hackett, T.P. and A.D. Weisman (1960). Psychiatric management of operative syndromes: II. Psychodynamic factors in formulation and management. *Psychosom. Med.* 22:356–72.

Heinrich, R.L. and C.C. Schag (1985). Stress and activity management: Group treatment for cancer patients and spouses. *J. Consult. Clin. Psychol.* 53:439–46.

Holland, J.C. and J.H. Rowland (1987). Psychological reactions to breast cancer and its treatment. In J.R. Harris, S. Hellman, I.C. Henderson, and D.W. Kinne (eds.), *Breast Diseases.* Philadelphia: Lippincott, pp. 632–47.

Jacobs, J.W., M.R. Bernhard, A. Delgado, and J.J. Strain (1977). Screening for organic mental syndromes in the medically ill. *Ann. Intern. Med.* 86:40–46.

Janis, I.L. (1958). *Psychological Stress.* New York: Wiley.

Jay, S.M., C.H. Elliot, M. Ozolins, R. Olson, and S. Pruitt (1985). Behavioral management of children's distress during painful medical procedures. *Behav. Res. Ther.* 23:513–20.

Johnson, J.E. (1973). The effect of accurate expectations about sensations on the sensory and distress components of pain. *J. Pers. Soc. Psychol.* 27:261–75.

Johnson, J.E. (1984). Coping with elective surgery. *Annu. Rev. Nurs. Res.* 2:107–32.

Johnson, J.E., J.M. Dabbs, Jr., and H. Leventhal (1970). Psychosocial factors in the welfare of surgical patients. *Nurs. Res.* 19:18–29.

Johnson, J.E. and H. Leventhal (1974). Effects of accurate expectations and behavioral instructions on reactions during a noxious medical examination. *J. Personality Soc. Psychol.* 29:710–18.

Johnson, J.E., H. Leventhal, and J. Dabbs (1971). Contribution of emotional and instrumental response processes in adaptation to surgery. *J. Pers. Soc. Psychol.* 20:55–64.

Katz, J., P. Ackerman, Y. Rothwax, E. Sachar, E. Weiner, L. Hellman, and F. Gallagher (1970). Psychoendocrine aspects of cancer of the breast. *Psychosom. Med.* 32:1–12.

Kendall, P.C., L. Williams, T.F. Pechacek, L.E. Graham, C. Sisslak, and N. Herzoff (1979). Cognitive-behavioral and patient education interventions in cardiac catheterization procedures: the Palo Alto Medial Psychology Project. *J. Consult. Clin. Psychol.* 47:49–58.

Kimball, C.P. (1969). Psychological responses to the experience of open heart surgery: I. *Am. J. Psychiatry,* 126:348–59.

Kornfeld, D.S., S.S. Heller, D.A. Frank, and R. Moskowitz (1974). Personality and psychological factors in postcardiotomy delirium. *Arch. Gen. Psychiatry* 31:249–53.

Kornfeld, D.S., S. Zimberg, and J.R. Malm (1965). Psychiatric complications of open heart surgery. *N. Engl. J. Med.* 273:287–89.

Layne, O.L. and S.C. Yudofsky (1971). Postoperative psychosis in cardiotomy patients: the role of organic and psychiatric factors. *N. Engl. J. Med.* 284:518–20.

Lindeman, C.A. and B. Van Aernam (1971). Nursing intervention with the presurgical patient: The effects of structured and unstructured pre-operative teaching. *Nurs. Res.* 20:319–32.

Massie, M.J. and J.C. Holland (1987). The cancer patient with pain: Psychiatric complications and their management. *Med. Clin. North Am.* 71:243–58.

Melamed, B.G. and L.J. Siegel (1975). Reduction of anxiety in children facing hospitalization and surgery by use of filmed modeling. *J. Consult. Clin. Psychol.* 43:511–21.

Mumford, E., H.J. Schlesinger, and G.V. Glass (1982). The effects of psychological intervention on recovery from surgery and heart attacks: An analysis of the literature. *Am. J. Public Health* 72:141–51.

Oberst, M.T. and R. James (1985). Going home: Patient and spouse adjustment following cancer surgery. *Top. Clin. Nurs.* 7:46–57.

Pack, G.T. (1962). Counselling the cancer patient: Surgeon's counsel. *The Physician and the Total Care of the Cancer Patient: A Symposium Presented at the 1961 Scientific Session of the American Cancer Society.* New York: American Cancer Society, pp. 56–61.

Penman, D.T., J.R. Bloom, S. Fotopoulos, M.R. Cook, J.C. Holland, C. Gates, D. Flamer, B. Murawski, R. Ross, U. Brandt, L.R. Muenz, and D. Pee (1986). The impact of mastectomy on self-concept and social function: A combined cross-sectional and longitudinal study with comparison groups. *Women and Health* 11:101–30.

Renneker, R. and M. Cutler (1952). Psychological problems of adjustment to breast cancer. *J.A.M.A.* 148:833–38.

Rosenberg, S.A. (1985). Principles of surgical oncology. In V.T. DeVita, Jr., S. Hellman, and S.A. Rosenberg (eds.), *Cancer: Principles and Practice of Oncology,* 2nd ed. Philadelphia: Lippincott, pp. 215–25.

Schmitt, F.E. and P.J. Wooldridge (1973). Psychological preparation of surgical patients. *Nurs. Res.* 22:108–16.

Schover, L.R. (1987). Sexuality and fertility in urologic cancer patients. *Cancer* 60:553–58.

Schover, L.R., A.C. von Eschenbach, D.B. Smith, and J. Gonzalez (1984). Sexual rehabilitation of urologic cancer patients: A practical approach. *CA* 34:66–74.

Scott, D.W. (1983). Anxiety, critical thinking, and information processing during and after breast biopsy. *Nurs. Res.* 32:24–28.

Scott, D.W., M.T. Oberst, and M.J. Dropkin (1980). A stress-coping model. *Adv. Nurs. Sci.* 3:9–23.

Scott, L.E., G.A. Clum, and J.B. Peoples (1983). Preoperative predictors of postoperative pain. *Pain* 15:283–93.

Seeman, R.G. and M.A. Rockoff (1986). Preoperative anxiety: The pediatric patient. *Int. Anesthesiol. Clin.* 24(4):1–15.

Seymour, D.G., P.J. Henschke, R.D. Cape, and A.J. Campbell (1980). Acute confusional states and dementia in the elderly: the role of dehydration/volume depletion, physical illness and age. *Age and Aging* 9:137–46.

Shimkin, M.B. (1977). *Contrary to Nature.* DHEW Publ. No. (NIH) 79-720. Washington, D.C.: U.S. Govt. Printing Office.

Sime, A.M. (1976). Relationship of pre-operative fear, type of coping, and information received about surgery to recovery from surgery. *J. Pers. Soc. Psychol.* 34:716–24.

Small, S.M. (1976). Psychological and psychiatric problems in aged and high-risk surgical patients. In J.H. Siegel and P.D. Chodoff (eds.), *The Aged and High Risk Surgical*

*Patient: Medical, Surgical and Anesthetic Management.* Orlando, Fla.: Grune & Stratton, pp. 307–28.

Solomon, S., J.R. McCartney, S.M. Saravay, and E. Katz (1987). Postoperative hospital course of patients with history of severe psychiatric illness. *Gen. Hosp. Psychiatry* 9:376–82.

Stehlin, J.S. and K.H. Beach (1966). Psychological aspects of cancer therapy. *J.A.M.A.* 197:140–44.

Strain, J.J. and S. Grossman (1975). Psychological Care of the Medically Ill. New York: Appleton-Century-Crofts.

Strain, J.J. (1985). The surgical patient. In R. Michels, J.O. Cavenar, Jr., H.K.H. Brodie, A.M. Cooper, S.B. Guze, L.L. Judd, G.L. Klerman, and A.J. Solnit (eds.), *Psychiatry*, Vol. 2. Philadelphia: Lippincott, Chapter 121.

Streltzer, J. and H. Leigh (1978). Psychological preparation for surgery: the usefulness of a preoperative psychotherapeutic interview. *Hawaiian Med. J.* 37:139–42.

Sugarbaker, P.H., I. Barofsky, S.A. Rosenberg, and F.J. Gianola (1982). Quality of life assessment of patients in extremity sarcoma clinical trials. *Surgery* 91:17–23.

Sutherland, A.M. and C.E. Orbach (1953). Psychological impact of cancer and cancer surgery: II. Depressive reactions associated with surgery for cancer. *Cancer* 6:958–62.

Sutherland, A.M., C.E. Orbach, R.B. Dyk, and M. Bard (1952). The psychological impact of cancer and cancer surgery: I. Adaptation to the dry colostomy: Preliminary report and summary of findings. *Cancer* 5:857–72.

Turk, D.C., D. Meichenbaum, and M. Genest (1983). *Pain and Behavioral Medicine: A Cognitive-Behavioral Perspective.* New York: Guilford Press.

Vernon, D.T.W. and D.W. Bigelow (1974). Effect of information about a potentially stressful situation on responses to stress impact. *J. Personality Soc. Psychol.* 29:50–59.

von Eschenbach, A.C. (1980). Sexual dysfunction following therapy for cancer of the prostate, testis, and penis. *Front. Radiat. Ther. Oncol.* 14:42–50.

Walsh, P.C. and H. Lepar (1987). The role of radical prostatectomy in the management of prostatic cancer. *Cancer* 60:526–37.

Watson, S. and P. Hickey (1984). Cancer surgery: Help for the family in waiting. *Am. J. Nurs.* 85:604–7.

Weddington, W.W., K.B. Seagraves, and M.A. Simon (1985). Psychological outcome of extremity sarcoma survivors undergoing amputation or limb salvage. *J. Clin. Oncol.* 3:1393–99.

Wells, J.K., G.S. Howard, W.F. Nowlin, and M.J. Vargas (1986). Presurgical anxiety and postsurgical pain and adjustment: Effects of a stress inoculation procedure. *J. Consult. Clin. Psychol.* 54:831–35.

Wilson, J.F. (1981). Behavioral preparation for surgery: Benefit or harm. *J. Behav. Med.* 4:79–102.

Wolfer, J.A. and C.E. Davis (1970). Assessment of surgical patients: Preoperative welfare. *Nurs. Res.* 19:402–14.

# 9

# Radiotherapy

Jimmie C. Holland

## HISTORICAL PERSPECTIVE

Roentgen's discovery of x rays in 1895 and the Curies' discovery of radium in 1896 were quickly followed by recognition of the biological effects of ionizing radiation and the potential for clinical application to medicine. The observation that some incurable neoplasms had responded to "Roentgen rays" and the first report of a patient cured by radiation therapy in 1899 led to excitement about a new potential treatment for cancer (Perez and Brady, 1987). Early efforts to use radium clinically were hampered by the absence of techniques to assure the ability to give a standardized and reproducible dose. This technical problem resulted in a highly variable dose and severe burns at times. Technical advances in machines were made rapidly, so that by the 1920s they were capable of giving deep therapy that yielded a standardized and reproducible dose. However, early successes were countered by the reports of the hazards of x rays as observed by the development of malignant epitheliomas on the exposed hands of the pioneer radiologists, evidence that radiation not only could cure, but could cause cancer as well. The field of clinical radiation therapy began in 1922 at the International Oncology Congress in Paris, where the first successful treatment of advanced laryngeal cancer was reported (Perez and Brady, 1987).

Knowledge of the biological aspects of radiation in that early period was slower to develop than the technical methods to deliver it. Workers at the Radium Institute in Paris observed early, however, that those tumor cells most sensitive to radiation were those that had a greater rate of reproduction, were in the mitotic phase of the cell cycle, and had less degree of differentiation (Shimkin, 1977). These principles, when combined in 1922 with the concept of fractionation of dose, became the basis for modern radiotherapy. The distribution of radium and radon, especially by Madame Curie in the early part of the century, to other medical centers, led to the establishment of radium institutes around the world and the rapid spread of its clinical application to cancer.

Janeway, a surgeon in New York, was placed in charge of radium therapy at the Memorial Hospital for Cancer and Allied Diseases in New York in 1912 soon after the first reports of clinical efficacy of radiation in cancer. He established the radium department in 1915, under the guidance and encouragement of Ewing, who was head of the hospital. The ability to treat patients in the United States was made possible through the efforts of Ewing, Douglas, and Kelly who, with the U.S. government as a partner, established the National Radium Institute, which mined carnotite deposits on lands leased in Colorado (Hilaris and Nori, 1984). From 1913 to 1917, 8.5 g of radium were produced and divided among the partners. Memorial Hospital was given 3.75 g, with which the early patients were treated. The beginning of brachytherapy in the United States dates to the work of the Janeway group in improving methods of radium application.

## PRESENT DAY RADIOTHERAPY PRACTICES

Radiation and surgery are the two primary treatments for localized cancer. Whereas the mechanism by which radiation affects biological tissues is not entirely clear, it is commonly accepted that damage to cellular DNA is an important part of the process. The radiation dosage and length of exposure affect the consequences. The challenge for the radiotherapist is to obtain maximal chance for cure or control of tumor growth while minimizing the risk of adverse effects of normal tissues. Figure 9-1 shows this principle by sigmoid curves representing the range of optimal dose

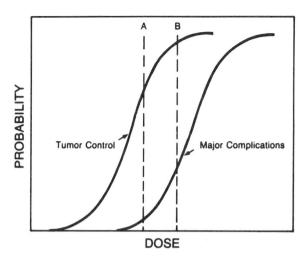

**Figure 9-1.** Range of optimal radiation dose for maximal tumor control and minimal complications. *Source:* Reprinted with permission from S. Hellman (1985). Principles of radiation therapy. In V. De Vita, Jr., S. Hellman, and S. Rosenberg (eds.), *Cancer: Principles and Practice of Oncology,* 2nd ed. Philadelphia: Lippincott, pp. 227–255.

that offers maximal tumor control with minimal complications (Hellman, 1985).

Radiotherapy is given after a treatment plan is developed that takes into account the location of the tumor volume, its relation to normal structures, histological tumor type, extent of disease, and other treatment modalities to be considered, before or after radiation. The treatment plan is then developed by the radiotherapist. Palliative treatment, about 50% of cases, is planned by dosimetry, and is followed by simulation. In primary treatment of a tumor, the radiotherapist, in consultation with the radiation physicist, uses computed data to assure the best approach, which is checked by simulation and the exact sites to be treated indicated by small tattoos to assure the proper application by the technician.

This preparation just described is used for external beam therapy, or teletherapy. It is the most commonly used form of radiotherapy, which is given in fractionated doses to achieve the total desired dose. Treatment is usually 5 days a week over 2 weeks for palliation or 4–6 weeks to deliver a curative dose. The older orthovoltage machines were limited by the maximum dose that the skin could tolerate. Supervoltage or megavoltage machines, given originally by cobalt and now by linear accelerators, produce high-energy beams that allow the radiation to be given at higher doses, which reach deeper tissues with a lower relative dose to the skin. Present-day research attempts to develop radiosensitizers to obtain even greater benefit by

making tumors more sensitive to radiation. Most approaches have attempted to decrease the anoxic cells in a tumor mass, which are known to be less sensitive. Radioprotector substances that may enhance the tolerance to radiation of organs and tissues previously shielded only by mechanical or surgical means, continue to be developed as a means of furthering the potential for use of radiotherapy.

The other form of radiation is brachytherapy, in which the isotope is placed in a body cavity near the tumor or within the tumor itself. Applicators or tubes to hold the isotope are usually inserted in the operating room, and patients are "afterloaded" with isotope in the radiotherapy suite or in their room after localization films have been taken and a computerized plan developed. The hospitalized patient may be isolated in a private room over several days while the radioisotope implant is in place until the desired dose is reached. Other implants are permanent, and the patient is discharged with low-energy seeds in the tumor.

Radiotherapy is used today in several ways. First, it is curative when used as a single modality in early-stage laryngeal cancer and in early-stage Hodgkin's disease. Radiotherapy contributed to one of the initial success stories of cancer therapy in the 1960s when Hodgkin's disease, previously universally fatal, began to be cured in its early stages by radiation alone. The remarkable ability to preserve the voice in a curative treatment for stage I carcinoma of the larynx contributed to its expanded role as primary therapy. Second, radiotherapy is used as curative treatment when combined with chemotherapy and surgery in many head and neck cancer patients, in pediatric tumors, and in ovarian cancer. It is used palliatively to control tumors of the bladder, uterus, ovary, lung, pancreas, and oropharynx. It has an increasingly important role in treatment of early breast cancer, permitting more conservative segmental resection to be done, which is followed by radiotherapy. Third, it is used as prophylaxis against brain metastasis, in lung cancer, and for symptom control, especially of pain due to bone metastases. It also may be used as an emergency treatment for control of superior vena cava compression, spinal cord compression, airway compromise, rapid neurological decompensation, and malignant cardiac tamponade (Dobelbower, 1987).

## PSYCHOLOGICAL PERSPECTIVE

### Attitudes Toward Radiation

Considering the wide range of clinical applications of radiotherapy in cancer, it is not surprising that over half of all patients treated for cancer receive radiation in some form as part of their treatment (Kramer et al.,

1984). The history also suggests several reasons why it is frightening to the patient contemplating treatment, because its early use was most often palliative and it often resulted in adverse side effects. The horrors related to radiation, beginning with Hiroshima, are well known. Three Mile Island, Chernobyl, and descriptions of inadequately controlled nuclear reactor plants cause fears about radiation effects in general, which contribute to concerns about voluntary exposure, even for therapeutic reasons. Some individuals fear even the exposure resulting from diagnostic radiological procedures.

Most individuals are aware of their exposure to ionizing radiation in the environment from many sources and that its hazard to health is inadequately understood. The success stories of curative treatment for radiation are recent; however, far clearer in the minds of older individuals are memories of the severe treatment side effects of friends and relatives who received radiation for palliation. The fears that many patients have when radiation is recommended are several: that their tumor is incurable; that the treatment will result in painful radiation burns; that the large, unfamiliar machine will fall upon them or emit excess radiation. A study done in 1961 showed that even among patients who received only sham radiation exposure in a controlled study, 75% developed symptoms of nausea and fatigue in anticipation of experiencing radiation sickness (Parsons and Webster, 1961). Gottschalk and colleagues (1969) also showed heightened anxiety prior to both sham and actual radiation.

Thus, the staff of a radiotherapy clinic should be aware of the patients' concerns and reactions to the treatments for many reasons: (1) to help them to accept the treatments, (2) to assure that patients adhere to the planned regimen to achieve total dose, and (3) to allay fears and distress of the patients, and provide support and enhance their quality of life during treatment. A knowledge of the commonly seen psychological reactions and their management constitute an important area of psychooncology that relates specifically to the psychological issues raised by treatment with radiotherapy. They are reviewed here in relation to pretreatment distress and its management, to psychological responses during radiotherapy, and to the long-term consequences that have significant psychological impact.

Special emphasis is placed first on the supportive role of the radiotherapist, nurse, and technician who constitute the critically important daily social environment of the patient during radiation treatments, along with the social worker whose role may vary depending on availability and need (Smith and McNamara, 1977). The fellow patients undergoing treatment be-

**Table 9-1** Psychological interventions

| Type of intervention | Specific intervention or provider |
| --- | --- |
| Psychosocial support | Radiotherapist |
| | Nurse |
| | Social worker |
| | Radiotherapy technician |
| | Clinic staff |
| | Patient-to-patient support |
| Psychiatric consultation | Evaluate pathological anxiety, depression, preexisting psychiatric disorders, and/or alcohol and drug abuse. |
| | Provide management of psychiatric problems requiring modification of usual treatment procedures. |
| | Assure family support through coordination with social worker and clinic staff. |

come informal but important sources of information and social support, because they are facing and coping with the same stresses. Table 9-1 outlines sources of psychosocial support and the indications for a psychiatric or mental health professional consultation.

## Referral for Radiotherapy

The first issue in psychological support for the patient facing radiotherapy is continuity. The primary physician with prior treatment experience with the patient should refer the patient to radiotherapy. The explanation to the patient should include the reason for the recommendation for radiotherapy, its goals, the general plan, and the reassurance that the physician will be in contact with the radiotherapist and that they will work together during this phase of treatment. Patients ask "Who is my doctor?" when gaps occur in referral. Ideally, patients should know that they remain generally under the primary doctor's care. However, in some situations today the radiotherapist becomes and remains the primary physician. For example, women who receive radiation after limited surgery for breast cancer often remain under the care of the radiotherapist. Mitchell and Glicksman (1977) found that 52% of patients felt that the referring physician had been of no help in preparing them for radiation. The patient who experiences care that has been delegated among many physicians without any one seemingly in charge of the total treatment is at high risk for distress as a result of the discontinuity.

The radiotherapist, like the surgeon with surgical patients, is the key individual to whom the patient looks for review of the medical data, review of physical findings, explanation of the treatment plan, and description of the expected side effects that must be tolerated to attain therapeutic benefit (Rotman et al., 1977). The explanation and subsequent discussion provide the basis for mutual trust and respect on which the doctor–patient relationship rests. The patient, whether referred for definitive treatment or palliation, deserves the same thoughtful, frank, but hopeful outline of the plan. The patient whose treatment is for palliation or symptom control presents the most challenging psychological problem in terms of how to present the information honestly yet preserve hope. Optimal management requires genuine concern and empathy combined with confidence in how to communicate the information. Many young doctors are fearful of what to say and leave the patient with vague explanations that are much more frightening for most patients than a clear review of "Where I am and what I can expect" (Kagan et al., 1984). Their resiliency, when they feel they will continue to be supported by the doctor, is far greater than often assumed.

Simulation allows further psychological preparation, discussion, and explanation of the skin tattoos that are necessary for treatment. Though less visible than the earlier identification markings, the small tattoos are still viewed by the patient as stigmatizing signs of receiving radiation. Questions about radiation raised at this time, even if they seem trivial, may reflect long-held myths and misbeliefs. Mitchell and Glicksman (1977) also found that 82% of the patients undergoing radiotherapy felt that neither the referring doctor nor the radiotherapist were individuals to whom they would bring their emotional problems, suggesting that more training of radiotherapy personnel in communication skills and management of psychological problems would be helpful.

Because many patients interviewed showed significant distress, they recommended that a mental health professional be available on a daily basis in a radiotherapy clinic. Although few radiotherapy clinics actually have this concept in practice, some do have a mental health professional available. It allows for more rapid identification and better diagnosis of problems in patients, and provides ready referral. Conferences can be organized regularly and directed toward exploring the various problems of patients in order to enhance the expertise of staff in understanding the emotional problems of the patients and their own stresses in dealing with them.

Much of the information for the patient about treatment and side effects is given by nurses in the form of booklets and videotapes supplemented by one-to-one sessions on the first clinic visits and before the first treatment. Keeping in mind that anxiety is high, the nurse extends the radiotherapist's explanations and gives details about anticipated weakness, fatigue, and (depending on site) anorexia and nausea. Skin care, medications, mouth care, and diet are areas requiring advice. Such interventions substantially enhance the ability to comply with the treatment, which in turn contributes to optimal treatment results (Herbert, 1977).

Cassileth and colleagues (1980) found that among 160 patients undergoing radiotherapy, many felt poorly informed and desired more information, preferably from the radiotherapist. They suggested that the uncertainty patients expressed appeared to reflect also a desire for more understanding from the doctor, as well as explanation of the treatment and anticipated results.

A study piloted by our group in 1976 randomly assigned women radiotherapy patients to receive an orientation to the clinic by the radiotherapist. Patients received a tour of the radiotherapy department, including a description of the machines and introduction to the technician, to the room, and to the procedure. A brief interview concluded the half hour with a discussion of concerns and answering questions (Holland et al., 1979). Verbal content analysis of speech samples revealed that women who received the intervention were less anxious at the time of the first treatment, when anxiety is highest.

The radiotherapy technicians, in another effort to reduce distress of radiotherapy patients at Montefiore Hospital, attended six sessions to learn how to monitor patients' psychological response as they positioned them each day and to report observations to the staff. They also learned supportive ways to intervene with the patients, enhancing their confidence in social interaction with the patient. Supportive sessions that examine and deal with the stresses of this important staff group can have a salutary effect on the social environment experienced by the patient.

Rainey (1985) conducted a controlled trial of the preparation of radiotherapy patients for treatment, examining an educational intervention. Patients assigned to the high-information group were individually shown a 12-minute slide–tape program that introduced the personnel, their role, the equipment, and the procedure; the program also included information about what the patient would experience (see, hear, and feel), and a discussion of some of the common misconceptions about the treatment. The staff was available to answer questions. The low-information group received a booklet. Patients in the high-information group were better informed and had less anxiety and mood disturbance at the first and last week of treatment, irrespective of coping style. These data demonstrate objectively the correctness of our clinical observations that providing better preparation for the

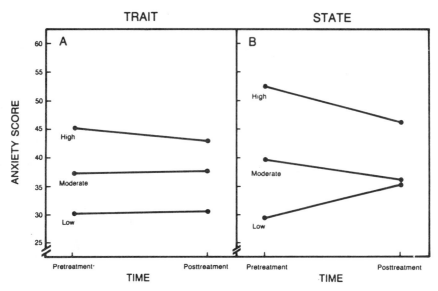

**Figure 9-2.** Data Pattern for significant three-way interaction. Panel A indicates stability of trait–anxiety scores across time for low, moderate, and high pretreatment anxiety groups. Panel B indicates significant interactions in state–anxiety scores across time for low, moderate, and high pretreatment anxiety groups. *Source:* Reprinted with permission from B.L. Anderson and H.H. Tewfik (1985). Psychological reactions to radiation therapy: Reconsideration of the adaptive aspects of anxiety. *J. Pers. Soc. Psychol.* 48:1024–32.

stressful nature of radiotherapy reduces distress immediately and throughout treatment.

Anderson and colleagues (1984) studied the pretreatment response of women who were receiving intracavitary radiation for gynecological cancer. This procedure entailed the positioning of an applicator that was later loaded with radioactive pellets, with the women remaining in an isolation room for 48–72 hours until their removal. Women reported becoming anxious and agitated, with physiological arousal and accelerated pulse 24–48 hours before the treatment. Anxiety scores were high and remained elevated after the treatment. The women who had to receive a second treatment did not "adapt" and experience less anxiety, although physicians perceived them as less distressed. Anderson and Tewfik (1985) found that those women with low initial anxiety experienced more disruption after treatment. Using the concept of Janis, which suggested that a moderate level of anxiety promotes the "work of worry" and better subsequent adaptation, they found that a pretreatment period of moderate anxiety likely facilitated adjustment, although in the case of cancer, anxiety continued higher than with a benign condition. The most anxious remained highest, those who were moderately anxious remained the same, and those who were lowest showed an increase in anxiety after treatment, perhaps reflecting lack of psychological preparation. Trait anxiety levels did not change. Anger and hostility were greatest in the high- and low-anxiety extremes and not in the moderate, suggesting that Janis' concept (1958) of adaptive level of anxiety may apply to the adjustment to radiotherapy as well as surgery (Fig. 9-2).

The social worker today plays a key role in identifying the distressed patient, reassuring and discussing fears with patients, and organizing support during and after treatment (Smith and McNamara, 1977). New patients at the Memorial Sloan-Kettering Cancer Center are encouraged to attend an orientation meeting run by a nurse and social worker, where patients and families can ask questions, become acquainted, and support one another.

## REACTIONS TO TREATMENT

It is surprising that few studies of patients' reactions to radiotherapy were done before the 1960s. Yonke (1967), a social worker, noted the pervasive fear of death among patients at the time that radiotherapy was still largely palliative. She also noted the salutary effect of creating an ambiance of warmth and support in the clinic.

Peck (1972) and Peck and Boland (1977) provided the first systematic interviews of patients undergoing radiation. They found the common reactions to be anxiety, depression, anger, and guilt. Patients used defense mechanisms of denial, displacement (concern for others), identification (joining the doctor's fight),

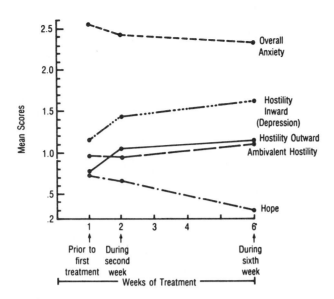

**Figure 9-3.** Mean scale scores for emotional responses prior to and during radiotherapy (Note: $p < .05$). *Source:* Reprinted with permission from J.C. Holland, J. Rowland, A. Lebovitz, and R. Rusalem (1979). Reactions to cancer treatment: Assessment of emotional response to adjuvant radiotherapy as a guide to planned intervention. *Psychiatr. Clin. North Am.* 2:347–58.

and dependence on the doctor and treatment. They were pessimistic about treatment and unprepared for it. Those interviewed after completion of the treatment showed higher levels of depression and anxiety, in part because treatment side effects were misinterpreted as irreparable damage. They also noted the impact of the lay view of the futility of radiation treatment.

A study of patients during their radiation treatments was undertaken at Montefiore Hospital in the 1970s (Holland et al., 1979). Following their mastectomy 20 women referred for radiation therapy were interviewed. Mean age was 62, with a range from 31 to 83. Slightly fewer than half (45%) were married. Most of the women were white.

On the patient's initial visit to the radiotherapy clinic and after seeing the radiotherapist, the patient was interviewed by a psychiatrist and a 5-minute sample of speech was obtained and analyzed by the Gottschalk–Gleser Content Analysis Scales, a technique that yields verbal projective information, similar to that obtained from visual projective tests. This was done at three points during the treatment by the cobalt-60 machine: prior to the first treatment, during the second week, and near the end of treatment.

Three characteristics of emotional distress were assessed: (1) overall anxiety and six subtypes, (2) hostility (which included depression), and (3) hope. Figure 9-3 shows the mean scores at each time period. There was an overall significant increase in internalized hostility (depression) over time and a significant increase

in externalized hostility (anger) over time. Decrease in overall anxiety and hope over time was seen, though not at a significant level.

The findings, consonant with clinical observation, indicated that patients were indeed most fearful and anxious when they began radiotherapy, a new treatment modality administered by large machines in radiation-shielded rooms. Adequate explanation, information, and reassurance given at this critical juncture by the radiotherapy technician and the radiotherapist likely contributed to the lessening of anxiety over time, as well as increasing familiarity with the room, the staff, and the routine. However, as the women neared the end of their treatment, they were paradoxically more—not less—depressed, and they expressed more overt anger and less hope. Patients also felt worse at the end of their treatment because of the side effects of anorexia, fatigue, and a general sense of malaise; therefore, they might have been more depressed and angry because they were feeling worse as a consequence of their therapy. The symptoms might also reawaken fears about the harmful effects of radiation.

The subscales of anxiety provided additional information showing that separation-related anxiety was increased. In a number of instances, women voiced concern about greater vulnerability to recurrence of the tumor when the treatment ended and their medical condition would no longer be closely monitored by the radiotherapists' frequent visits. They also anticipated a loss of the meaningful relationships that were established with the radiotherapy clinic staff. In a sense, the women felt "protected" both medically and emotionally as long as treatment continued. This reaction is seen clinically in other situations, such as the need for weaning from germ-free environments, and similar distress on the completion of chemotherapy.

Although high overall anxiety is expected and must be dealt with at the outset of treatment, these data suggest that additional attention should be directed to the patient's psychological state on reaching the end of the radiotherapy treatments. The staff often assumes that patients feel relief upon reaching the end of a lengthy, onerous treatment regimen. These data seem to suggest quite the contrary: women were significantly more depressed and angry at the end of their treatment and were also anxious about termination, with its consequences of the loss of the comfortable relationship with the staff, the loss of close monitoring, and the increased vulnerability to their disease.

Given the recognized levels of distress, few studies have tested interventions to reduce the distress of patients receiving radiation. Forester and colleagues (1978) carried out a controlled trial in patients receiving radiation of an educational–supportive psychotherapy model. They found less distress and fewer physical symptoms among those who received the brief weekly psychotherapy sessions. Such information, coupled with that of the salutary value of pretreatment education, suggest a need for more support built into the total care.

## Radiation Side Effects

In a study of patients interviewed weekly during radiotherapy and for 3 months after it ended, King and colleagues (1985) reported the common presentation and timing of treatment-related side effects. Used to plan nursing interventions, the critical time when initial significant symptoms began to appear was within the second and third weeks when anorexia, nausea, vomiting, fatigue, weakness, sore throat, and diarrhea became pronounced as acute signs of radiation sickness.

Changes in exposed skin may become uncomfortable or actually painful, although skin problems occur less with the use of supervoltage machines. Leukopenia, thrombocytopenia, and anemia develop acutely as well; the latter appears more severely with extensive bone marrow exposure. Immunosuppression also occurs with radiation. It is used for this reason in preparation of patients for bone marrow transplant to reduce the likelihood of rejection.

When radiation is applied to the brain or spinal cord, the edema of the tumor and adjacent tissues that occurs increases intracranial pressure and spinal cord compression, causing increased neurological symptoms that must be controlled by steroids. Although pain of cord compression is usually relieved, the effect of steroids on mental function (added to the distress related to the presence of the underlying medical condition), can be extremely stressful and requires psychiatric evaluation. The somnolence syndrome seen in children a few weeks after radiation is poorly understood. However, though related to dose, the impact of cranial radiation, even in a prophylactic dose in children with acute lymphocytic leukemia, produced a mean 10-point loss in children who also received intrathecal methotrexate (Rowland et al., 1984). The effect was greatest in younger children. Hypothalamic damage causes growth hormone reduction and results in small stature in children receiving cranial radiation for brain tumors by whole body irradiation for bone marrow transplantation (Duffner et al., 1985).

In adults in whom cranial radiation is given for prophylaxis against brain metastases from lung cancer, Johnson and colleagues (1985) found that among the few long-term survivors of small-cell lung carcinoma treated also with chemotherapy and chest radiation, three-fourths had significant neurological symptoms and diminished mental acuity, varying from mild to severe. (See Chapter 29 for a full description of radiation effects on the CNS.)

Alopecia occurs rapidly with cranial radiation and results in great distress in some patients. Lower dose of radiation used for prophylaxis in children with acute lymphocytic leukemia results in hair loss, which is replaced later by regrowth of normal hair. However, higher doses used for treatment of primary brain tumors and metastases results in permanent alopecia or scanty and irregular hair regrowth.

The acute symptoms usually begin to abate when treatments end. However, King and colleagues (1985) found that 3 months later, one-third of the patients had persistent symptoms, especially fatigue. Discouragement can be avoided by including information about possible protracted symptoms, even after treatment ends.

Silberfarb and colleagues (1980) also noted persistent distress in women receiving adjuvant radiotherapy after mastectomy, among whom many felt they needed help to carry out household tasks during and immediately following treatment.

The nature of specific acute symptoms depends on the radiation dose and site. For example, treatment to the mouth, pharynx, and neck causes changes in taste, saliva production, and oral mucosa that may make nutrition a major problem. The altered sense of taste and dental problems may be chronic. Pelvic radiation results in the side effect of troublesome diarrhea, which abates as treatment ends, but may continue for some time.

Delayed effects of radiation can be severe: radiation fibrosis causing chronic pulmonary distress; second malignancies, particularly acute leukemia, osteogenic and soft-tissue sarcomas, lung, thyroid, and skin cancer; intellectual impairment and growth problems with cranial radiation in children; dementia and progressive leukoencephalopathy in adults with cranial radiation (see Chapter 29). Among the most psychologically distressing delayed effects of irradiation is sterility. This has become a more apparent long-term adverse effect as more young patients have been cured of previously fatal neoplasms. (See Chapter 7 on psychological problems of survivors and Chapter 33 on sexual dysfunction for more detail.)

Children and adolescents pose particular problems because they may be too young to discuss the sexual sequelae of treatments or for boys to bank sperm. Cella and Cherin (1987) found that many of the children cured of Hodgkin's disease, interviewed as late teenagers and young adults, had not been given information about the status of their fertility, despite becoming sexually active. Parents and physicians, having not discussed it initially, found it difficult to find the "right" time to bring it up later. The issues of early and adequate explanation become more important as the number of children cured of leukemia by bone marrow transplantation mature with sterility resulting from the combination of whole-body radiation and chemotherapy.

Radiotherapists have given much attention to shielding of testes and ovaries to prevent damage to gonadal cells. Ovaries have been surgically moved to a protected pelvic area to prevent damage. Sperm banking is far more frequently offered young men today who receive radiation to the testes or pelvic area where shielding is impossible. Dosage also is a consideration in predicting the impact on fertility; this is information that can be more accurately given to patients today.

Irradiation with orchiectomy is the definitive treatment for seminoma of the testes, and it is used at times in treatment of nonseminomatous testicular tumors. Schover and von Eschenbach (1985) found that the nonseminomatous tumor patients (followed over the long term), who received retroperitoneal irradiation and orchiectomy, or retroperitoneal dissection and chemotherapy, had significantly greater erectile and orgasmic dysfunction. Despite the optimistic view of sexual function gained from small cross-sectional studies of seminoma patients, they found sexual dysfunction and infertility were important problems for a significant number of the 84 studied: a third were

childless, a half had decreased semen volume, a third had less intense orgasm, and low sexual interest, desire, and erectile problems were common (Schover et al., 1986). The men who had a greater paraaortic radiation dosage had more problems with erection and orgasm.

Irradiation and limited surgery have improved the possibilities for the preservation of the breast after treatment for breast cancer. See Chapter 14 for review of the psychological consequences of this treatment and the long-term radiation effects on breast tissue.

Long-term effects of definitive irradiation were examined in a large group of patients 3 to 10 years after completion of treatment. The questions of quality of life were broad, but in major domains of education, marriage, family, and job reactions they were near the norm, with some enhanced satisfaction with life in general (Danoff et al., 1983). Despite these general findings, more careful analysis of the patients' sense of well-being after cancer treatment, including radiotherapy, suggested subtle but significant areas of distress. (See Chapter 7 on psychological aspects of long-term survivors.)

## Abnormal Psychological Reactions to Radiotherapy

Excessive psychological distress with radiotherapy results from several causes, including the special meaning attached to the treatment of cancer by virtue of other concurrent events or prior experiences, and a preexisting psychiatric disorder that leads to exacerbation of psychiatric symptoms during radiotherapy treatment.

### SPECIAL MEANING ATTACHED TO THE TREATMENT

The association of radiotherapy with palliation has not been fully dispelled in the public's mind; indeed, many patients are still referred for radiation for the control of symptoms when the prognosis is guarded. Treatment oriented to palliation is associated with heightened anxiety and depression especially when the news of tumor spread or recurrence has recently been received. This distress may be compounded by concurrent life events and result in even greater distress or even failure to seek treatment, as described in the case that follows.

#### CASE REPORT

A 55-year-old businesswoman postponed medical consultation for vaginal bleeding over a 3-month period because of her husband's critical illness and death from heart disease. She sought care after his death and was found to have stage

III cervical carcinoma. External beam and intracavitary radiation treatment was recommended. Grieving for her husband, she was indecisive about agreeing to treatment, was disinterested in her health, had little hope for a meaningful life, had severe insomnia, and expressed suicidal wishes. Psychiatric evaluation was necessary to deal with her acute grief, which abated somewhat over four psychotherapy sessions, during which time sleep improved with a bedtime antidepressant. Engaging her adult children as supports, and working with the supportive radiotherapists, she agreed to the treatments and completed them. Over several months, her interest in her surroundings returned and she has not had further gynecological problems.

Heightened anxiety prior to the initial treatment is the most commonly encountered problem. Memories of a relative's death after irradiation, or of the painful side effects of treatment, make it difficult for some to accept treatment. For others, the room, the machines, or isolation present an overwhelming barrier because of prior association. Chapter 25 on anxiety describes a patient who as a child had heard her parents' stories of the holocaust. Her experience of being placed alone and isolated in a bare room for the treatment, followed by the sound of a switch and a whirring sound, caused her to panic. She later realized she had unconsciously associated the room with her parents' description of a gas chamber.

Another case illustrates the impact of special meaning resulting in adverse effects.

CASE REPORT

A 33-year-old young man referred for definitive treatment for Hodgkin's disease had no hesitation about consenting to treatment. However, when he saw the machine being lowered toward his chest, his anxiety was so great that the treatment was interrupted. On referral for his emotional difficulty, he recalled having a narrow escape from death when an automobile under which he was working fell and pinned him there until help arrived. Reliving the memories and being reassured about the fail-safe mechanism on the machine, combined with special attention by the technician to his comfort, allowed him to understand and control his fears.

## PRIOR PSYCHIATRIC DISORDERS

Many individuals have mild phobias of heights, enclosed spaces, or isolation, which are controlled by avoidance. Referral for radiotherapy may elicit an otherwise quiescent phobia by the nature of the rooms, the isolation with communication limited to a speaker, and the unfamiliar machines capable of emitting powerful rays. Patients with severe agoraphobia, who cannot tolerate distance from a familiar figure, may have severe panicky feelings when placed in the treatment room. Likewise, persons who have chronic high levels of anxiety, a generalized anxiety disorder, or a history

of panic attacks have difficulty, because they are prone to having an attack before or during treatments. Similarly, a patient with a severe personality disorder precluding cooperation, such as a paranoid personality disorder, or a patient with schizophrenia may have difficulty in cooperating. They should be evaluated before beginning treatment by radiotherapy to allow formulation of a treatment plan between the technician, radiotherapist, and psychiatrist.

CASE REPORT

A 45-year-old housewife had progressively confined herself to her home because of fears of travel and public places. She required a relative to be with her at all times, which was not noted as a difficulty because of a large extended family in the household. However, she had a 20-year history of significant psychiatric impairment based on chronic anxiety and intermittent panic attacks that led to her progressive reclusiveness. An episode of hemoptysis led to diagnosis of an inoperable lung cancer. Radiotherapy was recommended, which she and her family felt she could not tolerate. Consultation between the radiotherapist and psychiatrist led to a treatment plan in which she was given diazepam at home before leaving for the treatment. The psychiatrist accompanied her to the first treatment, which was scheduled for early morning to prevent her from waiting. The technician was given instructions about reassurance, especially in terms of frequent communication. Her husband was allowed to talk to her during the time she was alone in the treatment room, "talking" her through each phase. Over several treatments, with scheduled psychiatric visits weekly, she completed the series of treatments over 6 weeks.

## STRESSES ON RADIOTHERAPY STAFF

The radiotherapist and staff face significant stress since patients are often referred at the time of diagnosis of a tumor or its extension and they often lack extensive information about the patients' prior or current psychological state. Thus, they frequently do not have information about the patient's level of knowledge about the diagnosis, wishes to be informed, coping ability, or family support. More careful attention to this information in the referral by the primary doctor to the radiotherapist would address this problem. Nevertheless, the patient arrives distressed and it is the radiotherapist usually who must explain the reason for the treatments and the expectations. The radiotherapist will follow the patient through the several difficult weeks to months of treatment before returning the patient to the primary physician. The person referred for palliation addresses many painful questions to the radiotherapist, not only at the outset, but during the treatment when the guard is down and discouragement unmasks a previously cheerful exterior. "How long do I have?" or "What can I expect?" or "What are my chances?" The answers are as difficult as the questions and require honesty, though also offering realistic hope and attainable goals.

## PSYCHOLOGICAL INTERVENTIONS

Recommendations based on observations and research findings suggest several useful guidelines for psychological management of radiotherapy patients (Holland et al., 1979).

1. The provision of an "orientation" session for new patients will make them feel more comfortable. A tour conducted by the radiotherapist, nurse, or technician reviews the daily procedure and the rooms, allows an introduction to the technicians who will give the treatment, and briefly explains the type of machine from which they will receive therapy. Special attention to the bidirectional intercom and closed-circuit TV monitoring are important. Patients should be encouraged to ask any questions about their treatment or the procedure, because misperceptions are common.

The orientation session may also begin in a group, supplemented by videotapes. Weekly meetings held for patients in treatment are separate from those held for new patients, which also provide emotional support and encourages patient-to-patient support.

2. The increase in emotional distress, identified toward the end of the therapy, indicates that it is important to plan for and discuss the termination of treatment, allowing the patient to anticipate it well in advance. An abrupt end to treatment that does not allow psychological preparation for termination and "going it alone" without frequent contact with staff should be avoided.

3. The concern for the loss of medical surveillance can be alleviated in part by reassurance that the radiotherapist will be available, evidenced by scheduling of an early posttreatment visit that serves to diminish the sense of loss and eases fears about increased vulnerability to disease raised by the termination of active therapy. The simple information that they may telephone the clinic any time adds to patients' sense of security. Availability of the nurse or social worker may be sufficient.

4. A sense of continuity of care and emotional support is promoted by identifying a single staff person, in addition to the radiotherapist, who maintains a relationship with a particular patient, especially across the transitional period from the time the active treatment ends and the routine of daily activities is reestablished. This may be anyone among the staff, but it is important that one individual is identified.

5. The inclusion of psychological aspects of patient care in the training of radiotherapy technicians and staff can add to their ability, through "therapeutic use of self," to provide additional and continuous emotional support. This can be facilitated by weekly multidisciplinary rounds in which specific patients, the problems they present, and the staff's reactions are discussed. It is also fostered through special teaching programs for radiotherapy technicians separately, in which instruction in the psychological aspects of cancer patient care, using videotapes and interviews with patients, is given. Sensitization to the fluctuations that may occur in levels of anxiety and depression among patients enables the radiotherapy clinic staff to recognize and handle patients' emotional reactions. The psychological dependence that many patients develop on the clinic staff—and which is often perceived as a burden—can be better tolerated when its origin is understood.

The secretary in the radiotherapy office is often the first introduction to the clinic, and it is she or he who deals with the distressed, angry, or depressed patient. Often, the secretary receives little training or recognition for an exceptionally stressful job. Memorial Sloan-Kettering now has seminars for clinic secretaries on the importance of communication and recognition of problems which has diminished burnout in this critically important group (see Chapter 51).

6. Attention to the ambiance of a radiotherapy clinic is important, with small, pleasant waiting areas in which groups of patients with similar levels of illness can wait together. Too often hospitalized patients on stretchers are placed with ambulatory patients in large, single waiting areas. The lengthy wait for treatment, with the visual impression of a crowded, uncomfortable room (sometimes with acutely ill patients), reflects lack of adequate attention to the importance of physical surroundings.

## SUMMARY

As a modality used in half of all patients with cancer, radiotherapy requires careful attention with regard to the societal views that still harbor a stigma about its value and application: normal fears elicited by any unfamiliar treatment, especially utilizing large and powerful machines, and the immediate side effects that are best tolerated when anticipated and emotionally prepared for; the delayed effects that patients should know may occur, especially when preparation can diminish their impact, such as sperm banking; the psychological supports that should be built into care; and the stresses on radiotherapy staff that may negatively affect their ability to be sensitive to the human side of care. In addition to the social worker who monitors the responses of patients and families, a psychiatric consultant can assist in the care of patients who require special consideration by virtue of their psychological distress related to severe psychological reactions, based on prior or concurrent negative experiences, or prior psychiatric disturbance.

The steady daily care of such patients is a source of professional stress. Young radiotherapists need training in how to deal with patients' questions about prognosis, how to recognize the common psychological problems presented by patients, and how to handle their own responses to their work.

## ACKNOWLEDGMENT

The author expresses gratitude to Dr. Beryl McCormick, radiotherapist, for her critical review and contributions to this chapter.

## REFERENCES

Anderson, B.L., J.A. Karlsson, B. Anderson, and H.W. Tewfik (1984). Anxiety and cancer treatment: Response to stressful radiotherapy. *Health Psychology* 3:535–51.

Anderson, B.L. and H.H. Tewfik (1985). Psychological reactions to radiation therapy: Reconsideration of the adaptive aspects of anxiety. *J. Pers. Soc. Psychol.* 48:1024–32.

Cassileth, B.R., D. Volckmar, and R.L. Goodman (1980). The effect of experience on radiation therapy patients' desire for information. *Int. J. Radiat. Oncol. Biol. Phy.* 6:493–96.

Cella, D.F. and E.A. Cherin (1987). *Measuring Quality of Life in Patients with Cancer.* Paper presented at the American Cancer Society Fifth National Conference on Human Values and Cancer, San Francisco, March 1987.

Danoff, B., S. Kramer, P. Irwin, and A. Gottlieb (1983). Assessment of quality of life in long-term survivors after definitive radiotherapy. *Am. J. Clin. Oncol.* 6:339–45.

Dobelbower, R.R., Jr. (1987). Principles of radiation therapy. In R.T. Skeel (ed.), *Handbook of Cancer Chemotherapy* 2nd ed. Boston: Little, Brown & Co., pp. 35–47.

Duffner, P.K., N.E. Cohen, M.L. Voorhees, M.H. MacGillivray, M.L. Brecher, A. Panahon, and B.B. Gilani (1985). Long-term effects of cranial irradiation on endocrine function in children with brain tumors: A prospective study. *Cancer* 56:2189–93.

Forester, B.M., D.S. Kornfeld, and J. Fleiss (1978). Psychiatric aspects of radiotherapy. *Am. J. Psychiatry* 135:960–63.

Gottschalk, L.A., R. Kunkal, T.H. Wohl, E.L. Saenger, and C.N. Winger (1969). Total and half body irradiation: Effect on cognitive and emotional processes. *Arch. Gen. Psychiatry,* 21:574–80.

Hellman, S. (1985). Principles of radiation therapy. In V.T. DeVita, Jr., S. Hellman, and S. Rosenberg (eds.), *Cancer Principles and Practice of Oncology,* 2nd ed. Philadelphia: Lippincott, pp. 227–25.

Herbert, D. (1977). The assessment of the clinical signifi-cance of noncompliance with prescribed schedules of irradiation. *J. Radiat. Oncol. Biol. Phys.* 2:763–72.

Hilaris, B.S. and D. Nori (1984). Looking back. Brachytherapy Oncology Update. *Proc. Mem. Sloan-Kettering Cancer Center Symp.,* New York.

Holland, J.C., J. Rowland, A. Lebovits, and R. Rusalem (1979). Reactions to cancer treatment: Assessment of emotional response to adjuvant radiotherapy as a guide to planned intervention. *Psychiatr. Clin. North Am.* 2:347–58.

Janis, I.L. (1958). *Psychological Stress: Psychoanalytic and Behavioral Studies of Surgical Patients.* New York: Wiley.

Johnson, B.E., W.B. Goff II, N. Petronas, M.A. Krehbiel, R.W. Makuch, G. McDenna, E. Glatstein, and B.G. Ende (1985). Neurologic, neuropsychologic and computed cranial tomography scan abnormalities in 2-to-10 year survivors of small cell lung cancer. *J. Clin. Oncol.* 3:1659–67.

Kagan, A.R., P.M. Levitt, T.M. Arnold, and J. Hattem (1984). Honesty is the best policy: A radiation therapist's perspective on caring for terminal cancer patients. *Am. J. Clin. Oncol.* 7:381–83.

King, K.B., L.M. Nail, K. Kreamer, R.A. Strohl, and J.E. Johnson (1985). Patients' description of the experience of receiving radiation therapy. *Oncol. Nurs. Forum* 12(4): 55–61.

Kramer, S., G.E. Hanks, J.J. Diamond, and C.J. Maclean (1984). The study of patterns of clinical care in radiation therapy in the United States. *CA* 34:75–85.

Mitchell, G.W. and A.S. Glicksman (1977). Cancer patients' knowledge and attitudes. *Cancer* 40:61–66.

Parsons, J.A. and J.H. Webster (1961). Evaluation of the placebo effect in the treatment of radiation sickness. *Acta Radiol.* 56:129–40.

Peck, A. (1972). Emotional reactions to having cancer. *Am. J. Roentgenol. Radiat. Ther. Nucl. Med.* 114:591–99.

Peck, A. and J. Boland (1977). Emotional reactions to radiation treatment. *Cancer* 40:180–84.

Perez, C.A. and L.W. Brady (1987). Introduction. In C.A. Perez and L.W. Brady (eds.), *Principles and Practice of Radiation Oncology.* Philadelphia: Lippincott, pp. 1–55.

Rainey, L.C. (1985). Effects of preparatory patient education for radiation oncology patients. *Cancer* 56:1056–61.

Rotman, M., L. Rogow, G. DeLeon, and N. Heskel (1977). Supportive therapy in radiation oncology. *Cancer* 39:744–50.

Rowland, J.H., O.J. Glidewell, R.F. Sibley, J.C. Holland, R. Tull, A. Berman, M.L. Brecher, M. Harris, A.S. Glicksman, E. Forman, B. Jones, P.K. Duffner, and A.I. Freeman (for the Cancer and Leukemia Group B) (1984). Effects of different forms of central nervous prophylaxis on neuropsychologic function in childhood leukemia. *J. Clin. Oncol.* 2:1327–36.

Schover, L.R. and A.C. von Eschenbach (1985). Sexual and marital relationships after treatment for nonseminomatous testicular cancer. *Urology* 25:251–55.

Schover, L.R., M. Gonzales, and A.C. von Eschenbach (1986). Sexual and marital relationships after radiotherapy for seminoma. *Urology* 27:117–23.

Shimkin, M. (1977). *Contrary to Nature*. DHEW Publ. No. (NIH) 76-720. Washington, D.C.: U.S. Govt. Printing Office.

Silberfarb, P.M., L.H. Maurer, and C.S. Crouthmel (1980). Psychosocial aspects of neoplastic disease: I. Functional status of breast cancer patients during different treatment regimens. *Am. J. Psychiatry* 137:450–55.

Smith, L.L. and J.J. McNamara (1977). Social work services and radiation therapy patients and their families. *Hosp. Community Psychiatry* 28:752–54.

Yonke, C. (1967). Emotional response to radiotherapy. *Hosp. Top.* 43:107–8.

# 10

# Chemotherapy, Endocrine Therapy, and Immunotherapy

Jimmie C. Holland and Lynna M. Lesko

## CHEMOTHERAPY: DEVELOPMENT OF AGENTS

In the early 1900s, the first ''chemotherapy'' drug was used successfully by Paul Ehrlich to treat a parasitic infection; becoming the founder of modern chemotherapy. When one looks at the development of drugs, there are some striking historical parallels between the development of antiinfectious agents and anticancer drugs (DeVita, 1985). During the same period in which Ehrlich was working with rodent models for study of infectious diseases, George Clowes at Roswell Park Memorial Institute in Buffalo, New York, developed an inbred rodent tumor model in which the efficacy of new chemotherapeutic agents could be tested. Then came the observation that the alkylating agents developed for gas warfare in World Wars I and II caused bone marrow suppression and lymphoid hypoplasia. Experimental study of these agents in animals led to clinical trials in patients with lymphoma and Hodgkin's disease by the mid-1940s. Remissions of childhood leukemia after the application of a folic acid antagonist by Farber and co-workers suggested that wider trials of anticancer agents in human cancers would be worthwhile. (DeVita, 1985)

The steady development of cancer chemotherapy over the past four decades has produced a formidable array of drugs that are effective in treating both hematological malignancies and solid tumors (DeVita, 1985). In addition to the 35 noted in Fig. 10-1, mitoxantrone was added in 1987. Their clinical effectiveness has increased as the understanding of dose, timing, and mechanism of action has improved. The extensive exploration of the relationship between cell kinetics and pharmocokinetics increasingly led to the use in the mid-1950s of a single agent, methotrexate, to cure choriocarcinoma, and in the mid-1960s, cyclophosphamide for Burkitt's lymphoma.

Most cytotoxic drugs work by altering DNA synthesis and subsequent DNA function (see Fig. 10-2; Cohan, 1985). Cells in the resting phase of their cycle are usually not affected unless they are ready to divide. By studying treatment failures that resulted from drug resistance, either de novo or acquired, the use of combinations of non-cross-resistant cytotoxic agents developed. Between the 1960s and 1970s, acute lymphocytic leukemia, Hodgkin's disease, and testicular cancer began to be treated successfully with combination chemotherapy. Multiagent therapy began to be applied in combination with radiation and surgery, resulting in effective treatment of pediatric sarcomas and breast cancer (Chabner, 1986). Further elucidation of cytotoxic principles has led to the use of adjuvant therapies in solid tumors, such as breast, rectal, and lung cancer, where they are effective in delaying recurrence of disease (Krakoff, 1981). Table 10-1 summarizes the neoplasms and the chemotherapeutic agents that have been most effective in their treatment (Medical Newsletter, 1987).

## TOXICITY AND SIDE EFFECTS OF CHEMOTHERAPEUTIC AGENTS

Together with the remarkable impact on survival in some cancers and the frequent useful palliation in others, anticancer drugs produce significant side effects that must be tolerated in order to achieve the desired toxic effect on tumor cells. When the treatment is curative, patients can tolerate a great deal. When the chemotherapy is given for palliation, the quality of life and comfort become important issues. Much of the effort in quality-of-life research has addressed control of these side effects, particularly nausea and vomiting. However, there are several other common side effects identified by patients receiving treatment, such as al-

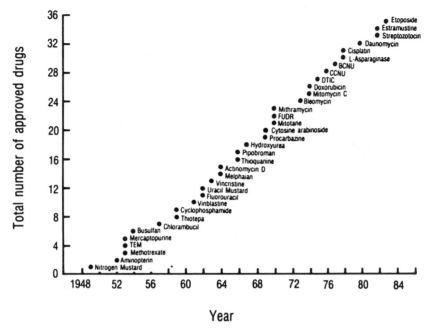

**Figure 10-1.** The developing pace of new anticancer drugs (excluding endocrines). Date of introduction refers to date of filing of new drug application with the Food and Drug Administration. *Source:* Reprinted with permission from V.T. DeVita (1985), Principles of chemotherapy.In V.T. DeVita, Jr., S. Hellman, and S.A. Rosenberg (eds.), *Cancer: Principles and Practice of Oncology,* 2nd ed. Philadelphia: Lippincott, pp. 257–85.

opecia, nausea and vomiting, fatigue, anorexia, peripheral neuropathies, stomatitis, diarrhea, and sexual problems (Table 10-2) (Penman et al., 1984). Side effects vary widely, however, depending on the particular drug or combination of drugs, the dosage, route, number of cycles of treatment, and, whether the agents are given in combination with radiotherapy. Nausea and vomiting usually occur soon after receiving treatment as a result of direct stimulation of the vomiting center, although some agents, particularly cisplatin,

**Figure 10-2.** Sites of action of commonly used cytotoxic agents. *Source:* Reprinted with permission from L.M. Cohan (1985). Principles of radiotherapy and chemotherapy. In D.A. Casciato and B.B. Lowitz (eds.), *Manual of Bedside Oncology.* Boston: Little, Brown & Co., p. 20.

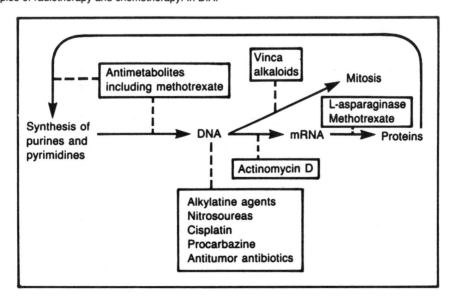

**Table 10-1**  Diseases in which chemotherapy has major activity

| Type | Drugs preferred | Type | Drugs preferred |
|---|---|---|---|
| Acute lymphocytic leukemia (ALL) | Induction: vincristine + prednisone ± asparaginase ± doxorubicin or daunorubicin | | Etoposide + cisplatin ± vincristine |
| | | | Cyclophosphamide + doxorubicin + etoposide (CAE) |
| | CNS prophylaxis: intrathecal methotrexate ± radiotherapy | | Methotrexate + doxorubicin + cyclophosphamide + lomustine (MACC) |
| | Maintenance: combination chemotherapy with methotrexate + mercaptopurine or other combinations | Non-Hodgkin's lymphoma; Burkitt's lymphoma | Cyclophosphamide |
| | | | Cyclophosphamide + vincristine + methotrexate |
| | BMT with cylophosphamide and total body irradiation | | Cyclophosphamide + high-dose cytarabine ± methotrexate with leucovorin |
| Acute myelocytic leukemia (AML) | Daunorubicin + cytarabine ± thioguanine | Diffuse histiocytic lymphoma | Cyclophosphamide + doxorubicin + vincristine + prednisone (CHOP) |
| | BMT with cyclophosphamide and total body irradiation | | Bleomycin + doxorubicin + cyclophosphamide + vincristine + prednisone + (BACOP) |
| Breast cancer* | Tamoxifen, progestins | | Bleomycin + doxorubicin + cyclophosphamide + vincristine + prednisone + methotrexate with leucovorin rescue (M–BACOP) |
| | Cyclophosphamide + methotrexate + fluorouracil ± prednisone (CMF or CMFP) | | Prednisone + methotrexate–leucovorin + doxorubicin + cyclophosphamide + etoposide–mechlorethamine + vincristine + procarbazine + prednisone (ProMACE–MOPP) |
| | Cyclophosphamide + doxorubicin ± fluorouracil (AC or CAF) | | |
| Choriocarcinoma | Methotrexate ± dactinomycin | | Bleomycin + doxorubicin + cyclophosphamide + vincristine + prednisone + procarbazine (COP–BLAM) |
| Embryonal rhabdomyosarcoma* | Vincristine + dactinomycin + cyclophosphamide (VAC) ± doxorubicin | | Methotrexate with leucovorin + doxorubicin + cyclophosphamide + vincristine + prednisone + bleomycin (MACOP–B) |
| | Vincristine + doxorubicin + cyclophosphamide | | |
| Ewing's sarcoma* | Cyclophosphamide + doxorubicin + vincristine (CAV) | | Cyclophosphamide + vincristine + methotrexate–leucovorin + cytarabine (COMLA) |
| Hairy-cell leukemia | Interferon or deoxycoformycin† | Osteogenic sarcoma* | Doxorubicin and/or high-dose methotrexate + leucovorin rescue ± cisplatin ± bleomycin ± cyclophosphamide ± dactinomycin |
| Hodgkin's disease | Mechlorethamine + vincristine + procarbazine + prednisone (MOPP) | | |
| | Doxorubicin + bleomycin + vinblastine + dacarbazine (ABVD) ± cyclophosphamide | Testicular | Cisplatin + vinblastine + bleomycin (PVB) |
| | MOPP alternated with ABVD | | Bleomycin + etoposide + cisplatin (BEP) |
| | Chlorambucil + vinblastine + procarbazine + prednisone (CVPP) ± carmustine | | Vinblastine + dactinomycin + bleomycin + cyclophosphamide + cisplatin (VAB-6) |
| | Mechlorethamine + vincristine + procarbazine + doxorubicin + bleomycin + vinblastine (MOP/ABV) | | |
| Lung, small cell (oat cell) | Cyclophosphamide + doxorubicin + vincristine (CAV) | | |

**Table 10-1** (*Continued*)

| Type | Drugs preferred |
|---|---|
| Wilms' tumor* | Dactinomycin + vincristine ± doxorubicin |

± = with or without.

*Drugs have major activity only when combined with surgical resection, radiotherapy, or both (adjuvant chemotherapy).

†Available only for investigational use.

*Source*: Adapted from Cancer chemotherapy (Editorial). (1987). *Med. Lett. Drugs Ther.* 29 (March 27):29–36.

can produce delayed nausea and vomiting 24–48 hours later. (See Chapter 34 for physiology of nausea and vomiting.) Nausea and vomiting may become the limiting reasons for patients' unwillingness to continue receiving chemotherapy. However, increasingly effective antiemesis regimens have significantly reduced this troublesome side effect. Major progress has also been made in understanding and controlling the conditioned or anticipatory response, which causes nausea and vomiting to develop before receiving the treatment (see Chapter 35).

Although subjective symptoms and visible physical changes are often most distressing to the patient, the more significant side effects are those that are life-threatening with an impact on normal cells. Rapidly proliferating cells, because of their frequent entry into the DNA-synthetic phase, become targets, along with the cancer cells, of the toxic effects of many chemotherapeutic agents. Bone marrow suppression and immunosuppression constitute the greatest threat to life (Hahn et al., 1978). Stomatitis and gastroenteritis are painful and may provide a portal of entry for bacterial or fungal invasion, particularly if myelosuppression exists at the same time. Interference with nutrition may

**Table 10-2** Side effects noted by patients receiving chemotherapy*

| Symptoms | Percentage |
|---|---|
| Hair loss | 84 |
| Nausea and vomiting | 71 |
| Tiredness and/or weakness | 70 |
| Anorexia | 53 |
| Numbness and/or tingling | 37 |
| Stomatitis | 36 |
| Diarrhea | 34 |
| Sexual difficulties | 20 |

*$n = 144$; >30 chemotherapy regimens.

*Source*: D. Penman, J.C. Holland, G. Bahna, G. Morrow, A. Schmale, and L. Derogatis, C.L. Carnrike, and R. Cherry (1984). Informed consent for investigational chemotherapy: Patients' and physicians' perceptions. *J. Clin. Oncol.* 2:849–55.

**Table 10-3** Disruptions associated with chemotherapy treatment*

| Disruptions | Percentage |
|---|---|
| Side effects | 66 |
| Wait in clinic or office | 36 |
| Interference with job or school | 29 |
| Transportation | 23 |
| Interference with family relationships | 16 |
| Concerns about uncertain benefits | 14 |

*$n = 144$; >30 different treatment regimens.

*Source*: D. Penman, J.C. Holland, G. Bahna, G. Morrow, A. Schmale, L. Derogatis, C.L. Carnrike, and R. Cherry (1984). Informed consent for investigational chemotherapy: Patients' and physicians' perceptions. *J. Clin. Oncol.* 2:849–55.

occur, as well as mild to severe diarrhea, which can cause fluid and electrolyte imbalance.

Alopecia is much dreaded by patients, yet it is temporary and reversible. On the other hand, the effects of gonadal dysfunction are not always reversible. Furthermore, other delayed effects, not appearing for weeks or months, may have adverse irreversible effects on the lungs, resulting in pulmonary fibrosis (bleomycin and alkylating agents), cardiomyopathy (anthracyclines and high-dose cytoxan), and leukoencephalopathy (methotrexate). In addition, some drugs produce second malignancies as part of their delayed effects, which is a concern for survivors as well. (See Chapter 7 by Tross.) It is this range of side effects, only some of which usually occur, that are often publicized more than the therapeutic effectiveness of the chemotherapeutic agents. The assumption that all the side effects may occur frightens many patients.

A patient contemplating chemotherapy must contend not only with the common negative impressions of chemotherapy and its effects, but with the disruptions of daily life that accompany committing to the treatment and adhering to it. Table 10-3 summarizes the common disruptions noted in a study of chemotherapy patients in three cancer centers. Not only are the physical side effects troublesome, but so are the repeated interference of the chemotherapy treatments with the job and family a cause of significant anguish (Penman et al., 1984).

## PSYCHOLOGICAL ISSUES

### Social Attitudes

Both radiotherapy and chemotherapy have been historically perceived as more frightening to patients than surgery. Radiotherapy and chemotherapy were both initially given for palliation or short-term control of tumor growth, and that meaning lingers in the minds of many. In earlier days, patients perceived that the risk to their life was great and treatment effectiveness was low; they often refused chemotherapy. Attitudes change slowly. Although there are still tumors for which chemotherapy has little or no effect, knowledge of the effectiveness in other diseases such as Hodgkin's disease and testicular cancer, contribute to changing attitudes. Positive results with breast, lung, colon, and ovarian cancer also support a view of constructive optimism. Continuing concerns result in part from ignorance or misconceptions about the effectiveness of chemotherapeutic agents. Thus, it is crucial that the patient and family be given information about the potential for benefit from chemotherapy to correct the myths that still lead some patients to say "I would rather die than take chemotherapy." Accurate information about the benefits and side effects of specific agents have begun to counter the public's fears, and the concerns of new patients are becoming more realistic (Lesko et al., 1986).

## Accepting Chemotherapy

News from the oncologist that chemotherapy is needed often comes as frightening information to the patient and family when they are still reeling from the impact of a cancer diagnosis, recurrence, or relapse. Of course, some patients accept it as welcome evidence that something further can be done. For most, however, anxiety, depressive symptoms, and difficulty in concentration make it difficult to hear and grasp the physician's discussion and treatment plan. An unhurried overview of the diagnosis and treatment under consideration is useful, but due to the inability to comprehend the information fully, more than one discussion may be necessary. An outline of the therapeutic goals and the side effects that must be tolerated to achieve the goals is an important source from which the patient gains a sense of trust—or lack of it—in the physician. Studies done by the Psychosocial Collaborative Oncology Group (Penman et al., 1984) and Lesko and co-workers (1988a) revealed that, irrespective of all other considerations, trust in the doctor was crucial in the decision of patients to accept treatment by investigational protocols. The same trust in the physician also underlies the successful conduct of standard chemotherapy. The role that the patient will play in the treatment must be emphasized, because chemotherapy regimens often last over several months. A strong sense of commitment to the treatment and cooperation with the physician are essential to assure the best outcome, which requires compliance to achieve the full dose prescribed.

The participation of a family member or trusted friend in the initial discussion between doctor and patient is very useful. It ensures that the patient and the family member (auditor) can later reflect on and further discuss what was said by the doctor. This also helps them to identify key questions for later discussion. Audiotaping the discussion, or giving the consent form to take home to read without pressure of time improves information and results in better adherence to the regimen, based on fuller understanding of the treatment. A range of books available to the public are also helpful in dispelling some of the fears (Bruning, 1985; Siegel, 1986). At Memorial Sloan-Kettering, patient education has been particularly well developed by chemotherapy nurses and the pharmacy. Patients receive detailed information about the particular drug(s) that they will receive on chemotherapy cards, which outline information about the drug's effects and side effects and offer nutritional advice.

After agreeing to chemotherapy, awaiting the first treatment is often the most anxiety-provoking period for patients. Anticipation associated with waiting to receive the first treatment is often later remembered as having been psychologically far worse than the actual treatment proved to be. In a study by Meyerowitz and colleagues (1983), 41% of women who received adjuvant chemotherapy for breast cancer reported that the treatment had been easier than they had expected. The waiting period is a time when prior personal associations with cancer or chemotherapy may cause distress. In some cases, psychiatric consultation may be needed to clarify the issues.

### CASE REPORT

A 42-year-old housewife, the mother of two small children, was referred for consultation following segmental resection for stage II breast cancer with 15 positive nodes. On being told that she required chemotherapy, she refused, saying, "It is hopeless—why bother." Her husband and oncologist together persuaded her to discuss her decision with a psychiatrist. She appeared for the interview reluctantly. She was depressed and withdrawn, and stated that she preferred that her children remember her as she was. An early death would be preferable to the lingering debilitation that would follow chemotherapy. On further review, she described her mother's diagnosis of breast cancer when she was 12 and that she had always feared that it would happen to her too. Her mother's mastectomy had been followed by painful bone metastases despite chemotherapy. She had distressing memories of her mother's suffering and had taken lengthy steps with her physicians to assure that mammograms and frequent breast examinations would allow her to be diagnosed early should breast cancer develop. Several calcification had been watched for a year. She now had anger toward her physician that her life was needlessly compromised by late diagnosis of something she had attempted to avoid for so long. The anger and hopelessness together were overwhelming. Clarification that she would be receiving adjuvant chemotherapy to prevent recurrence and awareness that her reason for refusing was based on memories of her mother, and assumptions about her own outcome, led the patient to reconsider. She was still well at the 3-year follow-up.

## Compliance

There are compelling reasons for receiving a full treatment course of chemotherapy. Patients with breast cancer who received a complete chemotherapy treatment program had survival rates better than those whose mean dose was attenuated (Bonadonna and Valagussa, 1981). Studies in the Cancer and Leukemia Group B (CALGB) showed similar results with osteogenic sarcoma and breast cancer. Similarly, in a study of adjuvant chemotherapy for breast cancer (Taylor et al., 1985), women who received less than 80% of the chemotherapy dose had poorer outcome. Patients are often aware of these data concerning full dose and survival. They become distressed and depressed when myelotoxicity makes it necessary to lower the dose or delay a treatment. Compliance is remarkably high, especially for those treatments that are given intravenously in hospital or at clinic. Noncompliance, however, may relate not only to patient behavior, but to physician behavior as well. Some physicians are reluctant to give the full scheduled dose because of unwillingness to incur side effects that might prove troublesome or life-threatening. The patient's optimal opportunity for survival can be compromised by lack of the physician's commitment to a full treatment dose (Barofsky and Sugarbaker, 1979; Lewis et al., 1983).

Among individuals who are unable to adhere to scheduled treatments, some have mild to severe psychiatric disorders that make it difficult for them to tolerate the frustrations and discomforts of treatment. A patient with a prior major mental illness, particularly schizophrenia, may have difficulty in attaining the level of cooperation needed. Similarly, individuals with an alcohol or drug abuse history are at risk for noncompliance. Adolescents and young adults, particularly adolescent boys and young men, may adhere poorly to a lengthy treatment schedule. A case is described in Chapter 59 of a teenager for whom chemotherapy for osteogenic sarcoma was potentially curative, yet he refused treatment and could not be persuaded by his parents or others to cooperate. These are especially painful cases for the staff, when cure is an expected outcome of treatment.

Largely unexplored, except in children, is noncompliance with oral chemotherapy taken at home (Smith et al., 1979). Using prednisone taken by mouth as a marker, compliance was found to be quite low in children whose parents were responsible for medication and among adolescents who were personally responsible for taking their medicine. This problem should be explored more fully in the adult cancer population.

## Chemotherapy and Quality of Life

Patients face a range of symptoms during chemotherapy, based on the side effects that develop. In a study by the Psychosocial Collaborative Oncology Group, patients in more than 30 chemotherapy protocols were studied at three centers. The patients ranked their most distressing symptoms as follows: hair loss, 84%; nausea and vomiting, 71%; and tiredness and weakness, 70% (Table 10-2). These symptoms, particularly diminished stamina, resulted in difficulty in meeting personal and work obligations. Patients also reported that major problems that interfered with function arose from side effects (66%), long waits in clinic (36%), interference with job or school (29%), transportation problems (23%), interference with family responsibilities (16%), and lingering concerns about uncertain benefits (14%) (Table 10-3). The side effects of treatment added to infringement on function take a toll on the quality of life.

More intensive therapies given in the hospital require stamina, compliance, and a grasp of future benefit. Chills, fever, sepsis, antibiotics, stomatitis, infusional feedings, transfusions, diarrhea, and confinement in bed with impaired ability to attend to personal needs are some of the physical aspects which result in dependence on caregivers. Hostility, anger at venipunctures, and anxiety about outcome characterize some of the essential emotions. In these patients, the quality of life during treatment is so poor that the equation must be balanced by hope for the results and by a desire to live.

Meyerowitz and colleagues (1983) studied women with breast cancer during chemotherapy treatment and for 2 years after completing it. Among those who were free of disease at 2 years, 23% described difficulty with their personal and family relationships during treatment, and 44% had continuing physical problems 2 years later. Despite these problems, 89% reported that they would recommend to a close friend that she definitely have the treatment. They suggested that they had coped with treatment by "staying busy," getting information about the treatment, and keeping a positive hopeful outlook. They also had lingering fears of recurrence and became "queasy" when they experienced reminders of their illness or treatment especially smells, such as alcohol.

Patients being treated for lymphoma were queried by Nerenz and colleagues (1982). They found that the presence of a greater number of side effects accounted for greater distress than the severity or duration of any single one. Weakness and fatigue were most troublesome. Patients coped best when they could see visible signs that the disease had regressed, for example, by reduction in size of lymph nodes. Objective signs of improvement in physical function were also heartening.

The question of quality of life in patients for whom treatment is palliative, not curative, raises important questions. Women with advanced breast cancer were studied by Coates and colleagues (1987) to determine whether continuous treatment administered until disease progression was evident was preferable to intermittent therapy in which treatment was stopped after three cycles and when there was evidence of disease progression. Contrary to expectations, a randomized trial showed not only better survival but also better quality of life in women receiving continuous therapy with doxorubicin plus cyclophosphamide or with cyclophosphamide, methotrexate, fluorouracil, and prednisone. Their data are important support for the role of anticancer drugs in palliation for metastatic breast cancer. The study underscores the need to measure quality of life in trials of treatment for palliation.

Several different measures have been developed to evaluate quality of life during treatment, some using patient self-report and others using observer's report (see Part III on research methods). In 1976, the CALGB was the first trials group to add psychosocial parameters to the assessment of treatment effects, especially chemotherapy, on quality of life and the patients' perceptions of their ability to function during treatment (Holland et al., 1986). These findings have added an important dimension to the evaluation of treatments, especially those that do not offer curative opportunity and in which palliation is the goal. In these patients, choosing the regimen with the least unpleasant side effects become important when length of survival is known to be limited. In a two-armed CALGB lung cancer protocol studying small-cell lung cancer, equal survival was found. Systemic toxicity was comparable for the two different regimens, both utilizing chemotherapy, chest radiation, and prophylactic cranial radiation. However, the treatment arm containing vincristine was associated with greater mood disturbance and depression (Silberfarb et al., 1983, 1986). Silberfarb emphasized the importance of considering quality of life in choosing a treatment regimen for patients receiving palliative care. Studies that include psychological evaluation provide a means of assessing the neurotoxic effects of chemotherapeutic agents, especially on mental function and mood (see Chapter 13 on lung cancer).

The importance of measuring treatment effects more broadly, to include cognitive function, was demonstrated in leukemic children. Poor school performance after finishing treatment was observed in some. Several studies showed that cranial radiation with intrathecal methotrexate adversely affected cognitive function. One study found a mean 10-point drop in intellectual achievement in the children treated with both therapeutic modalities, with greater impact on younger children (Rowland et al., 1984). The findings of several studies encouraged oncologists to develop treatment regimens that reduced the likelihood of this complication.

An important research area in psychooncology has been the development of rapid assessment tools to evaluate a patient's quality of life during cancer treatment. Part XII reviews these methods in detail. The Functional Living Index (FLIC) developed by Schipper and colleagues (1984) and the Quality of Life Index by Spitzer and co-workers (1981) represent important advances. The European Organization for Research in the Treatment of Cancer (EORTC) has also contributed valuable insights to this area (Aaronson and Beckmann, 1987). The cancer cooperative groups in the United States, especially the CALGB (Holland et al., 1986b), and the child cancer trial groups are pursuing innovative ways to evaluate patients during treatment. The hope is to identify the best instruments for use and to promote more uniform evaluation of quality of life.

## Responses to Alopecia

The ability of many patients to accept and tolerate chemotherapy is seriously affected by hair loss and anxiety about the possibility of baldness. Psychological preparation is essential. Helpful steps include: encouragement to buy a wig to match hair before it begins to thin and referral to a good wig maker, trimming longer hair (particularly important for male adolescents) to make the transition to a wig less dramatic, and talking to a veteran patient who has managed alopecia and who can give practical hints. Hair sometimes begins to grow back, even during treatment, which is reassuring. With adequate psychological preparation, the patient is not surprised or frightened when hair begins to fall out. Wig makers and hairdressers who work with chemotherapy patients often have considerable experience and expertise in offering help. Referral sources are available through oncology nurses, oncology social workers, and local American Cancer Society chapters.

Adriamycin, daunomycin, cyclophosphamide, vincristine, bleomycin, and radiotherapy are notable for causing alopecia. Combinations containing one of these is more likely than a single drug to cause alopecia. It is also dose dependent. Irrespective of helpful steps to reduce the impact, alopecia is an unmistakable stigma of chemotherapy, which may be particularly difficult to tolerate by individuals who feel that their work or position will be threatened by evidence of cancer treatments. For these individuals an ice cap to reduce scalp blood flow can be used during infusions to reduce the concentration of chemotherapeutic drugs reaching the scalp hair follicle. This may reduce hair loss at relatively low levels of drug, although it is uncomfortable during treatment.

## Cognitive Changes with Chemotherapy

The acute and chronic CNS effects of chemotherapeutic agents are reviewed in Chapter 29 on CNS complications of cancer. Chapter 7 on survivors also reviews the long-term cognitive effects. Most of the early research in this area focused on pediatric acute lymphocytic leukemia, in which children received intrathecal methotrexate and irradiation which led to a drop in intellectual function. Silberfarb and Lesko have called attention to the subtle changes in mental function that occur in patients receiving a range of chemotherapeutic agents. The findings may be interpreted as depression unless one is alert to their development. Neuropsychological testing can provide helpful confirmatory evidence (Silberfarb, 1983; Lesko et al., 1988c). A chart of the commonly used chemotherapeutic agents and the CNS symptoms they cause is presented in Table 10-4.

## Weight Changes and Psychological Consequences

Patients are fearful of cancer recurrence or progression. Weight loss is interpreted as evidence of advancing disease, even when an explanation, such as reduced intake, is apparent. Despite attempts to eat, the anorexia usually associated with advanced cancer leads to cachexia and the realization that the patient is wasting away. Allowing others to see him or her in a debilitated state is difficult for some, because fears of reactions of surprise, or worse, pity, are expected in others. Some patients become preoccupied with eating and maintaining normal weight to ward off the fears of tumor recurrence indicated by weight loss. They may actually gain weight from overeating; diminished exercise likely also contributes. Weight gain is seen particularly in women with breast cancer who are receiving adjuvant chemotherapy, and in women with metastatic breast cancer who receive hormonal therapy (Knobf, 1986). Megestrol acetate, for example, independent of its effect on tumor growth, increases appetite and weight gain of 10–20 pounds is not uncommon.

Alterations in appearance resulting from obesity or weight loss, particularly when coupled with alopecia, may result in humiliation about appearance and loss of self-esteem and self-confidence. From the outset of treatment, nutritional and fitness counseling can be helpful, especially when it deals constructively with these common problems. A structured exercise program has been shown to increase functional capacity of patients during treatment, as well as increasing a sense of well-being (MacVicar and Winningham, 1986).

## Disruption of Daily Routine

Side effects, together with generalized weakness and fatigue that interfere with work, may make it important to schedule treatments so that the worst side effects occur on the weekend. If more oncological clinics and offices offered flexibility of treatment hours for patients, it would allow full-time employed individuals to have treatments in the evenings or on weekends, avoiding loss of time from work. For some patients, the day immediately preceding a treatment is described as one filled with anxiety and apprehension as anticipation of the next treatment grows. In a study of women receiving cyclophosphamide–methotrexate–fluorouracil (CMF) adjuvant breast chemotherapy, Redd and colleagues found almost two-thirds experienced nausea as part of the anticipatory systems (see Chapter 35). Some patients vomited before the treatment.

Anticipation of chemotherapy with anxiety is reduced by using self-control methods such as progressive relaxation exercises to maintain a calmer feeling outlook. Daytime sedation and a bedtime hypnotic the night before also reduce anxiety.

## Psychological Consequences of Gonadal Effects

An additional source of emotional distress is the cytotoxic effect that chemotherapeutic agents have on gonadal cells in both men and women. Gonadal dysfunction is an especially unfortunate price to pay for cure in the young individuals who have benefited most in improved survival as a result of chemotherapy (Sutcliffe, 1979). In a review of the studies on gonadal dysfunction, the major group of drugs responsible for cytotoxic-induced gonadal dysfunction are the alkylating agents, particularly cyclophosphamide, chlorambucil, and busulfan (Itri, 1983). Other drugs, such as vinblastine, methotrexate, procarbazine, and cytosine arabinoside, also produce gonadal toxicity.

In men chemotherapeutic drugs affect the germinal epithelium and Leydig cells. Recovery of spermatogenesis is variable and is related to the specific agent and total dose necessary to produce germinal aplasia. Hormonal replacement is seldom indicated unless levels of serum testosterone are consistently low. In women there is a relationship between the age

**Table 10-4** Neuropsychiatric toxicity associated with major chemotherapeutic agents

| | Delirium | Lethargy | Hallucinations | Dementia | Depression | Personality change | Mania | Psychosis | Extrapyramidal symptoms | Ataxia |
|---|---|---|---|---|---|---|---|---|---|---|
| Methotrexate | + | | | + | | + | | | | |
| Fuorouracil | + | | | | | | | | + | + |
| Vincristine/vinblastine | + | + | | | + | | | | | |
| Bleomycin | + | | | | | | | | | |
| Carmustine (BCNU) | + | | | + | | | | | | + |
| Cisplatin | + | | | | | | | | | |
| Cyclophosphamide | + | | | + | | | | | | |
| Dacarbazine | | | | | | | | | | |
| Hydroxyurea | | + | + | | + | | | | | |
| Asparaginase | + | | + | | | | | | | |
| PALA | + | + | + | | + | | + | | | |
| Procarbazine | + | + | + | | + | + | + | + | | + |
| Prednisone | + | + | + | | + | + | + | + | | |
| Interferon | + | + | + | | | | | | | |

at the time of receiving the drug and the likelihood of ovarian dysfunction; older women have a greater incidence of ovarian failure and less drug is needed to produce it. Pregnancy outcomes of patients after treatment with cytotoxic chemotherapy have been inadequately studied, but the children appear normal (Erenson et al., 1984). Women frequently experience cessation of menstruation during chemotherapy, with premature menopausal symptoms caused by the abrupt reduction in normal hormonal levels.

It is important for men who hope to have children that they be informed about sperm banking and be informed about how to proceed with it prior to treatment. The banking of sperm appears to be psychologically important, although most men never make use of it. Banked sperm are often considered of poor quality by reproductive physiologists because of oligospermia. Viability of frozen human sperm is not fully known. Storage of fertilized ova in vitro for later attempts at implantation in a woman have been contemplated, but not yet reported.

There have been efforts to identify means by which ova and sperm might be spared by giving hormones to inhibit production during the time of the chemotherapy, but results have not been impressive. Treatment regimens for Hodgkin's disease that will be less toxic to germ cells are under study. In one trial, patients who received three or fewer cycles of MOPP (mechlorethamine–vincristine–procarbazine–prednisone) without pelvic irradiation experienced less treatment-induced azoospermia (da Cunha et al., 1984). The regime of ABVD (adriamycin, bleomycin, velban, and DTIC) appears to offer equal survival, (Canellos, 1988). Early CALGB data suggests less impact on fertility, from the same study.

All patients who agree to treatment with chemotherapy should be advised of possible changes in libido, sexual function, and fertility, based on data available. There have been a number of studies that indicate that women are not well prepared for the premature menopause and the loss of libido and sexual arousal associated with some chemotherapy regimens (see Chapter 33). Initial studies indicated a high rate of marital distress, discord, and even divorce in women who could not understand changes in their psychological state and their disinterest in sexual activity. Hormonal replacement is highly desirable with cyclic estrogen and progesterone, but the effect that sex hormones might have on some residual tumors is a concern. Oncologists have become more aware of the importance of accurate preparation, and women appear to be better informed about sexual changes than they were in the past. Clearly, psychological distress is considerably reduced when women anticipate the problems and are prepared when they occur. Loss of male libido during chemo-

therapy is rarely attributed to decreased testosterone levels. It can also be helpful for young couples to prepare for male infertility by sperm banking, or for infertility of either sex by planning for adoption.

In the study of survivors, it has been found that sexual issues continue to be a source of distress (see Chapter 7). Fobair and colleagues (1986) identified high divorce rates (32%), problems with fertility (18%), and less interest in sexual activity (20%) in a cross-sectional study of 403 Hodgkin's patients interviewed a median of 9 years after completion of treatment. The CALGB psychiatry committee has studied 186 Hodgkin's disease survivors a mean of 6 years after completion of treatment, including some individuals who were among the first cured by chemotherapy. Using a telephone interview and self-report measures, sexual difficulties of some type were reported by 47% (J. C. Holland, unpublished data). Decreased activity and interest in sex, and erectile problems in men were the most frequent complaints, present in about 20% of the cohort. Sexual functioning and satisfaction with sex were examined in 126 young men who had been treated for leukemia, lymphoma, or testicular cancer (Lesko et al., 1988c). Those men who were married and at high risk for infertility had greater distress, possibly because infertility was a greater issue to the young married man than to his single counterpart.

Companion studies of the gonadal effects of chemotherapy on boys and girls suggest that ovarian and testicular damage also occurs in children treated before puberty; there is no physiological protection associated with prepubertal status (Matus-Ridley et al., 1985; Nicosia et al., 1985). A review of the gonadal dysfunction resulting from chemotherapy by Schilsky and colleagues (1980) provides a description of the pathophysiological changes in children and adults associated with dysfunction. Cella and colleagues (personal communication), in unpublished studies of children cured of Hodgkin's disease, suggested that there is a great need for children to be counseled about their fertility, or infertility, as they reach sexually active ages. Discussion at that time about the adolescent's fertility status appears to be infrequently carried out by parents or physicians when the treatment was completed years before. Embarrassment of the teenager, and of the parent and doctor, about a delicate subject may make appropriate discussion difficult to initiate.

## Psychological Problems on Completion of Chemotherapy

Completion of chemotherapy often creates the unexpected psychological problem of paradoxical anxiety. Although one would anticipate that receiving the last cycle of chemotherapy after 6 months or a year of repeated treatment would be greeted with celebration; many patients are instead frightened to stop. They felt secure that the treatment was keeping the cancer cells growth in control; stopping treatment might allow their regrowth and relapse of disease. Even those who were barely able to conclude a scheduled regimen, or who stopped prematurely because of the severity of side effects, may suffer the same paradoxical anxiety. Furthermore, the frequent physical examinations and laboratory tests that monitored chemotherapy effects (and possible early recurrence) become less frequent. For these reasons, the patient should be prepared well in advance of the time when chemotherapy will be finished. There should be a discussion about the rationale for the length of time of the treatment and the decision to stop. The oncologist should point out that anxiety is normally greater for several weeks to months after the treatment has been discontinued. This special need for reassurance was noted by Meyerowitz and colleagues (1983) in 37% of women as long as 2 years after the completion of adjuvant chemotherapy for breast cancer.

The completion of chemotherapy also implies, though often incorrectly, that one has moved from ill to healthy status. Psychologically, this is not a sharp transition, but a continuum of responses from those of an ill person to those of the physically healthy. This transition or reentry phase, often requires weeks to months to achieve. The patient's concerns, dependent on the disease and stage, may shift from, "Will the treatment work?" to "When will the treatment benefit end?" The extension of "Will it go away?" is "When will it come back?" In addition, as patients move from illness to healthy, their families are making the same transition in perception of the previously ill member. A family is apt to be overprotective and may try to maintain the ill status at the same time that he or she is eager to be viewed as a former patient who is now healthy.

There are also reentry problems at work with concerns about being treated like someone who has "had cancer and who is going to die." Significant problems extend to employer and life insurance brokers, who continue to view the cancer survivor, even years later, as a poor risk. This leads to extreme difficulties in changing jobs (see Chapter 7 on survivors).

## Survivors

The increasingly large cohort of young survivors cured by chemotherapy and multimodality treatment is giving clinicians and researchers a clearer picture of the delayed effects of chemotherapy. The medical sequelae or delayed effects were noted first among chil-

dren and later in the young adult survivors. Second malignancies (solid tumors, leukemia, and lymphoma) and organ failure (particularly renal, cardiac, and pulmonary) were well documented early on (Li et al., 1975); subsequent reviews have described the delayed effects by organ system (Byrd, 1985). Longer follow-up of specific cancers for late toxicity is providing better answers about the effects of chemotherapy alone and in combination with irradiation, where the oncogenic potential is enhanced. For example, 15-year observations of Hodgkin's disease survivors from the Stanford cohort by Tucker and colleagues (1988) found that the cumulative risk for leukemia plateaus at 10 years, but the risk for development of solid tumors continues to rise.

Investigators are beginning to understand the long-term psychological and social morbidity of chemotherapy as well. (See Chapter 7 for a detailed discussion of survivors' psychological sequelae.) An important and repeated observation is that most survivors function well. However, whereas there are no gross psychological changes in survivors that would indicate severe psychiatric disorders, there is a subtle level of emotional distress that indicates a sense of vulnerability and uncertainty about the future, referred to as the Damocles syndrome. Individuals who show severe psychiatric disorders, such as major depression or suicidal behavior, usually have had antedating psychological problems. In terms of treatment-related symptoms that persist, specific cues, such as smells, sights, and sounds, continue to remind the individual of the chemotherapy treatment, producing transient anxiety and nausea longer than a decade later (Cella and Tross, 1986) (see Chapter 7).

## Education and Emotional Support

It is most important psychologically for patients to be given adequate information at each step of chemotherapy; including information about treatment side effects, being sure the patient understands all aspects of the informed consent, and providing psychological preparation and support in anticipation of treatment. The informed patient has less anxiety about "surprises." The nurse's attention to the discomforts of stomatitis, nausea and vomiting, and hair loss indicate concern for the patient as a person. The staff provides a sense that they (the oncology team) recognize the difficulties and are genuinely trying to reduce the associated discomforts that must be tolerated to get the benefits of the treatment. It is important for the receptionist, or anyone the patient meets in the course of repeated visits, to recognize that the patient needs to see a cheery countenance. A warm welcome coupled with a compassionate concern helps the frightened and uncomfortable patient tolerate the treatment (see Chapter 51).

It is important that secondary support services be made available to patients undergoing treatment, such as transportation and assistance in getting to appointments. This is the purview of family members, the social worker and service agencies; it should ideally not be a burden carried by the patient alone. It is easy to underestimate the confusion that results from keeping appointment dates, taking medications at home regularly, and managing multiple bills and insurance forms. The oncological team that assists with these aspects of treatment reducing strain on the patient, gains the best results. The positive transference of patient and family resulting from good service delivered well results in greater satisfaction, better compliance with treatment, less likelihood of inappropriate litigation.

It is important that the relationship to the oncology staff be one of trust and one in which there is a free and easy exchange of information. Patients should feel comfortable to ask questions about the treatments and potential problems; they should have no sense of fear in asking questions that might "offend the doctor." It is particularly important that they feel free to bring up issues about sexual dysfunction. The physician and nurse can do much by attitude and demeanor to encourage easy exchange. Questions about concurrent alternative therapies should be answered honestly. This subject is discussed further in Chapter 42.

Psychological support given within the context of a chemotherapy treatment is often provided by the nurse or social worker. However, some patients need referral for psychiatric consultation, psychotherapy, or pharmacological management of distress. These patients with severe distress often have had a preexisting psychiatric disorder or depression that is exacerbated by the stress of chemotherapy; they may require simply a crisis intervention model of psychotherapy and will do well once they have gotten comfortable with the treatment routine. Others require more extended support and treatment. The psychiatrist may choose to use other interventions—such as psychopharmacological agents (antidepressant or antianxiety medication), relaxation, hypnosis, and visual imagery—to reduce anxiety associated with the chemotherapy (and to reduce the anticipatory responses of nausea and vomiting before the treatment). Often, posttreatment distress and discomfort can be reduced by the use of these techniques. It is clear that combinations of psychotherapeutic, psychopharmacological, and behavioral interventions can be quite effective in reducing distressing side effects, thereby improving patient compliance with the full treatment protocol.

## ENDOCRINE THERAPY: PSYCHOLOGICAL ASPECTS

Historically, hormonal manipulations were observed to retard tumor growth, especially in prostate and breast cancer, before anticancer agents were found (Kennedy, 1982). It has long been recognized that administration of exogenous hormones, or removal of endogenous hormones, significantly alters tumor growth in carcinoma of the prostrate, breast, and endometrium. Adrenal corticosteroids also have a suppressive effect on lymphomas and leukemias, where they are important components of combination chemotherapy. The identification of an estrogen receptor, with methods to measure it clinically, is an example of the major advances made in relating tumor biology to potential hormonal therapy on a more rational basis. The development of hormonal antagonists that block physiological effects of the endogenous hormone has been important. Chapter 31 reviews the range of neuropsychiatric disorders that result from endocrine-related tumors and the side effects of corticosteriods.

Some of the sequelae of alterations in the sex hormones by castration, or by administration of pharmacological agents or of hormones of the opposite sex, produce significant psychological effects. In the early 1940s, both androgen deprivation by castration and estrogen administration were shown to be effective in management of carcinoma of the prostate. These two treatments have remained the mainstay of the treatment of metastatic prostate cancer. Bilateral orchiectomy results in prompt decline in serum testosterone level and is followed by impotence in nearly 100% after a few months. A smaller percentage experience hot flashes. Indirect suppression of testicular androgen production is accomplished by administration of estrogen, usually diethylstilbestrol (DES) or, more recently, by gonodotropin-releasing hormone (GnRH) agonists (Grayhack et al., 1987). All these measures that prevent testosterone synthesis result in some degree of objective tumor regression and subjective response. Relief of pain, increased ability to ambulate, and improvements in abnormal urinary function in about two in three cases, produce a considerable improvement in quality of life, which may last for years. After clinical failure and escape from testicular androgen control, aminoglutethimide suppression of adrenal androgen production, while the original treatment is continued, may induce a second remission.

Schover (1987) pointed out, however, that all treatments of prostate cancer—radical prostatectomy, radiotherapy, and conservative prostate surgery with hormonal therapy—result in varying degrees of sexual dysfunction. Hormonal treatment, by reducing testosterone, causes loss of the desire for sex, difficulty in achieving a full erection, a need for prolonged stimulation to reach orgasm, reduced semen volume, and a decrease in the intensity of pleasure produced during penile stimulation and orgasm. During estrogen administration, breast engorgement and changes in body fat, skin texture, and hair distribution result in fear of "becoming a woman." Depression is common and its treatment may be essential. Psychological distress was noted to be greater in those men treated by estrogen therapy than by other forms of castration (Bergman et al., 1984). The newer GnRH agonists cause no feminizing side effects and, aside from the expense and the bother of daily injections, may be preferred because of the absence of anatomical distortion and of feminization. A repository GnRH agonist is undergoing trial that requires only a monthly injection. Testicular prostheses are desired by many men; urologists, who generally endorse the surety of castration because it requires no concerns of compliance with medication, can insert artificial spheroids or create a mass out of the transected spermatic cord.

Endocrine therapy is the oldest systemic treatment of breast cancer, first evidenced by tumor regression following oophorectomy. Patients can be far more carefully selected today because of the ability to measure hormonal receptors and to predict the biological responsiveness of tumors. Most extensive use of hormonal therapy in the past has been in advanced stages of breast cancer. However, tamoxifen is being introduced at increasingly earlier stages of breast cancer treatment, including node negative women. Most of the forms of hormonal treatment used in metastatic breast cancer are about equally effective, resulting in response rates among unselected patients of about 21–36%: tamoxifen (an antiestrogen drug), oophorectomy, progestins, aminoglutethimide, estrogens, androgens, andrenalectomy, and hypophysectomy (Henderson, 1987). There are differences in response based on estrogen receptor status and on menopausal status. Those who are $ERP^+$ (positive for estrogen receptor protein) and $PRP^+$ (positive for progesterone) respond in progressively increasing percentage, so that high receptor values indicate 75–90% responsiveness. Megestrol acetate, a progestin, is also used in metastatic disease as an older agent that has been reintroduced for palliation. Partial responses to hormone therapies are often attained, but the median duration of each response is in the range of 12–18 months, rarely extending over years. Sequential use of hormonal therapies to inhibit ovarian, adrenal and pituitary hormonal contributions in metastatic disease can result in cumulative gains of as long as 10 years. The roles of estrogen deprivation, progestin administration, and androgen administration are not identical, but contribute as well to increased length of survival.

The psychological consequences of the masculinizing side effects of hoarseness, hirsutism, acne, and augmented sexual drive variably caused by androgens are difficult to accept for most women. Weight gain, with its changes in body image, may add to the problems. Unpleasant estrogen side effects include edema, breast engorgement, genital itching, and uterine bleeding. Because of these, tamoxifen, despite its greater cost, has largely replaced the equiactive DES. Tamoxifen may cause transient mild hot flashes, nausea at the outset, and decrease of vaginal secretions, but overall, it has very low toxicity and can be tolerated for long periods. Psychological preparation should be made before initiating the treatment for the changes that may occur. Support from the oncologist and the health care team is essential. Signs of depression or poor coping should be reasons to refer for counseling early, not late, after their appearance.

## IMMUNOTHERAPY

Another approach to cancer therapy involves attempts to enhance the host's immune response to the tumor. In 1943 Ludwig Gross showed such resistance in mice that had been immunized by intradermal inoculation of tumor cells to the transplant of a chemically induced murine sarcoma. The area of modern tumor immunology, however, did not develop until the late 1950s (Oettgen and Hellstrom, 1974). Evidence for immunosurveillance as a likely factor in tumor initiation and growth was derived from animal models. Examples were recognized in humans by the appearance of certain neoplasms in immunosuppressed individuals. In addition, evidence for cancer-associated antigens, even if not proven to be exclusively limited to them, added evidence to the possibility that immunotherapy might be applied therapeutically in human cancer. These tantalizing insights led to a major effort to develop for clinical trial the biological-response modifiers (BRM) and cytokines, particularly interferons, interleukins 1, 2, 3, 4, tumor necrosis factor (TNF), and growth factors (see Table 10-5). These substances represent an exciting departure from cytotoxic chemotherapy by utilizing biologically derived substances that appear to have therapeutically active anticancer effect when given in pharmacological doses. The BRM constitute a complex family of hormonelike cellular proteins (Kirkwood and Ernstoff, 1984).

The most extensive experience has been with $\alpha$-interferon (IFN-$\alpha$), which has demonstrated activity effective in the treatment of hairy-cell leukemia, chronic myelocytic leukemia, lymphomas, and Kaposi's sarcoma. IFN-$\alpha$ has shown limited clinical activity in myeloma, melanoma, and ovarian and renal cell carcinoma (Table 10-6) (Fauci et al., 1987).

**Table 10-5**  Cytokines and their functions

| Name | Function |
|---|---|
| Interleukin 1 (IL-1) | Product of monocytes and macrophages (and possibly others); activates lymphocytes |
| Interleukin 2 (IL-2); T-cell growth factor | Product of lymphocytes and lymphoid cell lines; stimulates growth and proliferation of cytotoxic T-lymphocytes after activation with mitogens or antigens; co-stimulates β-cell differentiation |
| Interleukin 3 (IL-3); mast cell growth factor | Product of T lymphocytes; stimulates most cell growth; multipotential hemopoietic cell growth factor |
| Interleukin 4 (IL-4); β-cell stimulatory factor | β-cell stimulation factor; stimulates T-cell growth |
| Interleukin 5 (IL-5); T-cell replacing β-cell growth factor; factor V; eosinophil differentiation factor; IgA-enhancing factor | Stimulates in vitro antibody responses; costimulates β-cell growth; enhances IgA production; enhances eosinophil differentiation |
| Granulocyt–macrophage colony-stimulating factor (GM-CSF) | Colony-stimulating factor for granulocytes and macrophages; induces outgrowth of granulocyte and macrophage colonies from bone marrow; distinct from IL-3 and CSF-1 |
| Granulocyte colony-stimulating factor (G-CSF) | |
| β-cell growth factor (β-CGF) | |
| β-cell differentiation factor (β-CDF) | |
| α,β,γ-Interferon (IFN-α, -β, -γ) | Product of stimulated lymphocytes; inhibits viral replication; activates human macrophages; inhibits all activities of IL-4 on β cells |
| Tumor necrosis factor (TNF); cachectin | Product of activated macrophages; inhibits lipoprotein lipase and causes cachexia |

*Source*: Adapted from J.P. Dutcher, N. Clobanu, E. Paletta, S. Marcus, J. Strausman, and P.H. Wiernik (1987). The clinical importance of Interleukin-2; 1987. *Einstein Q. J. Biol. Med.* 5:1–9.

The side effects of the interferons have been widely studied. They produce flulike symptoms, and the severity of side effects is related to dose (Clark and Longo, 1987) (Table 10-7). From 1 to 9 million units (MU) are well tolerated, more than 19 MU produce moderate side effects, and severe effects diminish performance status in doses above 36 MU (Quesada et al., 1986). In the higher dosage range, patients experience fatigue, aches, pains, headaches, a marked reduction in concentration, and depression so severe that at times suicidal ideation occurs. Confusion, somnolence, diffuse encephalopathy expressive aphasia, and psychotic episodes with hallucinations have also been described at doses of 100 MU (Quesada et al., 1986; Clark and Longo, 1987). Similar to other IFN side effects, CNS toxicity (with EEG changes) is reversible and resolves within a few days to weeks after discontinuation. A study of IFN in hepatitis B carriers in whom social class variables were controlled, conducted by McDonald and colleagues (1987) using the General Health Questionnaire (GHQ), found that IFN did increase psychiatric morbidity. Nonpsychotic symptoms of fatigue, poor concentration, anxiety, and depression were prominent. Preexisting psychiatric problems, such as phobias or obsessions, were accentuated in intensity during the treatment. Those patients who were HIV positive appeared to experience greater increase in psychiatric morbidity, although small numbers prevented a test of significance. This raises some interesting questions about the causes of psychiatric morbidity in the presence of HIV.

Interleukin 2 (IL-2) is a cytokine that can stimulate and maintain the proliferation of T cells in tissue culture. IL-2, produced by lymphocytes, can potentiate a range of intercellular activities. The antitumor activity of an IL-2 infusion appears to be mediated by lymphokine-activated killer lymphocytes (LAK cells), which are formed in vivo as well as outside the body. This combination of IL-1 and LAK cells appears to act as a mediator of tumor regression (Dutcher et al.,

**Table 10-6**  Antitumor effects of α-interferon

| Level of clinical activity | Disease |
|---|---|
| Significant (>30% response rate) | Hairy-cell leukemia<br>Chronic myelocytic leukemia<br>Non-Hodgkin's lymphoma (low grade)<br>Cutaneous T-cell lymphoma<br>Essential thrombocythemia<br>Kaposi's sarcoma (AIDS-related)<br>Carcinoid tumor<br>Bladder tumors (local therapy for superficial tumors) |
| Limited (10–30% response rate) | Multiple myeloma<br>Chronic lymphocytic leukemia<br>Melanoma<br>Renal cell carcinoma<br>Ovarian carcinoma |
| None (<10% response rate) | Breast cancer<br>Colonic cancer<br>Lung cancer |

*Source*: Reprinted with permission from A.S. Fauci, S.A. Rosenberg, S.A. Sherwin, C.A. Ginarello, D.L. Longo, and H.C. Lane (1987). Immunomodulators in clincial medicine. *Ann. Intern. Med.* 106:421–33.

**Table 10-7**  Side effects of interferons

| Frequency | Symptoms |
|---|---|
| Frequent | Fever and/or chills |
| | Myalgias |
| | Fatigue and/or weakness |
| | Anorexia and/or weight loss |
| | Lethargy and/or decreased ability to concentrate |
| Less common | Gastrointestinal |
| |   Nausea |
| |   Vomiting |
| |   Altered taste |
| |   Diarrhea |
| | Cardiovascular |
| |   Hypotension |
| |   Hypertension |
| |   Atrial and ventricular arrhythmias |
| |   Myocardial infarction |
| | Neurological |
| |   Headaches |
| |   Mood alterations (especially depression or irritability) |
| |   Dizziness |
| |   Lightheadedness |
| |   Peripheral neuropathy |
| |   Seizures (uncommon) |
| | Mucocutaneous |
| |   Local inflammation |
| |   Urticaria |
| |   Stomatitis |
| |   Reactivation of oral herpes simplex |
| |   Exacerbation of psoriasis |
| |   Enhanced radiation toxicity |
| |   Mild alopecia |
| |   Increased eyelash growth |

*Source*: Reprinted with permission from J.W. Clark and D.L. Longo (1987). Interferons in cancer therapy. In V.T. DeVita, Jr., S. Hellman, and S.A. Rosenberg (eds.), *Updates, Cancer: Principles and Practice of Oncology*, 2nd ed. Philadelphia: Lippincott, pp. 1–15.

1987). The treatment with IL-2 plus LAK cells, called adoptive immunotherapy, is carried out by obtaining lymphocytes by leukophoresis from the cancer patient. The cells are incubated in IL-2, and reinfused into the patient, who also receives IL-2 (Rosenberg et al., 1987). IL-2 may also be given alone.

Because side effects are severe, treatment is often given in a specialized or intensive care unit. Side effects are hypotension, fever, weight gain from fluid retention, and toxic effects on kidney, liver, skin, mucous membranes, and CNS. Delirium is common because of the encephalopathy produced, and may be the reason to interrupt treatment. Mental changes are transient and reversible but can be severe, with mood changes, disorientation, hallucinations, and delusions (Denicoff et al., 1987).

The effect of BRM on brain function represents a challenging area for study. Such studies may have application for better understanding of the origin of common mental changes accompanying flulike conditions. BRM are exciting, but they still represent a small area of chemotherapy that remains largely investigational.

## SUMMARY

Education, supportive care, psychotherapy, and the judicious use of psychopharmacological and behavioral interventions are important for the patient receiving cancer chemotherapy. These interventions are given by the physician and by the nurse and staff in the office or clinic, who monitor continuously the patient's emotional state and also show concern for the problems the patient is encountering. With full support from the staff, and added support from veteran patients and family members, it can be expected that patients will get through their chemotherapeutic regimens with a remarkable degree of equanimity. It is important that patients and families be told that the side effects *are* tolerable, that a single person rarely experiences *all* the side effects, that the treatment *benefits* often far outweigh the inconveniences and *risks,* and finally, that cooperation and commitment to complete the full treatment are important to achieve the best therapeutic results. Palliative chemotherapy must more carefully take into account quality-of-life issues. Because with palliation cure is not a goal, weighing the benefits in terms of the quality of survival against the discomfort that is likely to accompany a particular treatment is essential. Endocrine therapy remains a cornerstone of the management of advanced breast and prostate cancer, and is used, particularly as with corticosteroids, in many combinations for other diseases. Psychological sequelae can occur with all forms of hormonal manipulation. Immunotherapy, through introduction of the biological response modifiers, has opened a new field of cancer therapy. The neurotoxic effects of interferon treatment and interleukin 2 plus lymphocyte-activated killer cell (IL-2 plus LAK) treatments vary from the mild mood changes of depression and fatigue to severe and treatment-limiting confusion and depression. The neuropsychiatric side effects deserve careful study and attention to their management in patients receiving these agents.

## ACKNOWLEDGMENTS

The authors wish to express their thanks for the critique of this chapter by James F. Holland, M.D., medical oncologist.

# REFERENCES

Aaron, N.K. and J. Beckman (1987). *The Quality of Life of Cancer Patients*. New York: Raven Press.

Barofsky, I. and P.H. Sugarbaker (1979). Determinants of patients' nonparticipation in randomized clinical trials for the treatment of sarcomas. *Cancer Clin. Trials* 2:237–46.

Bergman, B., J-E. Damber, B. Littbrand, K. Sjogren, and R. Tomic (1984). Sexual function in prostatic cancer patients treated with radiotherapy, orchiectoomy or oestrogens. *Br. J. Urol.* 56:64–69.

Bloch, R. and A. Bloch (1985). *Fighting Cancer*. Kansas City: The Cancer Connection.

Bonadonna, G. and P. Valagussa (1981). Dose–response effect of adjuvant chemotherapy in breast cancer. *N. Engl. J. Med.* 304:10–46.

Bruning, N. (1985). *Coping with Chemotherapy*. New York: Dial Press/Doubleday.

Byrd, R. (1985). Late effects of treatment of cancer in children. *Pediatr. Clin. North Am.* 32:835–49.

Cancer chemotherapy (Editorial). (1987). *Med. Lett. Drugs Ther.* 29(March 27):29–36.

Canellos, G.P., K. Propert, R. Cooper, N. Nissen, J. Anderson, K.H. Antman, B. Santa Mauro, and A.J. Gottlieb (1988). MOPP vs. ABVD vs. MOPP Alternating with ABVD in Advanced Hodgkins Disease: A Prospective Randomized CALGB Trial. *Proc. Amer. Soc. Clin. Oncol.* 7:230, 888.

Casciato, D.A. and B.B. Lowitz (1983). *Manual of Bedside Oncology*. Boston, Little, Brown & Co., p. 20.

Cella, D.F., B. Orofiamma, J.C. Holland, P. Silberfarb, S. Tross, M. Feldstein, L.H. Maurer, R. Comis, M. Perry, and M. Green (1986). Relationship of psychological distress, extent of disease and performance status in patients with lung cancer. *Cancer* 60:1661–67.

Cella, D.F. and S. Tross (1986). Psychological adjustment to survival from Hodgkin's disease. *J. Consult. Clin. Psychol.* 54:618–22.

Chabner, B.A. (1986). The oncologic end game. *J. Clin. Oncol.* 4:626–38.

Clark, J.W. and D.L. Longo (1987). Interferons in cancer therapy. In V.T. De Vita, Jr., S. Hellman, and S.A. Rosenberg (eds.), *Updates, Cancer: Principles and Practice of Oncology*, 2nd ed. Philadelphia: Lippincott, pp. 1–15.

Coates, A., V. Gebski, J.F. Bishop, P.N. Jeal, R.L. Woods, R. Snyder, M.H.N. Tattersall, M. Byrne, V. Harvey, G. Gill, J. Simpson, J.F. Forbes, (1987). For the Australian–New Zealand Breast Cancer Trials Group. *N. Engl. J. Med.* 317:1490–95.

Cohan, L.M. (1985). Principles of radiotherapy and chemotherapy. In D.A. Casciato and B.B. Lowitz (eds.), *Manual of Bedside Oncology*. Boston: Little, Brown & Co., pp. 9–29.

da Cunha, M.F., M.L. Meistrich, L.M. Fuller, J.H. Cundiff, F.B. Hagemeister, W.S. Velasquez, P. McLaughlin, S.A. Riggs, F.F. Cabanillas, and P.G. Salvador (1984). Recovery of spermatogenesis after treatment for Hodgkin's disease: Limiting dose of MOPP chemotherapy. *J. Clin. Oncol.* 2:571–77.

Denicoff, K.O., D.R. Rubinow, M.Z. Papa, C. Simpson, C.A. Seipp, M.T. Lotze, A.E. Chang, D. Rosenstein, and S.A. Rosenberg (1987). The neuropsychiatric effects of treatment with interleukin-2 and lymphokine-activated killer cells. *Ann. Intern. Med.* 107:293–300.

DeVita, V.T. (1985). Principles of chemotherapy. In V.T. DeVita, Jr., S. Hellman, and S.A. Rosenberg (eds.), *Cancer: Principles and Practice of Oncology*, Philadelphia: Lippincott, pp. 257–85.

Dutcher, J.P., N. Coblanu, E. Paletta, S. Marcus, J. Strausman, and P.H. Wiernik (1987). The clinical importance of Interleukin-2. *Einstein Q. J. Biol. Med.* 5:1–9.

Erenson, D., Z. Arlin, S. Welt, M. Claps, and M. Melamed (1984). Male reproductive capacity may recover following drug treatment with the L-10 protocol for acute lymphocytic leukemia. *Cancer* 53:30–36.

Fauci, A.S., S.A. Rosenberg, S.A. Sherwin, C.A. Dinarello, D.L. Longo, and H.C. Lane (1987). Immunomodulators in clinical medicine. *Ann. Inter. Med.* 106:421–33.

Fobair, P., R.T. Hoppe, J. Bloom, R. Cox, A. Varghese, and D. Spiegel (1986). Psychosocial problems among survivors of Hodgkin's disease. *J. Clin. Oncol.* 4:805–14.

Grayhack, J.T., T.C. Keeler, and J.M. Kozlowski (1987). Carcinoma of the prostate. *Horm. Ther.* 60:589–601.

Hahn, D., S.C. Schempff, C.L. Fortner, A.C. Smith, V.M. Young, and P.H. Wiernick (1978). Infection in acute leukemia patients receiving oral nonabsorbable antibiotics. *Antimicrob. Agents Chemother.* 13:958–64.

Henderson, I.C. (1987). Endocrine therapy in metastatic breast cancer. In J.R. Harris, S. Hellman, I.C. Henderson, and D.W. Kinne (eds.), *Breast Diseases*. Philadelphia: Lippincott, pp. 398–428.

Holland, J.C., A.H. Korzun, S. Tross, P. Silberfarb, M. Perry, R. Comis, and M. Oster (1986a). Comparative psychological disturbance in patients with pancreatic and gastric cancer. *Am. J. Psychiatry* 143:982–86.

Holland, J.C., P. Silberfarb, S. Tross, and D.F. Cella (1986b). Psychosocial research in cancer: The Cancer and Leukemia Group B (CALGB) experience. In V. Ventafridda, F. van Dam, R. Yancik, and M. Tamburini (eds.), *Assessment of Quality of Life and Cancer Treatment: Proc. Int. Workshop on Quality of Life Assessment and Cancer Treatment*, Milan, December 11–13, 1985. New York: Elsevier, pp. 89–101.

Itri, L.M. (1983). The effects of chemotherapy on gonadal function. *Your Patient and Cancer* 3(3):45–49.

Kennedy, B.J. (1982). Principles of endocrine therapy. In J.F. Holland and E. Frei (eds.), *Cancer, Medicine,* 2nd ed. Philadelphia: Lea & Febiger, pp. 945–1027.

Kirkwood, J.M. and M.S. Ernstoff (1984). Interferons in the treatment of human cancer. *J. Clin. Oncol.* 2:336–52.

Kirkwood, J.M. and M.S. Ernstoff (1984). Interferons in the treatment of human cancer. *J. Clin. Oncol.* 2:336–52.

Knobf, T. (1986). Physical and psychologic distress associated with adjuvant chemotherapy in women with breast cancer. *J. Clin. Oncol.* 4:678–84.

Krakoff, I.H. (1981). *Cancer Chemotherapeutic Agents*. New York: American Cancer Society Education Publications.

Lesko, L.M., H. Dermatis, D. Penman, and J.C. Holland (1988a). Patients', parents', and oncologists' perception of informed consent for bone marrow transplantation (Submitted for publication).

Lesko, L.M., M.J. Massie, and J.C. Holland (1988b). Oncology. In A. Stoudemire and B. Fogel (eds.), *Medical Psychiatry*. Orlando, Fla.: Grune & Stratton.

Lesko, L.M., G. Mumma, and D. Mashberg (1988c). Psychological and psychosexual functioning of acute leukemia survivors treated with bone marrow transplantation and/or conventional chemotherapy. (Submitted for publication).

Lewis, C., M.S. Linet, and M.D. Abeloff (1983). Compliance and cancer therapy by patients and physicians. *Am. J. Med.* 74:673–78.

Li, F.P., J.R. Cassady, and N. Jaffe (1975). Risk of second tumors in survivors of childhood cancer. *Cancer* 35:1230–35.

MacVicar, M.G. and M.L. Winningham (1986). Promoting the functional capacity of cancer patients. *Cancer Bull.* (University of Texas M.D. Anderson Hospital and Tumor Institute, Houston) 38:235–39.

McDonald, E.M., A.H. Mann, and H.C. Thomas (1987). Interferons as mediators of psychiatric morbidity: An investigation in the trial of recombinant α interferon in hepatitis-B carriers. *Lancet* 11:1175–78.

Matus-Ridley, M., S.V. Nicosia, and A.T. Meadows (1985). Gonadal effects of cancer therapy on boys. *Cancer* 55:2353–63.

Meyerowitz, V.W., I.K. Watkins, and F.C. Sparks (1983). Psychosocial implications of adjuvant chemotherapy: A two-year follow-up. *Cancer* 52:1541–45.

Nerenz, D.R., H. Leventhal, and R.R. Love (1982). Factors contributing to emotional distress during cancer chemotherapy. *Cancer* 50:1020–27.

Nicosia, S.V., M. Matus-Ridley, and A.T. Meadows (1985). Gonadal effects of cancer therapy on girls. *Cancer* 55:2364–72.

Oettgen, H.F. and K.E. Hellstrom (1974). Tumor immunology. In J. F. Holland and E. Frei (eds.), *Cancer Medicine*. Philadelphia: Lea & Febiger, pp. 951–90.

Penman, D., J.C. Holland, G. Bahna, G. Morrow, A. Schmale, L. Derogatis, C.L. Carnrike, Jr., and R. Cherry (1984). Informed consent for investigational chemotherapy: Patients' and physicians' perceptions. *J. Clin. Oncol.* 2:849–55.

Quesada, J.R., M. Talpaz, A. Rios, R. Kurzrock, and J.U. Gutterman (1986). Clinical toxicity of interferons in cancer patient: A review. *J. Clin. Oncol.* 4:234–43.

Rosenberg, S.A., M.T. Lotze, L.M. Muul, A.E. Chang, F.P. Avis, S. Leitman, W.M. Linehan, C.N. Robertson, R.E. Lee, J.T. Rubin, C.A. Seipp, C.G. Simpson, and D.E. White (1987). A progress report on the treatment of 157 patients with advanced cancer using lymphokine-activated killer cells and interleukin-2 or high-dose interleukin-2 alone. *N. Engl. J. Med.* 316:889–97.

Rowland, J.H., O.J. Glidewell, R.F. Sibley, J.C. Holland, R. Tull, A. Berman, M.L. Brecher, M. Harris, A.S. Glicksman, E. Forman, B. Jones, M.E. Cohen, P.K. Duffner, and A.I. Freeman (1984). Effects of different forms of central nervous system prophylaxis on neuropsychologic function in childhood leukemia. *J. Clin. Oncol.* 2:1327–35.

Schilsky, R.L., B.J. Lewis, R.J. Sherins, and R.C. Young (1980). Gonadal dysfunction in patients receiving chemotherapy. *Ann. Intern. Med.* 93 (Part 1):109–14.

Schipper, H., J. Clinch, A. McMurray, and M. Levitt (1984). Measuring the quality of life of cancer patients: The functional index—cancer: Development and validation. *J. Clin. Oncol.* 2:472–83.

Schover, L.R. (1987). Sexuality and fertility in urologic cancer patients. *Cancer* 60:553–58.

Siegel, M.L. (1986). *The Cancer Patient's Handbook*. New York: Walker & Co.

Silberfarb, P.M. (1983). Chemotherapy and cognitive defects in cancer patients. *Ann. Rev. Med.* 34:35–46.

Silberfarb, P.M. (1986). Ensuring an optimal quality of life for lung cancer patients: A psychiatrist's perspective. In V. Ventafridda, F. van Dam, R. Yancik, and M. Tamburini (eds.), *Assessment of Quality of Life and Cancer Treatment: Proc. Int. Workshop on Quality of Life Assessment and Cancer Treatment*, Milan, December 11–13, 1985. New York: Elsevier, pp. 145–50.

Silberfarb, P.M., J.C. Holland, D. Anbar, G. Bahna, H. Maurer, A. Chahinian, and R. Comis (1983). Psychological response of patients receiving two drug regimens for lung cancer. *Am. J. Psychiatry* 140:110–11.

Smith, S.D., D. Rosen, R.C. Triceworth, and J.T. Lowman (1979). A reliable method for evaluating drug compliance in children with cancer. *Cancer* 43:169–73.

Spitzer, W.O., A.J. Dobson, J. Hall, E. Chesterman, J. Levi, R. Shepherd, R. Battista, and R. Catchlove (1981). Measuring the quality of life in cancer patients: A concise QL index for physicians. *J. Chron. Dis.* 34:585–87.

Sutcliffe, S.B. (1979). Cytotoxic chemotherapy and gonadal function in patients with Hodgkin's disease: Facts and thoughts. *J.A.M.A.* 242:1898–99.

Taylor, S.E., R.R. Lichtman, J.V. Wood, A.Z. Bluming, G.M. Dosik, and R.L. Leibowitz (1985). Illness-related and treatment-related factors in psychological adjustment to breast cancer. *Cancer* 55:2506–13.

Tucker, M.A., C.N. Coleman, R.S. Cox, A. Varghese, and S.A. Rosenberg (1988). Risk of second cancers after treatment for Hodgkin's disease. *N. Engl. J. Med.* 318:76–81.

# 11

# Bone Marrow Transplantation

Lynna M. Lesko

The past 20 years have witnessed major advances in transplantation medicine for the treatment of many cancers and metabolic abnormalities. It is rapidly changing from a controversial research procedure to a standard therapeutic modality as a result of progress in the fields of supportive and intensive care, histocompatibility typing, and immunosuppressive drugs.

Bone marrow transplantation (BMT) has emerged as the treatment of choice for ''severe'' aplastic anemia, immunodeficiency disease, some congenital hematological disorders such as Fanconi's anemia, Wiskott–Aldrich syndrome, and radiation accidents. Over the past 10 years, it has been used with increasing success for acute leukemia and is now being tried for patients with chronic leukemia, lymphomas, tumors sensitive to radiation (breast, testicular cancer), and genetic disorders of bone marrow such as thalassemia and sickle cell anemia (Appelbaum et al., 1984; Begg et al., 1984; Champlain and Gale, 1984; Dinsmore et al., 1983, 1984; Gluckman et al., 1984; Kadota and Smithson, 1984; Speck et al., 1984; Storb, 1981; Storb et al., 1981, 1984; Thomas et al., 1984).

Much of the progress in developing BMT has occurred at what are now the six largest American centers for bone marrow transplantation medicine and research: Memorial Sloan-Kettering Cancer Center in New York City, UCLA Medical Center in Los Angeles, the Fred Hutchinson Cancer Research Center in Seattle, M. D. Anderson Cancer Center in Houston, Johns Hopkins University in Baltimore, and Children's Hospital in Boston.

The transplantation procedure comprises several stages each of which makes its own psychological demands of the patient; these will be described in the next section. First the patient's immunologically deficient or malignant bone marrow is destroyed by high-dose chemotherapy (cyclophosphamide), alone or in combination with total-body irradiation (TBI). This mar-

row is then replaced by an infusion of marrow from an immunologically compatible donor (an ''allogeneic transplant'' from a parent or sibling) or from the patient (an ''autologous transplant'') harvested prior to chemoradiation and then ''purged'' of malignant cells by additional chemotherapeutic agents. The allogeneic procedure requires an extensive medical evaluation with human lymphocyte antigen (HLA)-histocompatability testing. Both allogeneic and autologous transplants necessitate a 2- to 3-month hospitalization in a reverse-isolation room or laminar-air flow (sterile) unit.

Complications that may arise from immediate and delayed effects of the transplant include graft rejection, infection, graft-versus-host disease (GvHD, in those receiving marrow from a donor), neurological and psychological problems. Convalescence, both physical and psychological, requires at least 1 year and can be profoundly stressful for patients and family, especially when it entails return to school or work.

The mortality in severe cases of aplastic anemia treated with conventional therapy is 75–90%. Most patients die within 6–9 months of diagnosis; the usual cause of death is graft rejection. BMT has resulted in 50% survival of aplastic anemia patients, from 1 to 6 years, with complete hematological restoration (Bortin et al., 1981).

Although children with acute lymphoblastic leukemia have benefited from advances in conventional treatment over the past decade, unfortunately this has not been the case for adults with acute leukemia. Although 80% of adult patients achieve complete remissions after conventional chemotherapy, long-term remission is usually not possible with the currently available chemotherapy when relapse occurs. The median survival of adult leukemics treated with standard chemotherapy without relapse is 12–20 months, with 25% of patients alive at 5 years. As a result, BMT is

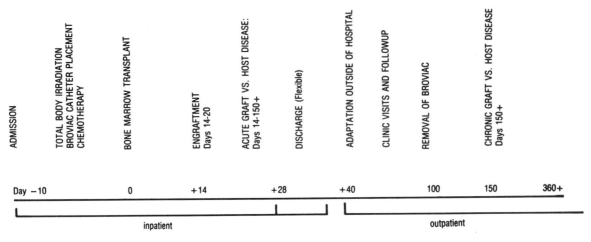

**Figure 11-1.** Bone marrow transplant schedule.

now increasingly used to cure this disease in adults. Current studies suggest that leukemics should be transplanted early, preferably during first remission, because patients receiving transplants in their second or third remission have a higher incidence of relapse. Approximately 60% of adults with acute leukemia who are treated this way survive without treatment from 1 to 5 years (Thomas et al., 1979a,b).

## PHYSICAL AND PSYCHOLOGICAL STATES OF BONE MARROW TRANSPLANTATION

The BMT procedure encompasses several stages of medical treatment, each with its own psychological effects (Brown and Kelly, 1976; Lesko and Hawkins, 1983). The medical stages are outlined in Fig. 11-1, while the corresponding psychological states are described in the following paragraphs.

The decision to accept the transplantation procedure is often made against a background of chronic illness and, at times, organ failure. Patients may have experienced months to years of feeling sick while relying on chemotherapy, medications, and transfusions for survival. During this time fear of death and uncertainty coupled with hope of possible cure pervade. The decision to have a transplant may be made many miles from the transplantation center and is often made quickly because of urgent medical complications, the physical status of the patient, and bed availability.

In contrast to leukemia or lymphoma patients, those with severe aplastic anemia often develop symptoms suddenly and are unacquainted with chronic illness and hospitalization. Whether or not the onset of cancer is rapid, the decision of patients and families to accept the recommendation for transplant is always preceded by the stresses associated with the batteries of physio-

logical tests and tissue typing of family members that determine if the transplantation is feasible.

The medical consultation usually takes place on an outpatient basis at the patient's own hospital and/or at the transplant center. Along with the physiological evaluations, some form of psychological assessment is often undertaken by a psychiatrist and/or psychologist and social worker to evaluate the patient's social supports and ability to cope with the procedure. This is a time when prospective patients, especially children, should be encouraged to visit the transplant unit and meet the staff who will care for them. Families should find housing, especially if they are a great distance from home, and learn what things may be brought from home to make the patient's hospital stay more pleasant. Ronald McDonald houses in several cities are invaluable aids to families, providing not only shelter but also a place where they can share experiences with other families in similar circumstances. Waiting and anticipation can be difficult; there is always the worry that relapse may occur before the treatment can be instituted due to lack of a transplant bed being available.

Hospitalization and preparation for the transplant require more tests and are accompanied by feelings of anxiety and hope. Patients enter the sterile germ-free or reverse-isolation room immediately to avoid infection. They then undergo a 10-day pretransplant conditioning regimen consisting of high-dosage immunosuppressive drugs and hyperfractionated TBI (given for several days in multiple sessions per day at levels lethal to bone marrow). A Broviac or Hickman catheter is put in place with a minor surgical procedure performed under local anesthesia. This is a central venous line that makes possible the drawing of blood samples and administration of blood products, medications, antibiotics, and total parenteral nutrition (TPN) without requiring frequent punctures of the patient's skin. These days are marked by episodes of nausea, vomiting, and fatigue secondary to the irradiation and chemotherapy. The patient's blood counts begin to fall as a result of the cytoreductive procedure. This is "the point of no return," because unlike kidney transplantation, there is no dialysis to fall back on.

The transplant is brief and anticlimactic compared to the lengthy pretransplant treatment and the convalescent period. It is usually uncomplicated and is paradoxically undramatic for patients, involving only an infusion of one or several packets of concentrated bone marrow. The donor, however, undergoes general anesthesia to permit harvest of his or her marrow by multiple aspirations over both iliac crests, similar to a bone marrow biopsy. Usually the donor is admitted to the hospital the night before and leaves the day after the procedure. Donors can return to a normal routine within a few days, experiencing only minor soreness and discomfort.

In the immediate convalescent period, the BMT recipient is concerned about marrow engraftment, transplant rejection, continuation of immunosuppressive drugs, the risk of infection, high fever, problems and side effects consequent to prolonged exposure to multiple antibiotics, and the specter of GvHD. This latter "turning of the transplant" against the recipient is poorly understood and causes great distress to the recipient, the donor, and staff when it occurs. Fortunately, researchers are virtually eliminating patients' risk of developing GvHD by employing newer techniques of T-cell depleted grafts. The requisite convalescent period in the hospital is usually 1–2 months, during which the patient must undergo weeks of hyperalimentation and antibiotic coverage. It is a trying time for the patient as well as for the families, who are usually asked to visit daily to provide important emotional support. Family disruption may be quite obvious at this time when the stresses of the ongoing—seemingly endless—procedure do not relent.

Preparation for discharge begins 1–2 months after transplantation, after the marrow is functioning adequately (WBC count >1000) and when the likelihood of infection is low. Patients have renewed hope of resuming their lives where they left off and show a heightened interest in the world outside the hospital. However, as they begin to learn the self-care procedures that will be necessary at home (Broviac or Hickman catheter care, and regimens of medication), the excitement over the anticipated discharge is mixed with fears of leaving the security of the isolation room and transplant unit. At this time patients commonly have difficulty with their appetite, particularly as they are being weaned from hyperalimentation. This transi-

tion period can also be complicated by side effects secondary to GvHD.

Convalescence and adaptation outside the hospital is protracted and can last almost 1 year. Transplantation does not guarantee total restoration of previous health status, and thus the transplant patient requires considerable support from staff throughout discharge and convalescence. Weekly visits to the transplant clinic occur for at least the first 2–4 months. With the passage of time, patients turn their concerns from "living as a patient" to "living as a survivor." They have profound fatigue and may show signs of difficulty or actual inability to "reenter" normal activities related to home and work. Young adults who have undergone BMT may in particular need help in managing their small, active children. Rehabilitation is as much a psychological process as a physiological process; the two must proceed simultaneously. Children, as compared to adults, resume normal life more rapidly.

## IMMEDIATE AND LONG-TERM EFFECTS OF THE BMT PROCEDURE

### Medical Complications

BMT demands a high level of commitment and extraordinary cooperation from patients. It is clear that having adequate information about illness and treatment reduces stress and improves most patients' ability to cope. Therefore, it is important to give an accurate explanation of the disease, a careful description of the BMT treatment, its desired effect, and information about side effects that must be tolerated to obtain the treatment's benefits. The transplant team, made up of the oncologist, the psychiatrist, the nurse, the social worker, and other professionals, must understand the psychological impact of not only the procedure itself, but also TBI, TPN (Broviac or Hickman catheterization), GvHD, and germ-free environments (Sullivan et al., 1984).

## TOTAL BODY IRRADIATION

Chemotherapy may be used alone or in combination with radiation and immunosuppressive drugs in the transplant protocol. Patients receive immunologically and hematopoietically lethal doses of TBI. TBI is given in the range of 800 to 1300 rads, usually divided into 12 hyperfractionated treatments over 3–4 days. The effects of this irradiation on the CNS may lead to transient or delayed neuropsychological sequelae. Gottschalk and his group (1969) have studied the impact of total and half-body irradiation on emotional and cognitive functions in a series of advanced-cancer patients. Transient impairment of intellectual function was found using a measure of verbal content analysis; no impairment was found employing the more commonly used Reitan neuropsychological test battery. The long-term neuropsychological effects of exposure to cranial irradiation used in combination with chemotherapy has been studied by Meadows and colleague (1981), and Rowland and co-workers (1984), as well as others. In their studies these authors found that children who receive cranial irradiation and intrathecal methotrexate as part of their CNS prophylaxis for leukemia developed mild learning and intellectual disabilities. The results of these studies have led some to argue that there could be a more rational basis for the timing and dosage of TBI with chemotherapy than is now being used, which would reduce these side effects (Santos and Kaiser, 1981).

## BROVIAC OR HICKMAN CATHETERIZATION AND TPN

Dudrick and colleagues introduced TPN in 1968, and it is currently used routinely in all BMT patients for nutrition in the hospital. The continuous infusion via intravenous catheter of a hypertonic solution of protein hydrolysates, glucose, vitamins, minerals, and lipids requires an indwelling catheter placed in the large vessels and right atrium (see Chapter 36 on anorexia). The catheter is used also as a route of administration for blood products, immunosuppressive drugs, and other medication. Patients may be maintained indefinitely on TPN. TPN is generally discontinued 2 weeks prior to discharge, but the catheters may stay in place for as long as 3–6 months after transplantation to maintain a venous access.

Complications of TPN and metabolic disorders such as hypoglycemia and hyperglycemia, hyponatremia, hypophosphatemia, hypokalemia, hypomagnesemia, prerenal azotemia, and osmotic diuresis with hyperosmolar dehydration can occasionally result in a metabolic encephalopathy with delirium (Ota et al., 1978). Hickman or Broviac line catheterization can cause profound anxiety, depression, fear, and negative body image (Malcolm et al., 1980; Price and Levine, 1977). The positive side, however, is that this special type of venous access decreases anxiety related to the multiple painful venipunctures that would otherwise be necessary.

TPN-related adjustment problems of transplant patients consist of four major areas: the temporary loss of the basic function of eating and controlling nutrition, dependence on nurses for TPN care resulting in separation anxiety on discharge, the high level of technical care of the catheter requiring maintenance for home use, and the psychological dependence on the line itself for food and fluids. Expressions such as, "Is it a chain, a life line, or an umbilical cord?" show the dependence, frustration, and problems for patients in adjusting to its presence and its removal.

## GRAFT-VERSUS-HOST DISEASE

Engraftment of donor bone marrow in the patient is a sign of partial success, but paradoxically it sometimes brings the life-threatening problem of GvHD. GvHD results when the engrafted competent lymphoid cells recognize the host antigens and react immunologically against them. Because the recipient is immunologically suppressed, his or her body is incapable of rejecting the hostile engrafted cells. Such a "turning of the the transplanted organ against the recipient" is unique to BMT. Approximately 50% of recipients develop mild to moderate GvHD; it is fatal in 20% of patients. GvHD has the clinical manifestations of an acute immune disease: enteritis, serositis, malar erythema, skin eruptions, polymyositis, and elevated liver enzymes (Deeg and Storb, 1984; Storb et al., 1981; Wick et al., 1983). Chronic GvHD may develop after 150 days, with chronic skin pigmentation and debilitating contractures. Both the acute and chronic forms add to the uncertainty of chronic illness, physical deformity, long-term medication, and altered lifestyle.

## GERM-FREE ENVIRONMENTS

Optimal care for BMT requires a germ-free environment. It is provided by a reverse-isolation room, which requires staff and visitors to wear mask, cap, gown, gloves, and booties, or by a sterile laminar-airflow unit where all items brought into the patient's room are first sterilized and all visitors perform a "surgical scrub" and put on a gown and mask before entering. Though useful in decreasing the risk of infection during bone marrow suppression, this milieu imposes prolonged physical isolation on the patient. The psychological ramifications of these special environments are described in more detail in the following section.

### Psychiatric Complications

The demands placed on the patient by the length and complexity of treatment may produce psychological as well as medical complications. Some may arise from preexisting sources, others may reflect problems related to the transplantation process or the treatments themselves. In all cases, prompt and effective intervention is important.

## PATIENTS WITH ANTEDATING OR CONCURRENT PSYCHIATRIC ILLNESS

Any BMT patient who has had a history of previous psychiatric illness is at high risk to have a recurrence of that illness during the course of transplantation. Presence of a major psychiatric disorder, such as schizophrenia, bipolar affective illness, or psychotic depression, is an indication for a psychiatric consultation *prior* to admission for transplantation. Severely disturbed patients may not be able to adapt to the rigors of the transplantation procedures. However, the psychological abnormality must be severe, and it is rare for a patient to be denied transplantation on this basis. We have found that even very disturbed patients can be maintained through the procedure with adequate psychiatric input, although input must be extensive in some cases. Psychiatric symptoms can at times compromise the transplant patient's care and endanger successful outcome. The role of the psychiatrist is to assure that the patient's disturbed behavior is controlled sufficiently to allow cooperation with the treatment. The use of psychopharmacological agents is often critical to management in this situation (see Part VII, Chapter 39).

Other patients, because of their personality or methods of coping, adapt poorly to transplantation. Common problems include excessive dependency, regressed behavior, excessive demands, manipulation of staff and family, and hostility toward staff. Management of these issues is discussed in the following section on long-term hospitalization in protected germ-free environments.

## EMOTIONAL DISTURBANCES RELATED TO ILLNESS AND TRANSPLANTATION

Transplantation is used in patients who usually are already dealing with a severe, chronic, or life-threatening disease. Coping mechanisms and psychological techniques (conscious and unconscious) to master or adapt to the stresses, such as repression, displacement, regression, and rationalization, are also means by which the individual copes with the transplant environment. Central to successful adaptation is the ability of the patient to delegate temporarily much of his or her control and authority to others, and the capacity to establish a close, trusting relationship with the staff (Viederman, 1974a). Psychological convalescence requires at least 1 year and is particularly difficult for those patients who have delayed or disrupted important developmental tasks. For example, young mothers find the return to caring for their small children very demanding.

Depression and chronic anxiety are by far the most common psychiatric sequelae of the transplantation procedure and the associated stresses of frequent outpatient visits, prophylactic medication for GvHD and infections, repeated blood tests and bone marrow biopsies, fatigue, decreased stamina, and concerns about relapse, and disability and job status. Many patients become disillusioned as they attempt to make the necessary philosophical transition from living 1 day at a time to anticipating the future. "Not looking beyond tomorrow" and "aiming at short-term goals," adaptations to the immediate stresses of relapse, can result in depression and difficulties in dealing with longer-term goals. Extreme depression and anxiety have led to suicidal gestures in a few successfully transplanted patients. Suicide may take the passive form of noncompliance, such as when a patient discontinues medication or develops eating problems. Health professionals should meet noncompliance with an attempt to understand the patient's motivations, to respect his or her wish for control, and to avoid a care provider–patient power struggle. Although studies are needed to assess the adjustment of these patients who have faced so much, it is encouraging to note that we have experienced little noncompliance on our BMT unit. This contrasts with reports from renal transplant units of a higher incidence of noncompliance (Armstrong, 1978).

Women who receive BMT experience premature menopause and attendant problems of sexual dysfunction, such as vaginal dryness, painful intercourse, and sterility. These symptoms are secondary to TBI and subsequent endocrine imbalances. In order to offer greatest relief, most women should begin receiving estrogen replacement. Men also experience infertility. Decreased sexual desire may also be related to depression and the patient's altered self-image; general debilitation, skin lesions caused by GvHD, and the prospect of sterility, all exact a physical and psychological toll.

## PSYCHOLOGICAL THEMES

Investigators have noted rebirth, changed body image, and psychological integration and/or rejection of the new organ as psychological themes expressed by transplant patients. Such themes are quite common in the transplantation of all solid organs (Abram, 1970, 1972, 1978; Basch, 1973; Schowalter, 1970; Cramond et al., 1967; Crombez and Lefebvre, 1972; Kemph, 1966; Lunde, 1969). Fantasies that one may take on physical or psychological characteristics of the donor are also common after receiving a transplanted organ. A young male recipient on our BMT unit hoped he would acquire some of his donor brother's athletic skills and good looks with the transplanted marrow. His mother added, on the transplantation day, that she hoped her recipient son would acquire the donor son's even-tempered personality. Psychological conflicts regarding sexual identity, noted in cases with kidney transplantation from a donor of the opposite sex, have not been seen with BMT.

After a transplant, patients often express a feeling of being reborn, of having a "new lease on life" or "a second chance." A similar response has been noted in patients who survive a cardiac arrest and is described as the Lazarus syndrome (Hackett, 1972). This life-extending view has received much attention on our BMT unit. Our institution has a ritual in which patients receive a birthday card and cake with candles on the day of their transplant. One aplastic anemia patient subsequently celebrated her birthday on the "new day" after her second BMT and spent time each year on that date visiting a BMT patient concurrently on the unit. There was much talk by staff, patients, and families about this "special" birthday party. One leukemic patient planned his wedding on the first anniversary of his transplant. Other rituals or themes are ongoing. For example, the day a pediatric patient receives back his or her own bacterial flora is celebrated with a "bug dance," with nurses and BMT fellows dressing up as insects to herald this event. It is often the attitude of the staff that makes the initiation of such rituals possible.

One obvious and striking difference between BMT and other transplants, such as kidney, is that the organ being transplanted is fluid and thus becomes integrated into the body; solid organs do not. This must have implications for patients' psychological adaptation to BMT and helps to explain why BMT patients have few of the difficulties in "integrating or assimilating" their own organ described in studies of kidney recipients (Muslin, 1971; Basch, 1973; Viederman, 1974b). Most people do not think of bone marrow as a true organ, and BMT patients generally perceive the actual transplant experience as being similar to a blood transfusion. Again, this stands in contrast to recipients of solid organs, who must undergo major and dramatic surgical procedures and are more apt to view their organ as an object capable of carrying donor-associated characteristics (Basch, 1973; Viederman, 1974b). Although our patient population to date has been small, we have not documented any problems in our patients about organ assimilation (Lesko and Hawkins, 1983). Even when patients develop GvHD, no patient has stated, "The graft is destroying or rejecting me."

## MEDICATION

Drugs used in the transplantation protocol may give rise to neuropsychiatric side effects. Such symptoms are distressing and many patients are reluctant to disclose them. However, not all psychiatric symptoms are drug induced; some are caused by an underlying reaction to the transplant itself. Therefore, it is wise for the physician and other health care providers to be familiar with those drugs that frequently lead to psychiatric complications, so that they may distinguish between those problems caused by drugs and those caused by functional issues.

Steroids in high doses are employed universally as immunosuppressive agents to prevent posttransplant rejection or GvHD. In addition to the physical side effects produced by prolonged administration such as cushingoid symptoms of moon face, acne, hyperphagia, obesity, insomnia, muscle atrophy, cataracts, diabetes, and (in children) stunted growth, steroids may produce psychiatric symptoms ranging from euphoria, lability of affect, and hypomania to depression and psychosis (Fine et al., 1979; Carpenter et al., 1972; Lewis and Smith, 1983). These disturbances are usually dose dependent but may occur at any dose and with abrupt increase or withdrawal of medication. Although most reactions respond to tapering and stopping the drug, discontinuation must be weighed against steroids' therapeutic immunosuppressive benefit. At times, neuroleptic treatment in low dosage is necessary for control of psychiatric sequelae (see Chapter 39).

The cytoreductive agents cyclophosphamide and methotrexate are used for marrow suppression and immunosuppression, and both cause fatigue, weakness, nausea, and vomiting. In addition, cyclophosphamide commonly causes significant transient CNS side effects such as delirium and encephalopathy (Young and Posner, 1980). Cyclophosphamide is thought to activate the chemoreceptor trigger zone (CRTZ) situated around the fourth ventricle. Thus antiemetic agents such as phenothiazines, especially prochlorperazine (Compazine) or thorazine, which act in diminishing impulses from the CRTZ, should be started about 6–8 hours before the patient receives chemotherapy. Tetrahydrocannabinol ($\Delta^9 -$ THC), the active component of marijuana, also has strong antiemetic effects and is becoming widely used clinically on an experimental basis. Metoclopramide (Reglan) is another drug now commonly used to prevent nausea (see Chapter 34). Besides the immediate side effects of nausea, vomiting, fatigue, and bladder irritation caused by high-dose cyclophosphamide and TBI, patients may experience late effects such as cataracts, bladder cancer, leukemia, and sterility, which can provoke psychological distress.

Methotrexate does not cross the blood–brain barrier, but when given intrathecally for prophylaxis against CNS leukemia, it can on rare occasion produce a leukoencephalopathy with focal signs of meningeal irritation, paraparesis, and mental confusion. This drug is given often in the post-BMT convalescent period to control GvHD.

## ROLE OF THE LIAISON PSYCHIATRIST

The psychiatrist working with the BMT team has responsibilities to the patient, donor, family, and transplantation team. Each of these will be briefly discussed here.

### Working with the Patient

One of the psychiatrist's tasks is to predict the prospective patient's emotional ability to tolerate the arduous transplant procedure and response to receiving a transplant. Information gathered should include assessment of prior psychiatric illness, psychological strengths and weaknesses, coping skills, personality, and responses to past emotionally stressful experiences. The patient's expectations with regard to the transplant are also of interest. The team should understand the threat as envisioned by the patient, the type and effectiveness of the patient's coping modes, and any predicted behavior that might impair his or her ability to cooperate.

The liaison psychiatrist must leave behind many of the guidelines useful in the usual psychotherapeutic situation and develop techniques that recognize the uniqueness of the BMT patient (Patenaude et al., 1979). Because patients are easily fatigued, visits of 15–30 minutes are appropriate. Flexibility of scheduling is mandatory, as large blocks of time are often needed to see a family member or patient. The psychiatrist must feel comfortable interviewing a BMT patient in a germ-free room while fully gowned and masked. Because a nurse is often in constant attendance, the psychiatrist must be prepared to deal with a lack of privacy. Meals, sleep, medical treatments, Broviac or Hickman line care, daily hygiene schedules, and patient discomfort often interrupt visits. A patient who is talkative one day may be delirious another; rapid changes in the patient's mental status are common.

The liaison psychiatrist is frequently asked to assist the team in managing side effects of drugs that result in a metabolic encephalopathy. Functional psychosis is rare and when it occurs is usually secondary to delirium or infection. The most common psychiatric problems seen in BMT patients are depression and anxiety that fluctuate with the patient's physical condition. During the weeks after transplant, the psychiatrist and staff monitor for depressed feelings of guilt over putting the donor through surgery and making him or her temporarily ill, fears that the transplant will not function, and anger at the staff related to unmet and unrealistic dependency needs. Patients should be allowed to express their feelings freely and be helped to understand their shifting moods of anxiety, depression, and guilt.

When discharge draws near, the patient must contend with feelings of separation from the staff and unit, and with feelings of dependency on them. The patient may try to work too soon or too hard and become exhausted or, conversely, do far too little. During clinic visits, the psychiatrist and social worker should see the patient and help with adjustment to the "different" life-style outside the transplant unit, giving special support through periods of infection, GvHD, or subsequent hospitalizations.

### Working with the Donor

Too often the "healthy" BMT donor receives little psychological attention. This is unfortunate because donor relatives do sometimes experience problems in connection with their donation. Left unaddressed, they may provide the seed for future psychological morbidity or lead to difficulties in interpersonal relationships between the donor, patient, and other family members.

Unlike donors of solid organs, the donor of bone marrow provides a body product that is easily regenerated within a few weeks. The psychiatrist needs to prepare the bone marrow donor for surgery by helping him or her understand the regenerative nature of the marrow and that the loss of such an organ will not have physiological consequences. Other issues that the psychiatrist needs to keep in mind when working with donors are their psychological stability, their degree of ambivalence, possible family pressure for donation and motivation for the donation ("ostracised family members who are often 'black sheep' try to redeem themselves by giving a lifesaving organ" [Abram, 1978]), and personality structure (for hospital management of the donor).

Donors are hospitalized for 2 days. Harvesting, which is performed under general anesthesia, is completed within 2 hours, and discharge follows 24 hours later. Unlike other organ donors, these donors do not become depressed, mourn the loss of a body part or usually resent those who suggested participation.

In studying kidney donors, Fellner and Marshall (1968) discovered that the decision-making process did not occur as the result of an extended period of deliberation; rather, it was "an instantaneous response." However, the donors still regarded the act of donation as positive, with few having any regrets. The authors identified three subsystems within the kidney donor selection process that are helpful in understanding the donation of bone marrow: "medical selection" involving HLA blood typing and other histocompatibility tests (most important in BMT); "donor self-selection" made by a potential donor without consulting family; "the family subsystem" of donor selection usually governed by family dynamics. Fellner observed that "the family subsystem" of donor selection is clearly at its most efficient level very early in the selection process and works primarily in the direction of trying to exclude some family members from participation. However, in the case of BMT, once the genetically potential donors have been tissue typed, the power of the family system to influence the medical selection process diminishes greatly.

In summary, the liaison psychiatrist may be asked to assist the team in screening and selecting the appropriate donor, prepare the donor for surgery, and attend to the donor's concerns, feelings, and fantasies after the transplantation.

## Working with the Family

Transplantation is difficult for the rest of the family as well as for the patient and donor. The repeated disappointments and stress of chronic chemotherapy, along with uncertainty about the future, are shared by parents, spouses, siblings, and children. Their worries are aggravated because the procedure itself is still somewhat experimental and because morbidity and mortality are high. The decision for transplantation may be more difficult when a child is the patient. Each family unit brings to the transplantation procedure its own marital conflicts, financial problems, school problems, and psychological concerns of the children. Some research suggests that even the most untroubled families suffer from the pressures of chronic illness, the transplant procedure, and dislocation from home and friends (Patenaude et al., 1979). Families often must travel hundreds of miles to a specialized unit, set up a new home away from home, and periodically take other children out of school. Even if the transplant center is in the same city, dislocation can be considerable because most BMT units encourage families to participate actively in caring for the patient, which often requires all-day trips to the unit.

On many transplant services, a psychiatrist or social worker and a nurse meet weekly with the patients' families. These professionals can assist families with airing concerns about donor selection (as selection of a living donor can create new and sometimes difficult relationships among siblings and family members), rearranging their life-styles (e.g., managing dislocation from home and friends and relocation to the transplant center), managing preexisting marital or family problems, coping with the strain of having the wage earner or the mother figure incapacitated, and dealing with signs of graft rejection or a transition into some terminal phase of illness. Our transplant team and others have recognized that a patient's positive response to hospitalization and treatment can be completely un-

done if the patient returns to an unstable marital or family situation.

## Working with the Transplant Team

Medical care, which entails intensive chemoradiation and difficult decisions, makes many psychological demands on the staff. The psychiatrist may be useful in helping the members of the transplant team to cope with the psychologically stressful tasks they must perform. Because BMT teams must work closely together with patients and families, an unusual sense of intimacy develops. This intimacy may lead the staff to become overly protective and possessive of their patients (especially when patients are transferred back to the referring physician), take on too many parental responsibilities when caring for their patients, become angry when a transplant patient does not return to a productive life, feel guilty and disappointed when a patient dies in spite of their efforts, and develop hostility toward patients who withdraw from posttransplant care even when the quality of care available to them is adequate. Staff meetings should review emotional reactions that are stressful and nonconstructive as part of patient care rounds.

Regular staff meetings with the team psychiatrist center on ethical aspects of decisions, psychological management of the patient, and communication with patients and families. The psychiatrist may interpret a patient's anger and maladaptive behavior for the staff. When conflicts arise among the members of the staff, the psychiatrist must balance the roles of participant, consultant, and arbitrator. Sometimes a consultant skilled in group therapy is asked to help resolve unusual team conflicts. Using psychotherapeutic skills requires precise judgment and balance by the BMT psychiatrist. When a team member shows signs of major psychological distress, these should be recognized and early referral should be made to another psychiatrist for consultation.

Bloom (1981) summarized the function of the liaison psychiatrist as "witness, bystander, and translator" of emotional events and "catalyst in promoting the best and most adaptive ways of interpersonal functioning." Patenaude (see Patenaude et al., 1979), a liaison psychiatrist on a pediatric bone marrow unit, views her role as a "lightening rod." The presence of a psychologically minded team member legitimizes certain topics that would otherwise be discussed less often or not at all.

## ETHICAL ISSUES

Although physicians disagree on whether BMT is an experimental or conventional treatment, it is still generally regarded more as experimental than as an established treatment modality. Determining its likely risks and benefits for each patient is difficult, and patients vary in their ability to understand all the procedure's ramifications. Thus common ethical concerns tend to intensify when BMT is involved (Levine et al., 1975; Gardner et al., 1977; Pfefferbaum et al., 1977; Popkin et al., 1977). First and foremost, physicians, patients, and families must weigh the decision to choose a procedure that may be fatal or, if curative, can profoundly and adversely affect quality of life. As a result, the informed-consent process is especially critical. In the case of transplantation between twins, which has moved from the experimental realm to a therapeutic reality, the question of how voluntary the donor twin's informed consent is can be raised. Other ethical concerns include donor risks, the allocation of a scarce resource, the thoroughness of the institutional review, and the safety of research protocols. Renee Fox (1970) has written extensively on the subject of ethical aspects of transplantation, and the interested reader may wish to consult her review article.

## SUMMARY

Bone marrow transplantation (BMT) is evolving from a controversial and innovative research procedure to a standard therapeutic modality. Advances in the field prolong the lives of some patients and cure others. New issues for the patient, family, and caregiver arise. The psychological issues have been studied by psychiatrists as members of the transplant team to provide new information about patients' responses to illness and stress in an unconventional setting.

The BMT procedures are divided into several stages, which have accompanying emotional problems. In providing psychological care for transplant recipients, donors, and families, caregivers must be familiar with the psychological stages of the procedure, the psychological themes such as body image, rebirth, and the patient's mechanisms of coping with the extreme stress of such protocols. BMT, with its complex medications, high-dose chemotherapy, total-body irradiation (TBI), germ-free environment, graft-versus-host disease (GvHD), Broviac or Hickman line catheterization, and total parenteral nutrition (TPN), can precipitate significant psychological sequelae with immediate and long-term consequences. In response to their illness, transplant patients may also develop emotional disturbances of anxiety, depression, agitation, suicidal thoughts, sexual dysfunction, and noncompliance. These reactions, and the occasional presence of concurrent psychiatric illness require recognition and development of guidelines for management. Finally, the liaison psychiatrist's role, as a team member, involves responsibilities to recipient, donor, family, and staff.

Future areas of psychological research in the area of BMT should include the assessment of long-term effects of BMT treatment (chemotherapy and radiation) on intellectual and sexual development, the study of immediate and delayed impact of BMT on psychological adaptation of patients, and the development and testing of materials to enhance information and reduce distress.

## REFERENCES

Abram, H.S. (1970). Psychological reaction to cardiac operations: An historical perspective. *Psychiatr. Med.* 1:227–94.

Abram, H.S. (1972). The psychiatrist, the treatment of chronic renal failure and the prolongation of life, III. *Am. J. Psychiatry* 128:1534–39.

Abram, H.S. (1978). Renal transplantation. In T.P. Hackett and N.H. Cassem (eds.), *Massachusetts General Hospital Handbook of General Hospital Psychiatry*. St. Louis: C.V. Mosby, pp. 365–79.

Appelbaum, F., R. Storb, R. Ramberg, H. Schulman, C. Buckner, R. Clift, H. Deeg, A. Fefer, I. Sanders, P. Stewart, K. Sullivan, R. Witherspoon, and E. Thomas (1984). Allogeneic marrow transplantation in the treatment of preleukemia. *Ann. Intern. Med.* 100:689–93.

Armstrong, S.H. (1978). Psychological maladjustment in renal dialysis patients. *Psychosomatics* 19:169–71.

Basch, S.H. (1973). The intrapsychic integration of a new organ. *Psychoanal. Q.* 42:364–84.

Begg, C.B., P.B. McGlave, J.M. Bennett, P.A. Cassileth, and M.M. Oken (1984). A critical comparison of allogeneic bone marrow transplantation and conventional chemotherapy as treatment for acute nonlymphocytic leukemia. *J. Clin. Oncol.* 2:369–78.

Bloom, V. (1981). Functions of a liaison psychiatrist in a kidney center: Personal reflections. *Dialysis Transplant.* 10:51–55.

Bortin, M.M., R.P. Gale, and A.A. Rimm (1981). Allogeneic bone marrow transplantation for 144 patients with severe aplastic anemia. *J.A.M.A.* 245:1132–39.

Brown, H.N., and M.J. Kelly (1976). Stages of bone marrow transplantation: A psychiatric perspective. *Psychosom. Med.* 38:439–46.

Carpenter, W.T., J.C. Strauss, and W.E. Bunney (1972). The psychobiology of cortisol metabolism: Clinical and theoretical implications. In R.I. Shader (ed.), *Psychiatric Complications of Medical Drugs*. New York: Raven Press, pp. 49–73.

Champlin, R.E. and P.R. Gale (1984). Role of bone marrow transplantation in the treatment of hematologic malignancies and solid tumors: Critical review of syngeneic, autologous and allogeneic transplants. *Cancer Treat. Rep.* 68:145–61.

Cramond, W.A., J.H. Court, B.A. Higgins, P.R. Knight, and J.R. Lawrence (1967). Psychological screening of potential donors in a renal homotransplantation programme. *Br. J. Psychiatry* 113:1213–21.

Crombez, J.C. and P. Lefebvre (1972). The behavioral responses of renal transplant patients as seen through their fantasy life. *Can. Psychiatr. Assoc. J.* 17(Special Suppl. II):5519–23.

Deeg, H.J. and R. Storb (1984). Graft versus host disease: Patholophysiological and clinical aspects. *Annu. Rev. Med.* 35:11–24.

Dinsmore, R., D. Kirkpatrick, N. Flomenberg, S. Gulati, N. Kapoor, J. Brockstein, B. Shank, A. Reid, S. Groshen, and R. O'Reilly (1984). Allogeneic bone marrow transplantation for patients with acute nonlymphocytic leukemia. *Blood* 63:649–56.

Dinsmore, R., D. Kirkpatrick, N. Flomenberg, S. Gulati, B. Shank, and R. O'Reilly (1983). Allogeneic marrow transplantation for acute lymphoblastic leukemia in remission: The importance of early transplantation. *Transplant. Proc.* 15:1397–1400.

Dudrick, S.J., D.W. Wilmore, H.M. Vars, and J.E. Rhodes (1968). Long term parenteral nutrition with growth development and positive nitrogen balance. *Surgery* 64:134–42.

Fellner, C.H. and J.R. Marshall (1968). Twelve kidney donors. *J.A.M.A.* 206:2703–7.

Fine, R.N., M.H. Malekzadeh, A.J. Pennisi, R.B. Henger, C.H. Uittenbogaart, V.F. Negrete, and B.M. Korsch (1979). Long term results of renal transplantation in children. *Pediatrics* 61:641–50.

Fox, R.C. (1970). A sociological perspective on organ transplantation and hemodialysis. *Ann. N.Y. Acad. Sci.* 169:406–28.

Gardner, G., C.S. August, and J. Githens (1977). Psychological issues in bone marrow transplantation. *Pediatrics* 60:626–31.

Gluckman, E., R. Berger, and J. Dutreix (1984). Bone marrow transplantation for Fanconi anemia. *Semin. Hematol.* 21:20–26.

Gottschalk, L., R. Kunkel, T. Wohl, E. Soenger, and C. Winget (1969). Total and half body irradiation: Effect on cognitive and emotional process. *Arch. Gen. Psychiatry* 21:574–80.

Hackett, T.P. (1972). The Lazarus complex revisited. *Ann. Intern. Med.* 76:135–36.

Kadota, R.P. and W.A. Smithson (1984). Bone marrow transplantation for diseases of childhood. *Mayo Clin. Proc.* 59:171–84.

Kemph, J.P. (1966). Renal failure, artificial kidney and kidney transplantation. *Am. J. Psychiatry* 122:1270–74.

Lesko, L.M. and D.R. Hawkins (1983). Psychological aspects of transplantation medicine. In S. Akhtar (ed.), *New Psychiatric Syndromes: DSM-III and Beyond*. New York: Aronson, pp. 265–309.

Levine, M.D., B.M. Cametta, D. Nathan, and W.J. Curran (1975). The medical ethics of bone marrow transplantation in childhood. *J. Pediatr.* 86:145–50.

Lewis, D. and R. Smith (1983). Steroid induced psychiatric syndromes. *J. Affect. Dis.* 5:319–32.

Lunde, D.T. (1969). Psychiatric complications of heart transplants. *Am. J. Psychiatry* 126:369–73.

Malcolm, R., J. Robson, T.W. Vanderveen, and P. Mahlen (1980). Psychosocial aspects of total parenteral nutrition. *Psychosomatics* 21:115–23.

Meadows, A., D.J. Massan, J. Gordon, K. Littman, J.

Glaser, and J. Ferguson (1981). Declines in IQ scores and cognitive dysfunctions in children with acute lymphocytic leukemia treated with cranial radiation. *Lancet* 2:1015–18.

Muslin, H.L. (1971). On acquiring a kidney. *Am. J. Psychiatry* 127:1145–48.

Ota, D.M., A.L. Imbembo, and G.D. Zuidena, (1978). Total parenteral nutrition. *Surgery* 83:503–20.

Patenaude, A.F., L. Szymanski, and J. Rappeport (1979). Psychological costs of bone marrow transplantation in children. *Am. J. Orthopsychiatry* 49:409–22.

Pfefferbaum, B., M.M. Lindamood, and F.M. Wiley (1977). Pediatric bone marrow transplantation: Psychological aspects. *Am. J. Psychiatry* 134:1299–1301.

Popkin, M.K., C.F. Moldow, R.C.W. Hall, R. Branda, and R. Varchoan (1977). Psychiatric aspects of allogeneic bone marrow transplantation for aplastic anemia. *Dis. Nerv. System* 38:925–27.

Price, B. and E. Levine (1977). Permanent total parenteral nutrition: Psychological and social responses of the early stages. *J. Parent. Ent. Nutr.* 1:24–28.

Rowland, J., O. Glidewell, R. Sibley, J. Holland, B. Tull, A. Berman, M.L. Brecher, M. Marris, A.J. Glicksman, E. Forman, B. Jones, M.E. Cohen, P.K. Duffner, and A.I. Freeman (1984). Effects of different forms of central nervous system prophylaxis on neuropsychologic function in childhood leukemia. *J. Clin. Oncol.* 2:1327–35.

Santos, G. and H. Kaiser (1981). Current states of autoiogous marrow transplantation. In J. Burchenal and H.F. Oettgen (eds.), *Cancer: Achievements, Challenges, and Prospects for the 1980s* Vol. 2. New York: Grune & Stratton, pp. 673–82.

Schowalter, J.E. (1970). Multiple organ transplantation and the creation of surgical siblings. *Pediatrics* 46:576–80.

Speck, B., A. Gratwohl, B. Osterwalder, and C. Nissen (1984). Bone marrow transplantation for chronic myeloid leukemia. *Semin. Hematol.* 21:48–052.

Storb, R. (1981). Bone marrow transplantation for the treatment of hematologic malignancy and of aplastic anemia. *Transplant. Proc.* 13:221–25.

Storb, R., K. Atkinson, L.G. Lun, K.M. Sullivan, T. Mangso, P.L. Weiden, and R.P. Witherspoon (1981). Graft-versus-host disease, immunologic reconstitution and graft-host tolerance in marrow graft recipients. In J.H. Burchenal and H.F. Oettgen (eds.), *Cancer: Achievements, Challenges, and Prospects for the 1980s*, Vol. 2. New York: Grune & Stratton, pp. 639–48.

Storb, R., E.D. Thomas, C.D. Buckner, F.R. Appelbaum, R.A. Clift, H.J. Deeg, K. Doney, J.A. Hansen, R.L. Prentice, J.E. Sanders, P. Stewart, K.M. Sullivan, and R.P. Witherspoon (1984). Marrow transplantation for aplastic anemia. *Semin. Hematol.* 21:27–35.

Sullivan, K.M., H.J. Deeg, J.E. Sanders, H.M. Shulman, R.P. Witherspoon, K. Doney, F.R. Appelbaum, M.M. Schubert, P. Stewart, S. Springmeyers, G.B. McDonald, R. Storb, and E.D. Thomas (1984). Late complications after marrow transplantation. *Semin. Hematol.* 21:53–63.

Thomas, E.D., C.D. Buckner, R.A. Clift, A. Fefer, F.L. Johnson, P.E. Neiman, G.E. Sale, J.E. Sanders, J.W. Singer, H. Shulman, R. Strob, and P.L. Weiden (1979a).

Marrow transplantation for acute nonlymphoblastic leukemia in first remission. *N. Engl. J. Med.* 301:597–99.

Thomas, E.D., R.A. Clift, and R. Storb (1984). Indications for marrow transplantation. *Annu. Rev. Med.* 35:1–9.

Thomas, E.D., J. E. Sanders, N. Flournoy, F.L. Johnson, C.D. Buckner, R.A. Clift, A. Fefer, B.W. Goodell, R. Storb, and P.L. Weiden (1979b). Marrow transplantation for patients with acute lymphoblastic leukemia in remission. *Blood* 54:468–76.

Viederman, M. (1974a). Adaptive and maladaptive regression in hemodialysis. *Psychiatry,* 37:68–77.

Viederman, M. (1974b). The search for meaning in renal transplantation. *Psychiatry* 37:283–90.

Wick, M.K., S. Moore, D.A. Gastineau, and H.C. Hoagland (1983). Immunologic, clinical and pathologic aspects of human graft versus host disease. *Mayo Clin. Proc.* 58:603–12.

Young, D.F. and J.B. Posner (1980). Nervous system toxicity of the chemotherapeutic agents. In P.J. Vinken and G.W. Bruyn (eds.), *Handbook of Clinical Neurology,* Vol. 39, *Neurological Manifestations of Systemic Diseases,* Part II. New York: Elsevier, pp. 91–129.

# 12

## Protected Environments

Lynna M. Lesko

Certain oncological and medical conditions, including aplastic anemia, severe combined immunodeficiency disease, leukemia, bone marrow transplantation, and aggressive administration of cancer chemotherapy may require treating a patient in a germ-free or protected environment. Although these environments decrease the risk and severity of infection in patients, they also impose prolonged physical and psychological isolation from family and staff (whether reverse isolation or sterile laminar airflow). This chapter describes the psychological consequences of such protected environments on patients and staff and suggests guidelines for dealing with them. Readers desiring a more extensive review are referred to the article by Lesko and colleagues (1984).

### OVERVIEW

Information from a variety of clinical and research sources provides insight into psychological issues similar to those experienced by patients treated in protected-isolation environments. These include literature on the intensive care unit (ICU) syndrome (Nahum, 1965; McKegney, 1966; Abram, 1965; Holland et al., 1973; Koumans, 1965; Kornfeld, 1971), social isolation in novel or extreme environments (Popkin et al., 1974), sensory deprivation (Hebb, 1955; Kenna, 1962; Zuckerman, 1964; Shurley, 1960; Ziskind, 1965; Lilly, 1956; Mendelson et al., 1958), parental separation from children (Bowlby, 1960), long-term isolation of children (Spitz, 1945; Spitz and Wolf, 1946; Nir et al., 1981; Lazar et al., 1983), and the importance of oral and maternal stimulation on early behavioral development (Harlow et al., 1963; Solkoff et al., 1969; Engel and Reichsman, 1956). In all of the clinical situations mentioned earlier, a range of cognitive, perceptual, and emotional alterations may occur in the affected adults and children.

Much of the work on the psychological consequences of isolation has been done in pediatrics, and opinion differs concerning the effects of therapeutic isolation on the pediatric patient (see Table 12-1). Although patients may at times exhibit symptoms of regression as well as affective, sensory, and behavioral changes, many researchers feel that these symptoms tend to be transient and isolation environments do not fundamentally interfere with normal development (Freedman et al., 1976; Kutsanellou-Meyer and Christ, 1978; Kellerman et al., 1976a,b; Kellerman et al., 1980). Others, however, have found that children in isolation exhibit a high level of anxiety, depression, and behavioral problems (Powazek et al., 1978). Still others indicate that young patients in isolation may suffer lasting cognitive impairment and learning disorders (Drotar et al., 1976; Simons, 1973; Teller et al., 1973). Greater awareness of the potential adverse sequelae of treatment in protected environments has resulted in special efforts to provide high levels of physical and intellectual stimulation and emotional support for patients of all ages in these settings. As a consequence, many of the problems observed in earlier studies are less commonly observed in patients treated today; the impact of the environment is mitigated by the increased support available. In addition, better controlled studies have shown that the problems that do occur are often transient and readily managed.

Most research on psychological aspects of adaptation of adults to protected environments was initiated with the expectation that severe psychological disturbances might result from prolonged isolation, a natural extension from earlier work on sensory deprivation and ICU psychosis (see Table 12-2). Indeed, depression, anxiety, irregular sleep, regression, withdrawal from one's surroundings, and occasional disorientation have been noted in adults (Kellerman et al., 1977). However, researchers found that although most pa-

**Table 12-1** Studies of pediatric patients in germ-free environments

| Reference | Type of germ-free environment | Number of patients | Length of stay | Remarks |
|---|---|---|---|---|
| Simons et al. (1973); Teller et al. (1973) | "Life island" (tent) | 2 | Birth to 28–32 months | Twins with cognitive impairment |
| Drotar et al. (1976) | Reverse-isolation room | 1 | Birth to 12 months | Below-age norm intellectual development with improvement in home environment |
| Freedman et al. (1976) | "Life island" | 1 | Birth to 52 months | Isolation compatible with normal development |
| Kellerman et al. (1976a,b, 1980) | "Life island", reverse-isolation room, laminar-airflow room | Up to 14 | Median stay 87 days | No cognitive impairment; no psychopathology; transient regression; transient behavioral changes |
| Kutsanellou-Meyer and Christ (1978) | Reverse-isolation room | 22 | 3–20 Months | Isolation compatible with normal development |
| Powazek et al. (1978) | Reverse-isolation room; laminar-airflow room | 123 | 37% treated <1 month | High levels of anxiety and depression |

tients were anxious and apprehensive before entering isolation, all adapted well despite the serious nature of their illnesses, their unusual environments, and their very different personalities. Cognitive and perceptual disturbances such as those described in sensory deprivation experiments were not found, nor was it necessary in any of these studies to remove a patient from the germ-free environment for psychological reasons. Only the severity of the patients' physical illness or the presence of a delirium, rather than isolation itself, exerted a profound influence on their psychological equilibrium. The loss of opportunities to touch and have physical contact was also a consideration in patients' adjustment.

**Table 12-2** Studies of adult patients in germ-free environments

| Reference | Type of germ-free environment | Number of patients | Length of stay | Remarks |
|---|---|---|---|---|
| Fine (1969) | "Life island" (tent) | 3 | Not stated | Patients were subjected to complex set of severe stresses. |
| Kohle et al. (1971) | "Life island" | 9 | 9 Patients whose total length of stay was 427 days | Isolation therapy is contraindicated in patients with previous psychopathology and those who could not care for themselves, creating dependency. |
| Graubert and Edmonson (1972) | "Life island" | 14 | 9–208 Days; average 60 days | All patients adapted well. |
| Gordon (1975) | "Life island" | 10 | 21–99 Days | In this controlled study, patients experienced anxiety, but viewed unit as special, altered sensory experience; unit creates dependency. |
| Holland et al. (1977) | Reverse isolation, laminar-airflow sterile unit | 52 | Average 30 days | Patients adapted well; psychological equilibrium is influenced by medical condition. |
| Kellerman et al. (1977) | "Life island" | Total of 260 patients from 13 units | 2–240 Days; average 35 days | Symptoms of depression, anxiety, irregular sleep, and withdrawal were noted; some patients were removed for psychological reasons; children appeared to adjust better than adults to environment. |

**Table 12-3**  Protected environment:
patient management guidelines

| Types of management | Reference |
|---|---|
| *Patient education* | |
| Knowledge about one's own illness | McKegney (1966); Holland et al. (1973) |
| *Preparation* | |
| Visiting the isolation unit | Kellerman et al. (1976a,b, 1980) |
| Meeting staff (nurses, social workers) | |
| Patient booklets | Lesko et al. (1984) |
| *Environmental manipulation* | |
| Access to windows, clocks, calendars, TVs, radios, natural light | Kellerman et al. (1980); McKegney (1966); Kornfeld (1971) |
| Personal belongings from home | Kellerman et al. (1980); McKegney (1966); Kornfeld (1971) |
| Stable daily schedule | Kellerman et al. (1980); McKegney (1966); Kornfeld (1971) |
| Single rooms, with monitoring equipment outside of room | Kellerman et al. (1980); McKegney (1966); Kornfeld (1971) |
| Patients participating in own care | Holland et al. (1977) |
| Liberal vising hours | Fine et al. (1969) |
| *Psychological support* | |
| Nurturing but structured support from all staff | Graubert and Edmonson (1972); Gordon (1973) |
| *Medication* | |
| Minor anxiolytics used to control anxiety; neuroleptics rarely indicated except for delirium | Graubert and Edmonson (1972); Holland et al. (1977) |

## PATIENT MANAGEMENT GUIDELINES

Several principles for managing the patient in a protected environment and his or her family can be drawn from the literature and from experience in working in these settings (Table 12-3).

## Patient Education and the Physician–Patient Relationship

Knowledge about one's illness, as well as its severity and treatment fosters emotional stability and cooperation under any condition and especially in restricted environments. The physician plays a key role here. A close, frank relationship between physician and patient allows the patient to gather more information about his or her illness and at the same time affords the physician an opportunity to get to know the patient and to learn

about his or her character style, psychological functioning, modes of coping with past illness, and capacity for dealing with stress.

## Preparation for Entry

It is recommended that all patients along with the family tour the isolation unit prior to entry. Meeting the unit's personnel, especially the nursing staff, can be comforting for children and will also provide an opportunity for patients and family members to ask questions. Many units have developed orientation pamphlets, which provide procedural as well as psychological preparation for confinement. These booklets are informative, help to decrease anxiety, and enable patients and families to generate more specific questions.

## Environmental Manipulation

Patients should be encouraged to bring personal belongings (books, paintings, posters, pictures, stereos, VCRs, radios, stuffed animals, albums, and clothes) to brighten up the isolation area, divert them, and promote a sense of familiarity. Access to windows, clocks, calendars, TV sets, and natural light can help in orienting patients to maintain a stable daily rhythm. In order to protect one patient from another's distress and discomfort, single rooms appear preferable. Monitoring equipment is best kept outside the patient's room when possible, and exposure to monotonous noises should be kept to a minimum. Psychological regression due to stress and illness can be minimized by encouraging patients to participate in their own care and to remain as self-sufficient as possible (e.g., managing their own hygiene, operating radios and TV sets). Liberal visiting privileges for the patient's family and friends are important in maintaining social support and ties with the world outside (Fine, 1969).

## Psychological Support

Clinical experience has shown that support from the staff is more valuable than psychotropic drugs in improving a patient's and family's capacity to cope with illness, physical concerns, and the stress of isolation. Kutsanellou-Meyer and Christ (1978) found that an open attitude of staff toward answering questions and listening to patients' concerns helped to alleviate patients' distress, although it was not sufficient by itself. They suggest that active exploration of patients' reactions to illness and treatment is important in relieving their distress in isolation therapy and is best done by a well-coordinated psychosocial team, consisting of a psychiatrist and/or psychologist, social worker, recreational therapist, specialized nurses, and hospital teachers as appropriate. This staff should meet regularly with the medical staff to assess how patients and families are coping and to devise interventions when appropriate.

## Preparation for Departure

Preparation for leaving the isolation unit should take place a few days before the actual move to a "stepdown" unit and eventual discharge. The staff should encourage patients to talk about the feelings of "reentering the world" and alert family members to possible behavioral and emotional reactions that could occur in the patient. Having left the germ-free room and hospital, patients may develop an anxiety about being out of that special environment. This may take the form of worries about breathing normal (uncleansed) air, fears of contagion from friends, pets, or family, and/or concerns about new aches, pains, and symptoms. Patients in isolation environments have become accustomed to being monitored and supervised very closely, with every symptom or change in their daily functions being brought to their attention. Consequently, upon discharge minor aches and pains can produce acute anxiety, and some patients may initially need constant reassurance that they are progressing as expected.

Paradoxically, other patients develop an unconcerned attitude toward their care and health when they return home and may become careless about Broviac catheter care, for example, or noncompliant about medication. This may be a form of rebellion against the hospital routine with which they needed to comply for so long. A few other patients develop depressive symptoms with their return to their regular room or home. These symptoms may represent an anxiety response to leaving a psychologically protected milieu and signal concerns about returning to a life-style similar to that lived before the illness. Patients tend to view their protected environments as "special," because there they develop closer relationships to staff and receive more attention and stimulation than patients in regular rooms. Kellerman notes that "children can endow the units (i.e. their rooms) with more potency than they deserve" (Kellerman et al., 1976a, 1976b). Adult patients at times state that "their room has pulled them through the ordeal" and protected them. It should be noted that the opposite may also occur; a room may be considered "jinxed" by some patients, especially if patients have died while being cared for in that particular isolation area.

Particular attention and support needs to be given to family members who are often required to visit daily and to participate in the patient's care. Family support issues are discussed at greater length in Chapter 11 on transplantation, because transplantation often requires lengthy stays in isolation.

## Medication

Anxiolytics can be used to modulate excessive anxiety, relieve insomnia, and serve as an adjunct in control of pain. Major tranquilizers (neuroleptics) are rarely indicated and could mask recognition of an acute confusional state secondary to metabolic abnormalities (see also Chapter 30). Antidepressants can and often should be utilized when patients experience major depressive symptomatology.

## STAFF SUPPORT

It is essential to monitor the psychological needs not only of patients and families but also of professional staff. Toward this end, regular counseling sessions should be arranged for all groups of health care providers. These sessions can focus on a particular patient and family, or on unit issues. Nursing staff need particular attention. Because they often must meet the patient's daily requirements for play (in the case of children), social interaction, and physical contact, they experience many of the same parental issues as the patient's own parents or spouse. Many, but not all, patients in protected isolation have lengthy hospital stays during the course of which patient dependence on staff can become an issue. Staff members who become overextended by assuming excessive nurturing responsibilities in these cases can use the counseling sessions to balance their caregiver and nurturing tasks more effectively.

## SUMMARY

Many clinicians and researchers have speculated about the psychological problems that germ-free environments create. In the past they hypothesized that responses to this therapy would be similar, if not identical to, behavior associated with sensory deprivation, social isolation, and parent–child separation paradigms. This has not been borne out. When it occurs, psychopathological behavior is usually a consequence of the underlying physical illness rather than an effect of the environment. Few patients require neuroleptics, and very rarely is it mandatory to discontinue isolation therapy for psychological reasons. Most researchers agree that a protected environment gives most patients a positive feeling of being attentively cared for and for some promotes feelings of becoming a privileged, "special" patient during the hospitalization. The feeling that isolation environments are adversely psychologically stressful may be more a reflection of the medical staff's projected reaction to this environment than of any real consequences of this treatment to the patient. The guidelines described in this chapter offer ways to minimize any adverse sequelae for patients and caregivers alike.

# REFERENCES

Abram, H.S. (1965). Adaptation to open heart surgery: A psychiatric study of response to the threat of death. *Am. J. Psychiatry* 122:659–68.

Bowlby, J. (1960). Separation anxiety: A critical review of the literature. *J. Child Psychol. Psychiatry* 1:251–59.

Drotar, D.D., R.C. Stern, and S.H. Polmar (1976). Intellectual and social development following prolonged isolation. *J. Pediatrics* 89:675–78.

Engel, G.L. and F. Reichsman (1956). Spontaneous and experimentally induced depressions in an infant with a gastric fistula: A contribution to the problem of depression. *J. Am. Psychoanal. Assoc.* 4:428–52.

Engel, G.L. and J. Romano (1959). Delirium, a syndrome of cerebral insufficiency. *J. Chron. Dis.* 9:260–77.

Fine, L., M. Wachspress, D.N. Grauber, et al. (1974). Psychological adaptation of patients during treatment of acute leukemia in life island isolator. *Ad. Exp. Med. Bio.* 3:27–34.

Freedman, D.A., J.R. Montgomery, R. Wilson, P.M. Bealmear, and M.A. South (1976). Further observations on the effect of reverse isolation from birth on cognitive and affective development. *J. Am. Acad. Child Psychiatry* 15:593–603.

Gordon, A.M. (1975). Psychological adaptation to isolator therapy in acute leukemia. *Psychother. Psychosom.* 26:132–39.

Graubert, D.M. and J.H. Edmonson (1972). Psychologic adaptation of patients isolated in protected environments. *N.Y. State J. Med.* 72:227–28.

Harlow, H.F., M.F. Harlow, and E.W. Hansen (1963). The maternal affectional system of the rhesus monkey. In A. Rheingold (ed.), *Maternal Behavior in Mammals*. New York: Wiley, pp. 260–85.

Hebb, D.O. (1955). The mammal and his environment. *Am. J. Psychiatry* 111:826–31.

Holland, J., S.M. Sgroi, S.J. Marwit, and N. Solkoff (1973). The ICU syndrome: Fact or fancy. *Int. J. Psychiatry Med.* 4:241–49.

Holland, J., M. Plumb, J. Yates, S. Harns, A. Tuttolomondo, J. Holmes, and J.F. Holland (1977). Psychological response of patients with acute leukemia to germ-free environments. *Cancer* 40:871–79.

Kellerman, J., S.E. Siegel, and D. Rigler (1980). Special treatment modalities: Laminar airflow rooms. In J. Kellerman (ed): *Psychological Aspects of Childhood Cancer*. Springfield, Illinois, C.C. Thomas, pp 128–154.

Kellerman, J., D. Rigler, S. Siegel, K. McCue, J. Pospisil, and R. Uno (1976a). Pediatric cancer patients in reverse isolation utilizing protected environments. *Pediatr. Psychol.* 1:21–25.

Kellerman, J., D. Rigler, S. Seigel, K. McCue, J. Pospisil,

and R. Uno (1976b). Psychological evaluation and management of pediatric oncology patients in protected environments. *Med. Pediatr. Oncol.* 2:353–60.

Kellerman, J., D. Rigler, and S.E. Sigel (1977). The psychological effects of isolation in protected environments. *Am. J. Psychol.* 134:563–65.

Kenna, J.C. (1962). Sensory deprivation phenomena: Critical review and explanatory models. *Proc. R. Soc. Med.* 55:1005–10.

Kohle, K., C. Simons, S. Weidlich, M. Dienich, and A. Durner (1971). Psychological aspects in the treatment of leukemia patients in the isolated bed system "Life Island." *Psychother. Psychosom.* 19:85–91.

Kornfeld, D.S. (1971). Psychiatric problems of an intensive care unit. *Med. Clin. North Am.* 55:1353–63.

Koumans, A.J.R. (1965). Psychiatric consultation in an intensive care unit. *J.A.M.A.* 194:163–67.

Kutsanellou-Meyer, M. and G.H. Christ (1978). Factors affecting coping of adolescents and infants on a reverse isolation unit. *Soc. Work Health Care* 4(2):125–37.

Lazar, R.M., M. Tamaroff, Y. Nir, B. Freud, R. O'Reilly, D. Kirkpatrick, and N. Kapoor (1983). Language recovery following isolation for severe combined immunodeficiency disease. *Nature* 306:54–55.

Lesko, L.M., J. Kern, and D.R. Hawkins (1984). Psychological aspects of patients in germ free isolation: A review of child, adult, patient management literature. *Med. Pediatr. Oncol.* 12:43–49.

Lilly, J.C. (1956). Mental effects of reduction of ordinary levels of physical stimuli on intact, healthy persons. *Psychiatr. Res. Rep.* 5:1–9.

McKegney, F.P. (1966). The intensive care syndrome. *Conn. Med.* 30:633–36.

Mendelson, J.H., P. Solomon, and E. Lindemann (1958). Hallucinations of poliomyelitis patients during treatment in a respirator. *J. Nerv. Ment. Dis.* 126:421–26.

Nahum, L.H. (1965). Madness in the recovery room from open heart surgery, or "they kept waking me up" (Editorial). *Conn. Med.* 29:771.

Nir, Y., M. Tamaroff, and N. Straker (1981). Psychological development of infants with severe combined immune deficiency in a reverse isolation environment. *Proc. Seventy-Second Annu. Mtg. Am. Assoc. Cancer Res. and Seventeenth Annu. Mtg. Am. Soc. Clin. Oncol.* Washington, D.C., April 30–May 2, 1981, 22:398 (Abstract C-259).

Popkin, M.K., V. Stillner, L.W. Osbor, C.M. Pierce, and J.T. Shurley (1974). Novel behaviors in an extreme environment. *Am. J. Psychiatry* 131:651–54.

Powazek, M., J.R. Goff, and J. Schyung (1978). Emotional reactions of children to isolation in a cancer hospital. *J. Pediatr.* 92:834–37.

Shurley, J.T. (1960). Profound experimental sensory isolation. *Am. J. Psychiatry* 117:539–45.

Simons, C., K. Kohle, V. Genscher, and M. Dietrich (1973). The impact of reverse isolation on early childhood development. *Psychother. Psychosom.* 22:300–309.

Solkoff, N.M., S. Yaffe, D. Weintraub, and B. Blase (1969). Effects of handling on the subsequent development of premature infants. *Dev. Psychol.* 1:765–68.

Spitz, R. (1945). Hospitalism: An inquiry into the genesis of psychiatric conditions in early childhood: I. *Psychoanal. Study Child* 1:53–74.

Spitz, R. and K.M. Wolf (1946). Anaclitic depression: An inquiry into the genesis of psychiatric conditions in early childhood: II. *Psychoanal. Study Child* 2:313–42.

Teller, W.F., W. Genscher, H.D. Flad, G. Hochapfel, R.P. Huget, D. Krieger, R. Wilson, K. Kohle, C. Simons, T.M. Flieoner, and F. Trepel (1973). Rearing of noniden-tical twins with lymphogenic hypogammaglobulinaemia under gnotobiotic conditions. *Acta Paediatr. Scand.* 240(Suppl.):5–45.

Ziskind, E. (1965). An explanation of mental symptoms found in acute sensory deprivation: Research 1958–1963. *Am. J. Psychiatry* 121:939–46.

Zuckerman, J. (1964). Perceptual isolation as a stress situation. *Arch. Gen. Psychiatry* 11:255–76.

# 13

## Lung Cancer

Jimmie C. Holland

Lung cancer has two psychological dimensions of particular concern: its devastating effect on the person and family, and its common relationship to a specific behavior—cigarette smoking. It is the single most preventable tumor and its control would substantially reduce the mortality from cancer in this country. However, cessation of smoking among smokers and prevention of the habit in young people has not been easy. It is estimated that 83% of lung cancer (85% in men, 75% among women) is related to cigarette smoking. Those who smoke two or more packs of cigarettes a day have 15–25 times greater lung cancer mortality than nonsmokers. In fact, smoking can be held accountable for 30% of all cancer deaths.

Lung cancer is the leading cause of cancer death in men aged 35 years or older. It has recently become the leading cause of cancer deaths in women, in some states surpassing breast cancer, which has been the leading killer for over 50 years. Age-adjusted lung cancer deaths in the United States are doubling approximately every 15 years. As evidence of the import of this neoplasm in twentieth-century America, Fig. 13-1 shows the precipitous rise in deaths since 1930, first in men and more recently in women (Minna et al., 1985). To provide effective psychological support, it is essential to have some knowledge of the disease, its prognosis, and treatment by histological type. A brief overview follows.

## MEDICAL BACKGROUND

Most cases of lung cancer arise from one of four cell types: epidermoid or squamous-cell carcinoma, small-cell (oat-cell) carcinoma, adenocarcinoma, and large-cell (anaplastic) carcinoma. Epidermoid or squamous-cell carcinoma is more prevalent in surgical series because it is subject to earlier detection by surgical resection and thus there is a better survival rate for the patient than with the other major cell types. Small-cell carcinomas are more often identified by biopsy and cytological specimens. Adenocarcinomas, becoming more frequent because of their increase in women, develop in the periphery and are missed on bronchoscopic examination.

For squamous-cell tumors, the origin can be traced largely to sites of segmental bifurcations, where repeated injury and chronic inflammation associated with smoking cause changes over many years. They are characterized first by metaplasia or dysplasia, carcinoma in situ, and, years later, by actual carcinoma. Other agents promote these changes as well, particularly asbestos. When chronic smoking and asbestos exposure are combined, they have a synergistic promoting effect on the malignant change.

The best prognosis is associated with squamous-cell tumors; adenocarcinoma has the next best prognosis, and large-cell tumors the poorest. Oat-cell carcinoma, with its characteristic small lymphocytelike cells, has responded well to chemotherapy in recent years, although it previously had a particularly poor prognosis because of its early hematological spread. In terms of overall 5-year survival, figures remain grim. With resection, the best survival with epidermoid carcinoma is 37% (Minna et al., 1985). Early diagnosis of a small (likely early) lesion offers the best prospect. Health professionals need to be alert for the common signs and symptoms of lung cancer, especially in patients who are smokers. Cough, hemoptysis, or dyspnea may be ignored or denied as significant by the individual, despite intellectually recognizing the symptom as one of the warning signs of cancer (Table 13-1). Symptoms outlined in Table 13-1 associated with spread should also be familiar to those working with lung cancer patients.

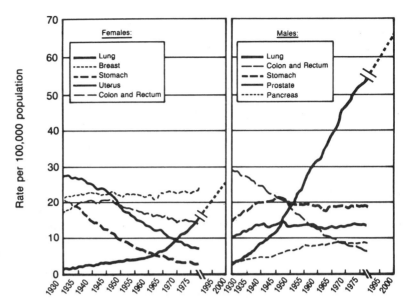

**Figure 13-1.** Age-adjusted cancer death rates for selected sites, United States. *Source:* Reprinted with permission from J.D. Minna, G.A. Higgins, and E.J. Glatstein (1985). Cancer of the lung. In V.T. DeVita, Jr., S. Hellman, and S.A. Rosenberg (eds.), *Cancer: Principles and Practice of Oncology,* 2nd ed. Philadephia: Lippincott, p. 508.

However, treatment in lung cancer of all types is limited in effectiveness because the majority of patients have inoperable tumors at the time of diagnosis. Even among those whose tumors are resectable, only 10% are cured; the remainder eventually develop local or distant metastases. In addition to surgery, treatment includes radiation, although it plays a largely palliative role for control of regional disease or an isolated metastasis. Recent successes have been seen in producing some long-term survivors of small-cell lung carcinoma by chemotherapy using vincristine, doxorubicin, and cyclophosphamide with and without radiation to the chest and cranial radiation, which is used often to prevent brain metastasis (Livingston, 1987). Interest in lung cancer treatment has also sparked new studies of the biology of the histological cell types; for example, small cell may arise from the amine precursor uptake and decarboxylation system (APUD tumors).

## NEUROPSYCHIATRIC AND PSYCHOLOGICAL ISSUES

### Neuropsychiatric Symptoms

There are two common medical complications that have neuropsychiatric manifestations. First, metastasis to brain is extremely common, occurring in 30–40% of patients with lung cancer. A sudden change in behavior or personality, forgetfulness, or slowed thinking should be cause for concern and neurological evaluation. Prophylactic cranial irradiation is now part of the treatment of small-cell carcinoma to prevent this common type of metastasis. However, among the few

long-term survivors of small-cell carcinomas who have had cranial irradiation, 75% have significant neurological and mental status changes with CT abnormalities (Johnson et al., 1985). Second, an aspect of lung cancer that bears attention of the mental health professional is the development with lung cancer of paraneoplastic syndromes, which affect other systems by indirect effects. Table 13-2 outlines the clinically manifest paraneoplastic syndromes, the systems affected, and the cell types associated with each. Of special interest are the endocrine syndromes, which account for 12% of paraneoplastic disorders and which produce neuropsychiatric symptoms [ectopic parathyroid hormone (PTH) and ectopic secretion of adrenocorticotrophic hormone (ACTH)]. The neurological-myopathic syndromes are only 1% of those observed, but the associated cortical degeneration produces mental changes of dementia. These interesting problems with psychiatric sequelae are reviewed in depth in Chapters 29 and 31.

### Psychological Reactions

#### DELAY AND DIAGNOSIS

Although chronic coughing, especially with hemoptysis, is a recognized danger sign of lung cancer, such a symptom is often ignored, especially by smokers. Fear also contributes to the delay in seeking a consultation for a symptom that might be from lung cancer. Pessimism and a fatalistic outlook about whether there is any effective treatment for lung cancer also contribute to delay. Other patients are asymptomatic, and a lesion

**Table 13-1**  Common signs and symptoms of lung cancer

*Symptoms secondary to central or endobronchial growth of the primary tumor*

Cough
Hemoptysis
Wheeze and stridor
Dyspnea from obstruction
Pneumonia from obstruction (fever, productive cough)

*Symptoms secondary to peripheral growth of the primary tumor*

Pain from pleural or chest wall involvement
Cough
Dyspnea on a restrictive basis
Lung abscess syndrome from tumor cavitation

*Symptoms related to regional spread of the tumor in the thorax by contiguity or by metastasis to regional lymph nodes*

Tracheal obstruction
Esophageal compression with dysphagia
Recurrent laryngeal nerve paralysis with hoarseness
Phrenic nerve paralysis with hemidiaphragm elevation and dyspnea
Sympathetic nerve paralysis with Homer's syndrome
Eighth cervical and first thoracic nerves with ulnar pain and Pancoast's syndrome
Superior vena cava syndrome from vascular obstruction
Pericardial and cardiac extension with resultant tamponade, arrhythmia, or cardiac failure
Lymphatic obstruction with pleural effusion
Lymphangitic spread through lungs with hypoxemia and dyspnea

*Source*: Reprinted with permission from J.D. Minna, G.A. Higgins, and E.J. Glatstein (1985). Cancer of the lung. In V.T. DeVita, Jr., S. Hellman, and S.A. Rosenberg (eds.), *Cancer: Principles and Practice of Oncology*, 2nd ed. Philadelphia: Lippincott, p. 517.

is found on a routine physical examination. Workup confirms the diagnosis. The initial response to such catastrophic news is disbelief and shock. This is followed by the recognition of the existential crisis, with anxious searching for the best treatment available. Periods of feeling depressed and hopeless alternate with others in which optimism supports the hope that all will be well. The diagnosis of cancer suddenly affects every aspect of life during the initial period, with continuing difficult adaptation over many weeks (Driever and McCorkle, 1984). A study from England found that 16% of patients, even prior to hearing the diagnosis, had symptoms of major depression, suggesting the likely awareness of the seriousness of their situation and anticipation of the diagnosis (Hughes, 1985).

The psychological management by the physician is critical at this juncture to encourage hope and pursuit of treatment. Hopelessness and a sense of having an incurable condition usually lead to major depression, apathy, withdrawal, and sometimes refusal of treatment for a possibly curable tumor.

## RESPONSES OF SMOKERS TO LUNG CANCER DIAGNOSIS

The emotional response to the diagnosis of lung cancer may be complicated by the self-inflicted origin of the disease with some patients who smoked. Some physicians, in expressing their frustration with individuals who continued smoking in the face of knowledge of the risk, become punitive, pointing out: "you brought it on yourself," or "it's too late now to discuss it." Nothing is gained and much is lost in the doctor–patient relationship by such attitudes when there is much

**Table 13-2**  Some clinically manifest paraneoplastic syndromes in lung cancer patients (histologic type of lung cancer predominantly associated with the syndrome)

*Systemic symptoms*

Anorexia–cachexia (31%)
Fever (21%)
Suppressed immunity

*Endocrine (12%)*

Ectopic parathyroid hormone hypercalcemia (epidermoid)
Inappropriate secretion of antidiuretic hormone: hyponatremia (small cell)
Ectopic secretion of ACTH: Cushing's syndrome (small cell)

*Skeletal*

Clubbing (29%)
Hypertrophic pulmonary osteoarthropathy: periostitis (adenocarcinoma) (1–10%)

*Neurologic-myopathic (1%)*

Myasthenic syndrome: Eaton–Lambert syndrome (small cell)
Peripheral neuropathy
Subacute cerebellar degeneration
Cortical degeneration
Polymyositis

*Coagulation-thrombotic (1–4%)*

Migratory thrombophlebitis, Trousseau's syndrome: venous thrombosis
Nonbacterial thrombotic (marantic) endocartitis: arterial emboli
Disseminated intravascular coagulation: hemorrhage

*Cutaneous (1%)*

Dermatomyositis
Acanthosis nigricans

*Hematologic (8%)*

Anemia
Granulocytosis
Leukoerythroblastosis

*Renal (<1%)*

Nephrotic syndrome
Glomerulonephritis

*Source*: Reprinted with permission from J.D. Minna, G.A. Higgins, and E.J. Glastein (1985). Cancer of the lung. In V.T. DeVita, Jr., S. Hellman and S.A. Rosenberg (eds.), *Cancer: Principles and Practice of Oncology* 2nd ed. Philadelphia: Lippincott, p. 525.

need on the patients' part for understanding and support. Some patients seek another doctor.

Most patients who are smokers are well aware of the role of their behavior in etiology. However, most seem to put it in perspective and do not experience painfully guilty feelings about it. Some, in whom the addiction is strong, continue to smoke. The smaller number who never smoked feel the unfairness of developing a tumor ordinarily associated with smoking. They may blame others who exposed them to side-stream cigarette smoke over many years, or they may be angry about an earlier occupational exposure, such as asbestos. Cooper (1984) quotes such a patient:

I feel some anger about the asbestos. I was a safety observer, a union steward, and I always fought it and the best I could do was to get them to x-ray our lungs each year. I wanted to completely get rid of asbestos. But you can't fight city hall, you know. I fought that a lot, but they never did anything about it. (p. 305)

Despite the resignation of the patient just described, a group of 38 patients who had pleural and peritoneal malignant mesothelioma associated with asbestos exposure had difficulty believing that their illness many years later was caused by their exposure to asbestos at work. Most had heard earlier about their increased risk but had not been concerned about it. Many had continued to smoke, despite being given information that it increased their risk of cancer (Lebovits et al., 1983).

A few patients suffer great regrets for having continued a habit that contributed to developing lung cancer.

### CASE REPORT

A 42-year-old housemaker and mother of two children, aged 8 and 10, had smoked heavily since her teenage years, in part because attempts to stop resulted in weight gain. Diagnosis of inoperable lung cancer led to profound guilt for what her children would experience by her premature death. She tearfully discussed wanting to make a videotape to tell young women about the risk of cigarette smoking "before it is too late."

## RESPONSES OF PATIENTS AND FAMILIES

Many patients are heartened by the knowledge of some celebrities, such as Arthur Godfrey, who had been cured of lung cancer. They are disheartened when famous people, such as Yul Brynner, die of lung cancer. The experiences of these individuals and their treatments are carefully assessed. Personal accounts of the struggle with lung cancer are far more frequently written today. Mack (1984), himself a surgeon, described his initial surgery for lung cancer, his complete remission for 2 years, and later recurrence. He found

positive aspects to the experience existing alongside the pain, as many others do.

One of the really ironic things about the human experience is that many of us have to face pain or injury, or even the possibility of death, in order to learn the real purpose of being and how best to live a rewarding life. My priorities, pleasures, and expectations began to change. I came to realize that I could have whatever aspiration I chose to have, in spite of the diagnosis of cancer. . . . I have spoken of my experience with cancer to many groups and have found that the insights into living with cancer that I have gained have become helpful to other people and to health-care workers responsible for such patients. (pp. 1642–43)

Most patients are reluctant to discuss their fears with their families. An outside source of psychological support is helpful initially to permit expression of the concerns about the future without upsetting other family members. However, the spouse may feel left out because emotions are not discussed and may need to be brought into discussions. The usual response to serious threat to life is greater closeness and a greater show of affection (Lieber et al., 1976). Chronic and severe symptoms of the ill family member often becomes a strain on the healthy member who must maintain other daily activities and care for an ill spouse.

Studies confirm that the next of kin, usually the spouse, experiences as many symptoms of distress as does the patient (Plumb and Holland, 1977). These include irritability, anger, nervousness, helplessness, and feelings of loneliness, vulnerability, and hopelessness. Adolescents may develop behavior problems in a family stressed by parental illness. Strong has provided an excellent guidebook for spouses (1988) and also has begun a vigorous, much needed national organization to address the needs of the spouses of chronically ill patients.

## INTERVENTIONS AND SYMPTOM CONTROL

Goldberg and Wood (1985) reported a controlled trial of psychotherapy with spouses of lung cancer patients, hypothesizing that this would also benefit the patient. They did not show any positive change on the psychosocial outcome measures chosen. The absence of benefit may have been due to methodological problems, or it may have been that the intervention that was given to every spouse was not needed by some; they would have shown no change in the levels of distress, masking the effect in those who were distressed and who benefited. Other studies have found that interventions are not needed or wanted by some patients and spouses, and likely should be offered only to those who have significant distress (see Chapter 38, "Psychotherapeutic Interventions").

The report by Goldberg and Wood also points out the complex design problem of control of variables, difficulty of giving a uniform intervention, and choice of outcome variables. It would appear to be a place where a therapeutic trial should be replicated because psychotherapy has been found helpful with other patients receiving largely palliative treatment for cancer, some of whom had lung cancer (Forester et al., 1985; Linn et al., 1982; Gordon et al., 1980; Bleeker, 1978).

After diagnosis, efforts to maintain equilibrium and hope are further frustrated by treatment side effects and disease symptoms, including weight loss, pain, anorexia, fatigue, cough, and shortness of breath. The crises continue unabated. Driever and McCorkle (1984) assessed lung cancer patients at 1, 2, and 6 months after diagnosis, comparing them to patients with myocardial infarction on qualitative measures of physical and psychological status. Even though patients with lung cancer had poorer physical status and more severe symptoms, they surprisingly maintained as positive an attitude as did the patients who had had a myocardial infarction.

Yates and colleagues (1980) followed a group of lung cancer patients who were managed at home during the advanced disease stage. They too largely remained optimistic despite advancing symptoms and diminishing physical status. Data showed that patients preferred care given at home, which was also less costly.

Advanced lung cancer requires careful attention to symptom control, particularly dyspnea, which is caused by obstruction, restrictions on breathing (e.g., pleural involvement), and, as a result of treatment toxicity, by pulmonary fibrosis and pneumonitis (Foote, et al., 1986).

An additional cause of dyspnea is emotional; efforts to breathe become absorbing and all attention is riveted on control of the breathlessness. Anxiety and panic develop, which increases the strain and makes the dyspnea worse. Many patients learn to use simple methods, with a nurse's help, to be more comfortable. A change in position, instruction in breathing, nasally administered oxygen, and drugs to relieve anxiety are efficacious (Brown et al., 1986). Time spent teaching both patient and family about simple management issues reduces distress. Arrangements for oxygen at home is also reassuring and helpful as needed for relief of hypoxia. Benzodiazepines in low doses reduce anxiety, as does morphine. Although concern for respiratory depression is appropriate, the sedation often is effective in reducing anxiety and respiratory suppression is not a problem in low doses. Steroids may reduce tumor edema; scopolamine is helpful to dry secretions and relax smooth muscles (Foote et al., 1986).

Management of terminal care at home is reviewed in Chapters 48 and 49 in detail. In lung cancer, however, communication to reassure patient and family of availability of a nurse on call who can consult with the doctor is essential because of the frightening nature of dyspnea.

Several rules for the mental health professional in managing advanced lung cancer are important. First, patients need to express fears, away from family; counseling visits are helpful for this. The visits allow for discussion of the difficulties in maintaining hope while fearful of the future, and having to weigh the potential risks and benefits of treatments offered. The sense that the therapist has a commitment to the patients, as does the medical staff, assures the patient of continued support, dispelling fears that the caretakers will lose interest as illness progresses. Second, communication, especially when the patient is being cared for at home, can become complicated as a result of the stress felt by the patient and the family. A psychiatric nurse clinician serves well in the liaison role connecting patient, family, doctor, and community resources (Chapter 49).

Third, family members should be monitored for how they are adapting to the altered family life, circumstances, and threat of loss. They should be seen, especially spouse and children, if symptoms suggest distress beyond normal levels. The ties that develop provide an important and immediately available resource for bereavement counseling when necessary (Chapter 50). Fourth, the patient must have frequent ongoing assessment of symptoms, both physical and mental, to control distress. Both depression and anxiety are common; pain and dyspnea require medication and assistance in tolerating them.

## QUALITY OF LIFE IN LUNG CANCER CLINICAL TRIALS

Chemotherapy is often given, and is particularly effective, in small-cell lung carcinoma. However, median survival remains short and for that reason, oncologists must give particular attention to quality of life, because most drug regimens are still largely palliative and are frequently not curative. Patients need to participate in the decision in such cases, in which the options are minimal or no treatment, a chemotherapy and radiotherapy combination known to be partially effective, or participation in a clinical trial of investigational agents through the National Cancer Institute (NCI). A study by Simes (1985) reviewed the Eastern Collaborative Oncology Group (ECOG) experience in non-small-cell lung cancer, in which median survival was 4.2 months, with 50% of the survival time spent on treatment by the protocol. He suggested that subgroups of patients could be identified who would likely receive no benefit, and he stressed the importance of obtaining a clear understanding of the patient's wishes in this situation in which encroachment on quality of life during expected short survival had to be weighed against the slight benefits.

The clinical trial, in situations in which the treatment is palliative, must include a measure of quality of life to assess the effectiveness of the treatments. A trial in the Cancer and Leukemia Group B (CALGB) randomly assigned patients to one of two chemotherapy regimens known to be active in treating lung cancer: (1) methotrexate, adriamycin, lomustine, and cyclophosphamide (MACC); or (2) adriamycin, lomustine, cyclophosphamide, and vincristine (CCV/AV). Identical chest and cranial irradiation was given to both groups (Maurer et al., 1985). Figure 13-2 shows equally poor survival of less than 25% at 36 months. However, quality of life measured by means of the Profile of Mood States (POMS) prior to treatment and at the end of induction at 15 weeks was the only outcome measure that differentiated the two treatments (Silberfarb et al., 1983). The psychological data showed that depression and fatigue were comparable on entry, but at 15 weeks, patients treated by the second regimen were more depressed (Table 13-3). This regimen contained vincristine. One interpretation is the neurotoxic effect of vincristine which altered biogenic amines. The vinca alkaloids may block the transport of dopamine β-hydroxylase, the terminal enzyme that converts dopamine to norepinephrine. The data show that it is important to measure quality of life in clinical trials, especially when treatments are palliative and comfort during treatment is important (Silberfarb, 1986).

An additional reason for measuring quality of life and psychosocial function in clinical trials is to permit

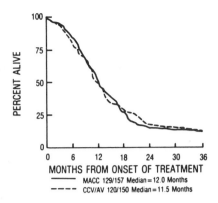

**Figure 13-2.** Survival comparison of MACC and CCV/AV regimens for all evaluable patients. Prognostic factor analysis influencing initial complete response and survival. *Source:* Reprinted with permission from L.H. Mauer, T. Pajak, W. Eaton, R. Comis, P. Chahinian, C..Faulkner, P.M. Silberfarb, E. Henderson, V.B. Rege, P.E. Baldwin, R. Weiss, S. Ratla, D. Prager, R. Carey, M. Perry, and N.C. Choi (1985). Combined modality therapy with radiotherapy, chemotherapy, and immunotherapy in limited small-cell carcinoma of the lung: a Phase III Cancer and Leukemia Group B study. *J. Clin. Oncol.* 3:969–76.

study of the interaction of psychological and physical variables. Cella and colleagues (1987) examined 45 patients treated in three CALGB protocols for limited (two protocols) or extensive (one protocol) small-cell lung carcinoma in whom the Profile of Mood States, a self-report of mood, was obtained on entry to the study and before the beginning of chemotherapy. It is of interest that whether patients' disease was extensive or limited, when their performance status was good, their total mood disturbance (distress) was equally low in both groups. It was only when extensive disease was

**Table 13-3** Mood change in 77 patients after receiving one of two cancer treatment regimens

| Mood‡ | Regimen 1* (n = 44) | | | Regimen 2† (n = 33) | | |
|---|---|---|---|---|---|---|
| | n | % | Significane§ | n | % | Significane§ |
| Depression | | | | | | |
| No change or decrease | 31 | 70 | p = .03 | 17 | 52 | N.S. |
| Increase | 13 | 30 | | 16 | 48 | |
| Fatigue | | | | | | |
| No change or decrease | 14 | 32 | p = .005 | 8 | 24 | p = .003 |
| Increase | 30 | 68 | | 25 | 76 | |

*A combination of methotrexate, adriamycin, lomustine, and cyclophosphamide given in two courses on days 1 and 21.

†A first course of cyclophosphamide, lomustine, and vincristine and a second course of adriamycin and vincristine.

‡Mood assessed according to the Profile of Mood States. Differences between the two regimens approached but did not reach statistical significance.

§Wilcoxon signed test.

*Source:* Reprinted with permission from P.M. Silberfarb, J.C. Holland, C. Anbar, G. Bahna, L.H. Maurer, A.P. Chahinian and R. Comis (1983). Psychological response of patients receiving two drug regimens for lung cancer. *Am. J. Psychiatry* 140:111.

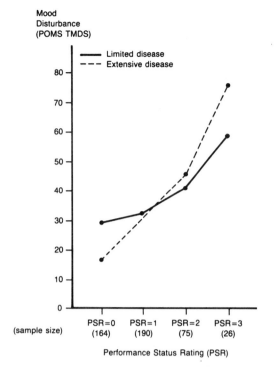

**Figure 13-3.** Mood disturbance as a function of performance status rating (PSR) in limited versus extensive disease. TMDJ = Total Mood Disturbance Scale. *Source:* Reprinted with permission from D.F. Cella, B. Orofiamma, J.C. Holland, P.M. Silberfarb, S. Tross, M. Feldstein, M. Perry, L.H. Maurer, R. Comis, and E.J. Orav (1987). Relationship of psychological distress, extent of disease, and performance status in patients with lung cancer. *Cancer* 60:1661–67.

accompanied by poor performance that distress became significantly greater than in those with equally poor performance, but with knowledge of limited disease status (Fig. 13-3). These data suggest that patients' knowledge of disease, even when it is extensive, is less distressing in the absence of disabling symptoms. When such symptoms occur, however, distress increases significantly more in patients who are aware of the extensive stage of their disease. Not surprisingly, the common concurrence of physical symptoms and knowledge of severe disease predicts greater distress in lung cancer patients.

## LONG-TERM SURVIVORS

There are few long-term survivors of lung cancer. Those who have survived often have a strong desire to help others. Their willingness to admit openly to having had lung cancer and to attempt to help others by description of their experience is enormously helpful to newly diagnosed lung cancer patients. Richard

Bloch, a philanthropist who was cured of lung cancer, has become an ardent crusader against cancer. He and his wife have written about the importance of seeking the best treatment, and maintaining a positive attitude (Bloch and Bloch, 1985). He joined in a venture with the NCI, which now provides a computer-generated list of current standard and investigational treatments for all tumors and where they are being used. Available now to physicians and patients as well by telephone, the Physician's Data Query (PDQ) is an outgrowth of a lung cancer survivor's commitment to assure treatment for others. (Telephone number 1-800-4-CANCER). Individuals who have survived a particularly lethal form of cancer often become important resources for help to others, particularly in encouraging constructive psychological responses (see Chapter 7).

Most long-term survivors are patients treated by combination chemotherapy and prophylactic cranial irradiation for limited small-cell lung cancers. The median survival for 21 such patients studied was 6 years after onset of therapy (range 2.4–10.6 years) (Johnson et al., 1985). Neurological symptoms were evident in 75%, 65% had abnormal neurological examinations, 65% had abnormal neuropsychological examinations, and 75% had abnormal CT scans. Progressive ventricular dilation or cerebral atrophy were major findings. Those at high risk of neurological complications were those patients who had high-dose induction chemotherapy at the time of cranial irradiation or who received greater radiotherapy fractions (>400 rad). Although risk of brain metastasis is reduced, long-term effects may significantly reduce mental acuity. Frytak and colleagues (1985) found magnetic resonance imaging superior to CT scanning to identify profound abnormalities in the periventricular white matter.

## SUMMARY

Lung cancer accounts for 30% of cancer deaths. The psychological dimension of lung cancer is greater than with other cancers because of the frequently self-introduced risk of cigarette smoking and because the psychological adjustment to a lung cancer diagnosis requires great resilience from the patient and family. Treatment today still leaves only a guarded prognosis for survival beyond 2 years. Existential concerns and coping with symptoms of fatigue, reduced activity, and dyspnea are difficult. Symptom control by skilled nursing is important, as is counseling for the patient and family. Paraneoplastic syndromes may cause unusual neuropsychiatric disturbance. Cranial radiation to prevent brain metastases, which are common, appears to cause significant changes in neurological function and mental acuity in the small group of survivors studied. It is important that treatments, especially those given in clinical trials, include measurement of quality of life to assess the negative effects on patients' lives of therapy that remains largely palliative.

## REFERENCES

Bleeker, J.A.C. (1978). Brief psychotherapy with lung cancer patients. *Psychother. Psychosom.* 29:282–87.

Brown, M.L., V. Carrieri, S. Janson-Bjerklie, and M.J. Dodd (1986). Lung cancer and dyspnea: The patients' perception. *Oncol. Nurs. Forum* 13:19–24.

Bloch, R. and A. Bloch (1985). Fighting Cancer. Kansas City, The Cancer Connection.

Cella, D.F., B. Orofiamma, J.C. Holland, P.M. Silberfarb, S. Tross, M. Feldstein, M. Perry, L.H. Maurer, R. Comis, and E.J. Orav (1987). The relationship of psychological distress, extent of disease, and performance status in patients with lung cancer. *Cancer* 60:1661–67.

Cooper, E.T. (1984). A pilot study on the effects of the diagnosis of lung cancer on family relationships. *Cancer Nurs.* 7:301–8.

Driever, M.J. and R. McCorkle (1984). Patient concerns at 3 and 6 months postdiagnosis. *Cancer Nurs.* 7:235–41.

Foote, M., D.L. Sexton, and L. Pawlik (1986). Dyspnea: A distressing sensation in lung cancer. *Oncol. Nurs. Forum* 13:25–31.

Forester, B., D.S. Kornfeld, and J.L. Fleiss (1985). Psychotherapy during radiotherapy: Effects on emotional and physical distress. *Am. J. Psychother.* 142:22–27.

Frytak, S., F. Earnest, B.P. O'Neill, R.E. Lee, E.T. Creagan, and J.C. Trautmann (1985). Magnetic resonance imaging for neurotoxicity in long-term survivors of carcinoma. *Mayo Clin. Proc.* 60:803–11.

Goldberg, R.J. and M.S. Wood (1985). Psychotherapy for the spouses of lung cancer patients: Assessment of an intervention. *Psychother. Psychosom.* 43:141–50.

Gordon, W.A., I. Freidenbergs, and I. Diller (1980). Efficacy of psychosocial interventions with cancer patients. *J. Consult. Psychol.* 48:743–59.

Hughes, J.E. (1985). Depressive illness and lung cancer: I. Depression before diagnosis. *Eur. J. Surg. Oncol.* 11:15–20.

Johnson, B.E., W.B. Goff II, N. Petronas, M.A. Krehbiel, R.W. Makuch, G. McKenna, E. Glatstein, and D.C. Inde (1985). Neurologic, neuropsychologic and computed cranial tomography scan abnormalities in 2- to 10-year survivors of small-cell lung cancer. *J. Clin. Oncol.* 3:1659–67.

Lebovits, A.H., A.P. Chahinian, and J.C. Holland (1983). Exposure to asbestos: Psychological responses of mesothelioma patients. *Am. J. Indust. Med.* 4:459–66.

Lieber, L., M.M. Plumb, M. Gerstenzang, and J.C. Holland (1976). The communication of affection between cancer patients and their spouses. *Psychosom. Med.* 38:379–89.

Linn, M.W., B.S. Linn, and R. Harris (1982). Effects of counseling for late-stage cancer patients. *Cancer* 49:1048–55.

Livingston, R.B. (1987). Carcinoma of the lung. In R.T. Skeel (ed.), *Handbook of Cancer Chemotherapy.* Boston: Little, Brown & Co., pp. 115–21.

Mack, R.M. (1984). Occasional notes: Lessons from living with cancer. *N. Engl. J. Med.* 311:1640–44.

Maurer, L.H., T. Pajak, W. Eaton, R. Comis, P. Chahinian, C. Faulkner, P.M. Silberfarb, G. Henderson, V.B. Rege, P.E. Baldwin, R. Weiss, S. Rafla, D. Prager, R. Carey, M. Perry, and N.C. Choi (1985). Combined modality therapy with radiotherapy, chemotherapy and immunotherapy in limited small-cell carcinoma of the lung: A Phase III Cancer and Leukemia Group B Study. *J. Clin. Oncol.* 3:969–76.

Minna, J.D., G.A. Higgins, and E.J. Glatstein, (1985). Cancer of the lung. In V.T. DeVita, Jr., S. Hellman, and S.A. Rosenberg (eds.), *Cancer: Principles and Practice of Oncology,* 2nd ed. Philadelphia: Lippincott, pp. 507–97.

Plumb, M.M. and J.C. Holland (1977). Comparative study of psychological function in patients with advanced cancer: 1. Self-reported depressive symptoms. *Psychosom. Med.* 39:264–75.

Silberfarb, P.M. (1986). Ensuring an optimal quality of life for lung cancer patients: A psychiatrist's perspective. In V. Ventafridda, F. van Dam, R. Yancik, and M. Tamburini (eds). *Assessment of Quality of Life and Cancer Treatment: Proc. Int. Workshop on Quality of Life Assessment and Cancer Treatment,* Milan, December 11–13, 1985. New York: Elsevier, pp. 145–50.

Silberfarb, P.M., J.C. Holland, D. Anbar, G. Bahna, L.H. Maurer, A.P. Chahinian, and R. Comis (1983). Psychological response of patients receiving two drug regimens for lung carcinoma. *Am. J. Psychiatry* 140:110–11.

Silverberg, E. (1987). Cancer statistics. *CA* 34:7–23.

Simes, R.J. (1985). Risk–benefit relationships in cancer clinical trials: The ECOG experience in non-small-cell lung cancer. *J. Clin. Oncol.* 3:462–72.

Strong, M. (1988). *Mainstay: For the Well Spouse of the Chronically Ill,* Boston: Little Brown & Co.

Yates, J.W., B. Chalmer, and F.P. McKegney (1980). Evaluation of patients with advanced cancer using the Karnofsky performance status. *Cancer* 40:2220–24.

# 14

# Breast Cancer

Julia H. Rowland and Jimmie C. Holland

Without question, breast cancer is the most widely studied cancer with respect to its psychological impact. In part this is because it is the most common cancer in women, affecting 1 in every 9; also, it is because this disease threatens an organ that is intimately associated with self-esteem, sexuality, and femininity, psychological issues of paramount concern to ill and healthy women alike. There is, however, another reason why breast cancer has featured so prominently in the psychological literature on cancer. Studies in this area serve as a paradigm for research in psychooncology: all three cancer treatment modalities are used in treating and controlling the disease (surgery, radiotherapy, and chemotherapy); major changes have occurred in the understanding and treatment of the disease, as well as in the type of rehabilitative options offered; increasing numbers of women are living longer with the disease controlled; the broad age range at time of diagnosis means that patients and their families cover the developmental spectrum; a large number of professionals are involved in the care of these patients; finally, social advocacy and local legislation have had a dramatic impact on patient management.

Breast cancer is a significant stress for any woman. Women vary widely, however, in their response to diagnosis and treatment. It is important for medical staff to understand both the normal emotional responses and the influences that contribute to them, as well as the range, nature, and types of abnormal responses and those characteristics that place women at high risk for poor adaptation. This chapter covers the issues of the influence of social context, psychological and medical variables that contribute to the psycholog-

ical response, and the usual responses of women to each phase of breast cancer from diagnosis through treatment and rehabilitation. In addition, the special problems of the impact of breast cancer on female relatives (especially children) and the debate about whether personality contributes to breast cancer risk or length of survival are reviewed.

## FACTORS CONTRIBUTING TO PSYCHOLOGICAL RESPONSE

### Sociocultural Context

#### HISTORICAL BACKGROUND

In order to understand the stresses on women facing breast cancer, it is helpful to view their experience from a historical perspective. Until the past decade, radical or modified radical mastectomy was the standard treatment for primary breast cancer in the United States and most of the Western world. In the earlier period, women were told at the time of diagnostic workup that they had something ''suspicious'' in the breast. They gave permission at the time of admission to the hospital for a biopsy to be performed under anesthesia and, if necessary, a mastectomy to be done at the same time—provided that results of the frozen specimen were positive. The woman did not know the outcome of the combined procedure until she awakened in the recovery room. Mastectomy often resulted in significant physical limitation due to lymphedema of the affected arm and a deformed ''washboard'' chest wall. Early psychological studies carried out at Memorial Sloan-Kettering Cancer Center and elsewhere showed that, following radical mastectomy, women had significant postoperative depression, anxiety, poor self-esteem, and impaired physical and sexual function (Bard and Sutherland, 1955; Schottenfeld and Robbins, 1970; Craig et al., 1974). In addition to confronting their major surgical defect,

---

1. This chapter was adapted from J.C. Holland and J.H. Rowland (1987). Psychological reactions to breast cancer and its treatment. In J.R. Harris, S. Hellman, I.C. Henderson, and D.W. Kinne (eds). *Breast Diseases*. Philadelphia: Lippincott, pp. 632–47.

these women had few social or psychological supports beyond those available from their own family. The taboos associated with cancer in general and the breast as a sexual organ, dictated that the diagnosis of breast cancer be kept a secret, largely precluding discussion of it with others. Nor was there likely detailed discussion between physician and patient concerning prognosis; often women were assured that all the malignant cells had been removed and only minimal follow-up was necessary. As a consequence of a number of major changes in the primary treatment of breast cancer largely brought about by greater public involvement in health care, women's experience with breast cancer today is very different.

In the early 1970s, a debate arose about the use of breast-conserving surgical procedures for the treatment of breast cancer; early data suggested that survival with this approach was comparable to that achieved with more radical surgery (Crile, 1974). Controlled clinical trials conducted under the auspices of the National Surgical Adjuvant Breast Project (NSABP) and under the leadership of Bernard Fisher provided data supporting an approach to primary breast cancer treatment aimed at achieving maximal opportunity for disease-free survival, best possible cosmetic effect, and absence of compromise of chance for cure (Fisher and Barboni, 1982). Fisher pointed out that recognition of breast cancer as a systemic disease eroded the premise on which radical breast surgery had been based and which had previously led surgeons in the past to attempt to remove "the last cancer cell."

In the past decade there has been a shift in the medical community away from mastectomy as the uniform and standard treatment for primary breast cancer (Veronesi et al., 1981; Harris et al., 1978). Newer approaches, though characterized by a greater degree of therapeutic uncertainty, have involved greater use of more breast-conserving procedures combined with irradiation. Comparable survival has been reported, although a thorough assessment of these newer treatment approaches is necessarily limited by a shorter follow-up period. This uncertainty, the widely reported differences of opinion among breast cancer "experts" about optimal treatment, and the survival statistics, which are less than desirable with either treatment regimen, have been widely shared with the public, and with women in particular, through the popular press. "Consensus" meetings about breast cancer treatment, which have helped in establishing policy, have emphasized to women that no currently available procedure is likely to ensure 100% survival, a fact not previously widely discussed in public.

These changes in the approach to medical management of primary breast cancer were paralleled by equally dramatic alterations in societal attitudes toward the disease during the 1970s. In 1974 Betty Ford and Happy Rockefeller publicly acknowledged having been treated for breast cancer. Mrs. Ford permitted disclosure that she had received adjuvant chemotherapy because of the presence of positive axillary nodes. In the wake of these revelations, women began to call their surgeons to inquire about details of their mastectomy, specifically wanting to know their definitive diagnosis, the extent of disease spread, and whether they also had positive axillary nodes. At about the same time, several autobiographical accounts of individual women's confrontation with breast cancer were published, bringing the disease further into the public eye (Kushner, 1975; Rollin, 1977). Reach to Recovery, the first woman-to-woman support program and an important self-help model, grew tremendously in the 1970s under the aegis of the American Cancer Society (Markel, 1971). These events occurred in the context of an increasingly active women's movement, which encouraged greater participation by women in decisions about their medical care in general, and about breast cancer treatment in particular. The more focused advocacy of women's groups was mirrored in the broader societal support for patients' rights to participate in treatment decisions. Both movements brought with them increasing emphasis on ethical issues and patient autonomy. Laws were introduced to assure this right. The proliferation of women's magazines served to underscore the responsibility of women to demand these rights. In addition to emphasizing women's need to take charge of their bodies, these publications in their health sections often advocated demanding specific treatments and being knowledgeable about current cancer treatments and the controversies about them.

The result of these changes is a vastly altered sociocultural climate for women dealing with breast cancer. Table 14-1 summarizes the change in focus of the problems faced by women 15–20 years ago as compared to those issues that are the focus today. The emotional problems are different today, but equally compelling. Although fears about breast loss and threat to body image and sexual function have decreased with the introduction of breast-conserving treatment techniques, fears and anxieties about having made the right treatment choice and about the likelihood of survival have increased. A change that is integral to the initial emotional burden today is the patient's increased level of participation in primary treatment decisions.

## DECISION-MAKING PATTERNS

Today, women diagnosed with breast cancer will likely be aware of the plurality of views about primary

**Table 14-1** Changes in the psychological issues in primary breast cancer treatment: past and present

| 15–20 years ago | The present |
| --- | --- |
| Fears of breast cancer and mastectomy | Fears of breast cancer and choice of treatment options |
| One-stage biopsy with or without mastectomy under anesthesia | Knowledge of two-stage procedure and two treatment options (mandated by law in some states) |
| Little participation in treatment decision | Full participation in care and choices made by patient |
| Little or no discussion of survival or prognosis | Full disclosure of survival prognosis |
| Full reassurance about future; minimal follow-up | Limited emphasis on reassurance about future; emphasis on frequent and long-term observation |
| Minimal social support or special rehabilitative programs | Access to self-help and support groups; availability of reconstruction; information that node negative women should receive chemo or hormone therapy |

breast cancer treatment. Most will recognize that no "best" treatment exists, but rather they have various options, and their preference with respect to each can be considered. Women now also have more access to precise survival statistics associated with each mode of treatment, although physicians consulted may offer quite different interpretations of the available data. Although the increased dialogue between physician and patient regarding diagnosis and care eases some of the stresses formerly faced by women, it also poses a new psychological burden, often at a time when anxiety is already great.

The steps through which a well-informed woman may go today before the primary breast cancer treatment begins to highlight these new psychological problems (Fig. 14-1). Most women consult their gynecologist or a trusted and accessible physician when they find a lump (80% of which are found by women themselves). A mammogram may then be ordered, and, depending on its outcome, the woman may be advised of "suspicious" findings and referred to a surgeon. In a growing number of states (including California, Massachusetts, Wisconsin, New Jersey, New York, and Virginia), the law and clinical practice dictates that the surgeon must inform the woman that she has the option of a two-stage surgical procedure, which separates the diagnostic biopsy from the primary treatment procedure allowing her time to adjust and consider options. In these six states listed, the two treatment options of mastectomy or lumpectomy with irradiation must be presented as well. Some insurance carriers

mandate a second opinion prior to the performance of any elective surgical procedure. Although these policies provide a valuable impetus for women to obtain thorough medical evaluation and information, they also serve to introduce yet another set of opinions.

During the diagnostic workup period, the woman must cope simultaneously with the need to keep her distressing emotions of anxiety and fear within tolerable limits while making the difficult decision about treatment for a disease that she knows may be fatal. To accomplish this, she must assimilate new medical information that, in itself, produces anxiety. One study has shown that before and after breast biopsy, anxiety and information overload compromise some women's decision-making ability, making informed decisions difficult, even at best (Scott, 1983). Valanis and Rumpler (1985) have provided a thoughtful review of the many issues faced by women in choosing among breast cancer treatment alternatives. They note that a woman's previous experiences, her personal and demographic characteristics, as well as those of her social support network (family and friends) and her physician influence her treatment selection. Research by Penman and colleagues (1984) emphasized the importance of the doctor–patient relationship in the decision-making process. In a multicenter study of patients' perceptions of giving informed consent for chemotherapy, they found that the information conveyed verbally by the doctor played a principal role in patients' efforts to arrive at a decision about treatment and that the written consent form contributed little. The primary reason cited for accepting the treatment outlined was "trust in the physician who discussed this treatment with me"; 86% said they relied strongly on the doctor's recommendations. This study also highlighted the apparent preference of some patients to assume a passive or acquiescent stance in making a decision.

The current climate which dictates that full and complete disclosure of information be given by the doctor, in a uniform manner to all women, fails to take into account the wide variation in women's reactions to the information and the range of ways of dealing with the decisions about treatment. Ideally, the method of giving information should be individualized for each patient. The emphasis on informed decision making places a heavy responsibility on the physician to be cognizant of the individual patient's physical and psychological needs, and to tailor the discussion and recommendations with that in mind. At least four response types among women (presented as extremes to highlight differences) can be delineated, each of which calls for an intervention or communication approach that is quite different.

**Type 1:** *"You decide for me, Doctor."* This is apt to be an older woman who has been accustomed

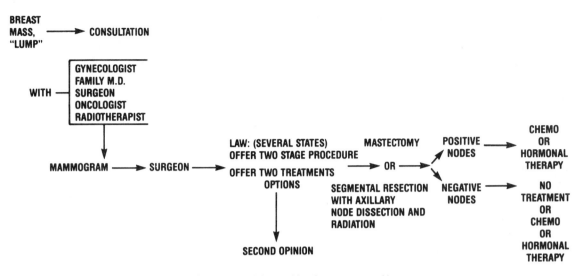

Figure 14-1  Steps in decision making for treatment of breast cancer.

to accepting the authority (and decisions) of the physician. She may be (or may choose to remain) less well informed about treatment options. She will cope best with a physician who outlines options but who accepts a strong role in the decision. She will do poorly with the "come back in a week and let me know your decision" stance. Because she relates to a generation taught to expect the physician to recommend treatment, such a stance is interpreted as "the doctor doesn't know what to do" and is seen as frightening.

**Type 2:** "*I demand you do the . . . procedure.*" This response is common among young women who are more medically sophisticated, have consulted all available resources, obtained all relevant materials, and have already made a decision, in keeping with their wish to assume an assertive role. These patients are often ready to assume an adversarial position if their requests are not heard or adopted. This response may be troublesome to the conscientious physician who may have to object to the patient's demands as inappropriate on sound medical grounds. Such a woman needs to be treated as a full participant in the decision process, and may need to be given a careful outline of the relevant medical data, often supplemented upon request by written materials from authoritative sources, with which she can assure herself of the facts. Discussing the op-

tions, listening and responding to questions, and detailing the limits of the available options, based on data, will maximize the possibility that *both* the patient's and the physician's points of view will be heard, and a relationship of mutual respect will be established, allowing a true, shared decision to be reached.

**Type 3:** "*I can't decide.*" This response is seen in women who feel overwhelmed by the knowledge that they have a breast lump and are frightened by its threat to life or its threat to their intact body; in such cases the options are often too painful to consider. These women are often referred for psychiatric consultation. It is helpful for them to have the pressure temporarily removed by postponing surgery and to be able to review the events and possible treatments in a setting where they feel secure in expressing concerns, recognizing that they must come to some closure. A useful procedure is to take them, step by step, through the consequences and ramifications of each treatment option, asking at each juncture "How would you respond to that?" By this approach, with reduced anxiety, it usually becomes clear that certain aspects of one or the other treatment are more acceptable to the patient. These women can then return to their surgeon ready to proceed with the therapy.

**Type 4:** "*Given the options, your recommendations*

*and my preferences, I choose. . . .''* This reaction suggests a mature patient who is anxious but who is able to engage in a constructive interaction with the physician to arrive at a thoughtful decision. The exposition of relevant facts with pamphlets and discussion of all facets of the treatment and outcome, leads to a decision.

Clearly, there is room for improvement in the present manner by which primary breast cancer treatment is presented. Some helpful ways that the current decision-making process could be improved are outlined.

1. *Information.* Attention should be given to developing videotapes and written materials that extend the information provided by those currently available.
2. *Breast diagnostic clinic.* Major cancer centers, where many second opinions are given, could organize weekly clinic hours during which the participation of a surgeon, pathologist, and radiotherapist was assured. This multispecialty consultation could occur over a period of hours rather than the usual weeks, thus eliminating the attendant prolonged lack of clear recommendations that currently occurs. The availability of a skilled counselor who is knowledgeable about breast cancer would assure needed emotional support.
3. *Nurse-specialist in breast cancer.* A nurse knowledgeable in breast cancer management who is sensitive to the psychological concerns of patients could provide an extremely valuable service in physicians' offices, expediting the discussion of options, listening to fears, assessing emotional stability in the decision-making process, supporting a doctor's recommendations, helping the patient to formulate questions, and correcting misinformation. The nurse could then convey information to the physician about the patient's psychological state, her ability to participate in the decision, and even her likely preferences, resulting in a more productive discussion between patient and physician.
4. *Research.* Studies of the decision-making process and the methods by which information about treatment options is conveyed to ensure effective communication while remaining sensitive to the needs of different patients are needed. As legal and ethical constraints change medical practice in this area, it is imperative that we learn more about the decision process—in part, to influence the legal authorities to develop laws that recognize individual differences and medical changes. Fisher points out that the mandate for a two-stage biopsy procedure, legislation that was originally intended

to safeguard patient's options, may now be a hindrance to optimal treatment (Fisher, 1985).

On a reassuring note, it should be mentioned that research by Ashcroft and co-workers (1985) revealed that, given the choice of mastectomy or limited resection plus radiotherapy, women opting for either type of treatment had done well. Levels of anxiety and depression for both groups were similar to those in other surgical patients. Evidence of profound anxiety and depression reported in other studies was also absent at 1-year follow-up. The authors point out, however, that women choosing one treatment or the other may focus on different needs and concerns, an issue discussed later in the chapter.

## Psychological Variables

In an excellent review of the published studies on the psychosocial correlates of breast cancer and its treatment, Meyerowitz (1980) identified the psychosocial impact of breast cancer as falling into three broad areas: psychological discomfort (anxiety, depression, and anger), changes in life patterns (consequent to physical discomfort, marital or sexual disruption, and altered activity level), and fears and concerns (mastectomy and death). Meyerowitz summarized the nature and direction of the impact of these variables on premorbid and postmastectomy adjustment. A commonality of opinion and observation emerges despite the fact that findings from most studies lacked a conceptual and historical framework. In addition to these variables which are important in psychological adaptation, the variables of the life stage at which the cancer occurs, previous emotional stability (personality and coping style), and the presence and availability of interpersonal supports should be included.

The point in the life cycle at which breast cancer occurs, and what social tasks are threatened or interrupted are of prime importance. The threat to a sense of femininity and self-esteem occurs in all women, but it may be more difficult for a young woman whose attractiveness and fertility are paramount, especially for those who are single and without a partner. In most instances, the meaning of the breast cancer is quite different for her than for the older woman who has a secure home and family, and for whom the risk to life may be predominant. However, that breast cancer occurs frequently in the older woman who is more apt to be experiencing other losses, particularly loss of a spouse, means that she will have to adjust not only to a concurrent major loss in her life, but also to a threat to her own life and body integrity. Preliminary reports by Fotopoulis and Cook (1980) of data from a multicenter study of the ''Psychological Aspects of Breast Cancer'' showed a high level of distress in older women.

The second variable contributing to adaptation relates to the patient herself, that is, her personality and coping patterns. Each woman has her own style of adaptation to stress, shown to be a remarkably abiding quality. In a study by Gorzynski and colleagues (1980) of women evaluated before biopsy for breast cancer and then 10 years later, coping styles and effectiveness in controlling emotional distress remained unchanged over time. The coping strategies that have been found to be most effective in managing the stresses of breast cancer have been identified by Penman (1980). Her research showed these strategies to be a cluster of behaviors, identifiable in the immediate postmastectomy period and characterized by a ''tackling stance'' to the problems raised by diagnosis and surgery. Those women who use avoidance and capitulation, rather than ''confrontational'' coping strategies, are more emotionally distressed in the early rehabilitative stages after mastectomy than are women who deal more directly with the stress. Moreover, women who have a sense of control over events, actively taking a role in rehabilitation, adjust better than those with a helpless outlook (Levy et al., 1985). A pessimistic response usually reflects prior psychological patterns of poor coping with stressful events. Women who have had prior psychiatric illness are at risk of not only exacerbation of previous symptoms but a more troubled and less adaptive response to breast cancer. Data from a large multicenter sample, compiled by Bloom and co-workers (1987) showed that when women with a preexisting psychiatric disorder were eliminated from a study of adaptation to breast cancer, there was an absence of serious psychopathological sequelae in the year following mastectomy. Schain (1985) found that poor adaptation was associated with previous unsatisfactory or negative sexual experiences, overly intense emotional investment in breasts, problems in body image, and difficulty discussing personal, especially sexual, problems.

Adaptation is also altered when a woman has a prior association with breast cancer. The memory of a mother or grandmother's death from breast cancer, or close friends, makes the diagnosis seem far more ominous. Some women with a high investment in their bodies cannot tolerate even the idea of loss or damage to a breast. Such women are at risk for delay in seeking consultation when a symptom occurs; they may also be at risk for problems in adaptation following treatment. Today, women who are at increased genetic risk of breast cancer or who have documented precancerous breast tissue changes must deal with the anxiety aroused by regular breast self-examination, routine physician visits, and regular mammography examinations. Reactions vary from denial of risk and noncompliance with surveillance measures to hypochondriacal preoccupation with checking the breasts repeatedly for lumps. Some of these women are candidates for a prophylactic mastectomy, after careful psychiatric evaluation.

Adjustment also depends on the response from other significant people—first and foremost from spouse or partner, but also from family and friends (Bloom, 1982; Peters-Golden, 1982; Wortman, 1984). In their study of men's adjustment to breast cancer, Wellisch and colleagues (1978) found that although they managed well overall, a subgroup remained distressed following their mate's mastectomy. Men who gave least support to their partners were those who had significant psychiatric problems, especially substance abuse, a history of infidelity, or abuse, an inability to tolerate the strain produced by their mate's increased dependency needs, or a chronic pattern of poor communication. It was helpful to the relationship when the partner participated in the decision about treatment, visited after the operation, saw the scar early, helped with dressings, and resumed sexual relations early. Sabo and colleagues (1986) found that the tendency for some men to assume a ''protective-guardian'' stance was sometimes detrimental to effective and open communication. These observations about better adaptation with adequate social support are of even greater interest in light of information that social support affects mortality (Marshall and Funch, 1983; see also Chapter 5 on social support and Chapter 60 on risk factors in cancer and survival).

Support from other women who had been through the experience of mastectomy served as the basis for the highly effective Reach-to-Recovery program which is now international in scope. The program has now been broadened to provide peer visitors who can offer advice and support for women undergoing breast reconstruction or segmental resection and irradiation. The closer the visitor's experience is to that of the patient, the better her ability to provide an effective role model for coping and to serve as a source of practical and emotional support. Many institutions are adopting programs that combine the use of peer and professional support in group counseling to promote optimal psychological and physical recovery during initial hospitalization (Euster, 1979; Scott and Eisendrath, 1985–1986).

Some women have phobias of anesthesia or surgery, and fear the operating room, loss of control, or death during surgery. These individuals may have greater psychological difficulties and require special psychological management for successful treatment. A careful medical, family, and psychiatric history will reveal these or other influences that put a woman at risk for greater emotional distress.

## Medical Variables

Psychosocial adjustment also depends on the stage of breast cancer found at the time of diagnosis, the treatment required, the likely prognosis, and the rehabilitative opportunities available. Central to all, however, is the relationship to a supportive surgeon, radiotherapist or oncologist who is sensitive to the concerns of the patient and who monitors emotional as well as physical well-being. The office or clinic nurse and hospital staff become the patient's "second family," at times buffering and compensating for the absence of a more substantive physician–patient relationship or family support. In a model developed at Montefiore Hospital, nurse clinicians were trained to provide not only continuity of care but also to serve as advocates for their breast cancer patients (Wieder et al., 1978). Faulkner and Maguire (1984) demonstrated that ward nurses, trained to monitor and manage psychological problems of their breast patients, were highly effective. Secretaries, as well as radiotherapy technicians, also contribute to the social environment which the patient experiences.

Changes in primary breast cancer treatment and rehabilitative options have changed the experience of women today so substantially that the extensive literature on adjustment to mastectomy, particularly radical mastectomy, applies to a far lesser degree. Newer treatments which conserve breast tissue, and the potential for breast reconstruction, have likely reduced fears somewhat, leading to the speculation that women seek early diagnosis and treatment more readily than in the past when they delayed seeking consultation out of anxiety. Reactions to each of the primary treatment options are discussed in greater detail.

## MASTECTOMY

Because mastectomy was for so long the standard of care in treating breast cancer, and still continues to be recommended for large numbers of women, early psychosocial literature on breast cancer was devoted almost exclusively to understanding the physical, social, and emotional consequences of the loss of one or both breasts. (For excellent reviews of this material, see Meyerowitz, 1980; Holland and Mastrovito, 1980; Lewis and Bloom, 1978–1979.) Studies of adaptation that have occurred, despite variability in approach and

design, have noted a remarkable consistency in the concerns of women undergoing mastectomy: threat of a fatal disease; impact of the loss of breast on body image, and appearance; diminished sense of femininity; decrease in sexual attractiveness and function; fears of recurrence; and shame and guilt. Mourning for the loss of a cherished body part and the threat to life are universal, but the extent to which they are experienced is highly variable. Some studies indicated that between 10 and 56% of women studied after mastectomy had some degree of impairment of social and/or emotional function (Maguire, 1976; Polivy, 1977).

However, in a large prospective study, Bloom and collaborators (1987) compared levels of psychosocial functioning in four groups of women among whom there was no history of prior significant psychiatric disturbance or medical illness. The groups consisted of women who had had a mastectomy for stage I or II breast cancer ($n = 145$), women who had had a cholecystectomy for gallbladder disease (removal of a less emotionally significant organ) ($n = 90$), women following biopsy for benign breast disease ($n = 87$), and, a group who had had no operation in the prior year (healthy controls, $n = 90$). Although women with breast cancer showed greater psychological distress, related to social and interpersonal relationships, these emotionally healthy women did not experience serious psychiatric sequelae, such as suicidal ideation. Thus, women who are well adjusted before they have a mastectomy, and whose disease is in an early stage, can expect at one year to have a quality of life equal to unaffected peers. However, women in this study with stage II disease who received adjuvant chemotherapy after mastectomy had more distress throughout the year and at 12 months. Other predictors of poorer adaptation were additional concurrent illness or stress, expectation of poor support from others, and a tendency to perceive events in life as less under one's own control (Penman et al., 1986). Recognizing early these vulnerable patients should lead to prompt referral for individual counseling or a peer–patient support group.

More recently, research has focused on the impact of breast-conserving and restoring procedures on women's adjustment which, while diminishing the loss of breast tissue, present different but equally difficult psychological issues. Ganz and colleagues (1987) found that women at 4–5 weeks after modified radical mastectomy or limited resection with or without axillary dissection experienced similar physical and psychological problems. However, while the mastectomy group had more difficulty with self-image and clothing, the limited resection group reported more problems with disrupted social and recreational activities.

**Table 14-2** Controlled studies of psychological response to mastectomy (M) versus limited resection and radiation (L–R)

| Study | Subjects L–R | Subjects M | Satisfaction with body image | Marital adjustment | Satisfaction with sexual function | Psychological adjustment | Fear of recurrence |
|---|---|---|---|---|---|---|---|
| Sanger and Reznikoff (1981) | 20 | 20 Modified | L–R More positive feelings | Equal | — | Equal | — |
| Schain et al. (1983) | 18 | 20 Modified | L–R Less negative feelings | Equal | Equal | Equal | Equal (M = 80%; L–R = 83%) |
| Steinberg et al. (1985) | 21 | 46 Modified | L–R More positive feelings | Equal | L–R Report husbands more sexual | Equal depression, anxiety; L–R better in general | Equal |
| Bartelink et al. (1985) | 114 | 58 Radical | L–R Less self-conscious | — | L–R Less sexually inhibited | — | M Greater |
| Taylor et al. (1985) | 26 | 31 Simple/ Modified 9 Radical | L–R Less concerns about disfigurement | Equal | L–R Report more frequent sex, more affectionate husbands | L–R Best overall adjustment | — |
| Haes and Welvaart (1985) | 21 | 18 Radical | L–R Less negative feelings | Equal | Equal | Equal | Equal (older patients less fearful) |
| Wellisch, Silverstein and Hoffman (In press) | 22 | 30 Modified | L–R More positive feelings | Equal | L–R Higher libido | Equal | Equal |
| Baider et al. (1986) | 32 | 32 Modified | — | M slightly less conflict than L–R | Equal | Equal | — |
| Fallowfield et al. (1986) | 48 | 53 Modified | — | — | Equal | M slightly fewer problems (32% vs. 38% for L–R) | L–R more (?) |
| Ganz et al. (1987)* | 19 | 31 Modified | L–R More positive feelings | Equal | Equal | Equal | Equal |

*One month after surgery (prior to radiation).

## LIMITED RESECTION RADIATION

With a clearer understanding of the biology of breast cancer which showed that radical surgery did not address the frequent early occurrence of micrometastases, support grew in the late 1970s for more breast conserving procedures. As data showed equal survival of women treated by breast-conserving procedures, the frequency of their use escalated. Women, increasingly active in decision making, began to ask for these less extensive procedures as they felt more confident of the therapeutic results offered, and as those who had breast-conserving procedures reported their perceived better psychosocial function as compared to women having a mastectomy. A number of studies have compared the impact of both procedures on psychosocial and sexual function.

Steinberg et al. (1985) reviewed six "first-generation" studies in which adaptation of women undergoing limited resection and radiation versus those undergoing mastectomy was compared. In general, the studies showed that women who receive more breast-sparing surgery are less self-conscious, have a better body image, manifest a somewhat better overall adjustment, and report greater satisfaction with sexual activity. The results of these studies along with those of three others, are presented in Table 14-2 and are discussed briefly later. Despite the small numbers of women studied, data suggest that women receiving limited resection and radiation have, as a group, adapted well. However, some researchers feel that the emotional benefit associated with breast-conserving surgery, relative to more radical surgery, has been less than expected (Zevon et al., 1987). The differences at one month following mastectomy or limited resection (and prior to beginning radiation) were minimal, as reported by Ganz and colleagues (1987). At a month, both groups were still focused on physical discomfort.

In addition, there is some indication that the differences between treatment groups may diminish over time.

The studies reported by Schain and colleagues (1983) and Fallowfield and co-workers (1986) are of particular interest in that the women studied had all participated in a randomized trial in which they were assigned to receive either mastectomy or limited resection and radiation. Schain's data showed more positive feelings about body image in the limited resection and radiation group, but little difference with respect to other parameters of mental well-being, psychological symptoms, and fears of recurrence. In contrast, the Fallowfield report found no differences on any parameters between the two procedures. If anything, women in the limited resection group fared slightly worse, exhibiting slightly more depressive symptoms. Bartelink and co-workers (1985) reported more fears of recurrence in women who had a mastectomy, but all patients in their study had undergone a radical mastectomy. Observations from our clinical practice indicated a high level of fears of recurrence among the early cohort of women who exercised the option for limited surgery, often over their physicians' and families' protests. Many were advised by skeptical surgeons that they might be saving the breast but putting their lives in jeopardy. As Steinberg and colleagues (1985) note, these women were choosing an unpopular treatment, and thus likely differed from women choosing mastectomy. As the procedure has been more widely recommended by surgeons, and as longer observation periods continue to support the chances of equal survival, fears about choice have diminished. Other factors which have an impact on the decision process are attitudes about cancer and about radiation. The thought of leaving any tumor cells in the breast is intolerable for some women who believe that mastectomy offers them greater assurance that the cancer has been removed. Other women fear radiation or, as exemplified by Nancy Reagan's choice of mastectomy, do not wish to devote six weeks to daily radiation therapy treatments. They prefer to "have it over with" by undergoing one procedure and getting back to their lives.

Research by Ashcroft and associates (1985) and Margolis and Goodman (1984) suggested that certain personality characteristics also influence a woman's decision. Both groups of researchers found that women selecting limited resection and radiation were more concerned about insult to their body image, were more dependent on their breasts for self-esteem, and believed that they would have difficulty adjusting to loss of the breast by mastectomy. In contrast, patients choosing mastectomy more often perceived the breast containing cancer as foreign, and wanted to have it removed; they were also more fearful of the side effects of radiation.

The largest prospective group studied to date suggests that of women given the option of limited resection and radiation or mastectomy as the primary treatment, 51% chose mastectomy (Wolberg et al., 1987). These figures are comparable to our experience at Memorial Sloan-Kettering Cancer Center. Although it may be expected that as more women gain confidence in the breast conserving procedures there will be further shift in that direction, it is nevertheless important to recognize that a significant proportion of women, if given a choice, will still prefer to undergo a mastectomy.

One of the disadvantages of the limited resection and radiation approach is the greater demands it places on patients over a longer period. The resection may be followed by the axillary node dissection as a second procedure. Following healing, consultation occurs with a radiotherapist and leads to beginning daily visits to a radiotherapy department for treatments. For some women, the time spent is a small burden in order to keep the breast. Most women who fear radiation are reassured by the explanations offered during simulation. Fear of carcinogenesis secondary to radiation, of delayed cardiac toxicity (particularly with left-chest wall radiation) and contralateral breast cancer are legitimate concerns. Finally, the long-term satisfaction of women with limited resection and radiation has not been systematically assessed. Certainly for most women, having the breast is of great emotional benefit, but the breast often lacks normal sensitivity, softness, consistency, and contour. Expectation of a healthy normal breast may be met with disappointment.

Clinical experience at Memorial Sloan-Kettering suggests that many women undergoing breast conservation do not begin to feel the true emotional impact of the experience until they begin the daily routine of radiotherapy. They are "numb" throughout the crises of diagnosis and surgery. It is with the daily visits to the clinic, seeing others who are ill, and experiencing the fatigue that accompanies radiation that the reactive anxiety and depression begins to be experienced (M.J. Massie, personal communication). There is also an impression that these women who "saved their breast" are perceived as having had a less severe psychological trauma than the mastectomy patient and therefore receive less sympathy from physicians, staff, partner and family. Few studies have prospectively followed these women to examine their specific problems and plan for appropriate interventions to meet them. However, experience is growing that they are at higher risk of psychological disturbance than might be assumed.

For many women undergoing radiation therapy, initial anxiety is usually allayed after a few treatments. It often returns, however, when the end of treatment is approaching. (See Chapter 9) We have found that women fear the possibility of tumor regrowth without treatment. They also fear the loss of frequent, reassuring visits to the doctor. The 5-year survival rate is known to have less meaning in breast cancer because a recurrence may develop many years later. Thus, the fears of recurrence remain high in many women who have had breast cancer; they seem to be more severe and even more disabling than with other cancer sites.

The primary treatment of breast cancer by surgery and radiation includes chemotherapy as well for women who are found to have positive axillary nodes. This means chemotherapy or hormonal therapy added to the already long period of surgery followed by radiation. A Clinical Alert from the National Cancer Institute (May 1988) was sent to inform physicians that even some node negative women are candidates for chemotherapy or hormonal therapy. It appears that the psychological impact associated with primary breast cancer will be substantially increased for the increasing numbers of women who will experience all three modalities of treatment, whether they have spread to axillary nodes or not.

For every woman, discussion of the relative risks, survival, side effects, cosmetic outcome, personal preference and the physician's recommendations must be reviewed before a choice is made about mastectomy or limited resection and radiation. In some cases, excision and radiation will not yield the best cosmetic result; mastectomy, particularly in light of technological advances in plastic and reconstructive breast surgery, is possible for some.

## RECONSTRUCTION

An increasing number of women consider breast reconstruction following mastectomy. Interest in this procedure has grown as a result of several developments. The increasing use of more tissue-sparing primary treatment procedures has resulted in better surgical candidates for reconstruction; also, rapid advances in the technological aspects of the reconstructive surgery itself have led to the development of procedures to correct defects from more radical surgeries, diminished complications, and the achievement of more optimal, "breastlike" outcomes. Finally, as noted earlier, there is an increasing demand by women for greater participation in their own health care. Although it is generally estimated that fewer than 10% of women undergoing mastectomy also undergo recon-

struction, data collected by the American Society of Plastic and Reconstruction Surgeons (ASPRS) suggest that this trend may be changing, especially for women treated a number of years ago. In a survey publicized in May 1985, they reported that an estimated 98,000 reconstructions were performed by their 2600 member surgeons in 1984, up from 20,000 recorded in 1981, just 3 years earlier (ASPRS, 1985). Research conducted in 1980 by the National Cancer Institute on attitudes about breast cancer found that almost 40% of the women interviewed indicated that they would be interested in breast reconstruction should they face a mastectomy (National Survey on Breast Cancer, 1980). It should be pointed out, however, that this survey was conducted at a time when the breast conserving procedure and radiation was not a commonly available choice, at least in this country. Thus, it is not clear what proportion of women who reported interest in breast reconstruction might have indicated a desire for breast-conserving primary surgery if given a choice. These studies clearly need to be repeated.

As Schain and colleagues (1984) noted in their excellent review, psychosocial issues in breast reconstruction fall into the five major areas of informational, economic, medical, intrapsychic or self-determined needs, and interpersonal or other-determined needs. Considerable progress has been made in the availability of information about breast reconstruction to women, in contrast to an earlier period when there was reluctance to inform women about the option and a tendency to discourage them from seeking out individuals who had undergone reconstruction. A number of woman-to-woman support groups sprang up around this latter issue (e.g. AWEAR—Ask a Woman to Explain About Reconstruction, RENU—Reconstruction Education for National Understanding). Although the cost of these procedures has not diminished, coverage by health insurance carriers has increased, largely in response to pressure from health consumer and women's groups to reclassify the surgery as rehabilitative, not cosmetic. In addition, far fewer medical problems now preclude a woman from being a candidate for reconstruction.

The psychological variables associated with who does and does not seek reconstruction, and women's response to reconstruction, were studied at Memorial Sloan-Kettering in a joint effort by the Psychiatry, Plastic and Reconstructive Surgery, and Breast Services (Jacobs et al., 1983; Rowland et al., 1984). At the time of initial consultation, 150 women seeking reconstruction after mastectomy were evaluated on a number of surgical and psychological parameters; 83 of the 117 women undergoing reconstruction were reassessed postoperatively. In addition, a matched-comparison sample of 50 women who had not sought reconstruction were also studied.

On the interview and self-report, women seeking consultation for reconstruction were psychologically well adjusted and functioning at a high level. Although they harbored some emotional pain related to cancer and the mastectomy, they were generally well informed about the nature of the surgery and approached reconstruction with realistic expectations of potential benefits to them both psychologically and physically. The reasons most frequently cited for seeking surgery were to be rid of the prosthesis, to "feel whole again," and to reestablish symmetry and thus diminish self-consciousness about appearance. Many pursued it despite their partner or families efforts to dissuade them from further surgery. These motives have been echoed in other samples studied (Goin and Goin, 1981; Clifford, 1979).

The study's results largely underscored the positive effects of breast reconstruction. With few exceptions, the net effect of the surgery was to increase both observed and stated satisfaction with levels of psychological, social, and sexual function. Most of the women (83%) stated they were happy or absolutely delighted with the overall results, and most found that the surgical results met or surpassed their expectations.

Response to reconstruction was found to be independent of a woman's age, social class, or her surgeon's estimate of the success of the procedure. However, women who pursued this surgery primarily to please others or with the expectation of improving sexual and social relations were at risk of disappointment. Amount of time after surgery also modified response. Although the time since the mastectomy increased satisfaction with the overall results, the time since completion of reconstruction increased the likelihood of a more critical response both to the physical aspects of the surgery and to the net effect. Finally, it was felt that a woman's ability to obtain clear and complete preoperative information about the surgery outlined for her, especially with respect to all surgery proposed to achieve symmetry for the remaining breast, and to have the opportunity postoperatively to express dissatisfaction or explore fears and concerns about results were also potentially important influences on later satisfaction.

When data derived from the study of women not seeking reconstruction were compared with that for women seeking reconstruction, results indicated that the two groups resembled each other in many aspects. No differences were seen between the groups in general satisfaction, or with the ability to resume daily activities after the mastectomy, levels of self-esteem, feelings of attractiveness, sexual functioning, or self-reported psychological symptoms. Nonreconstructed patients reported greater comfort with external prosthesis use, had less knowledge about reconstruction, and attached greater importance to their breasts. There was also a suggestion that women in the reconstruction group felt that their husband or sexual partner more frequently avoided touching or looking at the mastectomy site than did the husbands or partners of the nonreconstructed group.

Further comparisons between women who consulted and went on to have reconstruction and those who sought consultation but later refused surgery for nonmedical reasons revealed some interesting differences. Those who refused surgery for nonmedical reasons tended to be older and of lower socioeconomic status, and more often were single. They appeared to have experienced greater psychosocial dysfunction consequent to their mastectomy, were at greater risk for psychiatric symptoms, and were more likely to have seen a therapist for emotional problems. Finally, they tended to have undergone more radical treatment for their breast cancer and therefore, were poorer candidates for plastic surgery. The differences in psychosocial and physical status between groups indicated that women who were at increased risk for subsequent emotional or surgical disappointment following reconstructive procedures may select themselves out at the time of consultation.

Concerns that women who were seeking these procedures did so because of neurotic or psychotic needs were not supported by our own or other investigators' research (Goin and Goin, 1981; Clifford, 1979). Most women sought surgery for personal reasons. The importance of "personal" versus "public" body image was a consistent theme also echoed by patients in Daniel's study (1985). After reconstruction, many women found themselves less preoccupied with their health and that they had had cancer; they no longer had the constant reminder of the physical defect. Teimourian and Adham (1982) found increased sexual activity postreconstruction, and work by Gerard (1982) suggests that reconstructed patients achieve more sexual responsivity than do their mastectomy peers. Goin and Goin (1981) reported that in postclimacteric women the request for breast reconstruction may serve as a catalyst for more adequate adjustment to the midlife crises that are often complicated by a diagnosis of cancer.

Key concerns of women about reconstruction include the cost of the surgery, the safety of the techniques (used with respect to both potential for complications and risk of masking or promoting recurrent disease), and cosmetic results achievable. Surgeons differ in their approach to this latter concern. Some prefer to use written materials only; others show pictures of reconstructed breasts, while many use some combinations of these approaches and may at times refer a woman to a previously reconstructed patient for more details. In our own research and that of others, several additional issues seemed of importance in counseling women considering or undergoing these procedures (Schain et al., 1984; Winder and Winder, 1985). These issues were the need for discussion of all facets of the surgical steps (including number and length of hospitalizations, a thorough review of the surgical procedures planned to achieve symmetry of the breasts and to create a nipple; and consideration of timing of the procedure). The psychological impact of the timing of reconstruction has been the focus of additional studies.

## IMMEDIATE VERSUS DELAYED RECONSTRUCTION

While debate continues about the medical issues associated with immediate versus delayed reconstruction, the psychological literature indicates that early reconstruction prevents some of the emotional trauma associated with loss and disfigurement experienced by women undergoing mastectomy (Wellisch et al., 1985). Recent research with women undergoing immediate reconstruction has shown not only high levels of patient satisfaction with surgical results, but also significantly less psychosocial morbidity than those who undergo mastectomy alone (Dean et al., 1983; Noone et al., 1982; Stevens et al., 1984). Patients undergoing immediate reconstruction were less depressed and suffered less impairment of their sense of femininity, self-esteem, and sexual attractiveness than their peers who delayed or did not seek reconstruction. However, in their analysis of data from a large randomized comparison trial of patients undergoing immediate versus delayed reconstruction, Schain and her associates noted that initial differences in adjustment may be minimal and likely disappear over time (Schain et al., 1985). In addition, although the authors of the cited studies suggest that immediate reconstruction does not interfere with the necessary mourning process associated with threat to life and breast loss, some clinicians have reported this as a problem in long-term follow-up of these patients. It is an issue that bears further study.

The 1985 survey conducted by the American Society of Plastic and Reconstructive Surgeons (cited earlier) revealed that 34% of the breast reconstructions performed by member surgeons in 1984 were done at the same time as, or within a few days of mastectomy. As more women request these procedures, additional research will be needed to determine who will benefit from immediate reconstruction and who will be better served by having a waiting period between cancer surgery and repair.

A greater psychological burden is placed on women who are told that positive nodes were found at surgery and that chemotherapy must be added to their treatment. Treatment for these patients becomes significantly prolonged. Some women in this group describe their early weeks of treatment as having been characterized by ''one piece of bad news after another.''

## ADJUVANT CHEMOTHERAPY

The news that adjuvant chemotherapy is needed demands psychological adjustment to yet another treatment modality, a lengthened treatment period and awareness of the threat to life requiring a systemic therapy. While in the past adjuvant chemotherapy or hormonal therapy was reserved for Stage II disease, adjuvant therapy is now increasingly recommended for Stage I (node negative) disease. In May 1988, the National Cancer Institute alerted physicians of the results of three controlled randomized trials which were closed early because of the significant survival advantage of those node negative women who received chemotherapy or hormonal therapy (Clinical Alert, NCI, 1988). The survival advantage of almost 10% for women treated (increasing likely cure from 75 to 85%) has been widely publicized, causing all women with early breast cancer to recognize the far from fully reassuring statistics associated with either treatment. Release of these results also led to increased anxiety on the part of many women who had primary treatment only and who questioned seeking further treatment. Thus, more women face this treatment option today and its psychological concomitants. (See Chapter 10).

Anticipation of chemotherapy can be difficult. Women's fears of the potential adverse sequelae often arise from knowledge of other chemotherapeutic regimens. Women anticipating and undergoing adjuvant therapy should be told about the drugs that will be used and the side effects of each, with special emphasis placed on the transient nature of alopecia. At this point, counseling for reactive anxiety and depression can be helpful in reducing later distress. Despite these fears, few women refuse treatment and most comply with their regimen (Taylor et al., 1984b).

The nausea and vomiting associated with chemotherapy are generally well tolerated by the use of antiemetic drugs. The use of behavioral interventions provides a means of exercising self-control over symptoms while also reducing anxiety. Anticipatory nausea and vomiting are particularly susceptible to control by this means. (Chapters 34–35). The negative impact on the quality of life of patients undergoing chemotherapy of this conditioned response was stressed by Hughson and colleagues in their research (1986). Their work emphasizes the importance of early intervention for patients experiencing severe nausea and vomiting, and argues in favor of containing the course of treatment within 6 months. Their study also revealed significantly more depression among patients receiving adjuvant chemotherapy compared to those who underwent adjuvant radiotherapy alone, underscoring the value of providing early counseling for these women.

Another troublesome side effect of adjuvant therapy that has psychological consequences is weight gain. The cause of such weight changes remains unclear. A study by Huntington (1985) revealed that 50% of patients gained more than 10 pounds. No difference was found by treatment regimen (cyclophosphamide, methotrexate, and 5-fluorouracil versus these three drugs plus vincristine and prednisone), estrogen receptor status, age, or menopausal status, although a decrease in activity level was found in those who experienced weight gain. The added insult to self-esteem posed by significant weight gain suggests that more attention should be paid to this problem.

The 1985 NIH Consensus Conference on Adjuvant Therapy of Breast Cancer (Lippman, 1986) reviewed whether adjuvant therapy was effective and for whom, because in 50% of women with early breast cancer, disease has already spread to the lymph nodes (Kolata, 1985). There was support for the use of chemotherapy in premenopausal women with positive nodes. In addition, it was recommended that postmenopausal women with involved lymph nodes and tumors containing estrogen receptors receive tamoxifen. Although tamoxifen has few serious adverse side effects, its antiestrogen effects are distressing to some women. These changes in management approaches alter the treatment experience for older women. However, the need to encourage women to participate in clinical trials persists, because treatment for breast cancer is still far from as effective as it should be.

Psychological preparation for chemotherapy is essential and should incorporate patient educational materials, nursing input, and an outline by the physician of the disease and treatment-related expectations. (See Chapter 10 on psychological issues with chemotherapy). It is important to anticipate and plan for emotional reactions to ending treatment when, as with radiotherapy, fears of recurrence peak (Holland et al., 1979). Our clinical experience suggests that women experience more severe reactive anxiety and depression during this part of the treatment than in an earlier period, perhaps because of their greater awareness of the relative survival statistics.

## ADVANCED DISEASE

Supportive care for patients with advanced breast cancer is aimed at palliative management and control of symptoms (see also Chapter 6). Different metastatic sites, especially bone, lung, and brain, present special supportive problems. Bone pain must be controlled. Hypercalcemia causes mental changes that must be monitored and managed if a confusional state develops. The use of groups has been found to be an effective means of providing psychological support during this stage of illness (Spiegel et al., 1981). Advanced care is best provided at home with support from the family and, if needed, a homemaker, although a hospice setting with home care components also serves the needs of many patients well. Central to the success of a supportive program is a sense of continuity of care with physicians and staff and continued support of family and friends. (Chapters 48 and 49 review issues associated with home care).

Psychiatric consultation should be considered when distress is not responsive to the usual supportive measures. It is extremely helpful to have a psychiatric consultant who is knowledgeable about the problems faced by women with breast cancer available, ideally as a member of the multidisciplinary team. Hoffman (1988) described the role of the psychooncologist on such a team as falling into several areas: coordination of mental health team activities, liaison to other disciplines, education of patients, families, and staff, and consultation and research.

Among the psychiatric symptoms of most concern, anxiety and depression are most common and most disabling. Depression may reach significant proportions, and although suicide is unusual, suicidal ideation is common. Management that combines psychological support with psychopharmacological use of antidepressants is often helpful. Anxiety may be high and very distressing, especially in the presence of hypoxia or prolonged pain. Anxiolytic drugs are also helpful for control of symptoms. It is best to give these drugs at regular intervals initially to achieve control, thereafter tapering the dose or prescribing the drug on an as needed basis. In general, if given control of their own dose initially, women will take too little to be effective. Agitated behavior associated with a metabolic encephalopathy resulting often from hypercalcemia or from narcotic side effects may require control by administration of haloperidol in small doses.

## SPECIAL ISSUES

Experiencing the diagnosis and treatment of breast cancer in a friend or family member arouses intense feelings of threat and helplessness. (Lewis et al., 1985). Female relatives in particular find themselves worrying about their enhanced risk; and all involved wonder whether there is something they can do to reduce the risk of cancer in themselves or alter the course of it in their loved one. Although not always openly raised, these are issues that have ramifications for clinicians in their management.

## Children of Women with Breast Cancer

For all immediate female relatives, breast cancer in a sister, mother, or daughter is well known to mean heightened risk for all, particularly if the disease has occurred prior to premenopause. The increased need to monitor more closely for breast cancer in these survivors is becoming more widely appreciated. How best to support good health care practices without promoting fear is an area of needed research. The traumatic effect on children, both sons and daughters, is great when the mother develops breast cancer. Behavioral disorders, conflicts with parents, and regressive and acting-out behaviors in children have been seen to increase during a parental illness (Wellisch, 1979; Buckley, 1977; Litman, 1974). Lichtman and colleagues (1984) noted deterioration of the mother–child relationship in 12% of women with breast cancer whom he studied. Problems were more likely to arise in those situations in which the mother had a poor prognosis, extensive surgery, poor psychological adjustment, and to a lesser extent, difficulty adjusting to chemotherapy or radiotherapy. A prior history of parent–child conflicts also placed the relationship at risk during the mother's illness. Mothers' relationships with their daughters were significantly more stressed than those with their sons. Daughters were more likely to show signs of fearfulness, withdrawal, and hostility, emanating perhaps from their greater fears of developing the disease and the greater demands placed on the daughters. These findings parallel those reported by Litman (1974) and Wellisch (1979), who noted that mothers rely more often on daughters than sons during illness, and that adolescent daughters may be particularly vulnerable to disruption in their lives.

Support and intervention among daughters may be particularly important. These studies and experiences suggest that supportive measures should include a careful evaluation and discussion of hereditary risk, an explanation and demonstration of breast self-examination, and whenever possible, alleviation of additional burdens. The monitoring of all children, especially when the mother's breast cancer is advanced, is important.

## Risk Factors for Breast Cancer

### REPORTED FACTORS

There are a number of influences that have been found in epidemiological studies to increase the risk of breast cancer. They include the family history (as evidenced by breast cancer in immediate female relatives), nul-

**Table 14-3** Increased risk of breast cancer

Family history
Nulliparity or late first live birth
Early menarche
Late menopause
Benign hyperplasia
**Personal history** of contralateral breast cancer or prior colon, uterus, or ovarian cancer
Obesity
Cigarette smoking
Alcohol use
High-fat diet
Exposure to ionizing radiation
Caucasian race
Higher social class
Exposure to or use of exogenous hormones

liparity or late first live birth, early menarche, late menopause, benign hyperplasia, contralateral breast cancer (or prior colon, uterus, or ovarian cancer), obesity, cigarette smoking, alcohol consumption, high-fat diet, exposure to ionizing radiation (especially during adolescence), Caucasian race, higher social class, and use of or exposure to exogenous hormones (Table 14-3) (Senie et al., 1983; Hoover, 1977; MacMahon et al., 1973). These influences have received increased attention in the past decade as efforts have been directed first toward promoting early detection via encouragement of routine mammography and regular breast self-examination, and more recently toward fostering prevention. There is evidence of the success of these practices by the increase in diagnosis of early stage curable breast cancer (Breast Cancer Incidence, 1988).

Dietary and chemoprevention trials, using low-fat diet and administration of omega-three-fatty acids are among the research efforts being undertaken to reduce incidence of breast cancer in women at high risk. Studies at Memorial Sloan-Kettering have found that women at increased genetic risk of breast cancer are both interested in participating in prevention trials and are compliant with the medications offered (Rowland et al., 1987).

## PSYCHOLOGICAL FACTORS

It is within the context of the several already identified risk factors for breast cancer (see Table 14-3) that the possible role of psychological or social influences must be considered. Because breast cancer is a hormonally responsive neoplasm and one with great psychological impact, it has been the most extensively explored tumor site since the 1950s for possible psychological variables associated with risk and survival. As with the debate about breast cancer treatment, the controversy about the potential role of emotions in vulnerability to breast cancer and its progression has received much attention in the public press. The impact of this press coverage has not been studied directly, but in dealing with their illness, many women have expressed concern that they "brought it on themselves" or that their attitude is bad and that they may be making the cancer worse.

In a study of what women attributed to having caused their breast cancer, Taylor, Lichtman, and Wood (1984a) found that 41% of their well-educated sample felt that they were responsible for the development of the disease, and that stress was a major contributor in its development. The belief that they may be responsible for their own illness and its outcome has become an added psychological burden for many women; indeed, it is a hazard for those who, based on these beliefs, seek questionable and unproven therapies as primary treatment for their breast cancer, either never starting or discontinuing conventional treatments.

Thus, although the research into psychological factors and cancer risk and progression is an important pursuit on its own merit, publication in the public media of early and controversial findings about emotions in breast cancer is a growing concern. Therefore, it becomes important that oncologists know the status of psychosocial research in breast cancer risk and survival in order to answer their patients' questions on the subject and provide clarification and reassurance. The following is a brief review that outlines the pertinent issues as they relate to breast cancer. For a more extensive review of the research on psychological factors in cancer risk and survival, the reader is referred to Chapter 60, which reviews human studies, and Chapter 61, which primarily explores the animal data from psychoneuroimmunology studies that may be relevant to cancer. Fox (1978, 1983) has provided a continuing critique of the research in this emerging area for those who wish to pursue the topic. Cooper (1988) has written a monograph on the role of stress as it relates to breast cancer.

Data relating stress and illness have come from both animal and human studies. A series of studies in mice by Riley (1975, 1981) showed that cage conditions of crowding, noise, and manipulation caused elevated corticosterone levels which, in turn, caused involution of the thymus and enhanced mammary tumor growth. Other models of stress and other tumors have shown the opposite, protective effects or absence of an effect on carcinogenesis (Newberry, 1981). Miller (1985) has offered some hypotheses to explain the discrepancy in results related to the type of stress, timing (i.e., precarcinogen versus postcarcinogen exposure), type of tumor, and outcome measures used. However, irrespective of direction of change, perturbations of the

endocrine and immune systems result from stress. This may be particularly important in a tumor site such as breast, which is hormone dependent. Lippman (1985) has provided a model of the intricate links between the brain and the immune and endocrine systems whereby emotions could affect tumor growth (see Fig. 60-2). Weinstein (1982) has suggested that because carcinogenesis progresses via initiation to promotion and disease extension, psychosocial variables could act as one of many cocontributors influencing breast cancer development. Such influence might be particularly important when it occurs in young women prior to the first full-term pregnancy, an event that is known to lower risk.

Another model from animal studies was introduced by Sklar and Anisman (1979). They showed that tumor growth in mice implanted with P815 mastocytoma tumor cells was greatest in those mice that were yoked in a paradigm in which they received inescapable shock. Exposure to the "learned-helplessness" model was associated with norepinephrine depletion and suppressed lymphocytic stimulation to phytohemagglutinin (PHA) and concanavalin A (Con A) (Laudenslager et al., 1983). The animal studies by Ader (1981) have been provocative also, showing that the immune response can be conditioned to an immunosuppressive drug. These data, which show regulatory links between the brain and the immune and endocrine systems, provide a great challenge in exploring ways in which such perturbations could affect risk and growth of breast cancer.

Studies of personality factors in human breast cancer have focused on (1) the impact of personality on behavior that affects exposure to carcinogens or practice of optimal health care such as breast self-examination, and (2) the effect of emotions on hormonal or cellular mechanisms that could affect cancer risk. The first studies of women with breast cancer done in the 1950s used a retrospective approach in which premorbid personality patterns were deduced from anecdotal reports of women in whom breast cancer had already developed (see Fox, 1978, for review of studies). Because of the nature of the study design, evidence of repression, denial, and inhibition of emotions, especially anger, in the women interviewed could have been a reflection of response to disease, as well as prior personality. A controlled prospective study that would confirm a personality type associated with risk for breast cancer has not been reported as yet. However, one could hypothesize that a psychological state, or a stressful event, could act as a promoter in the presence of an initiator factor, particularly if the external or internal stressor occurred during a period when breast tissue is most vulnerable to abnormal change.

An increasing number of studies have examined

psychological factors that might influence survival from breast cancer. Pettingale and colleagues (1985) carried out a series of studies in England suggesting that recurrence-free survival is greater in women who show either denial or "fighting spirit," as compared to those who exhibit stoic acceptance or feelings of helplessness or hopelessness. When examined 10 years later, data on the survivors in the same study population indicated that traits or coping styles seen at time of diagnosis remained predictive of survival, even when controlled for eight other prognostic variables. However, significantly, the researchers did not have access to axillary nodal status, known to be the single most important predictor in breast cancer survival, nor did they follow women over the 10 years.

Derogatis, Abeloff, and Melisaratos (1979) found a positive correlation between survival and expression of negative emotions in a group of women studied from the time of initiation of chemotherapy for metastatic disease. Long-term survivors (those who survived for >1 year) showed more negative emotions and more symptoms of anxiety, depression, and hostility than those surviving for less than 1 year. A 1987 study by Jamison and colleagues using a selected sample of advanced breast cancer patients and instruments similar to those employed in the Derogatis study failed to replicate the association of an emotional state with survival. Similarly, Holland and colleagues (1986), studying women with stage II breast cancer on a clinical trials adjuvant protocol, failed to confirm a psychosocial variable associated with survival. Levy and colleagues (1985) have reported findings for a cohort of women studied at the time of mastectomy. Those patients with a greater number of positive axillary nodes showed "better" psychological adjustment (measured by fewer expressions of distress) and lower natural killer (NK)-cell activity than patients with few or no positive nodes. This careful study of the correlates of immune and psychological function represents a new level of sophistication within such studies in breast cancer, studies that have in the past suffered from small sample sizes and methodological flaws. Cella and Holland (1988) reviewed the methodological problems in prior studies and outlined criteria for a stringent trial of psychosocial influences on breast cancer development. Chapter 60 elucidates the additional studies in this area.

Gorzynski and co-workers (1980) conducted a follow-up study of 10-year survivors of breast cancer whose psychological state and cortisol production had been assessed at time of biopsy by Katz and colleagues (1970). At follow-up, women were found to have similar psychological coping responses and cortisol production as they had had 10 years earlier, suggesting that these represent stable traits. Mean cortisol production was higher in the group with breast cancer than in the group with benign biopsy results, both initially and 10 years later. Women who were alive at 10 years were compared to those who had died in the interim with respect to their prebiopsy characteristics. Psychological state was not significantly different; however, the mean weight of those who had died was significantly higher than that of survivors (Zumoff et al., 1982). These data support those of Donegan, Harts, and Rimm (1978), who reported a strong correlation between lower weight and longer survival, a relationship found to be secondary in significance to nodal status.

It may be that studies showing personality differences are actually measuring the association of personality with some behavioral variable, such as diet or weight. As increasing attention is being directed to dietary considerations—especially fat intake, which may correlate with greater caloric intake and obesity—and their role in risk and survival, these co-factors will need to be examined further. The studies to date evaluating psychological aspects of survival are provocative and suggest new directions for research. The "fighting spirit," described by Pettingale and co-workers (1985) in women with breast cancer, has received increasing interest as a psychological construct in adaptation which requires further research and definition. The impact of social support on morbidity and mortality is another area of interest.

Marshall and Funch (1983) examined survival in 352 women with breast cancer who completed crude social stress and social involvement measures at the time of diagnosis between 1958 and 1960. Records for 283 who had died were available for review. Using regression analysis, the researchers found that stage of disease at diagnosis was the most powerful predictor of the length of survival, accounting for 15–20% of the variance. However, 9% of the variance in survival in the younger group could be explained by the social variables; this was not true in the older group. Social stress was consistently found to have an adverse effect, and involvement with others was positively related to length of survival. Although the authors suggest that the significance of their findings is limited because of the crude measures used, their data are interesting in light of the large study of over 6000 elderly persons by Berkman and Syme (1979). In the latter study, the researchers found that longevity was associated with presence of social support. Although the number of subjects studied was not sufficient to separate out impact on cancer alone, early mortality from a range of diseases occurred more frequently in those who earlier had reported themselves to be isolated and lacking in social support.

In a study using some of the variables isolated in earlier investigations, Cassileth and co-workers (1985) tested the ability of seven social and psychological factors reported to be associated with longevity to predict survival: social ties, life satisfaction, job satisfaction, use of psychotropic drugs, subjective view of adult health, hopelessness or helplessness, and perception of adjustment required to cope with the diagnosis. Two groups of patients were followed: (1) those with irreversible cancer ($n = 204$), who were followed until death, and (2) those with stage II breast cancer or melanoma ($n = 155$), who were followed to disease recurrence. None of the factors delineated, either individually or in combination, was found by self-report data to influence survival or time to recurrence for women with either advanced or early stages of disease.

There remains a need for further research that uses a prospective multitiered design to identify possible predictors that could then be tested in a larger model. Psychological influences play an important role as they affect ability and willingness to obtain and comply with available treatment. Dietary patterns may also be important. In addition, psychological and social variables contribute to quality of life, if not directly to survival time. However, it is not clear whether there are psychosocial factors that influence the biology of breast cancer, in terms of either risk or survival. Fox (1978) has suggested that psychological influences, if they do play a role, may be salutary or detrimental, but that they likely constitute a small part of the variance in relation to the other known variables that relate to disease.

Advice to patients should reflect both the contradictory and preliminary nature of research findings. In addition, women with breast cancer should be encouraged to recognize that the available data do not support their fears that they caused their breast cancer to develop. "Fighting spirit" and active participation are desirable, but a period of distress associated with problems of illness is not, according to available data, likely to cause tumor progression as some women currently believe. Women who have a need for greater participation (and a sense of control) in their care that may be served by using alternative treatment methods should be encouraged to employ these methods, provided they do not interfere with conventional therapy and have no deleterious effect.

Women should be encouraged to participate in clinical trials of breast cancer treatment when they are available. The mortality from this disease is still too high, and much is to be learned about treatment and about the interaction of psychological and biological variables. It can be pointed out that the large multicenter studies compare the best present treatment with one that may be better. Women who agree to enter these trials are assured of care by physicians who constitute the cutting edge of science as it is applied to clinical trials. Participation in such studies also serves the altruistic goal of helping to reduce the toll that this disease takes on all women. Answers will only be found in large prospective studies in which the range of variables, well defined and controlled, can be assessed.

## SUMMARY

Breast cancer remains the most common tumor in women; it has a unique and, at times, complex psychological impact, but one to which psychologically healthy women respond well without developing serious psychological symptoms. Increased use in primary treatment of breast-conserving procedures is reducing the negative impact on self-image and body image. However, current ethical and legal constraints relating to treatment options have added significantly to decision-making dilemmas and to fears of recurrence, which, by virtue of the detailed information given about survival statistics, may persist for an indefinite period. Greater emphasis is needed on providing support to women during the decision-making period. Reconstruction has been shown to have a significant benefit in terms of quality of life in women who undergo mastectomy. Broader dissemination of information from the psychological studies of adaptation to the available treatment options will help in efforts to determine the best treatment to meet patients' physical and emotional needs.

Special attention must be directed to the psychological well-being of the immediate relatives of women with breast cancer, especially their daughters. Large prospective studies of the biological and psychological aspects of breast cancer are needed to understand the possible role of psychosocial influences in risk and outcome of breast cancer. At present, these influences appear to figure largely in issues of quality of life, although positive attitudes and "fighting spirit" are associated with responses and behaviors likely to enhance survival.

## REFERENCES

Ader, R. (ed.). (1981). *Psychoneuroimmunology*. New York: Academic Press.

American Society of Plastic and Reconstructive Surgeons. (1985). *Breast reconstructions quadruple* (News Release, May 16).

Ashcroft, J.J., S.J. Leinster, and P.A. Slade (1985). Breast cancer-patient choice of treatment: Preliminary communication. *J. R. Soc. Med.* 78:43–46.

Baider, L., S. Rizel, and A. Kaplan-DeNour (1986). Comparison of couples adjustment to lumpectomy and mastectomy. *Gen. Hosp. Psych.* 8:251–57.

Bard, M. and A.M. Sutherland (1955). Psychological impact of cancer and its treatment: IV. Adaptation to radical mastectomy. *Cancer* 8:652–72.

Bartelink, H., F. van Dam and J. van Dongen (1985). Psychological effects of breast conserving therapy in comparison with radical mastectomy. *Int. J. Radiat. Oncol. Biol. Phys.* 11:381–85.

Berkman, L.F. and L.S. Syme (1979). Social networks, host resistance and mortality: A nine year follow-up study of Alameda County residents. *Am. J. Epidemiol.* 109:186–204.

Bloom, J.R. (1982). Social support, accommodation to stress and adjustment to breast cancer. *Soc. Sci. Med.* 16:1329–38.

Bloom, J., M. Cook, S. Fotopoulis, D. Flamer, C. Gates, J.C. Holland, L. Muenz, B. Murawski, D. Penman, and R.D. Ross (1987). Psychological response to mastectomy: A prospective comparison study. *Cancer* 59:189–96.

Buckley, I.E. (1977). *Listen to the Children: Impact on the Mental Health of Children of a Parent's Catastrophic Illness.* New York: Cancer Care.

Cancer Letter (1988). Breast cancer incidence goes up most of it in early, local stages. 4:4–7.

Cassileth, B.R., E.J. Lusk, D.S. Miller, L.L. Brown, and C. Miller (1985). Psychosocial correlates of survival in advanced malignant disease? *N. Engl. J. Med.* 312(24): 1551–55.

Cella, D.F. and J.C. Holland (1988). Methodological considerations studying the stress-illness connection in women with breast cancer. In: C.L Cooper (ed.), *Stress and Breast Cancer.* New York: John Wiley, pp. 197–214.

Clifford, E. (1979). The reconstruction experience: The search for restitution. In N.G. Georgiade (ed.), *Breast Reconstruction following Mastectomy.* London: C.V. Mosby, pp. 22–34.

Clinical Alert, National Cancer Institute, May 16, 1988.

Cooper, C.L. (ed.) (1988). *Stress and Breast Cancer.* New York: John Wiley.

Craig, T.J., G.W. Comstock, and P.B. Geiser (1974). The quality of survival in breast cancer: A case–control comparison. *Cancer* 33:1451–57.

Crile, G. (1974). Management of breast cancer: Limited mastectomy. *J.A.M.A.* 230:95–98.

Daniel, E. (1985). Breast reconstruction postmastectomy: A psychosocial study. Doctoral dissertation, University of California, San Francisco, 1984. *Diss. Abstr. Int.* 46:1741B.

Dean, C., U. Chetty, and A.P.M. Forrest (1983). Effects of immediate breast reconstruction on psychosocial morbidity after mastectomy. *Lancet* 1:459–62.

Derogatis, L.R., M.D. Abeloff, and N. Melisaratos (1979). Psychological coping mechanisms and survival in metastatic breast cancer. *J.A.M.A.* 242:1504–8.

Donegan, W., A. Harts, and A. Rimm (1978). The association of body weight with recurrent cancer of the breast. *Cancer* 41:1590–94.

Euster, S. (1979). Rehabilitation after mastectomy: The group process. *Soc. Work Health Care* 4:251–63.

Fallowfield, L.J., M. Baum, and G.P. Maguire (1986). Effects of breast conservation on psychological morbidity associated with diagnosis and treatment of early breast cancer. *Br. Med. J.* 293:1331–34.

Faulkner, A. and P. Maguire (1984). Teaching ward nurses to monitor cancer patients. *Clin. Oncol.* 10:383–89.

Fisher, B. (1985). *Choice of Surgery in Early Breast Cancer.* Paper presented at the Conference on Early Breast Cancer: The Psychological Perspective sponsored by Long Island Jewish Medical Center and Memorial Sloan-Kettering Cancer Center, New York City, October 1985.

Fisher, B. and P. Barboni (1982). Breast cancer. In J.F. Holland and E. Frei III (eds.), *Cancer Medicine,* 2nd ed. Philadelphia: Lea & Febiger, pp. 2025–56.

Fotopoulis, S. and M.R. Cook (1980). *Psychological Aspects of Breast Cancer: Age.* Paper presented at the meeting of the American Psychological Association, Montreal, Quebec, September, 1980.

Fox, B. (1978). Premorbid psychological factors as related to cancer incidence. *Behav. Med.* 1:45–133.

Fox, B. (1983). Current theory of psychogenic effects on cancer incidence and prognosis. *J. Psychosoc. Oncol.* 1(1):17–31.

Ganz, P.A., C.C. Schag, M.L. Polinsky, R.L. Heinrich, and V.F. Flack (1987). Rehabilitation needs and breast cancer: The first month after primary therapy. *Breast Cancer Res. Treat.* 10:243–53.

Gerard, D. (1982). Sexual functioning after mastectomy: Life vs. lab. *J. Sex Marital Ther.* 8:305–15.

Goin, J.M. and M.K. Goin (eds.). (1981). Breast reconstruction after mastectomy. In J.M. Goin and M.K. Goin (eds.), *Changing the Body: Psychological Effects of Plastic Surgery.* Baltimore: Williams & Wilkins, pp. 163–89.

Gorzynski, J.G., J.C. Holland, J. Katz, H. Weiner, B. Zumoff, D. Fukushima, and J. Levin (1980). Stability of ego defenses and endocrine responses in women prior to breast biopsy and ten years later. *Psychosom. Med.* 42:323–28.

de Haes, J.C.J.M. and K. Welvaart (1985). Quality of life after breast cancer surgery. *J. Surg. Oncol.* 28:123–25.

Harris, J.R., M.B. Levine, and S. Hellman (1978). Results of treating stages I and II carcinoma of the breast with primary radiation therapy. *Cancer Treat. Rep.* 62:985–91.

Hoffman, R.S. (1988). The psycho-oncologist in a multidisciplinary breast treatment center. In C.L. Cooper (ed.), *Stress and Breast Cancer.* New York: John Wiley, pp. 171–93.

Holland, J.C., A.H. Korzun, S. Tross, D.F. Cella, L. Norton, and W. Wood (1986). Psychosocial factors and disease-free survival (DFS) in stage II breast carcinoma (Abstract). *Proc. Twenty-Second Ann. Mtg. Am. Soc. Clin. Oncol.* 5:237.

Holland, J.C. and R. Mastrovito (1980). Psychologic adaptation to breast cancer. *Cancer* 46:1045–52.

Holland, J.C., J. Rowland, A. Lebovits, and R. Rusalem (1979). Reactions to cancer treatment: Assessment of emotional response to adjuvant radiotherapy as a guide to planned interventions. *Psychiatr. Clin. North Am.* 2:347–58.

Hoover, R. (1977). *Breast cancer: Epidemiologic consid-*

*erations*. Reserpine and Breast Cancer Task Force. Washington, D.C.: Department of Health, Education and Welfare.

Hughson, A.V.M., A.F. Cooper, C.S. McArdle, and D.C. Smith (1986). Psychological impact of adjuvant chemotherapy in the first two years after mastectomy. *Br. Med. J.* 293:1268–71.

Huntington, M. (1985). Weight gain in patients receiving adjuvant chemotherapy for carcinoma of the breast. *Cancer* 56:572–74.

Jacobs, E., J. Holland, J. Rowland, N. Geller, G. Petroni, T. Chaglassian, D. Kovachev, and D. Kinne (1983). Who seeks breast reconstruction? A controlled psychological study (Abstract). *Psychosom. Med.* 45:80.

Jamison, R.N., T.G. Burish, and K.A. Wallston (1987). Psychogenic factors in predicting survival of breast cancer patients. *J. Clin. Oncol.* 5:768–72.

Katz, J.L., P. Ackman, Y. Rothwax, E. Sachar, H. Weiner, L. Hellman, and T.F. Gallagher (1970). Psychoendocrine aspects of cancer of the breast. *Psychosom. Med.* 32:1–18.

Kolata, G. (1985). Breast cancer consensus. *Science* 229(4720):1378.

Kushner, R. (1975). *Breast Cancer: A Personal History and Investigative Report*. New York: Harcourt Brace Jovanovich.

Laudenslager, M., S. Ryan, R. Drugan, R.L. Hyson, and S.F. Maier (1983). Coping and immunosuppression: Inescapable but not escapable shock suppresses lymphocytic proliferation. *Science* 221(4610):568–70.

Levy, S., R. Herberman, A. Maluish, B. Schliew, and M. Lippman (1985).Prognostic risk assessment in primary breast cancer by behavioral and immunological parameters. *Health Psychol.* 4:99–113.

Lewis, F.M. and J.R. Bloom (1978–1979). Psychosocial adjustment to breast cancer: A review of selected literature. *Int. J. Psychiatry Med.* 9:1–17.

Lewis, F.M., E.S. Ellison, and N.F. Woods (1985). The impact of breast cancer on the family. *Semin. Oncol. Nurs.* 3:206–13.

Lichtman, R.R., S.E. Taylor, J.V. Wood, A.Z. Bluming, G.M. Dosik, and R.L. Leibowitz (1984). Relations with children after breast cancer: The mother–daughter relationship at risk. *J. Psychosoc. Oncol.* 2(3/4):1–19.

Lippman, M.E. (1985). Psychosocial factors and the hormonal regulation of tumor growth. In S.M. Levy (ed.), *Behavior and Cancer*. San Francisco: Jossey-Bass, pp. 134–47.

Lippman, M.E. (1986). *National Institutes of Health Consensus Development Conference on Adjuvant Chemotherapy and Endocrine Therapy for Breast Cancer*. NIH Publication No. 86-2860. Department of Health and Human Services, U.S. Government Printing Office.

Litman, T.J. (1974). The family as the basic unit in health and medical care: A social behavioral overview. *Soc. Sci. Med.* 8:495–519.

MacMahon, B., P. Cole and J. Brown (1973). Etiology of human breast cancer: A review. *J. Natl. Cancer Inst.* 50:21–42.

Maguire, P. (1976). The psychological and social sequelae of mastectomy. In J.G. Howells (ed.), *Modern Perspectives in the Psychiatric Aspects of Surgery*. New York: Brunner/Mazel, pp. 390–421.

Margolis, G.J. and R.L. Goodman (1984). Psychological factors in women choosing radiation therapy for breast cancer. *Psychosomatics* 25:464–69.

Markel, W.M. (1971). The American Cancer Society's program for the rehabilitation of the breast cancer patient. *Cancer* 28:1676–78.

Marshall, J.R. and D.P. Funch (1983). Social environment and breast cancer: A cohort analysis of patient survival. *Cancer* 52:1546–50.

Meyerowitz, B.E. (1980). Psychosocial correlates of breast cancer and its treatment. *Psychol. Bull.* 8:108–31.

Miller, N. (1985). Effects of emotional stress on immune function. *Pavlov. J. Biol. Sci.* 20:47–52.

National Survey on Breast Cancer: A Measure of Progress in Public Understanding (1980). Bethesda, Md.: National Cancer Insitute.

Newberry, B.H. (1981). Effects of presumably stressful stimulation on the development of animal tumors: Some issues. In S.M. Weiss, J.A. Herd, and B.H. Fox (eds.), *Perspectives on Behavioral Medicine*. New York: Academic Press, pp. 329–50.

Noone, R.B., T.G. Frazier, C.Z. Hayward, and M.S. Skiles (1982). Patient acceptance of immediate reconstruction following mastectomy. *Plas. Reconstr. Surg.* 69:632–40.

Penman, D.T. (1980). Coping strategies in adaptation to mastectomy. Doctoral dissertation, Yeshiva University, 1979. *Diss. Abstr. Int.* 40:5825B.

Penman, D.T., J.R. Bloom, S. Fotopoulis, M.R. Cook, J.C. Holland, C. Gates, D. Flamer, B. Murawski, R. Ross, U. Brandt, L.R. Muenz, and D. Pee (1987). The impact of mastectomy on self-concept and social function: A combined cross-sectional and longitudinal study with comparison groups. *Women and Health* 11:101–30.

Penman, D.T., J.C. Holland, G.F. Bahna, G. Morrow, A.H. Schmale, L.R. Derogatis, C.L. Carnrike, and R. Cherry (1984). Informed consent for investigational chemotherapy: Patients' and physicians' perceptions. *J. Clin. Oncol.* 2:849–55.

Peters-Golden, H. (1982). Breast cancer: Varied perceptions of social support in the illness experience. *Soc. Sci. Med.* 16:483–91.

Pettingale, K.W., T. Morris, S. Greer, and J.L. Haybittle (1985). Mental attitudes to cancer: An additional prognostic factor. *Lancet* 1:750.

Polivy, J. (1977). Psychological effects of mastectomy on a woman's feminine self-concept. *J. Nerv. Ment. Dis.* 164:77–87.

Riley, V. (1975). Mouse mammary tumors: Alteration of incidence as apparent function of stress. *Science* 189(4201): 564–67.

Riley, V. (1981). Psychoneuroendocrine influences on immuno-competence and neoplasia. *Science* 212(4499): 1100–1109.

Rollin, B. (1977). *First You Cry*. New York: New American Library.

Rowland, J., H. Dermatis, J. Kerner, S. Tross, J. Miransky, M. Osborne, and J.C. Holland (1987). Psychosocial factors affecting consent to a breast cancer chemoprevention program (Abstract). *Proc. Twenty-Third Annu. Mtg. Am. Soc. Clin. Oncol.* 6:226.

Rowland, J., J.C. Holland, E.R. Jacobs, T. Chaglassian, N. Geller, G. Petroni, D. Kovachev, and D. Kinne (1984). Psychological response to breast reconstruction. *Continuing Med. Educ. Syllabus and Scientific Proc. 137th Annu. Mtg. A.P.A.* Paper Sessions No. 142.

Sabo, D., J. Brown, and C. Smith (1986). The male role and mastectomy: Support groups and men's adjustment. *J. Psychosoc. Oncol.* 4:19–31.

Sanger, C.K. and M. Reznikoff (1981). A comparison of the psychological effects of breast-saving procedures with the modified mastectomy. *Cancer* 48:2341–46.

Schain, W.S. (1985). Breast cancer surgeries and psychosexual sequelae: Implications for remediation. *Semin. Oncol. Nurs.* 1:200–205.

Schain, W., B.K. Edwards, C.R. Gorrell, E.V. de Moss, M.E. Lippman, L.H. Gerber, and A.S. Lichter (1983). Psychosocial and physical outcomes of primary breast cancer therapy: Mastectomy vs. excisional biopsy and irradiation. *Breast Cancer Res. Treat.* 3:377–82.

Schain, W.S., E. Jacobs, and D.K. Wellisch (1984). Psychosocial issues in breast reconstruction: Intrapsychic, interpersonal, and practical concerns. *Clin. Plast. Surg.* 11:237–53.

Schain, W.S., D.K. Wellisch, R.O. Pasnau, and J. Landsverk (1985). The sooner the better: A study of psychological factors in women undergoing immediate versus delayed breast reconstruction. *Am. J. Psychiatry* 142:40–46.

Schottenfeld, D. and G.F. Robbins (1970). Quality of survival among patients who have had radical mastectomy. *Cancer* 26:650–54.

Scott, D.W. (1983). Anxiety, critical thinking and information processing during and after breast biopsy. *Nurs. Res.* 32:24–29.

Scott, D.W. and S.J. Eisendrath (1985–1986). Dynamics of the recovery process following initial diagnosis of breast cancer. *J. Psychosoc. Oncol.* 3(4):53–66.

Senie, R.T., P.P. Rosen, and D.W. Kinne (1983). Epidemiologic factors associated with breast cancer. *Cancer Nurs.* 3:121–30.

Sklar, L. and H. Anisman (1979). Stress and coping factors influence tumor growth. *Science* 205:513–15.

Spiegel, D., J.R. Bloom and I. Yalom (1981). Group support for patients with metastatic cancer. *Arch. Gen. Psychiatry* 38:527–33.

Steinberg, M.D., M.A. Juliano, and L. Wise (1985). Psychological outcome of lumpectomy versus mastectomy in the treatment of breast cancer. *Am. J. Psychiatry* 142:34–39.

Stevens, L.A., M.H. McGrath, R.G. Druss, S.J. Kister, F.E. Gump, and K.A. Forde (1984). The psychological impact of immediate breast reconstruction for women with early breast cancer. *Plast. Reconstr. Surg.* 73:619–28.

Taylor, S.E., R.R. Lichtman, and J.V. Wood (1984a). Attributions, beliefs about control, and adjustment to breast cancer. *J. Pers. Soc. Psychol.* 46:489–502.

Taylor, S.E., R.R. Lichtman, and J.V. Wood (1984b). Compliance with chemotherapy among breast cancer patients. *Health Psychol.* 3:553–62.

Taylor, S.E., R.D. Lichtman, and J. Wood (1985). Illness related and treatment related factors and psychological adjustment to breast cancer. *Cancer* 55:2506–13.

Teimourian, B. and M. Adham (1982). Survey of patients' response to breast reconstruction. *Ann. Plast. Surg.* 9:321–25.

Valanis, B.G. and C.H. Rumpler (1985). Helping women to choose breast cancer treatment alternatives. *Cancer Nurs.* 8:167–75.

Veronesi, U., R. Saccozzi, M. Del Vecchio, A. Banfi, C. Clemente, M. De Lena, G. Gallus, M. Greco, A. Luini, E. Marubini, G. Muscolino, F. Rilke, B. Salvadori, A. Zecchini, and R. Zucall (1981). Comparing radical mastectomy with quadrantectomy, axillary dissection, and radiotherapy in patients with small cancers of the breast. *N. Engl. J. Med.* 305:6–11.

Weinstein, I.B. (1982). The scientific basis for carcinogen detection: Primary cancer prevention. *Ca* 32:348–62.

Wellisch, D.K. (1979). Adolescent acting out when a parent has cancer. *Int. Family Ther.* 1:230–41.

Wellisch, D.K., M.J. Silverstein, and R.S. Hoffman (1988). Psychosocial outcomes of breast cancer therapies: Lumpectomy versus mastectomy with and without breast reconstruction. *Psychosomatics* (In Press).

Wellisch, D.K., K.R. Jamison, and R.O. Pasnau (1978). Psychosocial aspects of mastectomy: II. The man's perspective. *Am. J. Psychiatry* 135:543–46.

Wellisch, D.K., W.S. Schain, B.R. Noone, and J.W. Little (1985). Psychosocial correlates of immediate versus delayed reconstruction of the breast. *Plastic Reconstruct. Surg.* 76:713–18.

Wieder, S., J. Schwartzfeld, J. Fromewick, and J.C. Holland (1978). Psychosocial support program for patients with breast cancer at Montefiore Hospital: Team effort. *Q.R.B.* 4:10–13.

Winder, A.E. and B.D. Winder (1985). Patient counseling: Clarifying a woman's choice for breast reconstruction. *Patient Educ. Counseling* 7:65–75.

Wolberg, W.H., M.A. Tanner, E.P. Romsaas, D.L. Trump, and J.F. Malec (1987). Factors influencing options in primary breast cancer treatment. *J.Clin. Oncol.* 5:68–74.

Wortman, C. (1984). Social support and the cancer patient. *Cancer* 53:2339–60.

Zevon, M.A., J.B. Rounds, and J. Karr (1987). *Psychological Outcomes Associated with Breast Conserving Surgery: A Meta-analysis.* Paper presented at the eighth annual meeting of the Society of Behavioral Medicine, Washington, D.C., March 1987.

Zumoff, B., J.G. Gorzynski, J.L. Katz, H. Weiner, J. Levin, J.C. Holland, and D.K. Fukushima (1982). Non obesity at the time of mastectomy is highly predictive of 10-year disease-free survival in women with breast cancer. *Anticancer Res.* 2:59–62.

# 15

# Gastrointestinal Cancer

Jimmie C. Holland

Special problems in psychological adjustment are posed when tumors develop in the gastrointestinal (GI) tract. Both patient and family may have to cope with a severe eating disorder, significant weight loss, nausea and vomiting, abdominal discomfort as well as other disease-related events that are difficult to manage. In addition, the disease attacks a part of the body that preoccupies many people.

Concern with the normal function of the GI tract is sometimes considered a national obsession of Americans. The variety of over-the-counter nostrums available for appetite control, dyspepsia, and regular elimination reflects this concern for healthy digestion. The release in 1982 of guidelines by the National Research Council's Committee on Diet, Nutrition and Cancer recommending specific dietary modifications to reduce risk of several cancers, in particular several in the GI tract, served to emphasize the role of diet in health and cancer in particular. The current enthusiasm for holistic health, with its focus on diet and exercise, adds further emphasis on personal responsibility for health. Thus the social context in which patients must cope with GI cancer makes them particularly vulnerable to psychological distress; the site is one of general preoccupation, and the cause of disease is often perceived as being within personal control.

In addition to the cultural emphasis on normal digestion, most individuals relate a sense of well-being to normal GI function. Loss of appetite, inability to taste or eat food, nausea, abdominal discomfort, diarrhea, or constipation, result in immediate emotional distress and concern. From earliest childhood, eating and GI function are intimately tied to psychological state; emotional distress produces eating problems and a range of GI symptoms. This known intimate interrelation of psyche and GI tract requires that the physician who cares for the patient with GI cancer be particularly attuned to the emotional component. For example, in the cancer patient, anorexia or difficulty eating may develop from pathophysiological changes related to cancer; it also frequently develops from anxiety about the status of the tumor.

Certain personality types are more vulnerable to emotional problems when they develop GI cancer. Those individuals who invest more of their self-esteem in body image than others are at increased risk of emotional distress. The person who places high value on the healthy appearance of his or her body will be especially disturbed by surgery that alters appearance, or by the weight loss that may occur. In addition, persons who are meticulous in their concern for normal body function and who have focused considerable attention on bowel control and elimination may be particularly psychologically distressed when a colostomy or ileostomy is required. These individuals need special attention in adjusting to a stoma and its care.

Beyond these general issues, there are particular problems associated with tumor at different sites in the GI tract. Cancer of the mouth, pharynx, and larynx is considered in Chapter 17.

## CANCER OF THE ESOPHAGUS AND STOMACH

Tumors of these two sites constitute 16% of GI neoplasms. Patients with these tumors have often experienced vague symptoms of discomfort and difficulty in keeping food down, experiencing unexplained regurgitation, vomiting, or ulcerlike symptoms. Common in middle age and often ascribed to "stress" or "eating the wrong foods," these symptoms are frequently ignored until they become troublesome. These individuals have usually been treated initially by a conservative approach involving prescription of an antacid, often with in relief of the symptoms in the early stages. The disruption imposed by diagnostic esophagoscopy and gastroscopy for a suspected neoplasm is significant, not infrequently followed by the news of a positive biopsy result. The need for an exploratory operation is explained by the surgeon, who usually describes a plan involving removal of the tumor and part of the esophagus and/or stomach. Finding evidence of spread at the time of exploration results in depression and decisions about use of radiotherapy or chemotherapy.

The emotional impact during this period is extreme for the patient and family, because each phase requires major decisions and new adjustments. Patients sometimes feel "numb" in the 2–3 weeks before surgery, and it is only after surgery that the import of the diagnosis and treatment begins to be felt and the stress experienced.

The surgical procedure itself is usually followed by a rapid postoperative recovery. However, the presence of diminished stamina for some time is an unexpected, though common consequence for many. During the postoperative period, patients are apprehensive about tumor recurrence and each minor symptom is viewed as a return of disease. Many minor discomforts and pains are experienced as the patient resumes a normal diet and as the pattern of meals becomes regular. Sometimes these are similar to or the same as symptoms that appeared as the first sign of illness. There are also occasionally postoperative pain syndromes that can be persistent and require careful workup to rule out cancer as their cause.

During this time patients may need particular reassurance about eating. Sometimes anorexia and nausea reflect fears about being able to eat sufficient amounts to maintain weight. In turn, weight loss triggers fears of cancer recurrence, creating a vicious cycle of concerns.

Successful management of these patients depends on adequate opportunities to address these common concerns. This includes having access to the surgeon when questions about symptoms arise. It is additionally important to have regularly scheduled checkups during which the physician provides an explanation about the cause of distressing symptoms and outlines the means for controlling them. Usually this is accomplished with antacids and mild sedation. It may be helpful to have the patient meet another patient who has undergone the same surgery (see Chapter 41 on self-help). Enlisting the support of the family is also important in assisting the patient's emotional rehabilitation and return to work. In the case of severe emotional distress, psychiatric consultation is warranted to provide diagnosis and management by psychotherapeutic and pharmacological intervention. Behavioral means are helpful at times for control of nausea and anorexia when it is related to anxiety.

Rehabilitation is often fully achieved within a few months, but the return to full work may take longer. Those patients who receive adjuvant chemotherapy or radiation face the problems confronted by all patients who complete major surgery and immediately undergo cycles of adjuvant therapy (see Chapters 9 and 10 on radiation therapy and chemotherapy).

Management of advanced disease, if the cancer recurs after the initial treatment, is outlined in Chapter 6.

## COLON AND RECTAL CANCER

Cancers of the colon and rectum produce psychological problems that relate primarily to concerns about the cancer itself and the impact of treatment on bowel function in relation to social and sexual activity. For patients whose bowel is reanastomosed after surgery, the problems are little different psychologically from those already described for gastric and esophageal cancer. Indeed, the remarkable recovery of President Reagan in 1985 from such surgery, with return to a full work load in the Oval Office, provided a great source of reassurance for colon cancer patients. Surgical treatment by abdominoperineal resection, however, still results in impotence in a high percentage of men, although those who have anterior resection alone generally retain sexual potency. Women undergoing these procedures remain sexually responsive, but many experience significant discomfort during coitus for considerable periods after surgery, resulting in diminished interest and arousal. Special techniques for dealing with the sexual sequelae in these surgical groups is covered in Chapter 33.

Two other small groups warrant special attention. Those patients who develop colon cancer after ulcerative colitis may have more significant difficulties than patients without prior medical history. This is due to both the added emotional effects of a long-standing chronic illness, often dating to childhood, and that some patients with ulcerative colitis have a history of psychological difficulties. A second group of patients with special psychological needs are those who come from a family at high genetic risk of colon cancer, especially familial polyposis, and those who are part of a "cancer family." The specter of being at high genetic risk and having seen family members die of the same tumor add to the fear, depression, and distress. Prophylactic colostomy recommended at an early age to prevent colon cancer is a common decision faced by these individuals.

All patients are concerned about the possibility of diversion of the fecal stream to the abdominal wall. Fears of spillage, noises, and odors often inhibit return to social and work settings, and concern about being sexually unacceptable is frequently significant in both men and women. Advice and counseling from other patients who have been through the experience, practical suggestions about covering the stoma, use of deodorants and perfumes, and routine care to prevent spillage have all been shown to be major methods of increasing self-confidence and in promoting return to normal activity. The Ostomy Society, which has chapters in most major cities, can also offer the patient a valuable source of support.

The stigma felt by individuals treated for rectal cancer was assessed by McDonald and Anderson (1984). In their study of 420 rectal cancer patients, of whom 265 had a permanent colostomy, stigma was defined as damaging social influences perceived by the patient. This represented one aspect of quality-of-life assessment in a self-report survey that covered physical, emotional, and social health. Half the patients showed signs of feeling stigmatized, as reflected in reports of increased self-consciousness (31%), decreased attractiveness (27%), avoidance of other people (14%), and feeling different (11%). More symptoms were seen in younger patients and those with a colostomy. Indication of these feelings correlated with poorer physical health and greater emotional distress. Although family interactions were retained, social isolation was a result in some cases, suggesting a need for preparation both before and after the operation to diminish this negative interpersonal dimension.

With the introduction in the early 1980s of modified abdominoperineal procedures, fewer patients with colon cancer will undergo permanent colostomy, and it is infrequently required for patients with rectal cancer. For those 15% of patients whose treatment necessitates a permanent ostomy, special psychosocial problems arise. These are reviewed in the context of other ostomies, which are less frequently performed, but which have similar sequelae.

## Psychosocial Sequelae of Ostomies in Cancer Patients[1]

Until the late 1940s patients were largely left on their own to adjust to both the practical and emotional problems resulting from colostomy. Toward the end of that decade, the American Cancer Society's visitor programs began to help ostomy patients by having other cured patients visit the new patient. Individual surgeons in the United States began to ask particularly well-adjusted patients to provide practical advice to the new patient with an ostomy (Hurny and Holland, 1985).

In 1947, C.E. Dukes, a British surgeon and pa-

thologist whose classification of colorectal cancer is still used, reported on "expert patients" who had been living with a colostomy, some for more than 30 years. He interviewed 100 patients in their homes, identifying the practical, social, psychological, and even sexual problems they described. He suggested counseling of new or future patients by these "expert patients," matched for age and social class. A similar study was done by James Ewing in 1950.

The first comprehensive study of psychosocial problems of the cancer patient with a colostomy was done in the early 1950s by Arthur Sutherland's pioneering group at the Memorial Sloan-Kettering Hospital for Cancer and Allied Diseases in New York (Sutherland et al., 1952; Dyk and Sutherland, 1956). They evaluated 57 patients with colostomies and their families. These patients, who had survived disease-free from rectal cancer for 5 or more years, had considerable impairment in both social (work, community, and family) and sexual (of both neurological and psychological origin) function. Depression, chronic anxiety, and a sense of social isolation were frequently observed. They also had difficulties in the practical management of the colostomy associated with the use of clumsy belts and cumbersome dressings to cover the colostomy. Significant problems occurred with spillage and odor despite lengthy irrigation procedures. Today, patients have vastly improved equipment available with which to manage the stoma. In addition, the placement of the stoma site is given attention to take into account skin folds and patient preference.

The practical management problems of early ostomy patients led to the formation of patient self-help groups in the early 1950s. The groups were supported by several surgeons who performed the procedure often and understood the psychological and practical problems. At about the same time, independent groups were formed in Philadelphia and Los Angeles, and at the Mount Sinai Hospital in New York City. The first stoma clinic was formed at Mount Sinai to help patients adapt both physically and emotionally to artificial intestinal openings (Lyons, 1952; Barr, 1982). The first ostomy newsletter appeared early in 1952; it was called the "QT Bulletin" named for the famous ward at Mount Sinai. Later it became the *Ileostomy Quarterly* and still thrives as the *Ostomy Quarterly*, serving as a forum for exchange of information among patients. In 1962 the local units of ostomy groups formed a national group, the United Ostomy Association of America (UOA), and the International Ostomy Association (IOA) now serves a worldwide advocacy role for these individuals.

In the late 1950s, enterostomal therapy emerged as a nursing specialty. Most of the first enterostomal thera-

1. This section is adapted from an article by Hurny and Holland (1985). Tables are reprinted with permission.

**Table 15-1** Incidence of different ostomies among 1.5 million people with ostomies in the United States and Canada

| Percentage | Type |
|---|---|
| 51.0 | Colostomy |
| 35.0 | Ileostomy (conventional) |
| 0.5 | Ieostomy (continent: Kock pouch) |
| 12.0 | Urostomy (mainly ileal conduits) |
| 1.5 | Two ostomies |

*Source*: Reprinted with permission from C. Hurny and J.C. Holland (1985). Psychosocial sequelae of ostomies in cancer patients. *CA*, 35:170–80.

pists themselves had ostomies. A school of enterostomal therapy was started in 1961, followed soon after by the first issue of the *Journal of Enterostomal Therapy*.

## INCIDENCE AND TYPES OF OSTOMIES

It is estimated that 1.5 million people have ostomies in the United States and Canada, with 100,000 per year performed, representing a number equal to mastectomy. Half are permanent. Table 15-1 shows 51% are colostomies, 35.5% ileostomies; 12% urostomies (mainly ileal conduits), and 1.5% both a colostomy and a urostomy. Table 15-2 outlines the types of ostomies, the diseases with which they are associated, as well as the sequelae and complications. By far the most

common stoma is the colostomy for colorectal cancer. Due to improvements in surgical techniques, however, only about 15–20% of patients with operable colorectal (mainly rectal) cancer require a permanent colostomy (Enker, 1982). There is a substantial hope that this number will decrease even further without compromising the high cure rate in early stages of the disease (Goligher, 1982).

Most patients cope well with both concerns about disease and the stoma when they have been given adequate information. On the other hand, Table 15-3 reveals the physical, emotional, and interpersonal problems that confront these patients (Dlin et al., 1969; Druss et al., 1969; Dempsey et al., 1975; Wirschung et al., 1975).

Practical management of the ostomy centers on learning to manage the stoma well, which often leads to development of a sense of pride. A special problem may be phantom rectum sensations following colostomy. Removal of the rectum and placement of a stoma often results in the sensation of an urge to defecate, which continues for some time. Common emotional issues involve loss of self-esteem and depression, and their consequences, as well as anxiety about ability to function adequately in social and sexual situations. The interpersonal dimension is often the most difficult to overcome, with persistent self-consciousness in the presence of others and avoidance and withdrawal being common problems.

Once the diagnosis of rectal cancer is established

**Table 15-2** Types of ostomies and possible sequelae and complications*

| Type of ostomy | Disease | Procedure | Excreta | Continence | Physical impairment of sexual function | Other complications |
|---|---|---|---|---|---|---|
| Colostomy | Colorectal cancer | Abdominoperineal resection | ± Formed stool | ± With irrigation | + | Skin irritation, bowel obstruction, prolapse or retraction of stoma, stenosis of stoma |
| Ileostomy | Inflammatory bowel diseases (ulcerative colitis, Crohn's disease) | Total colectomy | Fluid stool | − − With conventional care + With Kock pouch | ± | Renal stone formation† and the above |
| Urostomy (ileal conduit) | Bladder cancer | Radical cystectomy | Urine | — | + | Urinary infections and all the above |
| Colostomy and urostomy (ileal conduit) | Gynecological cancer (advanced and recurrent) | Pelvic exenteration | ± Formed stool Urine | ± With irrigation − − | + + | Combination of all the above |

*− −, Absent in all patients; ±, present in half; + +, present in all patients; + present in majority.

†Due to chronic asymptomatic water and salt depletion.

*Source*: Reprinted with permission. C. Hurny and J.C. Holland (1985). Psychosocial sequelae of ostomies in cancer patients. *CA* 35:170–80.

**Table 15-3**  Common psychosocial problems in ostomy patients

| Types of problems | Characterisitcs |
|---|---|
| *Physical* | Practical problems of handling the stoma and bowel or urinary function irrigation, changing bags, finding the adequate appliance, leakage |
| *Emotional* | Impaired self-esteem and psychological dysfunction with depression and anxiety; anxiety in social situations; fears of sexual undesirability |
| *Interpersonal* | Impaired sexual function or fears about sexual function, even if function is actually unimpaired |
|  | Strain on key relationships (partner, family, friends) |
|  | Strain in work situation imposed by stoma care and concerns about odors |
|  | Social isolation resulting from sense of stigma, low self-esteem, withdrawal because of depression and/or anxiety |

*Source*: Reprinted with permission from C. Hurny and J.C. Holland (1985). Psycholsocial sequelae of ostomies in cancer patients. *CA* 35:170–80.

and resection with possible ostomy is recommended, the patient has to deal with both the threat to life posed by the cancer and the threat to body integrity raised by the specter of ostomy and its consequences. The shock, anxiety, hopelessness, and helplessness are reduced by sharing the crisis with a close relative, friend, and or veteran patient. The patient who is unable to decide to undergo surgery will be helped by meeting and talking with an ostomate (Genzdilov et al., 1977). The extra time needed to make a decision is often valuable; the postoperative period is smoother when it follows adequate preoperative preparation. Table 15-4 outlines the important issues to be addressed at each stage of treatment.

Ostomy patients may initially refuse to look at the stoma; even thoughts about it evoke disgust, anger, embarrassment, and shame. The nurse may have to encourage participation in care. When the colostomy starts to work, the surgeon is pleased because normal bowel function has begun; the patient, however, is embarrassed. The guidance of an experienced nurse or enterostomal therapist helps the patient to become accustomed to the sight of the stoma and to learn to maintain it—even eventually being able to use humor in dealing with the stoma and the problems it produces.

Coping with a newly placed stoma in the hospital, where professional help is available, is one thing; coping at home is another. This is true not only for the patient, but even more so for the spouse or others close to the patient who are confronted with the burden of care that had previously been taken by the hospital staff.

Oberst and James (1985) studied 40 patients and their immediate families at 1 or 2 days prior to discharge and at 10, 30, and 60 days later, back in their home environment. All patients had been newly diagnosed with cancer of the large bowel or genitourinary system and had undergone surgical treatment for the cancer, with 50% requiring a stoma. According to their study, for the first 2 months concerns about the stoma

**Table 15-4**  Management of the cancer patient with an ostomy

| Stage of management | Characteristics |
|---|---|
| *Preoperative phase* | Adequate explanation of the actual medical situation, the needed surgical procedure, and possible (especially sexual) sequelae is crucial. Simple drawings are often of great help. Due to patient's anxiety, explanations may have to be given more than once. |
|  | Preoperative visit by a veteran patient with an ostomy and/or an enterostomal therapist, who functions as part of physician's team. |
|  | Physician should take time to listen to questions and concerns from patient and family |
| *Postoperative phase* | Postoperative care directed by enterostomal therapist or experienced surgical nurse. Self-care must be learned before discharge. Inclusion of significant other who will care for the patient at home is important, with adequate counseling of both by physician. |
| *Discharge home* | Detailed information to family physician about medical and emotional state of the patient should be available. |
|  | Offer of continued contact with patient and availability by phone of one team member (e.g., enterostomal therapist) is essential. |
| *Long-term adjustment* | At clinic visits after discharge, questions about emotional state and sexual function have to be addressed. |
|  | Coping of the patient's significant other should be explored. |
|  | Immediate referral to proper experts for care when emotional or sexual function is impaired and is of concern to the patient but cannot be handled by the family physician. |
|  | Information about ostomy groups in patient's community should be provided. |

*Source*: Reprinted with permission from C. Hurny and J.C. Holland (1985). Psychosocial sequelae of ostomies in cancer patients. *CA* 35:170–80.

are the central issue; life-and-death concerns begin to surface only later when the person has mastered the stoma's management. Although the stoma patients cope better with experience, their level of anxiety rises constantly from the day they leave the hospital through the first 2 months, in contrast to the nonostomy group in whom anxiety level, after peaking at 10 days at home, drops down and stays at the same relatively low level after 30 days.

The pattern for the partner is quite different. The spouse of an ostomy patient experiences even more distress and anxiety than the patient at home. After 10 days back at home, when the patient begins to cope relatively well, the spouse's ability to cope effectively diminishes, and by 2 months after discharge, his or her anxiety level is well above that recorded for hospitalized psychiatric inpatients. Typical partner comments include: "Nobody understands what I'm going through"; "He's feeling better and I keep feeling worse"; "Everyone pats him on the back and says how well he's managing, but no one asks about me"; "And no one, (including the patient) says, 'thanks'." It is clear that it is not only the patients who need assistance to cope; the closest relative needs it as well. As Oberst states, "Learning to live with someone else's cancer (and stoma) may be even more difficult, precisely because no one recognizes just how hard it really is" (Oberst and James, 1985).

Regarding long-term adjustment, there is a range of possible psychological outcomes. At one end of the spectrum is the patient who actually gets more out of life after the ostomy experience. This occurs with patients who have been chronically sick with inflammatory bowel disease, where the placement of an ileostomy marks the end of being chronically ill and marks the start of a healthier life. Such a positive response is less likely to occur when the ostomy is performed in an attempt to cure cancer in someone in previously good health. At the other end of the spectrum is the patient who actually is cured of cancer and is physically healthy, but who becomes an invalid for psychological reasons. The majority of patients are somewhere in the middle of these two extremes. In terms of quality of life, recent studies are more optimistic than earlier ones. Improvement is largely due to better surgical techniques and equipment available for care of the stoma.

## SEXUAL PROBLEMS

Besides the stigma of cancer and stomas, there is an additional problem confronted by the cancer patient who undergoes stoma surgery, that is, the sexual taboo. Although people speak more openly about sexual problems, it is still difficult for many physicians and patients to address the question that both are reluctant to ask.

In our study at Memorial Sloan-Kettering Cancer Center, about one-third of the patients with bladder and colon cancer (mean age 56.5) had completely stopped sexual activity after diagnosis, many with no physical impairment of sexual function. (Hurny and Holland, 1985). It is important to know why this group responded as they did, because their response is likely related to possible psychological changes. Two common misconceptions are that sex is not important if one is older or if one is physically ill, especially with cancer (Leiber et al., 1976). In interviewing those patients with advanced colorectal or bladder cancer, however, it was clear that some of them had rewarding means of sexual expression despite physical limitations and often in the absence of vaginal intercourse. This finding is helpful in dispelling the myth that vaginal intercourse is necessary for satisfaction and serves to caution against use of this as a sole criterion for assessing satisfactory sexual adaptation.

It has been recognized since the early 1950s that major surgical procedures in men that involve the pelvic area may lead to disturbance in sexual function. This occurs secondary to damage to the pelvic sympathetic nerves (L1, L2, and L3), which are responsible for ejaculation, and parasympathetic nerves (S2, S3, and S4), which are responsible for erection. A summary of the main effects on sexual function of abdominoperineal resection is given in Table 15-5. Although some information on women is provided, the majority of studies have involved men because the effects are more clear-cut and easier to describe.

In 1951 Goligher reported a study of sexual function in a selected sample of 81 men under the age of 60 with previously active sex lives, after the excision of the rectum for cancer. A total of 72% were still capable of having erections, which in 64% were adequate for intercourse. Of those having intercourse, 61% had normal ejaculation. In later series the incidence of sexual dysfunction was found to be somewhat higher (Goligher, 1951; Pruden, 1971; DeBernardinis et al., 1981), but some of these studies included patients who were sexually inactive before surgery.

It is safe to conclude that there is a 30–50% chance of impotence and a 50–75% chance of sterility after excision of the rectum. After total colectomy for inflammatory bowel disease (usually done in younger individuals with less damage to the pelvic nerves), the incidence of sexual dysfunction is lower, reported as 15% in men under the age of 35; this increases to 53% in those over 45. Sexual function after radical cystectomy (including prostatectomy and vesiculectomy) for bladder cancer has a much higher incidence of complete impotence (Bergman et al., 1979). Inability to

**Table 15-5**  Sexual function after abdominoperineal resection for colorectal cancer

| Sex | Functional Disruption* | | | | | |
|-----|-------|----------|-------------|-------------|--------|-----------|
|     | Drive | Erection | Ejaculation | Lubrication | Orgasm | Fertility |
| Men | + | ± | − | N.A. | + | − |
| Women | + | N.A. | N.A. | + | + | − |

*+, Present in majority; −, absent in majority; ±, present, in half; N.A., not applicable.

*Source*: Adapted from C. Hurny and J.C. Holland (1985). Psychosocial sequelae of ostomies in cancer patients. *CA* 35:170–80.

have an erection after pelvic surgery can be reversed by surgical implantation of a prosthesis, using either a rigid or an inflatable implant (Small, 1976) (see also Chapter 33 on sexual rehabilitation).

Less attention has been paid to physiological changes after abdominoperineal resection in women. One study describes decreased libido, decreased vaginal lubrication, and decreased incidence of orgasm after abdominoperineal resection for rectal cancer (Bergman et al., 1979). As with males, sexual disturbance seems to be less frequent in women treated with ileostomy after colectomy for inflammatory bowel disease (Bergman et al., 1979).

Sometimes the problem of physical and psychological dysfunction are so intertwined that they are difficult to separate. For instance, impotence and decreased libido may be symptoms of depression rather than the sequelae of the operation. Shame and embarrassment may interfere with pleasurable sex. For example, a 53-year-old man was completely impotent 2 years after cystectomy, but was able to enjoy orgasm through oral stimulation. He said that he could not expose his ileal conduit bag and covered it by wearing a shirt. Covering it was important to him, but not to his wife.

## IRRIGATION

In the United States in the 1950s and 1960s, there was a strong belief that for patients undergoing colostomy, irrigation was the only means to be in control and to have a reasonable life. Once bags became available to protect the patient from odor and spillage, irrigation became less important. Now it is up to the patient whether he or she wants to learn the procedure. In our study, fewer than 50% the patients with colostomies were irrigating on a regular basis.

In summary, in the last 30 years much has been done to improve the quality of life for patients with ostomies through better surgical techniques with fewer sequelae, improved technical devices for practical management of the stoma, better understanding of the accompanying psychosocial and sexual problems, and more available support through ostomy groups and enterostomal therapists. In spite of these improve-

ments, however, even today it is a difficult experience to face the diagnosis of cancer and to have a stoma. Adjusting to life with an ostomy involves physical, emotional, and interpersonal (especially sexual) problems. Although most patients cope well, they need considerable support and care by nurses, enterostomal therapists, the surgeon, an ostomate, and an understanding spouse. Guidelines for management of the cancer patient with an ostomy at each stage are given in Table 15.4.

## PANCREATIC CANCER

Adenocarcinoma of the pancreas is a tumor with an extremely poor prognosis; less than 1% survival at 5 years is currently obtained by any treatment. This is largely because the early symptoms are systemic and vague, and the spread of the disease beyond the pancreas has occurred in 85–90% of patients at the time of biopsy or surgical exploration. This condition is increasing in frequency in the United States, especially in women, with the sex ratio approaching 1 : 1 (Herman and Cooperman, 1979; Malagelada, 1979). There has been a long-held belief among clinicians that pancreatic cancer patients at times have a history of unexplained depression and distress that preceded the appearance of anorexia, weight loss, pain in the abdomen (often boring through to the back), and jaundice (Scholz and Pfeiffer, 1923; Yaskin, 1931; Latter and Wilbur, 1937; Savage et al., 1952; Savage and Noble, 1954; Perlas and Faillace 1964; Karlinger, 1967). Most early clinical case reports, beginning in the 1920s, described a triad of depression, anxiety, and premonition of impending doom. The question of whether this phenomenon is medical folklore or a psychiatric syndrome associated specifically with pancreatic cancer has been debated at length (Jacobsen and Ottoson, 1971; Holland, 1982; Sachar, 1975; Brown and Paraskevas, 1982). Most attention has focused on depressive symptoms, even though early accounts also reported anxiety as a prominent part of the mental disturbance.

Two retrospective chart reviews of pancreatic patients reported a prevalence of psychiatric symptoms in

**Table 15-6**  Median and range for profile of mood states (POMS) scores by disease site

| | Site | | | | |
| | Gastric ($n$ = 111) | | Pancreatic ($n$ = 107) | | |
| POMS scale | median | range | median | range | $p$ Value |
| --- | --- | --- | --- | --- | --- |
| Depression | 6 | 0–39 | 10 | 0–56 | .023 |
| Tension–anxiety | 10 | 0–31 | 13 | 1–35 | .003 |
| Anger–hostility | 4 | 0–35 | 4 | 0–37 | — |
| Fatigue | 7 | 0–30 | 11 | 0–28 | .0007 |
| Confusion–bewilderment | 5 | 0–17 | 7 | 0–22 | .01 |
| Vigor | 14 | 2–30 | 13 | 1–28 | — |
| Total mood disturbance | 21 | −28 to 123 | 38 | −19 to 152 | .003 |

*Source*: Adapted from J.C. Holland et al. (1986). Comparative psychological disturbance in patients with pancreatic and gastric cancer. *Am. J. Psychiatry*, 143, 982–86.

10–20% of the cases evaluated (Birnbaum and Kleesberg, 1958; Savage et al., 1952). A study at the Mayo Clinic done by Fras, Litin, and Pearson (1967) was the first to provide a prospective observation. They gave the Minnesota Multiphasic Personality Inventory (MMPI) to patients at the time they were admitted with symptoms suspicious of an abdominal neoplasm. Depression, anxiety, and loss of ambition were present in 76% of patients who received a diagnosis of pancreatic cancer at the time of surgery, as compared to 20% of patients who were found at operation to have other abdominal neoplasms. A similar prospective study by Klatchko and Gorzynski (1982) reported significantly higher depression scores at the time of admission among patients subsequently found to have pancreatic cancer, as compared to patients who received a diagnosis of abdominal tumors not of pancreatic origin.

A third prospective study, conducted in 1985, was part of a multidisciplinary collaborative effort with the Cancer and Leukemia Group B (CALGB) cancer clinical trials group. The question of presence of psychiatric morbidity in pancreatic cancer patients was addressed in a controlled study that compared a large cohort of patients with advanced pancreatic carcinoma ($n$ = 107) to a group of patients with advanced gastric cancer ($n$ = 111) who were about to undergo chemotherapy on one of two nearly identical chemotherapy protocols (Holland et al., 1986). All patients were stratified for key medical and sociodemographic variables, and assessed using the Profile of Mood States (POMS) prior to the beginning of drug treatment. Patient self-ratings of depression, tension–anxiety, fatigue, confusion–bewilderment, and total mood disturbance were significantly greater for the pancreatic cancer patients than for the gastric cancer group; the groups did not differ on vigor and anger–hostility (Table 15-6). These prospective data from a large cohort appear to confirm that significantly greater general psychological disturbance, which includes both depression and anxiety, occurs to a greater extent in patients with pancreatic cancer as compared to patients with another advanced abdominal neoplasm when matched for medical and demographic variables.

Although the consistency of these findings is compelling, several other issues must be considered in interpreting the emotional profile of these patients. The greater disturbance in the pancreatic cancer patients may simply reflect the psychological response to the knowledge of having a tumor whose extremely poor prognosis is well known. Moreover, the person may have had several months of systemic symptoms of an illness for which physicians could find no clear cause. When finally diagnosed by more definite symptoms, the person is told a diagnosis, often of advanced disease, for which depression is a well-known response (Bukberg et al., 1984; Plumb and Holland, 1977; Petty and Noyes, 1981). Anxiety is often present as well, as noted by Cassileth and colleagues (1984), especially in advanced disease.

The other more intriguing explanation for greater psychological distress in patients with this disease is that a biological, tumor-mediated paraneoplastic syndrome exists, similar to the unusual manifestations described by Schnider and Manolo (1979) that may alter mood in patients with advanced cancer through the production of a false neurotransmitter. The presence of extensive neuropeptides in the GI tract and brain suggest a range of possible interactions. Brown and Paraskevas (1982) proposed that some cases of depression in cancer could be caused by immunological interference with the activity of serotonin. They postulate a model in which serotonin, possibly mediated by an antibody induced against a protein released by the tumor, could cross-react with CNS tissue and bind to serotonin receptors and block them.

An alternative explanation could be antibody production, which stimulates antiidiotypic antibodies that act as an alternative receptor for serotonin and reduce its synaptic availability. Report of improvement of a treatment-resistant depression following surgical removal of a pancreatic tumor, in a patient who had a positive Dexamethasone Suppression Test (DST), suggests need for further study of the biological parameter (Pomara and Gershon, 1984).

## Diagnosis and Management

Individuals who are middle aged or older and who have affective symptoms without a clear precipitant, particularly when vegetative symptoms predominate, should be thoroughly worked up medically for an occult neoplasm of the pancreas. This is a poorly understood syndrome. Clinically we have seen several patients who had anxiety and agitation along with depression that responded poorly to all interventions including psychological support, medication, psychiatric hospitalization, and, in one case, electroconvulsive therapy. These are unusual case reports, but they support the need to study such cases closely.

The more common situation is one in which the patient shows reactive depression and distress in the context of increasing physical symptoms and where pain may be a primary, poorly controlled component. This is a visceral pain, often constant and poorly relieved by narcotic analgesics. Nerve blocks may be required and may give some relief. Anorexia is often also present. Given the known poor outlook, usually counted in months of survival and the burden of increasing symptoms, management centers on maximal comfort care and symptom control. Supportive care at home can be very meaningful to the patient and family. Psychotropic drugs are used as adjuvant for control of psychological symptoms and often insomnia. An antidepressant, such as desipramine, or a low-dose psychostimulant may enhance poor appetite. These patients and their families require active and aggressive support programs to cope with the hopelessness and sense of helplessness at altering the disease course and to cope with the patient's rapid decline (see also Chapters 48 and 49 on home care programs).

## REFERENCES

Barr, L.R. (1982). Psychiatric reactions to colectomy: A literature study. *Mt. Sinai J. Med.* 49:314–17.

Bergman, B., S. Nilsson, and I. Petersen (1979). The effect on erection and orgasm of cystecomy, prostatecomy, and vesiculectomy for cancer of the bladder: A clinical and electromyographic study. *Br. J. Urol.* 51:114–20.

Birnbaum, D. and J. Kleesberg (1958). Carcinoma of the pancreas: A clinical study based on 84 cases. *Ann. Intern. Med.* 48:1171–84.

Brovillette, J.N., E. Pryor, and T.A. Fox, Jr. (1981). Evaluation of sexual dysfunction in the female following rectal ressection and intestinal stoma. *Dis. Colon Rectum* 24:96–102.

Brown, J.H. and F. Paraskevas (1982). Cancer and depression: Cancer presenting with depressive illness: An autoimmune disease? *Br. J. Psychiatry* 141:227–32.

Bukberg, J., D. Penman, and J.C. Holland (1984). Depression in hospitalized cancer patients. *Psychosom. Med.* 46:199–212.

Cassileth, B.R., E.J. Lusk, R. Hutter, T.B. Strouse, and L.L. Brown (1984). Concordance of depression and anxiety in patients with cancer. *Psychol. Rep.* 54:588–90.

DeBernardinis, G., D. Tuscano, P. Negro, G. Flati, D. Flati, A. Bianchini, and M. Carboni (1981). Sexual dysfunction in males following extensive colorectal surgery. *Int. Surg.* 66:133–35.

Dempsey, G.M., H.J. Buchsbaum, and J. Morrison (1975). Psychosocial adjustment to pelvic exenteration. *Gynecol. Oncol.* 3:325–34.

Dlin, B.M., A. Perlman, and E. Ringold (1969). Psychosexual response to ileostomy and colostomy. *Am. J. Psychiatry* 126:374–81.

Druss, R.G., F. O'Connor, and L.O. Stern (1969). Psychologic response to colectomy: II. Adjustment to a permanent colostomy. *Arch. Gen. Psychiatry* 20:419–27.

Dukes, C.E. (1947). Management of a permanent colostomy: Study of 100 patients at home. *Lancet* 2:12–14.

Dyk, R.B. and A.M. Sutherland (1956). Adaptation of the spouse and other family members to the colostomy patient. *Cancer* 9:123–38.

Enker, W.E. (1982). Colorectal cancer? An ostomy is far from inevitable. *Your Patient and Cancer* 2:29–35.

Fras, I., E.M. Litin, and J.S. Pearson (1967). Comparison of psychiatric symptoms in carcinoma of the pancreas with those in some other intraabdominal neoplasms. *Am. J. Psychiatry* 123:1553–62.

Genzdilov, A.V., G.P. Alexandrin, N.N. Simonov, A.I. Evtjuhin, and U.F. Bobrov (1977). *J. Surg. Oncol.* 9:517–23.

Goligher, J.C. (1951). Sexual function after excision of the rectum. *Proc. R. Soc. Med.* 44:819–28.

Goligher, J.C. (1982). Current trends in the use of sphincter-saving excision in the treatment of carcinoma of the rectum. *Cancer* 50:2627–30.

Herman, R.E. and A.M. Cooperman (1979). Current concepts in cancer of the pancreas. *N. Engl. J. Med.* 301:482–85.

Holland, J.C.B. (1982). Psychological aspects of cancer. In J.F. Holland and E. Frei III (eds.), *Cancer Medicine*, 2nd ed. Philadelphia: Lea & Febiger, pp. 1175–1203.

Holland, J.C., A.H. Hughes, S. Tross, P. Silberfarb, M. Perry, R. Comis, and M. Oster (1986). Comparative psychological disturbance in patients and pancreatic and gastric cancer. *Am. J. Psych.* 143:982–86.

Hurny, C. and J.C. Holland (1985). Psychosocial sequelae of ostomies in cancer patients. *CA* 35:170–83.

Jacobsen, L. and J.O. Ottoson (1971). Initial mental disorder in carcinoma of the pancreas and stomach. *Acta Psychiatr. Scand.* 220:120–27.

Karlinger, W. (1967). Psychiatric manifestations of cancer of the pancreas. *N. Engl. J. Med.* 56:2251–52.

Klatchko, B. and J.G. Gorzynski (1982). *A Prospective Controlled Study of Depression in Patients with Pancreatic and Other Intra-abdominal Malignancies.* Paper presented at the annual meeting of the American Psychosomatic Society, Denver, March.

Latter, K.A. and D.L. Wilbur (1937). Psychic and neurological manifestations of carcinoma of the pancreas. *Proc. Mayo Clin.* 12:457–62.

Leiber, L., M.M. Plumb, M.L. Gerstenzang, and J.C. Holland (1976). The communication of affection between cancer patients and their spouses. *Psychosom. Med.* 38:379–89.

Lyons, A.S. (1952). An ileostomy club. *J.A.M.A.* 150:812.

MacDonald, L.D. and H.R. Anderson (1984). Stigma in patients with rectal cancer: A community study. *J. Epidemiol. Community Health* 38:284–90.

Malagelada, J. (1979). Pancreatic cancer: An overview of epidemiology: Clinical presentation and diagnosis. *Mayo Clin. Proc.* 54:459–67.

Oberst, M.T. and R.H. James (1985). Going home: Patient and spouse adjustment following cancer surgery. *Top. Clin. Nurs.* 7(1):46–57.

Perlas, A.P. and L.A. Faillace (1964). Case reports: Psychiatric manifestations of carcinoma of the pancreas. *Am. J. Psychiatry* 121:182.

Petty, F. and R. Noyes, Jr. (1981). Depression secondary to cancer. *Biol. Psychiatry* 16:1203–20.

Plumb, M. and J.C. Holland (1977). Comparative studies of psychological function in patients with advanced cancer: I. Self-reported depressive symptoms. *Psychosom. Med.* 39:264–76.

Pomara, N.P. and S. Gershon (1984). Treatment-resistant depression in an elderly patient with pancreatic carcinoma: Case report. *J. Clin. Psychiatry* 45:439–40.

Prudden, J.F. (1971). Psychological problems following ileostomy and colostomy. *Cancer* 28:236–38.

Sachar, E. (1975). Evaluating depression in the medical patient. In J. Strain and S. Grossman (eds.), *Psychological Care of the Medically Ill: A Primer in Liaison Psychiatry.* New York: Appleton-Century-Crofts, pp. 64–75.

Savage, C., W. Butcher, and D. Noble (1952). Psychiatric manifestations in pancreatic disease. *J. Clin. Psychopathol.* 13:9–16.

Savage, C. and D. Noble (1954). Cancer of the pancreas: Two cases simulating psychogenic illness. *J. Nerv. Ment. Dis.* 120:62–65.

Schnider, B. and A. Manolo (1979). Paraneoplastic syndrome's unusual manifestations of malignant disease. *Disease-a-Month* 25:1–59.

Scholz, T. and F. Pfeiffer (1923). Roentgenologic diagnosis of carcinoma of the tail of the pancreas. *J.A.M.A.* 81:275–77.

Small, P. (1976). Small-carrion penile prosthesis: A new implant for management of impotence. *Mayo Clin. Proc.* 51:336–38.

Sutherland, A.M., C.E. Orbach, R.B. Dyk, and M. Bard (1952). The psychological impact of cancer and cancer surgery: I. Adaptation to the dry colostomy: Preliminary report and summary of findings. *Cancer* 5:857–72.

Weissman, M.M. and J.K. Myers (1978). Affective disorders in a U.S.-urban community: The use of Research Diagnostic Criteria in an epidemiological survey. *Arch. Gen. Psychiatry* 35:1304–11.

Wirsching, M., H.U. Druner, and G. Herrman (1975). Results of psychosocial adjustment to long-term colostomy. *Psychother. Psychosom.* 7(1):46–57.

Yaskin, J.D. (1931). Nervous symptoms at earliest manifestations of carcinoma of the pancreas. *J.A.M.A.* 96:1664–68.

# 16

## Hematological Malignancies

Lynna M. Lesko

## CLASSIFICATION

### Leukemia

Since its first description by Donne in 1839, leukemia has been equated with hopelessness and a rapidly fatal outcome. The untreated median survival time is less than 2 months for acute leukemia; survival is longer with chronic leukemia, but it is also eventually fatal. Leukemias are classified according to the type of aberrant hematopoietic cell: lymphocytic leukemia or the nonlymphocytic leukemias comprising myeloid, monocytic, and erythroid cell types.

In the United States, 24,000 new cases of leukemia are diagnosed each year. The 16,000 deaths due to leukemia each year constitute 9% of all deaths related to cancer (Margolis and McCredie, 1983). Whereas many think of leukemia as a disease of childhood or adolescence, 89% of cases are adults over the age of 60.

Pediatric leukemia peaks at 7 cases per 100,000 in children under 5 years of age. Even though it is rare in children, it is the second most common cause of death after accidents. Acute lymphocytic leukemia is the most common form in children and accounts for 75% of all cases, with the acute nonlymphocytic forms making up the remainder.

Chronic and acute nonlymphocytic leukemia are the most common forms of the disease among adults (see Table 16-1). Table 16-2 summarizes current classification of the acute leukemias according to cell morphology, and gives their relative incidence. In the population of young adults from 15 to 35 years old, leukemia is the leading cause of cancer death in men and second in women after breast cancer. Although the cause of leukemia is unknown, chemotherapeutic agents, used to treat other cancers, can cause acute leukemia as one of the delayed effects.

### Lymphoma

Lymphoma is a general term for the group of neoplastic disorders involving the lymphoreticular tissue. First described by Hodgkin in 1832, the lymphomas were classified early in the twentieth century by Kundral-Brill. The cause or causes of this lymph node tumor are still unknown; however, histological, serological, and epidemiological evidence strongly suggest a viral or infectious origin. The lymphomas are usually separated into Hodgkin's lymphoma and the non-Hodgkin's lymphomas; the numerous subtypes within each group are identified by histopathological characteristics. Table 16-3 summarizes the histopathological classification of Hodgkin's and non-Hodgkin's lymphomas. Table 16-4 gives definitions of the stages of lymphomas, which is important in determining the extent of disease and treatment.

Lymphomas represent a relatively common form of malignancy in the United States. The incidence of Hodgkin's disease is approximately 3 cases per 100,000 per year (Table 16-5). Although rare in children under the age of 5, it is the most common form of lymphoma in children and has a bimodal age incidence with peaks between the ages of 15 and 34 and after age 50. Survival in the younger group is better than the older. Currently, 80% of all patients under age 35 with Hodgkin's disease are alive 5 years or more after treatment, making one of the significant successes in cancer treatment. The incidence of non-Hodgkin's lymphoma is close to 13 cases per 100,000 per year in the

**Table 16-1** Approximate annual incidence of leukemia

| Types of leukemia* | Age group | | Total |
|---|---|---|---|
| | Children | Adults | |
| ALL | 1,700 | 1,600 | 3,300 |
| ANLL | 250 | 8,000 | 8,250 |
| CLL | rare | 9,600 | 9,600 |
| CML | 50 | 4,600 | 4,650 |
| Total | 2,000 | 23,800 | 25,800 |

*ALL, Acute lymphocytic; ANLL, acue nonlymphocytic; CLL, chronic lymphcytic; CML, chronic myelogenous.
*Source*: Leukemia Society of America (1987). Facts about leukemia. National Office, 733 Third Avenue, New York, NY 10017.

United States, with a peak between the ages of 40 and 70. For the non-Hodgkin's lymphomas, 5-year survival is only 43% with current treatment.

## CLINICAL COURSE AND TREATMENT OF HEMATOLOGICAL MALIGNANCIES

### Clinical Course

Figure 16-1 outlines the several clinical courses that leukemia or lymphoma may follow. They determine

**Table 16-2** Classification of acute leukemias

| Class | Morphology | Percentage incidence in adults |
|---|---|---|
| M 1 | Acute myeloid leukemia without maturation | 35 |
| M 2 | Acute myeloid leukemia with maturation | |
| M 3 | Acute hypergranular promyelocytic leukemia | 10 |
| M 4 | Acute myelomonocytic leukemia (well differentiated) | 45 |
| M 5 | Acute monocytic leukemia (poorly differentiated) | 7 |
| M 6 | Erythroleukemia | 3 |
| L 1 | Acute lymphocytic leukemia (common childhood variant: homogeneous population | 20 |
| L 2 | Acute lymphocytic leukemia (common adult variant: heterogeneous population) | 80 |
| L 3 | Burkitt cell type | rare |

*Source*: Adapted from S. Schrier (1984). The leukemias and myeloproliferative disorders. In E. Rubenstein and D.D. Federman (eds.), *Scientific American Medicine*. Sec. 5, *Hematology*. New York: Scientific American, pp. 1–22; and H.R. Gralnick, D.A.G. Galton, D. Catovsky, et al. (1977). Classification of acute leukemia. *Ann. Intern. Med.* 87: 740.

the patient's psychological concerns and contribute to the adjustment to illness and treatment. The first stage begins often with seemingly minor symptoms. The presenting symptoms of leukemia vary but may include anemia with weakness and pallor, fatigue, dyspnea, palpitations, bleeding from gums, gastrointestinal tract, uterus, or bladder, petechiae, ecchymoses, increased susceptibility to infections, low-grade fever, and lymphadenopathy. In the case of lymphoma, similar symptoms of fatigue and lymphadenopathy appear. Loss of appetite and weight loss, accompanied by night sweats and pruritus, are more common with lymphoma. Usually the person seeks medical advice when these symptoms persist or worsen. People with leukemia usually seek medical attention earlier than those with lyphoma.

Leukemia is diagnosed by bone marrow aspiration. A histopathological diagnosis is made by subjecting the aspirate to cytochemical staining and identification of cell surface markers. To diagnose lymphoma, a pathological diagnosis is made from a lymph node biopsy. Staging of disease is done by physical examination to determine all involved lymph nodes, lung tomograms (to identify pulmonary involvement, hilar or mediastinal adenopathy), thoracic and abdominal CT scans (to identify thoracic or retroperitoneal adenopathy), and/or lymphangiography to outline nodes further. An exploratory laparotomy is often also necessary for staging in lymphomas (the staging criteria are included in Table 16-4). Later stages reflect more extensive disease, which necessitates lengthier treatment and more intense cycles of drugs.

Relating the diagnosis and treatment plan to the patient and family may take several sessions, because patients have such high anxiety that their recall of the facts is poor. Decisions must be made quickly, especially in patients with acute leukemia in whom rapid disease progression may occur if chemotherapy is delayed, even by a few days. Very few patients and families choose to accept *no* treatment. When this occurs, it is usually because of religious convictions about use of blood products, commitment to an alternative treatment, or the opinion that the treatment is too arduous for an older individual. However, most patients accept the treatment offered them, often participating in controlled clinical trials when treatment is in a cancer center. In fact, one study showed that children who participated in clinical trials had better survival rates than children who were treated without a protocol (Meadows and Evans, 1976).

In leukemia, induction chemotherapy is the first phase of treatment, followed by consolidation and possibly maintenance chemotherapy; the three phases require 2–3 years to complete. The lengthy treatment

**Table 16-3**  Histopathological classifications of non-Hodgkin's Lymphomas

|  | Immunologic phenotype | New formulation | Rappaport classification |
|---|---|---|---|
| Low grade | Predominantly B | Small lymphocytic (SL) | Diffuse, lymphocytic, well differentiated |
|  | B | Folliculular, Predominantly small cleaved cell (FSC) | Nodular, lymphocytic, poorly differentiated |
|  | B | Follicular, mixed small cleaved and large cell (FM) | Nodular, mixed, lymphocytic and histiocytic |
| Intermediated grade | B (mature) | Follicular, predominantly large cell (FL) | Nodular, histiocytic |
|  | B or T (mature) | Diffuse, small cleaved cell (DSC) | Diffuse, lymphocytic, poorly differentiated |
|  | B or T (mature) | Diffuse, mixed small and large cell (DM) | Diffuse, mixed, lymphocytic and histiocytic |
|  | B or T | Diffuse, large cell (DL): Cleaved or noncleaved cell | Diffuse, histiocytic |
| High grade | B or T | Immunoblastic (IBL) | Diffuse, histiocytic |
|  | T (thymocytic) | Lymphoblastic (LL): Convoluted or nonconvoluted cell | Diffuse, lymphoblastic |
|  | B | Small noncleaved cell (SNC): Burkitt's or non-Burkitt's | Diffuse, undifferentiated |
| Miscellaneous | Monocyte-macrophage | Histiocytic | — |
|  | T (mature) | Mycosis fungoides |  |
|  | B | Extramedullary plasmacytoma |  |
|  | B or T | Composite |  |
|  | B or T | Unclassifiable |  |

*Source*: S. Rosenberg and F. Stockdale (1984). Hodgkin's disease and other lymphomas. In E. Rubenstein and D.D. Dederman (eds.), *Scientific Medicine*. Sec. 5, *Hematology*. New York: Scientific American, p. 17.

involves many painful procedures and requires dedication and a high level of compliance on the part of patients. Cranial irradiation, intrathecal chemotherapy via an Ommaya shunt, venipunctures, bone marrow aspirations, and biopsies occur during clinic visits and

hospitalizations. Neutropenia and sepsis are frequent serious complications in the first few months of treatment. Some adults with acute leukemia do not respond to initial treatment; others go on to remission and then relapse.

At times of relapse or failure of conventional front-line treatment, families sometimes engage in frenetic efforts to find other treatments, second opinions, or alternative therapies. These are not their only options, however; they can also seek out other conventional approaches such as second-line chemotherapy, or participation in clinical investigative research trials. For the patient who does not relapse after initial treatment,

**Table 16-4**  Ann Arbor staging of the lymphomas*

| Stage | Site |
|---|---|
| I | Involvement of a single lymph node region (I) or of a single extralymphatic organ or site (I$_E$) |
| II | Involvement of two or more lymph node regions on the same side of the diagphragm alone (II) or with involvement of limited, contiguous extralymphatic organ or tissue (II$_E$) |
| III | Involvement of lymph node regions on both sides of the diaphragm (III), possibly including the spleen (III$_X$), or a limited, contiguous extralymphatic organ or site (III$_E$) or (III$_{ES}$) |
| IV | Multiple or disseminated foci of involvement of one or more extralymphatic organs or tissues, with or without lymphatic involvement |

*All cases are also subclassified to indicate the absence (A) or presence (B) of the systemic symptoms of significant fever, night sweats, and unexplained weight loss exceeding 10% of normal body weight.
*Source*: Ann Arbor Symposium (1971). Staging in Hodgkin's disease, Ann Arbor, Michigan. *Cancer Res.* 31:1707.

**Table 16-5**  Lymphoma statistics

|  | Annual Incidence per 100,000* |
|---|---|
| Hodgkin's lymphoma | 3.3 (Male) |
|  | 2.8 (Female) |
| Non-Hodgkin's lymphoma | 14.7 (Male) |
|  | 12.3 (Female) |

*Approximately 30,000 new cases diagnosed per year for all age groups.
*Source*: United States (1985) *Fact Sheet: Hodgkin's Disease and Non-Hodgkin's Lymphoma*. National Cancer Institute, Office of Cancer Communication, Washington, D.C.

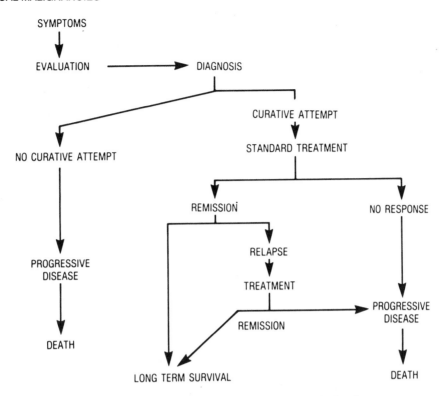

**Figure 16-1.** Clinical course of a patient with a hematological malignancy.

uncertainty about outcome and adjustment to the side effects of chemotherapy or irradiation are continuing problems.

## Treatment

More effective treatments for leukemia and lymphoma have occurred because of improved techniques in identifying pathological and histological subtypes of cells in leukemia, more precise staging of extent of disease in lymphoma, more effective supportive measures (antibiotics, blood products, protected environments, and intensive care units), and multimodal cytoreductive regimens along with allogeneic or autologous bone marrow transplantation (BMT) procedures. The treatment schemata for acute leukemia and lymphoma are outlined in Figs. 16-2 and 16-3.

## LEUKEMIA

The treatment of leukemia aims to eradicate all abnormal cells and to promote regeneration of normal cells. However, treatment often accomplishes only reduction of the cell population, and relapse follows as the remaining malignant cells regrow. Chemotherapy is the primary treatment; in select cases of young individuals, irradiation supplements intensive chemotherapy to eradicate a major sanctuary for leukemia cells.

Recently, allogeneic BMT has been utilized increasingly for patients under 45 years of age and in first remission for acute nonlymphocytic leukemia (ANLL), or in second remission of acute lymphocytic leukemia (ALL), and chronic myelogenous leukemia (CML) (see Fig. 16-4). Autologous BMT (i.e., transplantation of the individual's own purged or treated bone marrow) is being more extensively explored at many cancer centers especially for leukemia, lyphomas, and solid tumors. Protecting the patient during periods of immunosuppression and neutropenia through use of antibiotics is vital; germ-free environments and replacement of blood components are critically important in supportive care. The complex management required by these patients is best provided in major centers with the resources to give extensive supportive care.

The treatment of acute leukemia begins with *induction* chemotherapy, given in the hospital (Fig. 16-2). It is a multiagent regimen aimed at inducing a complete remission, defined as no clinical evidence of disease or less than 4% blast cells in the marrow. It usually requires 4–6 weeks of hospitalization at a cost (in 1986) of $30,000 or more. Only partial remissions are often achieved in older patients. Relapse can occur within

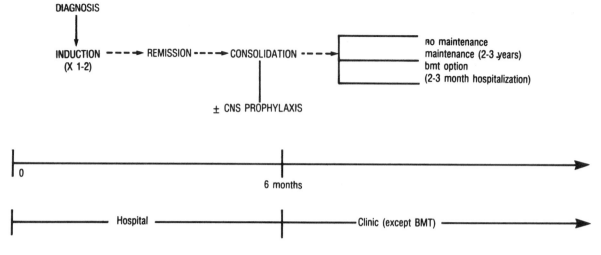

**Figure 16-2.**   Treatment course of acute leukemia.

weeks and is treated by chemotherapy again to accomplish reinduction. Chemotherapy, continuing into remission, is given in two phases: consolidation, possibly followed by maintenance. Consolidation chemotherapy requires hospitalization for one or two cycles employing the same cytoreductive agents used in the induction phase. *Maintenance* therapy, however, is given in the clinic or office over 1–2 years; lower doses of the same agents are used to prevent regrowth of residual leukemic cells. *Intensification* therapy is occasionally given after maintenance and involves administration of high doses of antileukemic drugs for 6 months. The optimal length of maintenance treatment is not known and its impact on survival is debated. Most ALL treatment schedules rely on vincristine, prednisone, and L-asparaginase, whereas those for ANLL use a combination of cytarabine and an anthracycline (Arlin and Clarkson, 1983; Clarkson et al., 1985).

Children and adults with ALL are at risk of developing leukemia in the central nervous system (CNS), even while in remission. This is because the CNS serves as a sanctuary for leukemic cells that are not destroyed by systemic chemotherapy, which does not effectively cross the blood–brain barrier. To reach these leukemic cells, intrathecal methotrexate, with or without cranial irradiation, is given as prophylaxis. Use of such therapy has reduced meningeal leukemia from greater than 40% to less than 10% incidence.

BMT is increasingly being utilized for acute and chronic leukemia and, more recently, lymphoma (O'Reilly, 1983) (see Fig. 16-3). Currently the three types of transplants used are syngeneic (bone marrow from a twin), allogeneic (bone marrow from a histocompatible sibling or parent), or autologous (the individual's own bone marrow that has been ''purged'' of neoplastic cells by chemotherapeutic agents and later

**Figure 16-3.**   Treatment course of lymphoma.

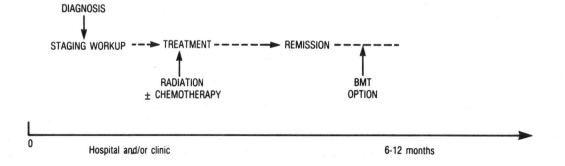

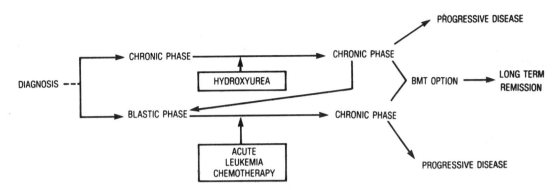

**Figure 16-4.**  Treatment course of chronic leukemia.

reinfused). In the 1970s BMT was an experimental therapy reserved for end-stage disease. Experience suggests that better results are attained when transplantations are done in the first or second remission of leukemia, while patients are medically stable, and when they are done early in the course of the disease (i.e., the chronic phase of CML, first remission of ANLL, and second or third remission of ALL) (Dinsmore et al., 1983, 1984). Unfortunately, BMT is an appropriate treatment for only 25% of patients, that is, for those under the age of 40 and those who have a histocompatible donor. Morbidity from this procedure may be as high as 50%, but BMT produces a disease-free survival in at least 75% of patients for periods of as long as 2–10 years. In contrast, standard chemotherapy results in 5-year disease-free survival in 20% of the adults with ANLL. Long-term sequelae of BMT are significant and include sterility, endocrine dysfunction, graft-versus-host disease (GvHD), interstitial pneumonitis, cardiomyopathy, cataracts, and immunosuppression.

## LYMPHOMAS

The histopathological diagnosis and sites of involved lymph nodes, above or below the diaphragm, determine the type and stage of lymphoma from which treatment is determined (see Tables 16-3 and 16-4). The sites of disease are also used to monitor response to treatment and to estimate prognosis. Treatment begins immediately after staging. Limited, localized, or early stages of disease are treated by radiotherapy alone to involved areas and regional lymph nodes. More extensive disease is treated by several multiagent combinations chemotherapy [i.e., MOPP (nitrogen mustard, vincristine, procarbazine, and prednisone) or ABVD (adriamycin, bleomycin, vinblastine, and darcarbazine) which is thought to produce less sterility]. Six

to eight cycles of the multiagents are usually given over 6 months. Adjuvant multiagent chemotherapy is used with radiotherapy in later stages of disease, in children, and in patients with large mediastinal tumors. Several classes of agents are employed, including vinca alkaloids, procarbazine, alkylating agents, nitrosoureas, bleomycin, doxorubicin, and corticosteroids (Straus et al., 1987).

## PSYCHOLOGICAL CONCERNS ASSOCIATED WITH DIAGNOSIS AND TREATMENT

Hematological malignancies are widely known to be rapidly fatal when untreated. Thus, when a patient or parent learns that leukemia or lymphoma has been diagnosed, the word alone strikes fear in their hearts. The psychosocial concerns associated with *all* cancers are intensified in these patients. The five *D*'s of psychosocial concerns outlined in Chapter 6 are particularly poignant in these diseases.

*Death* is a central fear, as is fear of discomfort from the medical procedures (bone marrow aspirations and lumbar puncture) as well as from the disease itself (pain secondary to leukemia infiltrates in joints or enlarged retroperitoneal nodes).

*Dependence* on family and physician is necessary during long hospitalizations for induction treatment and years of follow-up treatment.

A sense of *disfigurement* is consequent to changes in body appearance and function (hair loss, Broviac catheters, and infertility with lymphoma).

*Disruption* occurs in relationships during long and numerous hospitalizations.

*Disability* interferes with achievement of age-appropriate school, career, and personal goals.

Patients realize from the outset that the prognosis may be poor. Especially in adults, leukemia is generally known to be a worse diagnosis than lymphoma. The survival statistics, the physicians' tone during treatment discussions, and the rigors of treatment outlined all convey "bad news." It is during this period that patients and their families find the appearance of a "veteran" patient so helpful. The reassuring words that someone has "been there before" and "made it" are invaluable (see Chapter 41).

The supportive measures just described require the patient and family to assume a heavy responsibility for their maintenance, which adds an additional burden. Lengthy periods in germ-free environments are particularly difficult because of the fluctuation between isolation and overstimulation produced by such environments. Broviac or Hickman line catherization, providing access to the right atrium via the subclavian vein, is used for the administration of chemotherapy, blood products, antibiotics, and nutrition, and for obtaining blood samples for study (thus eliminating multiple venipunctures). Patients adjust well to these catheters, which are in place over months. However, they require daily care by patients including sterile dressing changes and flushing with heparinized solutions. Because the most common complication of indwelling catheters is infection, they require careful monitoring. Psychological issues that arise include overdependence on nurses for sterile techniques, the high level of mandatory technical self-care at home (a problem that may be particularly stressful for the adolescent or older individual), negative body image (an issue most apparent in young adults, who are often embarrassed in their intimate relationships by the presence of a catheter), and chronic loss of the ability to eat when total parental nutrition (TPN) is used for long periods. The impact on appetite makes it difficult to discontinue TPN at times and to reinstitute normal feeding.

## VARIABLES IN PSYCHOLOGICAL ADJUSTMENT

As with other forms of cancer, the variables that contribute to psychological adjustment to leukemia or lymphoma are medical and psychosocial. The medical variables are particularly important in leukemia, in which the clinical course is uncertain. The relapses, episodes of sepsis, hospitalizations, isolation, and treatment side effects can wear thin even strong psychological defenses (Lesko et al., 1983). Emotional exhaustion and demoralization are common. Different treatment modalities (Ommaya shunts, intrathecal chemotherapy, and multiple bone marrow aspirates) increase the stress; however, other measures can substantially reduce it, such as the use of a Broviac catheter access to eliminate painful venipunctures.

Profound fatigue and diminished stamina continue for long periods after treatment.

Young children adapt better psychologically than adults to long hospitalizations and germ-free environments, although extra time and assistance from parents and staff are often needed to reinforce precautions and instructions. Emotional stability of patient and family, as well as positive support form social and interpersonal resources, assist the patient in weathering the disappointments that are frequent throughout the course of the illness and in adjusting to the extensive treatment.

The financial burden of a catastrophic illness is an additional silent and unexpected problem. "Out-of-pocket" medical expenses—those not reimbursed by health insurance—are high with the longer hospitalizations required in leukemia. Specialized home care, administration of chemotherapy by infusion pumps, skilled nursing care, and TPN, are often not covered by insurance plans. The financial burden of nonmedical costs to the family of a child with leukemia is great and well documented (Cairns et al., 1979). Other hidden expenses with an afflicted child are wages lost as a result of need for child care of siblings and money spent on convenience foods, transportation to and from the physician's office or medical center, lodging for the parent or family member to stay near the hospital, wigs, clothing of several sizes to accommodate weight changes, baby-sitters, housekeepers, and supportive supplies for Broviac catheter care. Miscellaneous expenses that are often overlooked include telephone calls, special gifts, flowers, posters for the patient's room, toys, VCRs, air conditioners, and tutors for educational needs. According to Cairns et al., (1979), out-of-pocket costs can average 15% or more of a family's annual salary. The financial burden is felt long after the child has been cured or has died. Difficult choices about the use of financial resources must be made by parents when the education or financial needs of other children or the family are compromised.

Giving consent for the treatment when it involves fatal doses of radiation and chemotherapy that are countered only by BMT, is a difficult decision for patients and their families, especially parents. The consent process has been studied for both chemotherapy and BMT (Penman et al., 1984; Lesko et al., 1986a–d). Both studies confirm the value of the discussion with the doctor, as compared to the use of the informed-consent form only. The latter was helpful in investigational treatments, reaffirming the right to withdraw. It also appeared that better informed patients adjusted more positively to treatment.

Some patients adjust poorly to illness because they enter treatment with poor coping strategies. Poor coping is seen in the patient who does not confront these problems, assumes a passive "what will be, will be" stance, and employs abnormal levels of denial. Patients with a psychiatric disorder find it difficult to balance the self-care requirements with the need to be compliant and to relinquish overall care to others. Drug abuse and alcoholism are apt to be associated with noncompliance with treatment, in particular among those who must be involved in home administration of antibiotics, chemotherapy, or TPN.

Those patients who have good coping ability seem to adjust well to the treatment regimen. They become well informed about illness and treatment; they see illness as a challenge and solve problems one at a time, accepting limitations on their activities as well as their transiently altered appearance. In one of the studies on coping mechanisms in leukemic patients in remission, Sanders and Kardinal (1977) reported moderate levels of denial of illness as well as a strong identification with fellow patients and staff from the "hospital family." Grief over deaths of fellow patients was common.

## SURVIVORSHIP

The problems of cancer survivors are reviewed in Chapter 7. Those medical and psychological concerns specific to leukemia and lymphoma are outlined here (Table 16-6). Of considerable interest are the persistent problems with associations that remind the individual of the chemotherapy. In studies by Cella and colleagues (1986) and Lesko and colleagues (1987a,b) Hodgkin's disease and leukemia survivors were found to have conditioned nausea and anxiety as long as 12–17 years after chemotherapy had been completed when exposed to a reminder of their chemotherapy treatment.

### Medical Concerns

In the first major report on a large group of children with survival of 10 years or more treated at St. Jude's, half were survivors of Hodgkin's disease or leukemia. Although 90% judged that they had a good quality of life and social function, about 30% had problems specific to treatment, including infertility in the Hodgkin's patients and a decrease in IQ among the leukemia patients who received cranial irradiation (Thompson et al., 1987).

### NEUROLOGICAL PROBLEMS

Neurological toxicity from chemotherapy regimens has increased as toxicity from chemotherapy has increased, as more drugs are used together, and as they are more often combined in high dose with radiation

**Table 16-6** Common concerns in survivors of hematological malignancies

| Problem areas | Specific concerns |
|---|---|
| Medical concerns | Neurological and CNS dysfunction |
| | Occurrence of a second malignancy |
| | Organ failure (cardiovascular, pulmonary, renal, hepatic) |
| | Retardation or failure of maturation and growth |
| | Decreased stamina |
| | Relapse |
| Psychological concerns | Fears of minor physical symptoms |
| | Fears of termination of treatment |
| | Adjustment to accepting normal responsibilities; difficulty being on their own |
| | Difficulties in transition from being a patient to becoming healthy (Lazarus syndrome) |
| | Problem in revealing diagnosis when seeking jobs |
| | Awareness of job and health insurance discrimination |
| | Sense of vulnerability to illness and death (Damocles syndrome) |

(Young and Posner, 1980; Young, 1982). Intrathecal routes and aggressive treatment of relapses add to toxicity. In addition, as children and young adults treated for cancer survive longer, there is more opportunity for delayed CNS side effects to become apparent.

Immediate CNS side effects of chemotherapeutic agents include transient nausea, vomiting, anorexia, fatigue and weakness, confusion, and irritability (Goldberg et al., 1982; Weiss et al., 1974; Kaplan and Wiernik, 1982). Immediate side effects are seen transiently primarily with intrathecal administration of methotrexate in acute leukemia. Cognitive dysfunction and neurological impairment occur largely in children treated for acute leukemia by intrathecal methotrexate and cranial irradiation. Seizures, motor abnormalities, and language and behavioral difficulties have been reported (Meadows and Evans, 1976). Other studies found largely normal psychological and neurological development in spite of evidence of cerebral atrophy on CT scan (Soni et al., 1975; Obetz et al., 1979; Verosa and Rhomes, 1976). The clinical significance of CT scan abnormalities in children receiving various forms of CNS prophylaxis is unclear (Brecher et al., 1985). Subsequent research has revealed both structural abnormalities and cognitive deficits in 25–30% of childhood ALL survivors (Aur et al., 1978; Goff et al., 1980; Moss et al., 1981; Thompson et al., 1987).

## RELAPSE AND SECOND MALIGNANCIES

Patients with leukemia usually relapse because leukemia cells find sanctuary from chemotherapy in the CNS, testis, and ovary. Even though there have been improvements in the prevention of CNS relapse, testicular relapse still occurs in between 5 and 16% of males during initial remission and upward to 30–40% after treatment is discontinued (Bowman et al., 1984). Often early testicular relapse heralds subsequent (within 3 months) bone marrow relapse of drug-resistant leukemia.

Second malignant neoplasms (SMN) as a result of treatment are rare in leukemia; they most often appear as a secondary lymphoma or another type of leukemia (Mosijczuk and Ruymann, 1981). More often, SMN occur in patients with Hodgkin's disease treated with alkylating agents, with or without radiation (D'Angio, 1975, 1978; Meadows et al., 1985; Tester et al, 1984; Schomberg et al., 1984; List et al., 1985; Carey et al., 1984; Bartolucci et al., 1983; Kushner et al., 1988). The review of the large cohort of children treated at St. Jude's 10 or more years after treatment, identified SMN in only 2% of the children (Thompson et al., 1987). Sarcomas, thyroid carcinomas, and ANLL have developed as SMN in children with Hodgkin's disease 3 months to 21 years after termination of treatment. Solid tumors appear at a mean of 9.5 years after treatment in leukemia and 5.5 years after treatment for lymphoma in adults and children (Meadows et al., 1985). Hodgkin's disease adult patients are at increased risk for lung and breast cancer and secondary ALL, incidence of which may be as high as 10%.

## GROWTH AND ORGAN FAILURE

Most children with hematological malignancies grow and mature normally, although patterns of growth and growth hormone (GH) levels in children with acute leukemia who receive cranial irradiation along with chemotherapy are at greater risk of growth abnormalities. Impaired GH responses to provocative tests of GH release has been reported in children with acute leukemia treated with cranial irradiation for CNS prophylaxis (Shalet et al., 1977). Later, others noted only temporary impairment of growth in children receiving chemotherapy and cranial irradiation, with symmetrical loss in height (Sundermann and Pearson, 1969; Hakami et al., 1980). Unfortunately, there are conflicting studies about GH concentration, GH stimulation after provocative testing and linear growth patterns in children with acute leukemia after treatment by CNS prophylaxis. Voorhess and colleagues (1986) studied the hypothalamic–pituitary function of 93 children receiving CNS prophylaxis (intratecal methotrexate (IT-MTX), IT-MTX and 2400 rads cranial irradia-

tion, or IT MTX and intravenous intermediate dose MTX. Eleven patients had subnormal GH responses after pharmacologic stimulation of the pituitary however, long term linear growth patterns were unaffected. Children who are subsequently treated by bone marrow transplantation with additional high dose chemotherapy and total body irradiation appear to be a particularly high risk of endocrine abnormalities that adversely affect growth and development (Sanders et al., 1986).

Children with Hodgkin's disease and non-Hodgkin's lymphoma who received irradiation to specific sites (e.g., thoracic and pelvic areas), especially during rapid growth periods, experience maturation loss in the irradiated area. Unilateral irradiation to the thoracic area or growth centers of the long bones produces scoliosis and short stature.

Survivors also may experience delayed toxicity to the cardiovascular, endocrine, pulmonary, hepatic, renal, and the peripheral nervous systems. Patients may have permanent vincristine-associated peripheral neuropathy, anthracycline-related cardiomyopathy, hepatic fibrosis secondary to methotrexate, and antibiotic-related renal failure. Occasionally, when chemotherapy is given with irradiation, organ damage is enhanced. Some agents, such as methotrexate, are "radiation reactivators" and, when given weeks to months later, reactivate the radiation effects. Radiotherapy for Hodgkin's disease in the thorax can result in delayed pneumonitis, pericarditis, pleurisy, and thyroid dysfunction.

The delayed sequelae of hematological malignancy treatment on fertility and sexual function have been a particular focus of psychological studies (Horning et al., 1981; Cella and Tross, 1986; Lesko et al., 1987a,b). Young men who undergo chemotherapy and pelvic irradiation for Hodgkin's disease or rigorous induction leukemia chemotherapy often become aspermic and remain sterile. Sperm-banking is important to allow a later possibility for a natural child. Fertility in men with acute leukemia treated with standard chemotherapy is less well studied. Evenson et al. (1984) noted that men treated at Memorial Sloan-Kettering on the L-10 protocol for this disease remained fertile. Treatment consisted of a minimum of 3.5 years of continuous chemotherapy using adriamycin, vincristine, prednisone, intrathecal metotrexate, cytosine arabinoside (Ara-C), BCNU and dactinomycin. The fertility may have been spared by the use of intrathecal methotrexate rather than cranial irradiation as CNS prophylaxis, thereby sparing the hypothalamic-pituitary-gonadal axis.

Chemotherapy-related ovarian failure and subsequent amenorrhea, diminished libido, and sexual dysfunction have occurred in a number of young women who are Hodgkin's disease survivors. Radiation of less than 2000 rad and/or relocation of the ovaries during treatment for lymphoma may prevent reproductive damage. Siris and colleagues found that most young women aggressively treated for leukemia in childhood have a relatively good prognosis for normal CNS-controlled ovarian function (Siris et al., 1976). On a more optimistic note, it appears that for fertile couples in whom one survives cancer, neither chemotherapy nor radiation has an oncogenic or mutagenic effect on progeny (Li and Jaffe, 1974). However, many young adult survivors are unaware of or are unprepared for possible treatment-related sexual dysfunction, adding further stress and problems in adjustment.

## Psychological Concerns

Most early psychological studies of cancer survivors were retrospective reviews of children with leukemia and Hodgkin's disease. The need for longitudinal studies of adults and children was noted by several investigators who identified problems of survivors (Sherins and Devita, 1973; Chapman et al., 1979a,b, 1981; Sutcliffe, 1979; Li and Jaffe, 1974; Li and Stone, 1976). These studies highlighted several important psychological areas of concern that relate in large part to the medical concerns of physical damage, risk of a second neoplasm, relapse, survival, and psychological function. Remission brings a return to near-normal appearance, but stamina is slow to return (Bloom et al., 1987). Consequently, there can be a precarious balance between elation at achieving cure and fears of future disease. Depressive mood, anxiety, and a sense of diminished self-worth and control over events are frequently seen. (Table 16-6). Cure itself imposes a difficult task—that of discarding the patient role in separating from the hospital-family, reentering into job or school and actual family while continuing regular, if less frequent, clinic visits. Patients with hematological malignancies often have a transient enhanced level of psychological distress related to the uncertainty of how long maintenance treatment should continue, "how many cycles of treatment are enough?" Patients at this time are often concerned about the loss of close monitoring of their physical condition and experience a sense of increased vulnerability to relapse.

Follow-up visits with bone marrow aspirations or development of minor physical symptoms result in increased anxiety. As time goes by, anniversaries of diagnosis and treatment are reminders that cause transient distress. In a survey of 70 leukemia patients, they outlined issues that made their clinic visits difficult (Lesko et al., 1987a,b). Dislike of returning to the clinic environment and discomfort of the examination and diagnostic procedure were noted. Further sources of complaint were that clinic visits served to remind patients of the lack of certainty about cure, coupled with interference with work or school caused by the visits.

The inability to ignore everyday aches and pains adds to the survivors' preoccupation with physical symptoms and loss of control over their health and future. This is particularly evident in leukemia because relapse may occur without any warning, becoming apparent only by an abnormal bone marrow test result or development of frequent infections. Finally, these malignancies are "invisible" upon completion of therapy, leaving no physical manifestations. The invisibility of physical damage can aid in the patient's denial of being chronically ill and diminish the sense of being only precariously in good health. Other psychological sequelae of survivorship (e.g., Lazarus and Damocles syndromes, survivor guilt, job and insurance discrimination) are described in Chapter 7 by Tross and in research by Koocher and O'Malley (1981).

Systematic studies on the psychological adaptation of adults surviving hematological malignancies are increasing in numbers (Lesko et al., 1987a,b; Bloom et al., 1987; Fobair et al., 1987; Tross et al., 1987). Wolcott and colleagues (1986) reported on the adaptation of 26 patients with leukemia and aplastic anemia who were treated by BMT. At an average of 3.6 years after treatment, only 2.5% had some physiological sequelae secondary to disease or treatment. These authors reported that 25% or less of patients reported low self-esteem, less than optimal life satisfaction, and significant emotional distress.

The psychological profile of survivors and the long-term psychological impact of disease and treatment on patients are under active study. At Memorial Sloan-Kettering, research is being conducted among young adults with acute leukemia and Hodgkin's disease (Lesko et al., 1987a,b; Cella and Tross, 1986). Data from these studies reveal that survival is achieved without impairment of quality of life and psychological well-being of survivors. Survivors in both studies were at least 6–12 months off treatment. No differences were found between survivors and healthy controls. However, depending on the patient population, the cancer survivor demonstrated lower intimacy motivation, increased avoidant thinking about illness, numerous illness-related concerns, and prolonged difficulty returning to premorbid work status. Such data suggest that cancer and its diagnosis and treatment have some residual psychological effects.

## FAMILIES AND LEUKEMIA OR LYMPHOMA

Families, like patients, go through developmental life stages that influence the adjustment of the patient to illness. Stress on the family in which a member has hematological malignancy is particularly great, because the disease occurs at all ages and challenges the family in its early, middle, and/or older years to cope with issues of serious illness and treatment.

The young family is often ill-equipped because of a lack of experience or maturity to deal with leukemia in a child, yet they must face the pain of having a child with a life-threatening illness and the decisions parents must make about treatment. They must simultaneously manage the stresses of caring for the ill child and other healthy children at home. Young mothers, whether they themselves are the patient or are caring for an ill young child, find it particularly difficult to be away from their young children during extended hospitalizations, and to care for their other healthy children.

The middle-years family may have an adolescent with leukemia or Hodgkin's disease, or possibly a parent with lymphoma. Parents must deal with the ill adolescent who struggles with the age-appropriate drive toward identity and independence in the context of an illness that increases dependency and erodes self-esteem. When a parent in the middle years has a hematological malignancy, the adolescent child may appear unconcerned, uninvolved, cold, and callous, not unlike any other adolescent whose parent does not have a cancer diagnosis. These behaviors may serve as either protective or denial mechanisms.

The aging family in which leukemia or lymphoma develops is concerned with cost of medicines, hospitalization, dependency on adult children, and fears of loss of spouse—often after long years of marriage. The lengthy hospitalization, with its reverse isolation or protracted cycles of chemotherapy, intrudes on closeness to family members. Young adult children must share responsibility for treatment decisions and provide support while caring for their own young children at home.

## TEAM APPROACH TO MEDICAL AND PSYCHOLOGICAL CARE

Patients with hematological malignancies are intimately involved with a range of health care professionals, paraprofessionals, and support staff throughout their illness, treatment, and even later as survivors. Years later, patients talk about the team members who cared for them during precarious times of illness (Lesko et al., 1987a,b; Cella et al., 1986a; Cella and Tross, 1986). At the time of the yearly checkup, patients usually visit their favorite floor, clinic secretary, special nurse, attendant in the coffee shop, patient escort, or dietitian. The impact of the "team" on patient and family is often underestimated. A team member is remembered to have imparted a piece of medical infor-

mation, eased some physical or psychological discomfort, assisted and offered reassurance in a treatment decision, cajoled and nurtured during times of defeat, and provided a link to the world during long hospitalizations. Because of their extensive and rigorous treatment protocols, these patients develop a personal attachment to the treatment center and to its staff, who become an extended family. They are seen as resources not only for medically related concerns, but also for personal advice about school, career, family, and work.

The basic team in a teaching center usually consists of an oncologist, nurse, and social worker, with other support as needed from a psychiatrist, nurse-clinician, dietitian, and pharmacist. They work together in the hospital and clinic settings. However, home visits by a team member may also be used to ease the transition from hospital to home, to help control medication, to facilitate administration of chemotherapy at home, and to assist in providing a hospicelike care in the home setting. Each team member may serve as a resource when questions about fever, Broviac care, oral hygiene, dietary problems, or other concerns about physical or psychological well-being arise.

This team may fluctuate in its membership depending on the needs of the patient and family, the age of the patient, and the patient's stage of illness. Young patients may benefit from a child psychiatrist or psychologist whose function is to assist in facilitating adjustment with the return to school. At Memorial Sloan-Kettering, a social worker, upon the request of the child and family, will visit the child's school and classroom, providing information to teachers that eases the transition back to school. A special social worker is also available to address the concerns of healthy children of parents who have a cancer diagnosis. This is of particular importance when ill parents find it difficult to tell or prepare their young children about the present or potential complications consequent to their illness. In some cases, the role of the individual is to help ill parents understand the occasional "unconcerned" attitude of their adolescent children to illness. The complexities of the financial burden incurred through extensive hospitalization, hidden costs, management of home care, and auxilary personnel costs (homemakers, nurses) can be eased by input from nursing and social work team members. These team members can also "troubleshoot" such simple problems as what type of tape to use for catheter dressings, what to do when a fever develops, how to arrange for transportation to and from the hospital, or how to obtain special educational classes for the children recuperating at home.

When resources are available, a mental health professional, often a psychiatrist or psychologist, can be helpful. At Memorial Sloan-Kettering over several years, the gradual assignment of one psychiatrist was made as a consultant to work with the leukemia, lymphoma, and BMT groups on the inpatient floors and in the clinics. The responsibilities of this psychiatrist were to attend all weekly tumor board meetings of the services covered, to assess patients and family members before admission for treatment (especially when the patient or family member is at risk of inability to comply with the treatment because of the presence of a psychiatric diagnosis or mental retardation, psychiatric medications, or a serious drug abuse or alcohol problem), to provide monitoring of these "at-risk" patients and families, to assist in discussion of sensitive issues, and to evaluate the patients in the hospital who show psychological decompensation. Clinic hours are also kept so as to coordinate the three services covered, to allow patients who travel from a distance for clinic visits to manage all visits in one trip. The psychiatrist makes biweekly clinic multidisciplinary rounds with the hematology–oncology attending physicians, reviewing the status of patients, facilitating attention of psychosocial concerns, and helping to manage terminal care in and outside the hospital.

Meetings with nursing and house staff concerning their stresses in regard to management of patients (often their age peers), and communication among team members follow easily when there is close integration of the psychiatrist in the group. Often the most valuable opportunities arise from the impromptu discussions in the nursing stations and corridors.

## SUMMARY

The hematological malignancies have been among the first to respond to treatment, which has produced cures initially among children and young adults. However, to achieve a cure from leukemia or lymphoma, the required chemotherapy, irradiation, and bone marrow transplantation cause psychological stresses that are predictable on the basis of the treatment side effects. Transplantation particularly requires an intensive treatment regimen and long hospitalization in a germ-free environment. Maladaptive responses often require psychiatric evaluation and intervention to prevent inability to continue treatment. Because the hematological malignancies occur at all ages, it is necessary to have knowledge of the disease and treatment, as well as having an understanding of the common psychological responses. Optimal patient and family care for these diseases is best done in a center where a team of specialists who work together can maximize the patient's chance for the best physical and emotional outcome.

## REFERENCES

Ann Arbor Symposium (1971). Staging in Hodgkins disease, Ann Arbor, Michigan. *Cancer Res.* 31:1707–70.

Arlin, Z.A. and B.D. Clarkson (1983). The treatment of acute nonlymphoblastic leukemia in adults. *Adv. Intern. Med.* 28:303–23.

Aur, R., M. Verzosa, O. Hustu, J. Simone, and L. Barker (1978). Leukoencephalopathy during initial complete remission in children with acute lymphocytic leukemia receiving methotrexate. *Proc. Sixty-Sixth Annu. Mtg. Am. Assoc. Cancer Res. and Eleventh Annu. Mtg. Am. Soc. Clin. Oncol.* 16:92.

Bartolucci, A.A., C. Liu, J.R. Durant, and R.A. Gams (1983). Acute myelogenous leukemia as a second malignant neoplasm following the successful treatment of advanced Hodgkin's disease. *Cancer* 52:2209–13.

Bloom, J., R. Gorsky, P. Fobair, R. Cox, A. Varghese, D. Spiegel, and R. Hoppe (1987). *Proc. Am. Soc. Clin. Oncol.* 6:258 (Abstract No. 1016).

Bowman, W.P., R.J.A. Aur, H.O. Hustu, and G. Rivera (1984). Isolated testicular relapse in acute lymphocytic leukemia of childhood: Categories and influence on survival. *J. Clin. Oncol.* 2:924–29.

Brecher, M.L., P. Berger, A.I. Freeman, J. Krischer, J. Boyett, A.S. Glicksman, E. Foreman, M. Harris, B. Jones, M.E. Cohen, P.K. Duffner, J.H. Rowland, Y-P Huang, and S. Batnitsky (1985). Computerized tomography scan findings in children with acute lymphocytic leukemia treated with three different methods of central nervous system prophylaxis. *Cancer* 56:2430–33.

Cairns, N.V., G.M. Clark, J. Black, and S.B. Lansky (1979). Childhood cancer: Non-medical costs of illness. *Cancer* 43:403–8.

Carey, R., R.M. Linggood, W. Wood, and P.H. Blitzer, (1984). Breast cancer developing in four women cured of Hodgkin's disease. *Cancer* 54:2234–36.

Cella, D.F., A. Pratt and J.C. Holland (1986). Persistent anticipatory nausea, vomiting, and anxiety in cured Hodgkin's disease patients after completion of chemotherapy. *Am. J. Psychiatry* 143:641–43.

Cella, D.F. and S. Tross (1986). Psychological adjustment to survival from Hodgkin's disease. *J. Consult. Clin. Psychol.* 54:618–22.

Chapman, R.M., S.B. Sutcliff, and J.S. Malpas (1979a). Cytotoxic-induced ovarian failure in women with Hodgkin's disease: I. Hormone function. *J.A.M.A.* 242: 1877–81.

Chapman, R.M., S.B. Sutcliffe, and J.S. Malpas (1979b). Cytotoxic-induced ovarian failure in women with Hodgkin's disease: II. Effects on sexual function. *J.A.M.A.* 242:1882–89.

Chapman, R.M., S.B. Sutcliffe, and J.S. Malpas (1981). Male gonadal dysfunction in Hodgkin's disease: A prospective study. *J.A.M.A.* 245:1323–28.

Clarkson, B., S. Ellis, C. Little, T. Gee, A. Zalmen, R. Mertelsmann, M. Andreeff, S. Kempin, B. Koziner, R. Chaganti, S. Jhanwar, S. McKenzie, C. Cirrincione, and J. Gaynor (1985). Acute lymphoblastic leukemia in adults. *Semin. Oncol.* 12:160–79.

D'Angio, G.J. (1975). Pediatric cancer in perspective: Cure is not enough. *Cancer* 35:866–70.

D'Angio, G.J. (1978). Complications of treatment encountered in lymphoma–leukemia long-term survivors. *Cancer* 42:1015–25.

Dinsmore, R., D. Kirkpatrick, N. Flomenberg, S. Gulati, B. Shank, and R.J. O'Reilly (1983). Allogeneic marrow transplantation for acute lymphoblastic leukemia in remission: The importance of early transplantation. *Transplant. Proc.* 15(1,March):1397–1400.

Dinsmore, R., D. Kirkpatrick, N. Flomenberg, S. Gulati, N. Kapoor, J. Brochstein, B. Shank, A. Reid, S. Groshen, and R.J. O'Reilly (1984). Allogeneic bone marrow transplantation for patients with acute nonlymphocytic leukemia. *Blood* 63(3,March):649–56.

Evenson, D., Z. Avlin, S. Welt, M. Claps, and M. Melamed (1984). Male reproductive capacity may recover following drug treatment with the L-10 protocol for acute lymphocytic leukemia. *Cancer* 53:30–6.

Fobair, P., J. Bloom, R. Hoppe, A. Varghese, R. Cox, and D. Spiegel (1987). Work patterns among long-term survivors of Hodgkin's disease. *Proc. Am. Soc. Clin. Oncol.* 6:260 (Abstract No. 1023).

Goff, J.R., H.R. Anderson, and P.F. Cooper (1980). Distractability and memory deficits in long-term survivors of acute lymphocytic leukemia. *J. Dev. Behav. Pediatr.* 1:158–63.

Goldberg, I.D., W.D. Bloomer, and D.M. Dawson (1982). Nervous system toxic effects of cancer therapy. *J.A.M.A.* 247:1437–41.

Hakami, N., A. Mohammad, and J.W. Meyer (1980). Growth and growth hormone of children with acute lymphocytic leukemia following central nervous system prophylaxis with and without cranial irradiation. *Am. J. Pediatr. Hematol./Oncol.* 2:311–16.

Horning, S., R.T. Hoppe, H.S. Kaplan, and S.A. Rosenberg (1981). Female reproductive potential after treatment for Hodgkin's disease. *N. Engl. J. Med.* 304:1377–82.

Kaplan, R.S. and P.H. Wiernik (1982). Neurotoxicity of antineoplastic drugs. *Semin. Oncol.* 9(1):103–30.

Koocher, G. and J. O'Malley (1981). *The Damocles Syndrome: Psychosocial Consequences of Surviving Childhood Cancer.* New York: McGraw-Hill.

Kushner, B., A. Zauber, C.T.C. Tan (1988). Second malignancies after childhood Hodgkin's disease. *Cancer* 62:1364–70.

Lesko, L., H. Dermatis, D. Penman, and J.C. Holland (1986a). *Psychological Aspects of the Informed Consent Process in Adults Undergoing Allogeneic Bone Marrow Transplantation (BMT).* Paper presented at the Fourteenth International Cancer Congress, Budapest, August.

Lesko, L.M., H. Dermatis, D. Penman, and J.C. Holland (1988). *Patients', parents' and oncologists' perceptions of informed consent for bone marrow transplantation.* (submitted for publication).

Lesko, L., H. Dermatis, D. Penman, J.C. Holland, and S. Groshen (1986b). The influence of coping, psychological distress and physician–patient interaction on informed consent outcome in bone marrow transplantation (BMT) (Abstract). *Proc. Twenty-Second Ann. Mtg. Am. Soc. Clin. Oncol.* 5:240.

Lesko, L., H. Dermatis, D. Penman, J.C. Holland, S. Groshen, and R. O'Reilly (1986c). Parent and physician perception of informed consent for pediatric allogeneic bone marrow transplantation (BMT) *Proc. Am. Soc. Clin. Oncol.* 5:240.

Lesko, L., H. Dermatis, D. Penman, J.C. Holland, S. Groshen, and R. O'Reilly (1986d). Parental adjustment to child's bone marrow transplantation (BMT) as a function of coping, psychological distress and information retained at time of informed consent *Proc. Am. Soc. Clin. Oncol.* 5:240.

Lesko, L., J. Kern, and D.R. Hawkins (1983). Psychological aspects of patients in germ-free isolation: A review of child, adult and patient management literature. *Med. Pediatr. Oncol.* 12:43–49.

Lesko, L., G. Mumma, D. Mashberg, and J.C. Holland (1987a). Psychosocial adjustment and sexual functioning of acute leukemia survivors: A preliminary report, The Third National Symposium of the Leukemia Society of America. *Leukemia* 1(3):278 (Abstract No. 23).

Lesko, L., G. Mumma, and D. Mashberg (1987b). Psychosocial functioning of acute leukemia survivors treatment with bone marrow transplantation or standard chemotherapy. *Proc. Am. Soc. Clin. Oncol.* 6:255 (Abstract No. 1002).

Leukemia Society of America (1987). *Facts about Leukemia.* National Office, 733 Third Avenue, New York, N.Y. 10017.

Li, F.P. and N. Jaffe (1974). Progeny of childhood cancer survivors. *Lancet* 2:707–12.

Li, F.P. and R. Stone (1976). Survivors of cancer in childhood. *Ann. Intern. Med.* 84:551–53.

List, A., D.C. Doll, and A. Greco (1985). Lung cancer in Hodgkin's disease: Association with previous radiotherapy. *J. Clin. Oncol.* 3:215–21.

Margolis, C.P. and K.B. McCredie (1983). *Understanding leukemia.* New York: Scribner's.

Meadows, A.T., E. Baum, F. Fossati-Bellani, D. Green, R.D.T. Jenkin, B. Marsden, M. Nesbit, W. Newton, O. Oberlin, S.G. Sallan, S. Siegel, L.C. Strong, and P.A. Voute (1985). Second malignant neoplasms in children: An update from the late effects study group. *J. Clin. Oncol.* 4:532–38.

Meadows, A.T., and A.E. Evans (1976). Effects of chemotherapy on the central nervous system. *Cancer* 37:1079–85.

Mosijczuk, A.D. and F.B. Ruymann (1981). Second malignancy in acute lymphocytic leukemia. *Am. J. Dis. Child.* 135:313–16.

Moss, H., E.D. Nannis, and D.G. Poplack (1981). The effects of prophylactic treatment of the central nervous system on the intellectual functioning of children with acute lymphocytic leukemia. *Am. J. Med.* 71:47–52.

National Cancer Institute, Office of Cancer Communications (1983). *Fact Sheets on Hodgkin's disease and Non-Hodgkin's lymphoma.* Washington, D.C.: NCI.

Obetz, S.W., W.A. Smithson, R.V. Groover, O.W.

Houser, D.W. Klass, R.J. Ivnik, R.C. Colligan, G.S. Gilchrist, and E.O. Burgert, Jr. (1979). Neuropsychologic follow-up study of children with acute lymphocytic leukemia. *Am. J. Pediatr. Hematol. Oncol.* 1:207–13.

O'Reilly, R.J. (1983). Allogeneic bone marrow transplantation: Current status and future directions. *Blood* 62:941–64.

Penman, D.T., J.C. Holland, G.F. Bahna, G. Morrow, A.H. Schmale, L.R. Derogatis, C.L. Carnrike, and R. Cherry (1984). Informed consent for investigational chemotherapy: Patients' and physicians' perceptions. *J. Clin. Oncol.* 7:849–55.

Rosenberg, S. and F. Stockdale (1984). Hodgkin's disease and other lymphomas. In E. Rubinstein and D.D. Federman (eds.), *Scientific American Medicine.* Sec. 5., *Hematology.* New York: Scientific American.

Rowland, J.H., O.J. Glidewell, R.F. Sibley, J.C. Holland, R. Tull, A. Berman, M.L. Brecher, M. Harris, A.S. Glicksman, E. Forman, B. Jones, M.E. Cohen, P.K. Duffner, and A.I. Freeman (for the Cancer and Leukemia Group B) (1984). Effects of different forms of central nervous system prophylaxis on neuropsychologic function in childhood leukemia. *J. Clin. Oncol.* 2:1327–35.

Sanders, J.E., S. Pritchard, P. Mahoney, D. Amos, C.D. Buckner, R.P. Witherspoon, H.J. Deeg, K.C. Doney, K.M. Sullivan, F.R. Appelbaum, R. Storb, and D. Thomas (1986). Growth and development following marrow transplantation for leukemia. *Blood* 68(5):1129–35.

Sanders, J.B. and C.G. Kardinal (1977). Adaptive coping mechanisms in adult acute leukemia patients in remission. *J.A.M.A.* 238:952–54.

Schomberg, P.J., R.G. Evans, P.M. Banks, W.L. White, M.J. O'Connell, and J.D. Earle (1984). Second malignant lesions after therapy for Hodgkin's disease. *Mayo Clin. Proc.* 59:493–97.

Schrier, S. (1984). The leukemias and myeloproliferative disorders. In E. Rubinstein and D.D. Federman (eds.), *Scientific American Medicine.* Sec. 5, *Hematology.* New York: Scientific American, pp. 1–22.

Shalet, S.M., C.G. Beardwell, J.A. Twomey, P.H. Morris-Jones, and D. Pearson (1977). Endocrine function following the treatment of acute leukemia in children. *J. Pediatr.* 90(4):920–23.

Sherins, R.J. and V.T. DeVita (1973). Effect of drug treatment for lymphoma on male reproductive capacity: Studies of men in remission after therapy. *Ann. Intern. Med.* 79:216–20.

Siris, E.S., B.G. Leventhal, and J.L. Vaitukaitis (1976). Effects of childhood leukemia and chemotherapy on puberty and reproductive function in girls. *N. Engl. J. Med.* 294:1143–46.

Soni, S., G. Martin, and S. Pitner (1975). Effect of central nervous system irradiation on neuropsychologic function-ing of children with acute lymphocytic leukemia. *N. Engl. J. Med.* 293:113–18.

Straus, D.J., J.J. Gaynor, P.H. Lieberman, D.A. Filippa, B. Koziner, and B. Clarkson (1987). Non-Hodgkin's lymphomas: Characteristics of long-term survivors follow conservative treatment. *Am. J. Med.* 82:247–52.

Sunderman, C.R., and H.A. Pearson (1969). Growth effects of long-term antileukemic therapy. *J. Pediatr.* 75:1058–62.

Sutcliffe, S.B. (1979). Cytotoxic chemotherapy and gonadal function in patients with Hodgkin's disease: Facts and thoughts. *J.A.M.A.* 242:1898–99.

Tester, W.J., T.J. Kinsella, B. Waller, R.W. Makuch, P.A. Kelley, E. Glatstein, and V.T. DeVita (1984). Second malignant neoplasms complicating Hodgkin's disease: The National Cancer Institute experience. *J. Clin. Oncol.* 2:762–69.

Thompson, E., D. Fairclough, D. Crom, and J. Simons (1987). Normal physical and psychosocial function in the majority of childhood cancer patients surviving 10 years or more from diagnosis. *Proc. Am. Soc. Clin. Oncol.* 6:258 (Abstract No. 1013).

Tross, S., D. Cella, L. Lesko, and J.C. Holland (1987). General versus cancer-specific distress in cancer survivors. *Proc. Am. Soc. Clin. Oncol.* 6:255 (Abstract No. 1001).

Verosa, M. and J.A. Rhomes (1976). Five years after central nervous system irradiation of children with leukemia. *Int. J. Radiat. Biol.* 1:209–15.

Voorhess, M.L., M.L. Brecher, A.S. Glicksman, B. Jones, M. Hams, J. Krischer, J. Boyett, E. Forman, and A.I. Freeman (1986). Hypothalamic-pituitary function of children with acute lymphocytic leukemia after three forms of central nervous system prophylaxis. *Cancer* 57:1287–91.

Weiss, H.D., M.D. Walker, and P.H. Wiernik (1974). Neurotoxicity of commonly used antineoplastic agents: Part I. *N. Engl. J. Med.* 291:75–81.

Weiss, H.D., M.D. Walker, and P.H. Wiernik, (1974). Neurotoxicity of commonly used antineoplastic agents: Part II. *N. Engl. J. Med.* 291:127–33.

Wolcott, D.L., D.K. Wellisch, F.I. Fawzy, and J. Landsverk (1986). Adaptation of adult bone marrow transplant recipient long-term survivors. *Transplantation* 41(4): 478–83.

Young, D. (1982). Neurological complications of cancer chemotherapy. In A. Silverstein (ed.), *Neurological Complications of Therapy: Selected Topics.* New York: Futura Publishing, pp. 57–113.

Young, D.F. and J.B. Posner (1980). Nervous system toxicity of the chemotherapeutic agents. In P.J. Vinken and G.W. Bruyn (eds.), *Handbook of Clinical Neurology.* Vol. 39, *Neurological Manifestations of Systemic Diseases, Part II.* New York: Elsevier, pp. 91–129.

# 17

# Head and Neck Cancer

William Breitbart and Jimmie C. Holland

The patient with a neoplasm of the head and neck region must cope with the life-threatening diagnosis as well as the alteration of normal facial appearance, and possible loss or impairment of the important functions of speech, sight, taste, and smell. This enormous threat to self-image, confidence and identity, as well as survival, requires the individual to muster considerable emotional strength. Normal reactions before surgery and during rehabilitation are characterized by marked anxiety and depressive symptoms. Suicidal thoughts are not uncommon, especially in patients contemplating radical surgery. In addition, tumors of the aerodigestive tract frequently develop in individuals who have a history of chronic excessive use of alcohol and tobacco (Shedd, 1982). Psychological problems that predisposed the individual to chronic substance abuse, especially alcohol, are apt to complicate care and rehabilitation by poor treatment compliance. In the head and neck patient, the presence of chronic alcoholism often complicates recovery by continued drinking, withdrawal states, and poor comprehension of treatment issues due to dementia. Thus in head and neck patients, psychiatric issues arise frequently as a consequence of both the neoplasm and the predisposing problem of alcoholism.

This chapter outlines the common psychosocial issues confronting patients with head and neck neoplasms, their impact on rehabilitation, their management, and the common types of alcoholic complications.

## PSYCHOSOCIAL ISSUES

Psychological investment in the head and neck area is greater than any other part of the body because social interaction and emotional expression depend to a great extent on the integrity of the face, and especially the eyes. Communication of affection and closeness to spouse, children, and friends depends largely on facial expressiveness. It is thus not surprising that fears of isolation, rejection, and concerns about the reactions of others lead to indecision about surgery and depression in the postoperative period. The impact of facial disfigurement on normal sexuality has been studied little, but it likely is significant and exceeds that associated with the more documented problems associated with mastectomy and colostomy (Curtis and Zlotolow, 1980). The head and neck cancer patient cannot hide the structural changes, and must deal with their constant exposure as well as the reactions of others. The result is a strong negative impact on self-esteem and confidence (Scott et al., 1980).

## PHYSICAL DYSFUNCTION

The two separate parameters of impairment that patients with head and neck cancer face are structural and functional. They result from the defect produced by a surgical procedure, radiation, or tumor growth. They also determine the degree of body image change required of the patient in psychological adaptation; the greater the degree of structural change and/or dysfunction, the greater is the severity of emotional distress, particularly with radical operative procedures.

### Measurement of Structural and Functional Loss

The degree of structural and functional alteration is important to assess because of the relationship to emotional response. Dropkin and colleagues at Memorial Sloan-Kettering Cancer Center developed a scale of disfigurement and dysfunction to assist in postoperative care (Dropkin, 1983; Dropkin et al., 1983) (Fig. 17-1). Orbital exenteration resulting in the loss of the eye with radical maxillectomy was the

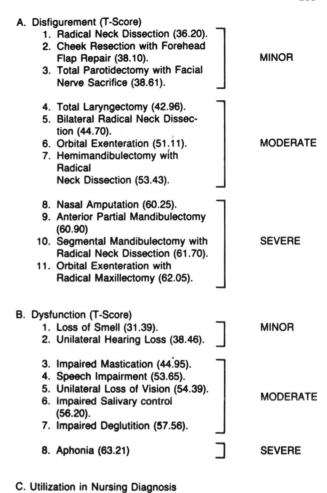

A. Disfigurement (T-Score)
1. Radical Neck Dissection (36.20).
2. Cheek Resection with Forehead Flap Repair (38.10).
3. Total Parotidectomy with Facial Nerve Sacrifice (38.61).

MINOR

4. Total Laryngectomy (42.96).
5. Bilateral Radical Neck Dissection (44.70).
6. Orbital Exenteration (51.11).
7. Hemimandibulectomy with Radical Neck Dissection (53.43).

MODERATE

8. Nasal Amputation (60.25).
9. Anterior Partial Mandibulectomy (60.90)
10. Segmental Mandibulectomy with Radical Neck Dissection (61.70).
11. Orbital Exenteration with Radical Maxillectomy (62.05).

SEVERE

B. Dysfunction (T-Score)
1. Loss of Smell (31.39).
2. Unilateral Hearing Loss (38.46).

MINOR

3. Impaired Mastication (44.95).
4. Speech Impairment (53.65).
5. Unilateral Loss of Vision (54.39).
6. Impaired Salivary control (56.20).
7. Impaired Deglutition (57.56).

MODERATE

8. Aphonia (63.21)

SEVERE

C. Utilization in Nursing Diagnosis

**Figure 17-1.** Disfigurement/dysfunction scale. (Mild/moderate/severe) alteration in body image related to (specific disfigurement or dysfunction) as evidenced by D/D scale. *Source:* Reprinted with permission from Dropkin, M.J., Malgady, G.R., Scott, D.W., et al. Scaling of disfigurement and dysfunction in postoperative head and neck patients. *Head Neck Surg* 8:559–579, 1983.

most disfiguring procedure on the scale (Fig. 17-1). Segmental mandibulectomy combined with radical neck dissection, anterior partial mandibulectomy, and nasal amputation were also considered to be severe. Hemimandibulectomy with radical neck dissection, orbital exenteration, bilateral neck dissection, and total laryngectomy were within the moderate range. Radical neck dissection alone and cheek resection with forehead flap repair and parotidectomy with facial nerve sacrifice were regarded as less disfiguring. In regard to the degree of dysfunction, the most severe loss was aphonia, followed by impaired deglutition and control of saliva; loss of smell and unilateral hearing loss were considered less severe.

In studies using the scale and the concept of a body reintegration model in predicting rehabilitative problems, more severe functional and/or structural loss was indeed associated with slower recovery, more prolonged social isolation, lower self-esteem, greater sense of worthlessness, and more severe depression (Fig. 17-2).

## PSYCHOLOGICAL REACTIONS AND PSYCHIATRIC COMPLICATIONS

The several common psychological responses and psychiatric complications with head and neck cancer that require careful attention in terms of recognition and management (Table 17-1 are the emotional reactions to diagnosis and treatment, preexisting personality and coping style, alcohol and tobacco-related disorders, and rehabilitation.

### Emotional Reactions to Diagnosis and Treatment

The threat to one's normal healthy life results in fear and dysphoria, which are manifested as anxiety and/or depression. Both reactions are normal at certain levels and represent a healthy means of adapting to the stress. In the course of head and neck cancer, however, these common emotions can become extreme, interfering with the patient's ability to cooperate with the complex

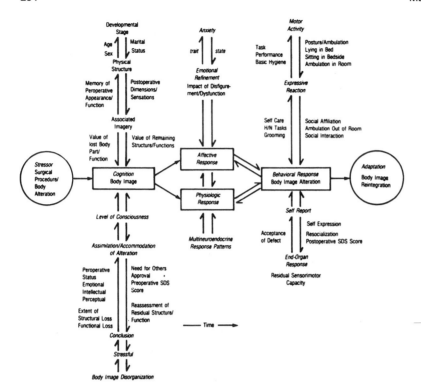

**Figure 17-2.** Body image reintegration with head and neck surgery. *Source:* Reprinted with permission from D.W. Scott, M.T. Oberst, and M.J. Dropkin (1980). A stress-coping model. *Adv. Nurs. Sci.* 3:9–23.

multimodal treatments that currently may entail chemotherapy, surgery, and irradiation.

## ANXIETY

Anxiety disorders seen in patients with head and neck neoplasms are either reactive to the stress of the illness (adjustment disorder with anxious or anxious and depressed mood) or preexisting the diagnosis of cancer and manifested by generalized anxiety, panic disorder, or phobias.

Adjustment disorder with anxious, depressed, or mixed mood was diagnosed in 50% of the head and neck cancer patients seen among 481 psychiatric consultations reviewed by the psychiatry group at Memorial Sloan-Kettering, confirming that this is the most common psychiatric disorder seen among cancer patients.

Preoperative anxiety is common in all surgical patients. The preoperative period for the head and neck cancer patient is particularly characterized by fears about the procedure and the extent of the anticipated postoperative deficit, especially in the procedures that result in the loss of a major function or a disfiguring facial alteration (Johnston, 1980). The anxiety (and resulting indecision about surgery) is often diminished by talking with a patient who has had the same procedure and adapted well. This has proved helpful, especially in patients anticipating laryngectomy. In the

postoperative period, concerns that provoke high anxiety include poorly controlled pain, inability to swallow or speak, and concerns about appearance, socialization, and adaptation to dysfunction.

### CASE REPORT

A 54-year-old married socialite sought psychiatric consultation because of several episodes of severe anxiety and panic attacks that developed 4 days after a radical maxillectomy, while receiving intravenous antibiotics. The patient was married to a wealthy businessman and maintained an active social life; she was a social drinker and a nonsmoker. She had a history of mild phobias, including claustrophobia and, after undergoing cosmetic surgery on two occasions in the past, transiently had developed panic attacks. According to her family, she had tolerated delayed diagnosis and uncertainty preoperatively about whether an orbital exenteration would also be required. The orbit was preserved, but the patient became distraught after the surgery and had difficulty tolerating the pain, difficulty breathing, and drooling. Infection required intravenous antibiotics; a full-blown panic attack ensued and occurred each time the infusion was given, until she refused the antibiotics and asked for psychiatric help to assist her in tolerating the needed treatment. She responded to alprazolam (0.5 mg po tid), cognitive-behavioral interventions, and psychological support.

## DEPRESSION

Depression occurs in approximately 25% of medically ill patients (Moffic and Paykel, 1975; Schwab et al.,

**Table 17-1**  Common psychiatric problems in head and neck cancer patients

| Problem areas | Components |
| --- | --- |
| Emotional reactions to diagnosis and surgery | Anxiety |
| | Depression |
| | Suicide risk |
| Preexisting personality and coping style | Unrelated to alcohol and tobacco use |
| | Related to alcohol and tobacco use |
| Alcohol and tobacco-related disorder | Alcoholism |
| | Alcohol withdrawal syndromes |
| | Delirium tremens |
| | Wernicke–Korsakoff's syndrome |
| | Alcohol-associated dementia |
| | Competency to sign consent forms |
| | Poor compliance |
| | Tobacco withdrawal syndromes |
| Rehabilitation | Difficulty adapting to structural change |
| | Delayed socialization |
| | Psychosocial concerns of rejection |
| | Psychosexual difficulties |
| | Difficulty adapting to dysfunction |
| | Self-care |
| | Use of prosthesis |
| | Use of artificial larynx |
| | Learning esophageal speech |
| | Continued smoking and drinking |

1967) and cancer patients (Derogatis et al., 1983; Bukberg et al., 1984; Plumb and Holland 1977). Head and neck cancer patients, as a result of the often mutilating surgery and frequent alcoholic history, are at an even higher risk of depression as well as suicide (Goodwin, 1982).

In a study by Farberow and co-workers (1971) of suicides among male cancer patients over an 8-year period, three sites that accounted for almost 50% of the total were lung, larynx, and tongue. This increased risk of suicide among patients with head and neck cancer was supported by findings in several other studies (Bolund, 1985; Farberow et al., 1963; Weisman, 1976). The explanation for this increased suicide risk may relate to the impact of adjusting to extensive surgical deficits, coupled with the underlying emotional problems in individuals who use alcohol and tobacco to an excessive degree and who have less ability to cope with the stresses of illness.

CASE REPORT

The same 54-year-old socialite's successful struggle to control her anxieties and phobias allowed for completion of anti-

biotic therapy; however, during the remainder of her hospitalization she had difficulty in looking in a mirror, undertaking self-care; socializing with others, and accepting the facial prosthesis. Problems with speech, control of saliva, and chewing became disheartening. After discharge she refused to see friends and had insomnia, anorexia, poor concentration, and depressed mood; she was withdrawn and wanted to die. Suicidal thoughts were frequent and troubling. She was seen frequently in crisis-oriented psychotherapy, using both individual and family sessions. Desensitization was used to help her view her face, socialize, and cope. She was given amitriptyline (150 mg po at bedtime) and alprazolam (0.5 mg qid). Her depression lifted rapidly, and she was able to return to normal activities.

## Premorbid Personality

Premorbid personality and emotional maturity influence both course of treatment and rehabilitation. A study in Norway of 188 laryngectomees found that premorbid adjustment was a strong predictor of the ability to adapt to loss of laryngeal speech and mastery of esophageal speech (Natvig, 1983). Other predictors of good vocational and social adjustment were high motivation of both patient and family, and realistic expectations in participating in speech rehabilitation (Goldberg, 1975). Among individuals who have abused alcohol and cigarettes before developing head and neck cancer, personality characteristics of dependence, inability to change habits, and poor adaptive coping skills contribute to poor outcome. Individuals whose identity is dependent on physical appearance or verbal communicative skills may require special attention and counseling. These patients should be referred early for psychiatric consultation in order to maximize preoperative and postoperative cooperation. The following case illustrates several of the issues.

CASE REPORT

A 58-year-old married attorney came to the hospital with a pharyngeal lesion with local spread. He had been aware of a mass but had refused to see a doctor until the pain became severe. History from his wife indicated that he had been a heavy drinker for 20 years, consuming large amounts of vodka daily; work impairment had occurred over the past 6 months. He had smoked a pack and a half of cigarettes each day since age 16. The patient complained that chronic nervousness required that he "steady his nerves" with alcohol, especially before a court appearance. Attempts at abstinence through both Alcoholics Anonymous and psychotherapy initiated at family urging had failed. Psychiatric evaluation found a bright, previously highly productive attorney who had a dependent immature personality with underlying anger toward obligations of family life. Upon discharge he continued to drink daily and cooperated poorly with his medical care throughout a stormy course, with recurrence and death.

## Psychiatric Disorders Related to Alcohol and Tobacco

Whereas around 20% of squamous-cell neoplasms of the aerodigestive tract tumors appear in individuals who do not drink or smoke, the majority do occur in individuals who have a history of excessive alcohol and tobacco use. While each of these habits alone increases risk, the two together have a synergistic, rather than a merely additive effect (Rothman and Keller, 1972). Because alcoholics are almost always heavy smokers, the combination places them at exceptionally high risk.

The alcohol-related mental disorders that may complicate treatment of cancer are alcohol intoxication, withdrawal, delirium tremens, hallucinosis, amnestic (Wernick–Korsakoff's) syndrome, and alcoholic dementia. In addition, marital and family disruption secondary to chronic alcoholism often reduces social resources. Work performance may have been poor, legal and financial difficulties may be long-standing, and decision-making ability may be impaired. The temptation to drink when confronted by cancer is great in such individuals. Abrupt alcoholic withdrawal may result from hospitalization, and delirium tremens may develop in the postoperative period. The cognitive impairment of mild to severe dementia may reduce understanding of the medical facts and cooperation with self-care. Alcohol-associated medical problems of malnutrition, hepatitis, cirrhosis, varices, pancreatitis, and cardiomyopathy predispose to impaired healing, treatment complications, and poorer prognosis after surgery.

It is important for those who work with head and neck cancer to be able to recognize alcohol withdrawal syndromes (Sellers and Kalant, 1976). When alcohol ingestion is abruptly discontinued or rapidly decreased by admission to the hospital, tremors, insomnia, and irritability may appear within 48 hours. The patient may appear calm following admission and before surgery, only to develop a postoperative delirium related to alcohol withdrawal. In a severe withdrawal reaction, delirium tremens is recognized by tremulousness, hallucinations (often visual), confusion, and seizures, appearing between 48 and 60 hours after cessation of drinking. The peak danger period for seizures is 30–48 hours after withdrawal. Delirium tremens develops in fewer than 5% of hospitalized patients during withdrawal, primarily among those predisposed by fever, malnutrition, or electrolyte disturbance. Mortality can be as high as 15%.

The goals in management of withdrawal reactions are relief of symptoms and control of complications, especially seizures, while preparing the patient for alcohol rehabilitation. Attention to fluid and electrolyte balance, infection, bleeding, and nutritional status are coordinated with specific pharmacotherapy for withdrawal. Benzodiazepines are most often used. Chlordiazepoxide is effective in large doses, ranging from 100 to 400 mg on the first day of treatment, but occasionally some individuals may need a higher dose. It is tapered at a rate of about 25% of the initial dose per day to avoid accumulation of the drug. Hallucinations usually can be managed with adequate benzodiazepine; however low-dose haloperidol (0.5–2.0 mg po, im, or iv qh or q2h) helps to control hallucinations. The extrapyramidal and hypotensive side effects of neuroleptics make them less desirable. Phenytoin should be given if there is a history of seizure disorder, or previous withdrawal seizures.

### CASE REPORT

A 48-year-old firefighter with a long history of alcohol abuse was seen in psychiatric consultation 4 days after hemiglossectomy and tracheostomy for carcinoma of the tongue. His behavior had suddenly become agitated and confused, and he had tried to walk off the unit. He had been admitted with alcohol on his breath and stated that he had been drinking up to the time of admission, despite the request of his surgeon to abstain from it at least a month before surgery. Postoperatively, he did well for several days, receiving chlordiazepoxide (25 mg po qid). On the evening of the third postoperative day, he became restless and unable to sleep, pacing the floor and the hallway. On the fourth day, he was more agitated, pulled out his feeding tube and was found wandering in the lobby. The patient's alcohol abuse began in his late teens, and he now drank 1–2 quarts of vodka and orange juice per day and 6–12 beers a day. He had cirrhosis, esophageal varices, and gynecomastia; also he had had one episode of upper GI bleeding, several bouts of alcoholic hepatitis, and seizures on two occasions. He had been hospitalized for alcohol detoxification 12 times, each time experiencing confusion, agitation, and hallucinations during withdrawal. Mental status examination revealed an agitated man whose speech was poor because of surgery, requiring that he write his answers to questions. He was irritable, tremulous, disoriented, had poor short-term memory, hallucinations, and marked distractability. He had mild fever, tachycardia, and elevated blood pressure, with normal laboratory values. His treatment consisted of 2.0 mg iv haloperidol initially, followed by chlordiazepoxide (80 mg po q4h) for the first day, then tapered over the next week.

The use of tobacco as a means of coping with stress results in greater anxiety and distress with discontinuation.

The common symptoms of tobacco withdrawal are irritability, restlessness, sleep disturbance, headache, impaired concentration and memory, anxiety, and craving for tobacco (Greden, 1985). These symptoms can be assuaged with nicotine given orally, but antianxiety drugs and relaxation techniques also can help to minimize the symptoms. Management of this difficult

**Table 17-2**  Rehabilitation management principles

| Stage of management | Principle |
| --- | --- |
| Preoperative psychosocial assessment | Prior psychological stability and coping strategies |
|  | History of alcoholism and its consequences |
|  | Presence of social resources |
| Preoperative counseling | Preparatory information |
|  | Early interaction with the rehabilitation "team" members |
|  | Social worker |
|  | Dental prosthetic consultant |
|  | Speech and communication therapist |
|  | Early training in coping skills |
|  | Patient volunteer |
| Postoperative | Early confrontation with loss (mirror, family) |
|  | Early social interaction on ward (patients, staff) |
|  | Postoperative socialization through group meetings |
|  | Family meetings |
|  | Special individual and group meetings of those with specific deficits, (e.g., laryngectomy patients) |
|  | Early use of prosthetics and/or artificial speech |
|  | Plastic reconstructive surgery |

problem in chronic heavy smokers may prevent their signing out or surreptitiously continuing to smoke.

## Rehabilitation

The primary psychosocial problems of rehabilitation are fears of socializing with others, difficulties in adapting to dysfunction and altered appearance, and continued use of tobacco and alcohol. Rehabilitation should start well before surgery with careful preoperative psychosocial assessment and planning to ensure continuity (Table 17-2). The goal of rehabilitation is to achieve maximal work and social rehabilitation through optimal use of the patient's remaining healthy function and capacity for psychosocial recovery.

## PREOPERATIVE PERIOD

The preoperative psychosocial assessment should identify strengths as well as weaknesses of the patient. Early recognition of marital, family, financial, and vocational problems allows for early intervention. Premorbid personality and coping skills, family supports, presence of alcohol history or alcohol-related disorders

(i.e., malnutrition, cognitive impairment, and recent drinking history to indicate likelihood of withdrawal complicating the preoperative period) are important. Evidence of memory impairment requires a careful assessment of cognitive capacity and ability to comprehend the nature and quality of the procedure planned. Competency to give consent may be a major question, as well as the ability to cooperate in selfcare. Preoperative counseling also prepares the patient for what to expect in the postoperative period. It should be given primarily by the surgeon and nurse, with details of the procedure and defects outlined. A consultation with the dentist who will later manage the prosthesis is a very useful form of continuity between the preoperative and postoperative periods. A speech therapist can also be introduced at this time. The meeting with a veteran patient can add a sense of confidence about the procedure. A psychiatric consultation is important in any patient with a history of alcoholic or psychiatric problems. Social work intervention should likewise begin in the preoperative period in order to anticipate psychosocial problems. Relaxation and cognitive techniques to help control anxiety and be an adjunct to pain control should be taught well before the actual surgery.

The preoperative period today increasingly includes the use of neoadjuvant chemotherapy, given to shrink the primary tumor before surgery to control systemic and local spread. The concerns about the control of nausea and vomiting, hair loss, and chemotherapy side effects must be dealt with and the full treatment course outlined. Alcoholics have been observed to experience less chemotherapy-related nausea and vomiting than other patients, even with highly emetic regimens. They may be managed on lower doses of antiemetic drugs (D'Acquesto et al., 1986). Radiotherapy is also frequently a part of the multimodal approach to head and neck tumors. Attention to psychological preparation for the treatments is important, with reassurance about shielding of critical areas. The radiotherapist and the technician who positions the patient and gives the treatment become important sources of emotional support to the patient during daily visits to the clinic, when adaptation can be monitored through these short but meaningful encounters.

## POSTOPERATIVE PERIOD

The postoperative period, which is critical to rehabilitative efforts, begins on a surgical floor that is geared to encouraging the patient toward early socialization with staff, other patients, and family. This includes early confrontation with facial appearance by looking in the mirror and discouraging avoidance of it, despite the difficulty in doing it. Patients who refuse to look at their face are often those who make a poorer adjustment and who may be less able to cooperate in their rehabilitation. Dropkin and co-workers (1983) found that the point 5 days after the surgery was critical in recovery in terms of acceptance of the defect, participation in self-care, and resocialization. It usually takes about 4 days of initial participation in self-care to recognize and accept the defect. Delay in undertaking self-care beyond 5–6 days is often predictive of poor coping and a poor rehabilitative outcome. Those with a high need of approval from others proceed more slowly. Patients at risk of poor rehabilitation can thus be identified early and interventions undertaken.

Early socialization is helped by encouraging attendance at group meetings of patients, families, and both together, often organized by social workers on the units. Harris, Vogtberger, and Mattox (1985) noted that weekly support meetings of patients and family members resulted in improved morale, compliance, support of one patient to another, and a diminished number of patients discharged against medical advice. The value continues after discharge because the family feels more confident in managing the psychological problems that may arise at home.

At most hospitals, group meetings for laryngectomees are held in the immediate postoperative period. They must use pads and pencils to communicate, but it is helpful to see others with the same problem attempt to communicate, and begin to plan for learning esophageal speech or use of a device. Postlaryngectomy patients who have mastered esophageal speech are available in most hospitals to counsel patients. These informal contacts have evolved into self-help groups, affiliated with the International Association of Laryngectomees, which assists patients and families with the practical problems of adaptation. Martin (1963) demonstrated the value of such groups by showing that emulation of well-rehabilitated laryngectomy patients provides a strong motivation to rehabilitation and acts as a buffer against the trauma of the loss of normal speech.

Willingness to move rapidly to rehabilitative measures and learning esophageal speech are good prognostic signs of emotional strength and adaptability (Nahum and Goldin, 1983). Goldberg (1975) showed that motivation and a realistic outlook were the best predictors of vocational and social adjustment. Over 95% of the laryngectomees studied in Holley's communications disorders center attained some form of oral expression (1983).

Among patients who experienced disfiguring surgery for cancer of the head and neck, adaptation to altered appearance is remarkably good. West (1977) surveyed 152 disfigured patients and found that 93% had adapted well socially, vocationally, and interpersonally. Recognition that they were cured of cancer was a major determinant in the ability to accept the losses.

## SUMMARY

In managing the patient with a head and neck tumor, the major psychosocial issues concern the emotional reactions to structural and functional deficits, and the recognition and treatment of the preexisting personality problems, especially those related to alcohol and tobacco abuse, which frequently complicate their treatment course. These issues influence the rehabilitation process that should begin in the preoperative period with careful attention to psychological and social assessment and psychiatric evaluation, if an alcoholic history is elicited. Important continuity in rehabilitation can be accomplished by contact with the rehabilitative team members *before* surgery.

Attention to appropriate adaptation to facial prostheses and dealing early with communication disorders require a specialized staff and a rehabilitative team that can call on a range of skills, including a psychiatric consultant. Although the ordeal of the head and neck cancer patient is psychologically difficult and challenging, most patients are able, with the proper help, to resume full and productive lives with a good quality of life.

## REFERENCES

Bolund, C. (1985). Suicide and cancer: II. Medical and care factors in suicides by cancer patients in Sweden, 1973–1976. *J. Psychosoc. Oncol.* 3(1):31–52.

Bukberg, J., D. Penman, and J. Holland (1984). Depression in hospitalized cancer patients. *Psychosom. Med.* 46:199–212.

Curtis, T.A. and I.M. Zlotolow (1980). Sexuality and head and neck cancer. *Front. Radiat. Ther. Oncol.* 14:26–34.

D'Acquesto, R., L.B. Tyson, R.T. Gralla, R.A. Clark, M.G. Kris, D.M. von Witte, and A. Cacavio (1986). The influence of chronic high alcohol intake on chemotherapy-induced nausea and vomiting. *Proc. Am. Soc. Clin. Oncol.* 5:257.

Derogatis, L.R., G.R. Morrow, J. Fetting, D. Penman, S. Piasetsky, A.M. Schmale, M. Henrich, and C.L.M. Carnicke, Jr. (1983). The prevalence of psychiatric disorders among cancer patients. *J.A.M.A.* 249:751–57.

Dropkin, M.J. (1983). Body image reintegration and coping effectiveness after head and neck surgery. *J. Official Publ. Soc. Otorhinolaryngol. Head and Neck Nurses* 2:7–16.

Dropkin, M.J., R.G. Malgady, D.W. Scott, M. Oberst, and E. Strong (1983). Scaling of disfigurement and dysfunction in postoperative head and neck patients. *Head Neck Surg.* 8:559–70.

Farberow, N.L., S. Ganzler, F. Cutter, and D. Reynolds

(1971). An eight-year survey of hospital suicides. *Life-Threatening Behav.* 1:184–201.

Farberow, N.L., E.S. Shneidman, and C.V. Leonard (1963). Suicide among general medical and surgical hospital patients with malignant neoplasms. *Med. Bull. Dept. Med. Surg. Veterans Admin. (Washington)* Washington, D.C.: U.S. Veterans Administration, MB-9, pp. 1–11.

Goldberg, R.T. (1975). Vocational and social adjustment after laryngectomy. *Scand. J. Rehabil. Med.* 7:1–8.

Goodwin, D.W. (1982). Alcoholism and suicide. In E.M. Patison and E. Kaufman (eds.), *The Encyclopedic Handbook of Alcoholism.* New York: Gardner Press, pp. 655–62.

Greden, J.F. (1985). Caffeine and tobacco dependence. In H.I. Kapland and B.J. Sadock (eds.), *Comprehensive Textbook of Psychiatry.* Baltimore, Md.: Williams & Wilkins, pp. 1031–33.

Harris, L.L., K.N. Vogtsberger, and D.E. Mattox (1985). Group psychotherapy for head and neck patients. *Laryngoscope* 95:585–87.

Holley, B. (1983). Counseling the head and neck cancer patient: Laryngectomy. In C. Mettlin and G.P. Murphy (eds.), *Progress in Clinical and Biological Research.* Vol. 121, *Progress in Cancer Control III. A Regional Approach.* New York: Alan R. Liss, pp. 215–25.

Johnston, M. (1980). Anxiety in surgical patients. *Psychol. Med.* 10:145–52.

Martin, H. (1963). Rehabilitation of the laryngectomee. *Cancer* 6:823–41.

Moffic, H.S. and E.S. Paykel (1975). Depression in medical inpatients. *Br. J. Psychiatry* 126:346–53.

Nahum, A.M. and J.S. Golden (1983). Psychological problems of laryngectomy. *J.A.M.A.* 186:70–80.

Natvig, K. (1983). Study No. 1: Social, personal and behavioral factors related to present mastery of the laryngectomy event. *J. Otolaryngol.* 12:155–62.

Plumb, M.M. and J.C. Holland (1977). Comparative studies of psychological function in patients with advanced cancer. *Psychosom. Med.* 39:264–76.

Rothman, K. and A. Keller (1972). The effect of joint exposure to alcohol and tobacco on risk of cancer of the mouth and pharynx. *J. Chron. Dis.* 25:711–16.

Schwab, J.J., M. Bialow, J.M. Brown, J.M. Brown, and C.E. Holzer (1967). Diagnosing depression in medical inpatients. *Ann. Intern. Med.* 67:695–707.

Scott, D.W., M.T. Oberst, and M.J. Dropkin (1980). A stress-coping model. *Adv. Nurs. Sci.* 3:9–23.

Sellers, E.M. and H. Kalant (1976). Alcohol intoxication and withdrawal. *N. Engl. J. Med.* 294:757–62.

Shedd, D.P. (1982). Cancer of the head and neck. In J.F. Holland and E. Frei III (eds.), *Cancer Medicine,* (2nd ed.) Philadelphia: Lea & Febiger, pp. 167–85.

Weisman, A.D. (1976). Coping behavior and suicide in cancer. In J.W. Cullen, B.H. Fox, and R.N. Isom (eds.), *Cancer: The Behavioral Dimensions.* DHEW Publ. No. (NIH) 76-1074. Washington, D.C.: National Cancer Institute, pp. 3-105–18.

West, D.W. (1977). Social adaptation patterns among cancer patients with facial disfigurements resulting from surgery. *Arch. Phys. Med. Rehabil.* 58:473–79.

# 18

# Psychological Adjustment in Testicular Cancer

Susan Tross, Ph.D.

Testicular cancer is characterized by a combination of clinical features that make psychological issues critically important even after treatment has been completed. It occurs in young men who have a good prognosis, but in whom sexual, reproductive and other long term treatment effects may pose difficulties in adaptation. Testicular cancer reaches peak incidence in early adulthood (i.e., ages 20–40) when impact on active work, sexual, and social functioning is most likely to be readily manifest (Graham and Gibson, 1972). It is generally a cancer with a good prognosis, with cure rates between 70 and 80%, thereby readily permitting the mobilization of future goals (Jacobs, et al., 1966; Ansfield et al., 1969; Vugrin et al., 1983; Bosl, 1984). Finally, the sexual-reproductive system is focally involved in the disease and its treatment, all at a time of life when fertility is a major concern (Kedia et al., 1975; Bracken and Johnson, 1976; Gorzynski and Holland, 1979).

The psychological impact posed by the onset of genital cancer during the peak phase of adult male experience is greatest in its assault on psychosexual integrity, body image, sense of masculinity, sense of generativity, and sexual desire and performance (Gorzynski & Holland, 1979). They also, along with other researchers (Weisman and Worden, 1976–1977), described the heightened risk of depression, anxiety, and anticipation of pain, mutilation, and death accompanying the diagnosis of any form of cancer, upon which site-specific psychosexual liability is superimposed. Even when cure has been achieved, the testicular cancer survivor may be prone to lingering fears of recurrence, hypersensitivity to somatic complaints, and transient anxiety over losing the protection of treatment and frequent follow-up. He may also experience transient social anxiety about reentering his non-cancer-related work and leisure life-style. In the following review, the two major areas of psychological vul-

nerability, namely, acceptance of infertility and of cure, will be discussed. Functional problems, due to the physical late effects of chemotherapy, will also be described. Recommendations for management by the primary care clinician at time of diagnosis and follow-up after cure has been achieved will be offered.

## IMPACT OF INFERTILITY

### Disease-Related Infertility

Infertility may be a problem for the testicular cancer patient as early as the prodromal phase of the disease. "Subfertility," in the form of diminished sperm concentration and motility, is an early consequence of the disease process. Rates of subfertility among newly diagnosed testicular cancer patients have been estimated to be between 52 and 96% (Thachil et al., 1981) when minimal requirements for sperm banking were used as fertility criteria (i.e., a minimum sperm concentration of 40,000 per milliliter and 60% motility). The rate of subfertility for healthy male controls is approximately 60% (Sanger et al., 1980). It is an acute phenomenon that is confined to the few months just prior to diagnosis. It is a secondary disorder that occurs in patients who generally have a primary history of successful fertility. Such subfertility can seriously limit the usefulness of banking sperm at the time of diagnosis for later use in artificial impregnation. However, the option to bank sperm, when there is reasonable hope for successful artificial insemination, is an important psychological support to the young man facing infertility.

There has been speculation about the putative existence of a lifelong hypothalamic-pituitary-gonadal defect that may be a risk factor for testicular cancer. However, no studies have confirmed the presence of such a defect in diagnosed patients. Clinical folklore at times has also labeled these patients as disturbed, low functioning, and psychosexually immature; they have often been perceived as more noncompliant than other young male cancer patients. This psychosexual profile has also not proved to be true. In fact, the only certain risk factors identified for testicular cancer are prior history of cryptorchidism (Campbell, 1959; Collins and Pugh, 1964) or testicular atrophy (Hausfeld and Schrandt, 1965; Melicow, 1965).

## Treatment-Related Infertility and Sexual Dysfunction

Standard primary treatment for testicular cancer has traditionally consisted of unilateral orchiectomy (i.e., removal of the testicle) if the tumor is contained, and retroperitoneal lymph node dissection, radiotherapy, and/or combination chemotherapy if it has spread to the abdomen or beyond. The research on surgery-related infertility is summarized in Table 18-1. Retroperitoneal lymph node dissection poses the greatest threat of temporary or, especially, permanent infertility. The loss of fertility is secondary to physical interference with ejaculation. Because seminal emission depends on the sympathetically controlled peristalsis of the muscles of the vas deferens and the seminal vesicle, damage or excision of the sympathetic ganglia or adjacent tissue during retroperitoneal lymphadenectomy impairs ejaculation (Tavel et al., 1963; Leiter and Brendler, 1967; Kom et al., 1971). In contrast with retroperitoneal lymph node dissection, unilateral orchiectomy does not compromise fertility.

The research on radiotherapy- and chemotherapy-related infertility is summarized in Table 18-2. Radiotherapy, alone or in combination with chemotherapy, may reduce sperm count for several years, if not permanently (Amelar et al., 1971; Clark and Resnick, 1978; Bracken, 1981; Hahn et al., 1982), especially if administered in higher doses to the paraaortic field (Schover, et al., 1986). The two standard combination-chemotherapy regimens for testicular cancer may present yet another source of reproductive damage. These are the VAB (cyclosphosphamide, bleomycin, vinblastine, dactinomycin, chlorambucil, and *cis*-platinum) regimen, developed at the Memorial Sloan-Kettering Cancer Center, and the VBP (vinblastine, bleomycin, and platinum) regimen, developed at Indiana University (Einhorn and Donohue, 1977). At least three agents in the VAB regimen place the patient at added risk for infertility, although this risk may be impossible to distinguish from that associated with surgery. In high (i.e., >11-g) doses cyclophosphamide may cause azoospermia and germ-cell aplasia; in lower doses, it may cause oligospermia. Were it not for compounded surgical damage, it is estimated that these

effects would reverse in 46% of these cases (Buchanan et al., 1975). High-dose (i.e., >400 mg) chlorambucil may cause azoospermia (Richter et al., 1970). In both VAB and VBP, vinblastine may lower sperm volume and motility (Cutts, 1961). The sterilizing potential of the remaining agents is unknown.

The relationship between treatment-related infertility and sexual impairment is less clear; the relevant research is summarized in Table 18-3. In general, sexual dysfunction is a rarer (i.e., a 38% maximum rate of impairment in any particular function assessed) and weaker (i.e., partially rather than absolutely compromised) outcome of treatment than infertility. The higher rates of impairment of the more recent studies reflect their introduction of more explicit, detailed sexual histories, in place of global questions. The major areas of impairment are decreased sexual activity (Rieker et al., 1985; Trump et al., 1985) and diminished intensity of orgasm (Schover and von Eschenbach, 1984; Tross, 1984; Schover et al., 1986). However, the former investigators did not include questions about orgasmic

**Table 18-1** Surgery-related infertility in testicular cancer patients

| Reference | Surgery | Results |
|---|---|---|
| Kedia et al. (1975) | RPLND* | Dry ejaculation (97%) |
| Bracken and Johnson (1976) | RPLND | Decreased to dry ejaculation (70%) |
| Narayam et al. (1982) | RPLND | Decreased ejaculation (55%) |
| Schover and von Eschenbach (1984) | RPLND | Decreased ejaculation (76%) |
| Rieker et al. (1985) | RPLND | Decreased ejaculation (47%) |
| Thachil et al. (1981) | Orchiectomy | Normal ejaculation |

*Retroperitoneal lymph node dissection.

**Table 18-2** Infertility in testicular cancer patients related to chemotherapy (C) and radiation (R)

| Reference | Treatment | Results |
|---|---|---|
| Clark and Resnick (1978) | R | Decreased ejaculation |
| Bracken (1981) | R | Decreased ejaculation |
| Schover et al. (1986) | R (especially paraaortic) | Decreased ejaculation (49%) |
| Buchanan et al. (1975) | C (cyclophosphamide) | Dry (high dosage) or decreased (low dosage) ejaculation |
| Richter et al. (1970) | C (chlorambucil) | Dry ejaculation |
| Cutts (1961) | C (vinblastine) | Decreased ejaculation |

**Table 18-3**  Treatment-related sexual impairment in testicular cancer patients

| Reference | Treatment | Results |
|---|---|---|
| Kedia et al. (1975) | RPLND* | Normal sexual function |
| Bracken and Johnson (1976) | RPLND | Slight ↓ in libido (18%) and performance (12%) |
| Thachil et al. (1981) | Orchiectomy | Normal sexual function |
| Schover and von Eschenbach (1984) | RPLND | Difficulty with: orgasm (6%), premature ejaculation (6%), erection (10%), no activity (11%), ↓ orgasm intensity (38%) |
| Tross et al. (1984) | RPLND | Cancer patients > benign genital surgery controls in global sexual dysfunction |
| Rieker et al. (1985) | RPLND | Mild to moderate difficulty with erection, orgasm, satisfaction, libido, ↓ frequency (25–33%) |
| Trump et al. (1985) | RPLND | ↓ Frequency |
| Schover et al. (1986) | Radiation | Difficulty with: climax (10%), libido (12%), premature ejaculation (14%), erection (15%), ↓ orgasm intensity (33%) |

*Retroperitoneal lymph node dissection.

intensity. Whenever they were included, this complaint was observed to be the most common. Thus, a thorough sexual history should include questions about frequency and intensity of sexual activity, desire, erection, orgasm, and satisfaction. Personal or medical characteristics that may jeopardize the sexual functioning of some infertile men, while protecting that of others, are not known. Whereas the determinants of sexual impairment per se are not known, the determinants of concern about such impairment are (Rieker et al., 1985). Taken together, ejaculatory impairment and years off treatment account for a highly significant amount (~60%) of the variance in this outcome variable. That is, men with ejaculatory impairment who have been off treatment as long as 6–10 years are at greatest risk for concern about sexual impairment. Ejaculatory impairment and (interval) history of unsuccessful attempts at fertilization account for 66% of the variance in concern about infertility.

## Impact of Physical Late Effects

The aggressive therapies for testicular cancer may cause residual dysfunction in nonreproductive organs as well. These physical late effects include peripheral neuropathy (from vinblastine), Raynaud's phenomenon (Vogelzang et al., 1981), cardiotoxicity (from bleomycin and vinblastine) (Vogelzang et al., 1980), pulmonary fibrosis (from bleomycin), nephrotoxicity (from *cis*-platinum) (Schilsky and Anderson, 1979), myelosuppression with possible increased risk of infection and bleeding (from dactinomycin, vinblastine, cyclophosphamide, and *cis*-platinum), and audiological impairment (from *cis*-platinum) (Bosl, 1984). Thus, the survivor may have diminished stamina and sensory acuity with which to

meet standard, full-time work demands. This may be a source of demoralization and frustration.

## Impact of Cure

Finally, there are compelling reasons to predict that the testicular cancer survivor might be at heightened risk for general psychological distress. These include the delayed physical complications of cancer therapies (known as late effects), the practical complications of having been labeled a cancer patient, and emotional fallout from having come so close to the prospect of death. Even after cure has been achieved, the survivor may experience an only tenuous sense of longevity, producing anxiety, depressive mood and ideas, damaged body image, and fears of recurrence. The transition from "patient" to "healthy" status may be problematic. The survivor may experience a new sense of vulnerability over having "graduated" from active treatment. His relationships may be complicated by a sense of uniqueness and estrangement in the social network. He may incur a sense of financial insecurity from difficulties in improving or changing employment or acquiring new health or life insurance. This has been called the Damocles syndrome (Koocher and O'Malley, 1981). The research on psychosocial sequelae in testicular cancer survivors is summarized in Table 18-4. There is general agreement that the cancer experience does not impair the major areas of function of the survivor's life, such as employment, marriage, or economic status. When explicit questions are asked about mood, especially depressed and anxious states, increased subjective distress is observed among these survivors, but it is subtle and nonimpairing.

**Table 18-4** Psychosocial sequelae in testicular cancer survivors

| Reference | Time since diagnosis | Results |
|---|---|---|
| Tross et al. (1984) | 2–4 Years | Cancer patients similar to benign general surgery patients in self-reported emotional and social adjustment but not in clinician-rated adjustment |
| Trump et al. (1985) | 6 Months | ↑ Anxiety, depression, work dysfunction |
| | 24 Months | Normal psychosocial adjustment |
| Rieker et al. (1985) | 2–10 Years | Normal mood, unemployment (7%), and divorce (10%) |

## Implications for the Care of Testicular Cancer Patients

When the stakes of a treatment are life and death, and the prognosis for recovery is excellent, it is easy to ignore the subtler considerations of psychological well-being that are central in the lives of healthy individuals. However, it is precisely because of this prognosis that psychological intervention with the testicular cancer patient is so important. If the excellent prospect for cure and functional recovery can be effectively communicated to the newly diagnosed patient, he will be far better equipped to cope with the serious side effects and disruption of life-style that go along with the therapy. At the same time, cancer diagnoses, treatment, and newly achieved cure are clearly transitional experiences during which the young-adult survivor is likely to take stock of himself, his relationships, and his accomplishments. They are therefore experiences in which the patient can benefit from both advance psychological preparation and continued support from the health professionals who follow him. If he expects to recover baseline functioning sooner than is realistic, he may compromise his potential for a more profound resolution of the problems posed by the illness and treatment. He may also find himself sharpening the differential between the way he feels privately and the feelings he is able to share with those who expect a prompt recovery.

Although Auchincloss covers some of the general principles of appropriate psychosexual rehabilitation in Chapter 33, several specific areas of concern are of note. In particular, the problem of damaged aspirations for paternity is a critical emotional issue that the patient

may not feel comfortable raising on his own. The primary care clinician should take the lead in eliciting the patient's cognitive grasp of and emotional response to this issue in a frank and sensitive way. Whenever limited disease (i.e., stage I) permits it, treatment by orchiectomy alone with regular follow-up should be seriously considered as a fertility-sparing option (Sogani et al., 1984). Even though sperm banking and artificial insemination may not ultimately prove to be viable methods for paternity, they can, at the very least, be crucial sources of psychological support to the young man facing infertility. The survivor who unsuccessfully tries to become a father needs professional support and clarification of alternative methods of fatherhood. Although their history of cancer may jeopardize eligibility, the option to adopt should be discussed. Although partner insemination with donor sperm should also be raised, these patients tend to reject this option. α-Sympathomimetic medication has also been suggested as a possible means of improving ejaculation (Nijman et al., 1982).

The obvious absence of a testicle may be expected to prompt feelings of self-consciousness, inadequacy, and defective body image, especially in men without primary partners at the time of diagnosis. To offset these reactions, the patient should be offered the option to insert surgically a comfortable and realistic silicone gel prosthesis into the scrotum.

The possibility of secret, subtle sexual impairment (chiefly in the forms of diminished orgasmic intensity or sexual activity) demands that serial sexual histories be obtained throughout the patient's course and follow-up. Such a history should include questions about frequency and intensity of sexual activity, desire, erection, orgasm, and satisfaction. Sex therapy, by a therapist with specialty training, can offer a vast repertoire of behavioral techniques for reducing performance anxiety and enhancing pleasure. Use of midodrin with patients' experiencing orgasm problems has also been reported in Europe (Jonas et al., 1979).

## SUMMARY

Dramatic progress in testicular cancer therapy has provided a new body of research data about the psychological experience of people who are living rather than dying with cancer. Successful treatment has sometimes some unfortunate side effects, that is, delayed physical, especially reproductive and sexual, complications from its aggressive therapies, and practical complications of having been labeled a cancer patient and psychological fallout from having come so close to the prospect of death. However, the consensus of existing research is that at the same time that newly achieved cure may reintensify the patient's confrontation with any (physical or emotional) vulnerability associated with his illness, it at least as readily offers him a sense of purpose, efficacy, and renewal.

# REFERENCES

Amelar, E.D., L. Dubin, and R.S. Hotchkiss (1971). Restoration of fertility following unilateral orchiectomy and radiation therapy for testicular tumors. *J. Urol.* 106:714–18.

Ansfield, F.J., B.C. Korbitz, H.L. Davis, Jr., and G. Ramirez (1969). Triple therapy in testicular tumors. *Cancer* 24:442–46.

Bosl, G.J. (1984). Status and prospects of the treatment of disseminated germ-cell tumors. *World J. Urol.* 2:38–42.

Bracken, R.B. (1981). Cancer of the testis, penis and urethra: The impact of therapy on sexual function. In A.C. von Eschenbach and D.B. Rodriquez (eds.), *Sexual Rehabilitation of the Urologic Cancer Patient.* Boston: G.K. Hall, pp. 108–24.

Bracken, R.B. and D.E. Johnson (1976). Sexual function and fecundity after treatment for testicular tumors. *Urology* 1:35–38.

Buchanan, J.D., K.F. Fairley, and J.U. Barrie (1975). Return of spermatogenesis after stopping cyclophosphamide. *Lancet* 2:156–57.

Campbell, H.E. (1959). The incidence of malignant growth of the undescended testicle: A reply and re-evaluation. *J. Urol.* 81:663–68.

Clark, S. and M. Resnick (1978). Infertility following radiation and chemotherapy. *Urol. Clin. North Am.* 5:531–35.

Collins, D.H. and R.C.B. Pugh (1964). Classification and frequency of testicular tumors. *Br. J. Urol.* 36:1–11.

Cutts, J.J. (1961). The effect of vincaleukoblastine on dividing cells in vivo. *Cancer Res.* 21:168–72.

Einhorn, L. and J.P. Donohue (1977). *Cis*-diaminedichloroplastinum, vinblastine, and bleomycin combination chemotherapy in disseminated testicular cancer. *Ann. Intern. Med.* 87:293–98.

Gorzynski, G. and J.C. Holland (1979). Psychological aspects of testicular cancer. *Semin. Oncol.* 6:25–29.

Graham, S. and R.W. Gibson (1972). Social epidemiology of cancer of the testis. *Cancer* 29:1242–49.

Hahn, E.W., S.M. Feingold, L. Simpson, and M. Batata (1982). Recovery from aspermia induced by low-dose radiation in seminoma patients. *Cancer* 50:337–40.

Hausfeld, K.F. and D. Schrandt (1965). Malignancy of testis following atrophy: Report of three cases. *J. Urol.* 94:69–72.

Jacobs, E.M., F.D. Johnson, and D.A. Wood (1966). Stage III metastatic malignant testicular tumors. *Cancer* 19:1697–1704.

Jonas, D., P. Linzbach, and W. Weber (1979). The use of midodrin in the treatment of ejaculation disorders following retroperitoneal lymphadenectomy. *Eur. Urol.* 5:184–87.

Kedia, K., C. Markland, and E.E. Fraley (1975). Sexual

function following high retroperitoneal lymphadenectomy. *J. Urol.* 114:237–39.

Kom, C., S.G. Mulholland, and M. Edson (1971). Etiology of infertility after retroperitoneal lymphadenectomy. *J. Urol.* 105:528–30.

Koocher, G.P. and J.E. O'Malley (1981). *The Damocles Syndrome: Psychosocial Consequences of Surviving Childhood Cancer.* New York: McGraw-Hill.

Leiter, E. and H. Brendler (1967). Loss of ejaculation following bilateral retroperitoneal lymphadenectomy. *J. Urol.* 98:375–78.

Melicow, M.M. (1965). New British classification of testicular tumors: A correlation, analysis and critique. *J. Urol.* 94:69–72.

Narayam, P., P.H. Lange, and E.E. Fraley (1982). Ejaculation and fertility after extended retroperitoneal node dissection for testicular cancer. *J. Urol.* 127:685–88.

Nijman, J.M., S. Jager, P.W. Boer, J. Kremer, J. Oldhoff, and H. Schraffordtkoops (1982). The treatment of ejaculation disorders after retroperitoneal lymph node dissection. *Cancer* 50:2697–2971.

Richter, P., J.C. Calamera, M.C. Morgenfeld, A.L. Kierszenbaum, J.C. Lavieri, and R.E. Mancini (1970). Effect of chlorambucil on spermatogenesis in the human with malignant lymphoma. *Cancer* 25:1026–30.

Rieker, P.P., S.D. Edbril, and M.B. Garnick (1985). Curative testis cancer therapy: Psychosocial sequelae. *J. Clin. Oncol.* 3:1117–26.

Sanger, W.G., J.O. Armitage, and M.A. Schmidt (1980). Feasibility of semen cryopreservation in patients with malignant disease. *J.A.M.A.* 14:12–19.

Schilsky, R.L. and T. Anderson (1979). Hypomagnesemia and renal magnesium wasting in patients receiving cisplatin. *Ann. Intern. Med.* 90:929–31.

Schover, L.R. and A.C. Von Eschenbach (1984). Sexual and marital counseling with men treated for testicular cancer. *J. Sex Marital Ther.* 10(1):29–40.

Schover, L.R., M. Gonzalez and A.C. von Eschenbach (1986). Sexual and marital relationship after radiotherapy for seminoma. *Urology* 27(2):117–23.

Sogani, P.C., W.F. Whitmore, Jr., H.W. Herr, G.J. Bosl, R.B. Golbey, R.C. Watson, and J.J. DeCosse (1984). Orchiectomy alone in the treatment of clinical stage I non-seminomatous germ-cell tumors of testis (NSGCaT). *J. Clin. Oncol.* 2:267–70.

Tavel, F.R., T.G. Osius, J.W. Parker, R.B. Goodfriend, D.J. McGonigle, M.P. Jassie, E.L. Simmons, M.I. Tobenkin, and J.W. Schulte (1963). Retroperitoneal lymph node dissection. *J. Urol.* 89:241–45.

Thachil, J.V., M.A.S. Jewitt, and W.D. Rider (1981). The effects of cancer and cancer therapy on male fertility. *J. Urol.* 126:141–45.

Tross, S., J. Holland, G. Bosl, and N. Geller (1984). A controlled study of psychosocial sequelae in cured survivors of testicular neoplasms. *Proc. Am. Soc. Clin. Oncol.* 3:74.

Trump, D.L., E.P. Pomsaas, K.C. Cummings, and J.F. Malec (1985). Assessment of psychologic and sexual dysfunction in patients following treatment of testis cancer: A prospective study. *Proc. Twenty-First Annu. Mtg. Am. Soc. Clin. Oncol.* 4:250 (Abstract No. C-975).

Vogelzang, N.J., G.J. Bosl, K. Johnson, and B.J. Kennedy (1981). Raynaud's phenomenon: A common toxicity after combination chemotherapy for testicular cancer. *Ann. Intern. Med.* 95:288–92.

Vogelzang, N.J., D.H. Frenning, and B.J. Kennedy (1980). Coronary artery disease after treatment with bleomycin and vinblastine. *Cancer Treat. Rep.* 64:1159–60.

Vugrin, D., W.F. Whitmore, and R.B. Golbey (1983). VAB-6 combination chemotherapy without maintenance in treatment of disseminated cancer of the testis. *Cancer* 51:211–15.

Weisman, A. and W. Worden (1976–1977). The existential plight in cancer: Significance of the first 100 days. *Int. J. Psychiatry Med.* 7:1–15.

# 19

# Skin Cancer and Melanoma

Jimmie C. Holland

Skin is the most common site of cancer; its cure rate exceeds 95%, yet the emotional distress related to its disfiguring effects can be high (Klein et al., 1973). It is interesting that skin cancers have always been identified to patients as cancers, even while the diagnosis of other sites of cancer were not being revealed to patients. This is likely because the threat to life is generally known to be low for the two common skin cancers, basal and squamous-cell carcinoma. Consequently, they have never carried the same stigma or produced the degree of fear associated with other cancers. However, the less common tumor arising in skin, malignant melanoma, is known by most individuals to pose a serious threat to life. The common skin tumors, basal cell and squamous cell, are discussed first for their broad medical and psychological implications; melanoma is reviewed separately.

## BASAL AND SQUAMOUS-CELL CARCINOMA

Basal-cell carcinoma represents 75% of skin cancers in southern states and 90% or more in northern states (Haynes et al., 1985). It appears on the head, neck, and trunk as a smooth, shiny, nontender, sometimes ulcerating lesion. It spreads, not by metastasis but by local invasion into bone, nerve, and blood vessels. Squamous-cell carcinomas appear on the sun-exposed areas of skin over the ears, nose, lower lip, and hands, and are usually erythematous. They too rarely metastasize, except in immunosuppressed individuals. The precancerous lesions that predispose to development of squamous-cell carcinoma are actinic keratosis, Bowen's disease (a form of in situ carcinoma), and keratoacanthoma.

Basal-cell and squamous-cell carcinomas arise from epidermal cells; they also share common epidemiological and etiological features (Haynes et al., 1985). The most commonly known causes are by chemical exposure. In 1775, these causes were noted first by Sir Percival Pott, who observed that scrotal tumors developed from chronic exposure to soot among chimney sweeps. Other chemical exposures that initiate skin tumors are pitch, croton oil, and benzopyrene. The carcinogenic effects of ionizing radiation on the skin were noted among the early radiologists who worked without protection of their hands. Exposure to ultraviolet (UV) radiation from the sun was later found to act as both initiator and promoter of these tumors. In fact, there is a direct relationship between incidence and geographic location in relation to the equator among light-skinned Caucasians. Darker-skinned individuals, whose skin contains more melanin, are thus protected from UV radiation effects and have a lower incidence.

Treatment is by biopsy, surgical excision with grafting (if needed), and radiotherapy. Keratoses are treated successfully by topical 5-fluorouracil (5-FU).

### Psychological Considerations

Considering the high incidence of skin tumors, it is surprising that so little has been written about related psychological issues. Freidenbergs (1981) described some of the important issues in dealing with patients with skin tumors. Some patients delay in seeking consultation because of the fear of cancer, assuming that skin cancers are as dangerous as tumors of the internal organs. This attitude leads to fatalism and fear in pursuing treatment. Physicians should be careful to include the actual prognosis and potential for spread in their discussion of the diagnosis and treatment. Irrational fears may be a problem, even when skin cancers are present. Misperceptions should be ascertained through questioning and corrected by factual information. This is most apt to occur through an earlier experience with cancer that colors reactions to the diagnosis of skin cancer, even if it is far less likely to be life-threatening. Good communication between doctor and patient is essential in dealing with these tumors.

Wide excisions or surgical procedures that disfigure, especially on the face, may require careful psychological preparation to encourage the patient to accept a curative procedure. Explanation about skin grafts and the possible use of facial prostheses is essential. Preoperative consultation with those who will be responsible for rehabilitation is important, including dentists, speech therapists, and plastic surgeons. Consultation with a mental health professional may be helpful when preoperative anxiety is interfering with rational decision making about treatment, and when emotional problems appear likely to impede rehabilitation. Postoperative problems most often relate to difficulties in socialization due to an altered appearance. These are discussed in detail in Chapter 17 on head and neck neoplasms.

The psychological problems associated with squamous and basal-cell tumors are essentially the same as those of other visible tumors, particularly on the head and neck. They share the common problems of producing unsightly lesions and altering appearance. The adverse consequences are fear of the negative emotional responses of others, impaired self-esteem, and social withdrawal. In addition, life-threatening metastases do occur with both basal and squamous-cell cancers which are at times aggressive and resistant to treatment, invading local tissues to produce fatal complications. The progression is slow and inexorable, requiring painful adjustment to an unresponsive tumor. Depression, anxiety, and problems in pain control are common.

## MALIGNANT MELANOMA

Melanoma is a neoplasm whose incidence has increased rapidly in recent years, most likely as a result of cultural patterns leading to increased recreational sun exposure. Melanoma is a malignant tumor that arises from the melanocytes in the skin; the cells originate in the neural crest and migrate to the skin and eye (Luce et al., 1973). Most melanomas arise in the skin, but about 10% occur first in other sites, primarily the eye, mucous membranes, and genitalia (Nathanson, 1986, 1987). The neoplasm is uncommon in dark-skinned races and occurs most often in fair-skinned individuals who are exposed to the UV spectrum of actinic radiation. It is of interest etiologically because it never occurs before puberty, suggesting hormonal influences on growth. Familial melanoma also occurs, suggesting a genetic influence. Nagle and colleagues (1970) reported simultaneous malignant growth of moles on the chest wall of identical twins within a set

of triplets in their fifties, further reflecting genetic influences. Psychological distress of the surviving twin whose melanoma did not metastasize in the surviving triplet and siblings was documented, showing the impact of a familial pattern of melanoma on survivors (Holland et al., 1971).

The primary lesions on the skin are, with increasing frequency of spread, lentigo, superficial spreading, nodular, and mucosal, palmar or plantar. Characteristic symptoms are itching, bleeding, and change in appearance of a mole. Malignant lesions most often lack hair follicles and have irregular margins and variegated coloring, as compared to benign nevi (Nathanson, 1986). Far more public information is available today to warn individuals at risk to be alert for suspicious changes in pigmented moles and freckles. Dermatologists today educate high-risk patients to carry out regular self-examination of skin surfaces; some use photographs of pigmented nevi in these individuals to identify changes more rapidly. Lesions on the back are most likely to go unnoticed and may be reported to the doctor, only after serious spread has occurred.

Because 30% of melanoma patients already have spread at the time of initial diagnosis, prognosis is guarded and uncertain. Depth of the lesion, by Clark classification, predicts 5-year survival; evidence of local and regional spread or distant metastases reduces prognosis precipitously (Table 19-1).

Wide excision with regional lymph node dissection is standard treatment. Regional treatment by perfusion chemotherapy has been used, utilizing alkylating agents. Systemic combination chemotherapy using Cisplatin, dacarbazine, carmustine, and tamoxifen has resulted in response in some patients. The sensitivity of some melanomas to both endocrine and im-

**Table 19-1** Staging and prognosis in malignant melanoma

| Stage | Site | Percentage 5-year survival |
|---|---|---|
| I | Primary tumor only (size, mm) | 85 |
| | <0.75 | 99 |
| | 0.76–1.5 | 92 |
| | 1.51–3.99 | 78 |
| | >4.0 | 40 |
| II | Local metastases | 50 |
| | <5 mm from primary melanoma) | |
| III | Regional metastases | 25 |
| | Lymph node | |
| | Soft tissue | |
| IV | Distant metastases | 10 |
| | Soft tissue | |
| | Visceral | |

*Source*: Reprinted with permission from L. Nathanson (1987). Melanoma and other skin malignancies. In R. T. Skeel (ed.), *Handbook of Cancer Chemotherapy*, 2nd ed. Boston: Little, Brown & Co., p. 183.

munological manipulation has led to trials of these treatments with encouraging results. Interferon has resulted in encouraging responses in metastatic melanoma; interleukin 2, with and without lymphocyte-activated killer cells, currently appears promising in trials, as is use of monoclonal antibodies. However, no treatment offers significant hope of cure as yet. Relapse in the brain is a common complication that responds poorly to treatment. Partial response is seen with cranial irradiation.

## Psychological Issues

There are several behavioral and psychological issues in melanoma. The first is the key role of behavior in prevention. Sunbathing is a current popular activity that increases risk of melanoma, particularly in fair-skinned individuals. To reduce this risk by changing behavior with public education is a high priority in cancer control. In addition, malignant melanoma has been the object of study for the psychological impact it has on patients and their families. It has also been studied for the role that psychological influences and behavior play in outcome, because the speed with which an individual seeks a consultation for a nonpainful skin lesion that may have changed in appearance may be the key to early diagnosis and curative treatment.

The nature of the seemingly insignificant change in a skin lesion often causes delay in seeing a physician. Temoshok and co-workers (1984) found that delay was greater with lesions on the back, which were less readily identifiable. Patients more easily detected the nodular melanomas, which have a poor prognosis. However, those with less knowledge of melanoma and its treatment, and those who failed to minimize the seriousness (thereby leading to paralyzing fear), were found to delay longer. Cassileth and colleagues (1982) reviewed charts of over 200 patients and found that the majority of melanomas were not recognized at an early and low-risk phase when tumor depth and elevation of the lesion were lowest. They raised the question of whether one can expect a major increase in identification of early curable lesions.

Melanoma poses some unique psychological problems at the time of diagnosis. The potential risk to life is well understood by patients, but after the initial treatment there is no evidence of the disease and the individual feels well. There are some psychological parallels to coronary heart disease, in which patients, in the absence of symptoms or signs of the disease, tend to minimize its meaning. Cassileth and colleagues (1982), using the Mental Health Well-Being Scale of the Rand Corporation, found melanoma patients who were returning for clinic visits to be well adjusted.

Others have found reactions to diagnosis similar to those with cancer in general, but with initial distress followed by a positive outlook toward treatment, family, friends, and life (Longman and Graham, 1986). These findings suggest that the major psychological problem following a diagnosis of melanoma is dealing with the sense of being a "walking time bomb." Handling the uncertainty results in anxiety that dominates the picture. F. Fawzy has found supportive psychotherapy to be extremely helpful in control of distress in this group (personal communication). Depression appears more clearly at the point when disease dissemination becomes evident.

The wide excision of a melanoma can leave a large defect with an unsightly appearance. Patients who were less distressed by the cosmetic surgery were those who were psychologically prepared for the size and depth of scars, and those who had primary closure of the incision (Cassileth et al., 1983). The same study found that women had more concerns about cosmetic appearance than men.

When melanoma becomes disseminated, the psychological issues are those of any other advanced cancer known to respond poorly to traditional treatments, as described in Chapter 6. Newer immunological and hormonal therapies are looked to with optimism, but most patients recognize that newer treatments are still needed for successful treatment of this tumor.

## PSYCHOLOGICAL INFLUENCES IN SURVIVAL

Some of the most provocative studies of psychosocial influences in survival have been done on melanoma, based on the hypothesis that because this tumor appears to be highly sensitive to hormonal and immunological influences, it might be most influenced psychosocially. The major studies are reviewed in Chapter 60. The findings by both Rogentine and colleagues (1979) and Temoshok (1985) have identified a coping style in individuals with melanoma whose survival is poorer. Temoshok has called it the Type C personality, in which the person objectively reveals the presence of negative affects, such as depression, anxiety, and anger, but fails to report awareness of the feelings. These individuals are cooperative, compliant, and uncomplaining. Melanoma provides a cancer site in which interaction of psychological and biological variables can be studied prospectively to answer some of these intriguing questions.

## SUMMARY

Skin is the most common site of cancer and has the best chance of cure. The two common types are basal-cell and squamous-cell carcinoma. Both are usually cured by surgical excision, but the site and nature of the incision and defect resulting from curative surgery may lead to emotional distress, self-consciousness about appearance, and social withdrawal. Preparation psychologically for surgery is a major influence in adaptation. Cutaneous malignant melanoma is a far more life-threatening neoplasm that is increasing in incidence, especially among fair-skinned people with extensive sun exposure. Early detection and surgical excision offer the best outlook. When melanoma disseminates in the body, it is highly aggressive and responds poorly to most treatment, although the biological response modifiers and monoclonal antibodies are of research interest. Psychological issues focus around adaptation to the diagnosis of a potentially fatal disease, surgical excision, and dealing with the uncertainty of recurrence. When melanoma recurs, the emotional issues are similar to those of other tumors in advanced disease stages. Melanoma, as a tumor responsive to hormonal and immunological influences, is a neoplasm that offers an interesting site in which interaction of psychological and biological influences can be studied.

## REFERENCES

Cassileth, B.R., W.H. Clark, R.M. Heilberger, V. March, and A. Tenaglia (1982). Relationship between patient's early recognition of melanoma and depth of invasion. *Cancer* 49:198–200.

Cassileth, B.R., E.J. Lusk, and A.W. Tenaglia (1983). Patients' perceptions of the cosmetic impact of melanoma resection. *Plast. Reconstr. Surg.* 71:73–75.

Freidenbergs, I. (1981). Psychosocial management of patients with cutaneous cancers: A preliminary report. *J. Dermatol. Surg. Oncol.* 7:828–30.

Haynes, H.A., K.W. Mead, and R.M. Goldwyn (1985). Cancers of the skin. In V. DeVita, S. Hellman, and S. Rosenberg (eds.), *Principles and Practice of Oncology.* Philadelphia: Lippincott, pp. 1343–69.

Holland, J., S. Harris, and J. Holmes (1971). Psychological response to death of an identical twin by the surviving twin with the same disease: concurrent malignant melanoma in identical twins of triplets. *Omega* 2:160–67.

Klein, E., G.H. Burgess, and F. Helm (1973). Neoplasms of the skin. In J.F. Holland and E. Frei (eds.), *Cancer Medicine.* Philadelphia: Lea & Febiger, pp. 1789–1822.

Longman, A.J. and K.Y. Graham (1986). Living with melanoma: Content analysis of interviews. *Oncol. Nurs. Forum* 13;58–64.

Luce, J.K., C.M. McBride, E. Frei, III (1973). Melanoma. In J.F. Holland and E. Frei (eds.), *Cancer Medicine.* Philadelphia: Lea & Febiger, pp. 1823–43.

Nagle, G.A., G. St. Arneault, and J.F. Holland (1970). Cell-mediated immunity against malignant melanoma in monozygous twins. *Cancer Res.* 30:1828–32.

Nathanson, L. (ed.) (1986). *Medical Management of Advanced Melanoma.* New York: Churchill-Livingstone.

Nathanson, L. (1987). Melanoma and other skin malignancies. In R.T. Skeel (ed.), *Handbook of Cancer Chemotherapy,* 2nd ed. Boston: Little, Brown & Co., pp. 182–91.

Rogentine, G.W., D.P. Van Kammen, B.H. Fox, J.R. Docherty, J.E. Rosenblatt, S.C. Boyd, and W.E. Bunney (1979). Psychological factors in the prognosis of malignant melanoma. *Psychosom. Med.* 41:647–58.

Temoshok, L. (1985). Biopsychosocial studies on cutaneous malignant melanoma: Psychosocial factors associated with prognostic indicators, progression, psychophysiology and tumor–host response. *Soc. Sci. Med.* 20:833–40.

Temoshok, L., R.J. DiClemente, D.M. Sweet, M.S. Blois, and R.W. Sagebiel (1984). Factors related to patient delay in seeking medical attention for cutaneous malignant melanoma. *Cancer* 54:3048–53.

# 20

## Malignant Bone Tumors

Eric Heiligenstein and Jimmie C. Holland

Bone tumors represent fewer than 1% of all malignant lesions and approximately 5% of tumors in children and adolescents (Schweisguth, 1982). The age of presentation is most frequently in the second decade of life, with discovery of the tumor resulting from pain, swelling, and rarely, spontaneous fracture. The primary tumors found are osteosarcoma and Ewing's sarcoma. Other less common types are fibrosarcomas, chondrosarcomas, and reticulum cell sarcomas. This chapter reviews the two most common types, osteosarcoma and Ewing's sarcoma, outlining the key facts about incidence, treatment, and the psychiatric considerations and management.

## OSTEOSARCOMA

Osteosarcoma is the most common type of bone tumor with a peak incidence from 10 to 25 years (Goorin et al., 1985). The sites are usually the femur, tibia, and humerus. Metastases are found in 23% of patients at the time of diagnosis; 85% of these are in the lungs. The prognostic considerations are extent of disease at diagnosis, histological type, age of the patient, site of the primary tumor, duration of symptoms, and serum level of the alkaline phosphatase (Rosen et al., 1979). Treatment consists of ablative surgery or limb salvage, with a combination of neoadjuvant (preoperative) and adjuvant (postoperative) chemotherapy, or surgery and adjuvant chemotherapy (Rosen, et al., 1976). The drugs commonly used are high-dose methotrexate, vincristine, doxorubicin, cyclophosphamide, cisplatin, bleomycin, and dactinomycin. The prognosis has dramatically improved in recent years; 2-year survival for localized tumors is 40–90%, while 2-year survival for metastatic disease is 30–60% (Goorin et al., 1985).

## EWING'S SARCOMA

Ewing's sarcoma is a rare bone tumor that occurs most often in the second decade of life (Schweisguth, 1982). The most common sites are the pelvis, femur, humerus, and ribs. Approximately 80% of those with apparent localized disease have occult metastases at the time of diagnosis. Prognostic considerations are location of the primary tumor and the extent of disease at diagnosis (Gehan et al., 1981). Treatment of Ewing's sarcoma has involved multidrug chemotherapy and radiation therapy. The role of surgery is limited to the initial biopsy of the tumor site and rarely is used for ablative treatment. Investigational drugs are frequently used, but standard agents include vincristine, doxorubicin, cyclophosphamide, and dactinomycin. Radiation therapy consists of doses of 400–6000 rad to the tumor site with reduced doses to the whole bone. Prognosis for localized disease is better than 50% for 5-year survival; for metastatic disease it is 20–50% for 5-year survival (Rosen et al., 1981).

## PSYCHIATRIC CONSIDERATIONS

The age of presentation of osteosarcoma and Ewing's sarcoma necessitates an awareness of adolescent development. The healthy adolescent faces developmental tasks that conflict directly with the demands of chronic illness (Hamburg and Wortman, 1985; Zeltzer, 1980). The emergence of adult cognitive abilities allows the adolescent to deal with the realities of cancer and also with the abstract uncertainty of survival. Age-appropriate concerns with pubertal body changes, peer relations, and social conformity are exacerbated by the diagnosis of cancer. During a period characterized by urges toward independence, cancer can lead to exaggerated wishes for dependence and nurturance or lead to denial, hyperindependence, acting out, and noncompliant behavior.

Issues of control are an expected part of adolescence, and the regressive pull of chronic illness intensifies this phenomenon. Specific symptoms or treatment can become a focal point expressed as "they can't force me, it's my body." The resultant oppositional stances noted both at home and in the hospital need to be understood in the context of normal adolescent strivings.

The diagnosis of a malignant bone tumor is associated with a period of mourning. Adolescents feel that they will miss being able to enjoy their best years as a result of cancer and its impending treatment. This is often expressed as "my life is at a pause and I'm missing out." Adolescents commonly deal with grief through withdrawal from their peer groups, feeling they "are not like everyone else." The attempt to minimize conflicts experienced in the area of self-image and peer acceptance unfortunately heightens concerns with independence and identity formation. Adaptive coping can be facilitated through a series of interventions involving the cancer treatment team (Nir, 1981). This can include preoperative preparation by the surgeon, psychosocial assessment of the adolescent and his or her family, development of comprehensive rehabilitation, and support groups. If maladaptive coping styles become apparent following diagnosis, short-term focused psychotherapy can be essential.

Cancer patients are at a high risk for organic mental disorders, particularly delirium (Silberfarb, 1983). Recognition is of great importance, as delirium is underdiagnosed in adolescents and in mild forms can be misinterpreted as behavior problems. Multidrug chemotherapy, fever, infection, malnutrition, and drug-induced metabolic or hematological disorders are all potential causes. Outcome generally depends on etiology, and recovery can be slow and variable in some instances.

Surgical treatment for bone tumors can involve amputation or limb-salvage procedures; each presents unique psychological issues. Amputation has been the foundation of treatment for osteosarcoma for many years. Psychological recovery from an amputation entails grieving similar to that experienced with traumatic loss of a body part or loss of a loved one. Preoperative psychological preparation by the treatment team should cover the extent of surgery, expected functional outcome, and rehabilitation available. This can facilitate anticipation of the loss, reduce the fears, and assist the adolescent in adjusting to the realities of treatment. Postoperative distress is greater when limb salvage had been anticipated but the decision to amputate is made during surgery.

Adolescents display resentment at the enforced dependency resulting from amputation, mourning the activities that are lost more than the limb itself. One commented that "not only don't I have hair but I have to learn to walk again." Amputation is a blow to developing sexual identity. The adolescents' developing body image is a reflection of the impression they make on others and how they appear to themselves. Not "being the perfect girl" anymore or fears of impaired masculinity can be expressed. Group support from other amputees and peer acceptance can assist the adolescent in regaining confidence that he or she can be a sexually attractive adult.

Phantom-limb phenomenon is extremely common following amputation (Lundberg and Guggenheim, 1986). It is an almost indefinable sensation of the presence of the amputated part and is usually not unpleasant. Patients may have phantom sensations continuously, intermittently, or not at all. An increase in awareness or intensity of the phantom phenomenon may occur during periods of stress. Psychological and physiological etiologies have been proposed. Psychological formulations attribute the sensations to the patient's enduring concept of a total body image. Physiological theories focus on overstimulation in the cortical area of the amputated limb. Most symptoms disappear in a proximal-to-distal sequence over a period of weeks. Long-term problems are rare.

Phantom pain is true pain experienced by a small percentage of amputees. Pain is usually due to peripheral nerve damage or excessive cortical stimulation of nerves in the stumps. Psychogenic origins need to be considered when a structural etiology cannot be found or rehabilitative treatment is not effective.

Long-term adjustment to amputation is related to an individual's background, interests, personality style, coping mechanisms, and support system (Boyle et al., 1982). Improvement in surgical techniques, prosthetic devices, and rehabilitation have enhanced quality of life. Most adolescents and young adults acknowledge problems around mobility but consider themselves independent. Long-term adaptation to school, employment, marriage, and family life appear to be successful in the majority of patients. Psychiatric morbidity is not increased by amputation, as specific psychopathological disorders occur at rates similar to those in the general population (Weddington et al., 1985). The problems, when they occur, are more subtle and are similar to those seen in other cancer survivors (see Chapter 7).

Limb salvage is a recent development in the initial treatment of osteosarcoma. It is an alternative surgical procedure that involves total ablation of the bone and adjacent tumor followed by replacement with an implant. This maintains a normal appearance and potential for growth in the affected limb. Local recurrence of tumor and survival appear to be similar to amputation (Malawer et al., 1982). Maximal functional results are achieved at about 1 year following surgery and maintained when comprehensive rehabilitation and reconstructive surgery is possible.

Limb salvage is a more complex operative procedure than amputation, and complications can impair good results. Infection can lead to additional surgery with possible removal of the implant and subsequent amputation. Rehabilitation can be impaired by loosening of the implant, fractures, or nonunion at the graft site. Emotional adjustment can be difficult because of the prolonged hospital course and variable outcome (Kagan, 1976).

In spite of these difficulties, limb salvage is being more frequently chosen at some centers in the belief that avoidance of loss of a body part improves psychological adaptation. It is controversial, however, whether outcome is ultimately better. A comparison of limb salvage and limb amputation patients found no significant differences in quality-of-life measures 1–3 years after surgery (Sugarbaker et al., 1982). Other research has found no difference between limb salvage and limb amputee patients in physical and psychological adjustment (Weddington et al., 1985). Further work needs to be performed before surgical decisions can be based solely on perceived quality-of-life differences.

Treatment-related issues can contribute to a wide range of psychological problems in adolescents. The consequences of scarification, alopecia, nausea and vomiting, and Broviac catheter placement are reviewed elsewhere.

Pain with cancer is a major concern. In addition to physician issues regarding pain assessment, adolescents can distort their degree of discomfort. Minimization of new bone pain often represents denial of metastatic disease. Inaccuracies in reporting pain can represent a developmental issue. The adolescent's sense of competence and ability to care for himself or herself is threatened with disclosure of uncontrolled pain. The decision to request treatment can be irrationally avoided in some instances. Patients with untreated or poorly controlled pain frequently have symptoms of depression, hopelessness, and helplessness (Kroetsch and Shamoian, 1983). The management of pain and the associated psychiatric morbidity is covered in Chapter 32.

Noncompliance is a considerable problem during adolescence and can be a vehicle for maladaptive coping. Research has demonstrated that up to 59% of adolescents do not comply with some aspect of their cancer treatment (Smith et al., 1979). This can in-

volve adjunctive medications, completion of protocol lengths, length of hospitalization, and unilateral decisions to stop treatment. Management should include listening and observing for these behaviors, with concerns presented to the adolescent in a nonjudgmental manner. Providing the adolescent a degree of control through collaborative decision making balanced with empathic limit setting can strengthen the therapeutic alliance.

Discontinuing treatment can be an appropriate and mutually reached decision in the management of cancer in some adolescents. In others, it can be a specific and self-destructive form of acting out resulting from a range of issues that must be explored. Psychiatric consultation may be requested to evaluate the behavior and recommend managements. It is essential to work with the adolescent, family, and staff, because each may have different expectations of the consultant. It is necessary to clarify the adolescent's issues and the family alignments, and to be aware of their interactions to intervene effectively.

## SUMMARY

The management of adolescents with bone tumors presents difficult issues for the staff, who must deal with normal adolescent behavior that is inconsistent and unpredictable. The presence of serious illness, treatment requiring a strong commitment, and altered appearance cause even more emotional turbulence. Knowing both the developmental issues for this age group and the common responses to diagnosis, chemotherapy, and surgery is essential for effective management.

## REFERENCES

Boyle, M., C.K. Tebbi, E.R. Mindell, and L.J. Mettlin (1982). Adolescent adjustment to amputation. *Med. Pediatr. Oncol.* 10:301–12.

Gehan, E.A., M.E. Nesbit, E.O. Burgert, T.J. Vietti, M. Tefft, C.A. Perez, J. Kissane, and C. Herpel (1981). Prognostic factors in children with Ewing's sarcoma. *Natl. Cancer Inst. Monogr.* 56:273–78.

Goorin, A.M., H.T. Abelson, and E. Frei (1985). Osteosarcoma: fifteen years later. *N. Engl. J. Med.* 313:1637–43.

Hamburg, B.A. and R.N. Wortman (1985). Adolescent development and psychopathology. In R. Michaels and J.O. Cavenar (eds.), *Psychiatry*, Vol. 2. New York: Basic Books, pp. 1–13.

Kagan, L.B. (1976). Use of denial in adolescents with bone cancer. *Health Soc. Work* 1:71–87.

Kroetsch, P. and C.A. Shamoian (1983). Pain and depression. *J. Psychiatr. Treat. Eval.* 5:417–20.

Lundberg, S.G. and F.G. Guggenheim (1986). Sequelae of limb amputation. *Adv. Psychosom. Med.* 15:199–210.

Malawer, M.M., H.T. Abelson, and H.D. Suit (1982). Sarcomas of bone. In V.T. DeVita, S. Hellman, and S.A. Rosenberg (eds.), *Cancer*. Philadelphia: Lippincott, pp. 1293–1342.

Nir, Y. (1981). Psychological support for children with soft tissue and bone sarcomas. *Natl. Cancer Inst. Monogr.* 56:145–48.

Rosen, G., A.G. Murphy, M. Gutierrez and R.C. Marcove (1976). Chemotherapy, en bloc resection and prosthetic bone replacement in the treatment of osteogenic sarcoma. *Cancer* 37:1–11.

Rosen, G., R.C. Marcove, B. Caparros, A. Niremberg, C. Kosloff, and A.G. Huvos (1979). Primary osteogenic sarcoma: The rationale for preoperative chemotherapy and delayed surgery. *Cancer* 43:2163–77.

Rosen, G., B.I. Caparros, A. Nirenberg, R.C. Marcive, A.G. Huvos, C. Kosloff, J. Lane, and M.L. Murphy (1981). Ewing's sarcoma: Ten year experience with adjuvant chemotherapy. *Cancer* 47:2204–13.

Schweisguth, O. (1982). *Solid Tumors in Children*. New York: Wiley.

Silberfarb, P.M. (1983). Chemotherapy and cognitive defects in cancer patients. *Annu. Rev. Med.* 34:35–46.

Smith, S.D., D. Rosen, R.C. Trueworthy, and J.T. Lowman (1979). A reliable method for evaluating drug compliance in children with cancer. *Cancer* 43:169–73.

Sugarbaker, P.H., I. Barofsky, S.A. Rosenberg, and F.J. Gianola (1982). Quality of life assessment of patients in extremity sarcoma trials. *Surgery* 91:17–23.

Weddington, W.W., K.B. Seagraves, and M.A. Simon (1985). Psychological outcome of extremity sarcoma survivors undergoing amputation or limb salvage. *J. Clin. Oncol.* 3:1393–99.

Zeltzer, L.K. (1980). The adolescent with cancer in J. Kellerman (ed.), *Psychological Aspects of Childhood Cancer*. Springfield, Ill.: Charles C Thomas, pp. 70–99.

# 21

## Acquired Immunodeficiency Syndrome (AIDS)

Susan Tross

The harsh medical idiosyncrasies of the acquired immunodeficiency syndrome (AIDS) have made it the primary American public health problem of the 1980s. These idiosyncrasies include its nearly uniform fatality, its rapid spread, its debilitating and dementing course, and the lack of vaccine, cure, or definitive treatment for it. Its epidemiological association with homosexual men and intravenous (iv) drug users has given rise to new discrimination toward groups who have been traditionally ostracized by society. Its association with the causal retrovirus HIV, or human immunodeficiency virus, has raised widespread fear of contagion, while presenting the American public with a mandate for radical change in sexual behavior and recreational drug use.

In this chapter, the basic medical and epidemiological features of AIDS and other HIV disease will be briefly reviewed. These features include the clinical definition and manifestations, relationship between infection and disease, incidence, mortality, modes of transmission, and treatment. The primary psychological problems posed by AIDS and other HIV disease will be outlined. These problems consist chiefly of reactive psychiatric symptoms, adjustment reactions to major social stressors, and/or bereavement reactions. The neuropsychological complications of the AIDS dementia complex (ADC), which may result from direct HIV brain infection, will be considered. The hypochondriacal and/or phobic symptoms that are signs of excessive fear of AIDS in the "worried well" who do not have AIDS will be described. Finally, major therapeutic interventions for these problems will be outlined. These interventions include psychotherapy, psychotropic medication, behavioral interventions, social services, and self-help interventions. Current recommendations for AIDS risk prevention in the forms of safer sexual practices and needle use precautions will be described.

## MEDICAL AND EPIDEMIOLOGICAL FEATURES OF AIDS AND HIV DISEASE

AIDS is a disease of the immune system that weakens the body's capacity to fight infection. According to the Centers for Disease Control (CDC, 1985), the diagnosis of AIDS can be made in the presence of certain rare opportunistic infections or cancers (indicative of an at least moderate defect in cell-mediated immunity), and laboratory evidence of HIV infection (on serum antibody testing or viral culture). The presence of any other preexisting cause for immunodeficiency must be ruled out. The cell-mediated immune defect is demonstrated by a reduced number of CD4 T ("helper") lymphocytes, or a low ratio of CD4 T to CD8 T ("suppressor") lymphocytes. AIDS is clinically characterized by a range of severe symptoms that may progress rapidly to more generalized debilitation. These symptoms include night sweats, diarrhea, fatigue, weight loss, fever, hacking cough, generalized ache and pain, and enlarged lymph nodes in the neck, axillary, or inguinal areas. Neurological complications—beginning with mental and/or motor slowing, forgetfulness and loss of concentration, and culminating in the ADC (Navia et al., 1986)—may also result from direct HIV brain infection.

There are two major types of presenting diseases of AIDS. The most common are the opportunistic infections (OI) that cause disease only in immunodeficient individuals. The four main types of OI are protozoal and helminthic infections (especially *Pneumocystis carinii* pneumonia or PCP, cryptosporidiosis, toxoplasmosis, and strongyloidosis), fungal infections (especially candidiasis, either *Candida* esophagitis or oral candidiasis or thrush), bacterial infections (especially *Mycobacterium tuberculosis, Mycobacterium avium* or *intracellulare, Mycobacterium kansasii* or salmonella), and viral infections (especially cyto-

megalovirus, herpes simplex, herpes zoster, or pa-
povavirus-related progressive multifocal leukoencephalopathy). The second major type of presenting
disease is cancer. The most common form is Kaposi's
sarcoma (KS), a cancer of the blood and/or lymphatic
vessels that is often distinguished by purplish skin lesions. AIDS–KS is similar to the aggressive form,
previously seen in African chidren, rather than the
classical form seen in middle-aged men of Jewish or
Mediterranean descent (Safai and Good, 1981). For as
yet undetermined reasons, the incidence of AIDS–KS
is declining; it has always been chiefly confined to
homosexual men (i.e., 95% of all cases). AIDS also is
associated with lymphoma.

However, frank AIDS and the associated infections
and neoplasms represent only the most advanced stage
of the spectrum of HIV infection, which begins with an
asymptomatic phase of variable length. A nomenclature for the classification of disorders has recently
been developed by the CDC (1986a) (Table 21-1).

A transient "mononucleosis-type" flu, consisting
of fever, rash, and fatigue, with or without aseptic
meningitis, may occur right around the time of acute
HIV infection (i.e., within a couple of weeks to a few
months) (group I) (Cooper et al., 1985). The number
of individuals with asymptomatic HIV infection
(group II) is suspected to be far greater than the number
of AIDS cases. However, the former can only be
roughly estimated. The number of individuals infected
with HIV has been estimated to be between 1 and 1.5
million [Public Health Service Plan for the Prevention
and Control of AIDS (PHS Plan), 1986]. The percentage of HIV-infected individuals who may be expected
to progress to frank AIDS during the 5-year period
between June 1986 and December 1991 has been estimated to be between 20 and 30% (PHS Plan, 1986).
However, this percentage is certain to increase with
longer periods of observation. The usual incubation
period between infection and onset of symptoms is
some time within 5 years, but it has been observed to
be longer. Persistent generalized lymphadenopathy
syndrome (group III) is the technical classification for
the condition more widely described as AIDS-related
complex (ARC). It consists of swollen lymph nodes
(lymphadenopathy), fever, night sweats, fatigue, diarrhea, and weight loss that persist for at least 3 months
(Metroka et al., 1983; Gold et al., 1984). The percentage of individuals with ARC who may be expected to
develop frank AIDS is not yet known. It has been
estimated at about 25–30% within 30 months of onset;
however, it is certain to increase with longer periods of
observation (Abrams et al., 1985). The broad range of
clinical disease that may be associated with HIV infection is classified under group IV. This may include
constitutional, neurological, neoplastic, or other dis-

**Table 21-1**  Summary of classification system for human
T-lymphotropic virus type III–lymphadenopathy-associated
virus

| Classification | Description |
|---|---|
| Group I | Acute infection |
| Group II | Asymptomatic infection* |
| Group III | Persistent generalized lymphadenopathy* |
| Group IV | Other disease |
| Subgroup A | Constitutional disease |
| Subgroup B | Neurological disease |
| Subgroup C | Secondary infectious diseases |
| Category C-1 | Specified secondary infectious diseases listed in the CDC surveillance definition for AIDS† |
| Category C-2 | Other specified secondary infectious diseases |
| Subgroup D | Secondary cancers† |
| Subgroup E | Other conditions |

*Patients in groups II and III may be subclassified on the basis of a labora-
tory evaluation.
†Includes those patiens whose clinical presentation fulfills the definition of
AIDS used by CDC for national reporting.
*Source*: CDC (1986). Classification system for HIV infections. *Morbid.
Mortal. Weekly Rep.* 35:334–39.

eases that may (i.e., subcategories C-1 and/or D) or
may not fit the CDC surveillance definition of AIDS.

Since the discovery of five AIDS cases in 1981
(CDC, 1981), its incidence has grown steadily and
rapidly. By the end of 1986, there were 35,000 AIDS
cases cumulatively diagnosed in the United States,
among whom 16,000 were diagnosed that year. For the
next 5-year period, ending in December 1991, the projected number of cumulative cases is 270,000; 74,000
of these were diagnosed during that year alone (PHS
Plan, 1986). AIDS has been diagnosed in all states of
the United States, and in 100 countries, especially in
central Africa, Haiti, and western Europe. AIDS has
remained a nearly uniformly fatal disease with a 75%
mortality rate at 2 years after the diagnosis. Prognosis
is the best for individuals with AIDS–KS only; there
are at least 100 survivors of several years in United
States. Prognosis is poorer for pediatric AIDS than for
adult AIDS (general mortality rates of 69% and 55%,
respectively: CDC, 1986b).

While the incidence of AIDS in the United States
has rapidly escalated since 1981, it has remained
largely confined to a few high-risk groups and the
people immediately linked to them through the known
modes of transmission. These modes include the exchange of semen and/or blood during sexual (especially anal or vaginal) intercourse, blood during
shared use of contaminated needles or "works" during iv drug use, blood during medical transfusions, and
blood products during coagulation treatment with Fac-

tor VIII concentrate. The majority of cases (66%) have occurred among gay or bisexual men. This risk group was originally thought to be restricted to a highly sexually active subgroup (Jaffe et al., 1983; Marmor et al., 1984). As etiological knowledge has increased, it has become apparent that a single viral exposure may be sufficient to produce HIV infection. The second largest risk group is iv drug users (17%); an additional 8% of AIDS cases are iv drug users who have also had gay male sexual experiences. Initially, recent Haitian immigrants were thought to be another distinct AIDS risk group. As a result of more explicit reporting, it is now known that they may be subsumed chiefly under the gay–bisexual or heterosexual contact risk groups (Pape et al., 1986). In 1985, 2% of AIDS cases received blood transfusions prior to the initiation of screening of the blood supply for HIV (Schorr et al., 1985). Another 1% of AIDS cases were treated for hemophilia A with Factor VIII concentrate, prior to the initiation of anti-HIV heat preparation. For another 3% of the cases, risk has been designated as "undetermined," either because there is insufficient documentation or because the sole "risk factor" is heterosexual contact with a female prostitute. An additional 471 children (i.e., 13 years old or younger) have acquired AIDS, primarily through in utero or perinatal transmission from an infected parent (80%) (Oleske et al., 1983; Rubinstein et al., 1983). Because first-generation heterosexual transmission between iv drug users or, less often, bisexual men and their heterosexual partners, represents the primary bridge to HIV infection in the general adult population, the small, but rapidly growing group of AIDS cases due to heterosexual contact (2%) is extremely important (Harris et al., 1983). Approximately 50% of these individuals have no known risk factor other than having emigrated from countries where heterosexual transmission is believed to be widespread. The other half are individuals who are the sexual partners of AIDS patients or risk group members; among them, the ratio of female to male cases is about 4 : 1.

There is no evidence that HIV can be spread through "casual contact," or touching, being near to, or sharing everyday objects with someone with AIDS or HIV infection. Studies of parents and siblings of children with AIDS have shown that even when they live in crowded and impoverished households with these children, they do not become infected with HIV (Friedland et al., 1986). A national study of health care personnel has shown that even accidental pricks with needles used with AIDS patients do not result in HIV infection. Among 100 health care workers, only two became infected with HIV, and infection by needle-prick could be proven for only one of these cases (McCray, 1986). However, a report in the *Mortality and Morbidity*

*Weekly Report* of the CDC presented presumptive evidence of HIV seroconversion in three health care workers following non-needle-prick exposures to the blood of HIV-positive patients (CDC, 1987). However, this is considered a highly improbable risk situation, if infection precaution guidelines are closely observed. Although HIV has been recovered from the saliva, sweat, and tears of people with HIV antibodies in their blood (Groopman et al., 1984), these fluids are not thought to be effective agents of transmission. New risk groups, resulting from these types of transmission, have failed to emerge in the 6 years since the discovery of AIDS. This is probably because entry into the bloodstream is critical for HIV infection.

At present, there is no vaccine, no cure, not even definitive treatment for AIDS. Although major vaccine research initiatives are currently in progress, serious biological and social obstacles make the development of a vaccine program within the next 5 years highly unlikely (Institute of Medicine, 1986). The following key biological issues remain unresolved (PHS Plan, 1986):

1. The relative utility of different forms of vaccine, including recombinant DNA-derived antigens, killed viruses, live recombinant or attenuated viruses, virus subunits, or synthetic peptides, must be determined.
2. A vaccine that will be broadly cross-reactive to the various strains of HIV must be developed.
3. In vitro and in vivo methods for assessing the immunogenicity, toxicity, and efficacy of the vaccine must be improved.

The following key social and practical issues also remain unresolved (Institute of Medicine, 1986):

1. An ethical plan for initiating vaccination incorporating conflicting needs for immediate protection of target populations, maintenance of participants' risk reduction behaviors, and controlled clinical trials, must be formulated.
2. A mechanism for providing government assistance to private industry to reduce the prohibitive costs of vaccine-related product liability should be planned.

Although there is no definitive treatment for AIDS, clinical benefits have been demonstrated for certain experimental antiviral agents. However, these agents tend to be expensive and difficult to obtain, and to cause serious side effects. At present, the most promising agent is AZT (azidothymidine), which appears to slow the rate at which HIV reproduces, to prolong the lives of AIDS patients, and to make them more comfortable (Mitsuya and Brader, 1986). During a 20-week placebo-controlled trial for patients with PCP, only 1 patient in the AZT arm died, while 16 patients died in the placebo arm (Institute of Medicine, 1986). Ribavirin has been shown to deter viral replication and to improve immunocompetence (Roberts et al., 1986). Current treatment strategies are chiefly aimed at managing the symptoms of the cancers and/or infections of AIDS. KS can be controlled with certain anticancer therapies, especially α-interferon (Krown et al., 1983). At higher doses, "flulike" side effects of lethargy, fever, and depression (Blalock and Smith, 1981) may be easily mistaken for a depression with vegetative signs. PCP can be treated with Bactrim (trimethoprim–sulfamethoxazole) or pentamidine isothiocyanate, but relapses may occur after treatment.

## PSYCHOLOGICAL RESPONSE TO AIDS

The potential for psychological distress in AIDS is enormous. Thorough and provocative discussion of this potential is still provided by early monographs of the American Psychological Association (Batchelor et al., 1984) and the American Psychiatric Association (Nichols and Ostrow, 1984), as well as more recent reviews (Bridge, Mirsky and Goodwin, 1988; Kaplan et al., 1987). The diagnosis of AIDS carries with it the combined psychological liabilities that belong to life-threatening illness, on the one hand, and to minority group discrimination on the other.

The traumatic impact of any life-threatening illness, or the "existential plight" of the first 100 days of diagnosis, is well established in the cancer psychiatry literature (Weisman and Worden, 1976–1977; see also Chapter). It is characterized by preoccupation with mortality, sense of personal vulnerability, and heightened emotional distress.

AIDS frequently forces catastrophic social change on its patients. Pervasive discrimination against AIDS patients has arisen out of long-standing societal homophobia (Altman, 1986) and prejudice against iv drug users, as well as acute fears of AIDS contagion. It is common for AIDS patients to have experienced prior and concurrent death of friends with AIDS, while confronting the prospect of their own death. Increased dependency imposed by the role of illness requires adaptation. Disability and prohibitive medical expenses often require early application for Medicaid and public assistance.

Apart from AIDS-specific hardship, the gay man with AIDS faces the concurrent social stress of maintaining a gay life-style in a not infrequently hostile heterosexual environment. The redefinition of homosexuality as an adult preference, not a psychiatric disorder, occurred in 1973, and in 1980 this appeared in the third edition of the *Diagnostic and Statistical Manual,* (DSM-III), the official U.S. psychiatric nomenclature (American Psychiatric Association, 1980). The

diagnosis of AIDS may force the gay man to precipitous confrontation with gay-related issues on which he may not otherwise have been psychologically prepared to act. These especially include pressure for complete personal resolution and for premature disclosure to others. Receiving a diagnosis of AIDS may be experienced as a "second coming out," thus reviving residual emotions associated with initial coming out (Nichols, 1985).

Facing comparable social ostracism in American society is the iv drug user. At the same time, the diagnosis of AIDS also forces them to confront the difficult process of detoxification, which may include physiological withdrawal, residential treatment, and abrupt disruption of drug-related friendships (Des Jarlais et al., 1985). Furthermore, the majority (i.e. 80%) of i.v. drug users with AIDS are inner city people of color–with multiple preexisting practical stressors, like poverty and unemployment (Mays and Cochran, 1987; Galea, Lewis and Baker, 1988).

As a result of these converging problems, the AIDS patient is vulnerable to reactive psychiatric symptoms, consisting of the triad of depression, anxiety, and preoccupation with illness. Diagnosis of progression of AIDS elicits a full range of existential depressive symptoms, which include dysphoric mood, hopelessness and helplessness, anhedonia, and abandonment or rejection sensitivity (see also Chapters 22–28). Passive suicidal ideation is common; suicidal plans or attempts are rare. Many patients have watched close friends die of AIDS. They often harbor thoughts of suicide or refusal of treatment or heroic measures as alternatives to a slow, deteriorating course, should it occur in the future. It is common for patients to experience regret, but it is usually over a future lost, rather than past deeds committed. General self-esteem may be lowered by the patient's experience of declining physical function, altered appearance, and/or thwarted personal goals. Anxiety may be manifested by tension, inability to sleep, agitation, lapses in concentration and attention, and persistent fears about the course of disease. Like other patients with grave illness, heightened sensitivity to physical symptoms is characteristic of AIDS patients. It is typical for the patient to live in a constant state of vigil for signs of disease progression. Most patients tend to increase their participation in health care, to contact physicians rapidly about physical complaints, and to seek information about medication and specialty referral. It is almost universal for patients to scrutinize their past sexual practices, drug use, and general recreational life-style, and to place spontaneous restraints on their present behavior. Often, vigorous mental effort is required to keep health concerns in perspective.

These symptoms generally take the form of adjustment disorders with depressed and/or anxious features. They are transient and situational with acute peaks of distress around significant medical events (Christ and Wiener, 1985). In particular, diagnosis evokes an acute stress response, which may continue for the next 4–6 weeks while the patient regroups his personal values and goals, and adapts his routine of daily activities to the illness. Like other patients with grave illnesses, the AIDS patient faces the central psychological tasks of coping with illness and anticipatory bereavement. This patient must come to terms with fear of an imminent death, closure on future goals and plans, and the challenge to maintain hope and purpose in his or her current life. Thereafter, the patient may sustain a residual form of this stress response, which results in fleeting distress, while permitting normal functioning. New physical symptoms, recurrent infection, or the discovery of treatment failure may throw the patient into a more serious depressive response in which suicidal features are more common. At this point more than ever before, the patient is confronted with the potential fatality of the disease.

Table 21-2 summarizes the published findings of psychiatric disorders in AIDS. This literature is chiefly restricted to case studies, clinical description, or psychiatric consultation data. The only two studies of rates of disorder found adjustment disorders to be quite common. Our own research on the psychological impact of AIDS in gay men, under the auspices of the National Institute of Mental Health, has detected DSM-III psychiatric disorders in approximately 50% of the 89 AIDS patients consecutively recruited from the Infectious Disease, Dermatology and Immunology Services of the Memorial Sloan-Kettering Cancer Center (Tross et al., 1986). Adjustment disorders with mixed emotional features accounted for approximately 75% of these diagnoses. These results are consistent with those of Dilley and his colleagues (1985) at the San Francisco General Hospital. The focus of most of this literature is the clinical presentation of neurological complications of AIDS as psychiatric symptoms. The problem of this differential diagnosis will be discussed in the section on the AIDS dementia complex. Without an empirical trial of antidepressant medication, differential diagnosis of major depression is difficult to make, because vegetative signs may be masked by AIDS symptoms.

## NEUROPSYCHOLOGICAL COMPLICATIONS IN AIDS

### AIDS Dementia Complex (ADC)

Neuropsychological complications are likely to be a common feature of AIDS. Early clinical studies, based on neurological examination, estimated that approx-

**Table 21-2** Psychiatric symptoms in AIDS patients

| References | Results |
|---|---|
| Tross et al. (1986) | 41% Have adjustment disorders; 13% depressive disorders |
| Dilley et al. (1985) | 38% Require psychiatric consultation |
| Donlou et al. (1985) | Decreased self-esteem, work and social impairment ($n = 17$) |
| Hoffman (1984) | Organic withdrawal ($n = 1$) and psychosis ($n = 1$) |
| Nurnberg et al. (1984) | Organic depression, delusions and command suicidal auditory hallucinations ($n = 1$) |
| Loewenstein and Sharfstein (1983–1984) | Organic depression and bizarreness ($n = 2$) |

imately 30% of the total AIDS population had CNS complications of their disease (Bredesen and Messing, 1983; Snider et al., 1983). However, when neuropathological methods were introduced into these studies, estimates of the scope of the problem increased. There is now compelling neuropathological evidence to support the contention that this rate is an *underestimate* of the true incidence of these complications. At autopsy, 78% of the patients studied showed evidence of CNS disease (Nielsen et al., 1984). Furthermore, approximately 40% of AIDS patients with dementia manifest cognitive impairment before or at the time of diagnosis of frank AIDS. In 10% of these patients, cognitive symptoms are the *sole* presenting AIDS-related complaint (Navia et al., 1986). Thus, the incidence of neurological complications in AIDS and other HIV disease is even higher than has been computed for cases meeting CDC surveillance criteria for AIDS proper.

Early clinical reports described the presence of diffuse organic brain syndromes (Horowitz et al., 1982; Britten et al., 1982; Herman, 1983) that were marked by highly variable intellectual, motor, and behavioral symptoms. Snider and colleagues (1983) identified ''subacute encephalitis (SE)'' in 18 of a series of 50 neurologically impaired patients as the most frequent neurological complications of AIDS. Nielsen and coworkers (1984) characterized SE as a progressive, deteriorating condition, leading form lethargy, social withdrawal, and decreased libido to psychomotor retardation and, finally, severe dementia. Because postmortem evidence of systemic cytomegalovirus (CMV) (Snider et al., 1983) or CMV-type inclusions (Nielsen et al., 1984) was detected in nearly 50% of both series of SE patients, it was initially thought to be the cause of SE.

However, a critical leap in our understanding of these complications has been provided by the detection of HIV, the etiological agent of AIDS, in the brain and/or cerebrospinal fluid of AIDS patients with neurological deficits (Shaw et al., 1985; Levy et al., 1985; Ho et al., 1985). Shaw and colleagues (1985) have cited two retrovirus models for the action of HIV in the brain. First, they likened HIV brain effects to those of visna virus, a lentivirus that causes a degenerative white-matter neurological disease in sheep. Second, they likened HIV-related dementia to the CNS lesions associated with simian T-cell virus III (STLV-III) inoculation in macaques. STLV-III is a simian retrovirus that is "antigenically, biologically, and neuropathologically" similar to HIV (Daniel, 1985; Kanki et al., 1985; Letvin et al., 1985).

ADC is now recognized as the most common neurological complication of AIDS (Navia et al., 1986; Rosenblum, Levy and Bredesen, 1988). It is characterized by general cognitive deterioration in the absence of impaired consciousness, caused by direct HIV brain infection (Shaw et al., 1985; Levy et al., 1985; Ho et al., 1985). Its clinical and neuropathological features have been well described by Dr. Richard Price and his colleagues (Navia et al., 1986; Tross et al., 1988) as part of a multidisciplinary research program in the neurological complications of AIDS at Memorial Sloan-Kettering Cancer Center. ADC was documented in the clinical histories of two-thirds of a series of 70 autopsied AIDS patients. In the majority of patients, the progression to general impairment was rapid, occurring with 2 months of the onset of any cognitive symptoms. In its early course, ADC is especially marked by cognitive symptoms, particularly mental slowing and deficits in recent memory and attention, which are manifested by the majority of patients. At the same time, approximately 33% complain of behavioral symptoms in the form of increased apathy and withdrawal. Neurological signs (detected by examination) are relatively limited to slowing and blunted affect (50%), gait problems and ataxia (50%), and hyperreflexia, especially in the lower extremities (33%). In its later course, ADC may resemble a full-blown, incapacitating geriatriclike dementia. General cognitive impairment was identified in 45 of 46 patients. Slowing, in both the verbal and motor modes, was detected in 38 patients. At this stage, motor symptoms were common, including ataxia ($n = 32$), hypertonia ($n = 22$), incontinence ($n = 21$), tremor ($n = 20$), frontal release signs ($N = 17$), and weakness, especially of the lower extremities ($N = 15$).

The concept of ADC has been validated by correlations between clinical diagnosis and neuropathological findings (Navia et al., 1986). In a series of 70 brains of AIDS patients, only 5 were neuropathologically normal; none of these had a history of ADC. ADC cases could be differentiated from nondemented AIDS cases by both lower brain weight and greater extent of atro-

phy (Britton and Miller, 1984). While mild to moderate atrophy was evident in 28 of 37 ADC brains, it was evident in only 2 of 18 nondemented brains. In the total series, white- and subcortical gray-matter involvement were most frequently detected. White-matter pathology was characterized by diffuse pallor ($n = 64$), vacuolation ($n = 36$), and focal rarefaction ($n = 13$). Gray-matter pathological findings most frequently involved the basal ganglia and the thalamus.

Subcortical dementia may be a compelling explanatory paradigm for ADC. It was first invoked by Albert et al. (1974) to characterize cognitive impairment in progressive supranuclear palsy, and by McHugh and Folstein (1975) to characterize Huntington's disease dementia. It has been described by Cummings and Benson (1984) as a clinical syndrome marked by

forgetfulness, slowing of mental processes, . . . impaired ability to manipulate acquired knowledge, and personality and affective changes, including apathy and depression [in which] elementary linguistic, calculation, and learning processes are intact, but spontaneous use of stored information, ability to generate problem-solving strategies, and insight are impaired [and in which] pathologic changes involve primarily, but not necessarily exclusively, the deep gray-matter structures, including the thalamus, basal ganglia, and related brain-stem nuclei.

Clinically, the prospect of neurological complications demands regular monitoring by the clinician, as well as referral for neurological, neuropsychological, and psychiatric consultation, should they be detected. The patient's capacity for daily functioning may be enhanced by behavioral techniques and practical assistance, used with other patients with cognitive impairment. These include maintenance of daily appointment logs and chore lists, taping of simple instructions to important household objects, and arrangements for a family member, friend, or volunteer buddy to check in with the patient on a daily basis (by visit or phone).

Relatively little is known about any possible patterns of differential deterioration or intactness that might implicate specific microscopic brain structures or material. Intensive multidisciplinary research, combining performance, neurodiagnostic, and neuropathological parameters, is indicated to pursue possible correlations between brain and behavior. Although it is likely that neurological complications may be present along the continuum of HIV infection, this remains an open question in critical need of prospective research.

## Other Neurological Complications

In addition to ADC, other specific CNS disorders may create neurological problems in patients with AIDS or HIV disease. These include CNS infections, lymphoma, vacuolar myelopathy, and peripheral neuropathies (Snider et al., 1983). Due to their specificity, these disorders are easier to diagnose. Preexisting specific therapies are available for some of them. The principal one of these disorders is CNS toxoplasmosis, an infection that presents as headache, focal dysfunction (i.e., hemiparesis, aphasia, central visual field deficit, etc.), and general mental status change (e.g., lethargy, confusion, and disorientation). Infection can be detected by CT scan and blood serology. When treated early, most patients respond dramatically to treatment with pyrimethamine plus sulfadiazine or clindamycin. Other CNS infections include cryptococcal meningitis, progressive multifocal leukoencephalopathy associated with papovavirus infection, and herpesvirus infection (especially herpes simplex, varicella zoster, and CMV, which may cause retinopathy and blindness). The major form of CNS neoplasm is primary CNS lymphoma, for which radiotherapy or chemotherapy may be used. Vacuolar myelopathy, which may be manifested by progressive motor symptoms of spastic-ataxic paraparesis and, eventually, mutism, myoclonus, and incontinence, has been identified in 20 of 89 consecutive brain and spinal cord autopsy samples of AIDS patients (Petito et al., 1985). Peripheral neuropathies manifest as burning paresthesias and numbness.

## PSYCHOLOGICAL RESPONSE TO ARC

Vulnerability to AIDS-related distress is at least as serious and widespread among ARC patients as it is among AIDS patients. In our comparative study of gay men with AIDS ($n = 89$), ARC ($n = 39$), and no physical symptoms ($n = 149$), ARC patients scored at least as high, if not higher than, AIDS patients on multiple parameters of both general and AIDS-specific distress (Tross et al., 1986). These parameters included depression, anxiety, somatization, interpersonal sensitivity, hostility, mental avoidance, and intrusive preoccupation with the subject of AIDS. Approximately 75% of the ARC group developed adjustment disorders in response to the stressor of diagnosis, while 50% of the AIDS group did so. Similar results have been documented for a sample of gay men in San Francisco (Temoshok, 1986). These data pinpoint the ARC group as the population at greatest risk for emotional distress, probably because of their persistent uncertainty about developing AIDS. These are individuals for whom each minor symptom, which might have previously gone unnoticed, now raises latent doubts of an impending diagnosis of AIDS. They are individuals who on a daily basis add to their personal census of friends lost to AIDS. They are individuals who typically experience themselves as "walking time

bombs" existing "in limbo," who lack the psychological resolution that a confirmed diagnosis of AIDS may afford.

## PSYCHOLOGICAL RESPONSE TO HIV INFECTION

Screening for HIV infection has been proposed as a method of primary prevention, especially among high-risk populations. Prevention of sexually transmitted diseases (STD), such as gonorrhea and syphilis, through screening of contacts of index patients or of (high-risk) STD clinic patients provides a model for this plan (Potterat and King, 1981). A number of investigators have reported that, at least for seropositive subjects, HIV testing and feedback is a trigger for sexual risk reduction in gay men (Valdessari et al., 1986), in blood donors who did not admit risk group membership (O'Reilly et al., 1986), and in needle-use risk reduction in iv drug users in treatment (Cox et al., 1986; Casadonte et al., 1986). However, preliminary reports from the March 1987 consensus conference on HIV testing highlight the disturbing fact that seronegative individuals seem to maintain, or even increase, their level of AIDS risk behavior after notification (D.C. Des Jarlais, personal communication, 1987). Furthermore, although there may be improvements in risk reduction as a result of HIV testing in seropositive individuals, they may be at the cost of serious emotional fallout (Frigo et al., 1986; O'Reilly et al., 1986; Casadonte et al., 1986). This fallout becomes especially critical when the relationship between health fears and health behaviors is considered. Communications theory suggests that a moderate level of threat arousal, which is strong enough to be motivating but mild enough to be reasonably tolerated, is the optimal level of fear required to support preventive health behaviors (Janis and Feshbach, 1954). Frigo and colleagues (1986) reported "significant adverse reactions" in the form of depression, anxiety, and preoccupation with AIDS in 48% of their sample of seropositive individuals; "serious difficulty" was observed in 10% of them. O'Reilly and colleagues (1986) reported an increase in interpersonal conflict with sexual partners, to whom the index seropositives were extremely likely to tell the results. Although Casadonte and co-workers (1986) noted few psychiatric symptoms in seropositive iv drug users after notification, he reported that 80% of those who spontaneously initiated condom use in their sexual relations lost their partners because of their disclosure of seropositivity. Furthermore, new mandates from the federal government for compulsory notification may make adjustment to testing more problematic. Prior researchers have identified both concerns about confidentiality and feared loss of insurance (Morin et al., 1986), and anticipated emotional distress (Williams et al., 1986; Valdessari et al., 1986), as reasons for test refusal, even under conditions of optional feedback. Although the asymptomatic seropositive individual has the advantage of better current health and prognosis, his or her psychological situation may be similar to that of the person with ARC.

## PSYCHOLOGICAL RESPONSE IN AIDS RISK GROUP MEMBERS

Despite the absence of the grave diagnosis of AIDS, the same range of psychological responses may characterize distressed individuals without physical symptoms in the AIDS risk group populations, whether or not they have been tested for HIV infection. These are preoccupation with physical symptoms, anxiety, and depression. Generally, these symptoms reflect brief reactions to the precipitants of minor physical symptoms, news of illness or death from AIDS in personal acquaintances, or news of AIDS reported in the mass media. Disappearance of the symptom, passage of time, advice from a physician, or any other form of clarification or reassurance may often be sufficient to resolve the individual's distress. Thereafter, the individual may sustain ongoing subclinical symptoms, which only escalate in the presence of further precipitants.

## PSYCHOLOGICAL RESPONSE IN THE GENERAL POPULATION

Individuals in the general population who are vulnerable to AIDS-related distress fall into two broad categories. The first category is the "worried well," which consists of people who, by virtue of anecdotal or media information, become hypersensitive to the possibility of having or getting AIDS (Forstein, 1984). Because of the recent emphasis on heterosexual transmission, this category is rapidly swelling with sexually active young adults who are concerned about their past and/or present life-style. The second, and less common category consists of individuals who are chronically preoccupied with the possibility of being ill, often with the current major illnesses receiving media attention. These individuals often harbor convictions of having cancer (see Chapter 2). Both categories of individuals may seek HIV testing as a means of gaining reassurance about their health. As described later in this chapter, HIV testing should only be carried out after the individual has undergone psychological screening and preparation by counseling.

## PSYCHOLOGICAL RESPONSE IN HEALTH CARE PERSONNEL

Dealing with the combined issues of contagion, fatality, social "deviancy," and the presence of organic mental disorders also requires extraordinary effort on the part of health care personnel. At most, fear of contagion may cause frank neglect of basic patient needs. Rooms may not be cleaned, food trays may be left in hallways, and physicians, nurses, and technicians may refuse to draw blood or handle body fluids during procedures. Phobic overreaction, in the form of inappropriate use of infection precautions (i.e., mask, gown, and gloves) in excess of CDC guidelines is more common. The vague and generalized symptoms of AIDS make it an easy target for overidentification, hypochondriacal complaints, "medical student" syndrome, and frequent visits to the employee health service for examination of minor symptoms. That AIDS patients are young, and sometimes come from the same social background as the staff, also makes identification likely. Spikes and Holland (1975) have described the emotional stress placed on the primary care clinician by the dying patient, who challenges his or her self-image as one who cures disease; therefore, the physician may feel a sense of failure when a patient dies. The terminal phase may evoke intense frustration, anxiety, and/or depression in the clinician. These emotions may lead to maladaptive behavior, including avoidance or transfer on the one hand, or false reassurance or inappropriately aggressive treatment on the other. The clinician's anxiety is likely to be especially heightened by the question from the patient or family about the probability of death. At the very time when the need of the patient and/or family for communication may be the greatest, the clinician may find it most difficult to shift emphasis from the modus operandi of biological treatment to that of supportive care, with major focus on amelioration of pain, providing emotional support, clarification of misconceptions, and reassuring patient and/or family that they will not be abandoned. Staff adaptation may be compromised by social prejudice against gay men or iv drug users, which may take the form of fear, anger, or excessive pity. At the extreme, the clinician may have religious or cultural convictions that disease is a just punishment for "deviancy," about which he or she may simultaneously feel guilty. When the diagnosis of AIDS brings gay or iv drug use out into the open, the clinician may inherit the same emotional strain that the patient and family experience. The clinician may be reluctant to discuss fears of contagion and health precautions related to AIDS, that are the common, urgent concerns of family members. Lovers or spouses may want advice about safer ways of sharing physical affection and safer sexual practices. Family members may ask whether they can touch the patient and share household objects with him or her, or whether they ought to be tested for HIV infection.

Staff response to the ADC is often limited by gaps in training and education in neurology and psychiatry. They may be reluctant to subject the patient to a mental status examination they perceive as particularly demoralizing, because it is associated with intellectual impairment. The patient's loss of continence, and of motor and impulse control may create serious management problems, which easily provoke staff frustration or anger (Spikes and Holland, 1975). The patient may become disruptive, apathetic, forgetful, irrational, and unappreciative of the special care that staff are providing. Even the most dedicated clinician may be prone to resignation and withdrawal.

Two major types of intervention are useful in facilitating staff adaptation to the care of AIDS patients. The first is the formulation and dissemination of a clear institutional policy regarding professional responsibility and safety in the care of these patients. In order for it to be effective, there must be a vigorous commitment to such policy at the chief executive level. The administrative consequences of refusal of care, including accountability to supervisors, intensive supervision, work transfer, or firing, should be made public. Guidelines for infection precaution must be clearly explained to all staff. The CDC has developed guidelines for infection precaution, based on standard practices for other, more easily transmissible viruses, especially hepatitis B (CDC, 1982). These guidelines are presented in Table 21-3. The provision of definite guidelines, per se, may alleviate staff anxiety and alarm, arising from a sense of uncertainty about HIV infection. The second type of intervention is staff education. This can take the form of educational conferences managed by outside experts, in-service training sessions, multidisciplinary and specialty rounds, and staff support groups. Educational programs for health care personnel are often available through the education departments or speakers' bureaus of local AIDS self-help organizations. Under the auspices of the New York City Department of Mental Health, the Social Work Department of Memorial Sloan-Kettering Cancer Center, and the Gay Men's Health Crisis have developed a model training program for this purpose.

## THERAPEUTIC INTERVENTIONS

The converging emotional, social, and practical complications of AIDS and HIV disease require a flexible multidisciplinary approach to the patient. The range of interventions that are required include psychotherapy,

**Table 21-3**  Infection precautions for the care of AIDS and HIV disease patients

- Avoid accidental wounds from contaminated instruments.
- Avoid contact with patient secretions on open skin lesions.
- Wear gowns and gloves to handle blood, body fluid, excretions, and secretions.
- Wash hands often, removing gowns and gloves.
- Wash hands if contaminated with blood.
- Label blood samples with "blood precautions" label.
- Clean blood spills with bleach.
- Label articles soiled with blood for reprocessing and disposal.
- Use disposable needles, and place them in puncture-proof containers for disposal.
- Assign private rooms to patients to ill to use good hygiene.

*Source*: CDC (1982). AIDS: Precautions for clinical and laboratory staffs. *Morbid. Mortal. Weekly Rep.* 3:577–80.

psychotropic medication, education and instruction, social services, and self-help interventions.

## Psychotherapy

Coping with AIDS may be strengthened by a range of psychotherapeutic techniques used with seriously ill patients. The techniques include crisis intervention, and supportive, cognitive-behavioral, existential, and psychoanalytically oriented therapies. Given appropriate clinical training, these techniques may be carried out by a psychiatrist, psychologist, social worker, psychiatric nurse-clinician, pastoral counselor, or peer counselor.

Contact with the AIDS patient in crisis should be initiated immediately upon referral, especially if significant depression is present. Whenever possible, a person important to the patient should accompany the patient to the initial visit to obtain a complete history and to reinforce treatment recommendations. If psychiatric hospitalization is necessary, it is critical to have a preexisting working relationship with a psychiatric unit accustomed to infection precaution practices sometimes necessitated by AIDS. During the acute crisis period, it is advisable that the outpatient live with another person, particularly if there is suspicion of neurological complications. The description of a treatment plan itself may have a therapeutic effect on the patient, in as much as it is a statement of treatability. The therapy should focus on the patient's immediate problem, resources for dealing with it, and options for resolution. Intervention should consist of face-to-face interviews three to five times per week and telephone interviews at a mutually agreed upon time on intervening days for a 2- to 3-week period. Thereafter, the frequency of the therapy can usually be reduced to once or twice a week and the period of therapy extended for an additional 6–8 weeks.

Individual, couple, group, or family sessions may be used with the patient with AIDS or other HIV disease. Group therapy may counter the patient's sense of isolation and alienation. The group can function as a source of camaraderie and personal validation that uniquely arises from common experience. Patients also welcome the opportunity to assume the role of helper to fellow patients. However, at the same time, the patient runs the risk of repeated exposure to painful mourning experiences, when fellow patients become progressively ill. Couples therapy may be used to enhance the adjustment of a couple to the impact of AIDS or other HIV disease in one or both of its members. Each partner may need to be seen individually as well as together.

The question of time frame in psychotherapy with AIDS patients is an open one. There are complementary advantages associated with time-limited and open-ended psychotherapy. Time-limited psychotherapy affords the patient a greater opportunity for sense of closure and mastery over immediate psychological issues, while minimizing demands for therapeutic introspection or ongoing regular meetings. The illness may make it difficult to keep appointments. Telephone interviews are very useful. Ongoing psychotherapy affords the patient a greater sense of consistent support which may be useful for dealing with the evolving illness. It may also give the patient greater freedom to pursue spontaneously emerging psychological issues of broader personal developmental scope, which are not strictly part of the AIDS-related complaints.

Supportive therapy has the widest applicability to the AIDS patient. In the context of the tangible problems of disease and medical treatment, the understanding and appreciation of the realistic stresses that the patient faces is the foundation for any technique. It may counter the patient's sense of despair, loneliness, and alienation, while minimizing guilt over imposing an emotional burden that may constrain his or her relationship with others. Cognitive-behavioral therapy may be used to supply the patient with a repertory of methods for symptom control. These methods may include mental techniques, such as thought suspension, or reframing of exaggerated pessimistic thoughts in more realistic terms (Beck et al., 1979). They may also include physical techniques, such as progressive relaxation (Bernstein and Borkovec, 1973). Existential therapy may be used to focus on the tasks of retrospective life review, separation from loved ones, and recognition of mortality that the patient with serious illness faces (Butler, 1974). Psychodynamically oriented therapy may be used to help patients integrate

their current response to illness into their understanding of personal identity and their general lifelong patterns of coping (Viederman and Perry, 1980).

## Psychotropic Medication

Anxious and depressive symptoms in patients with AIDS or HIV disease may require management with psychotropic medication. In general, as with other medically ill patients, medication may be effective at lower doses than is customary for physically healthy patients, with lower risk of significant side effects. Severe anxiety is treated with low-dose major or minor tranquilizers. Depression is treated with tricyclic antidepressants. When pain or insomnia complicate the picture, amitriptyline is highly effective because it has analgesic and sedative qualities. (See Chapter 39 on psychopharmacological management of cancer patients for detailed information.)

## Education and Instruction

Fear or despair commonly leads patients to exaggerate the pessimistic implications of new information in the mass media or of somatic symptoms they experience. The informed clinician can reduce distress by providing a balanced, realistic, and practical perspective. It is crucial for the clinician to maintain state-of-the-art knowledge of the prognosis and treatment of AIDS and HIV disease that is consistent with the information given by the patient's primary physician. Less often, the patient who minimizes the seriousness of illness may jeopardize his or her own or others' health by failing to learn or to observe preventive health recommendations for personal hygiene, sexual practices, and drug use. Providing the patient with these recommendations not only may promote the primary goal of prevention, but it may also enhance a sense of control. Current recommendations for safer sexual and needle-use precautions will be described later.

## Social Services

The combined impact of discrimination and disability may leave AIDS patients with catastrophic practical needs. Both the loss of employment and the rapidly mounting medical expenses may precipitously force them into poverty. Debilitation, from illness or treatment, may make it difficult for patients to take care of their homes or to go to clinics without assistance. There is a critical need for a social worker to act as a counselor, advocate, or resource for information concerning public assistance, health insurance, visiting nurse services, homemaker services, transportation, and gay advocacy and health service organizations that offer referral or direct service for AIDS-related problems.

## Self-Help Interventions

Approximately 60 organizations in 17 states, Puerto Rico, and western Europe offer referral or direct services for AIDS-related problems. These chiefly volunteer efforts are formed out of emergency response to local AIDS crises. The Gay Men's Health Crises (GMHC) in New York City, the San Francisco AIDS Foundation, the Shanti Project in San Francisco, and AIDS Project/L.A. are examples of self-help organizations that offer comprehensive services for patients with AIDS or other HIV disease. They are run by a core group of founding members and staffed by a large number of volunteers with a range of professional disciplines. Among the broad range of services that they offer are clinical services (including hotline, screening, crisis intervention, support and therapy groups for care partners and people with AIDS, and individual psychotherapy), social services (including buddy support, home health aide care, transportation, patient recreation, financial assistance, and legal advice), and educational services (including hotline, forums, training seminars, technical assistance, and publications). The PWA (People with AIDS) Coalition is a New York City-based national organization that serves as a social support network, information exchange, and political pressure group for people with AIDS. In New York City, ADAPT (Association for Drug Abuse Prevention and Treatment, Inc.) was formed by former and current iv users to initiate AIDS prevention and outreach programs within the drug user community. There are also numerous gay advocacy and health service organizations that offer referral or direct service for AIDS-related problems among their other aims. Under the auspices of the CDC, the American Social Health Association now operates a national hotline for information and referral regarding HIV disease-related concerns.

## TRANSFERENCE AND COUNTERTRANSFERENCE ISSUES

The development of a working relationship between the patient and therapist is complicated by the issues of overidentification, homophobia, and negative bias against iv drug users. The majority of AIDS patients are previously healthy, active, educated, urban men in their thirties, whose expectations, accomplishments, and values may be very close to those of the therapist. Therefore, it may be exceptionally difficult for the therapist to maintain the appropriate emotional dis-

tance; also the therapist's own fears of illness may be evoked, and he or she may be prompted to (avoidant or intrusive) overreaction. On the other hand, the discrepancy between the sexual life-styles of the heterosexual therapist and the gay patient may prevent the patient from believing that the therapist can empathize. Consequently, the AIDS patient may be more apt than other patients to test the therapist for attitudes toward or exposure of homosexuality; the therapist should thoughtfully determine what degree of self-disclosure is therapeutic. The therapist may actually harbor unresolved discomfort about homosexuality that may be mobilized by his or her work with AIDS patients. A therapist who cannot overcome discomfort or who is frankly homophobic should not attempt to work with these patients.

The therapist may also harbor negative stereotypes about iv drug users; it is imperative that this therapist relinquish these attitudes or refer the patient to someone else. The therapist should be prepared to refer these patients to drug treatment centers, so that their drug dependency can be managed and the use of contaminated needles prevented.

## HIV TESTING AND COUNSELING

A reasonably sensitive and specific procedure has been developed for detecting the presence of antibodies, or specific proteins, that develop in reaction to the presence of HIV in the blood (Gallo et al., 1984). This procedure starts with enzyme-linked immunosorbent assay (ELISA) testing; if HIV antibodies are detected, then it is repeated. If HIV antibodies are detected again, then a second test, the Western blot technique, is used to confirm these results. If HIV antibodies are also detected by this test, then the individual is considered seropositive. Like many procedures, this one has low, but acceptable, rates of "false negativity" (i.e., not showing antibodies when you are really infected with the virus) and "false positivity" (i.e., showing antibodies when you are really not infected with the virus). In particular, there may be a 6-month period of seroconversion following infection, during which an individual may be developing an HIV antibody response but not show it (Groopman et al., 1985). As long as this possibility exists, and as long as the relationship between virus and disease remains unclear, the use of test results for individual counseling is questionable. This procedure is available at local blood banks, AIDS research programs, and "alternative test sites" set up just for HIV testing. These programs are obligated to develop ways of giving the test and recording the results that are confidential, and to offer counseling to all participants before and after testing. Because of risk reduction and mental health concerns as described earlier, HIV testing should really not be initiated without counseling both before and after the test.

The several goals of pretest counseling include the following:

1. To screen testees for preexisting psychiatric symptoms or history that would make the testing procedure predictably traumatic. Of course, such screening should include gross symptoms such as suicidal intent, plans, or attempts, major depression, or psychosis. However, it should also include subtler conditions such as bereavement (resulting from a recent AIDS death), separation, or morbid preoccupation with the subject of AIDS.
2. To screen testees for exaggerated, unrealistic reasons for testing that would make it predictably traumatic. The most common, and most likely to produce distress, is the desire "to find out if I have AIDS."
3. To prepare testees for testing, by providing accurate and clear medical and risk reduction information, and practical and constructive counseling about how to deal with the possible emotional consequences of testing. Counseling should be centered around "walking" the individual through both the so-called best-case (i.e., learning of seronegativity) and worst-case (i.e., learning of seropositivity) scenarios.
4. To initiate the networking process between the AIDS health care system and the individual. At the outset referrals should be made to local resources (i.e., physicians, mental health professionals, and self-help organizations). In this way a safety net can be developed for the individual *before* there is an acute need for it.

Posttest counseling should follow up the same points. It is up to the counselor to be alert to the potential for crisis in the seropositive individual, particularly if the results were unexpected. Distortions of the meaning of test results should be actively elicited, so that they may be corrected. This may be done by actually posing some hypothetical questions that challenges certainty (e.g., "Some people think that being seropositive means you have AIDS, but . . ."). Individuals should be encouraged to enumerate all the regular coping skills that they have already acquired for dealing with the test results. These coping skills include rationalizing or talking oneself out of acute anxiety, meditation or relaxation techniques to short-circuit anxiety, confiding in a close friend, or seeking distraction in pleasurable activities (e.g., sports, movies, and meals). Emphasis should be placed on the details of maintaining risk reduction practices. Not only will this reinforce the goal of preventing HIV transmission, but it may also empower the individual

with some sense of personal control over what feels to be an uncontrollable situation. Just like any psychotherapeutic confidence, the counselor must be sensitive to the issue of privacy in HIV testing, especially because the price of disclosure of test results on employment, insurance, housing, schooling for children, and other basic aspects of daily life is not known. Test results should never be documented together with any recognizable identifier (e.g., name or social security number) without the individual's permission.

## AIDS PREVENTION

In the absence of a vaccine, preventive health behavior is the only means of reducing risk of HIV infection. There is little agreement among public health experts about what specific forms of behavior modification are sufficient and offer feasible protection against HIV infection. Abstinence from sexual intercourse or iv drug use is the most certain form of protection. However, sexual abstinence is not likely to be a feasible solution for the indefinite period required for AIDS prevention. In as much as the number of different partners increases the pool of individuals from whom it is possible to acquire infection, a reduction in number of sexual or needle-sharing partners has been recommended since the beginning of the epidemic. However, although such a reduction may decrease the risk of infection, it obviously offers no protection in those situations where sexual intercourse or needle use does occur. That HIV may be transmitted by unknowing, asymptomatic carriers dictates that it is not with whom he or she does it, but rather what the person does that can offer protection from infection. Short of abstinence, the single most effective, though not absolute, form of sexual risk reduction is the use of condoms during vaginal or anal intercourse. There is laboratory evidence that condoms are an effective barrier to HIV transmission (Conant et al., 1986). Condoms should be used with spermicides containing non-oxynol 9, which can destroy HIV. In the setting of serious debate about the risk of infection from oral sex, many experts recommend that condoms be used for this behavior as well. Print materials with explicit suggestions for sexual and verbal strategies for "Eroticizing Safer Sex" are available from the education department of the GMHC in New York City. Although HIV has been recovered from the saliva of seropositive individuals (Groopman et al., 1984), risk of infection from kissing is generally considered to be minimal.

Fear of AIDS had made abstinence slightly more compelling in terms of iv drug use. There has been a significant increase in the number of new applicants to drug treatment programs in major AIDS epicenters like the metropolitan New York–New Jersey area. Of the applicants in a New Jersey State Department of Health survey (J. French, personal communication, 1986), 50% cited fear of AIDS as their primary reason for entering drug treatment. Short of abstinence from iv drug use, using clean needles and personal "works," or sterilizing the equipment by soaking in alcohol, bleach, or boiling water, is the most effective form of iv drug use risk reduction. Clear and illustrated instructions for these preventive procedures can be obtained from HERO (Health Education and Resource Organization), the Baltimore, Maryland community-based AIDS organization. There has also been ongoing, volatile debate between government officials and public health experts in epicenters like New York City about the value of distributing free needles (Des Jarlais et al., 1985).

There is evidence of widespread, spontaneous risk reduction in gay male cohorts in San Francisco (Mc-Cusick et al., 1985), New York City (Martin, 1985), Chicago (Joseph et al., 1985), and other cities. Rates of behavior change, especially for the earliest recommendation to reduce the number of partners, generally fall around 80%. At the same time, objective corroboration of these self-report data may be found in the 75% decline in the rectal gonorrhea rates for San Francisco gay men from 1980 to 1984 (Puckett et al., 1985), and the 59% drop in rectal and pharyngeal gonorrhea rates for men enrolled in the sexually transmitted disease clinics of the New York City Department of Health from 1980 to 1983 (CDC, 1984). There is weaker evidence of initiation of condom use (Siegel et al., 1985), but this may be due to the relative lack of attention given to it by public health authorities at the beginning of the epidemic. Alternatively, in that condoms may demand unusual cooperation between partners and may make both erection and orgasm more difficult, and because they are popularly known to have a considerable failure rate in contraception, psychological constructs like perceived cost and preventive efficacy may provide better explanations of this lag. There is also evidence of spontaneous needle-use risk reduction among iv drug users. Virtually all iv drug users studied are aware of the risk of AIDS and the need to reduce needle use and sharing (Ginzburg, 1984; Des Jarlais et al., 1985; Selwyn et al., 1985). A majority report having initiated these drug use precautions on their own (Des Jarlais et al., 1985; Selwyn et al., 1985).

Although these reports are heartening, they must be tempered with the warning that radical and indefinite change in core adult pleasure-seeking and intimacy-seeking behavior cannot be maintained by education alone. Restraint in spontaneous sexual and/or drug use behavior may demand new social skills for negotiation, limit-setting, or partner rejection that the individual may not otherwise have developed. They may demand new psychological skills for frustration tolerance, anxiety reduction, peer rejection, self-assurance, and self-control. They may demand increased sexual openness to erotic methods, especially condom use, which may induce feelings of awkwardness or embarrassment.

For this purpose, comprehensive AIDS prevention programs are required that are aimed at enhancing skills for managing negative emotions, skills for social assertiveness, and limit-setting and risk reduction instruction. This caveat is a pervasive theme throughout the literature in more traditional areas of health promotion, such as smoking, eating disorders, and alcoholism. Direct precedents for this kind of program may be found in the intervention models of relapse prevention (Marlatt and Gordon, 1985), self-efficacy training (Bandura, 1977), and life skills training (Botvin, 1985; Botvin et al., 1980).

## SUMMARY

AIDS, whether actual or feared, has become a major mental health problem of the 1980s. It has given rise to a new generation of potential psychological problems at each of the key landmarks of its clinical course. These problems include HIV testing, notification of HIV seropositivity, development of HIV disease, diagnosis of frank AIDS, development of AIDS dementia complex, and terminal deterioration. It has given rise to a new generation of preventive health measures, including the adoption of safer sexual practices among homosexual and heterosexual adults, and needle-use precautions among iv drug users (Becker and Joseph, 1988). It has also given rise to a new generation of difficult practical and interpersonal demands, especially caretaking of and bereavement for primarily young adult patients. An ever-widening population including the people with AIDS, the best friends and families of AIDS victims, AIDS risk group members and their sexual partners, health care professionals, and the general public, is being forced to confront these issues in their daily lives. Mental health professionals already have a varied repertory of techniques, from the domains of behavioral medicine and consultation–liaison psychiatry, with which to meet the psychological needs of this population. However, the multiple harsh idiosyncrasies of AIDS and HIV disease demand new levels of flexibility, personal insight, and community outreach in the development of effective services.

## REFERENCES

Abrams, D.I., T. Mess, and P.A. Volberding (1985). Lymphadenopathy: End-point prodrome? Update of a 36-

month prospective study. *Adv. Exp. Med. Biol.* 187:73–84.

Albert, M.L., R.G. Feldman, and A.L. Willis (1974). The "subcortical dementia" of progressive supranuclear palsy. *J. Neurol. Neurosurg. Psychiatry* 37:121–30.

Altman, D. (1986). *AIDS in the Mind of America.* New York: Anchor Press.

American Psychiatric Association (1980). *Diagnostic and Statistical Manual of Mental Disorders,* 3rd ed. Washington, D.C.: American Psychiatric Association.

Bandura, A. (1977). Self-efficacy: Toward a unifying theory of behavioral change. *Psychol. Rev.* 84:191–215.

Batchelor, W.F., A.J. Ferrara, S.F. Morin, K.A. Charles, A.K. Malyon, J.G. Joseph, C. Emmons, R.C. Kessler, C.B. Wortman, K. O'Brien, W.T. Hocker, C. Schaefer, J.L. Martin, C.S. Vance, T.J. Coates, L. Temoshok, and J. Mandel (1984). AIDS: Psychology in the public forum (Monograph). *Am. Psychol.* 39:1277–1314.

Beck, A.T., A.J. Rush, and B.F. Shaw (1979). *Cognitive Therapy of Depression.* New York: Guilford Press.

Becker, M.H. and J.G. Joseph (1988). AIDS and Behavioral Change to Reduce Risk: a review. *Am. J. Public Health* 78:394–410.

Bernstein, D.A. and T.D. Borkovec (1973). *Progressive Relaxation Training: A Manual for the Helping Professions.* Champaign, Ill.: Research Press.

Blalock, J.E. and E.M. Smith (1981). Human leukocyte interferon (HuINF-A) potent endorphin-like opioid activity. *Biochem. Biophys. Res. Commun.* 101:472–78.

Botvin, G.J. (1985). The life skills training program as a health promotion strategy: Theoretical issues and empirical findings. *Spec. Serv. Schools* 1:9–23.

Botvin, G.J., A. Eng, and C.L. Williams (1980). Preventing the onset of cigarette smoking through life skills training. *Prev. Med.* 9:135–43.

Bredesen, D.E. and R. Messing (1983). Neurological syndromes heralding the acquired immune deficiency syndrome. *Ann. Neurol.* 14:141.

Bridge, T.P., A.F. Mirsky, and F.K. Goodwin (eds.). (1988) *Psychological, Neuropsychiatric, and Substance Abuse Aspects of AIDS.* New York: Raven Press.

Britton, C.B. and J.R. Miller (1984). Neurological complications in acquired immune deficiency syndrome (AIDS). *Neurol. Clin.* 2:315–39.

Britton, C.B., M.D. Marquard, B. Koppel, G. Garvey, and J.R. Miller (1982). Neurological complications of the gay immunosuppressed syndrome: Clinical and pathological features. *Ann. Neurol.* 12:80.

Butler, R.N. (1974). Successful aging and the role of the life review. *J. Am. Geriatr. Soc.* 22:529–35.

Casadonte, P.P., D. Des Jarlais, T. Smith, A. Novatt, and P. Hemdal (1986). Psychological and behavioral impact of learning HTLV-III/LAV antibody test results. *Proc. Second Int. Conf. Acquired Immunodeficiency Syndrome (AIDS),* Paris, p. 163 (Poster No. 444).

Centers for Disease Control (1981). Pneumocystis pneumonia—Los Angeles. *Morbid. Mortal. Weekly Rep.* 30:250–52.

Centers for Disease Control (1982). Acquired immune deficiency syndrome (AIDS): Precautions for clinical and laboratory staffs. *Morbid. Mortal. Weekly Rep.* 31:577–80.

C.D.C. (1984). Declining rates of rectal and pharyngeal gonorrhea among males—New York City. *MMWR* 33:295–97.

Centers for Disease Control (1985). Revision of the case definition of acquired immunodeficiency syndrome for national reporting—United States. *Morbid. Mortal. Weekly Rep.* 34:373–76.

Centers for Disease Control (1986a). Classification system for HIV infections. *Morbid. Mortal. Weekly Rep.* 35:334–39.

Centers for Disease Control (1986b). *Acquired Immunodeficiency Syndrome Weekly Surveillance Report.* Atlanta: CDC.

Centers for Disease Control (1987). Update: Human immunodeficiency virus infections in health care workers exposed to blood of infected patients. *Morbid. Mortal. Weekly Rep.* 36:285–88.

Christ, G. and L. Wiener (1985). Psychosocial issues for AIDS. In V. Devita, Jr., S. Hellman, and S. Rosenberg (eds.), *AIDS.* Philadelphia: Lippincott, pp. 295–97.

Conant, M., D. Hardy, J. Sernatinger, D. Spicer, and J.A. Levy (1986). Condoms prevent transmission of AIDS-associated retrovirus. *J.A.M.A.* 255:1706.

Cooper, D.A., J. Gold, P. Maclean, B. Donovan, R. Finlayson, T.G. Barnes, H.M. Michelmore, P. Brooke, and R. Penny (1985). Acute AIDS retrovirus infection: Definition of a clinical illness associated with seroconversion. *Lancet* 1:537–40.

Cox, C.P., P.A. Selwyn, E.E. Schoenbaum, M.A. O'Dowd, E. Drucker (1986). Psychological and behavioral consequences of HTLV-III/LAV antibody testing and notification among intravenous drug abusers in a methadone program in New York. *Proc. Second Int. Conf. Acquired Immunodeficiency Syndrome (AIDS),* Paris, p. 164 (Poster No. 698).

Cummings, J.L. and D.F. Benson (1984). Subcortical dementia—review of an emerging concept. *Arch. Neurol.* 41:874–79.

Daniel, M.D., N.L. Letvin, N.W. King, M. Kannagi, P.K. Schgal, R.D. Hunt, P.J. Kanki, W. Essex, and R.C. Desrosiers (1985). Isolation of T-cell tropic HTLV-III-like retrovirus from macaques. *Science* 228:1201–4.

Des Jarlais, D.C., S.R. Friedman, and W. Hopkins (1985). Risk reduction for the acquired immunodeficiency syndrome among intravenous drug users. *Ann. Intern. Med.* 103:755–59.

Dilley, J.W., H.N. Ochitill, M. Perl, and P.A. Volberding (1985). Findings in psychiatric consultations with patients with acquired immune deficiency syndrome. *Am. J. Psychiatry* 142:682–85.

Donlou, J.N., D.L. Wolcott, M.S. Gottlieb, and J. Landsverk (1985). Psychosocial aspects of AIDS and AIDS-related complex: A pilot study. *J. Psychosoc. Oncol.* 3(2):39–55.

Forstein, M. (1984). AIDS anxiety in the "worried well." In S.E. Nichols and D.G. Ostrow (eds.), *Psychiatric Implications of AIDS.* Washington, D.C.: American Psychiatric Press.

Friedland, G.H., C. Harris, C. Batkus-Small, D. Shine, B. Moll, W. Darrow, and R.S. Klein (1985). Intravenous drug abusers and the acquired immunodeficiency syndrome (AIDS): Demographics, drug use and needle sharing patterns. *Arch. Intern. Med.* 145:1413–17.

Frigo, M.A., J.S. Zones, D.R. Beeson, G.W. Rutherford, D.F. Echenberg, and P.M. O'Malley (1986). The impact of structured counseling in acute adverse psychiatric reactions associated with LAV/HTLV-III antibody testing. *Proc. 114th Annu. Mtg. Am. Public Health Assoc.* Las Vegas (Abstract No. 284).

Gallo, R.C., S.Z. Salahuddin, and M. Popvic (1984). Detection, isolation and continuous production of cytopathic retroviruses (HTLV-III) from patients with AIDS and pre-AIDS. *Science* 224:497–503.

Galea, R.P., B.F. Lewis, and L.A. Baker (eds.) (1988). *AIDS and IV Drug Users; Current Perspectives.* Owings Mills, Md.: National Health Publishing.

Ginzburg, H.M. (1984). A survey of attitudes concerning AIDS among clients in treatment. *Clin. Res. Notes.* National Institute on Drug Abuse, Rockville, Md.

Gold, J.W.M., C.L. Sears, S. Henry, M. Pollack, H. Donnelly, A.E. Brown, B. Wong, B. Koziner, S. Cunningham-Rundles, C. Urmachher, B. Safai, and D. Armstrong (1984). Lymphadenopathy syndrome in homosexual men and development of the acquired immune deficiency syndrome. *Clin. Res.* 31:363A.

Groopman, J.E., S.Z. Salahuddin, M.G. Sarngadharan, P.D. Markham, M. Gonda, A. Sliski, and R.C. Gallo (1984). HTLV-III in saliva of people with AIDS-related complex and healthy homosexual men at risk for AIDS. *Science* 226:447–49.

Groopman, J.E., P.I. Hartzband, L. Schulman, S.Z. Salahuddin, M.G. Sarngadharan, M.F. McLane, M. Essex, and R. Gallo (1985). Antibody seronegative human T-lymphotropic virus type III (HTLV-III)-infected patients with acquired immunodeficiency syndrome or related disorders. *Blood* 66:742–44.

Harris, C., C.B. Small, R.S. Klein, G.H. Friedland, B. Moll, E.E. Emeson, I. Spigland, and N.H. Steigbigel (1983). Immunodeficiency in female sexual partners of men with the acquired immunodeficiency syndrome. *N. Engl. J. Med.* 308:1181–84.

Herman, P. (1983). Neurologic complications of acquired immunologic deficiency syndrome. *Neurology (Minneap.)* 33(Suppl. 2):105.

Ho, D.D., T.R. Rota, R.T. Schooley, J.C. Kaplan, J.D. Allan, J.E. Groopman, L. Resnick, D. Felsenstein, C.A. Andrews, and M.S. Hirsch (1985). Isolation of HTLV-III from cerebrospinal fluid and neural tissues of patients with neurologic syndromes related to the acquired immunodeficiency syndrome. *N. Engl. J. Med.* 313:1493–97.

Hoffman, R.S. (1984). Neuropsychiatric complications of AIDS. *Psychosomatics* f25:393–400.

Horowitz, S.L., D.F. Benson, M.S. Gottlieb, I. Daves, and J.R. Bentson (1982). Neurological complications of gay-related immunodeficiency disorder. *Ann. Neurol.* 12:80.

Institute of Medicine, National Academy of Science (1986). *Confronting AIDS: Directions for Public Health, Health Care, and Research.* Washington, D.C.: National Academy Press.

Jaffe, H.W., K. Choi, P.A. Thomas, H.W. Haverkos, D.M. Auerbach, M.E. Guinan, M.F. Rogers, T.J. Spira, W.W.

Darrow, M.A. Kramer, S.M. Friedman, J.M. Monroe, A.E. Friedman-Kien, L.J. Laubenstein, M. Marmor, B. Safai, S.K. Dritz, S.J. Crispi, S.L. Fannin, J.P. Orkwis, A. Kelter, W.R. Rushing, S.B. Thacker, and J.W. Curran (1983). National case control study of Kaposi's sarcoma and *Pneumocystis carinii* pneumonia in homosexual men. Part 1: epidemiological results. *Ann. Intern. Med.* 99:145–51.

Janis, I.L. and S. Feshbach. (1954). Personality differences associated with responsiveness to fear-arousing communication. *J. Pers.* 23:154–66.

Joseph, J.G., C.A. Emmons, R.C. Kessler, D. Ostrow, and K. O'Brien (1985). Changes in sexual behavior of gay men: Relationship to perceived stress and psychological symptomatology. *Proc. First Int. Conf. Acquired Immunodeficiency Syndrome (AIDS),* Atlanta, p. 67.

Kanki, P.J., M.I. McLane, N.W. King Jr., N.L. Letxin, R.D. Hunt, P. Schgal, M.D. Daniel, R.C. Desrosiers, and M. Essex (1985). Serologic identification and characterization of a macaque T-lymphocyte retrovirus closely related to HTLV-III. *Science,* 228:1199–201.

Kaplan, H.B., R.J. Johnson, C.A. Bailey, and W. Simon (1987). The sociological study of AIDS: A critical review of the literature and suggested research agenda. *J. Health Soc. Behav.* 28:140–57.

Krown, S.E., F.X. Real, S. Cunningham-Rundles, P.L. Myskowski, B. Koziner, A. Mittelman, H.F. Oettgen, and B. Safai (1983). Preliminary observations on the effect of recombinant leukocyte A interferon in homosexual men with Kaposi's sarcoma. *N. Engl. J. Med.* 308:1071–76.

Letvin, N.L., M.D. Daniel, P.K. Schgal, R.C. Desrosiers, R.D. Hunt, L.M. Waldron, J.J. Mackey, D.K. Schmidt, L.V. Chalifoux, and N.W. King (1985). Induction of AIDS-like disease in macaque monkeys with T-cell tropic retrovirus STLV-III. *Science* 230:71–73.

Levy, J.A., J. Shimabukuro, H. Hollander, J. Mills, and L. Kaminsky (1985). Isolation of AIDS-associated retrovirus from cerebrospinal fluid and brains of patients with neurological symptoms. *Lancet* 2:586–88.

Loewenstein, R.J. and S.S. Sharfstein (1983–1984). Neuropsychiatric aspects of acquired immune deficiency syndrome. *Int. J. Psychiatry Med.* 13:255–60.

Marlatt, G.A. and J.R. Gordon (1985). *Relapse Prevention.* New York: Guilford Press.

Marmor, M., A.E. Friedman-Kien, S. Zolla-Pazner, R.E. Stahl, P. Rubinstein, L. Laubenstein, D.C. William, R.J. Klein, and I. Spigland (1984). Kaposi's sarcoma in homosexual men. *Ann. Intern. Med.* 100:809.

Martin, J.L. (1985). The impact of AIDS on New York City gay men: Changes in sexual behavior patterns (Abstract). *Proc. 113th Annu. Mtg. Public Health Assoc.* Washington, D.C.

Mays, V.M. and S.D. Cochran (1987). Acquired immunodeficiency syndrome and Black Americans: Special psychosocial issues. *Pub. Health Rep.* 102:222–31.

McCray, E. (1986). Occupational risk of the acquired immunodeficiency syndrome among health care workers. *N. Engl. J. Med.* 314:1127–32.

McHugh, P.R. and M.F. Folstein (1975). Psychiatric syndromes of Huntington's chorea: A clinical and phenomenologic study. In D.F. Benson and D. Blumer (eds.), *Psychiatric Aspects of Neurologic Disease*. New York: Grune & Stratton, pp. 267–85.

McKusick, L., W. Horstman, and T.J. Coates (1985). AIDS and sexual behavior reported by men in San Francisco. *Am. J. Public Health* 75:493–96.

Metroka, C.E., S. Cunningham-Rundles, M.S. Pollack, J.A. Sonnabend, B. Davis, R. Gordon, D. Fernandez, and J. Mouradian (1983). Generalized lymphadenopathy in homosexual men. *Ann. Intern. Med.* 99(5):585–91.

Mitsuya, H. and S. Brader (1986). Inhibition of the *in vitro* infectivity and cytopathic effect of HTLV-III/LAV by 21,31-dideoxynucleosides. *Proc. Natl. Acad. Sci. U.S.A.* 83:1191–95.

Morin, S.F., T.J. Coats, and L. McKusick (1986). AIDS antibody testing: Who takes the test? *Proc. Second Int. Conf. Acquired Immunodeficiency Syndrome (AIDS)*, Paris, p. 163 (Poster No. 446).

National Institute on Drug Abuse (1984). Clients in treatment. *Clin. Res. Notes*. Rockville, Md., National Institute on Drug Abuse.

Navia, B.A., E.S. Cho, C.K. Petito, and R.W. Price (1986). The AIDS Dementia Complex II. Neuropathology. *Ann. Neurol.* 19:525–35.

Navia, B.A., B.D. Jordan, and R.W. Price (1986). The AIDS dementia complex: I. Clinical features. *Ann. Neurol.* 19:517–24.

Nichols, S.E. (1985). Psychosocial reactions of persons with the acquired immunodeficiency syndrome. *Ann. Intern. Med.* 103:765–67.

Nichols, S.E. and D.G. Ostrow (1984). *Psychiatric Implications of AIDS*. Washington, D.C.: American Psychiatric Press.

Nielsen, L., C.K. Petito, C.D. Urmacher, and J.B. Posner (1984). Subacute encephalitis in acquired immune deficiency syndrome: A postmortem study. *Am. J. Clin. Pathol.* 82:678–82.

Nurnberg, H.G., J. Prudic, M. Fiori, and E.P. Freedman (1984). Psychopathology complicating acquired immune deficiency syndrome (AIDS). *Am. J. Psychiatry* 141:95–96.

Oleske, J., A. Minnefor, R. Cooper, Jr., K. Thomas, A. de la Cruz, H. Ahdieh, I. Guerrero, V.V. Joshi, and F. Desposito (1983). Immunodeficiency syndrome in children. *J.A.M.A.* 249:2345.

O'Reilly, K.R., L.L. Sanders, J. Ward, S.A. Allen, W. Cates, and A. Grindon, (1986). Sexual behavior change after positive HTLV-III antibody tests in blood donors: Report from a longitudinal study. *Proc. 114th Annu. Mtg. Am. Public Health Assoc.*, Las Vegas (Abstract No. 1035).

Pape, J.W., B. Liautaud, F. Thomas, J.R. Mathurin, M.M. St. Amand, M. Boncy, V. Pean, M. Pamphhile, A.C. Laroche, and W.D. Johnson, Jr. (1986). Risk factors associated with AIDS in Haiti. *Am. J. Med. Sci.* 29: 4–7.

Petito, C.K., B.A. Navia, E.S. Cho, B.D. Jordan, D.C. George, and R.W. Price (1985). Vacuolar myelopathy pathologically resembling subacute combined degenera-

tion in patients with the acquired immunodeficiency syndrome. *N. Engl. J. Med.* 312:874–79.

Potterat, J.J. and R.O. King (1981). A new approach to gonorrhea control: The asymptomatic man and incidence reduction. *J.A.M.A.* 245:578.

Public Health Service Plan for the Prevention and Control of AIDS (1986). *Public Health Rep.* 101:341–48.

Puckett, S., M. Bart, L.L. Bye, and J. Amory (1985). Self-reported behavioral change among gay and bisexual men—San Francisco. *Morbid. Mortal. Weekly Rep.* 34:613–14.

Roberts, R.B., D. Scavuzzo, J. Laurence, O. Laskin, Y. Kim, and H.W. Murray (1986). Effects of short-term oral ribavirin in high-risk patients for AIDS (Poster 567). *Proc. Second Int. Conf. on Acquired Immunodeficiency Syndrome (AIDS)*, Paris, p. 68 (Poster No. 567).

Rosenblum, M.L., R.M. Levy, and D.E. Bredesen (eds.) (1988). *AIDS and the Nervous System*. New York: Raven Press.

Rubinstein, A., M. Sicklick, A. Gupta, L. Bernstein, N. Klein, E. Rubinstein, I. Spigland, L. Fruchter, N. Litman, L. Haesoon, and M. Hollander (1983). Acquired immunodeficiency with reversed T4/T8 ratios in infants born to promiscuous and drug-afflicted mothers. *J.A.M.A.* 249:2351–56.

Safai, B. and R.A. Good (1981). Kaposi's sarcoma: A review and recent developments. *Cancer* 31(1):2–12.

Schorr, J.B., P.D. Berkowitz, P.D. Cummings, A.S. Katz, and S.G. Sandler (1985). Prevalence of HTLV-III antibody in American blood donors. *N. Engl. J. Med.* 313:384–85.

Selwyn, P.A., C.P. Cox, C. Feiner, C. Lipshutz, and R. Cohen (1985). Knowledge about AIDS and high-risk behavior among intravenous drug abusers in New York City. *Proc. 113th Annu. Mtg. Am. Public Health Assoc.*, Washington, D.C.

Shaw, G.M., M.E. Harper, B.H. Hahn, L.G. Epstein, D.C. Gaydusek, R.W. Price, B.A. Navia, C.K. Petito, C.J. O'Hara, E.S. Cho, J.M. Oleske, F. Wong-Stall, and R.C. Gallo (1985). HTLV-III infection in brains of children and adults with AIDS encephalopathy. *Science* 227:177–82.

Siegel, K., D. Hirsch, and G. Christ (1985). Adoption of modifications in sexual behavior among asymptomatic homosexual men (Abstract). *Proc. First Int. Conf. Acquired Immunodeficiency Syndrome (AIDS)*, Atlanta, p. 71.

Snider, W.D., D.M. Simpson, S. Nielsen, J.W.M. Gold, C.E. Metroka, and J.E. Posner, (1983). Neurological complications of acquired immune deficiency syndrome: Analysis of 50 patients. *Ann. Neurol.* 14:403–18.

Spikes, J. and J.C.B. Holland (1975). The physician's response to the dying patient. In J.J. Strain and S. Grossman (eds.), *Psychological Care of the Medically Ill: A Primer in Liaison Psychiatry*. New York: Appleton-Century-Crofts.

Temoshok, L. (1986). Psychosocial coping with a diagnosis of AIDS. Symposium: The acquired immune deficiency syndrome: Behavioral medicine research provides a paradigm for understanding and treatment. *Proc. Annu. Mtg. Soc. Behav. Med.*, San Francisco (Symposium VIII).

Tross, S., J. Holland, D.A. Hirsch, M. Schiffman, J. Gold,

B. Safai, and P. Myskowski (1986). Psychological and social impact of AIDS spectrum disorders. *Proc. Second Int. Conf. Acquired Immune Deficiency Syndrome (AIDS),* Paris, p. 157 (Communication 63S6c).

Tross, S., D.A. Hirsch, B. Rabkin, C. Berry, and J. Holland (1987). Determinants of current psychiatric disorder in AIDS spectrum patients. *Proc. Third Int. Conf. Acquired Immunodeficiency Syndrome (AIDS).* Washington, D.C.: Courtesy Associates, Inc., p. 60 (Abstract No. T.10.5).

Tross, S., R.W. Price, B. Navia, H.T. Thaler, J. Gold, D.A. Hirsch, and J.J. Sidtis (1988). Neuropsychological characterization of the AIDS Dementia Complex; A Preliminary Report. *AIDS* 2:81–88.

Valdessari, R.O., D.W. Lyter, and C.R. Rinaldo (1986). Factors influencing the decision to learn HTLV-III antibody results. *Proc. 114th Annu. Mtg. Am. Public Health Assoc.,* Las Vegas (Abstract No. 2159).

Viederman, M. and S. Perry (1980). Use of psychodynamic life narrative in the treatment of depression in the physically ill. *Gen. Hosp. Psychiatry* 3:177–85.

Weisman, A. and W. Worden (1976–1977). The existential plight in cancer: Significance of the first 100 days. *Int. J. Psychiatry Med.* 7:1–15.

Williams, A.G., R. D'Aquila, H. Kleber, L. Peterson, and A.E. Williams (1986). HTLV-III/LAV infection among intravenous drug abusers in New Haven, CT. *Proc. 114th Annu. Mtg. Am. Public Health Assoc.,* Las Vegas (Abstract No. 1025).

# PART IV

## Common Psychiatric Disorders and Their Management

# 22

# Overview of Normal Reactions and Prevalence of Psychiatric Disorders

Mary Jane Massie and Jimmie C. Holland

The influences that contribute to the emotional stress of receiving a diagnosis of cancer have been reviewed in relation to the social stigma attached to cancer (Part I), the characteristics of personality, coping, and social support that modify its impact (Part II), and the medical variables of stage, outcome, site of cancer, and treatment (Part III). Part IV examines normal reactions to cancer and the frequency and types of psychological disturbance that exceed the normal level of distress associated with a diagnosis of cancer. Guidelines for the recognition and management of these psychiatric disorders in cancer patients are given. When a psychiatric consultant should be called is also outlined.

## OVERVIEW OF NORMAL REACTIONS AND PREVALENCE OF PSYCHIATRIC DISORDERS

By far the most common types of psychological disturbance in cancer patients are depression and anxiety. Although both are expected emotions in response to the stresses of cancer, the person who faces cancer often asks the physician whether his or her emotional reactions are "normal." Patients sometimes question whether feelings represent "weakness" of character and whether they could avoid "giving in to their feelings" if they were "stronger." Often, reassurance that others have the same feelings is helpful. Increasingly, patients are concerned that their normal depressed feelings will contribute to a negative outcome of cancer treatment. This seems to be related to the emphasis given to emotions and cancer in the lay press, which has often reported stress, immunity, and cancer data uncritically. In fact, some patients ask for a "mental health checkup" before beginning treatment for cancer to be sure that they are responding emotionally in a way that will assure the best response of their tumor to treatment. We encourage the concept that patients'

optimism, personal participation, and commitment are vital contributions to treatment. However, we also point out that "down days" with depressed feelings are normal and unavoidable; variable moods are expected in healthy adaptation to illness and do not have an adverse effect on outcome. The impact of such worries on the search for alternative treatment methods is discussed in Chapter 42. Psychological and social influences in cancer risk and survival and the status of psychoneuroimmunological research are reviewed in Chapters 60 and 61.

Clearly, the clinicians' tasks in this area are to assess psychological responses and to differentiate those that are normal and will dissipate over time from those that may be pathological, that may interfere substantially with the patient's comfort, quality of life, and ability to make appropriate treatment decisions and adhere to treatment, and thus may have an effect on survival. Data showing the adverse impact on treatment outcome of receiving a reduced total dose of chemotherapy are readily available (Bonadonna and Valagussa, 1981). Thus, there is a sound clinical basis for sensitivity to this aspect of patient evaluation. Although significant psychiatric disorders are not common, some are frequently encountered and the clinician needs to know about their clinical picture and prevalence.

### Prevalence of Psychiatric Disorders

One of the earliest studies to provide objective data on psychiatric morbidity in cancer patients was done by Craig and Abeloff (1974). They gave a self-administered form of the Hopkins Symptom Checklist-90 (SCL-90) to 30 consecutively admitted patients to an oncology research unit. More than 50% showed moderate to high levels of depression, and 30% had elevated levels of anxiety. They noted that one quarter resembled patients seen by the psychiatric emergency service, suggesting the need to identify the significant subset of cancer patients who were likely to be under significant stress. Studies that followed focused largely on a single entity, such as organic brain disorders (Davies et al., 1973) (see Chapter 30) or depression (Plumb and Holland, 1977) (see Chapter 23).

The Psychosocial Collaborative Oncology Group (PSYCOG), the first cooperative group organized to study these issues, carried out a helpful study of the nature and prevalence of psychiatric disorders in cancer patients (Derogatis et al., 1983). In the cancer centers of Johns Hopkins, Rochester, and Memorial Sloan-Kettering Cancer Center, 215 ambulatory and hospitalized patients were randomly accessed and studied by a structured interview rated by interviewers

and by patient self-report scales. The clinical interviewers made a psychiatric diagnosis, using criteria of the third edition of the *Diagnostic and Statistical Manual* (DSM-III) of the American Psychiatric Association (1980). Table 22-1 shows the frequency of psychiatric disorders. Of the 215 patients interviewed, 53% were adjusting adequately to cancer without symptoms beyond those regarded as normal; however, 47% had sufficient psychiatric symptoms to warrant the diagnosis of a psychiatric disorder. Of the nearly 50% who had a psychiatric diagnosis, by far the most frequent disturbances were reactive depression, anxiety, or both. These moods were simply of greater intensity and duration than considered normal, and using the DSM-III criteria, were diagnosed as adjustment disorder with depressed, anxious, or mixed mood. This

**Table 22-1** Rates of DSM-III psychiatric disorders observed in 215 cancer patients from three cancer centers

| Diagnostic category | Number in specific category | Number in diagnostic class | Percentage of psychiatric diagnoses |
|---|---|---|---|
| *Adjustment disorders* | | 69 (32%) | 68 |
| Depressed mood | 26 (12%) | | |
| Mixed emotional features | 29 (13%) | | |
| Anxious mood | 12 (6%) | | |
| Emotion and conduct | 2 (1%) | | |
| *Major affective disorders* | | 13 (6%) | 13 |
| Unipolar depression | 8 (4%) | | |
| Bipolar depression | 1 (0.5%) | | |
| Atypical depression | 3 (1.5%) | | |
| Dysthymic disorder | 1 (0.5%) | | |
| *Organic mental disorders* | | 8 (4%) | 8 |
| Presenile dementia | 1 (0.5%) | | |
| Dementia with depression | 1 (0.5%) | | |
| Organic affective syndrome | 2 (1%) | | |
| Dementia | 1 (0.5%) | | |
| Atypical organic brain syndrome | 2 (1%) | | |
| Organic personality syndrome | 1 (0.5%) | | |
| *Personal disorder and alcohol abuse* | | 7 (3%) | 7 |
| Schizoid | 1 (0.5%) | | |
| Compulsive | 2 (1%) | | |
| Histrionic | 1 (0.5%) | | |
| Dependent | 1 (0.5%) | | |
| Other | 1 (0.5%) | | |
| Alcohol abuse (in remission) | 1 (0.5%) | | |
| *Anxiety disorders* | | 4 (2%) | 4 |
| Generalized anxiety disorder | 1 (0.5%) | | |
| Simple phobia | 1 (0.5%) | | |
| Obsessive-compulsive disorder | 2 (1%) | | |
| *Total psychiatric diagnoses* | | 101 (47%) | |
| *Psychiatric diagnosis absent* | | 114 (53%) | |

*Source*: Adapted from L.R. Derogatis, G.R. Morrow, J. Fetting, D. Penman, S. Piasetsky, A.M. Schmale, M. Henrichs, and C.L.M. Carnicke, Jr. (1983). The prevalence of psychiatric disorders among cancer patients. *J.A.M.A.* 249:751–57.

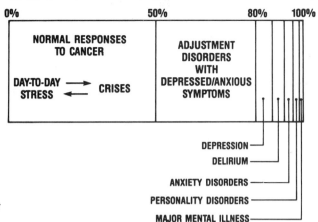

**Figure 22-1.** Spectrum of psychiatric disorders in cancer (derived from PSYCOG prevalence data).

category (adjustment disorder) is the closest approximation to the situational distress of patients with physical illness. However, the definition, which includes that the response is maladaptive, seems to make it less applicable and perhaps in need of revision in relation to diagnosing distress of individuals with life-threatening illness.

In this PSYCOG study, 13% of the patients had more severe depressive symptoms constituting major depression, 8% had CNS complications characterized by organic mental disorders, and only 11% had a preexisting psychiatric disorder, either a personality or an anxiety disorder. The combined diagnoses—adjustment disorder with depressed mood and major depression—represented the significant group of patients with symptoms in the depressive spectrum (see Chapter 23).

Using these data, we have developed a schema (Fig. 22-1) to illustrate the range of psychological responses one can anticipate among a large group of cancer patients. It can be assumed that 50% are experiencing normal responses in coping with cancer. These normal responses to stress include heightened levels of anxiety and depression at transition or crisis points, which occur in relation to disease or treatments. Symptoms abate as the crisis resolves and the individual returns to both normal mood and function. The remaining 50% of cancer patients experience distress that is more severe, primarily consisting of reactive anxiety and depression. The next most frequently encountered diagnosis is major depression, followed by delirium related to the effects of disease or treatment on the CNS. Preexisting psychiatric problems that worsen during treatment and complicate care constitute a small percentage of the whole. Indeed, by far the greatest majority of psychological problems relate to the efforts of psychologically stable individuals to adjust to cancer and its

treatment. Although only a small minority of problems are related to prior psychiatric illness, they may require lengthy evaluation and complex coordination of medical and psychiatric treatment.

In Part III of this book we reported studies that examined patients' distress by stage and site of disease. However, additional prevalence data from large samples, such as the PSYCOG study, are needed. The other major source of information on psychological distress in cancer patients, derived from consultation data, is discussed here.

## Psychiatric Consultation

As consultation–liaison psychiatry has developed in teaching hospitals, information has accumulated about cancer patients through surveys of psychiatric consultations. As diagnostic criteria have been refined, especially with use of the DSM-III and with the development of computerized data bases, more systematically accessed clinical information has become available. Using DSM-II criteria for psychiatric diagnoses, Levine, Silberfarb, and Lipowski (1978) reviewed 100 requests for psychiatric consultation in hospitalized patients with cancer at Dartmouth. The major reasons for referral were to evaluate depression and delirium. Of the patients seen, 56% were depressed and 40% had an organic mental disorder (delirium).

We have conducted a review of our psychiatric consultations on 546 patients (Massie and Holland, 1987) (Table 22-2). Similar to findings in the Dartmouth study, common reasons for patient referral were evaluation of depression and/or suicidal risk (59%) and assessment of delirium (18%). Using DSM-III diagnostic criteria, the largest diagnostic group was reactive distress, with 54% having adjustment disorder with depression, anxiety, or mixed mood. Major de-

**Table 22-2**  Psychiatric diagnoses in 546 consultations
by MSKCC psychiatry service (DSM-III criteria)

| Diagnoses | Number | Percentage |
|---|---|---|
| *Axis I* | | |
| Adjustment disorder | 295 | 54 |
| Depressed (140) | | |
| Anxious (62) | | |
| Mixed (93) | | |
| Major depression | 49 | 9 |
| Single episode (39) | | |
| Recurrent episode (10) | | |
| Organic mental disorder | 111 | 20 |
| Delirium (78) | | |
| Dementia (24) | | |
| Organic affective syndrome (9) | | |
| Major psychiatric disorder | 26 | 5 |
| Schizophrenia (21) | | |
| Manic-depressive (5) | | |
| Anxiety disorders | 22 | 4 |
| Other | 22 | 4 |
| Somatoform (20) | | |
| Mental retardation (2) | | |
| No mental disorder | 21 | 4 |
| *Axis II* | | |
| Compulsive | 19 | 20 |
| Dependent | 16 | 17 |
| Atypical mixed | 16 | 17 |
| Borderline | 12 | 12.5 |
| Histrionic | 12 | 12.5 |
| Schizotypal | 7 | 7 |
| Paranoid | 4 | 4 |
| Passive-aggressive | 4 | 4 |
| Narcissistic | 3 | 3 |
| Antisocial | 2 | 2 |
| Avoidant | 1 | 1 |

pression, usually the patient's first episode, was present in 9%. However, our psychiatrists are conservative in making the diagnosis of major depression because of the presence of confounding physical symptoms; 9% may be an underrepresentation (see Chapter 23). Organic mental disorders were diagnosed in 20% of the patients, usually manifesting as delirium; a small number of patients had dementia or organic affective syndrome related to steroids. Schizophrenia and manic-depressive illness constituted 5% of diagnoses, anxiety disorders 4% and mental retardation and somatoform disorder 4%.

Recognizing the spectrum of problems that patients are likely to experience, the normal responses to cancer and their differentiation from abnormal responses (see Part II for influences that contribute to adaptation) are reviewed next.

## Normal Responses to the Stress of Illness

Studies of the emotional reactions of individuals to a range of threatened and actual losses such as those experienced by survivors of concentration camps, Hiroshima, or natural disasters, or following extensive burns or limb amputations, have provided helpful information that has contributed to the understanding of the responses of psychologically healthy individuals to the diagnosis of cancer (Cobb and Lindemann, 1943; Adler, 1943; Lindemann, 1944; Lifton, 1967; Lifton and Olson, 1976; Hamburg et al., 1974; Chamberlain, 1980). The reactions of cancer patients are similar in nature to reactions of individuals to other catastrophic events. There are consistent patterns of response over time as adaptation occurs, but there are also wide variations in the degree of distress and disturbance manifested. Responses are modulated by the strength of inner resources, availability of social support, and the nature and meaning of the crisis in terms of life cycle tasks (see Parts I–III for a detailed discussion).

The emotional crisis presented by cancer was most widely studied in relation to adaptation to the diagnosis of cancer. Weisman and Worden (1976) described the adjustment of individuals to the first 100 days after diagnosis of cancer, terming it the period of "existential plight." Symptoms include acute distress that resolves as the impact is absorbed and the person returns to a normal pattern of function. Weisman (1976) developed an Index of Vulnerability that provides guidance for predicting those patients who have higher distress and greater vulnerability to poor psychosocial adjustment (Table 22-3).

Caplan (1981) conceptualized stress as a situation in which demands on the individual exceed the ability to respond, producing both physiological and psychological arousal. Mastery results in reduced arousal and a diminution of the stress. Using Caplan's model, receiving catastrophic news about cancer diagnosis or recurrence results in immediate cognitive problem-solving efforts. However, problem-solving ability is simultaneously reduced by virtue of physiological arousal that results in poor attention, concentration, judgment, and a sense of disorganization and erosion of self-concept. The inability to utilize adaptive skills results in transient dysphoria, manifested by anxiety and depression. Healthy adaptation in the normal person ultimately results in the use of effective coping mechanisms that reduce the psychological and physiological arousal.

The theoretical hierarchy of defense mechanisms provided by Vaillant's longitudinal study of healthy individuals (1986) is helpful in understanding the range of ways individuals have of coping with cancer.

**Table 22-3** Weisman's characteristics of high distress–high vulnerability to poor psychosocial adjustment

| | |
|---|---|
| Medical | More physical symptoms |
| | More advanced cancer at diagnosis |
| | Doctor perceived as less helpful |
| | Short-time perspecrive about survival |
| Social | Lower socioeconomic status |
| | More marital problems |
| | More background problems |
| | Expects and gets little support from others |
| | Little or no church attendance |
| Psychological and psychiatric | History of psychiatric problems |
| | High anxiety |
| | Low ego strength |
| | More suppression |
| | More concerns of all kinds |
| | Feels like giving up |
| | Alcohol abuse |
| | Coping less effective |

*Source*: Weisman, D. (1976). Early diagnosis of vulnerability in cancer patients. *Amer. J. of Med. Sci.* 271:187–196.

coming," "why bother with treatment, it's of no use."

This initial period, which usually lasts a few days, is followed by a period of turmoil and overt distress, anxiety, fears of the future, ruminative distressing thoughts, and difficulty sleeping, eating, and concentrating. Mood is often alternately anxious or sad, with a sense of hopelessness and despair. In the absence of crisis, these emotions would be considered pathological, but in this context they are signs of normal and adaptive coping.

These responses are managed best by the physician responsible for the patient's treatment, who understands the reactions and offers reassurance, support, and compassion while sensitively discussing the facts of the medical situation. The experienced clinician understands that the same information may have to be repeated several times because of the patient's anxiety and poor concentration. An unhurried discussion with a family member present, which outlines a new (or revised) treatment plan and encourages questions, helps the patient gain a sense of mastery of the situation and contributes to a supportive trusting relationship that will make future crises, should they develop, easi-

To cope effectively with stress, one gets help from others, makes conscious efforts of one's own, and uses the ego's unconscious adaptive mechanisms of defense. Individuals who cope well with cancer utilize many of the mature defenses Vaillant outlined: altruism, humor, suppression, anticipation, and sublimination. However, as Vaillant pointed out, the less mature defense, temporary denial, is so common that it can be viewed as normal in severe circumstances such as cancer.

The work of Horowitz and co-workers (1973, 1976), on stress response syndromes resulting from events unrelated to illness, has many logical applications to cancer. These concepts and our own observations of cancer patients have led to a model of phases of normal adjustment (Table 22-4), which is described here (see also Parts II and III).

The response to a crisis in cancer, either at the time of diagnosis or at some later transitional or crisis point, is characterized by an initial phase in which the person experiences either disbelief or temporary denial of the diagnosis. Patients describe a period of "numbness" or even derealization ("as if this isn't happening to me"). This permits a temporary emotional distancing from the full implication of the crisis. Some individuals do not experience disbelief, but describe experiencing an immediate sense of despair and demoralization that is often expressed as "I knew it was

**Table 22-4** Normal responses to the crises encountered with cancer

| Results of crisis | Symptoms | Time interval* |
|---|---|---|
| *Phase 1* | | |
| Initial response | Disbelief or denial ("wrong diagnosis," "mixed slide") *or* Despair ("I knew it all along," "no reason to take treatment") | Usually last less than a week |
| *Phase 2* | | |
| Dysphoria | Anxiety<br>Depressed mood<br>Anorexia<br>Insomnia<br>Poor concentration<br>Disruption of daily activities | Usually last 1–2 weeks, but varies |
| *Phase 3* | | |
| Adaptation | Adjusts to new information<br>Confronts the issues presented<br>Finds reasons for optimism<br>Resumes, activities (e.g., new or revised treatment plan, other goals) | Usually begins by 2 weeks |

*Approximations; may vary widely.

er to handle. Including family in discussions and encouraging their support of the patient are also important steps in assuring the patient's emotional well-being (see Part III).

While this normal response usually diminishes over a week to 10 days, occasionally it persists or is so severe that medication is indicated to control symptoms. A short-acting benzodiazepine such as lorazepam or alprazolam (0.25–0.50 mg tid) is useful for daytime anxiety. A hypnotic prescribed for a week or two may permit sleep and reduce fatigue related to insomnia. Patients ordinarily discontinue a drug when symptoms abate. Benzodiazepine dependence is a rare problem in cancer patients; more often, patients require encouragement to take a drug (see Chapter 39 on psychopharmacological management).

It is important to recognize how painful symptoms of distress at the time of diagnosis can be, and how frequently patients remember them and fear their return with another crisis. In this respect, the response is similar to a panic disorder in which anticipatory fear of a return of the symptoms comes to dominate the picture. Again explanation of the source of the fears and reassurance about recovery are usually adequate.

## REACTIVE ANXIETY AND DEPRESSION

### Adjustment Disorder with Depressed and Anxious Mood

At the borderline between normal and abnormal reactions lies the most common emotional disturbance seen in cancer patients: adjustment disorder with depressed and/or anxious mood (i.e., reactive depression and/or anxiety that exceeds that seen in the normal response to stress). While these symptoms are defined in DSM-III as a pathological state, psychiatrists question whether in the medically ill they are appropriately regarded as pathological. Indeed, one-third of patients showed this response in the 1983 Derogatis and colleagues study, and 50% received this diagnosis in our consultation series (Massie and Holland, 1987). These symptoms are an exaggeration of the emotions seen in the normal stress response; they are excessive in either *duration* (>7–14 days) or *intensity* (severity of symptoms sufficient to interfere with normal function). There have been no studies of the natural course of adjustment disorders in physically ill patients, including those patients with cancer.

The severity of symptoms in patients with adjustment disorders ranges from mild to severe (Fig. 22-1). Those with the most severe symptoms of adjustment disorder with depressed mood are difficult to distinguish diagnostically from patients with major depression. The diagnostic criteria do not easily differentiate these two categories in physically ill patients, especially patients with advanced cancer (see Chapter 23).

Symptoms of adjustment disorder are most often predominantly depressive in nature. Patients have a dysphoric mood, despair about the future, and feelings of guilt. Anxiety symptoms, often accompanying depression, or less often appearing alone, manifest sometimes as agitation and extreme fear. Insomnia is a common symptom; anorexia, often present, may be difficult to assess in cancer patients.

The treatment of patients with an adjustment disorder utilizes crisis-oriented psychotherapy alone or combined with the use of medication to reduce the level of distressing symptoms. Weekly visits, over 4–6 weeks, in which reassurance and support are combined with clarification of the medical situation and its implications are usually sufficient to assist the patient to regroup defenses and to cope. A family member may be included in some of the meetings. Time between visits is lengthened as the crisis resolves; however, most patients are encouraged to return if another crisis occurs.

The decision to prescribe a psychotropic drug depends on the level of distress and how significantly symptoms (anxiety or depression) impair daily function. Daytime sedation provided by low-dose alprazolam, lorazepam, or oxazepam helps in control of symptoms; bedtime sedation with a benzodiazepine (triazolam or tezmazepam) or antidepressant (amitryptyline, imipramine, or doxepin) ensures sleep and often reduces daytime symptoms of anxiety as well (see Chapter 39 on psychopharmacological management).

The following case report demonstrates both the diagnostic aspects of these problems and some of the therapeutic issues.

CASE REPORTS

A twenty-nine-year-old married businesswoman received a diagnosis of breast cancer with axillary lymph node invasion 1 week after her wedding. She immediately underwent a partial mastectomy with axillary node dissection. Her surgeon compassionately explained the diagnosis and outlined the necessary further treatment, which included both radiotherapy and chemotherapy.

On the first postoperative day, the nursing staff noted the patient had wide swings in mood and behavior, alternating between boisterous laughter and swearing, and uncontrollable weeping. She threatened suicide so that she would "not have to face the shame and humiliation of returning to work as half a person." The psychiatrist who saw the patient discussed with her that, although she described herself as an "intense" person, she had no serious psychological problems before and her fears that she was "out of control" were not justified. She lamented receiving a diagnosis of cancer so soon after a long-planned marriage to a man she loved and with whom she looked forward to sharing a full life. The psychiatrist acknowledged her profound distress while reassuring her that she could regain emotional control; she was told that her concerns were normal. The psychiatrist reinforced the surgeon's optimism, reviewed the treatment plan, and offered to see her through the coming weeks. Alprazolam (0.25 mg tid) was ordered; the psychiatrist made daily visits until the patient was discharged. The nursing and surgical staff approached her with compassion, support, and hopefulness about her outcome. Her husband was understanding and encouraging. By the time of discharge, the patient felt in control of her emotions, was committed to the treatment plan, and no longer had suicidal thoughts.

The psychiatrist saw her twice weekly during the first several weeks of chemotherapy, then once a week over several months. During these sessions, it became clear that part of her response related to the death of her father from cancer when she was 10 years old. He had died rapidly after a biopsy that had disclosed a cancer diagnosis, and the patient had been fearful of following a similar course.

The psychiatrist helped her to return to work and to anticipate the reactions of colleagues that she feared, and helped her to plan a work schedule that accommodated absences related to chemotherapy and radiotherapy. The patient adjusted to her new marriage and work, accepting the temporary disruption of her life related to treatment.

The other commonly seen psychiatric disorders in cancer patients are reviewed in the following chapters. Many disorders are evaluated and managed readily by nonpsychiatrist mental health professionals who commonly work in cancer centers. However, because the medical and psychiatric problems frequently overlap, making the two difficult to differentiate at times, there are occasions when a psychiatric consultant is needed. This often does not need to be a formal consultation. An informal ''curbside consultation'' is a common means of providing advice; this is particularly conveniently done by the liaison psychiatrist, who is known and trusted by the staff (see Chapter 56 on mental health professionals in oncology). Table 22-5 outlines the indications for requesting a psychiatric consultation, beginning with those that constitute an emergency.

## INDICATIONS FOR A PSYCHIATRIC CONSULTATION

### Suicidal Risk

When a patient makes suicidal statements, they should be taken seriously and explored further. If, however, the patient is depressed, feels hopeless, and describes plans or methods of suicide, a psychiatric consultation should be requested. The more clearly a plan is described the greater the risk (see Chapter 24). Depressed patients who are seriously ill and mildly confused or in

**Table 22-5** When a psychiatric consultation is indicated

- Suicidal risk or threat to others
- Altered or unusual behavior (often evidence of underlying delirium)
- Ability to consent to or refuse treatment
- Indecision about treatment
- Anxiety symptoms
- Depressive symptoms
- History of prior psychiatric or personality disorder
- Sexual disorders
- Pain
- Conflict between patient, family, and staff

pain are in a high-risk group for suicide because they have less control over impulses and may act on suicidal thoughts (see Chapter 24 for detailed discussion of suicide in cancer patients).

### Threat of Violence to Others

Patients and their families are under great stress during hospitalization. The stress for patients is often complicated by drugs that decrease impulse control and may produce confusional states with paranoid ideation. These states are best handled when recognized early (see Chapter 30 on delirium). Patients with prior psychiatric history of schizophrenia may experience exacerbation of symptoms of delusions and combative behavior during the stress of illness. Relatives are stressed, especially during the hospitalization of a dying family member. Self-medication of anxiety symptoms, sleep deprivation, and frustration contribute, in some individuals, to anger at staff and, at times, threats. A family member may lose control when death is announced, and may threaten a doctor viewed as responsible for their loss. These situations are best handled by early anticipation of the risks and request for intervention by a psychiatrist *before* the threat of violence is great. Chapter 30 outlines the way in which a situation with threat of harm should be handled, with the psychiatrist organizing staff and security presence to contain rapidly and defuse a dangerous situation. Guidelines for managing psychiatric emergencies need to be part of house staff and nursing orientation; a well-prepared staff working with a psychiatrist who is familiar with management principles can smoothly handle these situations without causing major disruption or fear in other patients (Perry and Gilmore, 1981).

### Altered or Unusual Behavior (Often Evidence of Underlying Delirium)

The psychologically healthy, cooperative hospitalized patient who seemingly, without cause, becomes irritable and angry or withdrawn and apathetic is cause for concern. Although these mood changes may have an emotional basis, they more often herald insidious onset of a delirium resulting from metabolic imbalance or drug side effect (especially steroids). Careful but rapid evaluation of mild cognitive changes is necessary to make an accurate diagnosis of encephalopathy and to start treatment.

## Ability to Consent to or Refuse Treatment

A psychiatric consultation may be needed, at times in emergency situations, to evaluate a patient's ability to consent to or refuse a procedure deemed critical to survival. An assessment must be made to determine if the patient understands the medical situation and the treatment proposed, and if he or she is able to assume responsibility for decision making. This decision is usually made in consultation with the patient's relatives. This judgment is not the determination of "competency," a judgment determined only by the courts. Rarely is legal advice or a judge's decision necessary to further treatment. However, when elective treatment is planned for a severely or chronically mentally impaired patient who has no family, a court direction may have to be sought.

An increasingly common concern is the patient who refuses a particular life-sustaining treatment, such as dialysis, as part of a decision to forego all further treatment. Physicians and nurses are often concerned about whether the patient is capable of understanding the circumstances relating to the decision. The complicating question of presence of depression biasing the decision must be assessed, as well as mental acuity. The psychiatrist can assist in assessing these issues. If ethical concerns persist, an ethics consultant should be called (see Chapter 49 on terminal care and Chapter 59 on ethical problems).

Sometimes a patient whose medical condition is precarious insists on leaving the hospital against advice, thus endangering his or her life. If this occurs, a psychiatric consultant should assess the patient's mental status for the presence of a confusional state related to illness, a psychotic state, or other psychiatric disorder (poor impulse control), to determine the etiology of the behavior and to make management recommendations to the staff.

## Indecision about Treatment

The decision to undergo a major operation or to agree to chemotherapy or radiotherapy is often logically and rationally made, but anxiety increases as the time for the actual procedure nears. Anxiety may result in last-minute indecision. If anxiety is not resolved with the patient's physician, a psychiatric consultation can often provide additional information and permit the patient to discuss specific fears of similar prior experiences. A preexisting anxiety disorder may need to be actively treated with medication and support to assist a patient to accept appropriate treatment (see Chapter 25).

## Anxiety Symptoms

Anxiety may vary from the normal and expected concerns about illness to significant and intolerable physiological symptoms, great emotional distress, and inability to tolerate treatment. Individuals who have had panic attacks, phobias, or generalized anxiety are vulnerable to exacerbation of symptoms in the hospital; symptoms must be evaluated and treated. Medication, behavioral interventions, and support should be initiated when the diagnosis becomes clear. Coordination by the psychiatrist of treatment of preoperative anxiety with the anesthesiologist, surgeon, and floor staff can make it possible for some patients to tolerate procedures they might otherwise refuse.

## Depressive Symptoms

Although mild depressive symptoms are common with cancer, severe ones are not. When severe symptoms (hopelessness, dysphoria, insomnia, isolation, and suicidal thoughts) are present, a major depression has developed that should be evaluated and treated. Severe depression is not normal, and psychiatric assessment should be requested. Data increasingly show that depressed patients respond to treatment with antidepressants, behavioral interventions, and psychotherapy. Rapid referral of depressed patients can reduce their distress (Holland et al., 1987).

## History of Prior Psychiatric or Personality Disorder

Psychiatric consultation should be requested to evaluate the patient with a history of a major psychiatric disorder (e.g., schizophrenia or manic-depressive illness) or severe personality disorder to assess the patient's current emotional status and ability to understand treatment recommendations and to comply with treatment decisions. Evaluation should be done ideally before hospital admission or the beginning of an outpatient treatment. This is especially important when the planned treatment (e.g., bone marrow transplantation or BMT) is lengthy, complex, and requires prolonged patient cooperation. At Memorial Sloan-Kettering Cancer Center all patients are evaluated psychiatrically before BMT to allow opportunity to prepare staff for the care of a person whose mental state may pose special problems. The psychiatrist can initiate treatment immediately on admission; many potential problems can be prevented by prior planning.

## Sexual Disorders

Sexual disorders and infertility are sometimes consequences of gynecological and genitourinary surgery. Sometimes medication side effects cause impotency or sexual dysfunction. Patients are often reluctant to report symptoms or ask for help for sexual dysfunction. The physician must introduce the topic and refer patients if necessary for evaluation and treatment. Because patients with sexual dysfunction often benefit from behavioral techniques that markedly improve sexual function, introducing a psychiatrist early during the course of treatment of gynecological, prostate, or bladder cancer can legitimize the patient's concerns and encourage later work with the psychiatrist or sexual dysfunction expert. This early referral, during cancer treatment, permits exploration of problems as the patient attempts to resume normal life including sexual activities (see Chapter 33).

## Pain

Pain is experienced in 60–90% of the patients with advanced cancer. Poorly controlled pain results in high levels of anxiety and depression. Suicide attempts, some successful, are made by the patient with poorly controlled pain. Psychiatric consultations are helpful to establish the origin of the psychological distress and to suggest adjunctive means of pain control such as psychotropic drugs and behavioral interventions (see Chapter 32).

## Conflict between Patient, Family and Staff

Some patients and their families create a conflict with staff. The source of conflict is often prolonged high stress caused by illness or a family's maladaptive methods of coping with stress or relating to staff. Contentious or angry families cause staff to become defensive and finally hostile. A psychiatric consultant is often able to assess the patient, family, and staff, to assume a liaison role, and to help clarify the contributions of each. A staff conference may help to clarify and resolve issues, or a family meeting with the patient present may help to ease family distress.

## SUMMARY

The variety of responses to cancer ranges widely. At one end of the spectrum are highly adaptive reactions similar to those of individuals reacting to *any* catastrophic situation, including physical illness. Adjustment disorders differ from these normal reactions by degree of severity or duration of symptoms, which may interfere with function or produce intolerable distress. Adjustment disorders represent the border between normal and abnormal, because they are essentially an exaggeration of normal responses. Patients with an adjustment disorder often have some prior family association with cancer or some concurrent life stress that enhances the meaning of the crisis.

Psychotherapy that uses a crisis intervention model—alone or with medication prescribed for symptomatic control of anxiety and depression—is highly effective at reintegrating the patient's own ability to cope again with stresses of illness and treatment. Whereas most mental health professionals are highly effective in dealing with emotional problems of cancer patients, some urgent and medically complicated cases are best handled by a psychiatric consultant, especially with regard to suicidal threat, threat of violence, behavior suggestive of delirium, ability to consent to or refuse treatment, indecision, severe anxiety or depression, prior psychiatric or personality disorder, sexual disorder, and conflicts between patient, family, and staff.

## REFERENCES

Adler, A. (1943). Neuropsychiatric complications in victims of Boston's Coconut Grove disaster. *J.A.M.A.* 123:1098–1101.

American Psychiatric Association (1980). *Diagnostic and Statistical Manual of Mental Disorders,* 3rd ed. Washington, D.C.: American Psychiatric Association.

Bonadonna, G. and P. Valagussa, (1981). Dose–response effect of adjuvant chemotherapy in breast cancer. *N. Engl. J. Med.* 304:10–46.

Caplan, G. (1981). Mastery of stress: Psychosocial aspects. *Am. J. Psychiatry* 138:413–20.

Chamberlin, B.C. (1980). The psychological aftermath of disaster. *J. Clin. Psychiatry* 41:238–44.

Cobb, S. and E. Lindemann (1943). Neuropsychiatric observations. *Ann. Surg.* 117:814–24.

Craig, T.J. and M.D. Abeloff (1974). Psychiatric symptomatology among hospitalized cancer patients. *Am. J. Psychiatry* 131:1323–26.

Davies, P.K., D.M. Quinlan, F.P. McKegney, and C.P. Kimball (1973). Organic factors and psychological adjustment in advanced cancer patients. *Psychosom. Med.* 35:464–71.

Derogatis, L.R., G.R. Morrow, J. Fetting, D. Penman, S. Piasetsky, A.M. Schmale, M. Henrichs, and C.L.M. Carnicke, Jr. (1983). The prevalence of psychiatric disorders among cancer patients. *J.A.M.A.* 249:751–57.

Hamburg, D.A., G.V. Coehlo, and J.E. Adams (1974). Coping and adaptation: Steps toward synthesis of biological and social perspectives. In D.A. Hamburg, G.V. Coelho, and J.E. Adams (eds.), *Coping and Adaptation.* New York: Basic Books, pp. 403–41.

Holland, J.C. G. Morrow, A. Schmale, L. Derogatis, M. Spefanek, S. Berenson, P. Carpenter, W. Breitbart and M. Feldstein (1987). Reduction of anxiety and depression in cancer patients by alprazolam or by a behavioral technique. *Proc. Twenty-Third Annu. Mtg. Am. Soc. Clin. Oncol.* 6:258 (Abstract No. 1015).

Horowitz, M. (1973). Phase-oriented treatment of stress response syndromes. *Am. J. Psychother.* 27:506–15.

Horowitz, M. (1976). *Stress Responses Syndromes.* New York: Jason Aronson.

Levine, P.M., P.M. Silberfarb, and Z.J. Lipowski, (1978). Mental disorders in cancer patients: A study of 100 psychiatric referrals. *Cancer* 42:1386–91.

Lifton, R.J. (1967). *Death in Life: Survivors of Hiroshima.* New York: Random House.

Lifton, R.J. and E. Olson (1976). The human meaning of total disaster: The Buffalo Creek experience. *Psychiatry* 39:1–18.

Lindemann, L. (1944). Symptomatology and management of acute grief. *Am. J. Psychiatry,* 101:141–148.

Massie, M.J. and J.C. Holland (1987). The cancer patient with pain: Psychiatric complications and their management. *Med. Clin. North Am.* 71:243–58.

Perry, S.W. and M.M. Gilmore (1981). The disruptive patient or visitor. *J.A.M.A.* 245:755–57.

Plumb, M. and J.C. Holland (1977). Comparative studies of psychological function in patients with advanced cancer 1. Self-reported depressive symptoms. *Psychosom. Med.* 39:264—76.

Vaillant, G. (1986). Adaptation and ego mechanisms of defense. *Harvard Med. School Ment. Health Lett.* 3:4–6.

Weisman, A.D. (1976). Early diagnosis of vulnerability in cancer patients. *Am. J. Med. Sci.* 271:187–96.

Weisman, A.D. and J.W. Worden (1976). The existential plight in cancer: Significance of the first 100 days. *Int. J. Psychiatry Med.* 7:1–15.

# 23

## Depression

Mary Jane Massie

Sadness and grief are normal responses to painful life events that are associated with actual or threatened loss; they are expected emotional reactions at the time of diagnosis of cancer and at transitional points of the illness, especially during advanced stages. Because sadness and depression are so commonly seen in cancer patients, it is important to be able to distinguish between "normal" degrees of sadness and "abnormal" levels of depression in cancer patients. Hopelessness and suicidal thoughts are common symptoms of severe depression, yet at times they are understandable responses to an incurable illness such as cancer (see Chapter 24 on suicide). No aspect of the psychological state is more difficult to assess than depression, yet none is more important for clinicians to be able to evaluate. Recognition of the pathological levels of depression for which consultation is needed and for which treatment should be instituted is a critical aspect of patient care. This chapter reviews the prevalence of depression in cancer patients, the types of depressive syndromes, and principles of management.

### PREVALENCE OF DEPRESSION

To put the prevalence of depression in patients with cancer in perspective, it may be compared with the prevalence of depression in the general population. According to a multicenter NIMH study in which 10,000 individuals in three cities were interviewed, the prevalence of depression in the general population was found to be 6% (Locke and Regier, 1985) (Table 23-1). Thus, a small number (~6%) of cancer patients can be expected to have a preexisting affective disorder, which places them at increased risk of depression during the course of cancer. Indeed, the studies of Plumb and Holland (1977, 1981) confirmed the presence of a history of prior depressive illness among a group of severely depressed patients with cancer.

The frequency of depression in cancer patients has been the subject of numerous studies, and the reported rates have ranged from as high as 58% (Hinton, 1972) to as low as 4.5% (Lansky et al., 1985). Table 23-2 shows results of nine studies of the frequency of depression in cancer patients who were assessed by clinician and/or self-report rating scales. In reviewing these nine studies of cancer patient populations that varied by stages and sites, the highest frequency of depression is reported in studies that depended on clinician reports of the spectrum of depressive symptoms with absence of defined diagnostic criteria for depression, in those that studied patients with advanced stages of disease, and in those that studied patients with more severe levels of illness (e.g., hospitalized patients). The symptom with the strongest relationship to clinical depression is physical performance measured by the Karnofsky scale (Bukberg et al., 1984). Bukberg and colleagues reported that of the patients who scored 40 or less on the Karnofsky scale (the most severely disabled), 77% met the criteria for major depression. Only 23% of those with scores above 60 (better physical function) had major depression (Table 23-3).

Derogatis and colleagues (1983) and Lansky and colleagues (1985) report the lowest rates of affective disorders: 13% and 4.5%, respectively. Both research groups utilized predefined criteria for diagnosis of major depression and adjustment disorder with depressed mood in patient populations that included ambulatory patients with good physical performance status.

The Derogatis and co-workers (PSYCOG) study randomly accessed 215 hospitalized and ambulatory patients at the three major cancer centers (Johns Hopkins, Rochester, and Memorial Sloan-Kettering Cancer Center). Trained clinical interviewers diagnosed psychiatric disorders using DSM-III criteria. Of the 47% who met the criteria for psychiatric disorder,

**Table 23-1** Prevalence of mental disorders in physically healthy individuals: NIMH multicenter study

| Disorder | Percentage |
|---|---|
| Anxiety disorders | 8.3% |
| Alcohol or drug abuse/dependence | 6.4 |
| Affective disorders | 6.0 |
| Schizophrenia | 1.0 |
| Antisocial personality | 0.9 |
| Severe cognitive impairment | 1.0 |

*Source*: Adapted from B.Z. Locke and D.A. Regier (1985). Prevalence of selected mental disorders. In C.A. Taube & S.A. Barrett (Eds.), *Mental Health United States* 1985, (pp. 1–6). Rockville, MD: National Institute of Mental Health.

68% had adjustment disorder with depressed or anxious mood and 13% had a major affective disorder including unipolar depression, bipolar depression, atypical depression, and dysthymic disorder. The remainder of patients with psychiatric disorder had organic mental disorder (8%), personality disorder (7%), and anxiety disorders (4%). Thus, depressive spectrum symptoms ranging from depressed mood to major depression constituted the most frequent diagnosis made, but major depression was less often diagnosed. Lansky and co-workers (1985) found an even lower rate of major depression (4.5%) among predominantly ambulatory female cancer patients, using carefully controlled Hamilton Depression Scale ratings to eliminate physical symptoms.

In the past, depression was generally thought to be greater in patients with cancer than in those with other medical illnesses. However, two studies of depression in hospitalized medical patients (including a few cancer patients) report a frequency of depression of 22–24% (Schwab et al., 1967; Moffic and Paykel, 1975) (Table 23-4), roughly comparable to the frequency of 20–25% found in several of the studies of hospitalized cancer patients, many with advanced disease (Bukberg et al., 24%; Plumb and Holland, 20–23%; Koenig et

**Table 23-2** Nine studies of depression in cancer patients

| Reference | Number | Site and stage | Method* | Percentage of depression | Special findings |
|---|---|---|---|---|---|
| Koenig et al. (1967) | 36 | Advanced bowel cancer; hospitalized | MMPI | 25 | |
| Peck and Boland (1972) | 50 | Ambulatory radiotherapy patients; all sites, all stages | Clinical interview | 10 Severe 32 Moderate 32 Mild | |
| Craig and Abeloff (1973) | 30 | All sites: advanced; hospitalized | SCL-90 | 50 | |
| Plumb and Holland (1977) | 97 | All sites; advanced stage; hospitalized | BDI | 23 | 19% Moderate severity 4% Severe |
| Plumb and Holland (1981) | 80 | All sites; advanced stage; hospitalized | Structured interview; Current and Past Psychologic Adjustment Scale | 20 | 12% Suicidal ideation; most severely depressed had prior history of depression |
| Derogatis et al. (1983) | 215 | All stages; half ambulatory, half hospitalized | DSM-III diagnostic criteria of major depression | 13 | Three-center study (Rochester, Johns Hopkins, Memorial Hospital) |
| Bukberg et al. (1984) | 67 | Hospitalized on medical oncology units | Modified DSM-III criteria (eliminating physical symptoms) | 24 Severe 18 Moderate 14 Some depressive symptoms 44 None | Correlation with more physical impairment; HDS correlated best with DSM-III diagnosis |
| Lansky et al. (1985) | 500 | Largely ambulatory; all women; gynecological cancer, stage I and II disease, breast, bowel, melanoma | DSM-III HDS (rated only for nonmedically-related symptoms) Zung Depression Scale | 4.5 (DSM-III) 5.3 (HDS and Zung) | |
| Evans et al. (1986) | 83 | All hospitalized women with gynecoogical cancer (excluding ovarian) | DSM-III HDS | 23 Major depression 24 Adjustment disorder depressed mood | |

*BDI, Beck Depression Inventory; HDS, Hamilton Depression Scale; SCL-90, Hopkins Symptom Checklist-90.

**Table 23-3** Rate of depression by physical performance status

| Karnofsky score | Depressed* | Not depressed |
|---|---|---|
| 0–40 | 10(77%) | 3(23%) |
| 41–60 | 8(57%) | 6(43%) |
| 61–100 | 8(23%) | 27(77%) |

*Comparison of Karnofsky scores for depressed and not depressed conditions was significant ($p < 0.001$).

*Source*: Reprinted with permission from J. Bukberg, D. Penman, and J.C. Holland (1984). Depression in hospitalized cancer patients. *Psychosom. Med.* 46:199–212.

al., 25%). These data strongly suggest that cancer patients are no more depressed than equally physically ill patients with other diseases.

Bukberg, Penman, and Holland (1984) conducted an extensive study of depression in hospitalized cancer patients that included opportunity to compare findings on different rating scales with clinical judgment. Using both DSM-III criteria that were modified to eliminate physical symptoms characteristic of cancer, and validated observer rating scales (Hamilton Rating Scale, Beck Depression Inventory), they found that 24% of the 62 patients studied were severely depressed, 18% were moderately depressed, 14% had some depressive symptoms. No depression at all showed in 44%, despite being hospitalized for treatment in a cancer research hospital. The depressive symptoms were a continuum from mild to severe, roughly comparable to criteria for adjustment disorder with depressed mood to major depression. Bukberg and colleagues also examined methodological issues in studying depression and found that the Hamilton Rating Scale for Depression most accurately correlated with clinical observation of depression, although in advanced illness it becomes extremely difficult to assign symptoms clearly to being of medical or psychological origin.

These studies suggest that among hospitalized patients with significant levels of physical impairment, at least 25% are likely to meet criteria for major depression or adjustment disorder with depressed mood. Thus a significant number of patients need to be recog-

nized by oncology staff as being depressed and needing therapeutic intervention. The myths that "*all* cancer patients are depressed" and "don't bother to treat depression, patients *should* be depressed" are not borne out by the data.

## DIAGNOSIS OF DEPRESSION IN PSYCHIATRIC CONSULTATIONS

The other major source of information about depression in the medically ill (Wallen et al., 1987), and specifically in cancer, comes from consultation studies (Hinton, 1972; Levine et al., 1978; Massie et al., 1979; Massie and Holland, 1987) (Table 23-5). Wallen and co-workers (1987) reviewed data on 263,000 patients hospitalized in 327 general hospitals and reported that approximately 24% of patients who received a psychiatric consultation were diagnosed as having depression. Data from cancer hospitals shows a somewhat higher frequency of diagnosis of depression made by psychiatric consultants. Hinton's early study (1972) of terminally ill patients found 58% with a diagnosis of depression. Levine and co-workers (1978) reviewed diagnoses of 100 hospitalized cancer patients with all stages and sites of diseases seen in psychiatric consultation and reported that 56% of patients were depressed. Massie and colleagues (1979) reported data on consultations on 334 hospitalized cancer patients. Using DSM-II criteria, 49% were diagnosed as having depression, and of this percentage, 70% had reactive depression. Patients with poorly controlled pain and patients in the advanced stage of the disease were the most depressed.

Massie and Holland (1988) have reviewed psychiatric consultations on 546 patients (446 inpatients, 100 outpatients) at Memorial Sloan-Kettering Cancer Center. Diagnoses were made using DSM-III criteria. The most common reason for referral for psychiatric consultation was depression and/or suicidal risk (59%). Advanced cancer (stage III or IV) was present in 77% of patients. Major depression was seen in 20% (single episode, 39 patients; recurrent episode, 10 patients) and adjustment disorder with depressed mood in 27%. Depressive-spectrum symptoms are the most frequent

**Table 23-4** Studies of depression in hospitalized medical patients

| Reference | Number | Patients | Method | Percentage of depression |
|---|---|---|---|---|
| Schwab et al. (1967) | 153 | Hospitalized; all diagnoses | Hamilton Depression Index; Beck Depression Inventory | 22 |
| Moffic and Paykel (1975) | 150 | Hospitalized; all diagnoses | Beck Depression Inventory | 24 |

**Table 23-5**   Psychiatric consultation studies of depression in cancer patients

| Reference | Number | Site and stage | Method | Percentage of depression | Special findings |
|---|---|---|---|---|---|
| Hinton (1972) | 50 | Terminally ill | Interview | 58 | 42% Anxious<br>10% Confusional state |
| Levine et al. (1978) | 100 | All stages; all sites; hospitalized | Interview; DSM-II criteria | 56 | Two times greater referral of patients with breast cancer |
| Massie et al. (1979) | 334 | All stages; all sites; hospitalized and ambulatory | Interview; DSM-II criteria | 49 | Includes adjustment disorder with depressed mood<br>DSM-II: 70% reactive depression |
| Massie and Holland (1987) | 546 | All stages; all sites; hospitalized and ambulatory | Interview; DSM-III criteria | 27 Adjustment disorder with depressed or mixed mood<br>20 Major depression<br>1 Bipolar | |

types of distress, and the most common reasons for asking for psychiatric consultation.

## VULNERABILITY TO DEPRESSION

With data from studies and extensive clinical observation, it is now possible to predict which patients are at highest risk for depression (Table 23-6).The influences that increase the risk of depression are history of affective disorder or alcoholism, advanced stages of cancer (especially pancreatic cancer) (Holland et al., 1986), poorly controlled pain (Massie and Holland, 1987), and treatment with medications or concurrent illnesses that produce depressive symptoms.

Numerous commonly prescribed medications can produce symptoms of depression, including methyldopa, reserpine, barbiturates, diazepam, and propranolol. Of the many cancer chemotherapeutic agents, depressive symptoms are produced by relatively few, including vincristine, vinblastine, procarbazine, L-asparaginase, amphotericin-B, interferon (Holland et al., 1974; Young, 1982; Weddington, 1982). The glucocorticosteroids prednisone and dexamethasone, which are widely used in cancer as a critical component of standard treatments, in cancer pain management, and to reduce edema from brain and spinal cord tumors, can cause psychiatric disturbances ranging from minor mood disturbances to steroid psychosis. Mood changes resulting from steroids include a sense of well-being, emotional lability, euphoria, or depression, sometimes with suicidal ideation (Hall et al., 1979). Depressive symptoms resulting from cancer chemotherapy and steroids can be severe, and because continuation of the drugs causing depression is

**Table 23-6**   Influences placing patients at greater risk of depression

| Category | Influence |
|---|---|
| Personal | History of depression (patient or family)<br>History of alcoholism |
| Illness and treatment | Advanced stages of cancer<br>Poorly controlled pain<br>Medications<br>  Corticosteroids<br>    Prednisone, dexamethasone<br>  Other chemotherapeutic agents<br>    Vincristine, vinblastine, procarbazine, L-asparaginase, interferon, amphotericin-B<br>  Other medications<br>    Cimetidine<br>    Diazepam<br>    Indomethacin<br>    Levodopa<br>    Methyldopa<br>    Pentazocine<br>    Phenmetrazine<br>    Phenobarbital<br>    Propranolol<br>    Rauwolfia alkaloids<br>    Estrogens<br>  Other medical conditions that cause depression<br>    Metabolic<br>    Nutritional<br>    Endocrine<br>    Neurological |

usually absolutely necessary, the psychiatrist often treats severe depressive symptoms with antidepressants. Steroids can cause an organic affective syndrome that mimics a psychotic depression but abates when steroids are stopped. In some cases treatment with neuroleptics and/or antidepressants is required.

Many metabolic, nutritional, endocrine, and neurological disorders produce symptoms that can be mistaken for depression (Hall et al., 1978). Cancer patients with abnormal serum levels of potassium, sodium, or calcium may appear depressed, as can patients who are febrile, anemic, or deficient in such vitamins as folate or $B_{12}$. Hypothyroidism, hyperparathyroidism, and adrenal insufficiency must be considered in the differential diagnosis of the depressed cancer patient; if they are present, appropriate treatment should be instituted.

## CLINICAL PICTURE

The normal response to hearing the diagnosis of cancer is sadness about the loss of health as well as about anticipated losses, including death. This normal response is part of a spectrum of depressive symptoms that range from normal sadness to adjustment disorder with depressed mood to major depression. Figure 22-1 (see overview, Chapter 22) outlines this spectrum, showing its continuous rather than categorical nature. There are variations in the levels of depressive symptoms at the "normal" end of the spectrum. Symptoms are minimal when stresses are few but may become severe when a crisis occurs. If the symptoms become more severe and interfere with daily activity, an adjustment disorder with depressed mood is diagnosed. If this reactive state evolves to include more severe symptoms, then criteria for a major depression may be met.

The clinical evaluation includes careful assessment of symptoms, mental status, physical status, treatment effects, and laboratory data. The clinician obtains a history of previous depressive episodes, family history of depression or suicide, concurrent life stresses, and the availability of social support. It is essential to assess what the illness means to the patient, as well as his or her understanding of the medical situation. In our experience, the dexamethasone suppression test (DST) and the thyrotropin-releasing hormone (TRH) test are not useful as screening tests for depression in cancer patients. Table 23-7 outlines the aspects of clinical evaluation of depression to be considered.

One major caveat for diagnosis of depression in cancer is important: the diagnosis of depression in physically healthy patients depends heavily on symptoms of anorexia, insomnia, loss of energy, fatigue, weight loss, psychomotor slowing, and decreased interest in

**Table 23-7** Evaluation of depression in the cancer patient

| Evaluative category | Findings |
|---|---|
| Family history | Depression |
| | Suicide |
| Personal history | Previous psychiatric illness (depression or manic episodes, alcoholism, drug abuse) |
| | Suicide attempt |
| Signs and symptoms | Psychological |
| |     Dysphoric mood (e.g., sad, depressed, anxious, crying); diurnal mood change |
| |     Feelings of hopelessness, helplessness |
| |     Loss of interest and pleasure |
| |     Guilt, burden on others, worthlessness |
| |     Poor concentration |
| |     Mood incongruent to disease outlook |
| |     Suicidal thoughts or plans |
| |     Delusional thoughts (psychotic symptoms rare, except in organic affective syndrome) |
| | Somatic (less value in more physically impaired patients) |
| |     Insomnia |
| |     Anorexia and weight loss |
| |     Fatigue |
| |     Psychomotor retardation or agitation |
| |     Constipation |
| |     Decreased libido |

sex. Of course these indicators have less value as diagnostic criteria for depression in a cancer patient because they are common to both cancer and depression. In the study by Plumb and Holland (1977), which utilized the Beck Depression Inventory, the contribution of possible cancer-related physical symptoms to total score was apparent when the somatic items were examined separately from the psychological items. Thus, depression in cancer patients is best evaluated by the severity of dysphoric mood, the degree of the feelings of hopelessness, guilt, and worthlessness, and the presence of suicidal thoughts.

Included in the following Chapter 24 is a discussion of the difficulty of evaluating suicidal statements in patients with advanced or terminal disease. Suicidal ideation always requires careful assessment to determine whether talk of suicide is a symptom of depression, or the talk of suicide is one way the patient expresses the wish to have ultimate control over intolerable symptoms. Individuals at higher risk of suicide include those with prior psychiatric history, personality disorder, a history of previous suicide attempts or a family history of suicide, a history of recent death of friends or spouse, a history of alcohol abuse, and few social supports. Poorly controlled pain is a significant contributor to risk, as is having just received information about a grave prognosis (Breitbart, 1987).

## MANAGEMENT OF DEPRESSION IN THE CANCER PATIENT

The cancer patient is most effectively managed through the consistent emotional support given by the physician with whom there is a trusting relationship. Psychiatric consultation should be considered when depressive symptoms last longer than a week, when they worsen rather than improve, or when they interfere with the patient's ability to function or to cooperate with treatment. The psychiatric intervention most often used is short-term supportive psychotherapy based on a crisis intervention model. The goals of psychotherapy are to help the patient regain a sense of self-worth, to correct misconceptions about the past and present, and to integrate the present illness into a continuum of life experiences. The patient becomes aware of and must adjust to the need to modify plans for the future and to accept new limitations. Psychotherapy emphasizes past strengths, supports previously successful ways of coping, and mobilizes inner resources. Between 4 and 10 sessions are usually sufficient to reduce symptoms to a tolerable level, but the length of therapy must be tailored to individual patient needs. Additional beneficial approaches involve having a family member in the therapy setting and having the patient attend a group with others who share similar problems (see Chapter 38).

Prolonged and severe depressive symptoms usually require treatment that combines psychotherapy with somatic treatment (medication or electroconvulsive therapy). The following case illustrates the treatment of depression in a patient just diagnosed as having cancer.

### CASE REPORT

A 45-year-old divorced executive was referred for psychiatric consultation by her surgeon while she was in the process of deciding whether to have bilateral mastectomy or breast conserving surgery and radiotherapy. She reported the onset of symptoms of depression (insomnia, anorexia, decreased libido, fatigue, irritability and decreased concentration) coincided with the diagnosis of having cancer. She had a history of one episode of major depression 15 years previously, when she was divorcing her husband. This episode had been successfully treated with amitriptyline and brief supportive psychotherapy.

Because of her symptoms of depression, she was having trouble deciding which treatment option was best. She was started on amitriptyline 50 mg. po qHS and her dose was increased to 125 mg Q.D. over 3 weeks. After one month of pharmacotherapy, psychotherapy and meeting with several

breast cancer specialists, her symptoms had improved; she was able to select her treatment (bilateral mastectomy) and underwent surgery. She continued amitriptyline for four months after all symptoms remitted; amitriptyline was then slowly tapered and discontinued. She continued psychotherapy for a year, considering other life problems (e.g., work, relationship problems) and preparing herself for bilateral breast reconstruction, which she underwent successfully.

The use of antidepressants is discussed fully in Chapter 39. The antidepressants most commonly used for cancer patients are the tricyclic antidepressants (e.g., amitriptyline, doxepin, imipramine, nortriptyline, and protriptyline). Tricyclic antidepressants are started in low doses (25–50 mg) given at bedtime, and are increased slowly over days to weeks until the symptoms improve (usually the peak dose is lower than that tolerated by physically healthy patients). Depressed patients with insomnia and psychomotor agitation often rapidly benefit from the effects of the sedating tricyclics; however, improvement in mood is often not noted for several weeks. Patients need continued encouragement, support, and understanding during the period before antidepressant effect is seen.

The family of the depressed cancer patient is often distressed by the patient's depressive symptoms, perceiving the patient to have "given up" or believing symptoms of depression indicate the cancer is worsening. Family members, as well as the patient, need to hear the psychiatrist explain both the biological (if present) and psychological influences contributing to the depressed mood, plans for interventions, and the anticipated timing of the response to treatment. Because continued family support is essential for the patient's well-being, the psychiatrist will need to inform, encourage, and reassure the family.

Most depressed cancer patients are treated as outpatients or on medical oncology units; rarely is transfer to a psychiatric unit necessary or feasible. In most hospitals, psychiatric units are for physically healthy ambulatory patients, and acutely medically ill depressed cancer patients cannot receive adequate medical or surgical care on such units. If suicidal risk is present in a hospitalized cancer patient, we arrange for 24-hour nursing companions to monitor suicidal thinking and provide continued observation of and support for the patient. The need for companions is evaluated daily; companions are discontinued when suicidal thinking is no longer evident.

The cancer patient who has had a depressive episode before or during cancer illness should receive special monitoring by the oncologist throughout cancer treatment. If symptoms of depression recur, the patient should be rapidly referred for psychiatric consultation.

## ELECTROCONVULSIVE THERAPY

Occasionally, but rarely, electroconvulsive therapy (ECT) is given to depressed cancer patients. The efficacy of ECT has been established most convincingly for the treatment of delusional and severe endogenous depressions (NIMH Consensus Development Conference Statement, 1985). ECT is not effective for patients with milder depressions (e.g., dysthymic disorder and adjustment disorder with depressed mood). Unfortunately, ECT still has an unfavorable reputation in the general public, and severely physically ill cancer patients (and their families) often are extremely reluctant to consider this form of therapy. Depressed cancer patients in whom ECT should be considered are those with life-threatening depressions (delusional or endogenous depressions) with symptoms that include refusal to eat, mutism, or severe suicidal ideation, and those who have responded well to ECT in the past and/or who are unable to tolerate the effects of antidepressant medication or in whom antidepressants are ineffective. The only absolute contraindication to ECT is increased intracranial pressure; space-occupying lesions in the brain and recent myocardial infarction are relative contraindications. The most troublesome side effect of ECT is short-term memory loss (both anterograde and retrograde amnesia), which can be minimized by the use of unilateral ECT on the nondominant hemisphere. Between 6 and 12 treatments are usually effective, and the usual frequency is three times weekly. ECT is sometimes given on an outpatient basis; however, most physically ill cancer patients are hospitalized to provide special monitoring of their condition while they are receiving ECT. Following ECT most patients are maintained on tricyclics or lithium to reduce relapse. Bidder (1981) and Dubovsky (1986) have comprehensively reviewed the usefulness of ECT in the medically ill, including its usefulness in patients with neurological disease.

## SUMMARY

The nature and prevalence of the spectrum of depressive disorders in cancer patients is now known. It is essential that clinicians accurately diagnose depressive disorders, correct (if possible) organic influences that contribute to a depressed mood, and utilize psychotherapeutic and psychopharmacological interventions for the depressed patient.

## REFERENCES

Bidder, T.G. (1981). Electroconvulsive therapy in the medically ill patient. *Psychiatr. Clin. North Am.* 4:391–405.

Breitbart, W. (1987). Suicide and cancer. *Oncology* 1:49–54.

Bukberg, J., D. Penman, and J.C. Holland (1984). Depression in hospitalized cancer patients. *Psychosom. Med.* 46:199–212.

Craig, T.J. and M.D. Abeloff (1974). Psychiatric symptomatology among hospitalized cancer patients. *Am. J. Psychiatry* 131:1323–27.

Derogatis, L.R., G.R. Morrow, J. Fetting, D. Penman, S. Piasetsky, A.M. Schmale, M. Hendricks, and C. Carnicke (1983). The prevalence of psychiatric disorders among cancer patients. *J.A.M.A.* 249:751–57.

Dubovsky, S.L. (1986). Using electroconvulsive therapy for patients with neurological disease. *Hosp. Commun. Psychiatry* 37:819–25.

Electroconvulsive therapy (1985). *Consensus Dev. Conf. Statement* 5(11), National Institute of Mental Health.

Evans, D.L., C.F. McCartney, C.B. Nemeroff, D. Raft, D. Quade, R. N. Golden, J.J. Haggerty, V. Holmes, J.S. Simon, M. Droba, G.A. Mason, and W.C. Fowler (1986). Depression in women treated for gynecological cancer: Clinical and neuroendocrine assessment. *Am. J. Psychiatry* 143:447–52.

Hall, R.C.W., M.K. Popkin, R.A. Devaul, L.A. Faillace, and S.K. Stickney (1978). Physical illness presenting as psychiatric disease. *Arch. Gen. Psychiatry* 35:1315–20.

Hall, R.C.W., M.K. Popkin, S.K. Stickney, and E.R. Gardner (1979). Presentation of the steroid psychoses. *J. Nerv. Ment. Dis.* 167:229–36.

Hinton, J. (1972). Psychiatric consultation in fatal illness. *Proc. R. Soc. Med.* 65:29–32.

Holland, J., S. Fasanello, and T. Ohnuma (1974). Psychiatric symptoms associated with L-asparaginase administration. *J. Psychiatr. Res.* 10:165.

Holland, J.C., A. Hughes Korzun, S. Tross, P. Silberfarb, M. Perry, R. Comis, and M. Oster (1986). Comparative psychological disturbance in pancreatic and gastric cancer. *Am. J. Psychiatry* 143:982–86.

Koenig, R., S.M. Levin, and M.J. Brennan (1967). The emotional status of cancer patient as measured by a psychological test. *J. Chron. Dis.* 20:923–30.

Lansky, S.B., M.A. List, C.A. Herrmann, E.G. Ets-Hokin, T.K. DasGupta, G.D. Wilbanks, and F.R. Hendrickson (1985). Absence of major depressive disorder in female cancer patients. *J. Clin. Oncol.* 3:1553–60.

Levine, P., P.M. Silberfarb, and Z.J. Lipowski (1978). Mental disorders in cancer patients. *Cancer* 42:1385–91.

Locke, B.Z. and D.A. Regier (1985). Prevalence of selected mental disorders. In C.A. Taube and S.A. Barrett (Eds.), *Mental Health United States 1985*, (pp. 1–6). Rockville, MD: National Institute of Mental Health.

Massie, M.J. and J.C. Holland (1984). Diagnosis and treatment of depression in the cancer patient. *J. Clin. Psychiatry* 45(3, Sec. 2):25–28.

Massie, M.J. and J.C. Holland (1987). The cancer patient with pain: Psychiatric complications and their management. *Med. Clin. North Am.* 71:243–48.

Massie, M.J. and J.C. Holland (1988). Consultation and liaison issues in cancer care. *Psychiatr. Med.* 5:343–359.

Massie, M.J., J.G. Gorzynski, R. Mastrovito, D. Theis, and J. Holland (1979). The diagnosis of depression in hospitalized patients with cancer. *Proc. Am. Soc. Clin. Oncol.* 20:432 (Abstract No. C-587).

Moffic, H. and E.S. Paykel (1975). Depression in medical inpatients. *Br. J. Psychiatry* 126:346–53.

Peck, A. and L. Boland (1972). Emotional reaction to having cancer. *Am. J. Roentgenol. Rad. Ther. Nucl. Med.* 114:591–599.

Peteet, J.R. (1979). Depression in cancer patients. An approach to differential diagnosis and treatment. *J.A.M.A.* 241(14):1487–89.

Plumb, M.M. and J. Holland (1977). Comparative studies of psychological function in patients with advanced cancer—I. Self-reported depressive symptoms. *Psychosom. Med.* 39(4):264–76.

Plumb, M.M. and J.C. Holland (1981). Comparative studies of psychological function in patients with advanced cancer: II. Interviewer-rated current and past psychological symptoms. *Psychosom. Med.* 43:243–54.

Rodin, G. and K. Voshart (1986). Depression in the medically ill: An overview. *Am. J. Psychiatry* 14:696–705.

Schwab, J.J., M. Bialow, J.M. Brown, and C.E. Holzer (1967). Diagnosing depression in medical inpatients. *Ann. Intern. Med.* 67(4):695–707.

Silberfarb, P.M., J.C.B. Holland, D. Anbar, G. Bahna, H. Maurer, A.P. Chahinian, and R. Comis (1983). Psychological response of patients receiving two drug regimens for lung carcinoma. *Am. J. Psychiatry* 140:110–11.

Wallen, J., H.A. Pincus, H.H. Goldman, and S.E. Marcus (1987). Psychiatric consultations in short-term general hospitals. *Arch. Gen. Psychiatry* 44:163–68.

Weddington, W.W. (1982). Delirium and depression associated with amphotericin B. *Psychosomatics* 23:1076–78.

Young, D.F. (1982). Neurological complications of cancer chemotherapy. In A. Silverstein (ed.), *Neurological Complications of Therapy: Selected Topics*. New York: Futura Publishing, pp. 57–113.

# 24

## Suicide

### William Breitbart

The health care professional in the oncology setting faces a dilemma when confronting the issue of suicide in the cancer patient. From the medical perspective, professional training reinforces the view of suicide as a manifestation of psychiatric disturbance to be prevented at all costs. However, from the philosophical perspective, many in our society view suicide in those who face the distress of an often fatal disease like cancer as "rational" and a means to regain control and maintain a "dignified death" (Kastenbaum, 1976; Roman, 1980; Siegel and Tuckel, 1984). An internal debate thus often takes place in the cancer care professional that is not dissimilar from the public debate that surrounds celebrated legal cases in which the rights of patients to terminate life-sustaining measures are at issue (Annas, 1984; Kane, 1985). Interest in these public issues, as well as heightened concern for the psychological needs of patients with advanced cancer raised by the thanatology and hospice movements, has served to focus new attention on the subject of suicide in cancer patients. The question for the clinician remains how reasonably and responsibly to identify and manage the cancer patient who is a suicide risk.

## SUICIDE AND CANCER

### Incidence

Although many cancer patients hold suicide as an option, often to retain some sense of control, there is a consensus that remarkably few actually commit suicide (Holland, 1978; Bolund, 1985a,b; Forman, 1979). In fact, there has been a misleading mythology about cancer patients suggesting that they never commit suicide. Adding to this confusion are various studies indicating that the incidence of suicide in cancer ranges from much the same as in the general population (Danto, 1972; Fox et al., 1982) to 2–10 times as

frequent (Campbell, 1966; Dorpat et al., 1968; Louhivuori and Hakama, 1979; Sainsbury, 1975; Whitlock, 1978). Early studies examined the prevalence of cancer among suicidal deaths and reported rates ranging from 1 to 23% (Dorpat, 1968; Pollack, 1957; Stewart and Leeds, 1960; Reich and Kelly, 1976; Marshall et al., 1983; Farberow et al., 1971; Achte and Vaukonnen, 1971a,b). In a Veterans Administration (VA) Hospital survey, Farberow and co-workers found cancer significantly overrepresented among suicides, accounting for 17% of all suicides, while a cancer diagnosis constituted only 6% of admissions (Farberow et al., 1971). Other recent studies from Finland (Louhivuori and Hakama, 1979), Connecticut (Fox et al., 1982), and Sweden (Bolund, 1985a,b) suggest that, while relatively few cancer patients commit suicide, they are at increased risk (see Table 24-1). The frequency of passive suicide and the degree to which noncompliance or treatment refusal represents a deliberate decision to end life is unknown. The actual incidence of suicide in cancer is likely underestimated, especially because families are reluctant to report death by suicide in those circumstances (Holland, 1978).

### Demographics

Men with cancer are clearly at increased risk of suicide relative to the general population, with a relative risk as high as 2.3 (Bolund, 1985a,b; Louhivuori and Hakama, 1979; Fox et al., 1982). Although Fox and co-workers did not find women to be at increased risk, Louhivuori's Finnish study found a relative risk of 1.9 in women and only 1.3 in men. In Scandinavian studies, suicide in men with cancer peaked at around age 70 (Louhivuori and Hakama, 1979; Bolund, 1985a,b). Farberow and co-workers (1963) found a bimodal distribution of age with one peak of cancer suicide con-

**Table 24-1** Studies on incidence of suicide among cancer patients

| Studies | Total suicides in cancer patients | Total cancer deaths | Risk relative to general population (1.0 = normal risk) Men | Women |
|---|---|---|---|---|
| Finland (Louhivuori and Hakama, 1979) | 63 | 28,857 | 1.3 | 1.9 |
| United States (Fox et al., 1982) | 192 | 144,530 | 2.3 | 0.9 |
| Sweden (Bolund, 1985a,b) | 22 | 19,000 | — | — |

**Table 24-2** Sites of cancer associated with suicide

| Studies | Primary sites |
|---|---|
| United States | |
| Weisman (1976) | Oral, urogenital |
| Farberow et al. (1971) | Tongue, larynx, lung |
| Farberow et al. (1963) | Lymphoma, leukemia (<45 years) Lung, bronchus, trachea, intestine (45–65 years) Pharynx, larynx (>65 years) |
| Breitbart (1987) | Kaposi's sarcoma/AIDS, urogenital, breast, lymphoma |
| Scandinavia | |
| Finland (Louhiuvori and Hakama, 1979) | Gastrointestinal, urogenital, breast |
| Norway (Olafssen, 1982) | Breast, prostate |
| Sweden (Bolund, 1985a,b) | Oral, pharyngeal, stomach, renal (men) Ovarian, breast (women) Gastrointestinal (both sexes) |

sisting of patients under 45 years of age and another 60 or older.

The choice of method of suicide is most often related to the methods that are available to an individual, and is characteristic of particular groups. Despite the early studies suggesting that cancer patients do not use analgesics and sedatives to commit suicide (Farberow et al., 1963), it is clear that this in fact is the most common method of suicide in the cancer patient (Bolund, 1985a,b). This method is used by more than 50% of women, but fewer than 25% of men. Men tend to utilize more violent methods, such as hanging, jumping, and shooting. Hospitalized patients use similar violent methods to a greater extent than those at home. Most cancer suicides take place at home, with the majority of cases being discovered by a family member or relative. A suicide note was found in 33% of the deaths in the Swedish study, using such phrases as "forgive me," "try to understand," and "cannot go on suffering" (Bolund, 1985a,b; Holland, 1978).

## Site of Cancer

The question of whether particular sites of cancer are associated with an increased risk of suicide has been the subject of considerable speculation (Farberow et al., 1963, 1971; Holland, 1978; Louhivuori and Hakama, 1979; Bolund, 1985a,b; Olafssen, 1982; Weisman, 1976) (Table 24-2). Indeed, growing evidence supports the finding of frequent oral, pharyngeal, and lung cancers among cancer suicides (Weisman, 1976; Bolund, 1985a,b). In an 8-year study of all suicides in men in VA hospitals, 50% had cancer of the larynx, tongue, or lung (Farberow et al., 1971). These sites of cancer are often associated with prolonged and heavy use of tobacco and alcohol, and also have profound psychological impact due to disfigurement and impaired function (Holland, 1978).

Heavy smoking and drinking may identify a vulnerable group who have limited coping skills and who may be more prone to use suicide as a coping strategy when faced with the stress of cancer. Gastrointestinal, urogenital, and breast cancers have also been reported to have increased incidence especially in Scandinavian studies (Louhivuori and Hakama, 1979; Bolund, 1985a,b; Olafssen, 1982; Weisman, 1976).

Age-specific, sex-specific, and culture-specific influences play a role in which sites of cancer are associated with increased risk of suicide. Farberow and coworkers (1963) found a distribution of sites among suicides based on age, with cancer of the pharynx and larynx predominating in those 65 or older, lymphomas and leukemias in those under 45, and lung and gastrointestinal cancers in the 45–64 age group. Perhaps reflecting more recent trends, a 1986 review of our psychiatric consultation data at Memorial Sloan-Kettering Cancer Center (MSKCC) of 71 suicidal patients revealed that Kaposi's sarcoma in patients with AIDS was the single most common cancer diagnosis (see Table 24-4). This suggests what we see clinically, that AIDS is viewed as a devastating disease often occurring in individuals who are grieving for friends who have died of the same disease. Those in the intravenous drug abuse group may have preexisting psychological difficulties that predispose them to maladaptive coping strategies.

Pancreatic cancer patients who are reported to have increased incidence of depression (Holland et al., 1986), and those with tumors that secrete hormones or

**Table 24-3**  Cancer suicide vulnerability variables

- Advanced illness and poor prognosis
- Depression and hopelessness
- Pain
- Delirium
- Control and helplessness
- Preexisting psychopathology
- Prior suicide history, personal or family
- Exhaustion and fatigue

other substances (e.g., serotonin-secreting carcinoid tumors, in light of recent evidence of serotonin's role in depression and suicide in particular), are surprisingly not overrepresented (Van Praag, 1982).

## IDENTIFYING THE CANCER PATIENT AT RISK

Identifying the cancer patient who is at increased risk for suicide is the first step in prevention, and allows for appropriate psychosocial interventions to be initiated (Forman, 1979). The constellation of variables that can influence suicidal behavior in cancer patients has been of great interest, and researchers have compiled lists of vulnerabilities that contribute to high suicide potential (Farberow et al., 1963; Weisman, 1976). Utilizing this body of information in addition to our clinical experience at Memorial Sloan-Kettering Hospital, the following characteristics (Table 24-3) are predictors of increased suicide risk in the cancer patient, especially when most or all are present. These characteristics should be incorporated into the assessment of suicide potential, and used as a framework for intervention in order to provide alternatives to suicide.

### Advanced Illness and Poor Prognosis

Cancer patients commit suicide most frequently in the advanced states of disease (Holland et al., 1978; Bolund, 1985a,b; Fox et al., 1982; Louhivuori and Hakama, 1979; Farberow et al., 1963). Of the suicides studied by Farberow, 86% occurred in the preterminal or terminal stages of illness, despite greatly reduced physical capacity (Farberow et al., 1963). Poor prognosis and advanced illness usually coincide, so it is not surprising that in Sweden those who were expected to die within a matter of months were the most likely to commit suicide. Of 88 cancer suicides, 8 had a good prognosis, 14 had an uncertain prognosis, and 45 had a poor prognosis (Bolund, 1985a,b). It is important to note that there may be a difference in the view of the prognosis between the physician and patient. Those

with advanced illness are in a particularly vulnerable position in regard to suicide risk because of the frequent coexistence of additional symptoms including pain, delirium, depression, and fatigue, as will be described (Foley, 1985; Massie et al., 1983; Bukberg et al., 1984).

### CASE REPORT

A 29-year-old white male musician with widely metastatic malignant melanoma developed spinal cord compression and was treated with high-dose steroids. Despite aggressive treatment the disease progressed, resulting in paraplegia, difficult-to-control pain, and steroid-related psychiatric symptoms (depression with psychotic features). Symptom control was pursued with difficulty, utilizing a coordinated team of pain specialists, oncologists, psychiatrists, social workers, and nurses. As the disease advanced, the patient became weaker and more debilitated. Shortly after the patient was informed that no further anticancer therapy was indicated because of his poor prognosis, he shot himself with a gun from his collection. Every effort had been made to remove all ammunition from the home. However, despite this and his extremely limited physical capacity, he committed suicide.

### Depression and Hopelessness

Depression is a symptom in 50% of all suicides. Those suffering from depression are at 25 times greater risk than the general population (Guze and Robins, 1970; Robins et al., 1959). The role depression plays in cancer suicide is equally significant. Approximately 25% of all cancer patients experience severe depressive symptoms, with about 6% fulfilling DSM-III criteria for the diagnosis of major depression (Bukberg et al., 1984; Plumb and Holland, 1977; Derogatis et al., 1983). Among those with advanced illness and progressively impaired physical function, symptoms of severe depression rise to 77% (Bukberg, 1984). Our consultation data at Memorial Sloan-Kettering Hospital on suicidal cancer patients showed that about one-third had a major depression, and more than half had an adjustment disorder, usually with depressed or anxious and depressed mood (see Table 24-4).

Hopelessness is the key variable linking depression to suicide, and is a significantly better predictor of completed suicide than depression alone (Beck et al., 1975; Kovacs et al., 1975). With the typical cancer suicide characterized by advanced illness and poor prognosis, hopelessness is a frequent variable (Holland, 1978). In Scandinavia, the incidence of suicide was significantly higher in cancer patients who were offered no further treatment and no further contact with the health care system (Louhivuori and Hakama, 1979; Bolund, 1985a,b). Being left to face illness alone creates a sense of abandonment that is critical to the development of hopelessness.

**Table 24-4**   MSKCC consultations regarding suicide risk patients

| Risk determinants | Number | Percentage |
|---|---|---|
| Consultations reviewed | 1080 | |
| Suicidal risk as reason for consultation | 93 | 8.6 |
| Suicide risk found | 71 | 6.5 |
| Among the 71 Patients: | | |
| Karnofsky rating | | |
| No special care needed | 27 | |
| Unable to work | 26 | |
| Unable to care for self | 18 | |
| Axis I psychiatric diagnoses | | |
| Adjustment disorder, depressed | 38 | 53.5 |
| Major depression | 22 | 30.9 |
| Delirium and organic brain syndromes | 14 | 19.7 |
| Alcoholism | 2 | |
| Mixed substance abuse | 1 | |
| Axis II psychiatric diagnoses | | |
| None | 34 | 47.8 |
| Mixed atypical | 16 | |
| Borderline | 5 | |
| Narcissistic | 4 | |
| Histrionic | 4 | |
| Dependent | 4 | |
| Compulsive | 4 | |
| Cancer sites | | |
| Kaposi's sarcoma/AIDS | 14 | |
| Urogenital | 8 | |
| Breast | 8 | |
| Lymphoma | 8 | |
| Colorectal | 6 | |
| Lung | 4 | |
| Head and neck | 3 | |
| Brain | 3 | |
| Leukemia | 3 | |
| Other | 5 | |
| No cancer | 6 | |

CASE REPORT

A 70-year-old Italian man with lung cancer that was metastatic to the thoracic vertebrae and left brachial plexus was transferred from a community hospital to Memorial Sloan-Kettering shortly after uncontrolled pain led to a nearly fatal suicide attempt. The patient's lung cancer led to severe chest and left arm pain. He underwent an extensive workup to diagnose the nature of his pain and received multimodal treatment for the pain, including narcotic analgesics, nerve blocks, and psychological support. After several changes in narcotic analgesics and several different nerve blocks, the patient was still in extreme pain. At that point his physician informed him that nothing more could be done for his pain. The patient explained later that he felt completely hopeless and saw no alternatives to relieving his pain but death. Shortly thereafter he took an overdose of his pain medications. Found by his family, he was rushed to the hospital, where he

remained comatose for several hours. After transfer to our center his treatment consisted of an aggressive approach to pain management, including psychiatric assessment. A tricyclic antidepressant was added after a diagnosis of clinical depression was established. With the relief of depression, though still in some pain, he felt more hopeful that his physicians would not give up until he was made more comfortable.

## Pain

Pain is a leading cause of morbidity in cancer (Foley, 1985). Some 15% of patients with nonmetastatic and 30% with metastatic cancer have significant pain (Daut and Cleeland, 1982; Kanner and Foley, 1981). In advanced cancer 60–90% of patients report debilitating pain, and up to 25% of all patients with cancer die in pain (Twycross and Lack, 1984; Cleeland, 1984; Foley, 1979).

Cancer is perceived by the public as an extremely painful disease relative to other medical conditions. A Wisconsin study revealed that 69% of the public agreed that cancer pain can get so bad that a person might consider suicide (Levin et al., 1985). The vast majority of cancer suicides had severe pain that was often inadequately controlled and tolerated poorly (Bolund, 1985a,b; Farberow et al., 1963). Clearly what may be an influence in cancer suicide is not merely the extent or degree of physical pain, but rather the suffering experienced as part of one's psychological reaction to illness and pain. Pain has adverse effects on patients' quality of life and sense of control, and it impairs the family's ability to provide support.

CASE REPORT

A 60-year-old immigrant chef from mainland China who spoke no English was working in an American Chinese restaurant when he developed an inoperable oat-cell carcinoma of the lung that had been unresponsive to therapy over 6 months. His daughter and son-in-law accompanied him to the clinic one day, explaining that their father had taken an overdose of pills the night before. He had written a suicide note asking that his family forgive him and understand that he could not take the pain any more. He had been disappointed when his attempt failed. When the psychiatrist evaluating this suicide attempt asked for more information about his pain, the patient revealed that he had been having extreme pain on the left side, especially in his ribs. No one, not his daughter, son-in-law (who interpreted), or his oncologist was aware that he was in pain. He was receiving no analgesics; the X-ray examination revealed bone involvement. When the patient was informed that there were medications for analgesia available that could diminish the pain, and that we would vigorously attempt to control his pain, he was no longer suicidal. The difficulty in communicating, combined with this patient's stoic nature, had led him to feel that there was no other way out of a controllable pain problem except death.

## Delirium

The prevalence of organic brain syndromes among cancer patients requiring psychiatric consultation has been found to range from 25 to 40% (Massie et al., 1979; Levine, 1978) and as high as 85% during the terminal stages of illness (Massie et al., 1983). Whereas earlier work (Farberow et al., 1963) suggested that delirium was a protective symptom in regard to cancer suicide, our clinical experience has found confusional states to be a major cause in impulsive suicide attempts, especially in the hospital. About 20% (see Table 24-4) of suicidal cancer patients seen at Memorial Sloan-Kettering had an organic brain syndrome at the time of their psychiatric evaluation. Patients with Kaposi's sarcoma and AIDS who were suicidal frequently had prominent signs of delirium superimposed upon an AIDS-associated dementia (Snider et al., 1983). Whereas a very dense confusional state may make it unlikely for a cancer patient to carry out effectively a completed suicide, the presence of mild delirium with loss of impulse control can set the stage for the acting out of suicidal thoughts in an already depressed, seriously ill individual.

### CASE REPORT

A 35-year-old homosexual white businessman with Kaposi's sarcoma (KS) and AIDS was admitted to Memorial Sloan-Kettering with *Pneumocystis carinii* pneumonia (PCP), his first serious infection in a 4-month illness. On the fourth hospital day, the patient informed the staff that he had taken an overdose of pills the night before in a suicide attempt. Psychiatric consultation revealed an irritable, hostile, disinhibited, and mildly paranoid man lying in bed with an intravenous infusion, appearing weak and extremely physically debilitated. He was disoriented as to time and place, confused, with impaired memory, concentration, attention, and ability to shift focus. He had a mild thought disorder with loosening of associations and visual hallucinations. A diagnosis of delirium related to hypoxia and septicemia was made and the patient was treated with a low-dose neuroleptic drug, 24-hour companion, and aggressive management of his pneumonia and multiple medical problems. After 24 hours, the patient was calm, coherent, alert, and no longer suicidal. He reported that he thought that he was dying and he was sure the doctors were about to place him on a respirator. Wanting to avoid this and feeling confused, he took several aspirin, anticipating that he would not awaken. Neuropsychological testing shortly before discharge showed no evidence of delirium or dementia; however, 6 months later he developed cognitive changes consistent with AIDS-associated dementia.

## Control and Helplessness

Loss of control and a sense of helplessness in the face of cancer is perhaps the single most important issue relating to suicide vulnerability. Control relates to both the extreme loss of control induced by symptoms or deficits due to cancer or its treatments, as well as an excessive need on the part of some patients to be in control of all aspects of living and dying. Farberow and colleagues (1963) noted that patients who were accepting and adaptable were much less prone to suicide than cancer patients who exhibited a need to be in control of even the most minute details of their care. This controlling trait may be prominent in some and cause distress with little provocation; however, it is not uncommon for cancer-related events to induce a great sense of helplessness even in those who are not particularly controlling. Deficit symptoms induced by cancer or cancer treatments include loss of mobility, paraplegia, loss of bowel and bladder function, amputation, aphonia, sensory loss, and inability to eat or swallow. It is most distressing for patients to sense that they are losing control of their minds, especially when they are confused or sedated by medications. The risk of suicide is increased in cancer patients with deficit symptoms, especially when accompanied by psychological distress and disturbed interpersonal relationships (Farberow, 1963).

### CASE REPORT

A 59-year-old white watchmaker with metastatic colon cancer developed severe radicular pain and weakness in his right arm due to epidural spinal cord compression. Treatment included narcotic analgesics, steroids, irradiation, surgery, and eventually experimental chemotherapy, all of which failed to halt the progression of the disease. Pain was being controlled, but at the expense of a clear sensorium at times. Progressive weakness of the arm and inability to concentrate forced the patient to stop work. He became demoralized and felt worthless and dependent. He was extremely distressed by his sense of complete helplessness. His children described him as a highly intelligent man who was a meticulous craftsman, but controlling to an extreme, and happy only when at work. With progressive disease came increasing weakness, bowel and bladder dysfunction, pain, depression, and periods of confusion. Desire for early death as well as thoughts of suicide were verbalized quite early and dramatically, just as deficit symptoms began to impair his function. Quite frank and graphic discussions of suicidal ideas and plans took place with his family and health care providers over a period of 6 months. Aggressive symptom control, psychological support of patient and family, and an acknowledgment that control was his, allowed the patient to delay acting on suicidal impulses. The patient eventually died at home surrounded by his family.

## Preexisting Psychopathology

Personality disorders, in which self-destructive behavior often occurs, drastically increase the risk of suicide. Borderline personality, alcoholism, substance abuse, and major mental illness (especially with psychoses) also increase risk. Alcohol abuse is second only to affective illness as an associated influence in up to 30% of suicides (Goodwin, 1982). Illicit drug abusers have a very high rate of suicide ranging from 82 to 350 per 100,000 (James, 1967). Schizophrenics also have a high rate of suicide, with 10% eventually taking their lives (Resnik, 1980). Holland advises that it is extremely rare for a cancer patient to commit suicide without some degree of preexisting psychopathology that places them at risk (Holland, 1978).

Farberow and colleagues referred to a large group of cancer suicides as the "dependent dissatisfied." These patients were immature, demanding, complaining, irritable, hostile, and difficult ward management problems. Staff often felt manipulated by these patients and were irritated by what they saw as excessive demands for attention. Suicide attempts or threats were often seen as "hysterical" or manipulative (Farberow et al., 1963). Our consultation data on suicidal cancer patients (see Table 24-4) showed that 50% had diagnosable personality disorders.

CASE REPORT

A 25-year-old unemployed messenger was admitted with bleeding secondary to recent diagnosis of acute leukemia. He had a history of substance abuse, poor work record, and erratic behavior. In the hospital, he was demanding of the nurses, uncooperative with required procedures, and noisy and unconcerned about the comfort of other patients. In an angry gesture he threatened suicide by turning on the oxygen jet and causing an explosion. His behavior was not manageable in a medical environment. He was transferred to a psychiatric unit with a diagnosis of borderline personality.

## Prior Suicide History and Family History

The frequency of suicide attempts in cancer patients has not been well studied. Suicidal thinking, however, is believed by some to occur frequently in advanced illness, and seems to act as a steam valve for feelings often expressed by patients as "If it gets too bad, I always have a way out" (Holland, 1978). Other published reports, however, suggest that suicidal thinking is relatively infrequent in cancer and is limited to those who are significantly depressed (Achte and Vaukonnen, 1971; Silberfarb et al., 1980). A Canadian study found that 10 of 44 terminally ill cancer patients in a palliative care service were suicidal or desired an early death, and all 10 were suffering from clinical depression (Brown et al., 1986). At Memorial Hospital, suicide risk evaluation accounted for 8.6% of psychiatric consultations, usually requested by the staff in response to the expression of a suicidal wish by a patient. Although the frequency of suicidal thinking in the cancer setting may be in question, its relationship to suicide attempts or completions is clearer. Bolund reports

that fully 50% of all Swedish cancer suicides had previously conveyed suicidal thoughts or plans to their relatives. In addition, many of the completed cancer suicides had been preceded by an attempted suicide (Bolund, 1985a,b). This is consistent with the statistics of suicide in general, which show that a previous suicide attempt greatly increases the risk of completed suicide (Ottosson, 1979; Murphy, 1977). A family history of suicide is of increasing relevance in assessing suicide risk. A significant genetic or biochemical vulnerability to suicide seems to exist that may be related to levels of the neurotransmitter serotonin in the brain (Asberg et al., 1987).

## Exhaustion and Fatigue

Fatigue with the exhaustion of physical, emotional, financial, spiritual, family, community, and health care resources increases the risk of suicide in the cancer patient. Cancer is now often a chronic illness. Increased survival is accompanied by increased complications, hospitalizations, and expense. Symptom control thus becomes a prolonged process with frequent advances and setbacks. The dying process also can become extremely long and arduous for all concerned. Both family members and health care providers at times withdraw prematurely from the cancer patient under these circumstances. A suicidal patient can feel even more isolated and abandoned. The presence of a strong support system that may act as an external control of suicidal behavior reduces the risk of cancer suicide significantly. It is important to note here that the spouse, parent, or other family member of a cancer patient may be at increased risk of suicide as well. In our experience, a successful suicide in a relative has usually been associated with pathological grief in an extremely dependent individual with prior depressive illness or personality disorder.

CASE REPORT

A 60-year-old white male dentist with unresectable lung cancer was being treated for symptoms of anxiety and depression utilizing medication, relaxation, and supportive psychotherapy that included his three children and his wife of 35 years. The wife was identified as having lifelong history of anxiety, depression, and extreme dependence. She had been in psychotherapy for 15 years. As the patient became progressively ill, the wife became more distressed. She repeatedly expressed that her husband "had to be cured," and that she was "unable to accept" his death. After becoming progressively depressed, the wife was started on antidepressant medication with subjective improvement. Shortly thereafter, on an afternoon when her husband was at a medical appointment, she ingested a lethal amount of her husband's pain medications.

## THE AFTERMATH OF SUICIDE: IMPACT ON FAMILY AND HEALTH CARE PROVIDERS

When suicide complicates bereavement, the loss can be especially difficult for the survivors left behind. When cancer has played a role in suicide, the loss is often difficult and elicits complex emotions. The intensity and nature of the survivors' reactions will depend on such variables as the age and physical condition of the deceased, the nature of the suicide, the relationship with the deceased, and the survivor's individual personality and cultural background. A pattern of reactions that include feelings of rejection, abandonment, anger, relief, guilt, responsibility, denial, identification, and shame is often seen in those left behind. Assisting survivors of suicide through the bereavement period is often necessary and rewarding. Mutual support groups have been developed to reduce isolation, provide opportunities for ventilating feelings, and find ways to deal with the aftermath of suicide.

Reactions to the suicide of a cancer patient in the staff are similar to those seen in family members, especially feelings of responsibility, guilt, shame, relief, and questioning of professional judgment. It is helpful for the team that cared for a patient who committed suicide to review the case by carrying out a "psychological autopsy," in an attempt to understand why and how it happened, the signs and signals of risk, and how routines might be altered to manage similar problems in the future. This type of meeting leads to discussion of personal feelings and allows for a sense of mutual support. Psychiatric colleagues can often be of help as participants in such a review, or to assist on an individual level.

## MANAGEMENT PRINCIPLES

Assessment of suicide risk and appropriate intervention are critical. Early and comprehensive psychiatric involvement with high-risk individuals can often avert suicide in the cancer setting (Dubovsky, 1978). A careful evaluation (Table 24-5) includes a search for the meaning of suicidal thoughts, as well as an exploration of the seriousness of the risk. The clinician's ability to establish rapport and elicit a patient's thoughts are essential as he or she assesses history, degree of intent, and quality of internal and external controls. One must listen sympathetically, not appearing critical or stating that such thoughts are inappropriate. Allowing the patient to discuss suicidal thoughts often decreases the risk of suicide. The myth that asking about suicidal thoughts "puts the idea in their head," is one that should be dispelled, especially when dealing with cancer (McKegney and Lange, 1971). Patients often

**Table 24-5** Evaluation of suicidal patient

- Establish rapport—empathic approach.
- Obtain patient's understanding of illness and present symptoms.
- Assess relevant mental status—delirium (internal control).
- Assess vulnerability variables.
- Assess support system (external control).
- Obtain history of prior emotional problems, or psychiatric disorders.
- Obtain family history.
- Record prior suicide threats, attempts.
- Assess suicidal thinking, intent, plans.
- Evaluate need for one-to-one nurse in hospital or companion at home; formulate immediate and long-term treatment plan.

reconsider the idea of suicide when the physician acknowledges the legitimacy of their option and the need to retain a sense of control over aspects of their death.

Table 24-3 outlines cancer vulnerability variables that can be utilized as a guide to evaluation and management. Once the setting has been made secure, the assessment of the mental status and the management of pain control can begin. Analgesics, neuroleptics, or antidepressant drugs should be utilized when appropriate to treat agitation, psychosis, major depression, or pain. Underlying causes of delirium or pain should be addressed specifically when possible. It is important to initiate a crisis intervention-oriented psychotherapeutic approach that mobilizes as much of the patient's support system as possible. A close family member or friend should be involved in order to support the patient, provide information, and assist in treatment planning. Psychiatric hospitalization can sometimes be helpful when there is a clear indication and the patient's medical illness is stable. Most frequently, however, the medical hospital or home is the setting in which management takes place. Although it is appropriate to intervene when medical or psychiatric reasons are clearly the driving force in a cancer suicide, there are circumstances when usurping control from the patient and family with overly aggressive intervention may be less helpful. This is most evident in those with advanced illness with whom comfort and symptom control are the primary concerns.

The goal of intervention should not be to prevent suicide at all costs, but to prevent suicide that is driven by desperation. Prolonged suffering due to poorly controlled symptoms lead to such desperation, and it is our role to provide effective management of such problems as an alternative to suicide in the cancer patient.

## REFERENCES

Achte, K.A. and M.L. Vaukonnen (1971a). Cancer and the psyche. *Omega* 2:46–56.

Achte, K.A. and M.L. Vaukonnen (1971b). Suicides committed in general hospitals. *Psychiatr. Fenn. Yearbook Psychiatr. Clin. Helsinki Univ. Gen. Hosp.*, pp. 221–28.

Annas, G.J. (1984). When suicide prevention becomes brutality: The case of Elixabeth Bouvia. *Hastings Center Rep.* 114:20–21.

Asberg, M., L. Traskman, and P. Thoren (1987). 5-HIAA in the cerebrospinal fluid: A biochemical suicide predictor? *Arch. Gen. Psychiatry* 33:1193.

Beck, A.T., M. Kovacs, and A. Weissman (1975). Hopelessness and suicidal behavior: An overview. *J.A.M.A.* 234:1146–49.

Bolund, C. (1985a). Suicide and cancer: I. Demographic and social characteristics of cancer patients who committed suicide in Sweden, 1973–1976. *J. Psychosoc. Oncol.* 3:17–30.

Bolund, C. (1985b). Suicide and cancer: II. Medical and care factors in suicides by cancer patients in Sweden, 1973–1976. *J. Psychosoc. Oncol.* 3:31–52.

Breitbart, W. (1987). Suicide in cancer patients. *Oncology* 1:49–54.

Brown, J.H., P. Henteleff, S. Barakat and C.J. Rowe (1986). Is it normal for terminally ill patients to desire death? *Am. J. Psychiatry* 143:208–11.

Bukberg, J., D. Penman, and J. Holland (1984). Depression in hospitalized cancer patients. *Psychosom. Med.* 46:199–212.

Campbell, P.C. (1966). Suicides among cancer patients. *Conn. Health Bull.* 80:207–12.

Cleeland, C.S. (1984). The impact of pain on patients with cancer. *Cancer* 54:235–41.

Danto, B.L. (1972). The cancer patient and suicide. *J. Thanatol.* 2:596–600.

Daut, R.L. and C.S. Cleeland (1982). The prevalence and severity of pain in cancer. *Cancer* 50:1913–18.

Derogatis, L.R., G.R. Morrow, J. Fetting, D. Penman, S. Piasetsky, A.M. Schmale (1983). The prevalence of psychiatric disorders among cancer patients. *J.A.M.A.* 249:715–57.

Dorpat, T.L., W.E. Andersson, and H.S. Ripley (1968). The relationship of physical illness to suicide. In H.L.P. Resnik (ed.), *Suicidal Behaviors*. London: Churchill-Livingstone.

Dubovsky, S.L. (1978). Averting suicide in terminally ill patients. *Psychosomatics* 19;113–15.

Farberow, N.L. and E.S. Schneidman (1961). The cry for help. New York: McGraw-Hill.

Farberow, N.L., S. Ganzler, F. Cutter, and D. Reynolds (1971). An eight year survey of hospital suicides. *Suicide Life-Threatening Behav.* 1:184–201.

Farberow, N.L., E.S. Schneidman, C.V. Leonard (1963). Suicide among general medical and surgical hospital patients with malignant neoplasms. *Med. Bull.* 9. Washington, D.C.: U.S. Veterans Administration.

Feigenberg, L. (1980). *Terminal Care: Friendship Contracts with Dying Cancer Patients*. New York: Brunner/Mazel.

Foley, K.M. (1979). Pain syndromes in patients with cancer. In J.J. Bonica, V. Ventafridda, R.B. Fink, L.E. Jones and J.D. Loeser (eds.), *Advances in Pain Research and Therapy*, Vol. 2. New York: Raven Press, pp. 59–75.

Foley, K.M. (1985). The treatment of cancer pain. *N. Engl. J. Med.* 313:84–95.

Forman, B. (1979). Cancer and suicide. *Gen. Hosp. Psychiatry* 1:108–14.

Fox, B.H., E.J. Stanek, S.C. Boyd, and J.T. Flannery (1982). Suicide rates among cancer patients in Connecticut. *J. Chron. Dis.* 35:85–100.

Goodwin, D.W. (1982). Alcoholism and suicide: Associated factors. In E.M. Pattison and E. Kaufman (eds.), *The Encyclopedic Handbook of Alcoholism*. New York: Gardner Press, pp. 655–62.

Guze, S. and E. Robins (1970). Suicide and primary affective disorders. *Br. J. Psychiatry* 117:437–38.

Holland, J.C. (1978). Psychological aspects of cancer. In J.F. Holland and E. Frei (eds.), *Cancer Medicine*, 2nd ed. Philadelphia: Lea & Febiger.

Holland, J.C., A.H. Hughes, S. Tross, P. Silberfarb, M. Perry, R. Comis, and M. Oster (1986). Comparative psychological disturbance in patients with pancreatic and gastric cancer. *Am. J. Psychiatry* 143:982–86.

James, I.P. (1967). Suicide and mortality amongst heroin addicts in Britain. *Br. J. Addict.* 62:391–98.

Kane, F.I. (1985). Keeping Elizabeth Bouvia alive for the public good. *Hastings Center Rep.* 15:5–9.

Kanner, R.M. and K.M. Foley (1981). Patterns of narcotic drug use in a cancer pain clinic. *Ann. N.Y. Acad. Sci.* 362:161–72.

Kastenbaum, R. (1976). Suicide as the preferred way to death. In E.S. Schneidman (ed.), *Suicidology: Contemporary Developments*. New York: Grune & Stratton.

Kovacs, M., A.T. Beck, and A. Weissman (1975). Hopelessness: An indication of suicidal risk. *Suicide* 5:98–103.

Levin, D.N., C.S. Cleeland, and R. Dar (1985). Public attitudes toward cancer pain. *Cancer* 56:2337–39.

Levine, P.M., P.M. Silberfarb, and Z.J. Lipowski (1978). Mental disorders in cancer patients: A study of 100 psychiatric referrals. *Cancer* 42:1385–1391.

Louhivuori, K.A. and M. Hakama (1979). Risk of suicide among cancer patients. *Am. J. Epidemiol.* 109:59–65.

Marshall, J.R., W. Burnett, and J. Brasure (1983). On precipitating factors: Cancer as a cause of suicide. *Suicide Life-Threatening Behav.* 3:15–27.

Massie, M.J., J.G. Gorzynski, R.C. Mastrovito, D. Theis, and J. Holland (1979). The diagnosis of depression in hospitalized patients with cancer. *Proc. Am. Assoc. Cancer Res. Am. Soc. Clin. Oncol.* 20:432–40.

Massie, M.J., J.C. Holland, and E. Glass (1983). Delirium in terminally ill cancer patients. *Am. J. Psychiatry* 140:1048–50.

McKegney, P.P. and P. Lange (1971). The decision to no longer live on chronic hemodialysis. *Am. J. Psychiatry* 128:47–55.

Murphy, G.E. (1977). Suicide and attempted suicide. *Hosp. Pract.* 12:78–81.

Olafssen, O. (1982). *Cancer and Suicide*. Report presented at the International Conference on Suicide, Paris.

Ottosson, J.O. (1979). The suicidal patient, can the psychiatrist prevent suicide? In M. Schon and P. Stromgrene (eds.), *Origin and Prevention of Affective Disorders*.

Plumb, M.M. and J.C. Holland (1977). Comparative studies of psychological function in patients with advanced cancer. *Psychosom. Med.* 39:264–76.

Pollack, S. (1957). Suicide in general hospitals. In E.S. Schneidman and W.L. Farberow (eds.), *Clues to Suicide*. New York: McGraw-Hill, Blakiston Div.

Reich, P. and M.J. Kelly (1976). Suicide attempts by hospitalized medical and surgical patients. *N. Engl. J. Med.* 294:298–301.

Resnik, H.L.P. (1980). Suicide. In H. Kaplan, A. Freedman, and B.I. Saddock (eds.), *Comprehensive Textbook of Psychiatry III*. Baltimore: Williams & Wilkins.

Robins, E., G. Murphy, R.H. Wilkinson, Jr., S. Gassner, and J. Kayes (1959). Some clinical considerations in the prevention of suicide based on 134 successful suicides. *Am. J. Public Health* 49:888–99.

Roman, J. (1980). *Exit House*. New York: Seaview Books.

Sainsbury, P. (1975). Suicide in London: An ecological study. In *Mandsley Monogr. No. 1*. London: Chapman & Hall.

Siegel, K. (1982). Rational suicide: Considerations for the clinician. *Psychiatr. Q.* 54:77–83.

Siegel, K. and P. Tuckel (1984). Rational suicide and the terminally ill cancer patient. *Omega* 15:263–69.

Silberfarb, P.M., L.H. Maurer, and C.S. Cronthamel (1980). Psychosocial aspects of neoplastic disease, I: Functional status of breast cancer patients during different treatment regimens. *Am. J. Psychiatry* 137:450–55.

Snider, W.D., D.M. Simpson, S. Nielson, J.W.M. Gold, C.E. Metroka, and J.E. Posner (1983). Neurological complications of Acquired Immune Deficiency Syndrome: Analysis of 50 patients *Ann. Neurol.* 14:403–18.

Stewart, I. and M.D. Leeds (1960). Suicide: The influence of organic disease. *Lancet* 2:919–20.

Twycross, R.G. and S.A. Lack (1984). *Symptom control in far advanced cancer: In Pain Relief*. London: Pitman.

Van Praag, H.M. (1982). Depression, suicide and the metabolism of serotonin in the brain. *J. Affect. Dis.* 4:275–90.

Weisman, A.D. (1976). Coping behavior and suicide in cancer. In J.W. Cullen, B.H. Fox, and R.N. Ison (eds.), *Cancer: The Behavioral Dimensions*. New York: Raven Press.

Weissman, M. (1974). The epidemiology of suicide attempts, 1960–71. *Arch. Gen.Psychiatry* 30:737–46.

Whitlock, F.A. (1978). Suicide, cancer and depression. *Br. J. Psychiatry* 132:269–74.

# 25

## Anxiety, Panic, and Phobias

### Mary Jane Massie

While it is relatively easy to diagnose anxiety in physically healthy individuals, it is far more difficult to assess it in physically ill patients, and especially those with cancer. The normal fears and uncertainties associated with cancer of possible death, disfigurement, dependence on others, disability, and disruption of new relationships are often severe (Chapter 22). Thus, there is often not a clear distinction between those normal fears and others that are simply more severe and appear, like depression, to represent a continuum of intensity of symptoms finally reaching the criteria for an anxiety disorder. Because the issue is clinically important, however, this chapter attempts to describe the anxiety disorders, their causes, and treatment in patients with cancer. The reader is referred to other sources for a review of the theories concerning anxiety and the neurophysiological mechanisms for its expression (Leigh and Reiser, 1985; Levi, 1975; Spielberger, 1972). Like other psychological problems in medically ill patients, anxiety disorders are in need of more systematic study (Dobson, 1985).

A word about measurement of anxiety is called for. As psychological distress is increasingly systematically examined and treated in medical patients, the methods of assessment become important. The most frequently used valid anxiety assessment methods were not devised for physically ill patients and may not be reliable in these situations. When one examines some of the tests for both anxiety and depression, there is considerable overlap in items that appear to measure both. We also know that these two emotions commonly occur together in cancer. An additional problem is the frequent lack of appropriate comparison groups for anxiety scales. Cella and colleagues (1987) have administered the Profile of Mood States (POMS) to 1000 cancer patients which now provides data to which other patients can be compared. Cella and Jacobsen have also developed a shortened form of the POMS

that is valid for total mood distress and is much easier to administer (see Part XII on research methods).

Table 25-1 outlines the types of anxiety most frequently encountered in cancer. They include reactive anxiety (situational) that is related to crises; anxiety related to medical influences that may be caused by pain, an abnormal metabolic state, hormone-producing tumors, or anxiety-producing drugs; and anxiety related to a preexisting anxiety disorder that is exacerbated by medical illness (phobias, panic, generalized anxiety-provoking situations in cancer treatment).

Irrespective of the cause of anxiety, the subjective and physical symptoms are similar. The person with anxiety describes a subjective feeling of fear that encompasses dread and apprehension. It may be vague and represent an ill-defined general emotion, but in the context of cancer, the focus is often a fear of death and body dysfunction. Physiological changes occur that result in the physical symptoms related to central and autonomic nervous system arousal and neuroendocrine responses (Leigh and Reiser, 1985). Table 25-2 outlines the physical signs and symptoms of anxiety, which may affect any system of the body. Primarily, however, changes in mood and behavior reflecting autonomic changes are accompanied by respiratory and cardiovascular symptoms. Anorexia is the most common gastrointestinal symptom in cancer that is related to anxiety; however, anxiety about gastrointestinal function and cancer may result in diarrhea, heartburn, air swallowing, and constipation (see Chapter 15). Fears associated with gynecological and genitourinary cancer produce the usual symptoms of anxiety, but in addition frigidity, impotence, dyspareunia, and dysuria may develop as result of anxiety about pelvic disease.

The signs of autonomic hyperactivity are common features of all anxiety states. When the anxiety occurs in episodes characterized by severe symptoms such as

**Table 25-1** Types of anxiety seen in patients with cancer

| Types of anxiety | Causes |
|---|---|
| Reactive anxiety (situational) related to crises | |
| Anxiety related to medical influences | Poorly controlled pain |
| | Abnormal metabolic states |
| | Hormone-secreting tumors |
| | Anxiety-producing drugs |
| Anxiety related to preexisting anxiety disorder | Phobias activated by some aspect of medical care |
| | Panic and generalized anxiety disorder |
| | Posttraumatic stress disorder |
| Special anxiety-provoking situations in cancer treatment | |

**Table 25-2** Symptoms and signs of anxiety

| | |
|---|---|
| Appearance and behavior | Flushed face |
| | Tense, worried expression |
| | Restlessness |
| | Signs of nail-biting; smoking |
| | Sweaty palms |
| | Diaphoresis |
| Neurological | Poor concentration and memory |
| | Little interest in usual activities |
| | Irritability |
| | Dizziness |
| | Weakness |
| | Exhaustion |
| | Fine tremor; tingling sensation of extremities; poor coordination |
| | Insomnia |
| | Nightmares |
| | Headaches |
| | Drowsiness |
| Cardiovascular | Palpitations |
| | Sinus tachycardia |
| | Elevated systolic blood pressure |
| | Precordial pain |
| Respiratory | Hyperventilation |
| | Dyspnea; feeling of suffocation |
| Gastrointestinal | Anorexia |
| | Diarrhea |
| | Heartburn |
| | Air swallowing |
| | Hyperphagia |
| Gynecological/genitourinary | Impotence |
| | Frigidity |
| | Urinary urgency and frequency |
| | Dysuria |
| | Menstrual changes and/or pain |

difficulty breathing, the person comes to dread a repeated episode so much that the fear of another attack results in a chronically anxious state as seen in patients with classical panic disorders. Patients with cancer who have long-standing generalized anxiety disorder or phobias activated by medical care are at most risk of severe anxiety having a medical illness superimposed on a preexisting disorder. The anxiety disorders that produce these common symptoms, vary in intensity and cause. They are discussed in the following sections.

## REACTIVE ANXIETY

By far the most commonly seen of these disorders is reactive anxiety. In the DSM-III R classification, this is called adjustment disorder with anxious mood, alone or combined with depressed mood. In Chapter 22, we reported one study of the spectrum of psychiatric disorders that showed that reactive depression and anxiety were present in one-third of cancer patients randomly interviewed (Derogatis et al., 1983). As shown in the schema of increasing levels of psychological symptoms (Fig. 22-1, Chapter 22), the level of reactive anxiety exceeds the level that is regarded as normal and adaptive and that is a part of response to crises related to illness. It is often a difficult judgment to determine when normal anxiety generated by a crisis in cancer or treatment is no longer normal and meets criteria for an anxiety disorder. The issues are similar to those discussed in regard to reactive depression. The present DSM-III R indicates that the adjustment disorder with anxious mood, the category most closely describing situational anxiety, is maladaptive.

In fact, in the survey mentioned earlier, only 45 of 215 patients interviewed had had a preexisting anxiety disorder. This reflects the overall prevalence of anxiety disorders seen largely as phobias in about 8% of the general population (Robins et al., 1984). Thus the major anxiety disorder seen in cancer is that of a reactive or situational nature; it is most often seen in conjunction with depressive symptoms (Chapter 23). Reactive or situational anxiety is seen at crisis or transitional points in the course of cancer, that is, at the time of diagnosis, awaiting a new treatment, prior to major surgery, on completion of a lengthy treatment, and in advanced and terminal stages of illness. The anxiety associated with advanced illness reflects the uncertainty of the future, the uncertainty of treatment effectiveness, the pursuit of new or alternative treatments with the fear of failing to find the right one, and the fears associated with actual poor respiratory function or chronic uncontrolled pain (see Chapters 48 and 49).

The management is often confined to receiving adequate information and support from the responsible physician. The anxiety about an operation and the expected problems in the postoperative period is substantially reduced by adequate preparation of the patient about what to expect. Mentally ''walking through'' events is very helpful. An important study done over two decades ago by Egbert and colleagues (1964) showed by the anesthesiologist's preoperative visit, when coupled with an explanation of events and a discussion of postoperative medication available, reduced both time in the recovery room and amount of medication needed. Unfortunately, this elegant study, which was done as a randomized trial, has changed clinical practice to only a minor extent. The counseling by the nurse, social worker, and veteran patient can be useful to reduce anxiety, particularly at the time of diagnosis or when a patient is awaiting major surgery or a new treatment. Referral of anxious patients depends on the causes and severity of distress. A mental health professional may be helpful to offer support and counseling. If an underlying medical cause must be ruled out, or if medication is likely necessary to control severe symptoms, referral to a psychiatrist is indicated both for diagnostic evaluation and management.

A study of reactive distress in 147 largely ambulatory patients with cancer undergoing chemotherapy or irradiation (with a Karnofsky score >60) were studied in a tricenter study that randomized patients with an identified elevated level of significant anxiety, depression, or both to receive either alprazolam (0.5 mg tid) or a relaxation tape to be used similarly for 10 days (Holland et al., 1987). After 10 days patients could then receive the other treatment or continue the same. The majority of patients, as judged by scores on the Hamilton Anxiety (HAS) and Depression Scale (HDS), Hopkins Symptom Checklist-90 (SCL-90), and Affects Balance Scale, experienced a significant drop in their levels of distress by about 50%, most clearly demonstrated on the HDS and HAS. Alprazolam was slightly more effective but both were highly effective with the majority of patients indicating a benefit. These data suggest that two cost-effective measures are available: for patients who prefer a drug, alprazolam is effective; for those who do not wish to take medication, an almost equally effective alternative relaxation is available. Oncologists can, with little effort, offer these types of assistance to reduce the distressing situational anxiety many patients experience during treatment.

In clinical management, brief psychotherapy for dealing with the crisis and a benzodiazepine (e.g., alprazolam, 0.25–0.5 mg po tid to qid) for daytime sedation, or a bedtime hypnotic (e.g., temazepam, 0.25–0.5 mg or triazolam, 0.25 mg po qhs) may be ordered. The benzodiazepines are readily discontinued

**Table 25-3**  Treatment of anxiety disorders

| Treatment modality | Components |
|---|---|
| Supportive psychotherapy | Providing information; rehearsal of feared events; reassurance |
| Behavioral | Relaxation |
| | Hypnosis |
| | Systematic desensitization |
| Psychopharmacological | Benzodiazepines |
| |   Short acting (alprazolam, lorazepam, oxazepam) |
| |   Long acting (diazepam, clorazepate) |
| | β Blockers |
| | Tricyclic antidepressants |
| | MAOI |
| | Antihistamines |
| | Neuroleptics |
| | Buspirone |
| Combination of all of the above | |

by patients when symptoms abate. In fact, more often these patients must be encouraged to take the medication long enough to be effective. Three interventions for anxiety, which are used alone or in combination (Table 25-3), are supportive psychotherapy, medications (which include the several classes of drugs with anxiolytic properties) (Liebowitz, 1985; Sheehan, 1985), and behavioral interventions and combinations of them. A severe form of anxiety before an operation that required a combination of treatments is illustrated by the following case.

CASE REPORT

A 54-year-old married businessman with no previous psychiatric history was admitted to the hospital for resection of the bowel for colon carcinoma. During the week prior to admission, he developed increasingly severe symptoms of anxiety (e.g., irritability, insomnia, diarrhea, palpitations, and hyperventilation), but he was too embarrassed to discuss his fear of the impending operation with his surgeon. On the evening of admission, when asked to sign the consent form for the operation, he panicked. He stated that he could not ''stand to spend the night in the hospital'' and demanded discharge. Although he was embarrassed by his behavior, which he felt was ''out of control,'' he could not tolerate the thought of having surgery the next day. The psychiatric consultant agreed that his level of anxiety was so high that surgery should be postponed. He was given twice-weekly appointments and started on diazepam (5 mg qid) and was also told to use audiotapes prepared for him to use as relaxation exercise at home.

Within 3 weeks he felt in control and asked to be rescheduled for surgery. He was able to undergo the procedure. His postoperative course was uneventful; diazepam was tapered and discontinued over 4 weeks. He had had no recurrence of either colon cancer or anxiety symptoms 5 years after the surgery.

The second case report of reactive anxiety shows the impact of prior experiences on the severity of situational anxiety.

CASE REPORT

A 28-year-old married childless businesswoman underwent limited breast resection and axillary dissection for stage II breast cancer. She tolerated surgery well, but upon viewing the surgical site, she became anxious and had an episode of hyperventilation with dizziness, tingling of her fingers and toes, and nausea. A consultation from psychiatry revealed that she had had a tendency in the past to fear accidents and she became anxious when she or her husband had an illness or an accident. She revealed that her parents were both survivors of concentration camps and she was sensitive to their suffering—sometimes as if it had been her own. She became able to look at her breast without severe anxiety, but she was anxious that radiation treatments were necessary. The psychiatrist accompanied her to the first treatment. Upon being placed in the treatment room with doors closed, the machine over her, and the technician outside the room communicating through the intercom, she became panicky when she heard the sound that signaled release of the radioactive load for treatment. She hyperventilated, and had tachycardia, tingling, and severe apprehension. After being removed from the room, she became calm and said that the swooshing sound reminded her of her parents' stories of the gas chamber. It activated her fears of death from radiation or from cancer. The consultant recommended mild sedation and that she use a tape player with headphones to avoid the sounds that were frightening to her. She managed the remaining treatments without further problems.

The anxiety of terminal illness, though in part situational and related to existential concerns, is often complicated by pain, nausea, and weakness that add to anxiety. Particularly, shortness of breath from chronic hypoxia is frightening and is often improved by control of the anxiety. Control of anxiety of the terminal state is reviewed in Chapter 49 and in Chapter 39 for pharmacological management.

The cured patient also has lingering anxieties about cancer that, though less overt, nevertheless are present and exacerbate at the time of annual checkup, or when minor symptoms appear. These are reviewed in Chapter 7 on survivors.

## ANXIETY RELATED TO MEDICAL INFLUENCES

In the patient having treatment for cancer, the second most frequent source of anxiety after situational anxiety is that caused by a metabolic state, a medication that produces anxiety as a side effect, or less frequently, a hormone-producing tumor. The efforts to

**Table 25-4** Anxiety related to common medical problems in cancer

| Medical problems | Examples |
| --- | --- |
| Poorly controlled pain | |
| Abnormal metabolic states | Hypoxia, pulmonary embolus, sepsis, delirium, hypoglycemia, bleeding, coronary occlusion and heart failure |
| | Cardiac arrhythmia |
| Hormone-secreting tumors (see Chapter 31) | Pheochromocytoma, thyroid adenoma or carcinoma, parathyroid adenoma, ACTH-producing tumors, insulinoma |
| Anxiety-producing drugs | Corticosteroids, neuroleptics used as antiemetics, thyroxine, bronchodilators, β-adrenergic stimulants, antihistamine (paradoxical reaction), withdrawal states (alcohol, narcotic analgesics, sedative-hypnotics) |

classify anxiety disorders in the 1980 DSM-III classification did not include a category for these common medically induced forms of anxiety. The revised classification in the DSM-III R (American Psychiatric Association, 1987) includes organic anxiety syndrome to describe the anxiety and panic attack associated with, for example, pheochromocytoma.

Organic anxiety syndromes are seen in cancer in several situations: with poorly controlled pain, with an abnormal metabolic state, with hormone-producing tumors, and as a side effect of medication (Table 25-4).

### Poorly Controlled Pain

The first and most commonly seen type of anxiety related to a medical cause is that associated with poorly controlled pain. The individual who has pain is tense, sweating, restless, and urgently requesting help (Sternbach, 1974). If there is not relief, agitation develops and the person may begin to express suicidal thoughts because this is an intolerable state in which to live (see Chapter 24). In the hospital, anxiety is heightened when pain medication is inadequate and staff have not recognized the level of poor control. Ordering analgesics on a prn basis contributes to anxiety by creating uneven control; better control could be attained more readily by ordering medication around the clock (atc) and thereby reducing the anxiety about getting the next dose. The patient's anger and insistent demanding may result in a call for psychiatric evaluation for the "control of anxiety." In our experience, one cannot evaluate anxiety until the pain has been controlled (Massie and Holland, 1987). Usually, the person becomes calm with relief of the pain and assurance that medication will be given on a regular schedule (see Chapter 32 on pain). If residual anxiety remains, it can then be assessed as to cause and a management plan instituted.

## Abnormal Metabolic States

Anxiety is often the first sign of an altered metabolic state or impending catastrophic event. Unexplained anxiety should be a signal to review the metabolic state for possible early changes. Sudden anxiety with chest pain may indicate a pulmonary embolus. The most common cause in cancer patients is hypoxia (from mild to severe); the patient senses it and becomes fearful that breathing is impaired. The anxiety makes breathing more labored but responds to a mild sedative that, by reducing the anxiety, improves breathing. The drug and dose should be chosen to have the least depressant effect on the respiratory center, such as an antihistamine or a short-acting benzodiazepine.

Sepsis is accompanied by chills and fever and often is associated with anxiety. Delirium related to a metabolic encephalopathy, irrespective of cause, may appear with anxiety, restlessness, and finally agitation. Hypoglycemia should be considered early because it may be life-threatening and may be manifested by anxiety or restlessness and only later confusion (see Chapter 29 on CNS complications). Hypocalcemia with hyperactive reflexes may be experienced by the patient as anxiety. Undetected bleeding may, in early stages, be accompanied by anxiety and unexplained restlessness. Both coronary occlusion and congestive failure, occurring in the course of cancer treatment, will have anxiety that must be controlled in the total management of the problem.

## Hormone-Secreting Tumors

Although the endocrine complications of cancer are described fully in Chapter 31, the hormone-secreting tumors are a source of anxiety and panic attacks that must be considered in a differential diagnosis. Pheochromocytoma often goes undiagnosed for many years, with the person being labeled as having functional anxiety. Thyroid and parathyroid tumors, as well as ACTH-producing tumors (most frequently associated with lung cancer and insulinoma), are tumors that may have associated episodic anxiety. Carcinoid has more recently been found to produce fewer neuropsychiatric symptoms, including anxiety, than previously assumed (see Chapter 31 on endocrine complications).

## Anxiety-Producing Drugs

Among the drugs commonly used in cancer, the corticosteroids most often produce anxiety, motor restlessness, and agitation. Dexamethasone, when given in a high dose for spinal-cord compression, causes a range of mental aberrations that may include restlessness. Prednisone in a usual dose does not produce anxiety; however, at high dosage or during a rapid taper, anxiety may develop.

An increasingly common form of anxiety in cancer patients is that caused by side effects of neuroleptic drugs given at high dose for emesis control, particularly metoclopramide. Akathesia, noted as motor restlessness with repetitive uncontrollable movement of legs, hands, or jaw, develops typically several hours to days after a chemotherapy treatment. The patient and family are bewildered by the ''anxiety'' and distress, which are initially explained as worry. Akathesia is rapidly controlled by a benzodiazepine or an antiparkinsonian agent. Patients should be warned of this possible side effect, which is frightening when they are unaware of its drug-related nature.

Other less common drug-related anxiety is seen with thyroid replacement when dosage is being adjusted. Bronchodilators and β-adrenergic stimulants used for complicating chronic respiratory states can cause severe and poorly controlled anxiety, irritability, and tremulousness.

Withdrawal states from alcohol, narcotic analgesics, and sedative-hypnotics produce anxiety and agitation. Alcohol, abruptly stopped by virtue of hospital admission, will cause a withdrawal state in 2–4 days, not uncommonly appearing in the postoperative period as an unexplained delirium. A full-blown delirium tremens may be averted by adequate medication (see Chapter 17 on head and neck cancer). Both narcotics and sedative-hypnotics should be tapered to prevent withdrawal symptoms that will occur with abrupt withdrawal. The increasing use of short-acting benzodiazepines, lorazepam, alprazolam, and oxazepam may be associated with rebound of anxiety between doses. Awareness of it should prompt change to a longer-acting drug or alteration of dose.

## ANXIETY RELATED TO PREEXISTING ANXIETY DISORDER

Anxiety caused by facing the stresses of illness and especially those of cancer, or anxiety secondary to a metabolic state or drug reaction, are common problems recognized and managed in a straightforward manner. However, there is a group of patients who, when they must undergo cancer treatment, experience activation of preexisting anxiety disorders that can interfere with or seriously complicate treatment. When that treatment might be curative or result in lengthy survival, management of the anxiety disorder becomes crucial. For this reason these disorders are described here. From the psychiatric side, these previously ill-defined disorders have been increasingly subcategorized because they appear to have different biological attributes, follow different clinical courses, and respond to different specific medications with relief of symptoms (Schuckit, 1987). This is most clearly seen in panic disorder. Panic disorder has come under special study since a genetic variable was found to be present and since it was found to respond specifically to antidepressant medication (Roy-Byrne and Katon, 1987).

For purposes of examining these disorders in cancer patients, they are outlined in the areas of simple phobias that are apt to be precipitated by treatment, panic and generalized anxiety disorder, and postraumatic stress disorders. While isolated phobias often are seen without any other emotional problems, they also are seen in the context of chronic anxiety and depressive symptoms. Agoraphobia, particularly while it may occur alone, may also be present with panic disorder. While panic disorder is most clearly delineated, generalized anxiety disorder is less clearly differentiated as a homogeneous group and may still represent a wider group to be further delineated. Most of these differentiations, including postraumatic stress disorder, have been the result of criteria for each defined in the DSM-III, in use in psychiatry since 1980. This has been a major step forward. Deficiencies that have become apparent, particularly in anxiety disorders, have been addressed in the DSM-III R (American Psychiatric Association, 1987).

## Phobias

While fears of cancer and AIDS dominate society's present fears of disease, most individuals respond to the information about both in a responsible manner. For individuals who have a true disease phobia (a nosophobia), however, the chronic preoccupation sometimes becomes disabling. Reviewed in Chapter 2, management is often difficult and only partially successful. This section deals with the phobias that arise and complicate care of those who have cancer. In this regard, the patient with a morbid fear of cancer who actually develops it has a high level of distress and fear of progression. Because this usually reflects an underlying somatoform disorder, particularly hypochondriasis, it is reviewed separately in Chapter 27.

Phobias complicate care of patients with cancer

when some aspect of the diagnostic workup or medical care leads to a confrontation with a feared situation that is otherwise controlled by avoidance of the stimulus. The primary phobias include agoraphobia, in which the individual cannot tolerate being alone or in an unfamiliar place; claustrophobia, which is activated by enclosure in a small space for diagnostic radiological scanning procedures (CT scan or magnetic resonance imaging) or radiation treatment; finally, fear of needles, the sight of blood, hospitals, and doctors.

These phobias usually occur in individuals who otherwise function well, who have insight into the unreasonableness of their fears and their inability to control them.

Because agoraphobia is the most common phobia in the general population, it is also the one most often found complicating medical care. The necessity to accept confinement in an unfamiliar hospital environment, coupled with anxiety elicited by awareness of serious illness, may be the precipitant for confrontation with an agoraphobia that otherwise was controlled by adaptation of family members to the individual's special needs. While agoraphobia may occur alone, it is often seen with panic disorder and generalized anxiety disorder, which is described later. When the treatment is elective such as a planned surgical procedure, the problem is usually brought up by the family and patient, who indicate the pattern of fears that may pose a substantial barrier to accepting and complying with treatment. An emergency medical problem will suddenly precipitate either the refusal of hospitalization or the necessity to modify hospital regulations to permit a relative to remain with the individual. The following case illustrates the issue in oncology.

### CASE REPORT

A 55-year-old woman, who attempted to reduce her severe chronic nervous tension with heavy smoking for many years, developed hemoptysis and was found to have an early operable lung cancer. She told the surgeon that since the birth of her second child 22 years ago she had developed fears of being alone that had resulted in the pattern of a relative always accompanying her away from home and staying, even while at home, near enough so that she could reach out or call to them. She and a devoted husband doubted that she could face the anticipation of a major procedure without assistance. The surgeon requested assistance in managing this patient's agoraphobia. The patient was seen by a psychiatrist for two visits prior to admission. A careful rehearsal of events with her and an anxiolytic drug along with planning with the anesthesiologist and with nursing staff followed. The floor nursing staff agreed to allow the husband to stay in his wife's room, and the anesthesiologist arranged for early preoperative sedation with attention to controlling an unusually high level of anxiety. She was placed first on the surgery schedule to avoid the wait in the morning; finally, a nurse from the floor walked with her to the operating suite so that she did not experience a period without someone familiar present. She tolerated the surgery well. The family, embarrassed by having to request modification of the routine, nevertheless, were grateful for care that recognized the special needs that, if not met, might have precluded the patient's surgery.

A second case outlines other phobias that complicate care.

CASE REPORT

A 60-year-old housewife required emergency admission to the hospital for surgical decompression of bowel obstruction resulting from metastatic ovarian carcinoma. She informed the staff that she had a lifelong history of fear of needles and the sight of blood, and an exposure to either was intolerable, resulting in a panic reaction. Her anxiety in the hospital was so intense that even 10 mg qid of diazepam did not reduce anxiety to allow her to tolerate the approach of the technician to obtain blood from a venipuncture. A phenothiazine was more effective in controlling anxiety, and she tolerated the required preoperative tests and surgery. Postoperatively, the frightening sight of intravenous tubes and a blood transfusion was minimized by keeping them away from her view and wrapping her arm containing the intravenous catheter as well as the tubing when she was given blood. Blood samples were limited as much as possible, and they were always obtained by a single surgical resident whom she trusted. Her lengthy hospitalization, which was beset with numerous postoperative complications, was managed well by the staff, who recognized the need to modify procedures to adapt to the specific phobias of the patient.

The following case illustrates the management of a patient with claustrophobia who required a brain scan.

CASE REPORT

A 47-year-old machinist developed a Horner's syndrome 3 years after surgical resection of a melanoma on his back. CT scan of the brain was ordered by the doctor to evaluate the possible presence of a brain metastasis. The patient, who had a long-standing claustrophobia, became anxious upon hearing about the cylinder in which he would be placed for the test, but he was too embarrassed to inform the doctor or admit his concerns. On arrival for the scan, he did not tell the technician about his fear of enclosed spaces. After 5 minutes of the procedure he screamed "I'm losing my mind—I've got to get out of here." He was flushed, diaphoretic, and hyperventilating. He was removed from the machine and given diazepam 10 mg po; this reduced his anxiety and he regained control. Although the technician suggested that he return another time, he chose to complete the scan, believing that his anxious state would only increase if he delayed the procedure.

Patients with claustrophobia who require magnetic resonance imaging, radiotherapy treatments or who must be confined in intensive care or reverse-isolation settings also experience distress (Brennan et al.,

1988). Behavioral interventions, including relaxation and distraction with music by earphones, are useful. Reassurance and an opportunity to rehearse mentally anticipated frightening events is helpful for reducing the anxiety.

## Panic and Generalized Anxiety Disorders

The panic disorder, as contrasted to phobias described earlier, is manifested by sudden and unpredictable attacks of intense discomfort and fear that are accompanied by shortness of breath, sense of smothering, choking, palpitations, sweating, trembling, and fears of dying. They last about 20 minutes and are followed by constant fear of recurrent attacks. In this context, the person may increasingly restrict activities to prevent recurrence, and a clinical picture of superimposed agoraphobia may evolve in which the person fears an attack in a public place, requires the presence of another, and becomes homebound.

The treatment of panic in the patient with cancer requires careful attention to the patient's overall medical and personal situation with supportive psychotherapeutic visits accompanied by pharmacological intervention.

The patient with a panic disorder, with or without agoraphobia, may respond to a tricyclic antidepressant, particularly imipramine. With some patients starting doses of 10–25 mg tid may be adequate; however, it may be necessary to increase this dose to 200–300 mg/day for therapeutic response in some patients (Liebowitz, 1985). The precise mode of action that accounts for the beneficial effects is not known; it may vary from patient to patient. The active biological property may be blocking of the uptake of norepinephrine and serotonin in the brain and periphery, or blocking the interaction of acetylcholine and histamine with their postsynaptic receptors (Schatzberg, 1987).

Successful treatment of panic has also been achieved with the use of monoamine oxidase inhibitors (MAOIs) in doses of 10 mg qid; phenelzine has been the most widely studied. β blockers are less effective in treatment of panic disorder than in management of acute situational anxiety. The triazolobenzodiazepine, alprazolam, is useful for both emergency treatment of panic disorder and for chronic management of mild to moderately severe symptoms. The usual starting dose is 0.25–0.5 mg tid, and the doses are increased every other day. Effective doses are usually in the range of 4–6 mg daily, and discontinuation of the drug must be gradual. Clonidine, an $\alpha_2$ agonist, has been reported as helpful. Buspirone is under study for panic disorder; the absence of undesirable sedating effect and addictive potential make it of interest.

Patients with a panic disorder who are under treatment for cancer require adequate control of anxiety by medication. However longer term management decisions must be postponed and a combination of drug management and behavioral or supportive psychotherapy should be considered (Marks, 1985). Although much interest has been generated about mitral valve prolapse and anxiety disorder, the relationship is unclear (Hickey et al., 1983; Shear et al., 1984; Levin, 1987).

From the outset, these patients require assurance that recognition of their psychological distress and its management will be integrated in their medical care.

The following case demonstrates the treatment of panic disorder in a patient with cancer.

### CASE REPORT

A 50-year-old woman realtor with stage II breast cancer adjusted to segmental resection and two cycles of chemotherapy in the hospital. She had a sudden anxiety attack that required sedation and reassurance by the nursing staff. This was followed by three more attacks prior to discharge home to begin radiotherapy. She asked for a psychiatric consultation because she feared more attacks and particularly her ability to tolerate the radiological diagnostic procedures and treatment where she felt a dreaded panic attack would occur. If she could not tolerate the radiation, she feared she would need a mastectomy, which she did not want. She had a 30-year history of minor phobias such as riding alone in elevators. This was embarrassing at times but had not interfered with her life. She did recall a period 20 years earlier when she had had two panic attacks but they had stopped. She also recalled that as a child she had witnessed the accidental death of a playmate who had been crushed when a tractor had overturned on him, which had remained a vivid memory. She was started on imipramine 10 mg tid; 1 week later she was able to complete the first treatment after premedication with alprazolam 2 mg. With continued staff support and treatment with imipramine, she completed radiotherapy and subsequent chemotherapy.

Generalized anxiety disorder, as outlined in the 1987 DSM-III-R classification, incorporates a constellation of symptoms previously called anxiety neurosis: chronic unrealistic worries with autonomic hyperactivity, apprehension, and hypervigilance. This category of anxiety disorders has overlap with other anxiety and depressive disorders; such patients may also develop other disorders over time. These individuals, when confronted by cancer, require conjoint management of the medical and psychiatric disorder with psychotherapeutic support and use of a benzodiazepine during medical treatment. Longer term management must be determined by the severity and the nature of the symptoms and may need to combine psychotherapy and antianxiety medication on a long-term basis.

## Posttraumatic Stress Disorder

Posttraumatic stress disorder (PTSD) is another anxiety disorder that may be activated by treatment for cancer in individuals who have experienced a close encounter with death in combat, by torture, in an accident, or in a natural disaster where many died. The experience of being treated for cancer with the underlying fears of death may, by some seemingly innocuous stimulus, set off a flashback in which they reexperience the traumatic event with terror and an overwhelming fear of dying. They often have chronic symptoms of startle reactions to minor sounds, nightmares, and chronic autonomic hyperactivity. Many survivors of the holocaust find treatment for cancer difficult because it elicits memories of their experiences in the concentration camp; the similarity is with the loss of the control over one's life by the action of others and with specific events, such as being enclosed in a bare room alone without clothes, which evokes panic with memories of gas chambers.

Treatment is directed toward providing support, encouraging abreaction of the traumatic event by eliciting memories of the event in the presence of a therapist, and using medication to reduce chronic anxiety when needed (Ettedqui and Bridges, 1985). The same drugs that are effective in other anxiety disorders are used, that is, benzodiazepines, tricyclic antidepressants, MAOI, β blockers, and neuroleptics.

The following case describes PTSD related to prior experience of combat and the activation of those memories by cancer treatment.

### CASE REPORT

A 35-year-old Vietnam War veteran began chemotherapy for diffuse histiocytic lymphoma; his uncle had died 3 years earlier of the same disease. He asked to speak to a psychiatrist because he had developed horrible dreams from which he awoke terrified, sweating and having trouble breathing. He could not get back to sleep. He had been in active combat during the Vietnam War and had seen his closest comrade die. He had never talked about the experience and had had only occasional flashbacks that he was able to tolerate and then they were gone. With beginning chemotherapy he had felt anxious and depressed. He reported having startle reactions, insomnia, nightmares of bombings and combat, and flashbacks of his first combat mission in Vietnam in which he was flown in by helicopter and his friend had been shot.

His extreme hyperarousal and flashbacks improved with repeated discussion of his memories, and administration of amitriptyline (50 mg po qhs) and thioridazine (10 mg bid). When he had improved, he related the similarities he had felt between having "fought for his life" in Vietnam and "fighting for his life now." With medications and support from oncology staff and psychotherapy, he successfully completed cancer treatment.

Although events related to treatment of physical illness are not currently included among the stimuli for PTSD in the DSM-III-R classification, painfully traumatic events that occur during treatment of cancer, especially in children, may cause PTSD symptoms later in life. Although this has not been systematically studied, PTSD related to some frightening event during cancer treatment has been described (Nir, 1986). Adults have described PTSD flashbacks when recalling being intubated for surgery while not fully anesthetized, with the frightening sensation of suffocation. A patient who experiences a long uncomfortable wait on a stretcher alone, in pain and awaiting a delayed procedure, may recall it with terror and become frightened that it may be repeated. The repeated venipunctures and procedures that children receive in the course of cancer treatment are often experienced with terror and extreme fright on their repetition. Long-term effects have not been systematically studied, but the incidence of PTSD may be elevated in these children.

## SPECIAL ANXIETY-PROVOKING ISSUES IN CANCER TREATMENT

Most of the conditions that induce anxiety have been reviewed, but there are several specific ones that have still to be noted.

### Anxiety with Termination of Treatment

Anxiety was highest prior to the first radiotherapy treatment in a study of women who were assessed over a 6-week period after mastectomy. They showed a paradoxical rise in anxiety specifically related to separation from staff at the end of treatment (Holland et al., 1979). Similarly, when finishing chemotherapy patients become fearful that without close surveillance and a protective treatment against the cancer, it may more readily recur. They need to be informed about this expected period of greater anxiety that will improve over time (see Chapter 10 on chemotherapy).

### Pancreatic Cancer and Anxiety

A large group of advanced pancreatic cancer patients were compared to a similar group with advanced gastric cancer. The pancreatic patients had greater total distress, anxiety, and depression than did the gastric group. Matched for level of illness, this study suggests a need to search for the secretion of a possible false neurotransmitter in this tumor of an endocrine gland (Holland et al., 1986).

### Patients Participating in Clinical Trials

Patients' adaptation to participation in randomized clinical trials has been studied by Cassileth and colleagues (1986), who studied the level of anxiety in individuals randomized to no treatment. Though not significantly different, those patients who were in the control (no-treatment) group had slightly greater anxiety than those women who received adjuvant chemotherapy for early breast cancer, suggesting that it is particularly stressful to tolerate the anxiety associated with no treatment, even though treatment in itself may be difficult.

### Anticipatory Nausea and Vomiting

Since anticipatory nausea and vomiting with chemotherapy has been studied, characteristics that predict vulnerability to it increasingly identify preexisting anxiety as a cause of the tendency to develop nausea easily. Although other influences contribute, such as the chemotherapy drugs and the antiemetic regimen used (Gralla et al., 1987), it is nevertheless a common problem, at least producing anxiety and nausea if not vomiting in up to 63% in some studies. Cella and coworkers (1986) found that it persisted up to 12 years later in cured Hodgkin's disease patients who, when reminded by a smell or a sight of the prior chemotherapy treatments, would experience a sense of acute anxiety and nausea. Although there are aspects of this phenomenon that resemble a PTSD, it has been conceptualized as a conditioned response and treated effectively by behavioral interventions (Redd, 1986). (See Chapter 35 on anticipatory nausea and vomiting.)

## SUMMARY

Anxiety is a ubiquitous emotion in cancer patients that can have various causes. Anxiety can be situational; it also can be produced by pain, by underlying medical conditions, by hormone-secreting tumors, by drugs directly, or as a side effect of medication. In addition, preexisting anxiety disorders are often activated by cancer or its treatment, such as phobias, panic disorders, generalized anxiety disorder, and posttraumatic stress disorder. Evaluation for cause can usually lead to immediate control of symptoms, with the long-term outcome dependent on etiology. Psychotherapy, drugs, and behavioral interventions are effective in the short term, but they are least effective in management of concurrent but long-standing anxiety disorders.

## REFERENCES

American Psychiatric Association (1987). *Diagnostic and Statistical Manual of Mental Disorders,* 3rd rev. ed. Washington, D.C.: American Psychiatric Association.

Brennan, S.C., W.H. Redd, P.B. Jacobsen, O. Schorr, R.T. Heelan, G.K. Sze, G. Krol, B.E. Peters, and J.K. Morrissey (1988). Anxiety and panic during magnetic resonance scans. *Lancet* 2:512.

Cassileth, B.R., M.W. Knuiman, M.D. Abeloff, G. Falkson, E.Z. Ezdinli, and C.R. Mehta (1986). Anxiety levels in patients randomized to adjuvant therapy versus observation for early breast cancer. *J. Clin. Oncol.* 4:972–74.

Cella, D.F. and E.A. Cherin (1987). Measuring Quality of Life in Patients with Cancer. In: *Proceedings of the Fifth National Conference on Human Values and Cancer—1987.* New York: American Cancer Society, pp. 23–31.

Cella, D.F., P.B. Jacobson, E.J. Orav, J.C. Holland, P.M. Silberfarb, and S. Rafla (1987). A brief POMS measure of distress for cancer patients. *J. Chron. Dis.* 40:939–942.

Cella, D., A. Pratt, and J. Holland (1986). Persistent anticipatory nausea, vomiting and anxiety in cured Hodgkin's disease patients after completion of chemotherapy. *Am. J. Psychiatry* 143:982–86.

Derogatis, L.R., G.R. Morrow, J. Fetting, D. Penman, S. Piasetsky, A.M. Schmale, M. Henricks, and C.M. Carnicke (1983). The prevalence of psychiatric disorders among cancer patients. *J.A.M.A.* 249:751–57.

Dobson, K.S. (1985). The relationship between anxiety and depression. *Clin. Psychol. Rev.* 5:307–24.

Egbert, L.D., G.E. Battit, C.E. Welch, and M.K. Bartlett (1964). Reduction of postoperative pain by encouragement and instruction of patients. *N. Engl. J. Med.* 270:825–27.

Ettedqui, E. and M. Bridges (1985). Posttraumatic stress disorder. *Psychiatr. Clin. North Am.* 8:89–103.

Gralla, R.J., L.B. Tyson, M.G. Kris, and R.A. Clark (1987). The management of chemotherapy-induced nausea and vomiting. *Med. Clin. North Am.* 71:289–301.

Hickey, A.J., G. Andrews, and D.E.L. Wilcken (1983). Independence of mitral valve prolapse and neurosis. *Br. Heart J.* 50:333–36.

Holland, J.C., A. Hughes Korzun, S. Tross, P. Silberfarb, M. Perry, R. Comis, and M. Oster (1986). Comparative psychological disturbance in patients with pancreatic and gastric cancer. *Am. J. Psychiatry* 143:982–86.

Holland, J.C., G. Morrow, A. Schmale, L. Derogatis, M. Spefanek, S. Berenson, P. Carpenter, W. Breitbart, and M. Feldstein (1987). Reduction of anxiety and depression in cancer patients by alprazolam or by a behavioral technique. *Proc. Twenty-third Annu. Mtg. Am. Soc. Clin. Oncol.* 6:258 (Abstract No. 1015).

Holland, J.C., J. Rowland, A. Lebovits, and R. Rusalem (1979). Reactions to cancer treatment: Assessment of emotional response to adjuvant radiotherapy as a guide to planned intervention. *Psychiatr. Clin. North Am.* 2:347–58.

Kolb, L.C. (1987). A neuropsychological hypothesis explaining posttraumatic stress disorder. *Am. J. Psychiatry* 144:989–95.

Leigh, H. and M.F. Reiser (1985). *The patient: Biological, Psychological and Social Dimensions of Medical Practice* 2nd ed. New York: Plenum.

Levi, L. (1975). *Emotions: Their parameters and Measurement.* New York: Raven Press.

Levin, B.H. (1987). Mitral valve prolapse, panic states and anxiety: A dilemma in perspective. *Psychiatr. Clin. North America* 10:141–50.

Liebowitz, M.R. (1985). Imipramine in the treatment of panic disorder and its complications. *Psychiatr. Clin. North Am.* 8:37–47.

Marks, I. (1985). Behavioral psychotherapy for anxiety disorders. *Psychiatr. Clin. North Am.* 8:25–35.

Massie, M.J. and J.C. Holland (1987). The cancer patient with pain: Psychiatric complications and their management. *Med. Clin. North Am.* 71:243–58.

Nir, Y. (1986). Post-traumatic stress disorder in children with cancer. In R.S. Pynoos and S. Eth (eds.), *Posttraumatic Stress Disorder in Children.* Washington, D.C.: American Psychiatric Press, pp. 121–32.

Redd, W.H. (1986). Use of behavioral methods to control the aversive effects of chemotherapy. *J. Psychosoc. Oncol.* 3:17–22.

Redd, W.H. and C.S. Hendler (1983). Behavioral medicine in comprehensive cancer treatment. *J.Psychosoc. Oncol.* 1(2):3–17.

Robins, L.N., J.E. Helzer, M.M. Weissman, H. Orvaschel, E. Gruenberg, J.D. Burke, and D.A. Reiger (1984). Lifetime prevalence of specific psychiatric disorders in three sites. *Arch. Gen. Psychiatry* 41:949–58.

Roy-Byrne, P.P. and W. Katon (1987). An update on treatment of the anxiety disorders. *Hosp. Commun. Psychiatry* 38:835–43.

Schatzberg, A.F. (1987). Anxiety disorders: Psychopharmacologic treatment strategies. *Mod. Med.* 55(Spec. Symp. Suppl., January), 7–14.

Schuckit, M.A. (1987). The diagnosis of generalized anxiety disorder and the hidden risk of treatment: An overview. *Mod. Med.* 55(Spec. Symp. Suppl., January):32–36.

Shear, K.M., R.B. Devereux, and R. Kramer-Fox (1984). Low prevalence of mitral valve prolapse in patients with panic disorder. *Am. J. Psychiatry* 141:402–3.

Sheenhan, D.V. (1985). Monoamine oxidase inhibitors and alprazolam in the treatment of panic disorder and agoraphobia. *Psychiatr. Clin. North Am.* 8:49–62.

Spielberger, C.D. (1972). *Anxiety: Current Trends in Theory and Research.* New York: Academic Press.

Sternbach, R.A. (1974). *Pain Patients: Traits and Treatment.* New York: Academic Press.

# 26

# Personality Disorders

Mary Jane Massie

Cancer patients with personality disorders are among the most difficult to treat. Their psychological problems often interfere with their care. They do not cooperate well with others or adapt to the stresses of cancer. Because they often try the patience of even the most tolerant of caregivers, early identification of these patients is essential for management planning. The reader is referred to several excellent papers that outline the special features of these individuals and guidelines for their care (Kahana and Bibring, 1964; Groves, 1978; Perry and Viederman, 1981).

The essential features of the personality disorders form a deeply ingrained, inflexible, maladaptive pattern of perceiving and relating to the environment that causes subjective distress and impairment in normal functioning (DSM-III R). The patient with a personality disorder is chronically impaired and is at increased risk of psychiatric symptomatology (Merikangas and Weissman, 1986).

The prevalence of personality disorders in the general population is estimated to be 7% (Robins et al., 1984). The sex ratio is about equal, although it varies by specific type (Merikangas and Weissman, 1986). The multicenter study of psychiatric disorders in cancer patients found 7% of those randomly interviewed had a personality disorder, which reflects the percentage in the general population (Derogatis et al., 1983). Among 546 patients seen in psychiatric consultation at Memorial Sloan-Kettering (MSKCC), 17% had a personality disorder. This is likely an underrepresentation, many individuals are too ill when seen to obtain sufficient history to make the diagnosis of a personality disorder unless it is severe and central to care (Massie and Holland, 1987) (Table 26-1). The personality disorders most commonly encountered were, in order of frequency: compulsive, dependent, borderline, histrionic, and mixed.

Although classification of personality disorders is

undergoing reconsideration and despite the considerable overlap in the criteria for specific disorders, the standard psychiatric diagnostic nomenclature (DSM-III R, 1987) lists 12 personality disorders that are clustered into four groups: odd or eccentric; dramatic, emotional, or erratic; anxious or fearful; atypical or mixed (Table 26-2). These broad descriptive terms identify core characteristics common to members of each group. In this chapter the disorders are briefly described, as are the problems posed by patients who have both personality disorder and cancer. A patient history is given to illustrate the clinical picture in each cluster of disorders and the management.

## "ODD OR ECCENTRIC" CLUSTER

This cluster of personality disorders consists of schizotypal, paranoid, and schizoid personality disorders. Characterized by an unusually constricted expression of emotion, mistrust of others, or aloofness of manner, they present an initially puzzling picture to an oncology unit. They are distant, unsociable, and—depending on subtype—suspicious or strange in their way of presenting information and perceiving treatment issues.

### Schizotypal Personality Disorder

Individuals with a schizotypal personality have unusual and odd ways of communicating and behaving. It is soon clear that this reflects unusual perceptions and ways of thinking. There may be paranoid, suspicious, or unusual beliefs present, such as clairvoyance that is not clearly delusional, but is similar in content. Their speech is often digressive, circumstantial, and metaphorical. They are often socially isolated, aloof, suspicious, and hypersensitive to real or imagined criticism. They desire little closeness and prefer their

**Table 26-1** MSKCC psychiatric consultations on 546 patients

| Axis II diagnoses* | Number | Percentage |
|---|---|---|
| Compulsive | 19 | 20 |
| Dependent | 16 | 17 |
| Atypical, mixed, other | 16 | 17 |
| Borderline | 12 | 12.5 |
| Histrionic | 12 | 12.5 |
| Schizotypal | 7 | 7 |
| Paranoid | 4 | 4 |
| Passive-aggressive | 4 | 4 |
| Narcissistic | 3 | 3 |
| Antisocial | 2 | 2 |
| Avoidant | 1 | 1 |
| Schizoid | 0 | 0 |
| Total | 96 | 100% |

*DSM-III diagnoses 1980.

**Table 26-2** DSM-III personality disorders

| Clusters | Personality disorders |
|---|---|
| "Odd" or eccentric | Paranoid |
| | Schizoid |
| | Schizotypal |
| Dramatic, emotional, or erratic | Histrionic |
| | Narcissistic |
| | Antisocial |
| | Borderline |
| Anxious or fearful | Obsessive compulsive |
| | Avoidant |
| | Dependent |
| | Passive-aggressive |

*Source*: Adapted from American Psychiatric Association (1987). *Diagnostic and Statistical Manual of Mental Disorders,* 3rd ed. revised Washington, D.C.: American Psychiatric Association.

privacy. They may have brief periods of bizarre behavior or thinking that approach delusional proportions. Although the oncology staff has concern about these strangely behaving individuals (fearing that they will have a psychotic decompensation when faced with the stress of cancer), they usually can cooperate. Some, however, delay in seeking consultation or have difficulty with the decision to accept treatment, at times compromising successful outcome (see Chapter 2).

CASE REPORT

A 46-year-old single unemployed college graduate first saw the dermatologist with a widespread basal cell carcinoma of the face. He had a lifelong history of isolated behavior, aloofness, suspiciousness, and several episodes of frank paranoid ideation as described by his sister. He dressed bizarrely, wearing four shirts at one time. He carried a duffle bag filled with completed crossword puzzles, which were his major avocation. His peculiar appearance and aloofness alarmed those in the clinic, and his suspiciousness of forms delayed hospital registration and the social worker's application for Medicaid.

When he was told his long delay in coming for medical treatment made it imperative that surgery be performed immediately, he became frightened and refused. A psychiatric evaluation found a guarded, suspicious patient. He slowly disclosed that the basal-cell tumors were the result of his having little religious faith. If he now "believed," the tumors would disappear. Weekly 15-minute supportive visits with him allowed the psychiatrist to check on medication for sleep. Crossword puzzles were the bridge to allow limited interaction.

After 2 months he was able to be admitted for surgery and skin grafting; the nursing staff tolerated his eccentricities in dress, permitting him to wear the four shirts in bed. He spent the day as he chose, bathing and eating on his own schedule. All information about procedures was given by one surgeon to minimize suspiciousness.

## Paranoid Personality

The person with a paranoid personality disorder is suspicious and mistrustful, but lacks the oddities of perception, behavior, and communication just described for the schizotypal patient. Being hypersensitive, this person is also easily slighted. Remarkable intensity and acuity of attention is a form of hypervigilance for problems in the environment (Shapiro, 1965). The paranoid individual with cancer often feels that other patients receive more attention and better care. Perceived slights in conversations with doctors or nurses result in anger and accusations. Many of these individuals are contemptuous in manner, and often threaten lawsuits. They are also apt to write critical letters to hospital administrators, news media, and politicians to draw attention to perceived wrongs.

Psychiatric intervention is best directed toward helping staff understand the patient's suspiciousness and mistrust. The staff needs to recognize the common impulse to retaliate in kind. However, ignoring the behavior may be equally deleterious. Limited intervention with the patient that avoids being intrusive may be tolerated and somewhat helpful. Medication usually is of no value.

## Schizoid Personality Disorder

Patients with a schizoid personality disorder have little desire for social involvement, preferring to spend time in solitude. They are reserved, withdrawn, and detached from the hospital staff and routine, and often have difficulty forming relationships with physicians and nurses. Allowing them distance, but explaining each unfamiliar routine allows them to tolerate the clinic or hospital. They are quiet and may not complain about problems, and hence they require more monitoring and questioning for problems.

## DRAMATIC, EMOTIONAL, OR ERRATIC CLUSTER

The second cluster of personality disorders are histrionic, narcissistic, antisocial, and borderline personality disorders. Individuals with these disorders have impulsive exaggerated behavior; they differ in their ability to form attachments to others.

### Histrionic Personality Disorder

The patient with a histrionic personality disorder has patterns of behavior that are animated, overly reactive, exhibitionistic, scattered, and diffuse. Minor environmental stimuli can cause intense emotional excitement leading to irrational or angry outbursts. Superficially they project a warm relationship to others by outgoing behavior, but they are actually vain, self-absorbed, and emotionally distant. Usually they are perceived by others as shallow, superficial, or insincere.

The cancer patient with a histrionic personality disorder usually will be known to hospital staff as a "colorful" patient. Their tendency toward dramatization of symptoms makes it difficult sometimes to distinguish a problem from an exaggeration. The initially appealing patient often becomes demanding, inconsiderate, and dependent. Seeking reassurance frequently from staff, they can become difficult management problems.

The following case demonstrates some of the management problems of histrionic patients.

CASE REPORT

A 37-year-old secretary with stage II breast cancer was referred to the cancer center for adjuvant chemotherapy following a mastectomy. She rapidly attempted to form a special relationship with the oncologist, behaving in a flirtatious manner and telling him how "special" he was to her. She effusively praised his brilliance and ability to cure her. She complained of dizziness and "fainting episodes" on her way home following the treatments, and she also became increasingly preoccupied with thoughts about possible cardiotoxic effects of chemotherapy because of her benign murmur. Finally she refused further treatments unless they were done in the hospital.

She was admitted to the hospital, but it was difficult to obtain a medical history because she said she could not be bothered by discussing "those problems." She attempted to form a friendship with the male intern, telling him about a recent romantic rejection. When the nurse came to administer chemotherapy, she became so anxious, frightened, and angry that the nurse had to repeat the venipuncture. The patient screamed "So you're the one who gives the lethal injections here." A psychiatrist was called to assist in the management of her flamboyant and sexually provocative behavior.

The psychiatrist helped the nursing staff and set firm limits on her unreasonable demands for time and attention. She constantly rang for their attention, complaining of "heart flutters and creepy feelings everywhere," yet their efforts to help were met with criticism.

The staff soon came to resent her exaggerated emotions and unconvincing complaints. They began to see that she was frightened and lonely, and that her behavior was a desperate and inappropriate attempt to get help from others. They worked out a schedule of visits to her room that made her feel more secure. The psychiatrist helped the patient to see how she "worked against herself" by her behavior with the nurses. She improved and was able to continue subsequent treatments in the clinic.

### Narcissistic Personality Disorder

The patient with a narcissistic personality disorder has a grandiose sense of self-importance or uniqueness; preoccupation with fantasies of unlimited success; exhibitionistic needs for constant attention and admiration, sense of entitlement in relationships that vacillate between extremes of over-idealization and devaluation (American Psychiatric Association, 1980). The cancer patient with a narcissistic personality disorder often has difficulties in relationships with staff, particularly with those they perceive as "beneath" them. They frequently have trouble recognizing or experiencing how others feel. Their sense of entitlement or the expectation of special favors may provoke angry responses on the part of the treatment staff. Their insatiable need for attention and admiration cannot be met. Their anger at a perceived criticism of themselves is expressed with vehemence. The narcissistic patient whose self-image is strongly based on physical appearance has great difficulty adjusting to amputation, surgical treatment of head and neck tumors, and radiotherapy or chemotherapy producing alopecia. The anger these patients generate among physicians and nurses is partially countered by understanding the origin of their behavior and their limited ability to tolerate an illness that assaults their appearance, physical integrity, or capability.

### Antisocial Personality Disorder

Individuals with an antisocial personality disorder have a limited capacity to respect the rights of others. They have poor work records, have either no or poor close relationships, and have often been convicted of assaults, theft, and felony.

Individuals with an antisocial personality disorder, most commonly young men, are a management problem when they develop cancer. Their impulsive behavior makes them tend toward poor cooperation and refusal of treatment—especially lengthy cycles of chemotherapy. The young man requiring treatment for testicular carcinoma, Hodgkin's disease, or osteogenic sarcoma who has this disorder may reduce his likelihood of cure by poor compliance. In the hospital, this individual may be demanding and noisy, and will show little sensitivity to the needs of others. Physical violence is rare, but threats, when behavior is questioned, are not. Demands for special consideration in terms of having visitors after hours, leaving the hospital, and excessive requests for pain medication are common. The care of these individuals centers around setting clear limits on behavior that will and will not be tolerated. When limits are clear to the patient and staff on all shifts, they can be enforced without becoming punitive. To avoid a vicious cycle, it is important for staff members to avoid becoming angry in response to a patient's provocation. Giving good medical care can be difficult in these young individuals who want help but resist it and alienate those they most need.

## Borderline Personality Disorder

Individuals with a borderline personality disorder are difficult to manage during illness because their behavior is apt to be unpredictable; their mood and pattern of reaction to others is also unstable. They often have a history of impulsive behavior that may include gambling, drug or alcohol use, or suicide attempts. Their ties to others are tenuous and unstable. They have changes in mood over short periods that vary from depressed to irritable or anxious. They have difficulty being alone and often have a pattern of self-mutilating acts or suicidal gestures. Borderline patients who receive a diagnosis of cancer will likely be able to exert even less control over erratic behavior because of the stress.

They may impulsively make a suicide attempt in the hospital in response to a restriction on their behavior or hearing stressful information from the doctors or their family. Similarly to the other personality disorders in this cluster, clear limits of tolerable behavior must be set and enforced firmly but kindly. They need psychiatric evaluation, however, in order to assess whether there is an affective disorder present that might be treatable. Studies have revealed a high frequency of affective disorders (between 25 and 60%) in individuals with borderline personality disorders far exceeding the 6–9% frequency in the general population (Docherty et al., 1986).

Borderline patients with concurrent affective disorders show roughly equivalent beneficial response to

antipsychotics, antidepressants, and lithium carbonate (Pope et al., 1983; Cole and Sunderland, 1982). Recommended guidelines for pharmacological treatment of borderline disorders include a tricyclic antidepressant or a monoamine oxidase inhibitor for those with depression as a prominent feature, lithium or the antipsychotic thioridazine for those with mood swings, antipsychotics for those with impulsive anger or chronic thought disorder, and stimulants for those with anger, restlessness, and short attention span as major symptoms.

## THE ANXIOUS OR FEARFUL CLUSTER

The third cluster of personality disorders consists of obsessive compulsive, avoidant, dependent, and passive-aggressive syndromes. These individuals, faced with cancer-related crises, may have difficulty making decisions, respond to any ambiguity with fear and mistrust, and experience severe anxiety symptoms. Persons with any one of these disorders are highly anxious and avoid anxiety-provoking situations such as decision making, social occasions, and confrontation with others.

## Obsessive Compulsive Personality Disorder

The individual with an obsessive compulsive personality disorder is preoccupied with details such as rules, order, organization, cleanliness, and efficiency. The "trees" are the focus; the "forest" is poorly conceived as a representation of the bigger whole. In dealing with cancer, the details of treatment are a preoccupation that helps to avoid the greater fear of the disease. There is a single way of doing things; despite devotion to work to the exclusion of pleasure, the individual does not accomplish as much as expected because of obsessive attention to detail and an indecisiveness.

The following case demonstrates the care of an individual with one of these personality disorders.

### CASE REPORT

A 54-year-old single accountant was admitted to the hospital for chemotherapy for adenocarcinoma of the colon with metastases to the liver. He delayed admission to the hospital until he was assured he would have a single room, because he could not tolerate another individual in the room and could not share a bathroom because of his need for privacy and cleanliness. His oncologist had outlined the series of tests planned for him in the hospital. The patient assumed that tests would be done immediately and in the order described to him. When they were not, he became anxious and demanded that the hospital operator call his doctor at midnight so he could "straighten out the impossible confusion" that worried him so that he could not sleep. He asked that the intern be taken off his case because his "sloppy behavior made him a threat to patients' lives" by not assuring the tests were done properly on his doctor's orders.

He kept a large flowchart of his weight, temperature, intake, elimination, and other pertinent information on the wall. The nurses noticed that he kept a notebook, recording dates and times of special procedures. On several occasions, he tape-recorded his interaction with the nurse by surreptitiously placing a tape recorder in the bedside-table drawer. The nurse felt angry and concerned when she had to care for him.

A psychiatric consultation revealed that, despite outstanding academic credentials, he could not keep a job because he could not tolerate the "ineptitude and stupidity" of his colleagues. He was exceptionally well informed about his illness and took pride in his efforts to read everything about colon cancer. The diagnosis of a liver metastasis had been devastating to him because his disease was now out of control. He became particularly anxious and angry when he was asked to participate in a study of pain control in which patients would randomly receive one of two analgesics.

The staff met with the psychiatric consultant and established several guidelines for his management, which included a daily inspection of the patient's chart with favorable comments, all communication about tests and medications provided only by the attending physician, the house staff and the patient's primary care nurse continually present when the patient's physician saw him to reduce the chance of distorted communication, and alprazolam (1.0 mg po qid). His daily dose of alprazolam and analgesic were given to him in the morning, and he was given responsibility to self-administer medication as ordered.

No attempt was made to have the patient examine his lifelong meticulous, demanding personality traits. The staff came to understand how the spread of cancer was an overwhelming emotional burden for a man who strived so hard to maintain control of his body and his environment. Their understanding care paid off, as evidenced by a reduction in the patient's irritability and demands over the remainder of the hospitalization.

## Avoidant Personality Disorder

Individuals who have an avoidant personality disorder are hypersensitive to rejection by others. They wish to be close to others but find it hard unless given a strong guarantee of acceptance. They have excessive concern about potential discomfort or danger in everyday situations and relationships that leads to inhibiting anxiety and painful shyness. These individuals, when faced with cancer, strive to be no trouble to others and may not ask for pain medication or help they need out of a fear of making the nurse or doctor angry. These seemingly model patients need to be recognized as being fearful, anxious, and unable to ask for care. The nursing staff and physician need to avoid being critical or short-tempered with them, because it will cause pain

and lead to withdrawal. Though rarely causing problems, they are more apt to suffer in silence. Understanding their timidity and establishing a warm relationship with them will encourage them to interact more openly.

## Dependent Personality Disorder

Individuals with a dependent personality disorder have a manner that demands that others assume responsibility for their decisions, and they require great emotional and practical support from those around them. They will often tolerate mistreatment to avoid being alone, and will act agreeably even when they believe that others are wrong (Siever and Klar, 1986). During a serious illness like cancer, these individuals are vulnerable to having decisions about their treatment made by the family. The doctor must take the time to be sure that they understand the treatments outlined and participate in the decisions (see Chapter 14 on breast cancer).

## Passive Aggressive Personality Disorder

Individuals with a passive aggressive personality disorder appear to be cooperative and pleasant, never straightforwardly asserting their demands. Yet they use behaviors that indirectly prevent them from meeting requests. They consistently procrastinate, "forget" to do things, and sulk in anger if they do not like demands placed on them (Siever and Klar, 1986). These individuals, when treated in the hospital or office for cancer, tend to be frustrating because of the covert anger and counterproductive behavior that are difficult to deal with directly. The underlying pattern, when understood, is easier to tolerate by the oncology staff. Each aspect of treatment requiring self-care and cooperation may need guidelines established to reduce the passive avoidance.

## GENERAL MANAGEMENT PRINCIPLES

Although patients with personality disorders vary in their distinctive characteristics—among them paranoid, eccentric, dramatic, self-absorbed, or anxious—all have personalities that are rarely modified by psychotherapy, particularly while under the stress of cancer. Their coping strategies and defenses are fixed in a single rigid pattern that denies them the ability to be flexible and use a range of strategies that may be needed to adapt successfully to illness (see Chapter 4 on coping). Because they have limited ability to adjust to unfamiliar routines, it is often necessary to make adjustments in the hospital or office routine to enable their treatment. This sometimes seems undemocratic to some staff members who feel reluctant to give in to a family member's overnight presence, or a request made in anger; still, these patients are unable to conform to the routine, so exceptions must be made to assure that they are treated. When demands infringe on the rights of others, however, a serious review may have to be undertaken regarding whether the individual can be treated or should be in a special medical-psychiatric unit that exists in some hospitals.

The following general principles can be applied to management of virtually all patients with personality disorder who must be managed during treatment for cancer:

1. Psychiatric evaluation should be requested early to determine the patient's personal issues and specific problems that are causing difficulties for staff. This should be followed by a meeting of staff about the patient in which a 24-hour management plan is organized, with plans to meet anticipated behavior and demands. When limits are placed on behavior, they must be consistently and firmly enforced.
2. Information about diagnosis, planned tests and treatments, and test results should be given by a single individual—preferably the responsible physician—to minimize miscommunication and heightened anxiety.
3. Daily patient rounds by the physician should include the responsible nurse and house officer; clinic visits should include family and nurse when instructions are given, to assure clarity of plans.
4. Some hospital rules may have to be modified for these patients in order to meet some request and allow them some sense of control; such modification may actually be required to keep the person in treatment. Relenting on minor restrictions (e.g., extending visiting hours by 30 minutes) may permit the patient to tolerate major requirements necessary for treatment.
5. Patients with borderline personality and poor impulse control are often less anxious when a nursing companion is present at bedside, especially with severe symptoms. The anxious patient is also reassured and symptoms often decrease. Close patient observation also decreases the nursing staff's concerns about possible unseen self-destructive behavior. Psychotropic medication may be indicated and should be employed with close psychiatric supervision.

## SUMMARY

About 10% of the population has a personality disorder. Among the 12 identified personality disorders, four clusters can be identified; each cluster has a core

of symptoms that characterize the individual's behavior, including odd or eccentric, dramatic, emotional, or erratic; anxious and fearful; and atypical or a mixed picture of several of the specific types. Each specific type of the 12 disorders creates its own problems for the individual who also has cancer. In all likelihood, the stress created by cancer will lead to the enhanced use of characteristic coping strategies and behavior, which will complicate treatment and interaction with the oncology staff. Because these patients do not respond well to attempts to help them understand their own behavior, management of these individuals during treatment for cancer focuses on helping staff members to understand the basis of the frustrating and unpredictable behavior, developing a 24-hour management plan for the hospitalized patient, and offering frequent supportive intervention to the patient. The limits of tolerable behavior should be applied firmly, kindly, and consistently by the staff. These patients can be managed with close collaboration of the treating staff and a psychiatrist or mental health professional.

## REFERENCES

American Psychiatric Association (1980). *Diagnostic and Statistical Manual of Mental Disorders,* 3rd ed. Washington, D.C.: American Psychiatric Association.

American Psychiatric Association (1987). *Diagnostic and Statistical Manual of Mental Disorders,* 3rd ed. revised. Washington, D.C.: American Psychiatric Association.

Cole, J.O. and P. Sunderland III (1982). The drug treatment of borderline personality disorder. *Arch. Gen. Psychiatry* 40:23–40.

Derogatis, L.R., G.R. Morrow, J. Fetting, D. Penman, S. Piasetsky, A.M. Schmale, M. Hendricks, and C.L. Carnicke (1983). The prevalence of psychiatric disorders among cancer patients. *J.A.M.A.* 249:751–57.

Docherty, J.P., S.J. Fiester, and T. Shea (1986). Syndrome diagnosis and personality disorder. In A.J. Frances and R.E. Hales (eds.), *Psychiatric Update: American Psychiatric Association Annual Review,* Vol. 5. Washington, D.C.: American Psychiatric Press, pp. 315–55.

Groves, J.E. (1978). Taking care of the hateful patient. *N. Engl. J. Med.* 298:883–87.

Kahana, R.J., and G.L. Bibring (1964). Personality types in medical management. In N. Zinberg (ed.), *Psychiatry and Medical Practice in a Medical Hospital.* New York: International Universities Press, pp. 108–23.

Massie, M.J. and J.C. Holland (1987). The cancer patient with pain: Psychiatric complications and their management. *Med. Clin. North Am.* 71:243–58.

Merikangas, K.R. and M.M. Weissman (1986). Epidemiology of DSM-III Axis II personality disorders. In A.J. Frances and R.E. Hales (eds.), *Psychiatry Update: American Psychiatric Association Annual Review,* Vol. 5. Washington, D.C.: American Psychiatric Press, pp. 258–78.

Perry, S. and M. Viederman (1981). Management of emotional reactions to acute medical illness. *Med. Clin. North Am.* 65:3–14.

Pope, H.G., J.M. Jonas, J.I. Hudson, B.M. Cohen, and J.G. Gunderson (1983). The validity of DSM III borderline personality disorder. *Arch. Gen. Psychiatry* 40:23–30.

Robins, L.N., J.E. Helzer, M.M. Weissman, H. Orvaschel, E. Gruenberg, J.D. Burke, and D.A. Reiger (1984). Lifetime prevalence of specific psychiatric disorders in three sites. *Arch. Gen. Psychiatry* 41:949–58.

Siever, L.J. and H. Klar (1986). A review of DSM-III criteria for the personality disorders. In A.J. Frances and R.E. Hales (eds.), *Psychiatry Update: American Psychiatric Association Annual Review,* Vol. 5. Washington, D.C.: American Psychiatric Press, pp. 279–314.

Shapiro, D. (1965). *Neurotic Styles.* New York: Basic Books.

# 27

# Somatoform Disorders and Cancer

Mary Jane Massie

The somatoform disorders constitute a group of psychiatric disorders in which the primary symptoms are physical, without an organic cause being present. They are not under voluntary control and hence are different from malingering and factitious disorder. They are assumed to be based on psychological conflicts. Identified as somatoform are the somatization disorder, conversion disorder, hypochondriasis, and somatoform pain disorder. Although these disorders are not commonly seen in cancer patients, they present difficult diagnostic and treatment issues. These disorders are seen more often in physically healthy individuals; patients with hypochondriasis often fear developing cancer. Chapter 2 outlines some of the problems of these disorders in physically healthy individuals. This chapter describes the somatoform disorders as they appear and may complicate treatment of cancer.

## SOMATIZATION DISORDER

Somatization disorder was formally described in 1980 in the psychiatric nomenclature (incorporating the terms hysteria and Briquet's syndrome) as a disorder of multiple, recurrent, unexplained symptoms for which some patients seek medical attention. Occurring in less than 2% of the population (more often in women), it is chronic and disabling. Physical symptoms usually begin before the age of 30; patients have a history of multiple physician visits and many surgical procedures. Complaints, presented in a vague and dramatic way, often suggest symptoms in several organ systems. Depression, anxiety, and substance use disorders involving prescription drugs are common. The per capita medical expenses of these patients are nine times the expected (Smith et al., 1986).

Although the comorbidity of cancer and somatization disorder is rare, the clinical problems may be quite complex to manage. The presence of a range of functional symptoms in an individual who has cancer or has been treated for cancer presents difficult issues. The physician must do an adequate workup to rule out an organic basis for symptoms. However, excessive tests and hospitalizations, which the patient may request for reassurance, should be resisted. Regular psychotherapy sessions with attention to symptoms and concern for distress, by a psychiatrist who collaborates closely with the oncologist, will often reduce anxiety and requests for evaluation of "new" functional symptoms. Care must be given by individuals familiar with the patient's history, because a new physician who does not know the history may order new tests and escalate the patient's anxiety unwittingly by concurring with the desire for more tests and attention. The success of this type of management was borne out by a randomized study of patients with somatization disorder. Patients treated by a psychiatrist who made recommendations for management to the primary physician had a 53% decline in quarterly health care charges, largely because of decrease in hospitalization (Smith et al., 1986). Although psychiatric treatment cannot cure this disorder, it is clear that careful attention, given in an outpatient setting, can reduce both the frequency and severity of functional symptoms that might otherwise result in expensive evaluations and hospitalization.

### CASE REPORT

An obese 50-year-old single clerical worker described herself as always "the sickly" child in her family. She was referred for psychiatric consultation when she was diagnosed with non-Hodgkin's lymphoma following a 33-year history of multiple multisystem symptoms (e.g., headache, facial pain, difficulty swallowing, nausea, dysphagia, bloating, diarrhea, constipation, dyspareunia, menorrhagia, muscle weakness, painful urination, shortness of breath, palpitations, chest pain, and dizziness). She was taking five cardiac medications, although her oncologist and cardiologist could not identify a need for these medications. Nonprescription analgesics, cold preparations, and muscle relaxants were also being taken. Though employed, she missed much work for doctors' appointments. Her family took her to all of the appointments; family leisure time was planned to respect her need for rest, to have alternating quiet and stimulating hours, and to satisfy her voracious appetite for specialty foods. Several difficult treatment problems emerged when her oncologist attempted to discontinue cardiac medications and regulate her analgesic dose while she was receiving chemotherapy and radiotherapy. She developed lumbar plexopathy, peripheral neuropathy, anemia of chronic disease, and multiple episodes of bronchitis and pneumonia. However, in addition, many episodes of palpitations, shortness of breath, tachycardia, and dizziness led to repeated evaluation for cardiac problems that could not be found. Each new symptom required careful attention to determine whether its origin was medical or psychiatric.

## CONVERSION DISORDER

Conversion disorder is not rare among medical patients. Engel (1970) estimated that 20–25% of patients admitted to a general medical service have had conversion symptoms at some time in their life. Posner (1982) reported a conversion disorder in 9 of 420 consecutive admissions to a neurological unit who were assumed to have a neurological disorder at the time of admission.

Conversion disorder is a functional disorder in which the loss or alteration in physical function resembles a physical symptom. Stress or conflict initiates or exacerbates the symptom, which is not under voluntary control; symptoms allow the individual to avoid conflict or gain support by secondary gain. Conversion symptoms can occur alone, as part of a psychiatric disorder, or as part of a medical or neurological disorder (Lazare, 1981). It is the latter category in which a conversion reaction may be seen in the course of cancer.

The conversion symptoms often appear to represent grave fears about progression of disease and may mimic extension of a previously present neurological deficit such as a partial paralysis. Patients with conversion symptoms may also appear depressed if they assume that the disease is progressing.

Amobarbital sodium infusion is a useful diagnostic test to assess suspected conversion symptoms, particularly in those with known neurological disease in whom an identified deficit or weakness becomes exaggerated in an inconsistent manner. Amobarbital sodium is infused intravenously (100–500 mg over 10–30 minutes) while the physician tests the neurological symptoms, noting their change (or disappearance), which commonly occurs in the patient with conversion disorder (Ward et al., 1979; Perry and Jacobs, 1982).

The following case demonstrates the usefulness of the amobarbital sodium interview as a diagnostic tool and facilitator of psychotherapy in a seriously ill cancer patient with acute onset of neurological symptoms.

### CASE REPORT

A 45-year-old woman with chronic myelogenous leukemia, blastic phase, was admitted for evaluation after 1 week of vertigo and inability to walk. These symptoms began 3 days after discharge from the hospital for a 2-week course of gentamicin for sepsis. She first noted vertigo upon rolling to the left in bed at home; several days later she became dizzy while attempting to walk. At first she could walk with a cane, but over the week she became unable to walk without assistance. Neurological examination revealed a narrow-based, unsteady, and weaving gait, with frequent lurches in all directions, but rarely falls. No nystagmus was elicited. Psychiatric consultation was requested. The psychiatrist found the patient to be a well-adapted and courageous woman with no previous psychiatric disorder or somatoform disorder. Despite 7 years of illness, she had managed her household until recently. After several days of examination, the neurologist and psychiatrist gave an infusion of 100 mg amobarbital sodium (Amytal); dizziness resolved and the patient was able to tandem-walk and hop on either foot. When the effects of Amytal lessened, the patient could recall that she had been able to walk without impairment during the Amytal infusion. She was puzzled about the cause of her gait disturbance. She asked the psychiatrist if ''emotional factors might have contributed to her problem''; as she asked the question, she said, ''Oh, my God, now I remember. I was in bed at home; my husband was writing checks, a job that always had been mine. I asked him why he was doing that, he said he needed to learn to handle our money in case I wasn't around. I was terrified and angry; I jumped out of bed, became dizzy and couldn't walk.'' The patient was relieved that her gait disturbance didn't mean that she had a brain tumor. She realized that she was terrified of dying, had never admitted her fears, and felt guilty that she was leaving household responsibilities to her husband. A psychiatric consultant worked with her until discharge. At home she resumed many of her household duties; although she continued to have occasional positional vertigo in bed, her gait remained normal. A month later, her white blood count climbed to 350,000; she became progressively obtunded and died.

## HYPOCHONDRIASIS

The hypochondriacal patient who has long feared cancer becomes far worse if the anticipated disease occurs. The normal fears of recurrence are greatly exaggerated, and fears develop around any minor symptom. These individuals appear to be particularly sensitive to physical sensations; the hypochondriacal cancer patient can become incapacitated by fears. These patients require joint management by an oncologist and psychiatrist who can evaluate every symptom for its origin. It is important that visits to many different physicians should be prevented, because patient suggestibility is so great; patients are susceptible to developing more symptoms after the inadvertent mention of possible problems. The presence of depression often complicates the picture as well, leading to concerns about the future as bleak and hopeless.

## CASE REPORT

A 50-year-old attorney was referred for psychiatric evaluation of severe fears of recurrence following a mastectomy for stage I breast cancer; no positive nodes had been found. Her fears were disabling and interfered with normal function. She had a history since her thirties of fears of physical illness and death. These fears had forced her to become panic-stricken at the development of skin rashes, bruises, minor pains, perceived muscle weakness, or swelling. The concerns often followed her having read about a disease such as leukemia or multiple sclerosis in which a minor symptom heralded the onset of a fatal disease. Diagnosis of breast cancer from a self-identified breast lump had led to great distress; however, the operation was tolerated quite well. The patient began to read about breast cancer 3 months after the operation and had many questions about the site of likely recurrence. She feared headache meant brain metastasis and could not rest until a CT scan of the brain was shown to be negative. A short respite was followed by fears of liver, spinal cord, and lung metastases. Panic was allayed only by evaluation and workup by the oncologist and a range of specialists. The psychiatrist finally became the "first line of defense" by discussing each new symptom, suggesting that an emergency medical workup was not indicated and reminding the patient that repeated medical tests did not allay anxiety. Weekly visits with the psychiatrist were instituted, with telephone calls scheduled in between as needed to discuss symptoms. An antidepressant also helped reduce distress; after 6 months of the treatment, the patient could resume her work.

## SOMATOFORM PAIN DISORDER

Somatoform pain disorder is often difficult to diagnose with certainty in a patient who has cancer and in whom pain may already be present as a result of direct tumor involvement, infiltration of nerves plexuses or meninges, or cancer therapy itself (see Chapter 32 on pain and cancer). In this situation the psychogenic component usually reflects the meaning of the pain, which includes tumor progression, hopelessness, and death. Pain becomes an aspect of general suffering. Much of pain management is geared to the alleviation of this psychological part of the pain. This management requires reassurance that the physician will alleviate the pain and that the despair of uncontrolled pain can be reduced (Moulin and Foley, 1984).

Somatoform pain disorder is also seen in individuals who have such tremendous fear of cancer recurrence that they amplify minor discomforts and identify them as signs of cancer. Hypochondriacal patients who have been treated for cancer and individuals with somatization disorder who fear cancer may have symptoms of pain that symbolize their fear and their need for attention and reassurance about its benign origin.

## SUMMARY

Individuals with cancer who have a history of somatoform disorder pose difficult management problems because their complaints focus on physical symptoms that have no organic basis. However, because patients who have cancer are vulnerable to disease progression and those who have had cancer previously may have disease recurrence, it is necessary to evaluate each symptom for its functional or medical origin. Persons who have had a long history of a somatoform disorder, especially hypochondriasis, are difficult to manage after treatment for cancer. The prognosis of these disorders is often poor, particularly when patients first appear (as they usually do) for psychiatric evaluation after years of having symptoms. Because having physical symptoms is the patient's way of communicating affective responses to the world, treatment requires patience and respect for the patient's suffering.

## REFERENCES

Engel, G.L. (1970). Conversion symptoms. In C.M. MacBride (ed.), *Signs and Symptoms*. Philadelphia: Lippincott, pp. 650–88.

Lazare, A. (1981). Current concepts in psychiatry. Conversion symptoms. *N. Engl. J. Med.* 305:745–48.

Moulin, D.E. and K.M. Foley (1984). Management of pain in patients with cancer. *Psychiatr. Ann.* 14:815–22.

Perry, C.P. and D. Jacobs (1982). Clinical applications of the amytal interview in psychiatric emergency settings. *Am. J. Psychiatry* 109:889–94.

Posner, J.B. (1982). Delirium and steroid psychosis: Differentiating neurological from psychiatric disorders. In *Current Concepts in Psychosocial Oncology: Effects of Cancer and Its Treatment on Patient, Family and Staff*. Syllabus of the postgraduate course, New York, Memorial Sloan-Kettering Cancer Center.

Smith, G.R., R.A. Monson, and D.C. Ray (1986). Psychiatric consultation in somatization disorder: A randomized controlled study. *N. Engl. J. Med.* 314:1407–14.

Ward, N.G., D.B. Rowlett, and P. Burke (1979). Sodium amobarbitone in the differential diagnosis of confusion. *Am. J. Psychiatry* 135:75–78.

# 28

## Schizophrenia

### Mary Jane Massie

Like cancer, schizophrenia bears a heavy stigma (Holden, 1987; Andreasen, 1986). The two diseases carry special meaning not only because of their consequences, but also because they appear without apparent cause and little is known about how to prevent their development. Thus, when they occur together in the same individual, the burden is particularly great for the patient and the family, as well as for those who must manage the medical and psychiatric care. Because schizophrenia occurs in less than 1% of the population, the frequency of schizophrenia and cancer occurring together is low. Among 564 patients surveyed who were seen for consultation in our hospital, only 4% had schizophrenia (Massie and Holland, 1987). Yet the problems presented by the dual diagnoses of schizophrenia as a comorbidity with cancer present so many critical problems that the area is given separate attention here.

### SCHIZOPHRENIA AND RISK OF CANCER

Studies of hospitalized psychiatric patients in the 1950s and 1960s explored the question of whether these individuals were protected against cancer by virtue of mental illness or treatment by psychotropic drugs, or whether they might have an increased incidence of cancer (Katz et al., 1967; Odegard, 1952; Csatary, 1972; Rassidakis et al., 1973). Fox and Howell (1974) reviewed these studies and found that authors reporting increased cancer mortality had found it among those recently admitted to the psychiatric hospital where age and physical disability were likely to be important influences in mortality. The patients with a lower cancer mortality were those who had had long hospitalizations. They had decreased mortality from cancer of the lungs and bronchi as well as gastrointestinal cancer and all sites combined. It appears likely that prolonged hospitalization at that time was associated with less exposure to cigarettes and that a simpler, lower calorie diet may have been protective for GI cancer; protection from environmental carcinogens may also have been contributory. One study showed no difference in mortality from cancer in a sample of ambulatory and hospitalized psychiatric patients (Babigian and Odoroff, 1969).

Suggestions that phenothiazines might be protective against cancer were not borne out. In addition, studies from the 1950s of patients who received high and prolonged doses of reserpine, one of the first psychotropic drugs available, did not show increased risk of breast cancer resulting from elevation of prolactin (Hoover, 1977). While mammary tumors in animals are affected by elevated prolactin, the same does not appear to be true in humans. This understanding has reduced concern about giving psychotropic drugs that elevate prolactin in breast cancer patients (see Chapter 6 on risk factors and cancer).

A study reported by Black and Winokur (1986–1987) offers useful data. In a major linkage of psychiatric diagnosis and mortality study done on 5412 psychiatric admissions to a mental hospital in Iowa, 46 died of cancer. This did not differ from expected mortality overall; however, there was an excess of cancer deaths within those who died in less than 2 years. At risk were women and those with organic mental disorders. Their results confirm the high-risk period found by Katz and colleagues (1967). The presence of a serious psychiatric disorder may have contributed to delay in seeking consultation and treatment for cancer. They suggested also that some of the variability in results reported in the past related to differences in the methods used for determining expected mortality.

### CLINICAL ISSUES

Schizophrenia has its usual onset in young adulthood. Characteristic disordered thinking, hallucinations, delusions, and social withdrawal are diagnostic. A family history of schizophrenia would also raise the level of concern about this diagnosis, because schizophrenia tends to appear disproportionately in some families. While some individuals have a single episode and recover, far more common is a chronic course that responds somewhat to psychopharmacological management, but in which a full level of prior function is usually not attained (Harding et al., 1987). However, in a survey of 50 postoperative patients with a history of severe psychiatric illness, including chronic schizophrenia, those patients who were in remission and who were not upset during the preoperative period had an uneventful postoperative course (Solomon et al., 1987). A first episode of schizophrenia rarely appears in the context of the treatment of cancer in a young adult. When it does, it is usually seen in those who have neoplasms common to that age group, such as Hodgkin's disease, leukemia, testicular cancer, and osteosarcoma. Far more common is the acute onset of bizarre thinking in a young cancer patient that relates to a CNS complication of cancer or treatment. Other disorders with psychotic features must also be considered in the differential diagnosis, such as drug intoxication (e.g., hallucinogens, amphetamines, and phencyclidine), organic hallucinosis, temporal-lobe epilepsy, and bipolar and schizoaffective disorder.

Individuals who have schizophrenia and develop cancer present problems in several areas. First, they respond poorly to warning symptoms of cancer and thus they appear often with more advanced stages of disease by virtue of delay in seeking consultation (see Chapter 2). Second, they often have difficulty in understanding the nature of their illness and the treatment proposed. Hence physicians must give special attention to issues of informed consent. Third, because they complain little of pain and discomfort, they are at risk of undiagnosed complications of treatment that can be life-threatening. And fourth, because they have limited ability to participate in their care, especially at home where noncompliance is more difficult to manage, they may compromise successful treatment outcome. Several case reports illustrate these issues.

The first case report describes the problems raised about informed consent by a withdrawn schizophrenic woman.

CASE REPORT

A 63-year-old housewife had a history of schizophrenia dating to her twenties. She had had many psychiatric hospitalizations and had been treated with electroconvulsive treatment and antipsychotic medication with limited success. Her psychotic symptoms were well controlled with perphenazine (20 mg/day) at the time she entered the hospital for treatment of vulvar cancer by radical vulvectomy. She had a blunted affect on admission and seemed disinterested in her condition, the proposed surgery, and her hospitalization.

It was determined that she did understand the medical problem and the treatment proposed in an evaluation by the psychiatric consultant. Her husband agreed to the treatment and felt that his wife, despite her flat affect and emotional withdrawal, understood and agreed with the plan. She underwent surgery and cooperated with postoperative care without any complaints. Perphenazine was restarted postoperatively when she could take fluids by mouth. She was discharged after an uneventful course.

The clinical problems posed by absence of normal response to pain in schizophrenic patients have long been recognized but infrequently studied. The mechanism for decreased perception of pain is unknown, but it has been suggested that dopamine and endorphins may affect this response. A review by Talbott and Linn (1978) described the unusual nature of chronic schizophrenic patients' inattention to and neglect of extensive neoplasms and unsightly ulcerating lesions that would be painful and intolerable to psychologically healthy individuals. They suggested the need for research into the reason for this response. On one hand, it might reflect the schizophrenic's decreased ability to filter input and focus attention, which leads to neglect of and inattention to somatic symptoms. Dopamine is known to potentiate morphine analgesia, and although it is attractive to hypothesize that a relationship between endogenous opioids and dopamine exists, at the present time, levels of endorphin cannot be measured well enough to give meaningful results (G.W. Pasternak, personal communication). This represents an interesting research question in the overlapping areas of pain and mental illness. The following case report describes the clinical problems that are encountered in patients who have inattention to pain.

CASE REPORT

A 25-year-old unemployed woman who had had undifferentiated schizophrenia since the age of 20 was admitted to the cancer center for segmental resection of an adenocarcinoma of the colon. Described by her psychiatrist as withdrawn and isolated, she was able to function at home while taking thioridazine (300 mg/day). She tolerated surgery well and had no complaints; the first 3 postoperative days were uneventful. She was noted by her mother to be increasingly less emotionally responsive over the first 4 postoperative days, but physical examination revealed no abnormalities. On the fifth day, she developed a temperature elevation (103°F), although she continued to walk the corridor several times a day and stated she had no pain. A leukocytosis was also present, and the physician examined her several times a day to find a focus of infection. Abdominal CT scan showed a large subphrenic abscess. The surgeons drained a very large abscess that ordinarily would be accompanied by incapacitating pain leading to early recognition and treatment. She never reported pain and never requested analgesics.

Because most schizophrenic patients with cancer must be managed on medical or surgical hospital units to receive the specialized treatment they require, it is preferable that a psychiatric evaluation be done before or shortly after admission to the hospital. The following case shows the difficulties in planning home care for a severely disturbed young man with schizophrenia who was noncompliant with recommendations.

## CASE REPORT

A 29-year-old unemployed man with recurrent diffuse, histiocytic lymphoma, stage IV, had been diagnosed as schizophrenia, paranoid type, at age 20. Before developing cancer, he had infrequently kept psychiatric appointments, had refused to take antipsychotic medication, and had been hospitalized briefly three times for acute severe psychotic symptoms of persecutory delusions with homicidal ideation. His family frequently called the police to take him to a psychiatric hospital when his vulgarity, threatening behavior, and refusal to bathe became intolerable to them. They would later relent and take him home. After diagnosis of cancer, the patient was briefly hospitalized on a medical unit to determine the extent of the disease. He found hospitalization intolerable, and most of his treatment had to be given as an outpatient.

His visits to the lymphoma clinic were often accompanied by similar behavior, shouting obscenities, threatening the doctor, and leaving the treatment room nude. With assistance from a psychiatric consultant, the clinic staff arranged for him to be seen quickly by a doctor and nurse whom he trusted and who understood his psychiatric problems. The strategy collapsed when the patient appeared unexpectedly or when his condition necessitated tests that he did not anticipate having. Absence of the doctor or nurse also led to problems. Nursing and medical staff feared him because of his disheveled appearance, hostile demands, and threatening statements. They worried also that the patient was unable to report complaints, and they feared follow-up was only marginally adequate because of his behavior. The psychiatric consultant evaluated him and attempted to give him medication, which he refused. The family frequently refused psychiatric hospitalization. His psychiatric illness almost precluded care of his lymphoma; it clearly led to less than ideal care and ability to monitor his disease.

## MANAGEMENT ISSUES

Although most of the common management issues have been illustrated by the case reports, several issues are useful to keep in mind.

First, schizophrenic patients cooperate best when they are managed solely by the same doctor and nurse. A social worker may be helpful to serve as liaison between the clinic or hospital staff, family, and patients. This liaison promotes trust and minimizes frightening confusion. Information should be kept to simple explanations with as little ambiguity as possible.

Second, it is helpful if a psychiatric evaluation is obtained early to assess potential problems, to inform the treating staff about expected behavior, and to provide an understanding of the illness and the degree to which staff should be concerned about disruptive behavior. Close work with nursing staff on management of abnormal behavior is enhanced in the hospital by close coordination of care especially when a special procedure (e.g., CT scan) may require alteration of medication or when medical complications such as fever, hypoxia, or electrolyte imbalance require medication changes.

Third, work with the family is critical because they must assume responsibility for care at home, giving medication, scheduling clinic visits, and monitoring symptoms. They need extensive support to manage the physically ill schizophrenic patient at home; the management may be best done by home visits from a psychiatric nurse and, at times, a psychiatrist (see Chapters 48 and 49). The family may need assistance to find a facility that can manage a patient with both cancer and a psychiatric illness when the relatives are unable to manage at home.

Fourth, it is important that the severely disturbed patient have a single person who is available for visits and telephone contact. Psychotherapy is supportive and often is important as a regularly scheduled contact, even when only day-to-day functioning and medical problems are discussed. This role may be assumed by any mental health professional so long as medication, if needed, is monitored by the psychiatrist. Close contact with the oncologist about medical issues by the one who maintains psychotherapeutic visits is important because ongoing monitoring of the complex medical and psychiatric care is necessary. Schizophrenic patients, while at times frustrating, are also rewarding in that they often develop strong ties that persist over many years, and they may be able to maintain a reasonable functional level with good support.

Finally, some patients require little or no medication, and they view efforts to prescribe as attempts to control their thoughts and behavior or deprive them of making their own decisions. However, most patients do require medication, and the psychiatrist should select the drug and dose schedule, especially in the periods before and after surgery and when the patient's metabolic status changes as a result of disease or treatment.

The pharmacotherapy depends on the nature and severity of the psychiatric symptoms and the issues related to cancer and its management. The decision to place the patient on phenothiazine medication is made after considering the patient's symptoms and the risks. Tardive dyskinesia, for example, is a significant possible longterm treatment side effect which would be of concern in the young individual who is likely to be cured of cancer.

Making changes in dosage and route of administration of medications to accommodate medical problems creates difficulties for the schizophrenic with stable functioning who is often psychologically dependent on medication, and who finds even small changes frightening.

## SUMMARY

Schizophrenia, like cancer, carries a strong stigma in society. It is feared, like cancer. Early suggestions of altered cancer mortality among psychiatric patients, primarily schizophrenics, appear to be related only to long psychiatric hospitalizations with reduced cigarette smoking, simpler hospital diet, and less exposure to environmental carcinogens. The management of the schizophrenic patient with cancer requires close coordination of medical and psychiatric care. Special issues arise in these individuals because they respond poorly to pain and warning symptoms of cancer. They often appear at advanced stages of disease, having failed to notice lesions that would be incapacitating in psychologically healthy individuals. They require special attention when giving informed consent, assuring they understand the nature of their illness and the treatment proposed. They may fail to report pain during treatment for cancer, and life-threatening complications may be detected later than in individuals who respond to pain normally. The ability to cooperate with self-care and home care is limited; attention to each of these potential problems, with closely coordinated efforts, can result in care that combines both medical and psychological support.

## REFERENCES

Andreasen, N.C. (1986). Schizophrenia: Forward. In A.J. Frances and R.E. Hales (eds.), *Psychiatric Update: American Psychiatric Association Annual Review*, Vol. 5. Washington, D.C.: American Psychiatric Press, pp. 5–6.

Babigian, H.M. and C.L. Odoroff (1969). The mortality experience of a population with psychiatric illness. *Am. J. Psychiatry* 126:470–80.

Barnes, D.H. (1987). Biological issues in schizophrenia. *Science* 235:430–33.

Black, D.W. and E. Winokur (1986–1987). Cancer mortality in psychiatric patients. The Iowa record-linkage study. *Int. J. Psychiatry Med.* 16:189–97.

Craig, T.J. and S.P. Lin (1981). Cancer and mental illness. *Compr. Psychiatry* 22:404–10.

Csatary, L.K. (1972). Chlorpromazine and cancer. *Lancet* 2:338–39.

Fox, B.H. (1978). Cancer death risk in hospitalized mental patients. *Science* 201:966–68.

Fox, B.H. and M.A. Howell (1974). Cancer risk among psychiatric patients: A hypothesis. *Int. J. Epidemiol.* 3:207–8.

Harding, C.M., J. Zubin, and J.S. Strauss (1987). Chronicity in schizophrenia: Fact, partial fact or artifact. *Hosp. Commun. Psychiatry* 38:477–86.

Holden, C. (1987). A top priority at NIMH. *Science* 235:431.

Hoover, J. (1977). *Breast Cancer: Epidemiologic Consideration.* Reserpine and Breast Cancer Task Force, Department of Health, Education and Welfare Publication.

Katz, J., S. Kunofsky, R. Patton, and N. Allaway (1967). Cancer mortality among patients in New York mental hospitals. *Cancer* 20:2194–99.

Massie, M.J. and J.C. Holland (1987). The cancer patient with pain: Psychiatric complications and their management. *Med. Clin. North Am.* 71:243–58.

Odegard, O. (1952). The excess mortality of the insane. *Acta Psychiatr. Neurol.* 27:353–67.

Rassidakis, N.C., M. Kelleponnis, and K. Goulis (1973). On the incidence of malignancy among schizophrenic patients. *Agressologie* 14:169–271.

Robins, L.W., J.E. Helzer, M.M. Weissman, H. Orvaschel, E. Gruenberg, J.D. Burke, and D.A. Reiger (1984). Lifetime prevalence of specific psychiatric disorders in three sites. *Arch. Gen. Psychiatry* 41:949–58.

Solomon, S., J.R. McCartney, S.M. Saravay, and E. Katz (1987). Postoperative hospital course of patients with history of severe psychiatric illness. *Gen. Hosp. Psychiatry* 9:376–82.

Soni, S.D. and J. Gill (1979). Malignancies in schizophrenic patients. *Br. J. Psychiatry* 134:447–48.

Talbott, J.A. and L. Linn (1978). Reactions of schizophrenics to life-threatening disease. *Psychiatr. Q.* 50:218–27.

# PART V

## Central Nervous System Complications of Cancer

# 29

# Cancer and the Nervous System

Roy A. Patchell and Jerome B. Posner

Cancer may affect the nervous system in several ways (Table 29-1). The tumor may arise from part of the nervous system itself (primary tumors) or originate outside the nervous system and metastasize to the brain or spinal cord. In addition, the cancer or its treatment can itself cause neurological damage in the absence of direct invasion.

Although cancer arising in the CNS accounts for only about 2% of all cancers, neurological disability occurring in patients with other cancers is common. Up to 20% of patients with systemic cancer develop neurological symptoms either as direct or indirect effects of their underlying disease (Posner, 1978). At Memorial Sloan-Kettering Cancer Center, approximately 30% of all inpatients are seen by the neurology consultation service for questions related to the effects of systemic cancer on the nervous system. This chapter will review the direct and indirect effects of cancer and its treatment on the nervous system.

## PRIMARY BRAIN TUMORS

Primary CNS tumors are neoplasms that arise from neural elements or supporting tissue in the CNS. These tumors have an annual incidence of about 10 per 100,000 population and account for about 3% of total cancer deaths. However, the problem is greater than the numbers suggest. Primary brain tumors cause more deaths than Hodgkin's disease and are the second most common tumor in children under the age of 15, accounting for about 20% of all childhood tumors (Walker and Posner, 1984).

Several characteristics make brain tumors unique among cancers.

1. They arise in the closed box of the skull and have only limited room to expand before causing death. Therefore, although CNS tumors may be relatively

slow growing, small tumors can cause serious neurological deficits and death. Even "benign" histological tumor types can be fatal if allowed to expand.
2. Primary CNS tumors do not usually metastasize out of the nervous system, and so the damage is due to direct destruction of brain tissue and indirect effects from increased intracranial pressure.
3. The brain has little capacity for regeneration once damage has occurred.

The cause of CNS malignancy is unknown, although in a few patients identifiable environmental or genetic influences can be identified (e.g., optic gliomas in patients with neurofibromatosis). In adults, the most common location is supratentorial, while in children infratentorial tumors are more common. Table 29-2 lists the overall frequency of each type of primary CNS tumor.

The symptoms of primary brain tumors depend on the site of involvement. Hemispheral tumors may bring about headache, seizures, dementia, visual loss (field cuts), aphasia, focal weakness, or sensory disturbances. Posterior fossa masses often cause symptoms of increased intracranial pressure with headache, nausea and vomiting, gait disturbances, and lethargy. The course of most brain tumors is one of progressive, gradual worsening of symptoms. Slow-growing tumors may become manifest only with signs of dementia. The differential diagnosis includes metastatic tumors, vascular malformations, strokes, and brain abscesses.

The diagnosis of primary brain tumor is made by CT scan in most cases. Magnetic resonance imaging (MR) is more useful in the detection of primary brain tumors, especially those located in the posterior fossa. Biopsy is needed to establish the exact tissue type and grade of malignancy.

**Table 29-1**  Classification of neurological complications of cancer

| Neurological complication | Examples |
|---|---|
| Primary tumors of the nervous system | Neuroectodermal tumors |
| | Mesodermal tumors |
| | Germ-cell tumors |
| Metastases to the nervous system | Intracranial |
| | Spinal |
| | Leptomeningeal |
| | Cranial or peripheral nerves, plexuses, or roots |
| Nonmetastatic neurological complications of cancer | Metabolic encephalopathy |
| | CNS infections |
| | Cerebrovascular disorders |
| | Side effects of treatment |
| | "Remote effects" |

The methods of treatment available for primary CNS tumors are the same as those available for tumors elsewhere in the body. These include surgery, radiation, chemotherapy, and biological response modification. Biological response modifiers (BRM) are agents that enhance the body's ability to resist tumor growth (e.g., immunotherapy). Most primary brain tumors are treated with combination therapy involving at least corticosteroids, surgery, and irradiation (Shapiro, 1982).

The treatment and prognosis of primary brain tumors depends in part on the histological type. Tumors are classified by their presumed tissue of origin. Neuroectodermal tumors are thought to arise from embryonic ectodermal tissue and are the most common type of primary brain tumor. The astrocytic series of tumors is the most common and includes three grades of malignancy: astrocytoma, malignant astrocytoma, and glioblastoma. These tumors may arise in any part of the brain; however, most originate in the cerebral hemispheres. Current treatment involves surgical re-

**Table 29-2**  Distribution of primary brain tumors by histological type

| Histological type | Percentage incidence |
|---|---|
| Glioma | 50 |
| Glioblastoma | (35) |
| Astrocytoma | (10) |
| Ependymoma | (2.5) |
| Oligodendroglioma | (2.5) |
| Meningioma | 20 |
| Pituitary adenoma | 10 |
| Neurinoma–schwannoma | 8 |
| Hemangioblastoma | 2 |
| Pineal region tumors | 1 |
| Other tumors | 9 |

section followed by radiation therapy. Chemotherapy has been shown to increase survival in some cases. Overall, the prognosis for glioblastomas is poor. The combination of maximal surgical resection, high-dose radiation therapy, and chemotherapy has increased the median survival to about 52 weeks (from about 14 weeks in patients who receive no treatment after surgery).

Other neuroectodermal tumors are oligodendrogliomas, medulloblastomas, and ependymomas. Oligodendrogliomas are slow-growing tumors that are usually located in the cerebral hemispheres. They are treated with surgery (either with or without irradiation), and long survivals are the rule. Medulloblastomas are the most common brain tumors in children and arise from the cerebellar vermis or roof of the fourth ventricle. These tumors are highly malignant and frequently metastasize through the cerebrospinal fluid (CSF) to sites within the spinal canal and more rarely spread outside the CNS. Initial symptoms are usually of midline cerebellar involvement and hydrocephalus. Patients with disease confined to the posterior fossa have much better prognoses than patients with disseminated disease. Treatment consists of surgery plus irradiation to both the posterior fossa and the spinal canal. The 5-year survival rate is about 50%. Ependymomas are also primarily tumors of children and arise from the ependymal lining of the ventricular system or filum terminale (in the spinal canal). These are slow-growing, infiltrating tumors that usually manifest with signs of increased intracranial pressure, and cerebellar and brainstem dysfunction. Treatment consists of surgical resection and local radiation therapy. Because spinal seeding occurs in up to 20% of patients, some investigators feel that spinal irradiation should also be given. The 5-year survival rate is about 25%.

The most common mesodermal tumor is the meningioma. These tumors arise from cells in the pia and arachnoid and occur in specific sites along the dorsal surface of the brain, the base of the skull, the falx cerebri, the sphenoid ridge, within the lateral ventricles, or within the spinal canal. Although these tumors usually do not invade the brain directly, they often reach large size and can compress vital structures. Treatment is by surgical removal with irradiation added if the tumor is not completely removed, is surgically inaccessible or recurs after removal. Long survival is the rule.

## METASTATIC COMPLICATIONS

### Brain Metastasis

Metastasis to the brain is the most common metastatic complication of systemic cancer. Autopsy studies show that as many as 25% of patients who die from cancer harbor intracranial metastases at the time of death. Of these, more than 66% will have had some neurological symptoms during life (Posner, 1979). There is evidence that as patients with systemic cancer live longer (as a result of improved treatment of the primary tumor), both the frequency and clinical importance of brain metastasis are increasing.

Most metastases reach the brain by hematogenous spread through the arterial circulation. This implies that pulmonary cancer will be an important source of brain metastasis and that if the primary tumor is not pulmonary, it has probably metastasized to the lung before seeding the arterial circulation and reaching the brain. Therefore, a careful chest x-ray examination is a fruitful diagnostic test and will show a lung lesion in the vast majority of patients with brain metastases. When the chest x-ray fails to demonstrate a lesion, computerized tomography (CT) of the lung may reveal metastases and suggest the cause of the neurological disorder. In the few patients with brain metastases but no identifiable lesions in the lung, the pathogenesis of the brain metastases may be spread through Batson's venous plexus, tumor embolus through a patent foramen ovale, or tumor filtered through the lungs with only local or microscopic growth.

Metastases may appear anywhere in the brain, but the distribution is, in general, in "watershed" areas of the cerebral hemispheres. Pelvic tumors often metastasize to the cerebellum (Delattre et al., 1988). Therefore, most metastases occur about equally in both hemispheres, with about 10–15% in the cerebellum and 2–3% in the brainstem. Brain metastases are multiple in 50% of patients, and certain tumor types such as malignant melanoma (and to a lesser degree lung cancer) have a greater tendency to produce multiple metastases. Metastases from colon, breast, and renal-cell carcinoma are more often single.

In most patients with brain metastases, the neurological history is one of headache followed over days to weeks by progressive focal neurological symptoms and signs (especially hemiparesis). Headaches may be mild and are often bilateral or diffuse, and rarely have localizing value. Early-morning headache, usually thought to be associated with increased intracranial pressure, occurs in only about 40% of patients who have headaches as the result of brain metastasis. Headaches are more common in patients with multiple metastases or with single metastases in the posterior fossa. Although headaches are often accompanied by increased intracranial pressure, papilledema is present only in about 25% of patients with brain metastases. Approximately 15% of patients have seizures as the first sign of the metastasis. An additional 5–10% of patients may present atypically with other acute neurological symptoms caused by the metastasis, and 1–2% of patients have a nonfocal encephalopathy as the

only sign of the brain metastasis. The best diagnostic tests for brain metastasis are the CT or MR scans. If the history is typical and the lesions are multiple, there is little doubt as to the diagnosis.

However, other diagnostic possibilities exist and should be considered. These include a primary brain tumor, a brain abscess, and a cerebral infarct or hemorrhage. Usually the CT scan can differentiate among these entities. Diagnostic accuracy of the CT scan can be increased by performing thin and overlapping tomographic sections or by increasing the amount of intravenous contrast material administered ("double-dose" contrast). Other diagnostic tests including MR scan, arteriography, or even biopsy may be needed to establish the diagnosis firmly.

Several methods of treatment are available for patients with intracranial metastases (Cairncross and Posner, 1983). Adrenocorticosteroids, radiation therapy, and surgery all have a place in the management of metastases. Chemotherapy is useful in some patients. In determining the optimal treatment for each patient, several considerations must be taken into account, including the patient's neurological status, extent of systemic disease, and the number and site of metastases. All patients should begin receiving steroids at the time of diagnosis. An approach to the management of brain metastases in neurologically stable patients is given in Fig. 29-1.

The occurrence of brain metastasis is associated with a poor prognosis. Untreated patients have a median survival of about 1 month, and with the addition of corticosteroid treatment the survival is increased to 2 months. Whole-brain radiation therapy (WBRT) increases the survival to 3–6 months, and data from large retrospective studies have shown that most patients so treated die ultimately from systemic cancer and not as a direct result of their brain metastases. In the small subgroup of patients who have single brain metastases and limited and controlled systemic disease, surgical treatment plus WBRT has been shown to increase survival more than WBRT alone. However, for most patients with brain metastases, corticosteroids followed by WBRT alone is the treatment of choice.

## Spinal Metastasis

Metastasis to the spinal cord (and its nerve roots) is the second most common neurological complication of systemic cancer and occurs in 5–10% of patients with cancer. Although spinal metastasis usually occurs in patients with advanced disease, it may complicate any stage of the illness, and in as many as 8% of patients who have spinal involvement it is the first manifestation of the underlying malignancy (Rodichok et al., 1981).

The spinal cord may be affected by metastases by

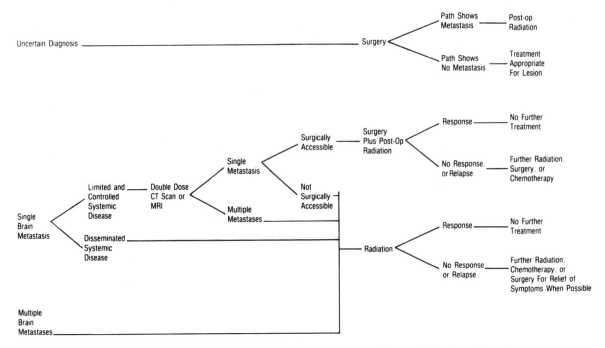

**Figure 29-1.** An approach to the management of brain metastasis in neurologically stable patients.

either spread to the spinal epidural space (with secondary compression of the spinal cord) or by direct invasion of the spinal cord parenchyma. Of the two, metastatic epidural spinal cord compression is by far the most common. Metastatic tumor reaches the epidural space and compresses the spinal cord in one of two ways. In most cases, there is a metastasis to the vertebral body and the tumor then grows into the epidural canal from the bony lesion. It is less common (but characteristic of lymphomas and neuroblastomas) that a paravertebral tumor grows into the spinal canal through an intervertebral foramen. Metastatic epidural cord compression damages the cord by direct compression (with demyelination and axonal damage) and secondary vascular compromise (causing ischemia, edema, and infarction).

The symptoms of spinal cord compression are the same regardless of the site of origin of the primary tumor. Back pain is the presenting symptom in more than 90% of patients with epidural spinal cord compression. Pain is usually present for days or weeks before other neurological signs and symptoms appear. There are two kinds of pain. Local pain is present in the midline (or slightly to the side) of the neck or back, near the site of the vertebral body involved. This pain is usually dull, aching, steady, and gradually increases over time. It is often exacerbated by lying down and may be partially relieved by sitting or standing. Radicular pain usually develops later and is particularly common when the cervical or lumbosacral spine is

involved. Cervical and lumbosacral radicular pain is usually unilateral, while thoracic radicular pain is usually bilateral and perceived by the patient as a tight, bandlike constriction around the thorax or abdomen. After weeks of pain only, the patients develop other neurological signs and symptoms, including weakness, sensory changes, and bowel and bladder failure. Once neurological symptoms other than pain develop, progression is often quite rapid, with a patient progressing to complete paraplegia in a matter of hours or days.

Occasionally patients develop progressive neurological signs and symptoms from epidural cord compression in the absence of pain. Weakness and sensory changes are usually symmetrical, and neurological function above the level of the lesion is unaffected, a finding that suggests spinal rather than brain involvement. More difficult is the diagnosis in the rare patient with ataxia of gait in the absence of either pain or motor or sensory changes. The patient is unsteady on his or her feet and has difficulty with point-to-point tests in the lower extremities; the upper extremities usually are normal, and there is no dysarthria or nystagmus. Although at first the symptoms suggest cerebellar dysfunction, cord compression must be kept in mind and appropriate diagnostic tests carried out to evaluate that possibility.

Once the diagnosis of cord compression is suspected, diagnostic tests should be carried out without delay. An approach to patients with suspected spinal

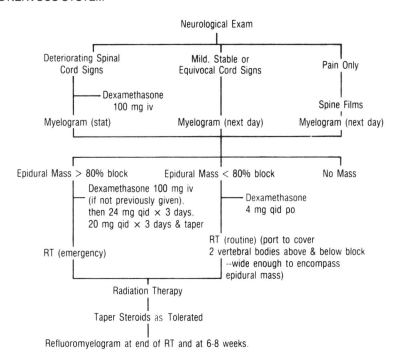

**Figure 29-2.** An approach to the management of metastatic epidural spinal cord compression.

cord compression is shown in Fig. 29-2. Although myelography remains the definitive test for detecting cord compression, MR will probably replace it in the future. Plain x-ray films of the spine are a useful screening procedure and show abnormalities in 85% of patients with epidural spinal cord compression. Loss of pedicles, destruction of the vertebral body, and vertebral body collapse are the most common abnormalities associated with cord compression that are seen on plain films. Myelography or MR should be performed on all patients with suspected cord compression, cauda equina lesions, or intramedullary lesions.

The differential diagnosis of epidural metastasis includes intramedullary metastasis, subacute transverse myelopathy, herniated disks, radiation myelopathy, epidural hematoma, and epidural abscess. The myelogram will rule out the first four of these possibilities; epidural abscesses and hematomas usually extend for more than one spinal segment on myelography, while epidural spinal cord compression from a tumor is usually only one segment long. Also, epidural abscesses and hematomas have a different clinical history (fever in the former and acute onset in the latter) from epidural spinal cord compression.

The treatment of cord compression involves the use of steroids and radiation therapy (Greenberg et al., 1980). The role of surgery is controversial (Slatkin and Posner, 1983). However, surgery has a clear place in several instances, including cord compression for unknown primary tumor (for diagnosis), relapse after maximum radiation therapy, and tumor progression while receiving radiation therapy. Laminectomy is probably not effective in most instances, but more radical procedures involving vertebral body resection have shown promise in preliminary studies. The prognosis depends on the neurological status of the patient when treatment is started. Patients who are ambulatory when they begin treatment will remain ambulatory, and patients who are not ambulatory before treatment do not regain function after treatment. This underscores the critical importance of early diagnosis and treatment.

## Leptomeningeal Metastases

Leptomeningeal metastasis is the diffuse or widespread multifocal seeding of the leptomeninges by systemic cancer. Although this disorder is not as common as solid metastasis to the brain or spinal cord, autopsy data show that it occurs in approximately 8% of patients with systemic cancer. The tumors that most commonly cause leptomeningeal metastases are carcinomas of the breast and lung, lymphomas, malignant melanomas, and adenocarcinomas of all types. Meningeal leukemia from acute lymphocytic leukemia (formerly a common complication of that disorder) is now much less common because of prophylactic treatment of the CNS.

The systemic tumor may reach the meninges by hematogenous spread or by direct extension from a preexisting metastasis. Once the leptomeninges have been invaded, the tumor spreads along subarachnoid pathways (probably carried by the flow of spinal fluid) to seed the subarachnoid space widely. The heaviest sites of infiltration are usually in the cisterns at the base of the brain, the sylvian and hippocampal fissures, and the cauda equina. Signs and symptoms of leptomeningeal metastases are produced in several ways:

1. There may be hydrocephalus and increased intracranial pressure from obstruction of the CSF absorption pathways by the tumor.
2. Cranial nerves and spinal nerve roots may be involved as they pass through the subarachnoid space.
3. Signs of focal brain or spinal cord dysfunction, including seizures, may be produced by direct invasion by the tumor.

Because the entire neuraxis can be seeded, signs and symptoms may involve any part of the nervous system. The hallmark of diagnosis is the finding of multiple, widely separated cranial nerve and spinal root lesions. A few clues should lead one to suspect the diagnosis of leptomeningeal metastases in a patient known to have systemic cancer. The first is that neurological symptoms are more widespread than can be explained by a single lesion (e.g., a patient may have diplopia from oculomotor nerve dysfunction and also have weakness or numbness in one extremity in a dermatomal distribution). The second clue is that although patients may have only unifocal complaints, careful neurological examination often reveals neurological signs not explainable by a lesion at the site of the major complaint. For example, a patient with a headache and papilledema suggesting increased intracranial pressure may be found to have an absent ankle jerk and weakness of plantar flexion of the foot, suggesting coexisting disease of the sacral roots.

Once the diagnosis is suspected from the clinical signs of multifocal involvement of the neuraxis, it can be confirmed by examination of the CSF (Glass et al., 1979). The CSF pressure is often elevated, and most patients have a pleocytosis caused by inflammation of the meninges by the tumor. The CSF protein is elevated in almost all cases, and in about 25% of patients the glucose concentration will be abnormally low. The diagnosis is established by finding malignant cells in the CSF. If no malignant cells are found on the first tap, two or three more spinal taps should be performed. In approximately 50% of the patients with leptomeningeal metastases, the first spinal tap will reveal the presence of malignant cells, and by the third tap over 90% of cases will be detected. The absence of malignant cells in the CSF does not, however, rule out the diagnosis of leptomeningeal metastases. In some patients, despite extensive leptomeningeal tumor at autopsy, multiple antemortem spinal taps have failed to demonstrate the tumor. If the diagnosis is suspected clinically and repeated spinal taps fail to make the diagnosis, a cisternal puncture should be considered. In the absence of malignant cells in the CSF, two other laboratory tests may strongly suggest the diagnosis. A CT scan may show hydrocephalus in the absence of a mass lesion (e.g., a cerebellar tumor) or contrast enhancement in the basilar cisterns (indicating a breakdown in the blood–brain barrier due to tumor infiltration). A myelogram may suggest the diagnosis by demonstrating small tumor nodules on multiple roots. The differential diagnosis includes multiple solid metastases and infective meningitis. Radiographic studies and CSF cultures (including fungal cultures and cryptococcal antigen studies) will rule out these other possibilities in most patients.

Treatment must be directed at the entire neuraxis (Wasserstrom et al., 1982). Whole-neuraxis radiation therapy usually cannot be given because of the severe bone marrow depression that results. Local irradiation to relieve hydrocephalus may be indicated in some cases. Current therapy involves intrathecal or intraventricular chemotherapy, and about 50% of the patients so treated will have stabilization or improvement of their symptoms. However, the median survival of patients with leptomeningeal metastases is 4–5 months, with less than 10% of patients alive 1 year after diagnosis. In addition, almost all long-term survivors have some evidence of leukoencephalopathy that is related to treatment.

## Metastases to Cranial or Peripheral Nerves, Roots, or Plexuses

Although systemic cancer can metastasize and compress or invade almost any nerve in the body, two frequently encountered clinical situations of particular importance are invasion of the brachial plexus and invasion of the lumbosacral plexus (Posner, 1979).

## METASTASES TO THE BRACHIAL PLEXUS

Metastases to the brachial plexus are particularly common when carcinoma of the lung involves the apex of the lung and infiltrates the lower part of the brachial plexus (Pancoast tumor), or when carcinoma of the breast metastasizes to axillary and supraclavicular nodes and either compresses or invades the plexus. In either case the symptoms are characteristic. Pain is almost invariably the first symptom. The pain usually begins in the shoulder or axilla and then radiates down the medial aspect of the arm toward the fifth finger. The pain is often localized to the medial aspect of the elbow, is usually severe and unremitting, and usually precedes other symptoms by several weeks. Paresthesia, the next symptom to appear, usually begins in the fifth finger and spreads to involve contiguous fingers. Weakness is usually the last symptom to appear. A Horner's syndrome may also be present if the lesion is situated medially.

The differential diagnosis includes radiation fibrosis of the brachial plexus (in patients who have received previous radiation therapy), metastases to the C7 and T1 vertebrae, herniated disks, and thoracic-outlet syndrome. In the patient with radiation fibrosis, the pain is usually less prominent or absent. Sensory loss and motor dysfunction are more prominent in the upper cervical roots, leading to numbness over the outer aspect of the arm and weakness of the shoulder girdle. Horner's syndrome is uncommon, but lymphedema of the arm is common. X-ray examination of the chest will often show an apical tumor. Myelography is also helpful in ruling out epidural disease. CT scan of the brachial plexus is the diagnostic test of choice to demonstrate tumor involvement. In some cases, none of the tests mentioned can establish the diagnosis, and surgical exploration of the plexus must be performed. The treatment of infiltration of the brachial plexus by tumor involves radiation therapy or surgical resection. Chemotherapy is occasionally effective.

## METASTASES TO THE LUMBOSACRAL PLEXUS

Lumbosacral plexus involvement is most often seen when tumors that originate in the pelvic area spread to invade the neurological structures of the posterior pelvis. As with brachial plexus involvement, pain is usually the first and most prominent symptom. The pain, located in the lower back and pelvic area and usually chronic, severe, and unremitting, is usually unilateral and frequently made worse by lying supine. In addition to the local pain, radicular pain is often present in the L5 and S1 distribution or may occasionally be present in an L3 or L4 distribution or the rectal area in the S2–S4 distribution. Paresthesias may also be present. Autonomic changes appear late in the course. CT scan is the diagnostic method of choice; myelography is usually helpful only in ruling out root or cord involvement. The differential diagnosis includes radiation fibrosis of the plexus. Treatment involves pain relief, usually with narcotic analgesics, and antitumor therapy with radiation therapy and/or chemotherapy.

## NONMETASTATIC COMPLICATIONS

Table 29-1 classifies nonmetastatic complications of systemic cancer. Except for metabolic encephalopa-

thy, nonmetastatic complications are less common than metastatic disease. Nonmetastatic complications frequently develop acutely; they are often fully reversible but may be fatal if not recognized and treated.

### Metabolic Encephalopathy

Metabolic encephalopathy refers to behavioral changes that result when a systemic cancer (or other systemic disease) indirectly alters cerebral metabolism (Lipowski, 1980). A well-known example of metabolic encephalopathy is that caused when cancer damages liver function (hepatic encephalopathy). Metabolic encephalopathy may complicate any stage of a patient's systemic illness but often occurs as part of the terminal events. Metabolic encephalopathies usually begin acutely or subacutely and produce a clinical picture dominated by evidence of confusion, thinking errors, behavioral abnormalities, disorders of consciousness, and abnormal motor signs (asterixis and multifocal myoclonus) (Plum and Posner, 1980). Therefore, metabolic encephalopathy is one cause of delirium (Chapter 30), although these terms are often used interchangeably. However, delirium can also be produced by brain metastasis and other nonmetastatic neurological complications of cancer described in this chapter. The clinical changes of metabolic encephalopathy are usually reversible if the underlying systemic metabolic abnormality can be treated successfully.

Metabolic encephalopathy is probably the most common neurological complication of systemic cancer. One study showed that delirium was present in 25% of hospitalized cancer patients who were seen for psychiatric consultation. Careful testing of the mental status of patients on medical wards of a cancer hospital showed that 15–25% had abnormalities of cognitive function that were not related to structural disease; these abnormalities were frequently not recognized by the patients' physicians.

The causes of metabolic encephalopathy are as many and varied as the illnesses that disturb body chemistry (Plum and Posner, 1980). However, in patients with systemic cancer, certain causes occur more frequently than in the general population (Table 29-3). In many cases no single metabolic abnormality is sufficient to cause delirium, but the patient suffers from multiple metabolic disturbances that, taken together, can produce the clinical symptoms. This confusing diagnostic problem has its happy therapeutic counterpart, because (at times) treatment of any one of the metabolic disorders may substantially restore normal cognitive function.

Mental status changes are the earliest and most subtle signs of metabolic brain disease. Early symptoms

**Table 29-3**  Some metabolic encephalopathies caused by cancer

| Type of encephalopathy | Examples |
| --- | --- |
| Destruction of vital organs | Liver (hepatic coma) |
|  | Lung (pulmonary encephalopathy) |
|  | Kidney (uremia) |
|  | Bone (hypercalcemia) |
| Elaboration of hormonal substances by tumor | Parathormone (hypercalcemia) |
|  | Corticotropin (Cushing's syndrome) |
|  | Antidiuretic hormone (water intoxication) |
| Nutritional deficits | Thiamine deficiency (Wernicke's encephalopathy) |
|  | $B_{12}$ and folate deficiency (dementia) |
|  | Tryptophan deficiency (carcinoid syndrome) |

can include alterations in the patient's usual behavior such as increased restlessness or lethargy, emotional lability, insomnia, or vivid nightmares. Some patients appear fearful and anxious; others are depressed. Patients may express the fear that they are going crazy. Usually, however, patients lie quietly or sleep when left alone, and rarely interact with the world around them. Occasionally, they become restless, irritable, and easily distractible. Disturbances of cognition characterized by difficulties with immediate recall and ability to abstract, as well as impairment of memory and orientation, also occur early. Later, perceptual errors occur and are usually followed by illusions and hallucinations. As the metabolic disturbances become more severe, patients become increasingly drowsy and eventually become stuporous or comatose. The mental status fluctuates so that marked changes occur from examination to examination. Patients who have underlying structural brain abnormalities will occasionally experience a worsening of preexisting focal findings that may wax and wane with the depth of the metabolic encephalopathy. Tremor, asterixis, and multifocal myoclonus are characteristic of metabolic brain disease, and the specificity of the last two makes them the most important physical signs that distinguish metabolic encephalopathy from psychiatric illness or structural brain disease.

The diagnosis of metabolic brain disease is based on the history and physical examination and augmented by laboratory studies. If the physical examination suggests focal brain dysfunction, then structural abnormalities must be ruled out by CT or MR scan. The electroencephalogram (EEG) is useful in evaluating patients with metabolic brain disease because the background activity is slower than normal, and the abnor-

mality is usually symmetrical. Other laboratory tests useful in determining the cause of the metabolic encephalopathy include serum electrolytes, calcium, blood gases, liver function tests, ammonia level, blood levels of sedative and narcotic agents, thyroid studies, and blood cultures.

The treatment of metabolic brain disease is the treatment of the underlying systemic metabolic abnormality. All attempts should be made to correct detectable metabolic abnormalities, and all drugs not essential for the treatment of the patient's systemic illness should be withdrawn. The patient should be kept in a quiet, well-lit room and have frequent contact with staff and family members. Haloperidol in small doses may calm the agitated patient and make management easier. Physical restraint is sometimes necessary to prevent self-injury.

## Infections

CNS infections are an infrequent but important cause of neurological disability in patients with systemic cancer. The anatomical sites of infection (e.g., the leptomeninges in meningitis and the brain in encephalitis and brain abscesses) are similar to the sites that are affected in the general population. However, many patients with cancer are immunosuppressed as a result of either their underlying disease or its treatment, and these patients are susceptible to a wider spectrum of infectious diseases than are normal people.

The brain, meninges, and subarachnoid space may be invaded by infectious agents through the bloodstream (during a septicemia), by metastasis (from a focal infection elsewhere in the body), or through direct extension from nearby structures (ears or sinuses). The usual manifestations of meningitis are fever, stiff neck, diffuse headache, and mental status changes. However, in severely immunodepressed patients, altered mental status may be the only indication of infection. Brain abscesses may bring about signs of a mass lesion or diffuse encephalopathy. A spinal tap is indicated in all cases of suspected neurological infection and in all instances of altered mental status for which no other cause can readily be determined. CT scans should usually be performed before the spinal tap to rule out mass lesions (metastases, brain abscess, etc.). Most CNS infections are treatable if they are diagnosed early. Table 29-4 lists the most common organisms associated with various types of CNS infections in cancer patients.

Neurological complications of acquired immunodeficiency syndromes (AIDS) represent a special category of infection (see Chapter 21). AIDS is caused by infection with the HIV virus, an organism that dis-

**Table 29-4** Nervous system infections associated with cancer

| Type of infection | Examples |
|---|---|
| *Meningitis* | |
| Bacterial | *Listeria monocytogenes* (lymphomas) |
| | *Streptococcus pneumoniae* (lymphomas, postsplenectomy) |
| | Gram-negative rods (head and spine tumors, low WBC) |
| | Staphylococci (head and spine tumors, patients with ventricular shunts or reservoirs) |
| Fungal | *Cryptococcus neoformans* (lymphomas) |
| | *Candida albicans* |
| *Abscess* | |
| Bacterial | Any organism (head and spine tumors) |
| | *Nocardia asteroides* (lymphomas) |
| Fungal (post-chemotherapy, antibiotics, low WBC) | *Aspergillus* spp. |
| | *Mucor* spp. |
| Protozoan | *Toxoplasma gondii* (Hodgkin's disease) |
| *Encephalomyelitis* | |
| Viral | Herpes zoster (lymphomas) |
| | Progressive multifocal leukoencephalopathy |
| Protozoan | *Strongyloides stercoralis* (lymphomas, patients on steroids) |
| | *Toxoplasma gondii* (lymphomas) |

**Table 29-5** CNS/Vascular disease in cancer patients

| Type of disease | Example |
|---|---|
| *Cerebral infarction* | |
| Thrombotic | Atherosclerotic thrombosis |
| | Intravascular coagulation |
| | Venous sinus occlusion |
| | Tumor invasion or compression |
| | Nonmetastatic thrombosis |
| Embolic | Nonbacterial thrombotic endocarditis |
| | Septic emboli |
| | Tumor emboli |
| Granulomatous angiitis (associated with herpes zoster and lymphomas) | |
| *Intracranial hemorrhage* | |
| Intraparenchymal | Metastatic tumor (melanoma and germ-cell tumors) |
| | Thrombocytopenia |
| | Coagulation disorders |
| Subarachnoid | |
| Subdural | |
| Epidural | |
| *Spinal infarction, septic* | |
| *Spinal hemorrhage secondary to lumbar puncture* | |

rupts T cells; this leads to the development of both opportunistic infections and immunodeficiency-related cancers (particularly Kaposi's sarcoma and lymphomas). Most patients suffering from AIDS develop substantial neurological complications, often as the first sign (Snider et al., 1983). The most common brain disorder in AIDS is a subacute encephalopathy characterized by slowly progressive dementia with evidence of brain atrophy on CT scan, small areas of demyelination in the white matter, and sometimes glial nodules (Price et al., 1988). This disorder is believed to be caused by direct invasion of the brain by the virus. In addition, patients may suffer infection of the brain and meninges from a number of opportunistic organisms, including *Toxoplasma*, cryptococcus, herpes simplex and zoster, and JC virus (progressive multifocal leukoencephalopathy). The brain may also harbor lymphoma, either metastatic from a primary lymphoma located elsewhere in the body or arising in the brain itself. The diagnosis of many of these disorders is made by CT scan and CSF evaluation. In some instances, the diagnosis can only be made by cerebral biopsy.

## Vascular Disorders

Cerebrovascular pathology is present in about 15% of cancer patients and is the second most common neuropathological finding in autopsy series of patients with systemic cancer (Graus et al., 1985). Symptoms from vascular disease are less common and occur in about 7% of patients during life. Cerebral infarction and hemorrhage are the most important vascular complications. The causes of cerebrovascular disorders in patients with cancer are classified in Table 29-5.

### CEREBRAL INFARCTION

Cerebral infarction can result from either thrombosis of vessels or embolism. Atherosclerosis is the most frequent cause of infarction found upon autopsy of deceased cancer patients; however, only about 25% of infarctions due to atherosclerosis are symptomatic during life.

The most common cause of symptomatic cerebral infarction is nonbacterial thrombotic endocarditis (NBTE). In this condition, sterile vegetations consisting of fibrin and platelets are present on otherwise normal heart valves. NBTE is most often associated with adenocarcinomas, but it can complicate any systemic cancer. CNS manifestations usually follow one of three patterns. About 33% of patients have a progressive encephalopathy without any focal neurological deficits, 33% have acute focal neurological signs suggesting a stroke, and 33% have acute multifocal neurological disease due to involvement of more than one major cerebral vessel. The antemortem diagnosis is difficult because there are usually no heart murmurs, echocardiographic abnormalities, or other stigmata of endocarditis. The diagnosis may occasionally be made by two-dimensional echocardiography, and cerebral angiography may demonstrate evidence of embolic occlusion of small vessels. Anticoagulation may be helpful in some patients, but no controlled clinical trials have demonstrated the effectiveness of any treatment.

Disseminated intravascular coagulation (DIC) is an important complication of cancer and is the second most common cause of symptomatic cerebral infarction in cancer patients. This disorder may complicate any type of cancer but is frequently seen in leukemia and lymphomas. The condition is marked pathologically by occlusion of small cerebral vessels by fibrin and platelet thrombi. There are multiple small infarcts and petechiae. The clinical course is characterized by the acute onset of a fluctuating encephalopathy, often complicated by focal or generalized seizures and transient or mild focal signs. Laboratory studies are of help in making the diagnosis. Early in the course there may be a falling platelet count, and later fibrinogen and fibrin split products are usually elevated. Anticoagulation is the recommended treatment.

Occlusion of cerebral veins or dural sinuses may also cause infarction. This problem is most frequently encountered in patients with leukemia or lymphomas but is also seen in patients with other types of solid tumors. Superior sagittal sinus thrombosis is most often related to infiltration by tumor but may also occur as a nonmetastatic complication. The clinical presentation is characterized by the acute onset of focal or generalized convulsions sometimes preceded by hours or days of headache. Occasionally the only abnormality will be a diffuse encephalopathy. Patients may or may not have papilledema. The diagnosis is made by arteriography. Treatment is controversial. Anticoagulation may be useful in certain cases. In general, treatment of the underlying disease usually is the best treatment.

## INTRACRANIAL HEMORRHAGE

Hemorrhages and infarctions occur in roughly equal numbers in cancer patients. However, cerebral hemorrhages are more likely to be symptomatic than infarcts.

The most common cause of spontaneous intracerebral hemorrhage is coagulopathy associated with leukemia or hemorrhage into a metastasis (especially melanomas and germ-cell tumors). Intracerebral hemorrhages are characterized by the acute onset of headache, focal neurological deficits, and the rapid development of coma and death. Subdural hematomas are another less frequent example of intracranial bleeding. These are also usually associated with either leukemia or dural metastases. Hypertensive intracerebral bleeding is very uncommon in cancer patients. The diagnosis of intracerebral hemorrhage is usually made by CT scan. Angiography is rarely needed to confirm the diagnosis.

## SPINAL HEMORRHAGE

Spinal subdural hematomas are almost always associated with spinal taps in patients with low platelet counts ($<20,000$ per mm$^3$). Most are probably asymptomatic. When they are clinically evident the symptom is back pain that may radiate into the legs. Progressive paraparesis rarely occurs. The treatment is platelet transfusions to allow a clot to form. Steroids may be helpful in cases with progressive weakness.

## Neurological Complications Due to Cancer Treatment

### RADIATION THERAPY

Permanent neurological damage from radiation therapy (RT) is generally rare. The likelihood of neurological disability is related to the dose of RT delivered, the volume of the nervous system irradiated, and other variables such as the vascularity of the irradiated tissue and the biological susceptibility to radiation of the individual patient (Berger, 1982). RT can produce damage to the brain, spinal cord, or peripheral nerves. Damage can become apparent acutely or up to several years after treatment (Table 29-6).

Radiation-induced encephalopathy is the most common complication of RT to the brain. Three main clinical syndromes have been described. An acute encephalopathy may occur in patients with increased intracranial pressure who receive large doses of RT. This syndrome is more likely to occur in patients who are not receiving steroids at the time of RT. The symptoms, which usually begin immediately following the first radiation fraction and may recur with less severity after each subsequent treatment, include headache, nausea and vomiting, fever, sleepiness, and occasionally worsening of preexisting focal neurological signs. In severe cases these symptoms may progress to herniation and death. The cause is probably an increase in intracranial pressure due to an acute radiation-induced

**Table 29-6**  Radiation-induced injury to the nervous system

| Organ affected | Time after injury | Clinical findings |
|---|---|---|
| Brain | Immediate (minutes–hours) | Signs of increased intracranial pressure |
| Brain | Early-delayed (6–16 weeks) | Somnolence, focal signs |
| Brain | Late-delayed (months–years) | Dementia, focal signs Hydocephalus |
| Spinal cord | Early-delayed (2–37 weeks) | Lhermitte's sign |
| Spinal cord | Late-delayed (months–years) | Transverse myelopathy |

change in the blood–brain barrier. The syndrome is treated with steroids.

An early-delayed encephalopathy may begin 6–16 weeks after treatment but can ensue within 24 hours or as long as 2 months. Major symptoms consist of lethargy, headache, and nausea and vomiting. In children who have received RT prophylactically for acute leukemia and do not have focal neurological damage, the symptoms usually consist of somnolence and headache. However, in patients who have been irradiated because of focal lesions (or whose radiation port has affected the brain focally), symptoms of focal neurological disease suggesting recurrence or continued growth of the brain tumor may be added to the generalized signs of sleepiness and headache. The exact cause of the early complications of RT are not known. It may be related to edema or demyelination. Most cases are self-limited and resolve spontaneously 1–6 weeks after onset. Steroids may be of help both as treatment after the syndrome develops and as prophylaxis in patients pretreated with steroids before and during RT.

A more severe late-delayed radiation encephalopathy may develop after a latency of 6–41 months (median 14 months). The syndrome is characterized by the gradual onset of headache, personality change, and focal neurological deficits. Seizures may also occur. These symptoms suggest a focal neurological lesion, and the major differential diagnosis involves recurrent (or residual) tumor, abscess, or infarct. CT scans often show a hypodense lesion in white matter that may or may not be enhanced by contrast. Biopsy samples show necrosis with changes in blood vessels and connective tissue. Treatment with steroids helps, but often surgical resection of the necrotic mass is necessary.

The spinal cord may be irradiated as part of treatment to a spinal tumor or as an "innocent bystander" when radiation is applied to other sites (lung or breast). Radiation myelopathy also occurs in early and late

forms. A transient myelopathy consisting entirely of Lhermitte's sign is a very common occurrence 2–37 weeks after RT (median 16 weeks). Lhermitte's sign consists of electric shocklike sensations below the neck, frequently confined to the lumbosacral area. These are brought on by neck flexion and are made worse with exercise. No other abnormal physical signs are present. Symptoms gradually resolve in 3–5 months, and the presence of this syndrome is not associated with progressive spinal cord dysfunction. No treatment is necessary. The cause of the acute syndrome is probably reversible demyelination in the posterior columns of the spinal cord.

Chronic progressive radiation myelopathy is a devastating late-delayed complication that usually occurs about 1 year after RT (range 5–60 months). The clinical features are marked by paresthesias and sensory loss, spastic motor weakness, bowel and bladder dysfunction, and painful dysesthesias. Often a Brown–Sequard syndrome will be present. The disease usually progresses to a complete transverse myelopathy, although occasionally patients stabilize short of paraplegia. Because the differential diagnosis includes recurrent (or new) spinal tumor, myelography is indicated in all cases of suspected chronic radiation myelopathy. The myelogram is usually normal; however, there may be atrophy or swelling of the cord. Treatment with steroids may be of some benefit, but the prognosis for full recovery of spinal cord function is poor. The most likely cause of the syndrome is vascular damage and demyelination.

## CHEMOTHERAPY

A variety of chemotherapeutic agents may produce neurotoxicity in the central or peripheral nervous system (Kaplan and Wiernik, 1984; Young, 1982). The nervous system may be affected by direct neurotoxicity or by indirect involvement due to toxicity of other organs (e.g., hepatic encephalopathy caused by liver failure from chemotherapy). Neurotoxicity from chemotherapy often resembles other neurological complications of cancer, especially metastases and remote effects, and must be differentiated from these entities. Syndrome recognition is important because the side effects of chemotherapy are often reversible. Table 29-7 lists the major syndromes associated with various neurological complications of chemotherapy. Several important drugs deserve special mention.

### Methotrexate

Methotrexate may produce both acute and chronic neurotoxicity. The most common acute reactions are meningeal irritation and transverse myelopathy, both of

**Table 29-7** Neurological complications of chemotherapy

| Major syndrome | Causative agent |
| --- | --- |
| Encephalopathy | Methotrexate |
| | Hexamethylmelamine |
| | 5-FU |
| | Procarbazine |
| | BCNU |
| | Cis-Platinum |
| | Cyclophosphamide |
| | 5-Azacytidine |
| | PALA |
| | Spirogermanium |
| | Misonidazole |
| | Ara-C |
| Acute cerebellar syndrome–ataxia | 5-FU |
| | Ara-C |
| | Procarbazine |
| | Hexamethylmelamine |
| | Spirogermanium |
| | BCNU |
| Arachnoiditis–myelopathy | Intrathecal methotrexate |
| | Intrathecal Ara-C |
| | Intrathecal thiotepa |
| Neuropathy | Vinca alkaloids |
| | Cis-Platinum |
| | Hexamethylmelamine |
| | Procarbazine |
| | 5-Azacytidine |
| | VP-16 |
| | VM-26 |
| | Misonidazole |
| | Methyl-G |
| | Ara-C |

which are associated with intrathecal (it) administration. Meningeal irritation occurs about 2–4 hours after intrathecal methotrexate administration and lasts for 12–72 hours. The symptoms are stiff neck, headache, nausea and vomiting, fever, and lethargy. CSF pleocytosis is often present, and the syndrome is clinically indistinguishable from acute bacterial meningitis. The diagnosis is made by the temporal relation between the intrathecal treatment and the development of symptoms. The syndrome is very common, and in some series more than 50% of patients treated with intrathecal methotrexate were affected. The symptoms are self-limited, and there is no specific treatment. The cause is unknown.

A more serious acute side effect of intrathecal methotrexate is transverse myelopathy. This is a rare complication with a clinical presentation consisting of paraplegia, sensory loss, leg pains, and neurogenic bladder dysfunction. Symptoms usually begin 30 minutes to 48 hours after intrathecal treatment but may be delayed for as long as 2 weeks. There is no

specific treatment for this condition. Improvement may occur after several days or may be delayed several months. Complete recovery is unusual. The cause is not known but probably represents an idiopathic reaction.

The most serious chronic complication of methotrexate is leukoencephalopathy. This entity occurs more frequently in patients who have received cranial irradiation before or during treatment with methotrexate. The clinical presentation is one of progressive diffuse encephalopathy, often with dementia, ataxia, dysarthria, and focal findings. The syndrome usually develops insidiously during the first year after treatment. CT scan will sometimes show areas of decreased density in white matter. Discontinuing methotrexate results in improvement or arrest in some patients; however, in others the damage is permanent. The cause is not known. However, it is suspected that prior irradiation damages the blood–brain barrier, and subsequent administration of methotrexate results in higher levels of methotrexate in the brain. Cerebral atrophy is also a complication of chronic methotrexate therapy.

## Platinum (DDP)

Cis-platinum is a relatively new antitumor drug that now has widespread use. The major neurotoxicity is tinnitus and hearing loss. Tinnitus occurs in about 9% of patients treated with cis-platinum and hearing loss in about 6%, although audiographic abnormalities have been found in up to 25%. Some reversal of deafness may occur with termination of the drug, but audiographic abnormalities rarely disappear. An encephalopathy may also complicate cis-platinum use. This is probably related to electrolyte disturbances and is usually self-limited. Peripheral neuropathy is a less common complication of platinum therapy. The neuropathy is primarily sensory and is usually reversible when the drug is discontinued.

## Vinca Alkaloids

Vincristine, vinblastine, and vindesine are the vinca alkaloids in use at the present time. All are associated with peripheral neuropathy that may also involve cranial nerves and the autonomic nervous system. The neuropathy is symmetrical and distal, and it resolves when the drug is discontinued.

## Fluorouracil (5-FU)

Currently used treatment regimens with 5-FU rarely produce neurotoxicity. However, a subacute cerebellar syndrome consisting of gait ataxia, incoordination of the extremities, dysarthria, and nystagmus is occasionally seen. The syndrome almost always remits 1–6 weeks after 5-FU therapy is stopped. There is no specific treatment. The differential diagnosis includes cerebellar metastasis and paraneoplastic cerebellar degeneration. Encephalopathy may also complicate treatment with 5-FU.

## Adrenocorticosteroids

Adrenocorticosteroid hormones (steroids) are widely used in the treatment of several cancers. The drugs, particularly in high doses, may have important effects on brain function and behavior. Some of the side effects are salutary; most patients feel a sense of well-being and develop an increased appetite. However, most of the neurological side effects of steroids are undesirable. Patients often become tremulous, slightly hyperactive, and often have difficulty sleeping. In some instances, these mild behavioral abnormalities may become florid (steroid psychosis). Psychotic reactions due to steroids were more common when naturally occurring hormones (e.g., cortisol) were used, and are much less common with synthetic steroids (e.g., dexamethasone). The incidence of psychosis is related not only to the drug but also to the dosage.

The most common psychotic manifestation of steroid drugs is mania. The clinical manifestations are no different from standard manic psychosis. Less common is depression appearing either during the course of steroid administration or during their withdrawal; this disorder likewise has no distinguishing characteristics. The least common psychotic reaction associated with steroids is delirium. Hallucinations occurring alone may be more common than generally realized, and patients may often only admit to having them on direct questioning. The diagnosis of steroid psychosis can only be made when the characteristic manic psychosis appears during the course of steroid therapy or when other metabolic or structural causes of behavioral abnormalities are ruled out by physical examination and laboratory tests.

## Remote Effects of Cancer on the Nervous System: Paraneoplastic Syndromes

The rarest nonmetastatic neurological complications of systemic cancer are the ''remote effects,'' or paraneoplastic syndromes (Clark and Posner, 1984). The phrases ''remote effects of a cancer on the nervous system'' and ''paraneoplastic syndromes'' are often used interchangeably. However, paraneoplastic syndromes are clinical abnormalities caused by cancer but not resulting from direct invasion of the involved organ by cancer. Remote effects of cancer on the nervous system are neurological disorders of unknown cause

**Table 29-8** Remote effects of cancer on the nervous system

| Site | Examples |
|---|---|
| Brain | Encephalomyelitis |
| | Carcinomatous cerebellar degeneration |
| | Opsoclonus–myoclonus syndrome |
| | Optic neuritis |
| | Retinal degeneration |
| Spinal cord | Subacute necrotizing myelopathy |
| | Motor neuronopathy |
| Roots and peripheral nerves | Subacute sensory neuropathy |
| | Sensorimotor polyneuropathy |
| | Guillain–Barré syndrome |
| | Autonomic neuropathy |
| Neuromuscular junction | Eaton–Lambert syndrome |
| | Myasthenia gravis (associated with thymoma) |
| Muscle | Polymyositis |
| | Dermatomyositis |
| | Carcinoid myopathy |
| | ''Muscle weakness'' |

that occur exclusively or with increased frequency in patients with cancer. Therefore, all nonmetastatic effects of cancer on the nervous system described in this chapter and some nonnervous system effects of cancer (e.g., cachexia and anemia) can be considered paraneoplastic syndromes. Remote effects of cancer are a subgroup of paraneoplastic syndromes as indicated in Table 29-8.

In about 50% of cases, the nervous system symptoms may precede or follow the discovery of the cancer and usually run a course that is independent of that of the tumor. Although the neurological disorders may be separated into anatomical categories (Table 29-8), there is often overlap. This is particularly true of the dementias that are often lumped together with brain stem, cerebellar, and spinal cord lesions under the rubric of ''carcinomatous encephalomyelitis.'' The term ''carcinomatous neuromyopathy'' has been used to describe all the remote effects of cancer on the nervous system as well as the disorders of peripheral nerves and muscle associated with cancer.

The cause and pathogenesis of the paraneoplastic syndromes are not known; suggestions for their cause have included autoimmune reactions, viral infections, toxins secreted by the tumor, and nutritional deprivation. Recent evidence including the finding of antineuronal autoantibodies in the serum of some patients supports the autoimmune hypothesis (Anderson et al., 1987). It is possible that different mechanisms are responsible for the several types of remote effects. The clinical problem is twofold. Either the patient is known to have cancer and the question is whether the neurological symptoms are due to a remote effect or to metastatic disease, or the patient is not known to have cancer and the questions are whether there is a paraneoplastic syndrome present and whether the patient should be carefully evaluated for an occult cancer.

In the first instance, remote effects are so rare and metastatic disease so common that in patients with known cancer, the physician is obligated to consider and rule out all of the other neurological complications of systemic cancer before arriving at a diagnosis of paraneoplastic syndrome. Neurological symptoms that may cause diagnostic difficulty include dementia, cerebellar dysfunction, and weakness of the extremities. Dementia, particularly with memory loss, is one of the well-described remote effects of cancer on the nervous system. However, similar symptoms may occur in patients with multiple cerebral metastases or in patients with leptomeningeal metastases. The former are usually visible on CT scan, and with the latter, one usually sees hydrocephalus on CT as well as abnormalities in the CSF. Also, if the patient has become acutely demented, metabolic brain disease is a possible diagnosis. In patients with lymphoma, infections of the nervous system, including progressive multifocal leukoencephalopathy and fungal meningitis, must also be considered.

If cerebellar dysfunction develops in a patient with a known cancer, it is more likely that the patient is suffering from a metastasis in the cerebellum than from a remote effect. Clinically, subacute cerebellar degeneration as a remote effect is characterized by bilateral appendicular signs (point-to-point test difficulties in both upper and lower extremities) and by dysarthria, usually without nystagmus. Dementia is common as well. Metastatic disease of the cerebellum usually causes difficulties with gait without involvement of the upper extremities or speech (midline lesion), or it causes unilateral ataxia without gross dysarthria (hemispheral lesion). A CT scan usually establishes the diagnosis.

The most serious diagnostic problems arise in patients developing weakness of the lower extremities with absent reflexes and with or without bladder or bowel dysfunction. The physician may suspect a paraneoplastic peripheral neuropathy, but invasion of the cauda equina by leptomeningeal tumor is more likely. The diagnosis can usually be established by careful examination of the CSF.

Most paraneoplastic neurological diseases, such as sensorimotor peripheral neuropathy, dementia, and acute transverse myelopathy, occur only slightly more commonly in patients with cancer than in the general population. In such patients, a careful search for an underlying neoplasm is unlikely to be fruitful and is probably not warranted. However, several neurological syndromes occur exclusively or with a much higher frequency in patients with cancer. These syndromes include dermatomyositis in middle-aged and elderly men, subacute cerebellar degeneration, subacute sensory neuropathy, and a subacute motor neuropathy. Any patient who shows one of these neurological syndromes should have a careful evaluation for an occult cancer. If the initial search is negative, a tumor should still be suspected until a definitive diagnosis is established. The search for tumor should include chest x-ray examination, sputum cytology, careful pelvic examination, intravenous pyelogram, upper and lower GI series, and serum samples for measurement of biochemical abnormalities and tumor markers.

Dermatomyositis (polymyositis) is characterized by the subacute development of proximal muscle weakness, with or without pain and muscle tenderness, but usually associated with a skin rash. Its occurrence in men over 40 is associated with a high incidence of underlying cancer, especially carcinoma of the lung, and a search for cancer is warranted.

Subacute cerebellar degeneration appears as a subacutely developing symmetrical ataxia of the arms and legs, usually associated with dysarthria and sometimes associated with nystagmus. The CSF may contain 10–40 lymphocytes and increased protein. The disorder is usually inexorably progressive. Carcinomas of the lung and ovary head the list of tumors most responsible for this remote effect. Occasionally the subacute cerebellar degeneration is associated with opsoclonus (i.e., rapid, chaotic, and uncontrollable movement of the eyes).

Subacute sensory neuropathy is characterized by the progressive loss of all sensory modalities and the deep tendon reflexes in all four extremities. Because of loss of position sense, ataxia is common. Motor power may be unimpaired and motor nerve conduction velocities may be normal. Many patients are mildly demented, and the CSF protein is usually elevated. This syndrome, when severe, warrants a careful search for an underlying neoplasm.

Subacute neuronopathy is associated with lymphomas and is characterized by gradual lower motor neuron weakening, usually without sensory changes, that waxes and wanes over months and generally improves spontaneously. The patients frequently recover after several months to years. The cause in unknown, although viral infection has been postulated as a possible cause. Patients with Hodgkin's disease and lymphoma have a higher incidence of acute polyneuritis (Guillain–Barré syndrome) than does the general population. However, the Guillain–Barré syndrome is so common and its association with lymphoma sufficiently rare that the diagnosis of this neurological disease does not require the physician to search for an underlying lymphoma.

# REFERENCES

Anderson, N.E., J.M. Cunningham, and J.B. Posner (1987). Autoimmune pathogenesis of paraneoplastic neurological syndromes. *CRC Crit. Rev. Neurobiol.* 3:245–99.

Berger, P.S. (1982). Neurological complications of radiotherapy. In A. Silverstein (ed.), *Neurological Complications of Therapy*. Mount Kisco, N.Y.: Futura Publishing, pp. 137–85.

Cairncross, J.G. and J.B. Posner (1983). The management of brain metastases. In M.D. Walker (ed.), *Oncology of the Nervous System*. Boston: Martinus Nijhoff, pp. 341–77.

Clark, A.W. and J.B. Posner (1984). Remote effects of cancer. In T.M. Bayless, M.C. Brain, and R.M. Cherniack (eds.), *Current Therapy in Internal Medicine*. Philadelphia: B.C. Decker, pp. 1362–67.

Delattre, J.Y., G. Krol, H.T. Thaler, and J.B. Posner (1988). Distribution of brain metastases. *Arch. Neurol.* 45:741–44.

Ehrenkranz, J.R.L. and J.B. Posner (1980). Adrenocorticosteroid hormones. In L. Weiss (ed.), *Brain Metastasis*. Boston: G.K. Hall, pp. 340–63.

Glass, P.J., M. Melamed, N.L. Chernik, and J.B. Posner (1979). Malignant cells in the cerebrospinal fluid (CSF): The meaning of a positive CSF cytology. *Neurology* 29:1369–75.

Graus, F., L.R. Rogers, and J.B. Posner (1985). Cerebrovascular complications in patients with cancer. *Medicine* 64:16–35.

Greenberg, H.S., J.H. Kim, and J.B. Posner (1980). Epidural spinal cord compression from metastatic tumor: Re-

sults with a new treatment protocol. *Ann. Neurol.* 8:361–66.

Kaplan, R.S. and P.H. Wiernik (1984). Neurotoxicity of antitumor agents. In M.C. Perry and J. Yarbro (eds.), *Toxicity of Chemotherapy*. Orlando, Fla.: Grune & Stratton, pp. 365–431.

Lipowski, Z.J. (1980). *Delirium: Acute Brain Failure in Man.* Springfield, Ill.: Charles C Thomas.

Plum, F. and J.B. Posner (1980). *The Diagnosis of Stupor and Coma,* 3rd ed. Philadelphia: F.A. Davis.

Posner, J.B. (1978). Neurological complications of systemic cancer. *Disease-a-Month* 25(2):1–60.

Posner, J.B. (1979). Neurological complications of systemic cancer. *Med. Clin. North Am.* 63:783–800.

Price, R.W., B.A. Navia, and E.S. Cho (1988). AIDS encephalopathy. *Neurol. Clin. North Am.* In press.

Rodichok, L.D., G.R. Harper, J.C. Ruckdeschel, A. Price, G. Robertson, K.D. Barron, and J. Horton (1981). Early diagnosis of spinal epidural metastases. *Am. J. Med.* 70:1181–88.

Shapiro, W.R. (1982). Treatment of neuroectodermal brain tumors. *Ann. Neurol.* 12:231–37.

Slatkin, N.E. and J.B. Posner (1983). Management of spinal epidural metastases. *Clin. Neurosurg.* 30:698–715.

Snider, W.D., D.M. Simpson, S. Nielsen, J.W.M. Gold, C.E. Metroka, and J.B. Posner (1983). Neurological complications of acquired immune deficiency syndrome: Analysis of 50 patients. *Ann. Neurol.* 14:403–18.

Walker, R.W. and J.B. Posner (1984). Central nervous system neoplasms. In S. Appel (ed.), *Current Neurology,* Vol. 5. New York: Wiley, pp. 285–322.

Wasserstrom, W.R., P.J. Glass, and J.B. Posner (1982). Diagnosis and treatment of leptomeningeal metastases from solid tumors: Experience with 90 patients. *Cancer* 49:759–72.

Young, D.F. (1982). Neurological complications of cancer chemotherapy. In A. Silverstein (ed.), *Neurological Complications of Therapy*. Mount Kisco, N.Y.: Futura Publishing, pp. 35–113.

# 30

# Delirium and Dementia

## Stewart Fleishman and Lynna M. Lesko

Delirium is common in patients with cancer. It occurs both as a transient CNS complication of disease and as a side effect of treatment. Dementia, while much less common, is a far more devastating complication because of its irreversible nature. In early stages both are often mistaken for depression or an emotional response to stress. Yet early recognition of the symptoms and a workup to establish the cause and treatment can prevent progression of delirium to coma and death, and progression of dementia may be slowed. Thus, recognizing diagnostic symptoms and signs, and managing the psychological and behavioral consequences (e.g., psychotic state, self-destructive or aggressive behavior) are central to good patient care in cancer.

This chapter reviews the key issues related to delirium and dementia first in general and then as they apply in cancer, with greater emphasis placed on delirium. It covers definitions and diagnostic criteria, prevalence, etiology, and clinical evaluation and management of the psychiatric component (organic mental disorders).

## DEFINITION AND DIAGNOSIS

Bonhoeffer (1910) was among the first to describe transient delirious states as "toxic" psychoses, suggesting their exogenous origin. Engel and Romano (1959) did much to clarify delirium in the modern era. They pointed out that delirium is the clinical picture resulting from general impairment of mental function; accompanied by diffuse slowing of EEG patterns; it can result from a range of pathophysiological causes that disrupt normal mental function. Plum and Posner (1972) described delirium as a clinical state characterized by clouded consciousness, disorientation, suspiciousness, fears, irritability, misperception of sensory stimuli, and often, delusions and visual hallucinations.

Lipowski (1980, 1983, 1987) has provided the most

scholarly reviews of organic mental syndromes. He proposed a taxonomy in 1980 (Table 30-1), of delirium and dementia based on mental symptoms, signs, and behavior; these categories served as the basis for the current DSM-III classification. He proposed that the two types of general cognitive impairment are delirium and dementia. Other forms of impairment appear in which cognition is relatively intact (as in organic personality syndrome), or in which there is selective memory loss (as seen in the amnestic syndrome and in organic hallucinosis). In the latter disorder, mental functions are largely intact but exist in the presence of visual, tactile, or auditory hallucinations. Such disorders are seen most often in drug-induced toxic or withdrawal states (e.g., alcohol and steroids). Another type of dysfunction is characterized by relatively intact cognition and symptoms that closely resemble a functional disorder: organic delusional syndrome (seen in drug- or metabolism-induced states) or organic affective syndrome, in which mood is the predominantly changed aspect of mental function, with symptoms of mania or depression.

Table 30-2A gives the DSM-III diagnostic criteria used for differentiating the symptoms of general impairment of delirium from the selective impairment seen with the amnestic syndrome, organic delusional syndrome, organic hallucinosis, and organic affective syndrome. They all represent mental changes that are the results of different patterns of impaired perception of the environment, faulty processing, storage and retrieval of information, and impairment of insight and judgment. The present classification allows for differentiation by description of the clinical symptoms that are characteristic of each specific syndrome.

At times it is difficult to differentiate between delirium and early dementia, which has a profound impairment of memory. Level of consciousness and patterns of the appearance of symptoms are helpful. Delirium is

**Table 30-1** Organic mental disorders

| Symptoms | Syndrome |
|---|---|
| General cognitive impairment | Delirium |
| | Dementia |
| Personality changes (cognition relatively intact) | Organic personality syndrome |
| Selective or circumscribed cognitive abnormalities | Amnestic syndrome |
| | Organic hallucinosis |
| Resemble functional disorders | Organic delusional syndrome |
| | Organic affective syndrome |

*Source*: Modified from Lipowski (1980).

characterized by fluctuating levels of consciousness (attention) and disordered orientation, with symptoms worsening at night, whereas dementia appears in a relatively alert individual and is associated with a less profoundly disordered sleep–wake cycle with impaired memory, judgment, and abstract thinking (see Table 30-2B). In older individuals who are physically ill, both delirium and dementia may be present, and manifest clinically as delirium superimposed on a pre-existing dementia. Liston (1984) has outlined the major diagnostic differences in the clinical picture of delirium and dementia, and these are presented in Table 30-3. A further consideration in the differential diagnosis of disorders of cognition, in older patients, is the presence of depression that presents as pseudodementia (Wells, 1979).

## PREVALENCE IN CANCER

Transient delirium often occurs in hospitalized cancer patients undergoing active and palliative treatment; dementia, however, is uncommon. In Table 30-4, 11 studies of organic mental disorders in cancer patients (alone or combined with other groups) are summarized. While the prevalence of delirium ranges from 8 to 85% in these studies, which were carried out since 1972, it is readily apparent from the evaluated populations that there are three groups in particular at risk for increased incidence of delirium: patients with more advanced or terminal disease (85%), those under treatment in the hospital, and those in older age groups (Seymour et al., 1980). Hospitalized patients are at an especially high risk of developing a narcotic or steroid-induced confusional state, or a metabolic encephalopathy related to the consequences of disease or treatment. At our hospital, Posner (1979) estimates that 15–20% of patients on medical oncology units may be experiencing some degree of cognitive impairment, usually not recognized unless it becomes severe or is accompanied by behavioral changes. Studies of these states are difficult because diagnosis depends largely on a

constellation of symptoms. Quantification of these symptoms is also difficult. However, the more refined criteria of the DSM-III and the screening instruments presently available have improved the reliability of data collected in more recent studies of prevalence.

The prevalence of dementia, usually from unusual remote effects on the CNS or from radiation, is so low that studies similar to those in Table 30-4 have not been carried out, except as they relate to special treatment or sites of cancer.

## CAUSES OF DELIRIUM AND DEMENTIA

The causes of delirium and dementia are outlined only briefly here and in Table 30-5 because they are reviewed by Patchell and Posner in their chapter on cancer and the nervous system. Posner (1978) outlines two major areas of causation in CNS complications. *Direct effects* are related to a primary brain tumor or metastatic spread by local extension, or by hematogenous or lymphatic routes, which may result in both delirium and permanent intellectual loss or dementia. *Indirect effects* are far more frequent, more commonly causing delirium as a consequence of metabolic encephalopathy, vital organ failure, electrolyte imbalance, drug or radiation side effects, infection, vascular complications, nutritional changes, and paraneoplastic syndromes (Table 30-5).

Failure of a vital organ, particularly liver, kidneys, lung, thyroid, and adrenals, is a common source of mental status change in patients with advanced disease. Respiratory compromise causes cerebral hypoxia and confusion; hepatic encephalopathy produces a neuropsychiatric disorder that may vary from a slightly altered mental state to coma (Fraser and Adrieff, 1985). Uremia produces a confusional state, and thyroid and adrenal gland dysfunction can also produce mental changes. The most common metabolic causes of mental status alterations are fluctuations in blood glucose (e.g., poor control of diabetics on steroids), calcium (hypercalcemia, especially in bone metastases or myeloma), or sodium and potassium.

Among treatment side effects, narcotic analgesics and cimetidine are a common cause of clouded consciousness and psychotic states. These frequently resemble functional disorders and are characterized by delusional and affective organic syndromes. Anticholinergic drugs can produce psychotic states, as can drugs commonly used in the cancer setting, such as amphotericin B, and acyclovir. Among the chemotherapeutic agents, steroids are the worst offenders, producing organic affective syndromes and psychosis. Transiently altered mental function, with altered attention, level of consciousness, cognition, and mood change are seen at times with particular cytotoxic

**Table 30-2A**  Criteria for differential diagnosis of delirium

*Diagnostic criteria for delirium*

A. Clouding of consciousness (reduced clarity of awarness of the environment), with reduced capacity to shift, focus, and sustain attention to environmental stimuli
B. At least two of the following:
   (1) perceptual disturbance: misinterpretations, illusions, or hallucinations
   (2) speech that is at times incoherent
   (3) disturbance of sleep–wakefulness cycle, with insomnia or daytime drowsiness
   (4) increased or decreased psychomotor activity
C. Disorientation and memory impairment (if testable).
D. Clinical features that develop over a short period of time (usually hours to days) and tend to fluctuate over the course of a day.
E. Evidence, from the history, physical examination, or laboratory tests, of a specific organic factor judged to be etiologically related to the disturbance.

*Diagnostic criteria for amnestic syndrome*

A. Both short-term memory impairment (inability to learn new information) and long-term memory impairment (inability to remember information that was known in the past) are the predominant clinical features.
B. No clouding of consciousness, as in delirium and intoxication, or general loss of major intellectual abilities, as in dementia
C. Evidence, from the history, physical examination, or laboratory tests, of a specific organic factor that is judged to be etiologically related to the disturbance

*Diagnostic criteria for organic delusional syndrome*

A. Delusions are the predominant clinical feature.
B. There is no clouding of consciousness, as in delirium; there is no significant loss of intellectual abilities, as in dementia; there are no prominent hallucinations, as in organic hallucinosis.
C. There is evidence, from the history, physical examination, or laboratory tests, of a specific organic factor that is judged to be etiologically related to the disturbance.

*Diagnostic criteria for organic hallucinosis*

A. Persistent or recurrent hallucinations are the predominant clinical feature.
B. No clouding of consciousness, as in delirium; no significant loss of intellectual abilities, as in dementia; no predominant disturbance of mood, as in organic affective syndrome; no predominant delusions, as in organic delusional syndrome
C. Evidence, from the history, physical examination, or laboratory tests, of a specific organic factor that is judged to be etiologically related to the disturbance

*Diagnostic criteria for organic affective syndrome*

A. The predominant disturbance is a disturbance in mood, with at least two of the associated symptoms for manic or major depressive episode.
B. No clouding of consciousness, as in delirium; no significant loss of intellectual abilities, as in dementia; no predominant delusions or hallucinations, as in organic delusional syndrome or organic hallucinosis
C. Evidence, from the history, physical examination, or laboratory tests, of a specific organic factor that is judged to be etiologically related to the disturbance

*Source: Diagnostic and Statistical Manual III (APA, 1980).*

**Table 30-2B**  Criteria for differential diagnosis of dementia

A. A loss of intellectual abilities of sufficient severity to interfere with the social or occupational functioning
B. Memory impairment
C. At least one of the following:
   (1) Impairment of abstract thinking as manifested by concrete interpretation of proverbs, inability to find similarities and differences between related words, difficulty in defining words and concepts, and other similar tasks
   (2) Impaired judgment
   (3) Other disturbances of higher cortical function, such as aphasia (disorder of language due to brain dysfunction), apraxia (inability to carry out motor activities despite intact comprehension and motor function), agnosia (failure to recognize or identify objects despite intact sensory function), "constructional difficulty" (e.g., inability to copy three-dimensional figures, assemble blocks, or arrange sticks in specific designs)
   (4) Personality change (i.e., alteration or accentuation of premorbid traits)
D. State of consciousness not clouded (i.e., does not meet the criteria for delirium or intoxication, although these may be superimposed)
E. Either of the following:
   (1) Evidence from the history, physical examination, or laboratory tests, of a specific organic factor that is judged to be etiologically related to the disturbance
   (2) In the absence of such evidence, an organic factor necessary for the development of the syndrome can be presumed if conditions other than organic mental disorders have been reasonably excluded and if the behavioral change represents cognitive impairment in a variety of areas.

*Source: Diagnostic and Statistical Manual III (APA, 1980).*

**Table 30-3**  Frequency of clinical features of delirium contrasted with dementia*

| Feature | Delirium | Dementia |
|---|---|---|
| Impaired memory | +++ | +++ |
| Impaired thinking | +++ | +++ |
| Impaired judgment | +++ | +++ |
| Clouding of consciousness | +++ | − |
| Major attention deficits† | +++ | + |
| Fluctuation over course of a day | +++ | + |
| Disorientation† | +++ | ++ |
| Vivid perceptual disturbances | ++ | + |
| Incoherent speech† | ++ | + |
| Disrupted sleep–wake cycle† | ++ | + |
| Nocturnal exacerbation† | ++ | + |
| Insight‡ | ++ | + |
| Acute or subacute onset§ | ++ | − |

*Always present (+++); usually present (++); occasionally present (+); usually absent (−).

†More frequent in advanced stages of dementia.

‡Present during lucid intervals or upon recovery from delirium; present in early stages of dementia.

§Onset may be acute or subacute in some dementias (e.g., multiinfarction, hypoxemia, certain reversible dementias).

*Source: Reprinted with permission from E.H. Liston (1984). Diagnosis and management of delirium in the elderly patient. Psychiatr. Ann. 14:109–18.*

**Table 30-4** Prevalence of organic mental syndromes in cancer patients

| Reference | Number of patients | Site and stage | Percentage of delirium | Method |
|---|---|---|---|---|
| Hinton (1972) | 50 | Cancer, all sites; terminally ill patients | 10 | Psychiatric consultations; interview, clinical diagnosis |
| Davies et al. (1973) | 46 | Cancer, all sites; advanced disease, inpatients | 27 | Consecutive patients; clinical diagnosis, standardized scales |
| Bergmann and Eastham (1974) | 100 | Geriatric medical inpatients: cancer and noncancer diagnoses | 16 | Screen admissions by interview; clinical diagnosis |
| Shevitz et al. (1976) | 1000 | Cancer and noncancer; general hospital | 16 | Consultations; interview; clinical diagnosis |
| Levine et al. (1978) | 100 | Cancer, all stages, inpatients | 40 | Psychiatric consultations; review of organic brain disorders |
| Massie et al. (1979) | 334 | Cancer all stages, inpatients | 25 | Consultations; clinical diagnosis |
| Seymour et al. (1980) | 71 | Medical inpatients; cancer and noncancer | 16 | Screen of all admissions; interview and clinical diagnosis |
| Massie et al. (1983) | 13 | Hospitalized terminally ill cancer patients | 85 | Patients *not* to survive current admission. Lowy Scale of Cognitive Impairment; Brief Psychiatric Rating Scale |
| Derogatis et al. (1983) (PSYCOG) | 215 | All stages cancer; hospitalized and ambulatory | 8 | Randomly accessed, hospitalized and ambulatory; interrater reliability on DMS-III criteria; Symptom Checklist-90 |
| Folstein et al. (1984) | 83 | Cancer, all stages; inpatients | 27 | One day prevalence to measure *cognitive impairment* by Mini-Mental Status Examination |
| Massie and Holland (1988) | 546 | Cancer, all stages; predominantly hospitalized | 15 | consultation data; clinical diagnosis using DSM-III |

**Table 30-5** Causes of delirium in cancer patients

| Causes | Examples |
|---|---|
| Metabolic encephalopathy due to vital organ failure | Liver, kidney, lung, thyroid, adrenal |
| Electrolyte imbalance | Sodium, potassium, calcium, glucose |
| Treatment side effects | Narcotics |
|  | Anticholinergics (narcotics, phenothiazines, antihistamines) |
|  | Chemotherapeutic agents; steroids |
|  | Radiation therapy |
| Infection |  |
| Hematological abnormalities | Microcytic and macrocytic anemias, coagulopathies |
| Nutritional | General malnutrition, thiamine, folic acid, $B_{12}$ |
| Paraneoplastic syndromes | Remote effects |
|  | Tumors |
|  | Hormone-producing tumor |

*Source*: Modified from Posner (1978).

agents including methotrexate (given intrathecally or in high dose), 5-fluorouracil, the vinca alkaloids, bleomycin, cisplatin, L-asparaginase, and procarbazine (Young and Posner, 1980). In general, however, with the exception of those already mentioned, most chemotherapeutic agents do not cross the blood–brain barrier and thus cause relatively few CNS side effects.

Cranial irradiation produces mild to severe immediate side effects and may also be associated with delayed effects. Radiation effects can range from a time-limited "somnolence syndrome," to (at times) a mild to moderate cognitive loss (seen in children given CNS prophylaxis for acute lymphocytic leukemia), to dementia in some patients who receive irradiation for brain tumors or CNS prophylaxis for lung cancer. A study by Johnson and colleagues (1985) suggested that those patients who received high-dose chemotherapy concurrent with cranial irradiation or large radiotherapy fractions (400 rad) were at greatest risk for abnormalities on neuropsychological tests.

Infections of the CNS produce an encephalopathy secondary to bacterial, viral, or fungal invasion of the brain. Toxic delirium occurs at times with sepsis and hyperpyrexia. Some of the nutritional deficiencies seen in cancer and associated with mental status changes are thiamine deficiency, which produces Wernicke–Korsakoff syndrome, and folic acid–vitamin $B_{12}$ deficiency, which can also produce progressive cognitive impairment and dementia.

Paraneoplastic syndromes are the clinical abnormalities caused by cancer but not resulting from direct invasion of the organ involved. Whereas this definition implies any nonmetastatic effect of cancer on the nervous system, it is usually used to refer to the remote effects of cancer (e.g., multifocal leukoencephalopathy and cerebellar degeneration) and the effects on mental and neurological function of the hormone-producing tumors (e.g., lung and adrenal) (see also Patchell and Posner, Chapter 29; Brietbart, Chapter 31).

## Multiple Etiological Agents

In actual clinical practice, patients with cancer who are seriously ill often are found to have multiple causes for delirium present, and establishing a single etiology may prove difficult (Adams, 1984). In research by Massie and colleagues (1983), 85% of patients studied during hospitalization for advanced and terminal cancer had a delirium at some point. In only one case was there only a single cause, hepatic encephalopathy. The remaining patients' delirium reflected multiple causes, including failure of a vital organ, electrolyte imbalance, narcotic analgesic side effects, sepsis, and direct CNS invasion. These data confirm the high frequency of confusional states in very ill hospitalized patients and highlight the generally multiple contributory causes for delirium seen in these patients that make definitive assignment of etiology at times impossible.

## CLINICAL EVALUATION

### Clinical Picture

When patients with cancer are being actively treated in the hospital, subtle changes in mental status are apt to go unnoticed or to be attributed, when recognized, as being due to the stress of illness. The mental changes may remain unnoticed if the patient's behavior remains quiet and unobtrusive. Overt behavioral and personality changes often must occur before the possibility of a delirium is recognized. Yet changes in mental status may be the first sign of a medical complication, warranting a close monitoring of mental function in a hospitalized cancer patient.

**Table 30-6**  Behavioral symptoms of delirium in cancer patients

| Stage | Symptom |
|---|---|
| Early, mild | *Change* in sleep pattern with restlessness and transient periods of disorientation |
| | *Increased* irritability, anger, temper outbursts |
| | *Withdrawal*, refusal to talk to staff or relatives |
| | *Forgetfulness*, not previously present |
| Late, severe with behavioral changes | *Refusal* to cooperate with reasonable requests |
| | *Angry*, swearing, shouting, abusive |
| | *Demanding* to go home; pacing corridor |
| | *Illusions* (misidentifies staff, visual and sensory clues) |
| | *Delusions* (misinterprets events, usually paranoid, fears of being harmed) |
| | *Hallucinations* (visual and auditory) |

### Pertinent History

Table 30-6 outlines the early signs and symptoms of delirium, and those that appear late, when severely disordered mental function has developed. The earliest signs are often readily identified from the nurses' progress notes about behavioral changes at night, such as unaccustomed restlessness and episodes of disorientation. Irritability, anger, and temper outbursts may be noted during the day; withdrawal and refusal to speak to staff or relatives are seen at times, and forgetfulness, previously unnoticeable, becomes apparent.

When the delirium develops further and marked mental changes occur, symptoms may resemble a functional psychotic state with compromise of cooperativeness with treatment and, at times, risk of harm to self or others. The person may become uncooperative, angry, abusive, and demanding, attempting to leave the hospital if not detained. Perceptual misconceptions (illusions) of persons and objects usually have a suspicious, paranoid association; delusions that result from misinterpretation of events, again, usually reflect fears of being harmed, especially when associated with auditory and visual hallucinations. A frequent delusion is that of being in a prison or being tortured, with no insight into the presence of disordered thinking. Patients can at times incur serious injury, even attempting to jump from a window in their efforts to escape, requiring close monitoring of their behavior. Although such a mental state in a physically healthy person would be treated in a protected environment provided by a psychiatric unit, the level of physical illness in these patients usually precludes transfer to such a unit, and they must be managed on the oncology unit with psychiatric consultation.

The clinical picture of delirium must be evaluated by comparing it to the patient's prior level of mental function, obtained by outside history from family members, and from the patient's medical chart, which will indicate mental state on prior visits or admissions. Review of notes from social workers may pick up changes noted by relatives. This review must include obtaining a history of prior drug or alcohol abuse and mental illness.

Of critical importance is a review of the doctor's order sheet for medications that were *ordered*. However, the additional crucial step is to review the nurses' medication chart to determine the drugs that the patient actually *received*. Orders written sometimes are not picked up, and drugs assumed to be given regularly may not have been given to the patient. Inadvertently discontinuing a drug may result in unexplained withdrawal symptoms (e.g., narcotics and analgesics).

## Mental Status Examination

The patient's mental state should be tested, when delirium is suspected, by conducting a full mental status examination. All major aspects of mental function must be tested to identify selective or subtle circumscribed dysfunction. The clinical examination covers the four major areas of the patients' appearance and behavior, mood and affect, thought content, and intellectual function. A report should be organized to allow a reader to review these clinical facts rapidly and understand the basis for the differential diagnosis considered and the diagnostic impression. The following aspects of the examination are pertinent in examining a patient with cancer in whom the question of delirium or dementia exists.

### GENERAL APPEARANCE AND BEHAVIOR

Note the patient's level of alertness in the interview, attention to questions, state of dress, body movements (quiet or agitated), facial expression, manner (cooperative or uncooperative), and speech (rapid, slowed down, blocking, searching for words).

### MOOD AND AFFECT

Note the patient's emotional state (cheerful, sad, irritable, anxious, hostile) and the affect elicited by the discussion. Is there an inappropriate cheerfulness, euphoria, or mania? Is there a depressed mood, sense of worthlessness, suicidal thoughts? Suicidal risk? Is there fear or anger at imagined recent events (e.g., illusions or delusions)? Is there an aggressive tendency or homicidal risk? Is there an inappropriate or flat response to discussion of issues that should elicit an emotion?

### THOUGHT CONTENT

When asked questions, can the patient answer directly or is there circumstantial or tangential thinking, or flight of ideas? Are thoughts logical, rapid, or slow? Is there evidence of illusions, misinterpretation of the place, objects, or persons in the room (e.g., "lines on the ceiling are snakes," "someone in the hall is trying to hurt me")? Are there frank paranoid delusions with fear of harm to the self by others? Are there visual (most common), auditory, or tactile hallucinations?

### COGNITIVE FUNCTION

Does the patient know the hospital's name, his own name, address, telephone number, date, length of time in the hospital? Check short-term memory (remember three objects over 5 minutes and digit span), long-term memory (prior events), general information (current events), calculations (serial 7's, simple arithmetic), and copying of figures. Insight, judgment, and abstract ability are evidenced by awareness of illness, reasons for treatment, explanation of meaning of proverbs, judgment (e.g., about finding a stamped letter or what to do in case of fire in a theater).

With profoundly disturbed patients, poor attention will preclude full testing. Awareness of educational level and native language also alter the level of questions asked, and evaluation of answers must take this into account. Likewise, patients who have been quite ill in the hospital may miss the exact day or date. Markedly slowed mentation may result in answers preceded by long silences. The slowed thinking may be due to sedation from narcotics, or it may reflect a response to distracting hallucinations. A delusion of being poisoned may result in the patient speaking in a whisper while suspiciously watching the door.

### MENTAL STATUS ASSESSMENT SCALES

Several assessment scales of mental status have been developed to screen for the presence of deficits and to provide a more standardized clinical measure. The Cognitive Capacity Screening Examination (CCSE) developed by Jacobs and colleagues (1977), and the Mini-Mental State Exam (MMSE) by Folstein and colleagues (1984) have been widely used (Figs. 30-1 and 30-2). They, too, however, must be interpreted in light of the patient's educational level and language. They often pick up gross changes but miss subtle ones that

Examiner _____ Date _____

Addressograph Plate

Instructions: Check items answered correctly. Write incorrect or unusual answers in space provided. If neccesary, urge patient once to complete task.

Introduction to patient: "I would like to ask you a few questions. Some you will find very easy and others may be very hard. Just do your best."

1) What day of the week is this? _____
2) What month? _____
3) What day of month? _____
4) What year? _____
5) What place is this? _____
6) Repeat the numbers 8 7 2. _____
7) Say them backwards. _____
8) Repeat these numbers 6 3 7 1. _____
9) Listen to these numbers 6 9 4. Count 1 through 10 out loud, then repeat 6 9 4. (Help if needed. Then use numbers 5 7 3.) _____
10) Listen to these numbers 8 1 4 3. Count 1 through 10 out loud, then repeat 8 1 4 3. _____
11) Beginning with Sunday, say the days of the week backwards _____
12) 9 + 3 is _____
13) Add 6 (to the previous answer or "to 12"). _____
14) Take away 5 ("from 18"). _____
   Repeat these words after me and remember them, I will ask for them later: HAT, CAR, TREE, TWENTY-SIX.
15) The opposite of fast is slow. The opposite of up is_____

16) The opposite of large is _____
17) The opposite of hard is _____
18) An orange and a banana are both fruits. Red and blue are both _____
19) A penny and a dime are both _____
20) What were those words I asked you to remember? (HAT) _____
21) (CAR) _____
22) (TREE) _____
23) (TWENTY-SIX) _____
24) Take away 7 from 100, then take away 7 from what is left and keep going: 100 - 7 is _____
25) Minus 7 _____
26) Minus 7 (write down answeres; check correct subtraction of 7) _____
27) Minus 7 _____
28) Minus 7 _____
29) Minus 7 _____
30) Minus 7 _____

TOTAL CORRECT (maximum score = 30)

Patient's occupation (previous, if not employed) _____ Education _____ Age _____
Estimated intelligence (based on education, occupation, and history, not on test score):

Below average, Average, Above average _____

Patient was: Cooperative _____ Uncooperative _____ Depressed _____ Lethargic _____ Other _____

Medical diagnosis:_____
IF PATIENT'S SCORE IS LESS THAN 20, THE EXISTENCE OF DIMINISHED COGNITIVE CAPACITY IS PRESENT. THEREFORE, AN ORGANIC MENTAL SYNDROME SHOULD BE SUSPECTED AND THE FOLLOWING INFORMATION OBTAINED.

Temp. _____   BUN _____   Endocrine dysfunction? _____
B.P. _____   Glu _____
Hct _____   $Po_2$ _____    $T_3$,   $T_4$,   Ca,   P,   etc.
Na _____   $Pco_2$ _____   History of previous psychiatric difficulty _____
K _____   Drugs: _____
Cl _____       Steroids?   L-Dopa?   Amphetamines?   Tranquilizers?   Digitalis?
$CO_2$ _____
EEG_____   Focal neurological signs: _____
ECG_____   Diagnosis: _____

**Figure 30-1.** Cognitive Capacity Screening Examination. *Source:* From J.W. Jacobs (1977). Screening for organic mental syndromes in the medically ill. *Ann. Intern. Med.* 86:40–46, with permission.

are important in recognizing mild delirium and dementia. The advantages to routine use of these tests, nevertheless, are several. They assure testing in all areas and provide a quantitative evaluation that helps in monitoring changes in mental state. They require only a few minutes to administer, can be given by any staff member, and encourage obtaining baseline mental status on patients at time of admission (Beresford et al., 1985).

Pauker and co-workers (1978) developed a rapid assessment using a hand-held tachistoscope that measures reaction time to a visual stimulus. Although it is simple and fast, it too will fail to identify early defects (Strain et al., 1988). A newer screening instrument, the Neurobehavioral Cognitive Status Examination (NCSE), was developed by Kiernan and colleagues (1987) to provide a rapid cognitive assessment of medically ill patients. It assesses level of consciousness, orientation, and attention as well as five major ability areas: language, constructions, memory, calculations, and reasoning. Because these last areas are independently assessed, and not summed to a global score, the clinician has a "differentiated profile of the patients cognitive status." The NCSE has a false negative rate of 7% compared to 53% for the CCSE and 43% for the MMSE (Schwamm et al., 1987). Its apparent sensitivity lies in its use of independent tests to assess skills within the five major areas of cognitions and the use of "graded" tasks within those domains. It may prove a useful screening tool for confusional states, isolated cognitive deficits, and dementias. When discrete deficits need to be assessed, by far the most preferable approach is to refer a patient for neuropsychological testing in which the areas of dysfunction can be delineated, and level of general dysfunction specified.

Patient ____________
Examiner ____________
Date ____________

"MINI-MENTAL STATE"*

| Maximum score | Score | |
|---|---|---|
| | | **Orientation** |
| 5 | ( ) | What is the (year) (season) (date) (day) (month)? |
| 5 | ( ) | Where are we: (state) (county) (town) (hospital) (floor)? |
| | | **Registration** |
| 3 | ( ) | Name 3 objects: 1 second to say each. Then ask the patient all 3 after you have said them. Give 1 point for each correct answer. Then repeat them until he learns all 3. Count trials and record. |
| | | **Attention and Calculation** |
| 5 | ( ) | Serial 7's. 1 point for each correct. Stop after 5 answers. Alternatively spell "world" backwards |
| | | **Recall** |
| 3 | ( ) | Ask for the 3 objects repeated above. Give 1 point for each correct. |
| | | **Language** |
| 9 | ( ) | Name a pencil, and watch (2 points)<br>Repeat the following "No ifs, ands or buts." (1 point)<br>Follow a 3-stage command:<br>"Take a paper in your right hand, fold it in half, and put it on the floor" (3 points)<br>Read and obey the following:<br>**Close your eyes (1 point)**<br>Write a sentence (1 point)<br>Copy design (1 point)<br>Total score<br>ASSESS level of consciousness along a continuum<br>Alert Drowsy Stupor Coma |

INSTRUCTIONS FOR ADMINISTRATION OF MINI-MENTAL STATE EXAMINATION

**Orientation**

(1) Ask for the date. Then ask specifically for parts omitted, e.g. "Can you also tell me what season it is?" One point for each correct.

(2) Ask in turn "Can you tell me the name of this hospital?" (town, county, etc.) One point for each correct.

**Registration**

Ask the patient if you may test his memory. Then say the names of 3 unrelated objects, clearly and slowly, about one second for each. After you have said all 3, ask him to repeat them. This first repetition determines his score (0-3) but keep saying them until he can repeat all 3, up to 6 trials. If he does not eventually learn all 3, recall cannot be meaningfully tested.

**Attention and calculation**

Ask the patient to begin with 100 and count backwards by 7. Stop after 5 subtractions (93, 86, 79, 72, 65). Score the total number of correct answers.

If the patient cannot or will not perform this task, ask him to spell the word "world" backwards. The score is the number of letters in correct order. e.g. dlrow" ' 5, dlorw ' 3.

**Recall**

Ask the patient if he can recall the 3 words you previously asked him to remember. Score 0-3.

**Language**

*Naming:* Show the patient a wrist watch and ask him what it is. Repeat for pencil. Score 0-2.

*Repetition:* Ask the patient to repeat the sentence after you. Allow only one trial. Score 0 or 1.

*3-Stage command:* Give the patient a piece of plain blank paper and repeat the command. Score 1 point for each part correctly executed.

*Reading:* On a blank piece of paper print the sentence "Close your eyes", in letters large enough for the patient to see clearly. Ask him to read it and do what it says. Score 1 point only if he actually closes his eyes.

*Writing:* Give the patient a blank piece of paper and ask him to write a sentence for you. Do not dictate a sentence, it is to be written spontaneously. It must contain a subject and verb and be sensible. Correct grammer and punctuation are not necessary.

*Copying:* On a clean piece of paper, draw intersecting pentagons, each side about 1 in., and ask him to copy it exactly as it is. All 10 angles must be present and 2 must intersect to score 1 point. Tremor and rotation are ignored.

Estimate the patient's level of sensorium along a continuum, from alert on the left to coma on the right.

**Figure 30-2.** Mini-Mental State Examination. *Source:* From M.F. Folstein, S.E. Folstein, and P.R. McHugh (1975). "Mini-mental state," a practical method for grading the cognitive state of patients for the clinician. *Source: J. Psychiatr. Res.* 12:189–98. Copyright 1975, Pergamon Press, Ltd.

## Neurological Workup

The diagnosis of delirium relies heavily on the history and altered mental state with identification of the general or selective cognitive impairment present. The neurological examination usually fails to elicit focal diagnostic signs, and the diagnosis of a nonfocal encephalopathy must be clarified further by seeking a cause. Table 30-7 lists some diagnostic signs that aid in identifying etiology (e.g., vital signs; changes in skin, pupils, and extremities).

Table 30-8 (Posner, 1979) lists the tests that should be done as emergency measures (in a life-threatening metabolic crisis): blood samples drawn for measurement of glucose, $Na^+$, $Ca^{2+}$, blood urea nitrogen (BUN), pH, $Pco_2$, $Po_2$; and a lumbar puncture to rule out infection or hemorrhage. As soon as these vital metabolic functions have been checked, tests that follow should be liver enzyme function, therapeutic drug or narcotic screens, CSF and blood cultures, other electrolytes, coagulation profile, EEG, and CT scan. The EEG is used considerably less often today unless

**Table 30-7** Signs and symptoms that help identify the cause of delirium

| Change | Causes |
|---|---|
| Level of consciousness | |
| clouded and fluctuating | Cardinal sign of metabolic encephalopathy; eliminates dementia |
| Vital signs | |
| hypotension; tachycardia | Sepsis and/or hemorrhage |
| dyspnea–tachypnea | Hypoxia |
| Skin | |
| Moist, cold | Hypoglycemia |
| Dry, warm | Hyperglycemia |
| Dry and red (vasodilatation) | Anticholinergic toxicity |
| Pupils | |
| Miosis | Narcotic toxicity |
| Mydriasis | Anticholinergic toxicity |
| Extremities | |
| Asterixis | Hepatic failure |
| Myalgias, arthralgias, proximal muscular weakness | Steroids |

**Table 30-8**  Laboratory evaluation of delirium

| Test | Reason for test |
| --- | --- |
| Emergency (life-threatening) | |
| Blood drawn for | |
| Glucose | Hypoglycemia, hyperosomlar coma |
| Na+ | Osmolar abnormalities |
| Ca²⁺ | Hypercalcemia or hypocalcemia |
| BUN | Uremia |
| pH, $P\text{co}_2$ | Acidosis, alkalosis |
| $P\text{o}_2$ | Hypoxia |
| Lumbar puncture | Infection, hemorrhage |
| As soon as possible: | |
| Liver function tests | Hepatic coma |
| Sedative drug screen | Overdose |
| Blood and CSF culture | Sepsis, encephalitis, meningitis |
| Full electrolytes, including Mg²⁺ | |
| Coagulation profile | Intravascular coagulation |
| EEG | Confirm diagnosis by presence of diffuse slow waves |
| CT Scan | Rule out structural change |

*Source*: Modified from Posner (1979).

**Table 30-9**  Management of delirium with psychotic or behavioral changes

- Prompt recognition and diagnosis
- Prompt treatment of underlying cause
- Psychiatric consultation—*early*, not late
- One-to-one nurse or companion
- Oral neuroleptics, when needed
- Alert all shifts about change in behavior (i.e., often worse at night)

there is a differential diagnosis between a functional origin and a delirium that is characterized by minimal cognitive changes and primary affective or psychotic symptoms.

## MANAGEMENT AND TREATMENT OF MILD DELIRIUM

Management of the patient with delirium is first directed to determining the underlying cause. Despite confusion many patients remain quiet and show only a memory or attentional deficit. In others behavior is profoundly altered in response to psychotic thinking, at times becoming extreme. Violent or self-destructive behavior requires attention to the safety of the patient, family, and staff. Because the cancer patients who develop a delirium are likely to be the most seriously ill physically, transfer to a psychiatric unit is not possible and the ability of an oncology staff to be able to handle both the emergency and the more common non-emergency situation is important. Table 30-9 gives principles of management.

When a patient shows signs and symptoms of delirium with mild psychotic or behavioral changes, prompt recognition and diagnosis, with treatment of the underlying medical cause, is crucial. Emergency situations are avoided when the confusional state is recognized and treated early.

Treatment of a mild delirium should maximize the comfort and support of the patient while the etiology of the delirium is sought (Table 30-9). Environmental manipulation, the judicious use of oral antipsychotic medication, and staff and family instruction in management all help to calm the patient and reassure family members.

Environmental manipulation is important because patients with delirium are especially sensitive to their environment. Rooms should be quiet and well lit during the daytime. The use of a night-light reduces disorientation that worsens during the evening and night hours when visual cues are reduced. Frequent, short contacts with a supportive family member or a familiar staff member who speaks in a calm, reassuring voice set a quiet and orderly tone. One or two family members who consistently visit provide an added sense of continuity and stability for the patient. The addition of a calendar, clock, and even a few small, familiar objects from home help reorient the forgetful, mildly confused patient. Sensory input should not be excessive. Many different individuals entering the room with requests or procedures add to the sense of confusion. The familiar companion or nurse becomes the monitor of both the patient and the environment, providing stable day and night schedule, and explanation for noises or unfamiliar equipment. Encouragement of walking, reading, and participation in personal care promotes awareness of reality and reduces response to delusional ideas.

Oral antipsychotic medications are the drugs of choice, because other sedatives (benzodiazepines, barbiturates and antihistamines) can worsen confusion (see Chapter 39 on psychopharmacology). Hospitalized cancer patients usually respond to low doses (e.g., 0.5 mg haloperidol or 10 mg thioridazine or chlorpromazine bid or tid). Haloperidol and chlorpromazine can be given orally as tablet or liquid concentrate, or parenterally as intramuscular or intravenous injection. Antipsychotics are not commercially prepared in suppository form, but they can be prepared by a hospital pharmacist upon request. Absorption, however, is not reliable. Haloperidol, which has a higher antipsychotic potency than other medications mentioned, produces less orthostatic hypotension and anticholinergic effects per milligram equivalent of antipsychotic activity. Although patients with only mild symptoms of a delirium will rarely need the faster acting parenteral route, nausea and vomiting from chemotherapy, gastric tumors, NPO orders, malabsorption states, or immediate postoperative treatment may require that medication be given in an injectable form. Patients who are already receiving a structurally similar drug, such as prochlorperazine or metaclopramide as antiemetics, are at greater risk for dyskinesias.

The ability of the staff on a unit to manage a delirious patient optimally is related to their tolerance for managing patients whose behavior is unpredictable, frustrating, and at times frightening. It is helpful to identify one or two staff members on a unit who are interested in psychiatric problems and disturbed patients. However, all staff members should know the legal and ethical issues, as well as how to handle a patient in a psychiatric emergency situation when behavior is unpredictable.

Monitoring the patient's behavior daily or several times a day when it is changing rapidly is essential. Visits at different times of the day are essential, particularly if medication dosage is being titrated against the patient's behavior. A psychotropic drug should be given at the lowest effective dose. A progress note indicating the time the mental status was assessed helps to convey this information to staff on all shifts. Integration of nurses' and physicians' progress notes is particularly valuable when managing patients with neurological complications of cancer, to assure easy and frequent review of changes in mental state. Use of standardized mental status scales, such as the Mini-Mental State or Cognitive Capacity Screening examinations, provides a charted record of standardized observations.

Outpatient follow-up of patients who have had an acute delirium while being treated in the hospital is essential. Patients often fear that they ''lost their mind'' in the hospital and feel distressed that they ''lost track'' of a period of time. They need to discuss their recall of events and be assured that their medical illness or treatment was the cause. The family too is reassured by such information and by being included in visits. They serve the purpose of making the transition to the home environment easier. If a psychotropic drug was given, it must be monitored and slowly tapered at home.

## EMERGENCY MANAGEMENT OF SEVERE DELIRIUM WITH PSYCHOSIS

Although emergency situations happen infrequently, they are highly distressing to the fearful patient, to other patients, and to the visiting family members. For this reason, it is important to have a plan that is known to all staff members by which a situation can be effectively and rapidly contained with maximal patient safety and minimal disruption of the floor activities. We have developed with head nurses and medical staff a psychiatric emergency plan for the management of emergency psychiatric complications encountered in cancer patients; this plan is included in the core course for house staff. Such a situation most often arises when a confused patient becomes belligerent, assaultive, and unable to respond to reasonable requests. The first step is to call the psychiatrist, who evaluates the situation and organizes, if needed, a team composed of the floor staff. Assistance of a security officer or guard is requested if there is a danger of extremely belligerent behavior. Security staff receive instruction as part of their training about the sensitive management of patients in these situations. They may be asked only to be present unobtrusively should the situation escalate, or if a dangerous staircase or exit pose a hazard.

Every effort must be made to assure the patient that he or she is safe and secure. Explanation to the family member present is important to ensure their understanding and cooperation with a request that he or she remain in the room as a person trusted by the patient. The hospital room is familiar, and bringing a trusted staff member to the room is helpful; otherwise, moving the patient to a quiet area away from others is desirable. This is often sufficient to induce a calmer state where observation by a familiar nurse can be instituted. The room should be cleared of potentially dangerous objects if the risk warrants it. If needed, the patient should be encouraged to take an oral sedative in the form of a liquid concentrate, which produces rapid absorption. If the patient refuses oral medication, or if the oral route is inadvisable for medical reasons (e.g., low platelet count in a leukemia patient or a coagulopathy), parenteral medication should be considered. Haloperidol is used because of the low frequency of hypotension as a side effect, minimal sedation, and short half-life, allowing close titration of dosage with behavior (Donlon et al., 1979) (see Chapter 39 on psychopharmacology).

The use of parenteral haloperidol (0.5–2.0 mg iv or im) is recommended as an initial dose; by the intravenous route, it is given at 1 mg/min. The psychiatrist should monitor behavior carefully after the initial dose and determine if additional doses are needed. Haloperidol may be repeated in 30–60 minutes if agitation has not subsided. Usually, one to three doses are sufficient. When the acute agitation resolves, the patient should be switched to an oral form of haloperidol at a dose of about one-half to one and one-half times the parenteral dose. Extrapyramidal side effects are not common at these dose levels. They are usually controlled by intravenous or oral diphenhydramine (25–50 mg po or iv bid), or benztropine (0.5–1 mg po or iv bid).

Most patients can be calmed by environmental changes; others can be encouraged to take medication. However, it is occasionally necessary to restrain the patient temporarily to prevent harm (e.g., the assaultive patient who has thrombocytopenia). With the psychiatrist directing a team that has previously been instructed in applying physical restraint, the situation is explained to the patient and to the relative who must understand and agree that the medication is indicated. If needed, minimal restraint is applied to each extremity while the medication is given. Similarly, the patient may have to be restrained for a diagnostic lumbar puncture required for diagnosis of etiology of the encephalopathy. These confusional states are usually not recalled later by the patient, who finds it difficult to believe that they occurred.

When any physical restraint is used, the "least restrictive" type is indicated. We find that one-to-one nursing observation is adequate in almost all situations. Occasionally a "posey" nylon vest or limb restraints that consist of loosely applied cotton padding and soft gauze are used to prevent a confused patient from removing catheters or tubes. Nylon mesh "sheets" that attach to the fixed parts of a hospital bed are a safer and less restrictive method of restraint. Use of any restraint should be for the shortest possible period and accompanied by careful and close monitoring of vital signs, behavior, intake, and output by a companion in constant attendance. Restraint of cancer patients requires special consideration in the presence of thrombocytopenia, fever, or dehydration.

## SPECIAL DIAGNOSTIC AND MANAGEMENT PROBLEMS

### Anticholinergic Toxicity

A wide range of drugs with anticholinergic properties that block cholinergic neurotransmission are used in cancer patients (Table 30-10). Antiemetics, antihistamines, antiparkinsonian drugs, antipsychotics, atropine to dry respiratory secretions during surgery, narcotic analgesics, tricyclics, and scopolamine are among those used. An anticholinergic delirium can occur from any of these drugs. However, the more common problem in cancer patients occurs when several drugs with these properties have been given for different reasons. The potential for additive anticholinergic side effects must be kept in mind. It is particularly important to watch for this complication in the postoperative period when several of the agents

**Table 30-10**  Drugs with anticholinergic effects often used in cancer treatment

| Drug category | Specific drug |
|---|---|
| Antiemetics | Prochlorperazine |
|  | Metaclopramide |
| Antihistamines | Diphenhydramine |
|  | Hydroxyzine |
| Antiparkinsonians | Benztropine |
|  | Trihexyphenidyl |
| Antipsychotics | Chlorpromazine |
|  | Thioridazine |
|  | Haloperidol |
| Atropine |  |
| Antispasmodics | Clidinium |
|  | Diphenoxylate |
|  | Hyoscyamine |
| Narcotic analgesics | Codeine |
|  | Hydromorphone |
|  | Levodromoran |
|  | Meperidine |
|  | Methadone |
|  | Morphine |
| Tricyclic antidepressants | Amitriptyline |
|  | Nortriptyline |
|  | Imipramine |
|  | Desipramine |
|  | Doxepin |
|  | Maprotoline |
|  | Trazodone |
| Scopolamine |  |

may have been ordered concurrently. If the problem is not recognized, seizures, coma, and death can ensue. The picture is characterized by a delirium accompanied by hyperpyrexia, mydriasis, dehydration, vasodilatation, hypertension, tachycardia, constipation, and urinary retention. The delirium and cardinal symptoms of fever, flushing, and mydriases can be remembered by the well-known mnemonics given in Table 30-11.

Treatment is to discontinue or taper *all* anticholinergic agents when possible. The use of physostigmine, a reversible peripheral anticholinesterase is required when tachycardia or resulting arrhythmias make the situation life-threatening. Physostigmine is administered (0.5–1.0 mg im or iv) at no more than 1.0 mg/min, repeated at intervals of 10–30 minutes. It is administered only when resuscitation equipment is available in case of cardiac arrest or respiratory failure due to obstruction by a sudden overabundance of secretions.

If sedation is necessary, antipsychotic medication at the lowest doses and with the lowest anticholinergic properties (haloperidol), or short-acting barbiturates (amobarbital sodium), or benzodiazepines (intra-

**Table 30-11** Anticholinergic syndrome ("parasympathetic paralysis")

| Syndrome | Mnemonics |
|----------|-----------|
| Hyperpyrexia | "Hot as a hare" |
| Mydriasis | "Blind as a bat" |
| Dehydration | "Dry as a bone" |
| Vasodilatation | "Red as a beet" |
| Delirium | "Mad as a hatter" |
| Hypertension | |
| Tachycardia | |
| Constipation | |
| Urinary retention | |

**Table 30-12** Common psychological changes with steroids administration

| Time | Change |
|------|--------|
| During treatment | • Sense of well-being or mild depression<br>• Optimism<br>• Increased appetite; weight gain<br>• Insomnia |
| During withdrawal | • Mild depression<br>• Irritability<br>• Anorexia<br>• Headache and myalgias |

venous lorazepam) should be used as a "STAT" dose. Caution must be used because these agents themselves may worsen behavioral signs and symptoms in a paradoxical fashion, or make clinical assessment of the anticholinergic state more difficult. Environmental alteration, physical restraint, and constant observation are best used until the anticholinergic drugs are metabolized.

## Steroids

Corticosteroids are used frequently in cancer as primary chemotherapeutic agents in leukemia and lymphoma, as a means to reduce edema associated with brain and spinal cord lesions, and increasingly as an antiemetic in combination with metaclopramide, haloperidol, diphenhydramine, or lorazepam (see also Chapter 29 on CNS complications).

The behavioral response to steroids is independent of the dosage used. More severe effects are seen with higher doses, but they can occur at small doses. Although a sense of well-being and increased appetite are useful initial side effects, obesity and proximal motor weakness are adverse effects that occur over time, along with insomnia, restlessness, hyperactivity, and depression. When steroids are withdrawn, a mild depression or irritability may be noticeable (see Table 30-12).

Severe mood disturbances are far less common than those just outlined. They are characterized by mania, severe depression, or delirium with affective changes. These drug-induced changes, termed organic affective syndromes, may be accompanied by frank hallucinations, delusions and may be clinically indistinguishable from a primary affective illness. The actual frequency of covert mental aberrations is not known, because few systematic studies have been undertaken in patients with cancer. It appears that some patients experience illusions and hallucinations but do not report them, recognizing that they are drug-related. Severe mood disturbances usually occur when the steroid dosage is abruptly changed, either by increasing, tapering, or discontinuing. During withdrawal, myalgias or arthralgias appear that help to confirm the physiological effects of the dosage reduction.

Patients on steroids may develop delirium secondary to an infectious process. However, the steroids have antipyretic properties that may mask the fever associated with infection and sepsis. These patients often appear confused, lethargic, and withdrawn but lack the usual signs of sepsis. The behavioral change may be an important sign of sepsis.

A history of drug abuse, alcohol dependence, or prior psychiatric illness is not a reason to withhold steroids. Mood and mental status should be carefully monitored; an antidepressant and/or antipsychotic should be given if early affective signs appear. We have not found that lithium given prophylactically prevents affective complications.

Treatment of steroid-induced psychosis involves the same management as a delirium of other causes, utilizing the same psychotropic drugs. The exception is those reactions relating to a rapid steroid tapering. In this instance, the treatment, as with other withdrawal states occurring with barbiturates or narcotics, may be to raise the steroid dose and lower it again gradually, while also instituting an antipsychotic medication if symptoms are severe.

## AIDS

Neurological complications from acquired immunodeficiency syndrome (AIDS) are increasingly recognized as a frequent and major source of dysfunction, which may appear as subtle neurological changes or cognitive impairment (Snider et al., 1983) (see Chapters 21 and 29 on AIDS and on CNS complications for more detailed review). The most common neurological complication is the AIDS-related dementia, a subacute encephalopathy characterized by a slowly progressing dementing illness with evidence of atrophy on the CT scan, small areas of demyelination in the white matter and sometimes glial nodules (Price, 1988). It is believed to be caused by direct invasion of the brain by the HIV. In addition, patients with AIDS develop CNS infections from Toxoplasma, cryptococcus, herpes simplex, herpes zoster, and Jakob–Creutzfeld (JC) virus (progressive multifocal leukoencephalopathy). Primary lymphoma in the brain occurs more often in AIDS patients, as well as metastatic spread from elsewhere in the body. These disorders can usually be diagnosed by CT scan and lumbar puncture. However, sometimes the only definitive method is cerebral biopsy.

In its early stages, AIDS-related dementia complex resembles depression, with poor concentration, slowed mentation, and short-term memory deficits. Similar disease changes in the spinal cord produce gait disturbance and weakness. Generalized seizures and coma appear as late changes.

## SUMMARY

This chapter has reviewed the definition, prevalence, and characteristics of delirium and dementia commonly seen in cancer. The early symptoms and signs, the characteristics of severe delirium as well as the psychotic behavior that endangers the patient and others, are reviewed. The steps in the diagnostic workup and in the management of the disturbed patient, to be carried out while seeking the cause of the confusion, are described. Guidelines for managing the delirious cancer patient, using pharmacological interventions and environmental manipulation, are outlined. This frequent complication of cancer compromises treatment and causes significant distress to the patient and family. It requires prompt management in the oncology unit, because transfer to a psychiatric unit is usually precluded by the serious level of medical illness. The fully competent staff of an oncology unit must be able to recognize and treat this complication.

## REFERENCES

Adams, F. (1984). Neuropsychiatric evaluation and treatment of delirium in the critically ill cancer patient. *Cancer Bull. Univ. Texas M.D. Anderson Hosp. Tumor Inst.* 36:156–60.

American Psychiatric Association (1980). *Diagnostic and Statistical Manual of Mental Disorders,* 3rd ed. Washington, D.C.: American Psychiatric Association.

Beresford, T.P., R.E. Holt, R.C.W. Hall, and D.L. Feinsilver (1985). Cognitive screening at the bedside: Usefulness of a structured examination. *Psychosomatics* 26(4):319–24.

Bergmann, K. and E.J. Eastham (1974). Psychogeriatric ascertainment and assessment for treatment in an acute medical ward setting. *Age and Aging* 3:174–88.

Bonhoeffer, K. (1910). *Die symptomatischen Psychosen in Gefolge von akuten Infectionen und inneren Erkrankungen.* Leipzig: Franz Deuticke, p. 94.

Davies, R.K., D.M. Quinlan, F.P. McKegney, and C.P. Kimball (1973). Organic factors and psychological adjustment in advanced cancer patients. *Psychosom. Med.* 35:464–71.

Derogatis, L.R., G.R. Morrow, J. Fetting, D. Penman, S. Piasetsky, A. Schmale, M. Henricks, and C.L. Carnicke, Jr. (1983). The prevalence of psychiatric disorders among cancer patients. *J.A.M.A.* 249:751–57.

Donlon, P.T., J. Hopkin, and J. Tupin (1979). Overview: Efficacy and safety of the rapid neuroleptization method with injectable haloperidol. *Am. J. Psychiatry* 136:273–78.

Engel, G.L. and J. Romano (1959). Delirium: A syndrome of cerebral insufficiency. *J. Chron. Dis.* 9:260–77.

Folstein, M.F., J.H. Fetting, A. Lobo, U. Niaz, and K. Capozzoli (1984). Cognitive assessment of cancer patients. *Cancer* 53(Suppl. May 15):2250–55.

Fraser, C.L. and A.I. Arieff (1985). Hepatic encephalopathy. *N. Engl. J. Med.* 131:865–73.

Hinton, J. (1972). The psychiatry of terminal illness in adults and children. *Proc. R. Soc. Med.* 65:1035–40.

Jacobs, J.W. (1977). Screening for organic mental syndromes in the medically ill. *Ann. Intern. Med.* 86:40–46.

Johnson, B.E., B. Becker, W.B. Goff, N. Petronas, M.A. Krehbiel, R.W. Mukuch, G. McKenna, E. Glatstein, and D.C. Ihde (1985). Neurologic, neuropsychologic and computed tomography scan abnormalities in 2- to 10-year survival of small-cell lung cancer. *J. Clin. Oncol.* 3:1659–67.

Kiernan, R.J., J. Mueller, J.W. Langston, and C. Van Dyke (1987). The neurobehavioral cognitive status examination: A brief but differentiated approach to cognitive assessment. *Ann. Intern. Med.* 107:481–85.

Levine, P.M., P.M. Silberfarb, and Z.J. Lipowski (1978). Mental disorders in cancer patients: A study of 100 psychiatric referrals. *Cancer* 42:1385–91.

Lipowski, Z.J. (1980). A new look at organic brain syndromes. *Am. J. Psychiatry* 137:674–78.

Lipowski, Z.J. (1983). Transient cognitive disorders (delirium, acute confusional states) in the elderly. *Am. J. Psychiatry* 140:1426–36.

Lipowski, Z.J. (1987). Delirium (acute confusional states). *J.A.M.A.* 285(2):1789–92.

Liston, E.H. (1984). Diagnosis and management of delirium in the elderly patient. *Psychiatr. Ann.* 14:109–18.

Massie, M.J., J.G. Gorzynski, R. Mastrovito, D. Theis, and J. Holland (1979). The diagnosis of depression in hospitalized patients with cancer (Abstract). *Proc. Am. Assoc. Cancer Res. Am. Soc. Clin. Oncol.* 20:432.

Massie, M.J., J. Holland, and E. Glass (1983). Delirium in terminally ill cancer patients. *Am. J. Psychiatry* 140:1048–50.

Massie, M.J. and J.C. Holland (1988). Psychiatric diagnoses among patients with cancer. In P. Silberfarb (ed.), *Psychiatric Medicine*. In press.

Navia, B.A., B.D. Jordan, and R.W. Price (1986). The AIDS dementia complex: I. Clinical features. *Ann. Neurol.* 19:517–24.

Navia, B.A., E-S. Cho, C.K. Petito, and R.W. Price (1986). The AIDS dementia complex: II. Neuropathology. *Ann. Neurol.* 19:525–35.

Pauker, N.E., M.F. Folstein, and T.H. Moran (1978). The clinical utility of the hand-held tachistiscope. *J. Nerv. Ment. Dis.* 166:126–29.

Plum, F. and J.B. Posner (1972). *The Diagnosis of Stupor and Coma,* 2nd ed. Philadelphia: F.A. Davis, p. 4.

Posner, J.B. (1978). Neurologic complications of systemic cancer. *Disease-a-Month* 25:1–60.

Posner, J.B. (1979). Delirium and exogenous metabolic brain disease. In P.B. Beeson, W. McDermott, and J.B. Wyngaarden (eds.), *Cecil Textbook of Medicine*. Philadelphia: W.B. Saunders, pp. 644–51.

Price, R.W., B. Brew, J. Sidtis, M. Rosenblum, A.C. Scheck, and P. Cleary (1988). The brain in AIDS: Central nervous system HIV-1 infection and AIDS dementia complex. *Science* 239:586–92.

Schwamm, L.H., C. Van Dyke, R.J. Kiernan, E.L. Merrin, and J. Mueller (1987). The neurobehavioral cognitive status examination: comparison with the cognitive capacity screening examination and the mini-mental state examination in a neurosurgical population. *Ann. Intern. Med.* 107:486–91.

Seymour, D.G., P.J. Henschke, R.D. Cape, and A.J. Campbell (1980). Acute confusional states and dementia in the elderly: The role of dehydration/volume depletion, physical illness and age. *Age and Aging* 9:137–46.

Shevitz, S.A., P.M. Silberfarb, and Z.J. Lipowski (1976). Psychiatric consultations in a general hospital: A report of 1000 referrals. *Dis. Nerv. Syst.* 37:295–300.

Snider, W.D., D.M. Simpson, S. Nielson, J.W.M. Gold, C.E. Metroka, and J.B. Posner (1983). Neurological complications of Acquired Immune Deficiency Syndrome: Analysis of 50 patients. *Ann. Neurol.* 14:403–18.

Strain, J.J., G. Folop, A. Lebovits, B. Ginsberg, M. Robinson, A. Stern, P. Charap, and F. Gany (1988). Screening devices for diminished cognitive capacity. *Gen. Hosp. Psychiatr.* 10:16–23.

Wells, C.E. (1979). Pseudodementia. *Am. J. Psychiatry* 136:859–900.

Young, D.F. and J.B. Posner (1980). Nervous system toxicity of the chemotherapeutic agents. In P.J. Viken and G.W. Bruyn (eds.), *Handbook of Clinical Neurology,* Vol. 39, *Neurological Manifestations of Systemic Diseases, Part II*. New York: Elsevier Biomedical Press, pp. 91–129.

# 31

## Endocrine-Related Psychiatric Disorders

### William Breitbart

Endocrine complications of cancer, though uncommon, present challenges in diagnosis and treatment. The behavioral disturbances and neuropsychiatric symptoms caused by cancer-related endocrine disorders are of particular relevance to those who work with cancer patients. Whereas an altered mood or behavior in a cancer patient is frequent, as part of the normal "psychological response" to illness, endocrine disorders can often mimic these responses as well as other functional psychiatric disturbances. The importance of this differentiation is reflected in the *Diagnostic and Statistical Manual of Mental Disorders* (DSM-III) criteria for major depressive episode, which require that an organic basis for symptoms be ruled out (American Psychiatric Association, 1980). A depressive syndrome, phenomenologically identical to a major depressive episode, may be caused by hypothyroidism or hypercortisolism and would more accurately be diagnosed as an organic affective syndrome. This chapter reviews the psychiatric manifestations seen with endocrine complications of cancer in order to facilitate more accurate diagnosis and treatment (Table 31-1).

Cancer-related disorders of endocrine function are caused by endocrine gland tumors, by ectopic endocrine syndromes, and by some cancer therapies. Tumors of the endocrine glands are uncommon; excessive hormone secretion may be the earliest and most significant sign of such a cancer's existence. In fact, excess secretion of hormone often poses a more immediate threat to life than does the cancer itself, as with parathyroid cancer or insulinoma. Neoplasms of several types produce ectopic humoral substances. Table 31-2 lists the hormones, hormone precursors, and peptides secreted by tumors arising from nonglandular tissues that are responsible for the most common ectopic endocrine syndromes (Odell, 1980).

The synthesis of biologically active peptides within the endocrine system and ectopically is associated with the amine precursor uptake and decarboxylation (APUD) system. Tumors derived from neuroectodermal origin that share a common ability for APUD also share the ability to synthesize and secrete many of the same peptides. Neoplasms derived from the APUD system include parathyroid adenoma, pheochromocytoma, carcinoid, islet cell tumors of the pancreas, medullary carcinoma of the thyroid, and pituitary adenoma (Pearse and Polak, 1978). Cancer therapies including surgery, irradiation, and chemotherapy are also a source of endocrine dysfunction (Bajorunas, 1980).

Endocrine complications in the cancer patient have such diverse etiologies that a review of their psychiatric manifestations is best approached by examining endocrine system disorders rather than specific endocrine gland neoplasms. Thus, the cancer-related disorders of cortisol, thyroid, calcium, glucose, and sodium regulation are presented here with emphasis on the neuropsychiatric features. The psychiatric manifestations of carcinoid tumor and pheochromocytoma are also discussed.

## CORTISOL

### Hypercortisolism (Cushing's Syndrome)

The syndrome of hypercortisolism, or Cushing's syndrome, in the cancer setting can be due to tumors of hypothalamic-pituitary origin, steroid-producing adrenal tumors, ectopic adrenocorticotropic hormone (ACTH) production, or exogenous administration of corticosteroid medication. Adrenal cancer itself is quite rare, and only about 20% of adrenal cancers produce Cushing's syndrome (Soffer et al., 1961). The ectopic production of ACTH by cancers has attracted much attention (Table 31-3). Cushing's syndrome caused by cancer production of ACTH was the first

**Table 31-1**  Psychiatric manifestations of common endocrine complications seen in cancer patients

| | Organic affective syndrome | | Organic brain syndrome | | Psychoses | Anxiety and/or panic attacks | Personality change |
|---|---|---|---|---|---|---|---|
| | Depression | Mania | Delirium | Dementia | | | |
| Hypercortisolism | +++ | ++ | ++ | + | +++ | + | + |
| Hypocortisolism | ++ | | + | + | + | | + |
| Hyperthyroidism | + | + | ++ | + | ++ | +++ | + |
| Hypothyroidism | +++ | | ++ | + | ++ | | |
| Hypercalcemia | ++ | | ++ | ++ | ++ | | + |
| Hypocalcemia | + | + | +++ | ++ | + | +++ | |
| Hyperglycemia | | | + | ++ | | | |
| Hypoglycemia | ++ | + | +++ | ++ | ++ | +++ | + |
| Hyponatremia (SIADH) | ++ | | ++ | ++ | + | | |
| Carcinoid | + | | + | | | | |
| Pheochromocytoma | | | | | | +++ | ++ |

ectopic endocrine syndrome described. Clinically such patients often do not exhibit the full Cushing's syndrome, but findings such as hypokalemia, abnormal glucose tolerance, weakness, and psychoses are present (Odell, 1980). Only a small percentage of patients with the tumors noted in Table 31-3 actually develop Cushing's syndrome. Among patients with oat-cell cancer of the lung, only 2.8% had hypercortisolemia (Kato et al., 1969).

Cushing's syndrome is the endocrine disorder with the highest frequency of mental changes. Abnormal behavioral symptomatology with prominent changes in affect and cognition occur in 40–90% of cases. Psychotic symptoms including confusion, paranoia, and hallucinations occur in 10–20%. Suicidal ideation or action accompanying depressive symptoms complicates 10% of cases of Cushing's syndrome. The signs and symptoms of depression interestingly may precede the appearance of obesity, hirsutism, striae, moon facies, or muscle wasting seen with hypercortisolism. Whereas euphoria and increased motor activity are observed early in the course of hypercortisolism, depression, emotional lability, insomnia, fatigue, loss of libido, and cognitive deficits are more common later (Carroll, 1977; Pepper and Krieger, 1984; L.M. Cohn and M.E. Moltich, 1984).

By far the most common psychiatric manifestation of Cushing's syndrome is affective disturbance. It was believed that hypercortisolism of hypothalamic or pituitary origin was more associated with mood disturbance (depression) than when due to adrenal adenoma or ectopic ACTH production. Exogenous steroid medications were thought to cause depression rarely and more likely to be characterized by euphoria or acute

**Table 31-2**  Ectopic hormones and peptides secreted by tumors

| | |
|---|---|
| Adrenocorticotropin (ACTH) | Prolactin |
| Corticotropin-releasing hormone (CRH) | Estradiol |
| Antidiuretic hormone (vasopressin), inappropriate (ADH) | Human chorionic gonadotropin (hCG) |
| Thyroid-stimulating hormone (TSH) | Human placental lactogen (HPL) |
| Melanocyte-stimulating hormone (MSH) | Carcinoembryonic antigen (CEA) |
| Growth hormone (GH) | α-Fetoprotein (AFP) |
| Growth hormone-releasing hormone (GHRH) | Insulin |
| Parathyroid hormone (PTH) | Hypoglycemic-producing factors |
| PTH-like factors | Glucagon |
| Osteoclast-activating factor (OAF) | Erythropoietin |
| Prostaglandins (PG) | Renin |
| Transforming growth factor | 5-Hydroxytryptophan (5HT) |
| Colony-stimulating factor (CSF) | Serotonin |
| Calcitonin | Histamine |
| Hypophosphatemia-producing factor | Bradykinins |
| | Vasoactive intestinal peptide (VIP) |

**Table 31-3**  Tumors associated with ectopic ACTH production

Lung, small cell and oat cell
Thymus
Pancreas, islet cell, carcinoid
Medullary thyroid
Bronchial adenoma (carcinoid)*
Pheochromocytoma
Neuroblastoma
Paraganglioma
Ganglioma

*Occasionally secretes corticotropin-releasing hormone (CRH) (Upton and Amatruda, 1971).

toxic psychosis. Recent attempts to categorize psychiatric disturbances in Cushing's syndrome (Haskett and Rose, 1981; S.I. Cohen, 1980; Haskett, 1985) demonstrate that more than 75% of patients meet criteria for the diagnosis of major affective disorder regardless of pituitary, hypothalamic, adrenal, or ectopic origin. Haskett demonstrated that 25 of 30 patients with Cushing's syndrome had a major affective disorder, including 16 with unipolar depression, 9 with bipolar mania, and only 5 with no psychiatric disorder. The natural history of manic symptoms was either spontaneous remission or switch into depression (Haskett, 1985). S.I. Cohen (1980) reported that 25 of 29 patients he studied were depressed, with a family history of depression or suicide in 12. Physically healthy individuals who suffer an episode of major depression have a persistent increase in adrenocortical function that may reflect a central dysregulation of the hypothalamic-pituitary-adrenal axis similar to the dysfunction in Cushing's syndrome. These psychiatric and endocrine disorders probably share a common limbic system disturbance.

Cognitive disturbances in Cushing's syndrome are also quite common. Increased levels of cortisol and ACTH cause impairment of memory and concentration. Up to 33% of patients may show moderate to marked deficits in language and nonlanguage tests of higher corticol function, as well as impairment of motor and sensory function involving visual processing (Starkman et al., 1981; Whelan et al., 1980).

Exogenously administered corticosteroids are widely utilized in the treatment of cancer and its complications. They are the most common cause of hypercortisolism in the cancer setting. Whereas severe steroid-induced neuropsychiatric disturbances are relatively uncommon, at times they constitute a major clinical problem that can inhibit cancer therapy. The incidence of minor cognitive and mood disturbances has not been documented, but is likely high in patients receiving high doses of steroids. Higher dosages of steroid appear to correlate with increased risk of neuropsychiatric disturbance; however, symptoms can occur at any dose and there may be a ceiling effect with respect to dosage (BCDSP, 1972).

The incidence of major mental disturbances related to exogenous administration of corticosteroids ranges from 3 to 57% for noncancer populations (BCDSP, 1972). The spectrum of disturbances includes affective disorders (mania or depression), cognitive impairment (reversible dementia), and delirium (steroid psychosis). In many studies, especially the early reports of marked mental changes, affective and psychotic reactions were common (Hall, 1979; Ling et al., 1981). Depression and mania are the most common mental

disturbances, with almost 50% of those on steroids developing manic symptoms (Lewis and Smith, 1983). Some investigators have noted predominantly cognitive impairment. Varney and co-workers (1984) reported six cases of reversible steroid dementia in which patients demonstrated deficits in attention, concentration, memory retention, mental speed, and occupational performance that improved with the discontinuation of steroids. Other changes noted included subtle alterations in sensation, perception, mood lability, and sleep disturbance (Henkin, 1970; Wolkowitz et al., 1986).

The onset of mental disturbance is most often within the first 2 weeks on steroids in patients who develop such problems, but it can range from 1 day to 3 months. Steroid-induced neuropsychiatric side effects are often rapidly reversible upon dosage reduction or discontinuation (Ling et al., 1981). There have been case reports of a "steroid withdrawal" phenomenon, in which depression, agitation, anxiety, and psychotic reactions are observed during the taper period (Morgan et al., 1973). Some investigators suggest a higher disturbance rate among females, while others disagree. There is also controversy over whether prior psychiatric illness, or prior disturbance on steroids is a predictor of susceptibility to, or the nature of, steroid-induced neuropsychiatric effects (BCDSP, 1972; Hall et al., 1979; Ling et al., 1981).

## Hypocortisolism (Adrenal Insufficiency)

Cancer-related adrenal insufficiency can be caused by anatomical destruction of the adrenal gland through invasion or surgical removal, suppression of the hypothalamic-pituitary axis via exogenous steroid administration or ectopic secretion of ACTH, hypopituitarism related to cancer or cancer treatment, and rarely, metabolic failure in hormone production secondary to cytotoxic agents such as 5-fluorouracil (5-FU) (Bajorunas, 1980). Adrenocortical insufficiency is characterized by slowly progressive weakness, fatigue, anorexia, weight loss, nausea and vomiting, hypotension, and in the classic Addisonian picture, cutaneous pigmentation.

It is not surprising that mental symptoms as well as changes in behavior and personality have been noted since Addison first described adrenocortical deficiency. Early psychiatric manifestations of hypocrotisolism include depression, apathy, fatigue, lack of motivation, negativism, and irritability (Whybrow and Hurwitz, 1976). Addisonian encephalopathy has been described, characterized by memory impairment, clouding of consciousness, an organic psychosis, or delirium that can progress to coma. Profound perceptual disturbances including lowered threshold of sensitivity to smell, taste, touch, and hearing have been reported (Henkin, 1970).

## THYROID

### Hyperthyroidism

Thyroid cancer is quite rare, with a prevalence of 0.2–0.8%. Radiation and prolonged high levels of thyroid-stimulating hormone (TSH) contribute to the incidence of thyroid neoplasms. Radiation-associated thyroid cancer, an unfortunate result of use of radiation in the treatment of thymic hyperplasia and acne, is the most common thyroid malignancy. Thyroid cancer can also present as a late secondary malignancy after radiation treatment for Hodgkin's disease. Hyperthyroidism secondary to a hyperfunctional thyroid nodule rarely occurs as part of a malignant process. Choriocarcinomas and embryonal carcinoma of the testis can also be ectopic sources of TSH (see Table 31-2) (Odell, 1980).

Hyperthyroidism is almost always associated with mental symptoms including mild to severe anxiety, affective symptoms, cognitive-intellectual impairment, psychosis and delirium (Table 31-1). Mild hyperthyroidism usually presents with anxiety, motor restlessness, irritability, emotional lability, and sleep disturbance. Panic attacks are rare. A delirium with psychosis, which is sometimes seen as an agitated delusional syndrome, can occur. In toxic states this delirium can progress to severe encephalopathy and coma. Organic brain damage may persist in a minority of patients even after hyperthyroidism is controlled (Whybrow and Ferrell, 1974). Affective syndromes can also occur. Apathetic forms of hyperthyroidism in the elderly may present as depression (Taylor, 1973). Manic syndromes have also been reported in hyperthyroid states (Corn and Checkley, 1983).

### Hypothyroidism

Surgery, ablative doses of $^{131}$I, radiotherapy, and some chemotherapy agents can all impair thyroid function and cause frank hypothyroidism. Patients receiving radiation therapy to the neck after hemithyroidectomy had a high incidence of hypothyroidism (Murken and Duvan, 1972). Patients with Hodgkin's and non-Hodgkin's lymphomas have a higher incidence of hypothyroidism than head and neck cancer patients, who received higher doses of neck radiation. This may be related to the use of lymphangiogram contrast containing iodide (Fuks et al., 1976). Unreported data from J. Redman and D.R. Bajorunas show elevated TSH lev-

els in 44% of lymphoma patients following chemotherapy alone. L-Asparaginase has been associated with low levels of $T_4$ (thyroxine) (Garrick and Larsen, 1979), and aminoglutethimide used to treat adrenal cancer can cause goiterous hypothyroidism (Fishman et al., 1967).

The onset of hypothyroidism is frequently accompanied by evidence of neuropsychiatric disturbance. Cognitive impairment, sometimes referred to as a subcortical dementia, can appear strikingly, with difficulty in concentration, slowed response time, and deficits in short-term memory. Patients frequently develop a facetious demeanor, resembling features of frontal lobe disturbance. Brain damage that results from the hypothyroid state is, for the most part, reversible.

Affective disturbance typically takes the form of depression and can be severe. "Myxedema madness" resembles depression or melancholia with psychotic or paranoid features (Touks, 1974). The full DSM-III syndrome of depression can be produced by hypothyroidism, and indeed, depression and hypothyroidism share many signs and symptoms. Approximately 14% of psychiatric patients with depression have evidence of hypothyroidism and often improve with thyroid replacement (Sternbach et al., 1983). Adequate evaluation of thyroid function with measurements of $T_4$, triiodothyronine, T3RU, and TSH is essential when faced with evaluation of depressive symptomatology.

## CALCIUM REGULATION

### Hypercalcemia

Hypercalcemia is one of the most common metabolic complications of cancer. The estimated incidence of the hypercalcemia of cancer is 150 new cases per million persons per year. The clinical features of hypercalcemia such as nausea, vomiting, anorexia, lethargy, confusion, stupor, and eventual coma may be confused with the terminal stages of cancer or with the effect of chemotherapy or irradiation. It is important to recognize that these symptoms can be reversed by lowering the serum calcium. Table 31-4 lists the types of cancer associated with, and the mechanisms of, hypercalcemia. Cancer of the lung (squamous cell) and breast are the most common cancers associated with hypercalcemia, and accounting for well over 50% of all cases.

Mundy and colleagues (1984) divided patients with the hypercalcemia of cancer into three groups based on different pathogenic mechanisms. Hematological cancers, particularly multiple myeloma and certain lymphomas (Burkitt's lymphoma, T-cell lymphoma, and lymphosarcoma), have the capacity to secrete a soluble

**Table 31-4**   Hypercalcemia of cancer

| Common tumors associated with hypercalcemia | Causes of hypercalcemia |
|---|---|
| Multiple myeloma | Hematological |
| Lymphomas | Osteoclast-activating factor (OAF) |
| Lung | 1,25-Dihydroxyvitamin D |
| Breast | Solid tumors with bone metastases |
| Pancreas | Direct bone erosion |
| Lung (squamous cell) | PG |
| Kidney | Solid tumors without bone metastases |
| Bladder | Ectopic PTH |
| Prostate | PTH-like factors |
| Ovarian | PG |
| Cervix | Transforming growth factor |
| Uterine | Colony-stimulating factor |
| Liver | |
| Esophagus | |
| Pancreas | |
| Head and neck | |
| Pheochromocytoma | |

*Source*: Adapted from Mundy et al. (1984).

**Table 31-5**   Types of multiple endocrine neoplasia (MEN)

| MEN type | Tumors included |
|---|---|
| I | Parathyroid hyperplasia, adenoma |
| | Pancreatic insulinoma, vipoma glucagonoma |
| | Pituitary: prolactinoma ACTH-secreting tumor eosinophilic adenoma |
| | Thyroid nodules |
| | Bronchial carcinoids |
| | Adrenal adenomas |
| IIa | Medullary thyroid carcinoma |
| | Pheochromocytoma |
| | Hyperparathyroidism |
| IIb | Marfanoid habitus |
| | Mucosal neuromas |
| | Bowel abnormalities |
| | Typical facies |
| | Pheochromocytoma |

factor that stimulates osteoclasts to resorb bone that is similar to osteoclast-activating factor (OAF), a lymphokine that is released by normal activated lymphocytes. Solid tumors with bone metastases cause hypercalcemia by direct bone erosion in conjunction with local factors such as protaglandins and OAF that increase osteoclast stimulation (Mundy et al., 1984).

Solid tumors without bone metastases that cause hypercalcemia are the least common but attract the most scientific interest. Hypercalcemia in these patients is due to increased bone resorption caused by the ectopic secretion by tumor cells of humoral factors that stimulate bone resorption systematically (Mundy and Martin, 1982). Factors noted to be involved include ectopic parathyroid hormone (PTH), PTH-like factors that bind to PTH receptors, prostaglandins (PG), colony-stimulating factor (CSF), and transforming growth factors (Stewart et al., 1980; Jacobs et al., 1983).

The secretion of PTH and the resulting unremitting severe hypercalcemia is the most threatening feature of parathyroid adenoma or hyperplasia. Of the patients with hyperparathyroidism, 40% have mental symptoms; in fact the psychiatric manifestations are the presenting feature in 12% of cases (Karpati and Frame, 1964). Mental disturbances are related only to the level of serum calcium. Parathyroid hyperplasia is the component most frequently seen that is common to all forms of multiple endocrine neoplasia (MEN) (see Table 31-5). The syndromes of MEN are familial and are transmitted as autosomal dominant traits with high penetrance and variable expressivity. MEN type I con-

sists of adenomas of the pituitary, pancreatic islet cell, and parathyroid gland, while MEN type IIa is characterized by the coexistence of medullary thyroid carcinoma, pheochromocytoma, and parathyroid adenoma or hyperplasia (Eberle and Grun, 1981).

Calcium ion is necessary for normal neural membrane function and synaptic transmission, and so it is not surprising that abnormalities in calcium regulation would have profound neuropsychiatric consequences (see Table 31-1). Mental symptoms vary with serum calcium levels. Elevated calcium levels of between 12 and 16 mg/100 ml are associated with primarily affective disturbance, typically depression with apathy and slowed thinking. Symptoms of depression begin to merge with those of delirium as calcium levels rise to between 16 and 19 mg/100 ml. An organic psychosis can manifest as disorientation, confusion, delirium, paranoia, and even hallucinations. Calcium levels above 19 mg/100 ml are marked by somnolence and eventually coma (Smith et al., 1972).

### CASE REPORT

A 49-year-old woman with breast cancer widely metastatic to the bone developed intractable hypercalcemia. Her initial complaints included depressed mood, dysphoria, irritability, and difficulty concentrating. Serum calcium levels were approximately 13 mg/100 ml. As serum calcium rose to between 14 and 15 mg/100 ml, she developed symptoms of paranoia with disorientation, confusion, and agitation. These symptoms were controlled with haloperidol in low doses while attempts to lower calcium levels were accelerated. When serum calcium levels progressed to 16 mg/100 ml, she became obtunded with brief periods of agitated wakefulness. Eventually the patient's hypercalcemia was controlled, resulting in complete resolution of all neuropsychiatric symptoms. A recurrence of hypercalcemia shortly thereafter produced interestingly very similar mental disturbances.

## Hypocalcemia

Hypocalcemia occurring in the cancer setting is often the result of surgical hypoparathyroidism, renal insufficiency, or malabsorption due to drug or other cancer-related complications, and finally as a result of drugs given to lower calcium levels, such as mithramycin or calcitonin. L-Asparaginase has been reported to cause hypocalcemia in 37% of children and 60% of adults receiving this chemotherapeutic agent (Oettgen et al., 1970). Calcitonin, which is normally produced by parafollicular cells of the thyroid, is secreted by some medullary carcinomas of the thyroid as well as some solid tumors, such as breast, pancreas, colon, and lung (K.E. Schwartz et al., 1979). However, hypersecretion of calcitonin by these tumors does not seem to produce symptoms of hypocalcemia.

In hypocalcemic states, the tetany and neuromuscular twitching can manifest as anxiety. However, the most common mental change is intellectual impairment, which occurs in 33% of patients (Smith et al., 1972). Organic brain syndrome clinically similar to delirium tremens has also been seen in approximately 33% of patients. Cases of hypomania and depression have been described, as well as clinical syndromes resembling a diverse range of psychiatric disorders (Denko and Kaebbing, 1960). The variety of psychiatric symptomatology with hypocalcemia is quite great (see Table 31-1), and so it is vital to measure serum calcium when evaluating mental disturbances in the cancer setting, remembering that these symptoms generally improve completely with calcium replacement.

## GLUCOSE

### Hyperglycemia

Hyperglycemia is generally not a problem specific to the cancer setting. Very high levels of glucose can be seen in untreated or uncontrolled diabetics, particularly under the stress of infection or with associated renal impairment. Patients who have had surgical pancreatectomy require careful attention to blood glucose levels and do well with appropriate insulin replacement therapy. Several chemotherapeutic agents can impair glucose regulation through effects on $\beta$ cells of the pancreas. Streptozotocin has a cytotoxic effect on $\beta$ cells (Junod et al., 1967), vincristine can impair glucose-induced insulin release (Shah et al., 1979), and L-Asparaginase can interfere with insulin synthesis (Whitecar et al., 1970) (see Table 31-6). Excessive secretion of glucagon by a glucagonoma can cause a modest hyperglycemia that is rarely clinically significant. Hyperosmolar states caused by hyperglycemia can result in an encephalopathy leading to coma that

**Table 31-6** Cancer and glucose regulation

| Condition | Mechanism |
|---|---|
| *Hypoglycemia* | |
| Insulinoma | Insulin excess |
| Bronchial carcinoid | Ectopic insulin |
| Liposarcoma | |
| Mesenchymal tumors | Hypoglycemia-producing factors |
| Mesotheliomas | Nonsuppressible insulin-like factors (NSILF) |
| Fibrosarcomas | |
| Rhabdomyosarcomas | Insulin-like growth factors (IGF) |
| Leiomyosarcomas | somatomedins |
| Neurofibromas | |
| Spindle cell sarcoma | |
| Hepatomas | Excessive glucose consumption |
| Adrenal carcinomas | |
| *Hyperglycemia* | |
| Chemotherapy | |
| Streptozotocin | Cytotoxic effect on $\beta$ cells |
| Vincristine | Impaired insulin synthesis |
| L-Asparaginase | Impaired insulin release |
| Surgical: pancreatectomy | Insulin deficiency |
| Glucagonoma | Glucagon excess |

may be fatal. Recovery of intellectual function after this insult may often be incomplete.

## Hypoglycemia

Hypoglycemia of clinical significance occurs in a wide variety of metabolic disorders, including hepatic insufficiency, adrenocortical insufficiency, or through the unmonitored use of exogenous insulin or oral hypoglycemic agents.

Cancer-associated hypoglycemia can have diverse etiologies (see Table 31-6). Insulinomas are rare $\beta$-cell tumors of the pancreas that hypersecrete insulin in a nonregulated fashion. The diagnosis is often made by determining the presence of fasting or inappropriate hypoglycemia accompanied by high plasma insulin levels. Tumors reported to secrete ectopic insulin include malignant bronchial carcinoids and liposarcomas (Shames et al., 1968). A number of neoplasms have been associated with hypoglycemia without elevations of immunoreactive insulin. These include the mesenchymal tumors, hepatomas, and adrenal cancer. A number of humoral mechanisms have been suggested through which these tumors cause hypoglycemia, as well as the concept of their excessive glucose consumption (Megyesi et al., 1975; Gorden et al., 1981; Carey et al., 1966).

The clinical presentation of hypoglycemia depends on the rate of fall in plasma glucose as well as on the absolute level. Gradually developing neuroglycopenia may imitate symptoms of depression. Similarly, chronic hypoglycemia may appear as depression, dementia, or even with schizophreniform symptoms. Acute drops in glucose levels are usually associated with such symptoms as tachycardia, sweating, pallor, tingling of fingers; with severe falls in glucose levels, myoclonic twitching and seizures occur. A drop in blood glucose levels from normal range to about 70 mg/100 ml can result in symptoms of hypoglycemia that primarily resemble anxiety. Changes in mental function follow as glucose levels fall, so that progressive impairment of cerebral function is seen at levels of 30–40 mg/100 ml that are typical of a mild delirium. At levels below 10 mg/100 ml coma can result, and the neurological or cognitive deficits resulting from such intense hypoglycemia may not be reversible (Sachs, 1973).

CASE REPORT

An emergency psychiatric consultation was requested at 11 P.M. by a distraught house staff physician who explained that a 29-year-old hispanic male with localized bladder cancer had unexplicably become agitated, bizarre, and delusional. The patient had apparently been doing well, ready for discharge the next day with no active medical problems. The only medications he was aware of the patient taking were mild analgesics. Upon examination, the patient was indeed agitated with euphoric mood, maniclike pressured speech, loosening of associations, and apparently psychotic. He felt that he had spoken to God, who told him he was cured, and that was why he was so happy. He also was disoriented to time and had apparent difficulty concentrating. A brief review of his chart showed that in addition to analgesics, the patient had been taking an oral hypoglycemic agent prescribed for mild diabetes. He continued to receive these agents while drastically lowering his sugar intake on a restricted diet in the hospital. His serum glucose had been normal on admission, but a bedside check of serum glucose revealed a level of 30 mg/100 ml. The patient was given two ampules of 50% dextrose–water intravenously, with almost immediate return to his normal mental state. In retrospect, the patient had been feeling anxious and sweaty for several days, and wondered if he was hypoglycemic.

## HYPONATREMIA

### Sustained Inappropriate Antidiuretic Hormone (SIADH)

Ectopic secretion of antidiuretic hormone (ADH) by tumors is the fourth most common ectopic endocrine syndrome. First described in 1957 as the Schwartz–Bartter syndrome, it is a tumor-caused humoral syndrome consisting of hyponatremia, renal sodium loss, hypervolemia, and inappropriately high urine osmolality (W.B. Schwartz et al., 1957). Lung cancers are the most common type of neoplasm associated with

ectopic secretion of ADH. Of patients with oat-cell carcinoma of the lung, 40% had SIADH (Gilbey et al., 1975). Other neoplasms such as prostate, adrenocortical cancer, and Hodgkin's disease can cause the syndrome, as can cerebral metastases of any origin. Of the chemotherapeutic agents, vincristine and cyclophosphamide have both been reported to cause SIADH (Table 31-7).

The physical symptoms associated with hyponatremia include anorexia, nausea, vomiting, and lethargy. The initial psychiatric manifestation of a sodium and water imbalance such as hyponatremia may be depression (Sandifer, 1983). Serum sodium levels that drop to 120 mEq/L or lower can be associated with confusion, cognitive impairment, and development of delirium, sometimes with psychotic features (Burnell and Foster, 1972). Seizures occur with levels close to 110 mEq/L.

**Table 31-7**   Causes of SIADH in cancer patients

| Cause | Examples |
|---|---|
| Ectopic ADH secretion | Lung cancer (oat cell) |
| | Prostate cancer |
| | Adrenocortical cancer |
| | Hodgkin's disease, lymphosarcoma |
| | Thymoma |
| | Carcinoma of duodenum |
| | Pancreatic cancer |
| Drug-Induced SIADH | Chemotherapy |
| |    Vincristine |
| |    Cyclophosphamide |
| | Psychotropics |
| |    Amitriptyline |
| |    Nortriptyline |
| |    Haloperidol |
| |    Thioridazine |
| |    Thiothixene |
| |    Fluphenazine |
| | Other drugs |
| |    Chlorpropamide |
| |    Carbamazepine |
| |    Narcotics |
| |    Barbiturates |
| |    Thiazide diuretics |
| |    General anesthesia |
| Pulmonary disease | Pneumonia |
| | Tuberculosis |
| | Lung abscess |
| CNS disorders | Metastases |
| | Tumor |
| | Trauma |
| | Cerebrovascular accidents |
| | Encephalitis |
| | Meningitis |
| | Pain |

## CASE REPORT

A 63-year-old white male with oat-cell cancer of the lung developed hyponatremia secondary to SIADH. As the serum sodium fell to levels as low as 113 mEq/L, he became quite lethargic and listless with difficulty in motor coordination, disorientation, and severe confusion. Efforts to raise sodium levels were quite successful, but at serum sodium levels of 120–125 mEq/L the patient's behavior became bizarre. His speech and thinking were quite slow with associated difficulties in concentration, attention, orientation, and short-term memory. The patient experienced episodes of depersonalization and dissociation accompanied by visual hallucinations. In addition, he developed a delusional belief that he was locked in a bare prison cell and was a prisoner of God. Without any psychiatric intervention, the patient's mental status cleared completely as the serum sodium returned to 132–136 mEq/L level. An EEG done during the period of abnormal behavior demonstrated diffuse slowing. A CTT scan and MRI of the head as well as repeated CSF examinations were all normal. A repeat EEG was also normal.

## PHEOCHROMOCYTOMA

Malignant or benign functional pheochromocytomas have the capacity to secrete excessive amounts of epinephrine and norepinephrine. Among these tumors of the adrenal medulla, 10–15% are malignant. Pheochromocytomas are derived from the APUD system, and familial pheochromocytoma is a component of type II MEN (Sipple, 1961). Diagnosis of functional pheochromocytoma is aided by measuring urinary metanephrines and plasma catecholamines.

It is the excessive secretion of catecholamines that is responsible for the physical symptoms and psychiatric manifestations of pheochromocytoma. Paroxysmal episodes of hypertension, and palpitations, headache, sweating, weight loss, tachycardia, and postural hypotension are only a few of the possible physical manifestations of pheochromocytoma. Often there is a family history of pheochromocytoma or a hypertensive response to anesthesia induction (DeQuattro and Compese, 1979). Psychiatric symptoms seen with pheochromocytoma include personality changes, anxiety, and panic disorders; their prominence can lead to misdiagnosis as a psychiatric disorder.

## CARCINOID

Carcinoid tumors are rare and arise from enterochromaffin cells that are part of the APUD system. They can occur throughout the gastrointestinal tract, lung, pancreas, testis, and ovary. Carcinoid tumors are rarely symptomatic and are most commonly discovered incidentally at autopsy. Only 6.7% of patients with carcinoid tumor develop carcinoid syndrome. Symptoms are a result of the secretion of PG, his-

tamine, bradykinins, vasoactive intestinal peptide (VIP), 5-hydroxytrytophan (5HI), and serotonin (5-hydroxytryptamine). Carcinoid tumors are capable of producing a large amount of serotonin, which is synthesized from tryptophan. The half-life of serotonin is short (<1 minute) because it is almost completely metabolized in one pass through the pulmonary circulation.

Massive amounts of serotonin must be produced by the tumor in order to produce the signs and symptoms of the carcinoid syndrome, which are flushing, diarrhea, dyspnea, bronchospasm, hypotension, glucose intolerance, arthropathy, vasomotor instability, pellagra (niacin deficiency), and endocardial fibrosis. Flushing, dyspnea, and vasomotor instability are often mistaken for anxiety or panic attacks (Trivedi, 1984). The psychiatric manifestations most often thought to be associated with carcinoid tumors (and serotonin metabolism) are depression and encephalopathy, although the frequency is unclear. This is of interest because a low level of CNS serotonin is thought to be the fundamental neurotransmitter abnormality in depression (Schildkraut, 1978). In carcinoid syndrome it is possible that the tumor may consume all available tryptophan in the periphery. A paradoxical situation thus occurs in which there is an excess of serotonin in the serum but a profound deficiency of serotonin in the brain.

Major and colleagues (1973) reported that in a retrospective chart review of 22 patients with carcinoid, 50% had depression and 35% had signs of delirium. Patchell and Posner (1986) reviewed the neurological complications of 219 patients with carcinoid seen in a 10-year period at Memorial Sloan-Kettering Cancer Center. In their study, only 1% of all patients had depression, whereas 11% of patients with evidence of hypersecretion of serotonin had depression. They felt that there was no suggestion of increased incidence of depression in patients with carcinoid tumors. Encephalopathy has also been reported with carcinoid tumors and has improved after tryptophan and niacin were replaced in the diet (Trivedi, 1984; Major et al., 1973).

## MANAGEMENT ISSUES

Correct diagnosis and treatment of endocrine complications of cancer is, of course, key in management of patients whose psychological symptoms have an organic origin. Medical and psychiatric interventions generally need to be combined and coordinated. Indeed, psychiatric management may be necessary in order to facilitate the medical workup. Initial medical management attempts to correct the resulting metabolic disorders proceeding from the most acutely life-threatening to those that can be addressed over several days. Water and sodium balance must be restored, glucose regulated, and calcium levels corrected as attempts to restore the body's normal homeostasis are made. Treatments that have specific endocrine effects are undertaken, such as thyroid replacement, insulin therapy, reduction of steroid dosage, and administration of demethylchlortetracycline (for SIADH). Drugs such as cyproheptadine (a serotonin antagonist), bromocriptine, and sodium valproate are used in the treatment of carcinoid syndrome and hypercortisolism (Cavagnini et al., 1984). Hypercalcemia is treated with saline infusion, furosemide, and occasionally with drugs such as mithramycin or calcitonin. Chemotherapy, surgery, or irradiation designed specifically to treat neoplasms that secrete various substances responsible for the endocrine and metabolic disturbances is often essential.

The psychopharmacological management of psychiatric symptoms and disorders that have an organic or medical origin is discussed fully in Chapter 30 on delirium and dementia. These disorders, which phenomenologically resemble functional psychiatric disorders, do respond to the standard psychopharmacological treatments usually reserved for those psychiatric disorders and should be employed.

Whereas the use of psychotropic drugs in the setting of medical illness is complicated by impaired metabolism, altered pharmacokinetics, drug–drug interactions, and unwanted side effects, the dangers of untreated psychiatric symptoms often outweigh those concerns (Breitbart and Holland, 1988). (See Chapter 39, Psychopharmacology). It is well accepted that the agitation and psychotic symptoms of a delirium are best treated with neuroleptic drugs such as haloperidol or the phenothiazines. These neuroleptic drugs have also been used successfully to treat steroid psychosis. Organic affective syndromes have also been successfully managed with psychotropic medication. Tricyclic antidepressants are effective in treating both emotional lability and major depressive episodes secondary to neurological and endocrine-related disorders (Schiffer et al., 1983; Lawson and MacLeod, 1969). Psychostimulants with amphetamine-like effects are safe and effectively used to treat depression in the medically ill (Kaufman et al., 1982). Occasionally patients with severe delusional depression secondary to high-dose steroids have responded to combinations of tricyclic antidepressants and neuroleptic drugs.

Electroconvulsive therapy (ECT) has been successfully used to treat steroid-induced depressions, as well as delusional depression complicating Cushing's syndrome (Fink, 1980). Lithium therapy, effective in ameliorating manic symptoms, has been reported useful in preventing steroid-induced psychosis (Goggans et al., 1983). Falk and colleagues (1979) found lithium prophylaxis useful in preventing corticotropin-induced psychoses among patients with multiple sclerosis. Of those patients on lithium with serum levels of 0.8–1.2 mEq/L. none developed mental symptoms compared to 14% in the comparison group without lithium prophlaxis. Our clinical experience in cancer has not supported the use of lithium prophylactically (Breitbart and Holland, 1988) (Chapter 39 on psychopharmacology).

## SUMMARY

This chapter outlines the common neuroendocrine complications of cancer, with emphasis on the psychiatric manifestations in terms of diagnosis and management. The understanding of these disorders in cancer is rapidly advancing and the need for studies of the neuropsychiatric aspects is great, because many available reports have depended on retrospective review. The increasing attention to prospective studies that correlate psychological and hormonal abnormalities will bring more sophisticated psychiatric information to bear on the subject. Reports of the efficacy of psychotropic drugs in treating organic affective syndromes have been for the most part anecdotal, with some outstanding exceptions. Clearly, more information through prospective, well-controlled studies of the efficacy of psychopharmacological intervention in such disorders is needed to place these management principles on firmer ground.

## REFERENCES

American Psychiatric Association, Committee on Nomenclature and Statistics (1980). *Diagnostic and Statistical Manual of Mental Disorders,* 3rd ed. Washington, D.C.: American Psychiatric Association.

Bajorunas, D.R. (1980). Disorders of endocrine function following cancer therapies. *Clin. Endocrinol. Metab.* 9:405–30.

Ballard, H.S., B. Frame, and R. Hartsock (1964). Familial multiple endocrine adenoma–peptic ulcer complex. *Medicine* 43:481–516.

Boston Collaborative Drug Surveillance Program (BCDSP) (1972). Acute adverse reactions to prednisone in relation to dosage. *Clin. Pharmacol. Ther.* 13:694–98.

Breitbart, W. and J.C. Holland (1988). Psychiatric complications of cancer. In M.C. Brain and P.P. Carbone (Eds.), *Current Therapy in Hematology Oncology-3.* Toronto: B.C. Decker, Inc.

Burnell, G.M. and T.A. Foster (1972). Psychosis with low sodium syndrome. *Am. J. Psychiatry* 128:133–34.

Carey, R.W., T.G. Pretlow, E.Z. Ezdinli, and J.F. Holland (1966). Studies on the mechanism of hypoglycemia in a patient with massive intraperitoneal leiomyosarcoma. *Am. J. Med.* 40:458.

Carroll, B.J. (1977). Psychiatric disorders and steroids. In E.

Usdin, D.A. Hamburg, and J.D. Barchas (Eds.). *Neuroregulators and Psychiatric Disorders*. New York: Oxford University Press.

Cavagnini, F., C. Invitti, and E.E. Polli (1984). Sodium valproate in Cushing's disease. *Lancet* 2:162–63.

Corn, T.H. and S.A. Checkley (1983). A case of recurrent mania with recurrent hyperthyroidism. *Br. J. Psychiatry* 143:74–76.

Cohen, L.M. and M.E. Moltich (1984). Psychiatric aspects of pituitary tumors. In T.C. Manschrech and O.B. Murray (eds.), *Medicine Update: Massachusetts General Hospital Review for Physicians*. New York: Elsevier.

Cohen, S.I. (1980). Cushing's syndrome in psychiatric study of 29 patients. *Br. J. Psychiatry* 136:120–24.

Denko, J.D. and R. Kaebbing (1960). The psychiatric aspects of hypoparathyroidism. *Acta Psychiatr. Scand.* 38:1–70.

DeQuattro, V. and V.M. Compese (1979). Pheochromocytoma: Diagnosis and therapy. In L.T. DeGroot (ed.), *Endocrinology, Vol. 2*. New York: Grune & Stratton.

Eberle, F. and R. Grun (1981). Multiple endocrine neoplasia, type I (MEN I). *Ergeb. Inn. Med. Kinderheilkd.* 46:75–150.

Falk, W.E., M.W. Mahnke, and D.C. Poskanzer (1979). Lithium prophylaxis of corticotropin-induced psychosis. *J.A.M.A.* 241:1011–12.

Fink, M. (1980). Neuroendocrinology and ECT: A review of recent developments. *Compr. Psychiatry* 21:450–59.

Fishman, L.M., G.W. Liddle, D.P. Island, N. Fleisher, and O. Kuchel (1967). Effects of aminoglutethimide on adrenal function in man. *J. Clin. Endocrinol. Metab.* 27:481–90.

Fuks, Z., E. Glatstein, G.W. Marsa, M.A. Bagshaw, and H.J. Kaplan (1976). Long-term effects of external radiation on the pituitary and thyroid glands. *Cancer* 37:1152–61.

Garrick, M.B. and P.R. Larsen (1979). Acute deficiency of thyroxine-binding globulin during L-asparaginase therapy. *N. Engl. J. Med.* 301:252–53.

Gilbey, E.D., L.H. Rees, and P.K. Bondy (1975). Biology and characterization of human tumors. In M. Davisco and C. Malroni (eds.), *Advances in Tumor Prevention, Detection and Characterization, Vol. 3. Proc. Sixth Int. Symp.* New York: Elsevier.

Goggans, F.C., L.J. Weisberg, and L.M. Koran (1983). Lithium prophylaxis of prednisone psychosis: A case report. *J. Clin. Psychiatry* 44:111–12.

Gorden, P., C.M. Hendricks, C.R. Kahn, K. Megyesi, and J. Roth (1981). Hypoglycemia associated with non-islet cell tumor and insulin-like growth factors. *N. Engl. J. Med.* 305:1452–55.

Hall, R.C.W., M.K. Popkin, S.K. Stickney, and E.R. Gardner (1979). Presentation of the steroid psychoses. *J. Nerv. Ment. Dis.* 167:229–36.

Haskett, R.F. (1985). Diagnostic categorization of psychiatric disturbance in Cushing's syndrome. *Am. J. Psychiatry* 142:911–16.

Haskett, R.F. and R.M. Rose (1981). Neuroendocrine disorders and psychopathology. *Psychiatr. Clin. North Am.* 4:239–52.

Henkin, R.I. (1970). The neuroendocrine control of perception. In D. Hamburg (ed.), *Perception and Its Disorders*. Baltimore: Williams and Wilkins.

Jacobs, J.W., E. Simpson, S. D'Souza, K. Ibbotson, and G.R. Mundy (1983). Identification of transforming growth factors associated with the humoral hypercalcemia of malignancy. *Clin. Res.* 31:502A.

Junod, A., A.E. Lambert, L. Orci, R. Pictet, A.E. Bonet, and A.E. Renold (1967). Studies of the diabetogenic action of streptozotocin. *Proc. Soc. Exp. Biol. Med.* 126:201–5.

Karpati, G. and B. Frame (1964). Neuropsychiatric disorders in primary hyperparathyroidism. *Arch. Neurol.* 10:387–97.

Kato, Y., T.B. Ferguson, D.E. Bennett, and T.H. Burfor (1969). Oat cell carcinoma of the lung. A review of 38 cases. *Cancer* 23:517–24.

Kaufman, M.W., G.B. Murray, and N.H. Cassem (1982). Use of psychostimulants in medically ill depressed patients. *Psychosomatics* 23:817–19.

Lawson, I.R. and R.D.M. MacLeod (1969). The use of imipramine and other psychotropic drugs in organic emotionalism. *Br. J. Psychiatry* 115:281–85.

Lewis, D.A. and R.E. Smith (1983). Steroid-induced psychiatric syndromes: A report of 14 cases and a review of the literature. *J. Affect. Dis.* 5:319–32.

Ling, M.H.M., P.J. Perry, and M.T. Tsung (1981). Side effects of corticosteroid therapy. *Arch. Gen. Psychiatry* 38:471–77.

Major, L.F., G.L. Brown, and W.P. Wilson (1973). Carcinoid and psychiatric symptoms. *South. Med. J.* 66:787–89.

Megyesi, K., C.R. Kahn, J. Roth, and P. Gorden (1975). Circulating NSILA's in man: Basal and stimulated levels and binding to plasma components. *Clin. Res.* 23:388A.

Morgan, H.G., J. Boulnois, and C. Burns-Cox (1973). Addiction to prednisone. *Br. J. Med. Psychol.* 2:93.

Mundy, G.R. and T.J. Martin (1982). Hypercalcemia of malignancy: Pathogenesis and management. *Metabolism* 31:1247–77.

Mundy, G.R., K.J. Ibbotson, S.M. D'Souza, E.L. Simpson, J.W. Jacobs, and J.T. Martin (1984). The hypercalcemia of cancer: Clinical implications and pathogenic mechanism. *N. Engl. J. Med.* 310:1718–27.

Murken, R.E. and A.J. Duvan (1972). Hypothyroidism following combined therapy in carcinoma of the laryngopharynx. *Laryngoscope* 82:1306–14.

Odell, W.D. (1980). Humoral manifestations of cancer. In R.H. Williams (ed.), *Textbook of Endocrinology*, 6th ed. Philadelphia: W.B. Saunders.

Oettgen, R.F., P.A. Stephenson, M.K. Schwartz, R.D. Leeper, G. Tallal, C.C. Tan, B.D. Clarkson, R.B. Golbey, I.H. Krakoff, D.A. Karnofsky, M.L. Murphy, and J.H. Burchenal (1970). Toxicity of *E. coli* L-asparaginase in man. *Cancer* 25:253–78.

Patchell, R.A. and J.B. Posner (1986). Neurologic complications of carcinoid. *Neurology* 36:745–49.

Pearse, A.G.E. and J.M. Polak (1978). The diffuse neuroendocrine system and the APUD concept. In S.R. Bloom (ed.), *Gut Hormones*. Edinburgh: Churchill-Livingstone.

Pepper, G.M. and D.T. Krieger (1984). Hypothalamic-pituitary-adrenal abnormalities in depression: Their possible relation to central mechanisms regulating ACTH release. In R. Post and J. Ballenger (eds.), *Neurology of Mood Disorders.* Baltimore: Williams & Wilkins.

Sachs, W. (1973). Disorders of glucose metabolism in brain dysfunction. In G.E. Guall (ed.), *Biology of Brain Dysfunction.* New York: Plenum, p. 143.

Sandifer, M.G. (1983). Hyponatremia due to psychotropic drugs. *J. Clin. Psychiatry* 44:301–3.

Schiffer, R.B, J. Cash, and R.M. Herndon (1983). Treatment of emotional lability with low-dosage tricyclic antidepressants. *Psychosomatics* 24:1094–96.

Schildkraut, J.J. (1978). Current status of catecholamine hypothesis of affective disorders. In M.A. Lipton, A. DiMascio, and K.F. Killiam (eds.), *Psychopharmacology: A Generation of Progress.* New York: Raven Press, pp. 1223–34.

Schwartz, K.E., A.R. Wolfsen, B. Forste, and W.D. Odell (1979). Calcitonin in non-thyroidal cancer. *J. Clin. Endocrinol. Metab.* 49:438–44.

Schwartz, W.B., W. Bennett, S. Curelops, and F.C. Bartter 1957). A syndrome of renal sodium loss and hyponatremia probably resulting from inappropriate secretion of antidiuretic hormone. *Am. J. Med.* 23:529–43.

Shah, J., B. Stevens, B. Sorensen, C. Hurks, G. Edwards, and R. Kaplan (1979). Dissociated effect of vincristine on insulin release and Beta cell micro-tubular content in the intact rat. *Diabetes* 28:372A.

Shames, J.M., N.R. Dhurandha, and W.G. Blackard (1968). Insulin-secreting bronchial carcinoid tumor with widespread metastasis. *Am. J. Med.* 44:632.

Sipple, J.H. (1961). The association of pheochromocytoma with carcinoma of the thyroid. *Am. J. Med.* 31:163–66.

Smith, K.C., J. Barish, J. Corren, and R.H. Williams (1972). Psychiatric disturbance in endocrinologic disease. *Psychosom. Med.* 34:69–86.

Soffer, L.J., A. Iannaccone, and J.L. Gabrilove (1961). Cushing's syndrome. *Am. J. Med.* 39:129–46.

Starkman, M.N., D.E. Schteingart, and M.A. Schork (1981). Depressed mood and other psychiatric manifestations of Cushing's syndrome: Relationship to hormone levels. *Psychosom. Med.* 43:3–18.

Stewart, A.F., R. Horst, L.J. Deftos, E.C. Cadman, R. Lang, and A.B. Broadus (1980). Biochemical evaluation of patients with cancer-associated hypercalcemia: Evidence for humoral and non-humoral groups. *N. Engl. J. Med.* 303:1377–83.

Sternbach, H.A., M.S. Gold, A.C. Pottash, and I. Extein (1983). Thyroid failure and protirelin (thyrotropin-releasing hormone) test abnormalities in depressed outpatients. *J.A.M.A.* 249:618–20.

Taylor, J.W. (1973). Depression in thyrotoxicosis. *Am. J. Psychiatry* 132:552–53.

Touks, C.M. (1974). Mental illness in hypothyroid patients. *Br. J. Psychiatry* 110:706–10.

Trivedi, S. (1984). Psychiatric symptoms in carcinoid syndrome. *J. Indian Med. Assoc.* 82:292–94.

Upton, G.V. and T.T. Amatruda, Jr. (1971). Evidence for the presence of tumor peptides with corticotropin-releasing-factor-like activity in the ectopic ACTH syndrome. *N. Engl. J. Med.* 285:419–24.

Varney, N.R., B. Alexander, and J.H. MacIndoc (1984). Reversible steroid dementia in patients without steroid psychosis. *Am. J. Psychiatry* 141:369–72.

Whelan, T.B., D.E. Schteingart, and M.N. Starkman (1980). Neuropsychological deficits in Cushing's syndrome. *J. Nerv. Ment. Dis.* 168:753–57.

Whitecar, J.P., Jr., G.P. Bodey, C.S. Hill, Jr., and N.A. Samaan (1970). Effect of L-asparaginase on carbohydrate metabolism. *Metabolism* 19:581–86.

Whybrow, P. and R. Ferrell (1974). Thyroid state and human behavior: Contributions from a clinical perspective. In A.J. Prange, Jr. (ed.), *The Thyroid Axis, Drugs and Behavior.* New York: Raven Press, p. 5.

Whybrow, P.C. and T. Hurwitz (1976). Psychological disturbance associated with endocrine disease and hormone therapy. In E.J. Sachar (ed.), *Hormones, Behavior and Psychopathology.* New York: Raven Press, p. 125.

Wolkowitz, O.M., D.R. Rubinow, A. Breier, A.R. Doran, and D. Packar (1986). Steroid effects in normals: A prospective study (Abstract). *Consult.–Liaison Symp.–A.P.A.,* May 13.

# PART VI

# Special Issues in the Psychological Management of Cancer

# 32

# Management of Cancer Pain

Russell K. Portenoy and Kathleen M. Foley

## SCOPE OF THE PROBLEM

A sense of dread experienced by many patients when the diagnosis of cancer is first made is intertwined with an anticipatory fear of pain. Unfortunately, this concern that the progression of the disease will be punctuated by episodes of pain is all too often the reality. A review of the available data suggests that in patients with far-advanced cancer of all types, 70% have significant pain at some time in the course of their illness (Foley and Sundaresan, 1985). Some authors have indicated that approximately 25% of cancer patients die without adequate pain relief (Twycross and Lack, 1983). With cancer accounting for approximately 10% of the 50 million deaths worldwide each year (WHO, 1979), it is clear that the management of pain in the cancer population is an enormous challenge.

Significant pain occurs in approximately 33% of the adult and pediatric patients receiving active therapy, varying with tumor site and extent of disease (Foley, 1979a). A breakdown by diagnosis reveals significant pain in only 5% of patients with leukemia, in 50–75% of those who have cancer of the lung, colon, gastrointestinal tract, and genitourinary tract, and finally, up to 85% of patients who have bone or cervical cancer.

The true scope of the problem, however, is not reflected in prevalence data. For the individual patient, pain is enervating and demoralizing; it produces profound affective and behavioral changes that augment the suffering of the patient and his or her family, particularly in the setting of a terminal illness. Cancer patients who have pain have greater psychological disturbance than those without pain, resembling more the patient with nonmalignant pain than those with cancer and no pain (Sternbach, 1974). Higher levels of depression and hypochondriasis are found repeatedly (Bond, 1979; Bukberg et al., 1984). Friends, family, and physicians often draw away, unable to deal with the patient's seemingly insoluble complaints. These realities emphasize the need to provide early and adequate pain management to the cancer patient at all stages of therapy.

The goals of therapy will vary. For the patient with pain in the early stages of disease, adequate pain therapy should allow the patient to function as normally as possible. For the terminally ill patient, comfort more than functional status is often the goal. In all cases effective pain control is imperative. To achieve this it is necessary to have an understanding of the nature of pain and the application of the available medical approaches to pain management.

## THE NATURE OF PAIN

### Subjective Experience

Pain is an intensely personal experience, a subjective response communicated by words and actions. The two major aspects are the sensation of a noxious stimulus, termed nociception, and the affective response, which together yield the perception of pain.

One widely accepted definition of pain attempts to clarify these components of the pain experience and has been accepted by the International Association for the Study of Pain (IASP). Pain is "an unpleasant sensory and emotional experience associated with actual or potential tissue damage, or described in terms of such damage" (IASP, 1980). Although this definition implies that a nociceptive stimulus need not be present for pain to occur, clinical experience suggests that the pain complaint of the cancer patient must be considered to have a contributing organic lesion until one is convincingly ruled out. Purely psychogenic pain is rare in this group of patients.

The perception of pain thus encompasses a broader scope than nociception alone and has been divided into three hierarchical elements (Melzack and Dennis, 1978). The sensory-discriminative aspect involves nociception and is related to the ability of the known pain pathways to transmit spatial and temporal information about a noxious stimulus. The affective-motivational component has a substrate of dense interconnections between the limbic system and pain-modulating systems in the brain. This element of the pain experience is in part stereotyped, in that acute pain generates anxiety, while chronic pain is often associated with depression. Finally, there is a cognitive-evaluative component to the pain experience, clinically apparent by the changes in pain that can occur when its meaning is altered. For example, in a study of women with metastatic breast cancer, the level of pain was predicted by the degree of mood disturbance and beliefs about the meaning of the pain in relation to the illness, but not by the site of metastasis (Spiegel and Bloom, 1983a,b). A second example is provided by Beecher (1959), who noted that soldiers wounded in battle complained of little or no pain while on the battlefield but escalated their pain complaints in the setting of a medical care facility. Thus, it is not simply the nociceptive stimulus alone, but also the patient's prior experience with pain, the setting within which it occurs, and the significance attributed to it, that influence how it is perceived.

Recognition of the role of contextual information in nociception raises an additional aspect of the pain experience, that of suffering. The patient's suffering reflects a general response to all perceptions, only one of which is pain. This implies that the approach to suffering extends beyond the relief of pain, and conversely, that the treatment of pain will not in all patients relieve suffering. A study by Stam et al. (1984) of cancer patients whose pain was successfully treated with radiotherapy confirms this distinction. Although pain diminished significantly, psychometric testing revealed no reduction in various measures of psychological distress. Thus, the optimal approach to the patient in pain includes an evaluation of those influences producing nociception, augmenting pain perceptions, and perpetuating suffering. In the patient with a terminal illness, these contributing influences may become blurred both to the patient and the physician.

The definition of pain requires further clarification on a temporal basis. Pain may be acute or chronic. The onset of acute pain is usually well defined. It is associated with the affect of anxiety and signs of sympathetic nervous system hyperactivity. As the pain persists, these concomitants are replaced by the affect of depression and vegetative signs, such as sleep disturbance, poor appetite, lassitude, poor concentration, and diminished libido. Acute pain is usually self-limited and responds to a wide variety of approaches, including resolution of the organic cause or control with analgesics. In contrast, chronic pain, which is often defined as pain lasting longer than 6 months, commonly leads to a decrease in functional status, personality changes, and disruption of work and social behavior. As correlates of these clinical differences, there is growing evidence that the physiological mechanisms of acute and chronic pain transmission and modulation also differ.

## Neural Mechanisms

The classification of pain patients and common pain syndromes derives in part from an understanding of the neural mechanisms of pain. Recent advances in pain research have led to a clearer understanding of both the neuroanatomical and neuropharmacological components of pain (Payne, 1987).

Information about noxious stimuli is transmitted from the periphery to the highest levels of the nervous system. Nociceptors are primary afferent neurons that respond selectively to noxious events. The cell bodies of these neurons are located in the dorsal root ganglia, and their peripheral extensions comprise either thinly myelinated A-delta or unmyelinated C fibers. The larger fibers conduct more rapidly and transmit spatial and temporal information about the stimulus, whereas the smaller fibers mediate the more prolonged, unpleasant sensations that persist after injury and are known as "second" pain.

With tissue damage, nociceptors undergo changes that are collectively known as sensitization. This is defined by a decrease in threshold and enhancement of the response to stimuli; it is probably due to both peripheral and central changes in neural function. Where a peripheral lesion is present, the process involves the local release of the products of inflammation, such as the prostaglandins (PG) and other substances whose origin is the nerve terminal itself. Interruption of these peripheral processes by inhibition of PG synthetase may be responsible for the analgesic effects of both the nonsteroidal antiinflammatory drugs and the corticosteroids.

Most primary nociceptive afferents terminate ipsilaterally within one or two segments of their entrance into the dorsal horn of the spinal cord. The dorsal horn represents a processing area where information about the noxious stimulus can be enhanced or suppressed. This was modeled in the gate control theory of Melzack and Wall (1965), which hypothesized a dynamic interaction of segmental and supraspinal pain-modulating systems ultimately influencing the transmission of nociceptive information through the dorsal horn. This interaction is enormously complex. On a segmental level, there is good evidence that substance P is involved as a neurotransmitter for the primary afferent. Adenosine triphosphate (ATP), glutamate, somatostatin, cholecystokinin, and vasoactive intestinal peptide (VIP) have been suggested for this role as well. Inhibitory interneurons, which act presynaptically or postsynaptically on the primary afferent, most likely contain either enkephalin (an opiate peptide) or γ-aminobutyric acid (GABA). Multiple descending pathways, which originate in the brain stem and use as neurotransmitters serotonin and norepinephrine, among other compounds, also synapse in this region and modulate the rostral transmission of nociceptive information.

Multiple pathways in the spinal cord carry nociceptive information to the reticular formation, thalamus, and cortex. A lateral, direct fiber bundle to the ventrobasal region of the thalamus (known as the neospinothalamic tract) is probably involved in the discriminative aspects of pain. Several medial pathways (the paleospinothalamic tracts) project to the medial thalamus, with some relaying through the brain stem, and are involved in the associated autonomic and affective components of pain. Finally, direct bidirectional connections between the thalamus and the cerebral cortex have been identified. These may provide the substrate for the cognitive-evaluative component of the pain experience described previously.

Perhaps the most important advances in pain research have involved the elucidation of endogenous pain-modulating systems. Multiple pain-modulating systems have now been identified (Mayer and Watkins, 1984). These systems operate at both segmental and supraspinal levels and have great pharmacological and anatomical complexity.

The discovery that either electrical stimulation or microinjection of morphine into select brainstem regions causes analgesia in animals was the initial step in unraveling the physiology of the descending supraspinal pain-modulating systems. The periaqueductal gray, a region of the midbrain rich in opioid peptides and receptors, plays a crucial role in these phenomena. This region has direct connections with the rostroventral medulla, which contains groups of neurons whose activation also produces analgesia (Basbaum and Fields, 1984). The dorsolateral funiculus of the spinal cord carries these medullary projections down to the dorsal horn. One of these projections is serotoninergic, whose activation, most likely through an enkephalinergic intermediary, inhibits pain transmission. This finding has led to the widespread use of medications that alter monoamines, particularly those that increase levels of serotonin, as analgesics.

Present at every level of the nervous system are the endorphins, a group of peptides that are clearly important in endogenous analgesia. They are involved both in the function of the descending system that originates in the periaqueductal gray, and the local processing that occurs at the level of the dorsal horn. Not surprisingly, studies with morphine have demonstrated that maximal analgesia occurs with activation of both the descending and segmental opioid systems.

Numerous endorphins have been identified thus far, including β-endorphin, the enkephalins, and the dynorphins. Their distribution throughout and outside the nervous system, their affinity for the opioid receptors, and the role they play in analgesia all vary widely. Adding to this complexity is the existence of multiple opiate receptors. Recent studies have demonstrated that certain receptors mediate the analgesic effects of opioids, while others are responsible for different actions, such as respiratory depression (Pasternak, 1981). Receptor-selective opioids are currently being evaluated in clinical trials to determine if analgesia can be obtained with fewer adverse effects. The finding of opioid receptors in the spinal cord provided the impetus for the development of intermittent and continuous epidural and intrathecal administration of opioids. Further investigation of these systems will undoubtedly add to their clinical import.

Other pain-modulating systems do not require endorphinergic mechanisms, and the analgesia produced is not reversed by naloxone, a specific opioid antagonist. For example, analgesia provided by stimulation of peripheral nerves, such as transcutaneous nerve stimulation or acupuncture, may or may not be altered by naloxone, depending on the parameters of stimulation. Similarly, stress analgesia functions through two independent mechanisms, one opioid and one nonopioid (Mayer and Watkins, 1984). Biofeedback, hypnosis, relaxation techniques, and cognitive-behavioral techniques appear to function through activation of nonopioid systems, although the specific anatomical basis for these approaches is not clearly understood.

In the cancer patient with pain, the putative mechanisms underlying pain can usually be determined from the patient's symptoms and signs. The most common mechanism involves tumor infiltration of bone or soft tissue, leading to activation and sensitization of peripheral nociceptors, or nociceptive pain. Other pains appear to depend on central changes in neuronal function. This follows peripheral nerve injury (e.g., tumor infiltration of the brachial plexus) (Kanner et al., 1982) and produces a pain syndrome characterized by dysesthetic burning and lancinating pain. These are referred to as deafferentation pains (Tasker, 1984) and are a significant problem in cancer patients with tumor infiltration of nerve plexus or in patients with postsurgical pain syndromes secondary to nerve injury.

## TYPES OF CANCER PATIENTS WITH PAIN

Pain patients may be classified by the chronology, etiology, and clinical setting of their pain complaint (Bonica, 1982; Foley, 1979a). In addition, five types of cancer pain patients have been described (Foley,

1984), incorporating an understanding of the psychological needs of the patient with characteristics of the pain complaint:

## Patients With Acute Cancer-Related Pain

These patients can be divided into those with pain caused by cancer and those with pain due to anticancer therapy. In the former group, the pain may be the first symptom of cancer or the first sign of recurrent disease. Defining the cause of the pain may present a diagnostic problem, but effective treatment of the cause (e.g., radiation therapy to bone metastases) is usually possible and effective, with dramatic pain relief in the majority of patients. In patients with acute cancer-related pain associated with cancer therapy (e.g., postoperative pain or pain secondary to the acute effects of chemotherapy, such as oral ulceration), the cause of pain is readily identified and its course predictable and self-limited. This group of patients endures significant pain for the promise of successful treatment of their cancer.

## Patients With Chronic Cancer-Related Pain

The progression of acute pain to chronic pain can be a subtle and ill-defined process. In nonmalignant pain syndromes, an arbitrary duration, usually 6 months, is applied for diagnostic purposes (Sternbach, 1974). In those with cancer, this group can be subdivided into patients with chronic pain from tumor progression and those with chronic pain related to cancer treatment. In patients with chronic pain associated with the progression of disease, the pain escalates in intensity, and pharmacological, anesthetic, neurosurgical, and psychological interventions are all employed with varying success. Psychological influences play a significant role in the experience of pain for this group of patients, in whom palliative therapy may be of little value and is physically debilitating. The pain is often one aspect of the patient's suffering, to which isolation, loss of function, and fear of death contribute. Those caring for this group of patients must be concerned with all aspects of distress and discomfort if the perception of physical pain is to be alleviated. The chronicity of the pain is associated with disturbances in sleep, reduction in appetite, impaired concentration, and irritability; these signs and symptoms may mimic a depressive disorder.

In contrast, patients with chronic pain due to cancer therapy experience persistent discomfort that, while not associated with progression of disease or impending death, is often difficult to treat because of the lack of available methods to remove the cause (e.g., a traumatic neuroma). This group closely parallels those patients in the general population with intractable non-

malignant pain. The recognition that cancer is not the cause of the pain markedly alters the patient's therapy, prognosis, and psychological state. All approaches to maintain the functional status of the patient should be employed. Alternative methods to therapy, rather than drug therapy alone, represent a major management approach.

## Patients With Preexisting Chronic Pain and Cancer-Related Pain

Patients with chronic nonmalignant pain have a high incidence of psychological disturbance (Sternbach, 1974), often compounded by numerous failed attempts at treatment in the past. With the diagnosis of cancer and the onset of cancer pain, these patients are at high risk to develop further functional incapacity and escalating chronic pain symptoms. Nonetheless, the past history of chronic pain should not be used in a punitive way to minimize present complaints. Rather, it should serve to identify this group of high-risk patients and emphasize the need to employ early psychological intervention in the management of their pain.

## Patients With Preexisting Substance Abuse and Cancer-Related Pain

Patients with a history of substance abuse may pose special difficulties in cancer pain management. On a physiological level, the chronic use of opioids will produce physical dependence and tolerance. The former predisposes the patient to an abstinence syndrome should the drugs be abruptly withdrawn in the hospital, and the latter may necessitate very high doses of analgesics in order to achieve effective pain management. Patients on methadone maintenance, for example, may be significantly undertreated if their tolerance to analgesics is not taken into account in prescribing opioid analgesics. Patients with a history of opioid abuse also appear to be more likely to escalate their dose of analgesics than those without this history. This may represent a more rapid development of tolerance, but may also result from purely psychological influences.

Adequate assessment of the pain complaint in these patients is colored by the confusion between pain symptoms and drug-seeking behavior. Attention to their medical and psychological needs requires individualization of therapy and consultation with health care professionals who are expert in drug-related problems. Experience suggests that patients with a past history of substance abuse and those on methadone maintenance can usually be readily managed, recognizing that the psychological stresses consequent to their pain and cancer may place them at higher risk for recidivism. In contrast, patients who are actively abusing drugs represent a major management problem, one that strains the most tolerant of medical care systems. Manipulative behavior can at times be handled through a pain medication contract, which presupposes that communication, unified purpose, willingness to define boundaries, and availability for reassessment on the part of the health care providers exists. One physician should be identified to provide analgesic therapy, and open communication between the patient and the physician should be encouraged.

## Dying Patients With Pain

For this group of patients, all efforts are directed toward the maintenance of comfort. Pain treatment should provide sufficient relief to allow the patient to function at the level they choose and to die relatively free of pain. The issues of hopelessness, death, and dying become prominent, and the suffering component must be addressed. Inadequate control of pain exacerbates suffering and demoralizes both the family and the caregivers, who feel that they have failed in treating the patient's pain at a time when adequate treatment may have mattered most. Rapid escalation of analgesic drug therapy, if needed, and sensitivity to the concerns and fears of the individual patient and his or her family are crucial at this time. Greater willingness on the part of both the patient and physician to tolerate the side effects of medication, such as sedation, confusion, or respiratory depression may be apparent as symptomatic relief becomes the overriding priority.

## PAIN SYNDROMES

An alternative method of classification is based on the etiology of the pain (Bonica, 1982; Foley, 1979a; Twycross and Fairfield, 1982). A number of well-defined pain syndromes have been identified (Table 32-1). Most are due to direct tumor involvement; this accounted for 78% of inpatient and 62% of outpatient pain complaints in separate surveys of these populations (Foley, 1979a; Kanner and Foley, 1981). Tumor invasion of bone, compression or infiltration of nerves, and obstruction of hollow viscus are the most common causes; tumor infiltration or occlusion of blood vessels, stretching of fascia or periosteum, and damage to mucous membranes or other soft tissues occur less commonly.

Cancer therapy was the cause of pain in 19% of inpatients and 25% of outpatients surveyed in the aforementioned studies. Surgery, chemotherapy, and radiation therapy can each have painful sequelae, and a large number of specific syndromes have been described (Foley, 1979a).

Finally, less than 10% of cancer pain patients have

**Table 32-1** Specific pain syndromes in patients with cancer

| Pain syndromes | Examples |
|---|---|
| Associated with direct tumor infiltration | Tumor infiltration of bone |
| | Base of skull syndromes |
| |   Jugular foramen metastases |
| |   Clivus metastases |
| |   Sphenoid sinus metastases |
| | Vertebral body syndromes |
| |   C2 Metastases |
| |   C7, T1 Metastases |
| |   L1 Metastases |
| | Sacral syndrome |
| | Tumor infiltration of nerve |
| |   Peripheral nerve |
| |   Peripheral neuropathy |
| | Plexus |
| |   Brachial plexopathy |
| |   Lumbar plexopathy |
| |   Sacral plexopathy |
| | Root |
| |   Leptomeningeal metastases |
| | Spinal cord |
| |   Epidural spinal cord compression |
| Associated with cancer therapy | Postsurgery syndromes |
| |   Postthoracotomy syndrome |
| |   Postmastectomy syndrome |
| |   Postradical neck syndrome |
| |   Phantom limb syndrome |
| | Postchemotherapy syndromes |
| |   Peripheral neuropathy |
| |   Aseptic necrosis of femoral head |
| |   Steroid pseudorheumatism |
| |   Postherpetic neuralgia |
| | Postradiation syndromes |
| |   Radiation fibrosis of brachial and lumbar plexus |
| |   Radiation myelopathy |
| |   Radiation-induced second primary tumors |
| |   Radiation necrosis of bone |
| Not associated with cancer or cancer therapy | Cervical and lumbar osteoarthritis |
| | Thoracic and abdominal aneurysms |
| | Diabetic neuropathy |

*Source*: From Foley (1979a).

pain that is unrelated to the disease or its therapy. This group included patients with arthritis, osteoporosis, and painful diabetic neuropathy.

A survey of patients with far-advanced disease (Twycross and Fairfield, 1982) found that 80% complained of more than one pain and 34% had four or more. Of 303 pains reported by 100 patients, 67% were caused by the cancer, 5% were directly related to therapy, and 28% were unrelated to either. In this last group, 6% were considered to be associated pains, such as constipation, while 15% were musculoskeletal and 7% were due to other diseases. Thus, the typical cancer pain patient does not develop one of the cancer pain syndromes in isolation. Recognition of these syndromes is a prerequisite to accurate diagnosis, and treatment often involves the evaluation and management of the multiple, separate pains.

## ASSESSMENT OF THE CANCER PATIENT WITH PAIN

The general principles involved in the assessment of patients with pain and cancer have been previously described (Foley, 1979b, 1984). These principles include the following:

1. Believe the patient's complaint.
2. Take a detailed history.
3. Assess the psychosocial status of the patient.
4. Perform a careful medical and neurological examination.
5. Order and personally review the appropriate diagnostic procedures.
6. Evaluate the patient's extent of disease.
7. Treat the pain to facilitate the diagnostic workup.
8. Consider alternative methods of pain control during the initial evaluation.
9. Reassess the pain complaint during the prescribed therapy.

A detailed history is the most important step in the assessment of the cancer patient with pain. This must include description of the location, quality, exacerbating and relieving influences, and timing of the pain. Functional disability should be evaluated, including interference with self-care, work, family life, sexual relationships, and recreation. The patient should be specifically questioned about the past and present use of prescription and nonprescription drugs, including alcohol. The psychological status of the patient should be queried; confirmation may need to come from the family. In particular, anhedonia and the presence of vegetative signs should be sought. Finally, in light of the evidence of cultural (Sternbach and Tursky, 1965) and religious (Lambert et al., 1960) differences in experimental pain perception and the benefit some patients derive if these affiliations are nurtured during the course of the disease, these influences should be noted as well.

The medical and neurological examinations require knowledge of pain referral patterns (Kellgren, 1939) and the common pain syndromes experienced by cancer patients. Diagnostic studies confirm clinical suspicions and assess the extent of disease. Pain should be treated early and aggressively during the initial evaluation in order to allow these tests to be done with a minimum of discomfort. Continuity of care with frequent reassessment is crucial after therapy begins, both encouraging an open and trusting relationship with the health care provider and permitting a continual evaluation of the treatment efficacy and the progression of the disease. Recurrence of pain in the cancer patient should initiate a process of assessment very similar to the original evaluation; some change in organic pathology, such as recurrence or new metastasis, should be presumed and explored. This posture will minimize such mistakes as attributing increased pain to drug tolerance while missing an unexpected new lesion.

## TREATMENT OF CANCER PAIN

The first step in the management of cancer pain is the identification of the underlying cause, followed by primary therapy directed at this lesion if appropriate and feasible. Surgery, chemotherapy, and radiation therapy treat the primary tumor and may lead to pain relief (Pannuti et al., 1979; Sundaresan and DiGiacinto, 1987). Radiotherapy is most reliable and is often used solely for the treatment of pain in cases of disseminated disease. A report by Stam and co-workers (1984) found that radiotherapy for bony metastases gave complete pain relief in 52% and partial relief in 37% of patients.

A detailed discussion of the oncological approaches for cancer pain is beyond the scope of this chapter. However, every physician caring for the patient with cancer and pain should know how to use analgesic drugs effectively and should be familiar with the other available therapeutic approaches to cancer pain management.

### Pharmacological Approaches

Drug therapy is the mainstay approach in the management of cancer pain. Analgesic drugs can be broadly divided into three groups: the nonnarcotic analgesics (including aspirin, acetaminophen, and the nonsteroidal antiinflammatory drugs or NSAID), the opioid analgesics (including the narcotic agonist and agonist–antagonist drugs), and the adjuvant analgesic drugs. This last category comprises a variety of unrelated compounds that are used to manage symptoms other than pain but that have been found to provide pain relief in certain settings, either alone or in combination with opioids.

### NONNARCOTIC ANALGESICS

The analgesic activity of these drugs is most likely due to inhibition of PG synthetase activity (Beaver, 1965). They appear to act at the site of pain in the periphery, where PG play a role in the activation and sensitization of the primary nociceptors. These drugs are most

**Table 32-2** Nonnarcotic analgesics for mild to moderate pain

| Type of analgesic | Comments |
|---|---|
| Aspirin | Standard for nonnarcotic comparison; use in cancer population limited by hematological and GI side effects |
| Acetaminophen | Less antiinflammatory effect than aspirin and fewer side effects |
| NSAID | Reversibly inhibit production of PG. Most, with the exception of indomethacin and the pyrazole group, have lesser toxicity than aspirin. Failure to respond to one drug warrants trial of another in a different class. |
|   Salicylates | |
|     Choline magnesium trisalicylate | |
|     Salsalate | |
|     Diflunisal | |
|   Propionic acids | |
|     Ibuprofen | |
|     Fenoprofen | |
|     Naproxen | |
|   Acetic acids | |
|     Indomethacin | |
|     Tolmetin | |
|     Sulindac | |
|   Fenamates | |
|     Meclofenamate | |
|     Mefenamic acid | |
|   Oxicams | |
|     Piroxicam | |
|   Pyrazoles | |
|     Phenylbutazone | |
|     Oxyphenylbutazone | |

useful for mild to moderate pain and, when combined with an opioid drug, provide additive analgesia in the treatment of severe pain. They are particularly useful in patients with bone pain, presumably because of the important role PG play in the development of bone metastases. A list of the commonly used drugs in this class is provided in Table 32-2.

## OPIOID ANALGESICS

This class comprises a diverse group of compounds that bind to specific opioid receptors (Table 32-3). They can be divided into several groups. The agonist drugs bind to opioid receptors and produce analgesia. The antagonist drugs, such as naloxone, block the effect of agonists at the receptor. A third group of drugs, referred to as the agonist–antagonists, has both analgesic and antagonist properties. These drugs are seldom used in cancer pain management because dose escalation is often associated with psychotomimetic effects (particularly true of pentazocine), and most (including butorphanol, nalbuphine and buprenorphine) are only available for parenteral use. Buprenorphine, a partial agonist without significant psychotomimetic ef-

fects, also exists as a sublingual preparation (not available in the United States) that may offer special advantages to the cancer patient with pain who is unable to take oral opioids. All agonist–antagonist drugs may produce withdrawal when administered to patients dependent on other opioids (Houde, 1979), which is an additional potential problem in the cancer population.

At the present time the narcotic agonists are the preferred drugs for moderate to severe pain. In contrast to the nonnarcotic analgesics, these medications do not have ceiling effects; increasing the dose will yield added pain relief until intolerable side effects supervene. The clearest indication for chronic administration of these drugs is in the cancer population, in which guidelines for use have been recently reviewed (Foley, 1979b; Inturrisi and Foley, 1984). Important considerations include the following:

1. *Choose a specific drug for a specific type of pain.* For moderate pain, codeine or oxycodone preparations (with aspirin or acetaminophen) are most often used. Moderate to severe pain is usually best managed with a morphine-like agonist drug, such as morphine, hydromorphone, methadone, oxycodone, or levorphanol. The use of meperidine should be discouraged, particularly in chronic administration. An active metabolite, normeperidine, can accumulate with repetitive administrations and can result in such signs of CNS excitability as myoclonus and seizures (Kaiko et al., 1983).

2. *Know the duration of the analgesic effect.* The average duration of effect varies among the different opiates (Table 32-3). In any patient, however, these norms may be influenced by individual differences in drug absorption and disposition. Oral administration generally results in a longer duration of effect, while parenteral administration yields an earlier onset of action and shorter duration.

3. *Know the pharmacokinetics of the drug.* Morphine, hydromorphone, and oxycodone have relatively short half-lives and require administration intervals of 3–4 hours in order to maintain analgesia. Although methadone and levorphanol usually have half-lives of 15–30 hours and 12–16 hours, respectively, administration intervals need to be much shorter, with most patients requiring a dose every 4 hours. This type of regimen must be instituted cautiously, because these drugs will initially accumulate, potentially leading to delayed toxic effects. For this reason, methadone in particular is usually begun on an as-needed basis (Sawe et al., 1981) and should be prescribed with special caution to the elderly and to those with impaired renal or hepatic function.

4. *Know the equianalgesic dose of the drug and its route of administration.* Equianalgesic doses for the various opioids are noted in Table 32-3. Clinical expe-

**Table 32-3**  Oral and parenteral narcotic analgesics for severe pain

| Drug | Route | Equianalgesic dose* | Duration of effect (hr) | Plasma half-life (hr) | Comments |
|---|---|---|---|---|---|
| *Narcotic agonists* | | | | | |
| Morphine | im | 10 | 4–6 | 2–3.5 | Standard for comparison; available in slow- |
| | po | 60 | 4–7 | 2–3.5 | release tablets |
| Codeine | im | 130 | 4–6 | 3 | Biotransformed to morphine; useful as initial nar- |
| | po | ≥200 | 4–6 | 3 | cotic analgesic |
| Oxycodone | im | 15 | — | — | Short acting; available as 5-mg dose in combi- |
| | po | 30 | 3–5 | — | nation with aspirin and acetaminophen |
| Heroin | im | 5 | 4–5 | 0.5 | Illegal in United States; high solubility for pa- |
| | po | (60) | 4–5 | 0.5 | renteral administration |
| Levorphanol | im | 2 | 4–6 | 12–16 | Good oral potency; requires careful titration in |
| (Levodromoran) | po | 4 | 4–7 | 12–16 | initial administration because of drug |
| | | | | | accumulation; more soluble than morphine |
| Hydromorphone | im | 1.5 | 4–6 | 2–3 | Available in high-potency injectable form (10 |
| (Dilaudid) | po | 7.5 | 4–6 | 2–3 | mg/ml) and rectal suppositories for cachectic |
| | | | | | patients |
| Oxymorphone | im | 1 | 4–6 | 2–3 | Available in parenteral and rectal suppository |
| (Numorphan) | pr | 10 | 4–6 | 2–3 | forms only |
| Meperidine | im | 75 | 4–5 | 3–4† | Contraindicated in patients with renal disease; |
| (Demerol) | po | ≥300 | 4–6 | 3–4† | accumulation of active toxic metabolite nor- |
| | | | | | meperidine produces CNS excitation |
| Methadone | im | 10 | | 15–30 | Good oral potency; requires careful titration in |
| (Dolophine) | po | 20 | 4–6 | 15–30 | initial dosing to avoid drug accumulation |
| *Mixed agonist–antagonists* | | | | | |
| Pentazocine | im | 60 | 4–6 | 2–3 | Limited use in cancer pain; psychotomimetic |
| (Talwin) | po | ≥180 | 4–7 | 2–3 | effects with dose escalation; available only in |
| | | | | | combination with naloxone, aspirin or |
| | | | | | acetaminophen; may precipitate withdrawal |
| | | | | | in tolerant patients |
| Nalbuphine | im | 10 | 4–6 | 5 | Not available orally; fewer psychotomimetic |
| (Nubain) | po | — | | 5 | effects than pentazocine; may precipitate |
| | | | | | withdrawal in tolerant patients |
| Butorphanol | im | 2 | 4–6 | 2.5–3.5 | Not available orally; psychotomimetic effects; |
| (Stadol) | po | — | | 2.5–3.5 | may precipitate withdrawal in tolerant pa- |
| | | | | | tients |
| *Partial agonists* | | | | | |
| Buprenorphine | im | 0.4 | 4–6 | ? | Available in United States in parenteral form; |
| (Temgesic) | sl | 0.8 | 5–6 | ? | no psychotomimetic effects; may precipitate |
| | | | | | withdrawal in tolerant patients |

*Based on single-dose studies in which an im dose of each drug listed was compared to morphine to establish relative potency. Oral doses are those recommended when changing from parenteral to oral routes.

†Normeperidine half-life 12–16 hours.

*Source*: From Foley (1985).

rience has suggested that cross-tolerance between these drugs is not complete. For this reason, the equianalgesic dose should be reduced by 1/3–1/2 when switching from one drug to another. Special note should also be made of the differences in oral to parenteral administration of the various opioids. For example, a parenteral dose of levorphanol is twice as potent as an oral dose, while parenteral hydromorphone provides five times the analgesia of an oral dose.

5. *Administer the analgesic regularly.* Opioid medications should be administered to the cancer patient on a fixed around-the-clock basis, including nocturnal doses, following the initial titration phase. It is generally more effective to prevent the exacerbation of pain than to treat it when it occurs. Opioids with long half-life started on an as-needed basis should be given at fixed intervals after the analgesic regimen has been tailored to the needs of the patient.

6. *Use a combination of drugs.* Additive analgesia has been demonstrated from the combination of an opioid and a nonnarcotic analgesic (Beaver, 1965), the antihistamine hydroxyzine (Beaver and Feise, 1976), and the stimulants methylphenidate and dextroamphetamine (Bruera et al., 1987; Forrest et al., 1977). Studies comparing the analgesic efficacy of an opioid plus either a benzodiazepine or a phenothiazine revealed increased sedation without additional analgesia (Houde and Wallenstein, 1955).

7. *Gear the route of administration to the patient's needs* (Portenoy, 1987). The oral route is preferred for the chronic administration of analgesic drug to the cancer patient. Rectal administration and repetitive parenteral bolus injections are alternatives if this is not possible. An innovation in repetitive parenteral administration is patient-controlled analgesia, in which the frequency of intravenous injections is controlled by the patient. Results are promising in studies of the postoperative period; trials with cancer patients have recently begun. Refinements in the use of continuous opioid infusions have also occurred, including acceptance of continuous subcutaneous infusion (Campbell et al., 1983).

The discovery of opioid receptors in the dorsal horn of the spinal cord has led to trials of opioids administered directly into the epidural or intrathecal spaces. Repetitive bolus injections and continuous infusions via an implanted pump have been used in the cancer population. Results have generally been favorable, with pain relief attained with relatively low doses of morphine.

8. *Treat side effects appropriately.* The use of a particular opioid is most often limited by the side effects it produces in the individual patient. Once an opioid is selected, its dose should be increased until either analgesia occurs or intolerable side effects preclude its use. Anticipation and treatment of side effects often permit higher, and thereby more effective, doses to be employed. Sedation is a frequent problem, for which a low dose of dextroamphetamine or methylphenidate one or two times daily can be beneficial, as can a change to a different opioid. Nausea and vomiting should be prevented with antiemetics. The common problem of constipation requires aggressive treatment, most often with a combination of a senna derivative and stool softener; administration of these drugs should be initiated concurrently with chronic administration of the narcotic analgesia. The more serious side effect of respiratory depression is fortunately rare if initial doses in the opioid-naive patient are low and if relative potencies are considered when switching drugs or routes of administration. It is axiomatic that respiratory depression occurring in the setting of chronic opioid use indicates the onset of additional pathology, usually cardiac or pulmonary. Finally, signs of CNS irritability, including myoclonus, tremulousness, and seizures, can occur with high doses of opioids. This has been best described with meperidine (Kaiko et al., 1983), where it is most common in patients with impaired renal function.

9. *Watch for the development of tolerance.* Tolerance is defined by diminishing effects with prolonged drug administration. Although the need for escalating doses during chronic administration of opioids relates in part to this phenomenon, the progression of disease and/or psychological influences may also play an important role in the cancer patient. The most rapid escalation of dose typically occurs in the terminal phase of the disease (Kanner and Foley, 1981). The first sign of tolerance is usually a reduction in the duration of the effect after a dose; this often mandates shortening of the administration interval. If this is not possible, or analgesia soon after a dose is inadequate, the dose itself should be increased. The absolute size of a dose is irrelevant; additional drug should be given until analgesia is adequate or intolerable side effects occur.

The concept of tolerance should be distinguished from those of physical dependence and addiction. Physical dependence is a physiological response to opioid exposure, which is manifest as the occurrence of an abstinence syndrome on abrupt withdrawal of the drug. Psychological dependence, or addiction, is defined by drug craving and intense involvement with its acquisition. Psychological dependence is rare in patients receiving opioid for medical indications (Porter and Jick, 1980). Fear of psychological dependence is a common and unjustified cause of the undertreatment of pain (Marks and Sachar, 1973).

10. *Respect individual differences among patients.* There is great variability in the response of individuals to various opioid effects. The overall response is a result of a complex interaction between drug metabolism, receptor sensitivity, status of disease, and psychological influences. These cannot be predicted in advance, and successful therapy can only be accomplished by frequent reassessment of the patient, followed by changes in medication regimen when appropriate.

11. *Do not use placebos to assess the nature of pain.* Approximately 33% of pain patients obtain short-lived analgesia from a placebo (Beecher, 1959). This response presumably derives in part from the activity of an endorphinergic endogenous pain-modulating system, because naloxone has been reported to induce partial reversal of the effect (Levine et al., 1978). Placebo analgesia therefore indicates nothing about the nature of the pain but reveals only whether the patient is a placebo responder. There is

essentially no role for the placebo in the management of cancer pain.

## ADJUVANT ANALGESICS

A large number of medications with primary uses other than analgesia have been found empirically to be useful in the management of cancer pain. Several produce analgesia, either alone or in combination with opioids; others counteract the side effects of the opioids, allowing higher and more effective doses to be used.

The tricyclic antidepressants are very useful adjuvants. Although controlled studies in the cancer population are lacking, several of these drugs are proven analgesics in a variety of chronic nonmalignant pain states (Watson et al., 1982; Walsh, 1983) and can be very useful in the management of the sleep disturbances that frequently accompany chronic pain. The doses used are typically below antidepressant levels, although escalation of a dose should be considered where depressed affect and vegetative signs are prominent. The analgesic effects of these medications presumably involve the alteration of biogenic amines important in pain-modulating systems, particularly serotonin. Those tricyclics with greatest effect on serotonin reuptake, such as amitriptyline and doxepin, are empirically the most useful.

Of the neuroleptics, only methotrimeprazine has been demonstrated to be independently analgesic (Beaver et al., 1966). As noted earlier, studies of chlorpromazine have shown no analgesic effect and enhanced sedation when this drug was combined with morphine (Houde and Wallenstein, 1955). Nausea, agitation, and delirium, often associated with opioid use, are other indications for these medications.

The anticonvulsants appear to have efficacy against lancinating pain (Swerdlow, 1984). As such, they are useful in the management of neuralgias due to tumor infiltration or related to therapy, such as stump pain. Carbamazepine and phenytoin are most often used, titrating to full anticonvulsant doses, and valproate and clonazepam can be effective as well.

Many other medications have been salutary in the appropriate settings. As noted earlier, hydroxyzine was shown to have independent analgesic effect in a single-dose assay employing 100 mg im (Beaver and Feise, 1976). In clinical practice, 25–50 mg four to six times daily has benefited an analgesic regimen when anxiolytic and/or antiemetic effects are desired. The stimulants methylphenidate and dextroamphetamine also enhance morphine analgesia (Bruera et al., 1987; Forrest et al., 1977). Cocaine potentiated the mood effects of the opioids, without providing added analgesia (Kaiko et al., 1984). Corticosteroids can have dramatic analgesic effects in tumor involvement of bone and nerve trunk (Twycross and Ventafridda, 1980; Schell, 1972), often permitting reduction in the dose of narcotics below that causing side effects. In addition, many patients will develop enhanced mood and appetite when treated with these drugs. L-Dopa has been reported to be of use in patients with pain from bony metastases (Tolis, 1975). Finally, the cannabinoids, such as $\Delta^9$-tetrahydrocannabinol and levonantradol, have been shown to have analgesic effects, often limited however by significant toxicity (Harris, 1979). Further studies of these compounds are needed.

### Anesthetic Approaches

These techniques comprise trigger point injection, temporary and permanent neural blockade, and nitrous oxide inhalation. These methods have been extensively reviewed (Travell and Simons, 1983; Cousins and Bridenbaugh, 1988). Trigger-point injection with a local anesthetic is a simple and often effective therapy for the myofascial pains that often complicate pain syndromes due to other etiologies in the cancer patient. As noted earlier, nearly 15% of the pains reported by cancer patients were musculoskeletal in type (Twycross and Fairfield, 1982).

Neural blockade, which can be temporary or neurolytic, includes peripheral nerve block, autonomic nerve block, and epidural or intrathecal block. These techniques are useful for localized pain. In general, permanent blocks should be performed only after temporary blocks have proved efficacious and other nondestructive methods of analgesia have failed. A possible exception to this is celiac plexus neurolytic block. Several reports have described excellent results with minimal risks, justifying early treatment of patients with pain due to carcinoma of the pancreas or upper abdominal viscera. Local anesthetics administered epidurally, both by repetitive bolus injections and by continuous infusion, have been useful for the short-term therapy of intractable pelvic and lower extremity pain (Pilon and Baker, 1976; Cousins and Bridenbaugh, 1988). Neurolytic block using phenol or alcohol epidurally or intrathecally is also effective in relieving tumor-induced pain, but carries a significant risk to both motor and autonomic nerve function.

### Neurosurgical Approaches

These techniques have a long history in cancer pain therapy and are important alternatives when antitumor therapy and nondestructive methods of analgesia have failed. They are most effective in treating patients with well-defined localized pain. Neuroablative procedures are usually performed late in a patient's illness, and full evaluation of their efficacy and duration of action is often limited by the patient's overriding medical problems. It is accepted, though, that neuroablation is not very effective in deafferentation pain (Tasker, 1984). More likely to respond are various types of somatic or visceral pain in which nerve injury has not occurred.

With one exception, surgical procedures fall into the two general categories of those that attempt to interrupt pain pathways, and those that relieve suffering without specific antinociceptive action. The latter techniques are seldom used; of those available, prefrontal leukotomy has been replaced by mesial frontal leukotomy and cingulotomy (White and Sweet, 1969).

Procedures that interrupt pain pathways have been designed for every level of the nervous system. Neurectomy is rarely useful, because few painful lesions are limited to the distribution of a single nerve. Dorsal rhizotomy has significant disadvantages, in that a laminectomy is required, multiple roots often need to be sectioned, and sectioning of the roots at the cervical or lumbar enlargement will impair the function of the involved extremity because of loss of proprioception (Loesser, 1973). Cordotomy is the most common procedure used to manage cancer pain. It involves the placement of a lesion in the spinothalamic tract and can be performed percutaneously or as an open surgical procedure. It is most useful in the treatment of unilateral pain to the level of C5 (Levin, 1983; Rosomoff et al., 1966). Up to 90% of patients have pain relief initially, with a favorable outcome in less than 66% at 1 year, and complications such as leg weakness persisting in 2–3% of patients. Midline myelotomy divides the spinal cord longitudinally, severing crossing spinothalamic tract fibers and disrupting medial ascending pain fibers. This is an alternative to bilateral cordotomy in the treatment of pelvic or bilateral leg pain. Experience with the procedure is limited at this time. Finally, procedures in which spinothalamic pathways in the medulla or midbrain are sectioned, as well as stereotactic destruction of other regions in the midbrain or thalamus, have been attempted in the treatment of intractable pain. The risk of significant complications and the need for a surgeon skilled in these techniques limit their utility.

A final neuroablative technique is hypophysectomy, which can be performed surgically or chemically. This procedure is capable of reducing the pain from disseminated cancer in 33–66% of patients, with a median duration of 6–7 weeks and a maximum of 20 weeks (Lloyd et al., 1981). Hormonal ablation of the pituitary is not required for analgesia (Miles and Lipton, 1976), and the tumor need not be hormone dependent for the procedure to be effective. Studies by Yanagida et al. (1984) have suggested that activation of a pituitary-related endogenous pain-modulating system may be involved in the analgesia produced by the procedure.

## Neuroaugmentative Approaches

These techniques can be applied peripherally (e.g., transcutaneous nerve stimulation and acupuncture) or centrally (as in dorsal column or deep brain stimulation). An intermediate step in all cases is believed to be activation of an endogenous pain-modulating system.

Transcutaneous nerve stimulation may be transiently effective in 70–90% of patients with acute pain, although controlled studies are lacking. Patients with chronic pain have less impressive results, with less than 50% of those with cancer pain reporting any relief. Dorsal column stimulation has yielded variable results in the decade since the procedure was devised. Relatively poor long-term outcome and fairly significant risks, including myelopathy, have generally limited the value of this technique. Deep brain stimulation has been performed via depth electrodes implanted into the medial thalamus, thalamic relay nuclei, internal capsule, or brain stem (Hosobuchi et al., 1977). Nearly all reported cancer patients achieved some level of relief, often significant. Although complications appear to be uncommon, a notable proportion of patients appear to develop tolerance to the effects of stimulation. As yet, these techniques, though promising, remain unproven.

## Psychological Approaches

Psychological issues are important in every patient with cancer-related pain. Recognition of these influences and appropriate intervention will facilitate the treatment of pain and help reduce the suffering of the patient and family. Every patient needs support and requires both empathy and direction. The successful treatment of pain often depends on the patient's perception that he or she has access to a concerned physician who will respect the pain complaint and manage it carefully and responsibly.

Patients may also benefit from one of several psychologically oriented techniques. These include such cognitive approaches as hypnosis, relaxation training, biofeedback, distraction, imagery, and sensation redefinition. Several specific indications can be inferred. Predictable pain, such as that associated with procedures or the incident pain reliably precipitated by certain movements, may be controlled using these approaches. Significant muscle spasm is often responsive to relaxation techniques. Finally, patients in whom a prominent component to pain and suffering relates to a loss of personal control may benefit. The latter is the thread that binds these techniques together.

They offer patients a method by which they may influence their own therapy and improve their own status. By doing so, they diminish the helplessness and demoralization that often accompany progression of disease and the fruitless attempts to treat it. (For reviews of the role and use of behavioral techniques in cancer, see Chapters 40 and 46.)

Numerous case reports have documented the utility of hypnosis in the management of pain and anxiety in the cancer patient (Barber and Gitelson, 1980). A controlled study by Spiegel and Bloom (1983a) revealed that training in self-hypnosis therapy combined with group therapy yielded greater pain relief than the group therapy alone. The degree of success with this technique is correlated with the underlying sensitivity of the patient to hypnosis (Barber, 1960). This requirement, combined with the need for trained personnel and the interference with cognitive function during the trance state, are the major disadvantages. Predictable pain is probably that most amenable to this approach.

Biofeedback training utilizes equipment that quantifies selected physiological responses. Although specific responses, such as muscle tension or fingertip temperature, are altered, the net response is often generalized relaxation. A review by Turk et al. (1979) cites mixed results in patients with chronic pain and concludes that equivalent results at less cost would accrue from various other cognitive-behavioral approaches.

Other cognitive approaches that have been applied to the treatment of pain include distraction, sensation redefinition, and imagery (Tan, 1982). In experimental and acute pain, all these techniques have some documented efficacy. A study of chronic pain (Rybstein-Blinchik, 1979) revealed that neutral imagery reduced reported pain intensity without affecting observer ratings of pain behavior. Because training in these methods is within the capability of most patients, their use can be encouraged for whatever improvement in pain and personal control they can confer. Some of these techniques require skilled health care providers and special equipment. Others can be more simply taught and readily learned by patients, who can then use them without additional medical supervision. Relaxation techniques, for example, should be widely prescribed by physicians and nurses.

## SUMMARY

Pain in cancer continues to represent a significant problem for both the patient and the caregiver, despite the extraordinary advances in pain research and therapy. That many of cancer patients die with pain unrelieved is a humbling reminder of the need for further progress. When cure is impossible, every effort must be employed to provide comfort. The treatment of cancer pain should have the highest priority in the overall care of the patient.

## REFERENCES

Barber, J. and J. Gitelson (1980). Cancer pain: Psychological management using hypnosis. *CA* 30:130–36.

Barber, T.X. (1960). "Hypnosis," analgesia and the placebo effect. *J.A.M.A.* 172:680–83.

Basbaum, A.I. and H.L. Fields (1984). Endogenous pain control system: Brainstem spinal pathways and endorphin circuitry. *Ann. Rev. Neurosci.* 7:309–38.

Beaver, W.T. (1965). Mild analgesics: A review of their clinical pharmacology. *Am. J. Med. Sci.* 250:517–604.

Beaver, W.T. and G. Feise (1976). Comparison of the analgesic effects of morphine, hydroxyzine, and their combination in patients with postoperative pain. In J.J. Bonica and D.G. Albe-Fessard (eds.), *Advances in Pain Research and Therapy*, Vol. 1. *Proc. First World Congr. Pain*, Florence. New York: Raven Press, pp. 553–57.

Beaver, W.T., S.L. Wallenstein, R.W. Houde, and A. Rogers (1966). A comparison of the analgesic effect of methotrimeprazine and morphine in patients with cancer. *Clin. Pharmacol. Ther.* 7:436–46.

Beecher, H.K. (1959). *Measurement of Subjective Responses; Quantitative Effects of Drugs*. New York: Oxford University Press.

Bond, M.R. (1979). Psychologic and emotional aspects of cancer pain. In J.J. Bonica and V. Ventafridda (eds.), *Advances in Pain Research and Therapy*, Vol. 2. *Int. Symp. Pain of Advanced Cancer*. New York: Raven Press, pp. 81–88.

Bonica, J.J. (1982). Management of cancer pain. *Acta Anaesthesiol. Scand.* 74(Suppl.):75–82.

Bromage, P.R., E.M. Camporesi, P.A.C. Durant, and C.H. Nielsen (1982). Rostral spread of epidural morphine. *Anesthesiology* 56:431–36.

Bruera, E., S. Chadwick, C. Brenneis, J. Hanson, and R.N. MacDonald (1987). Methylphenidate associated with narcotics for the treatment of cancer pain. *Cancer Treat. Rep.* 71:67–70.

Bukberg, J., D. Penman, and J.C. Holland (1984). Depression in hospitalized cancer patients. *Psychomsom. Med.* 46:199–212.

Campbell, C.F., J.B. Mason, and J.M. Weiler (1983). Continuous subcutaneous infusion of morphine for the pain of terminal malignancy. *Ann. Intern. Med.* 98:51–52.

Cousins, M.J. and P.C. Bridenbaugh (eds.) (1988). *Neural Blockade in Clinical Anesthesia and Management of Pain*. Philadelphia: Lippincott.

Foley, K.M. (1979a). Pain syndromes in patients with cancer. In J.J. Bonica and V. Ventafridda (eds.), *Advances in Pain Research and Therapy*, Vol. 2. *Int. Symp. Pain of Advanced Cancer*. New York: Raven Press, pp. 59–75.

Foley, K.M. (1979b). The management of pain of malignant origin. In H.R. Tyler and D.M. Dawson (eds.), *Current Neurology*. New York: Wiley, pp. 279–302.

Foley, K.M. (1984). Assessment of pain. In R.G. Twycross

(ed.), *Clinics in Oncology: Pain Relief in Cancer* (Vol. 3, No. 1. London: W.B. Saunders, pp. 17–31.

Foley, K.M. (1985). The treatment of cancer pain. *N. Engl. J. Med.* 313:84–95.

Foley, K.M. and N. Sundaresan (1985). The management of cancer pain. In V.T. DeVita, S. Hellman, and S.A. Rosenberg (eds.), *Cancer: Principles and Practices of Oncology,* 2nd ed. Philadelphia: Lippincott, pp. 1940–61.

Forrest, W.H., B.W. Brown, C.R. Brown, R. Defalque, M. Gold, H.E. Jordan, K.E. James, J. Katz, D.L. Mahler, P. Schroff, and G. Teutsch (1977). Dextroamphetamine with morphine for the treatment of postoperative pain. *N. Engl. J. Med.* 296:712–15.

Harris, L.S. (1979). Cannabinoids as analgesics. In R.F. Beers and E.G. Bassett (eds.), *Mechanisms of Pain and Analgesic Compounds.* New York: Raven Press, pp. 467–73.

Hosobuchi, Y., J.E. Adams, and R. Linchitz (1977). Pain relief by electrical stimulation of the central gray matter in humans and its reversal by naloxone. *Science* 197:183–86.

Houde, R.W. (1979). Analgesic effectiveness of the narcotic agonist-antagonists. *Br. J. Clin. Pharmacol.* 7 (Suppl. 3):297s–308s.

Houde, R.W. and S.L. Wallenstein (1955). Analgesic power of chlorpromazine alone and in combination with morphine. *Fed. Proc.* 14:353 (Abstract No. 1141).

International Association for the Study of Pain (1979). IASP Subcommittee on Taxonomy Pain Terms: A list with definitions and notes on usage. *Pain* 249–52.

Inturrisi, C.E. and K.M. Foley (1984). Narcotic analgesics in the management of pain. In M. Kuhar and G.W. Pasternak (eds.), *Analgesics: Neurochemical, Behavioral and Clinical Perspectives.* New York: Raven Press, pp. 257–88.

Kaiko, R.F., K.M. Foley, and P.Y. Grabinski (1983). Central nervous system excitatory effects of meperidine in cancer patients. *Ann. Neurol.* 13:180–85.

Kaiko, R.F., R.M. Kanner, K.M. Foley, S.L. Wallenstein, A. Canel, C. Anderson, A.G. Rogers, and R.W. Houde (1984). Cocaine and morphine in cancer patients with chronic pain. *Pain* 20(Suppl.): Abstract No. S203.

Kanner, R.M. and K.M. Foley (1981). Patterns of narcotic drug use in a cancer pain clinic. *Ann. N.Y. Acad. Sci.* 362:161–72.

Kanner, R.M., N. Martini, and K.M. Foley (1982). Incidence of pain and other clinical manifestations of superior pulmonary sulcus (Pancoast) tumors. In J.J. Bonica, V. Ventafridda, and C.A. Pagni (eds.), *Advances in Pain Research and Therapy,* Vol. 4. *Management of Superior Pulmonary Sulcus Syndrome (Pancoast Syndrome).* New York: Raven Press, pp. 27–39.

Kellgren, J.G. (1939). On the distribution of pain arising from deep somatic structures with charts of segmental pain areas. *Clin. Sci.* 4:35–46.

Lambert, W.E., E. Libman, and E.G. Poser (1960). The effect of increased salience of a membership group on pain tolerance. *J. Pers.* 28:350–57.

Levin, A.B. (1983). Techniques and results of cordotomy in patients with pain of benign and malignant origin. In R.

Rizzi and M. Visentin (eds.), *Pain Therapy. Proc. Second Int. Postgrad. Practical Course Pain Ther.* Amsterdam: Elsevier Biomedical Press, pp. 357–365.

Levine, J.D., N.C. Gordon, and H.L. Fields (1978). The mechanism of placebo analgesia. *Lancet* 2:654–57.

Lloyd, J.W., W.A.L. Rawlinson, and R.J.D. Evans (1981). Selective hypophysectomy for metastatic pain. *Br. J. Anaesth.* 53:1129–33.

Loeser, J.D. (1973). Dorsal rhizotomy. In J.R. Youmans (ed.), *Neurological Surgery.* Philadelphia: W.B. Saunders, pp. 3664–70.

Marks, R.M. and E.J. Sachar (1973). Undertreatment of medical inpatients with narcotic analgesics. *Ann. Intern. Med.* 78:173–81.

Mayer, D.J. and L.R. Watkins (1984). Distraction and coping with pain. *Psychol. Bull.* 95:516–33.

Melzack, R. and P.D. Wall (1965). Pain mechanisms: A new theory. *Science* 150:971–79.

Miles, J. and S. Lipton (1976). Mode of action by which pituitary alcohol injection relieves pain. In J.J. Bonica and D.G. Albe-Fessard (eds.), *Advances in Pain Research and Therapy,* Vol. 1. *Proc. First World Congr. Pain,* Florence. New York: Raven Press, pp. 867–69.

Pannuti, F., A. Martoni, A. Rossi, and E. Piana (1979). The role of endocrine therapy for relief of pain due to advanced cancer. In J.J. Bonica and V. Ventafridda (eds.), *Advances in Pain Research and Therapy,* Vol. 2. *Int. Symp. Pain of Advanced Cancer.* New York: Raven Press, pp. 145–65.

Pasternak, G.W. (1981). Opiate, enkephalin, and endorphin analgesia: Relations to a single subpopulation of opiate receptors. *Neurology* 31:1311–15.

Payne, R. (1987). Anatomy, physiology, and neuropharmacology of cancer pain. *Med. Clin. North Am.* 71:153–68.

Pilon, R.N. and A.R. Baker (1976). Chronic pain control by means of an epidural catheter. *Cancer* 37:903–5.

Portenoy, R.K. (1987). Novel methods of opioid administration. *Cancer Nurs.* 10(Suppl. 1):138–42.

Porter, J. and H. Jick (1980). Addiction rate in patients treated with narcotics. *N. Engl. J. Med.* 302:123.

Rosomoff, H.L., P. Sheptak, and F. Carroll (1966). Modern pain relief: Percutaneous chordotomy. *J.A.M.A.* 196:108–12.

Rybstein-Blinchik, E. (1979). Effects of different cognitive strategies on chronic pain experience. *J. Behav. Med.* 2:93–101.

Sawe, J., J. Hansen, C. Ginman, P. Hartvig, P.A. Jakobsson, M.I. Nilsson, A. Rane, and E. Anggard (1981). Patient-controlled dose regimen of methadone for chronic cancer pain. *Br. Med. J.* 282:771–73.

Schell, H.W. (1972). Adrenal corticosteroid therapy in far-advanced cancer. *Geriatrics* 27:131–41.

Snyder, S.H. (1978). The opiate receptor and morphine-like peptides in the brain. *Am. J. Psychiatry* 135:645–52.

Spiegel, D. and J.R. Bloom (1983a). Group therapy and hypnosis reduce metastatic breast carcinoma pain. *Psychosom. Med.* 45:333–39.

Spiegel, D. and J.R. Bloom (1983b). Pain in metastatic breast cancer. *Cancer* 52:341–45.

Stam, H.J., C. Goss, L. Rosenal, and S. Ewens (1984). Cancer pain and distress in patients undergoing radiotherapy. *Pain* 20(Suppl. 2):S181 (Abstract No. 273).

Sternbach, R. (1974). *Pain Patients: Traits and Treatments*. New York: Academic Press.

Sternbach, R. and B. Tursky (1965). Ethnic differences among housewives in psychophysical and skin potential responses to electric shock. *Psychophysiology* 1:241–46.

Sundaresan, N. and G.V. DiGiacinto (1987). Antitumor and antinociceptive approaches to control cancer pain. *Med. Clin. North Am.* 71:329–48.

Swerdlow, M. (1984). Anticonvulsant drugs and chronic pain. *Clin. Neuropharmacol.* 7:51–82.

Tan, S-Y. (1982). Cognitive and cognitive-behavioral methods for pain control: A selective review. *Pain* 12:201–28.

Tasker, R.R. (1984). Deafferentation. In P.D. Wall and R. Melzack (eds.), *Textbook of Pain*. Edinburgh: Churchill-Livingstone, pp. 119–32.

Tolis, G.J. (1975). L-Dopa for pain from bone metastases. *N. Engl. J. Med.* 292:1352–53.

Travell, J.G. and D.G. Simons (1983). *Myofacial pain and dysfunction: The trigger point manual*. Baltimore: Williams & Wilkins.

Turk, D.C., D.H. Meichenbaum, and W.H. Berman (1979). Application of biofeedback for the regulation of pain: A critical review. *Psychol. Bull.* 86:1322–38.

Twycross, R.G. and S.A. Lack (1983). *Symptom Control in Far Advanced Cancer: Pain Relief*. London: Pitman.

Twycross, R.G. and V. Ventafridda (1980). *The Continuing Care of Terminal Cancer Patients*. New York: Pergamon.

Walsh, T.D. (1983). Antidepressants in chronic pain. *Clin. Neuropharmacol.* 6:271–95.

Watson, C.P., R.J. Evans, K. Reed, H.J. Merskey, L. Goldsmith, and J. Warsh (1982). Amitriptyline vs. placebo in post herpetic neuralgia. *Neurology* 32:671–73.

White, J.C. and W.H. Sweet (1969). *Pain and the Neurosurgeon: A Forty-Year Experience*. Springfield, Ill.: Charles C Thomas.

World Health Organization (WHO) (1979). *Cancer Statistics*. (Tech. Rep. Ser. No. b32). Geneva: World Health Organization.

Yanagida, H., G. Corssen, A. Trouwborst, and N. Erdmann (1984). Relief of cancer pain in man: Alcohol-induced neuroadenolysis vs. electrical stimulation of the pituitary gland. *Pain* 19:133–41.

Yeung, J.C. and T.A. Rudy (1980). Sites of antinociceptive action of systematically injected morphine: Involvement of supraspinal loci as revealed by intracerebroventricular injection of naloxone. *J. Pharmacol. Exp. Ther.* 215:626–32.

# 33

# Sexual Dysfunction in Cancer Patients: Issues in Evaluation and Treatment

Sarah S. Auchincloss

The field of sexual rehabilitation of cancer patients might be described as the young offspring of a seemingly unlikely but successful match between two parent areas of study, namely psychosocial oncology and human sexuality. In the past two decades, a heightened awareness of the likelihood of long-term survival with improved cancer therapy has led to greater study of quality-of-life issues for cancer survivors. Over roughly the same time span, the study of human sexuality and sexual dysfunction has resulted in significant advances in the evaluation and treatment of sexual disorders in healthy persons (Masters and Johnson, 1966, 1970; Kaplan, 1974, 1979, 1983) as well as in those with medical illness (Wise, 1983). The result of the blending of these two areas of interest is a growing body of literature concerning the nature, prevalence, and treatment of sexual problems occurring in the context or aftermath of cancer treatment.

In this chapter some of the available literature on cancer and sexuality will be summarized, with particular emphasis on the sites of cancer that have direct impact on sexual functioning, including the breast, urological, gynecological, and colorectal areas. Despite the growing literature in the field, a central problem remains with the tendency of oncology clinicians to avoid discussing sexual concerns with their patients; some possible reasons for this persisting difficulty are considered. General guidelines are set forth for the clinical evaluation of sexual problems arising in the course of a cancer treatment. Treatment issues associated with management and rehabilitation of disorders of sexual desire, excitement, and orgasm in both sexes are described, including some practical suggestions the health professional can offer both the patient and his or her partner. Finally, implications for future research and clinical endeavors in this developing field of study are outlined.

## HISTORICAL BACKGROUND

The literature in the area of sexual evaluation and rehabilitation in cancer reflects the difficulties faced by a young field of study, emerging at a time when criteria for scientific credibility are more stringent than ever. A series of reports (Wise, 1978; Schain, 1980; Bullard et al., 1980; Derogatis and Kourlesis, 1981; Lamb and Woods, 1981; von Eschenbach and Schover, 1984; Walbroehl, 1985; Andersen, 1985; Vaeth, 1986, and others) charts the two endeavors of this new area of treatment and research, which include providing quickly a spectrum of descriptive information of immediate clinical usefulness, and conducting well-designed research efforts to determine the nature and prevalence of, and effective solutions for, the sexual problems of cancer patients.

A number of authors have contributed to the clinical evolution of the field. Sutherland and colleagues (1952) were among the first to study sexual sequelae of cancer treatment in colorectal and uterine cancer patients. Since that time a number of papers have appeared, highlighting specific issues in the assessment and treatment of sexual problems in cancer. Donahue and Knapp (1977) focused attention on the need for careful recording of previous sexual experiences and beliefs of cancer patients. They noted the importance of the role of cancer myths in inhibiting sexual activity, and demonstrated the efficacy of simple, practical solutions in managing common sexual problems following gynecological cancer. Wise (1978) emphasized the role of cancer site, life stage, previous sexual function, and disease prognosis in evaluating the sexual sequelae of cancer treatment. Lamont, DePetrillo, and Sargent (1978), among others, advocated a team approach to sexual rehabilitation, with surgeon, oncologist, nurse, social worker, ostomy specialist, and psychologist or psychiatrist all contributing to an optimal outcome. They underscored the usefulness of reconstructive surgery for some patients, until recently an often neglected option.

Wellisch, Jamison, and Pasnau (1978) studied the male partners of mastectomy patients with respect to the sexual impact on them after their mates' surgery. Bullard and co-workers (1980) suggested that patients at increased risk for sexual dysfunction included single patients and patients with pelvic or genital cancer. Derogatis and Kourlesis (1981) pointed out the influence of the oncology team members' beliefs on their avoidance of discussions of sex with their patients (e.g., staff member's belief that cancer patients were not concerned with sexual matters). Von Eschenbach and Schover (1984), incorporating the triphasic model of sexual response (desire, excitement, and orgasm) into their approach to sexual evaluation, found that male patients with cancer are more likely to lose the erection response (excitement phase), while females are more likely to lose interest in sex (desire phase). Schover and Fife (1985) have provided an excellent summary of the unique effects of specific pelvic or genital surgeries on male and female sexual physiology and underscored the importance of using this information to tailor counseling.

Two valuable reviews are provided by Schain and Howards (1985) and Andersen (1985). Schain and Howards offer a useful historical and clinical review of issues in the development and treatment of sexual problems in cancer patients, especially those with breast, gynecological, and genitourinary tumors, covering both current medical therapy and the psychological significance of these sites. Andersen (1985) has contributed a lucid critique and summary of current research issues in the field, highlighting limitations of current methodological techniques and offering thoughtful suggestions for future research efforts. This is discussed further shortly.

As the field has evolved, few models have been proposed that might aid the oncology professional in offering sexual counseling to the cancer patient. Taking into consideration the team structure of modern health care and the varying expertise brought by team members to the goal of psychosexual rehabilitation, a number of authors have supported the usefulness of the PLISSIT model first described by Annon (1976) as an approach to this goal. In theory, with the PLISSIT model each health professional participates in providing sexual information and counseling up to his or her own level of comfort or competence. In a stepwise manner, the health professional moves from giving permission (P) to the patient for having and asking about any sexual feelings, thoughts, and behaviors in the context of a medical illness, to providing limited

information (LI) that is essentially education about sexual function in the context of a particular illness, to specific suggestions (SS) based on a full evaluation of the presenting problem, to intensive therapy (IT) that is essentially a referral for psychotherapy or sex therapy or further medical and/or surgical treatment. Lack of formal data in regard to the efficacy of this approach makes critical evaluation difficult, but its delineation has provided a helpful first step in formulating a systematic approach to psychosexual rehabilitation.

The impediments to successful research in this area are daunting. Sexuality, by virtue of its physically and psychologically private nature, presents numerous obstacles to any formal research effort. Not surprisingly, many studies in the area of sexuality and cancer are hampered by methodological limitations. These include small samples, lack of controls, variable diagnosis by site, stage of disease, and variable cancer treatment modalities (different surgical approaches, chemotherapeutic agents, and irradiation regimens), which also change over time. Further difficulties have included variable time elapsed since treatment, variable (or absent) operational definitions of facets of sexual function studied, the use of retrospective analyses, inadequate study of partners, and the derivation of data largely from self-report, while utilizing instruments to assess sexual function that were sometimes inappropriate or not validated for use in cancer patients.

A comparison of the incidence of sexual dysfunction in cancer patients with that in the "normal" or general population would be helpful, but reliable data for this comparison are quite sparse and at times conflicting. E. Frank, C. Anderson, and D. Rubinstein (1978), studying 100 couples (predominantly white, well-educated, and happily married) by questionnaire, stated that 40% of the men reported erectile or ejaculatory dysfunction and 63% of the women reported arousal or orgasmic difficulties. Cognizant of all these limitations, Andersen (1985), in her excellent review, cites an overall incidence of sexual dissatisfaction and/or dysfunction after cancer treatment ranging from 20 to 90% in reports of groups surveyed. In an effort to refine future descriptive and research efforts, she has conceptualized the type of research design needed, as well as a series of clearly defined questions to be posed in any research effort undertaken in this area: What disease and treatment context produces what kind of sexual difficulties? For which subgroups of cancer patients? Over what time course? and, What are the etiological components? Using this framework she makes several valuable points (Anderson, 1987).

1. Research studies must take into account that both cancer site and treatment affect the incidence data

of sexual dysfunction, and that cancer treatments themselves produce differential sexual morbidity.

2. The specific, cancer-related sexual dysfunctions need to be defined in greater detail, along both psychological and behavioral parameters. The self-report data obtained from psychometrically sound instruments should ideally be correlated with those obtained from psychophysiological techniques available to quantify sexual excitement (e.g., vaginal photoplethysmography and penile volumetric plethysmography). Parallel data from partners, using self-report or questionnaire, should also be obtained.

3. Patients at risk for development of sexual dysfunction should be defined according to demographic, personal, and sexual characteristics. The hypotheses that younger or partnerless patients or those with a preexisting sexual dysfunction are at increased risk require validation.

4. More longitudinal studies would clarify the true time course over which sexual problems develop in cancer patients. The impact of treatments extended over time (chemotherapy) and of treatments with long-lasting side effects (irradiation and chemotherapy) is inadequately documented.

5. Although it appears that a number of approaches to sexual rehabilitation have a positive effect on patients' sexual functioning (Lamont et al., 1978; Capone et al., 1980), the application of sex therapy techniques to the multiply determined sexual problems of cancer patients remains unstudied.

The challenges presented by research and treatment efforts in this area have been addressed at an American Cancer Society Symposium on psychosexual and reproductive issues (ACS 1987). The difficulties involved in applying standard sex therapy techniques to the problems of the cancer patient population have been: few trained staff, motivational issues for staff and patients, combined physical and psychological making treatment longer, scheduling problems during treatment, difficulty in arranging ongoing couple treatment during or after treatment when one spouse is employed, patients at great distance from the medical center, financial concerns, and lack of appropriate facilities for such counseling efforts. Meanwhile, as well-designed and controlled research endeavors continue, such as described by Andersen (1986), the specific needs of specific subgroups of the cancer population are being clarified so that more effective treatments may be offered.

Although carefully controlled research is at present still limited, there are, nevertheless, important clinical reports available that are helpful in working with cancer patients with sexual problems. What follows is a review of several cancer diagnoses by site, with comments on the treatments commonly employed, the sexual dysfunctions commonly associated with the cancer or its treatment, and the rehabilitative measures with which the sexual problems may be addressed. The sites discussed include those most likely to have direct impact on sexual response. Although it is helpful to be familiar with the possible sexual outcomes of any given cancer treatment, it is important to remember that the responses outlined do not serve to predict the nature of the sexual response of any one individual.

## PREVALENCE AND TYPES OF SEXUAL DYSFUNCTION BY TUMOR SITE

### Cancer Sites in Men

Surprisingly little has been written about the powerful social and psychological influences in a man's response to the diagnosis of genitourinary cancer. Shipes and Lehr (1982) speculate on the difficulties brought to sexual recuperation by masculine sex role expectations of strength, impassivity, self-reliance, and control. (For a brief and excellent review of the practical concerns of patients with urological cancer regarding sexual rehabilitation, see Schover et al., 1984; Shover, 1987).

## PROSTATE CANCER

Cancer of the prostate is the most common cancer in men and is diagnosed in approximately 73,000 men over age 50 each year. It is usually treated with surgery and/or with irradiation to the pelvis. While this cancer tends to occur in older men whose sexual function may already be partially compromised by age and preexisting medical conditions, it is unwise to assume an absence of sexual interest or capacity in this group; the impact of prostate cancer treatment on sexual function should not be underestimated.

A nearly 100% incidence of erectile impotence results from radical prostatectomy. However, it is now reported that approximately 10–15% of men so treated will eventually recover a normal erection response; in men younger than 60, the rate of recovery of potency may be even greater (von Eschenbach and Schover, 1984). The dysfunction probably results from surgical damage to autonomic nerve pathways, and may require 6–12 months or longer for recovery. Treatment with external-beam radiation produces essentially the same sexual outcome (100% impotence), probably as a result of fibrosis of the arteries of the pelvis (Goldstein et al., cited in Stoudemire et al., 1985). Irradiated patients may also complain of painful ejaculation secondary to irritation of the posterior urethra. Treatment of prostate cancer with implant of $^{125}$I as reported by Herr (1979) may preserve potency to a greater degree and may be suitable for some candidates.

In more advanced illness hormonal therapy may be utilized. With orchiectomy (removal of the testes) and/or administration of estrogen, as many as 80% of men may experience loss of erectile function. It is important that in men treated with surgery or irradiation, sexual desire and capacity for orgasm may be retained (even though less likely with concurrent estrogen therapy) and, despite the loss of the erection response, a continuing sex life can be built around this, given a supportive partner.

Patients treated for prostate cancer benefit from knowing about the likely course of their sexual recovery, including the possibility of the gradual return of erectile response over a year, the continuation of desire, capacity for orgasm, and the availability of penile prosthesis implantation should posttreatment impotence not remit. Counseling the couple with regard to sexual practices (other than intercourse) that can provide intimacy and gratification is often helpful. Many couples who understand that the impotence is organic and not psychogenic choose not to have prosthetic implantation performed, finding themselves able to have comfortable and gratifying sexual relations regardless of the absence of intercourse.

## PENILE CANCER

Squamous-cell carcinoma of the penis accounts for less than 1% of cancer in men, and occurs primarily in men over 50. Unless the lesion is early and noninvasive, it is usually treated with surgery involving either partial penectomy or total penectomy with perineal urethrostomy. In either case, sexual desire continues to be maintained by normal testosterone secretion. With partial penectomy, the remaining penile tissue retains its erectile capacity and may be sufficient for masturbation and vaginal penetration. Orgasm and ejaculation are usually unchanged. With complete penectomy, excitement may occur with stimulation of erotically sensitive areas around the mons, scrotum, perineum, and anus, and orgasm may follow with ejaculation through the perineal urethrostomy (Witkin and Kaplan, 1982). The patient or couple will benefit from counseling that acknowledges feelings of mourning for the loss of the penis, but that emphasizes the man's continued normal desire and his ability to satisfy his partner in a variety of ways without intercourse. The couple should be encouraged to explore the man's body for his own particular sensitive areas that may lead to heightened pleasure and orgasm for him, and they should continue to do so, because these areas may

appear and change over time. Witkin and Kaplan (1982) have described the treatment of a couple in which the man had undergone radical penectomy. Witkin's intervention and support, using a standard sex therapy approach, resulted in a very successful sex life for both.

## TESTICULAR CANCER

Testicular cancer is the most common cancer in men aged 15–34 years. Treatment varies depending on the type and stage of the cancer and may involve surgery and chemotherapy for nonseminomatous tumors or surgery and radiation therapy for seminomas. Although orchiectomy is the treatment of choice, it may also be necessary to perform a retroperitoneal lymphadenectomy (removal of pelvic and abdominal lymph nodes) for staging and debulking purposes. Those patients who are found to have positive nodes at the time of surgery receive chemotherapy with agents that are cytotoxic to germinal cells.

After retroperitoneal dissection, the majority of patients experience retrograde ejaculation, probably due to surgical damage to paraaortic sympathetic nervous system pathways (Bracken and Johnson, 1976). Usually desire, erections, and orgasms remain otherwise unchanged. However, Schover and von Eschenbach (1984) found in a survey of 121 men treated for nonseminomatous testicular cancer with retroperitoneal lymphadenectomy that 10% complained of erectile dysfunction, which is a high rate for this young group, and 38% noted decreased pleasure with orgasm. A further 11% were not sexually active, and 9% had sexual activity less than once a month. The psychological impact of testicular cancer treatment may affect sexual desire and result in a pattern of sexual avoidance that is best treated by seeing the couple together in therapy.

Treatment for testicular cancer often results in infertility; many of these men have been found to have low sperm counts even prior to diagnosis. Surgery, chemotherapy, and retrograde ejaculation compound the problem. However, antegrade ejaculation may return spontaneously over the months or years following surgery, and when it does not, recent reports indicate that administration of sympathomimetic drugs (imipramine and others) can convert retrograde to antegrade ejaculation, resulting in successful impregnation (Narayan et al., 1982).

In addition to organic influences, the psychological impact of a genital cancer diagnosis in a young man in his prime can be felt in sexual activities, relationships, and marital distress. (See Chapter 18 by Tross for a detailed review of these issues.) Living with uncertainty about the return of fertility after treatment, anxiety about potential birth defects in a child conceived after treatment, ambivalence about artificial insemination and adoption, and changes in the wife's role during illness are all issues for the young couple who face testicular cancer (Schover and von Eschenbach, 1984). The availability of sperm banking should be discussed with the patient and partner before undertaking treatment, even if it means a brief delay in beginning treatment to permit this to be accomplished.

The man who has been treated for testicular cancer should know that desire, erections, and orgasm will probably remain normal; that he may expel little or no semen at orgasm; that normal ejaculation may possibly return spontaneously (perhaps over years after treatment), or with the use of sympathomimetic medication; finally, that fertility may also return after chemotherapy, raising optimism about parenthood as well as concerns about the desirability of childbearing after chemotherapy. The impact of treatment on fertility, sexuality, and relationships should be discussed in depth at the start of therapy and at intervals thereafter; the spouse should be included in these discussions.

## Cancer Sites in Women

### BREAST CANCER

Although surpassed as the leading cause of cancer deaths in 1986 by lung cancer, breast cancer remains the most prevalent site of cancer in women. It is presently estimated that 1 in 11 women will develop breast cancer in her lifetime. Although treatment, particularly of early lesions, remains controversial, initial treatment is usually surgical, ranging from radical to simple mastectomy and to lumpectomy with irradiation. Thereafter, treatment may include irradiation, chemotherapy, or hormone therapy, or a combination of these over the sometimes protracted course of the disease. Although the general psychological impact of breast cancer has received considerable research attention (for reviews see Lewis and Bloom, 1978–1979; Meyerowitz, 1980; and Chapter 14 of this volume), the more specific effects on sexuality of this cancer and its treatment have received attention only recently.

The findings reported in the literature on breast cancer and sexual functioning are conflicting, and the studies themselves are vulnerable to critical analysis. As Bransfield (1983) points out in her excellent review, many important variables are vaguely defined, not assessed, or not reported, including age of the patient, stage of disease at diagnosis, treatment modality used, extent of disease at time of study, time elapsed since treatment (or type of treatment ongoing

at time of study), presence or absence of partner, pre-existing sexual status, clear definition of sexual functioning variables, and extent of sexual counseling, if any. Several studies, however, support the idea that the first several months after surgery is a time of impaired sexual response for a large proportion of women. Smaller subgroups within this group will not have returned to their preoperative baseline level of function or satisfaction even a year afterward. Whether breast cancer treatment represents a different experience in this regard from gynecological, or colorectal, or other cancer treatment remains to be clarified. Certainly the impact of the diagnosis and initial treatment of breast cancer on sexual functioning can be seen in the research reported. Maguire and colleagues (1978) found in studying 75 women who were 65 years old or younger, and free of disease after treatment, that 27% indicated severe sexual problems 4 months after surgery as compared with 6% of controls (women with benign breast disease). At 1 year, 33% of the cancer patients indicated moderate or severe problems compared with 8% of controls. Other authors similarly report finding diminished sexual self-esteem (Abt et al., 1978) or sexual responsiveness (D. Frank et al., 1978) after mastectomy. By contrast, studying a population consisting largely of older, stably married women, Battersby, Armstrong, and Abrahams (1978) reported little change in sexual functioning after mastectomy. Jamison, Wellisch, and Pasnau (1978) reported that a small proportion of women studied (12%) experienced improved sexual relationships after mastectomy.

The impact of breast cancer on issues of body image, sexual identity, femininity, and mood, and thus on sexual functioning as well, remains an area of continued interest and little consensus (Derogatis, 1980). Although it is clear that breast cancer has impact on how a woman feels about herself, her body, and her sexuality, these concepts are defined and measured quite variably by different authors. In addition, a diagnosis of breast cancer, like any other cancer, brings fear of death or disfigurement, of loss of the partner, and of becoming a burden to one's loved ones. These and other concerns must also influence sexuality in ways that have not yet been clarified. The roles of the patient's partner and of her cultural background, both of obvious significance to the clinician, remain similarly largely unexamined. Although these issues are really of interest across cancer diagnoses, the paucity of research endeavors including such important concerns, even for the better-studied sites (e.g., the breast) indicates the early stage of work in this field.

With breast reconstruction, particularly if done at surgery or soon after, the psychological impact of breast loss appears to be lessened (Rowland et al.,

1984; Schain et al., 1985). This augurs well for sexual recuperation after breast cancer treatment.

## GYNECOLOGICAL CANCER

Gynecological cancers compose the fourth most common form of cancer diagnosed in women (after lung, breast, and colorectal); approximately 73,000 women receive a diagnosis of gynecological cancer annually. The tumors included in the gynecological cancers are, in order of frequency, those of the cervix, endometrium, ovary, vagina, and vulva. Treatment varies with tumor type and stage. With aggressive multimodal treatment, life expectancy with these tumors has improved. In recent years the literature on psychological and sexual impact of gynecological cancers, previously quite limited, has begun to expand.

As with the breast cancer literature, the literature of the last two decades regarding sexual impact of gynecological cancer is vulnerable to criticism from a methodological viewpoint, showing insufficient attention to a number of central variables, including cancer site and stage, nature of treatment, sexual history and function prior to treatment, partner response, and the influence on adaptation of personality and cultural variables. However, the literature also supports the picture of the first months after diagnosis and treatment as a time when sexual desire and functioning are impaired, probably for a variety of reasons, including treatment aftereffects and psychological recuperation (Good and Capone, 1980).

If anything, even less is known about the status of the sex life of the long-term survivor of gynecological—as opposed to breast—cancer. This is an area that deserves, and is currently receiving, greater clinical and research interest. The studies that are reported indicate that a significant proportion of women experience long-standing sexual difficulty or impairment after gynecological cancer treatment, and that women with treatment-related sexual difficulties want and benefit from appropriate sexual counseling. A number of authors document the use and helpfulness of a range of sexual counseling approaches in the gynecological cancer population (Weinberg, 1974; Cobliner, 1977; Donahue and Knapp, 1977; Lamont et al., 1978; Capone et al., 1980). Without intervention, sexual dysfunction in this population may persist despite good psychological and marital adjustment posttreatment (Brown et al., 1972; Dempsey et al., 1975; Sewell and Edwards, 1980). This is not for lack of interest in such counseling on the part of patients. Vincent and colleagues (1975) found in studying cervical cancer patients that 80% desired more information about sex from their doctors; however, 75% said they would not bring it up themselves, a finding that emphasizes the

need for staff to take the initiative in discussions of the sexual impact of treatment. At this writing research efforts are under way at several centers that focus on providing prevalence and descriptive data regarding sexual dysfunction after gynecological cancer treatment, as well as intervention studies aimed at reducing the high rates of sexual dysfunction currently reported.

### Cervical Cancer

Cervix cancer, excluding carcinoma in situ, may be treated with radical hysterectomy, with radiation therapy, or by both in combination. A higher incidence of sexual dysfunction (variably defined) after radiation therapy than after surgical treatment has been reported by a number of authors (Decker and Schwartzman, 1962; Abitbol and Davenport, 1974; Vincent et al., 1975; Seibel et al., 1982). Some but perhaps not all of this dysfunction may be attributed to fibrosis, vaginal stenosis, and decreased lubrication associated with radiation (Seibel et al., 1980). However, a considerable portion of this dysfunction should be preventable or treatable. Treatment for surgical and radiation-induced changes in the vagina should include support, education, and use of lubricants. Trying different positions for sex to maximize comfort is essential; the woman-on-top position offers the woman greater control over the timing and degree of penetration, which helps her to feel less anxious and respond more easily. A regimen of regular vaginal dilatation with vaginal dilators is easily learned and practiced, and may be of great help to women with moderate stenosis, in combination with lubricants. Attention to adequate time for foreplay, to permit an excitement response (often slowed by treatment) to develop fully, is an additional important measure.

### Endometrial and Ovarian Cancer

Few studies have been done on the sexual impact of endometrial and ovarian cancer treatment, but unpublished reports indicate an incidence of sexual dysfunction comparable to that for other gynecological cancer treatments, with 75% of the women in one sample reporting sexual difficulties after treatment for endometrial cancer, and 33% reporting complete cessation of sexual behavior after treatment.

Treatment for ovarian cancer involves surgical excision or "debulking" of the tumor, which usually includes hysterectomy and oophorectomy, followed by chemotherapy incorporating a combination of chemotherapeutic agents for periods extending up to a year and more. Chemotherapy is often delivered by intraperitoneal injection in patients with minimal peritoneal residual disease. Clinical evidence suggests that, as with other demanding cancer treatment regimens that include chemotherapy, recuperation may extend over months. Sexual desire may be diminished for an extended period while health is gradually regained and issues of survivorship are addressed. The issues of surgically induced menopause, loss of childbearing capacity, and impact of a major life-threatening illness figure prominently in the psychological recuperation from ovarian cancer. However, with time, normal sexual desire and response are physiologically entirely possible.

Pelvic exenteration, in which the bladder, vagina, uterus, rectum, and associated structures are removed en bloc, with ostomies created for urinary and fecal excretion, is the recommended treatment for some advanced pelvic cancers. Obviously such radical surgery entails a major psychological adjustment. Not infrequently the response may start with a postoperative depressive syndrome (Knorr, 1967), but ultimately it can progress to good or satisfactory psychosocial and marital adjustment (Brown et al., 1972; Dempsey et al., 1975; Vera, 1981). For most patients with exenteration, sexual function is seriously disrupted afterward (Andersen and Hacker, 1983a), with 11 of 15 (Brown et al., 1972), 7 of 10 (Dempsey et al., 1975), 5 of 6 (Fisher, 1979), and 12 of 15 (Vera, 1981) women studied reporting *no* sexual activity after surgery. Construction of a neovagina, with the special attention to sexual rehabilitation entailed, enhances the sexual outcome significantly (Morley et al., 1973); in the study of Lamont and co-workers (1978), 6 of 8 women with vaginal reconstruction and special rehabilitative assistance became sexually active and orgasmic within 6 months of surgery. The role of the partner and of the patient's own motivation is not to be underestimated in such recuperative efforts (Andersen and Hacker, 1983a).

## Vulvar Cancer

Carcinoma of the vulva is rare, occurs primarily in older women, and is treated with wide local excision or with radical vulvectomy, entailing removal of the labia majora and minora, and the clitoris, as well as the inguinal lymph nodes. This procedure evokes a major psychological response on a par with pelvic exenteration (Andersen and Hacker, 1983b), with feelings of depression (Stellman et al., 1984) and isolation predominating. The need for continuing support, education, and realistic sexual counseling is great. Sexual recuperation is aided by continued capacity for normal sexual desire, as adrenal androgens and ovarian hormone function are unaffected. The patient may experience some changes in the sensation evoked by intercourse and orgasm. Problems with local numbness,

and indubitably psychological responses to genital change must be addressed (Di Saia et al., 1979; Morley, 1981; Andersen and Hacker, 1983b). In younger patients, instances of successful pregnancy and vaginal delivery following treatment have been reported (Weinberg, 1974). Schultz and co-workers (1986) found sexual recuperation less likely in vulvectomy patients over 60 and emphasized motivation as an unstudied variable in regaining sexual function.

In summary, the sexual toll on women treated for gynecological cancer is great, even where their emotional, marital, and social health is relatively good. It seems, however, that with sexual counseling, even women sustaining the most extreme pelvic cancer treatments (including exenteration) are able to regain acceptable pretreatment levels of sexual desire, arousal, and orgasm. The need for greater study of this group in an effort to prevent or treat sexual dysfunction is apparent. Andersen and Hacker (1983c) offer useful guidelines for future research on sexual adjustment of gynecological oncology patients.

## Cancer Sites in Both Sexes

### BLADDER CANCER

Carcinoma of the urinary bladder accounts for 2% of all malignant tumors. Incidence increases with age; it occurs in a 3:1 male–female ratio. This tumor is normally treated with surgery, sometimes with additional radiation therapy, more rarely with radiation alone. Radical cystectomy has an impact on sexual response in men similar to that of radical prostatectomy; virtually 100% erectile impotence occurs, as a result of surgical transsection of the nerves governing erection. Sexual desire can continue unchanged, as testosterone secretion is unimpaired. Orgasm occurs with retrograde ejaculation. However, cystectomy necessitates formation of a stoma; ileal loop diversion above the radiation field, with creation of a permanent stoma, is usually the procedure of choice. Sexual issues raised by the presence of an ileal conduit include concerns about odor, leakage, spills, and embarrassment. Impact on the partner is of great concern, with patients often reporting worries about being found offensive, repulsive, or sexually unattractive because of the ostomy.

A number of measures, detailed by Schover and co-workers (1984), help to diminish these worries. The patient or couple may bathe before sex; the appliance should be emptied; a pouch cover may help the appliance look better; tucking the pouch into a belt or otherwise keeping it out of the way helps too. Some couples place a towel on the bed in case of leaks; others bathe and continue sex if a leak occurs. Intercourse positions may be changed so that pressure or friction on the stoma is avoided.

When cystectomy is performed in a woman, the innervation of the perineum may be impaired, resulting in loss of sensation or numbness. The vaginal vault may become narrowed or shortened, and scarring may develop, resulting in dyspareunia. As a result of surgery, irradiation, scarring, or of the experience of pain with intercourse, the woman's excitement and orgasm may be impaired, with subsequent loss of lubrication and absence of gratification perpetuating the cycle.

When radical cystectomy is performed in the female patient, a hysterectomy and bilateral salpingo-oophorectomy are also performed and the anterior vaginal wall is removed. The vagina may therefore be much narrower or shallower than before, as well as less lubricated as a result of estrogen depletion consequent to oophorectomy. Appropriate treatment measures include liberal use of a water-based lubricant or of an estrogen cream; however, should dyspareunia persist, as is not uncommon, a change in intercourse positions can be helpful. In the female superior position, as mentioned previously in instances of gynecological surgery, the woman has much greater control over the rate of penetration and the depth and rate of thrusting. This extra control helps women treated for pelvic cancer to feel better able to protect themselves from pain during sex, leading to increased ability to relax and respond more freely. Some women benefit from a course of vaginal dilatation, as used for treating vaginismus, in which the woman daily inserts gradually larger plastic dilators while learning how to relax her pubococcygeal muscles (Kegel exercises). These techniques permit the woman to refamiliarize herself with her vagina under safe and pain-free circumstances and can markedly facilitate her sexual responsiveness. The impact of radical cystectomy on female desire, excitement, and orgasm deserves greater research interest.

It should be noted that patients who undergo repeated cystoscopies for follow-up of more superficial bladder tumors may lose the desire for sex and describe pain with erection and ejaculation in men, or with coitus in women (Schover et al., 1984). The negative feelings that treatment or repeated follow-up procedures for pelvic lesions induce in the patient call for extra support, as well as education, from staff.

## COLORECTAL CANCER

Cancer of the colon is one of the most common cancers in both men and women; approximately 140,000 people receive a diagnosis of colorectal cancer each year, the majority in older age groups. Surgical treatment with abdominoperineal resection, introduced in 1908 (Sutherland et al., 1952), continues to be the mainstay

of treatment. Reports in the literature on the impact of this surgery on sexual function in men yield varying estimates of postoperative erectile dysfunction, ranging from 33 to 100%. Influences affecting outcome include extent of surgery, age, prior level of sexual functioning, and psychological disposition. The disruption at surgery of the parasympathetic nerves governing erection and of the sympathetic nerves governing ejaculation may produce either partial or complete loss of erectile function, and ejaculation that is retrograde or diminished in amount of forcefulness (Bernstein and Bernstein, 1966; Bernstein, 1972; Yaeger and van Heerden, 1980). Desire continues, maintained by normal testosterone secretion. Erectile function is less likely to be impaired in men 50 or younger, or where less extensive surgery is required. As with urological cancers, sexual function postoperatively may improve gradually over about a year.

The impact of colon cancer surgery on sexual response in women is less well studied. Dlin, Periman, and Ringold (1969) describe some impairment of orgasm in the women they assessed, and mention other concerns such as depression, poor body image, and worry about leaks and smells. The incidence of postoperative problems with desire, excitement, orgasm, or dyspareunia in this population is undetermined and awaits further study.

In addition to surgery, the patient with colorectal cancer—whether male or female—must usually contend with the psychological and practical consequences of a colostomy for his or her life and sexual functioning. The initial response to a colostomy may be shock, numbness, or denial. Sutherland and colleagues (1952) found in studying psychological responses to colostomy that sexuality in both sexes may be restricted "far beyond the physical limitations necessitated by the colostomy." Feelings of depression, anger with no one to blame, and being mutilated are common. Fears of becoming repugnant or being helplessly unable to keep clean must also be addressed (Druss et al., 1969). The supportive response of staff and gradual mastery of colostomy care are crucial; talking with experienced colostom-mates can be an invaluable aid to self-esteem. Adjustment to the colostomy extends over the first postoperative year (Druss et al., 1969) and sometimes longer (Hurny and Holland, 1985).

With time, support, and the opportunity to resolve practical problems, sexual function may return to normal. When erectile functioning is impaired, counseling should initially focus on obtaining pleasure and gratification without erections or intercourse. Many men with postsurgical impotence are able to have orgasms with manual or oral stimulation; many partners are similarly satisfied with sex without intercourse. If erectile function does not improve over time, but the desire for intercourse remains, a penile prosthesis should certainly be considered; acceptance and satisfaction rates with the prosthesis are high (Blake et al., 1983).

An increasing number of patients have a temporary colostomy with later closure and reanastomosis of the bowel. For this group, while colostomy issues are resolved, sexual function may still require attention.

## Other Cancer Sites

Some of the principal psychosexual concerns by cancer site are summarized in Table 33-1. However, a number of cancer sites with obvious significance for sexual functioning have been studied little or not at all. This reflects both the youth of the field and the magnitude of the challenge presented. Head and neck cancers present a combination of difficulties for those addressing sexual functioning and rehabilitative efforts. These include a frequent history of alcoholism, aging issues, and the personal, social, and practical problems surrounding disfiguring facial surgery, as well as management of feeding and tracheostomy tubes (Metcalf and Fischman, 1985). Lung cancer deserves study, not the least because it is currently the most common form of cancer, affecting approximately 150,000 people annually. Lymphomas and leukemias similarly merit further study, in particular as they commonly affect young adults who are usually in the early, less stable years of relationships or career and family building, and may experience greater distress over the threat to sexual functioning posed by their disease and treatment. Chapman and colleagues (1979) have studied the consequences of ovarian failure secondary to chemotherapy for Hodgkin's disease, and found depressed libido (mild or none) in 73% of women studied, as well as separation or divorce in 30% of couples (four times greater than the comparable national average for Britain). Sutcliffe has also reported sequelae and management with lymphoma (1987). Although hormonal replacement therapy alleviates symptoms of chemically induced menopause in these women, further work in this area is greatly needed. The loss of fertility caused by many chemotherapy regimens for lymphoma and leukemia treatment represents a major psychological stress with direct bearing on sexual self-esteem and functioning and is as yet little explored. Other tumor sites or treatment regimens similarly need consideration from the vantage point of impact on sexuality, for example, osteogenic sarcoma and other tumors affecting adolescents.

As health professionals become aware that sexual sequelae of cancer are to some degree predictable and very often treatable, that treatment can be brief and

**Table 33-1** Special issues by cancer site

| Site | Issues |
| --- | --- |
| Breast | Large number of patients |
| | Significance of breast—emotional, sexual |
| | Appearance concerns—scar, prosthesis, reconstruction |
| | Surgical treatment—loss of breast |
| | Chemotherapy—loss of ovarian function |
| | Young patients—childbearing possible after treatment |
| Gynecological | Patients of all ages |
| | Significance of gynecological organs—emotional, sexual, reproductive |
| | Surgical treatment—loss of uterus, ovaries, vagina, or external genitals |
| | Chemotherapy—loss of ovarian function, appearance concerns |
| | Radiation therapy—fibrosis and scarring of vagina |
| | Sexual dysfunction—fear of pain with intercourse, other concerns |
| | Loss of childbearing capacity |
| Testicular | Young men |
| | Significance of testes—emotional, sexual, reproductive |
| | Appearance concerns—prosthesis, chemotherapy-related |
| | Treatment (surgery, chemotherapy) may cause sterility, changes in ejaculation |
| | Sperm banking |
| Bladder, prostate | Older men—effect of aging on erection |
| | Surgical treatment—high incidence of impotence |
| | Impact of ostomy, even temporary |
| Colon and rectal | Older patients |
| | Surgical treatment—high incidence of impotence |
| | Impact of ostomy, even temporary |
| Lymphoma, leukemia | Young patients |
| | Long, stressful treatment |
| | Appearance concerns—chemotherapy-related |
| | Treatment (chemotherapy, radiation) can cause sterility, loss of ovarian function |

effective, and that problems can be minimized with ongoing information, counseling, and support, management of sexual dysfunction will then become integrated into cancer treatment and follow-up of cancer survivors.

The following sections provide some guidelines for evaluation of sexual dysfunction and for sexual rehabilitation of the cancer patient, with illustrative treatment case vignettes.

**Table 33-2**   Staff attitudes leading to avoidance of sexual issues

---

It's not my job.
It takes special training.
It takes a lot of time.
Sex therapy is weird.
Sex therapy is only for healthy people.
There isn't any treatment, so it's cruel even to bring it up.
He or she should be grateful to be alive.
What if he or she falls apart when I ask?
I'm too uncomfortable talking about sex.
I would bring it up if this patient were married.
I might bring it up if this patient were younger.
I should bring it up, but I think this patient is gay.
If it's a real problem, he or she'll mentioned it.
It'll probably take care of itself with time.
If he or she brings it up again, I'll do something about it.

---

## EVALUATION: GENERAL GUIDELINES AND MODEL

### Learning to Ask: Staff's Responsibility

The cancer patient's need for sexual information and counseling from the health care team is obvious. In practice, however, the ability of the team to provide such help may be compromised in a number of ways, including embarrassment, the belief that nothing can be done, other fixed preconceptions about sexual functioning, and lack of time (see Table 33-2). Because avoidance is the first obstacle to successful sexual rehabilitation, a brief discussion of the various influences that contribute to staff and patient avoidance of sexual issues is in order.

There are many reasons why health professionals may hesitate to offer sexual counseling in the context of cancer treatment. First, many professionals may define their responsibilities as solely treatment-centered, with a simple goal of preserving life or managing illness. The sexual consequences of cancer treatment constitute predictable side effects of therapy, and, like any other side effect, should be evaluated and managed appropriately by the health care team, using known treatments or through referral. Second, the lack of information about what can be done for sexual problems may prevent the issue from being raised. Because sex therapy has developed rapidly over the last decade, many professionals may just be learning that effective treatment is available for problems like impotence, painful intercourse, and loss of sexual desire. The old belief that ''nothing can be done'' or that the only treatment is a vague, lengthy, ineffective talk therapy are only gradually being replaced. Health professionals are increasingly becoming aware that with bet-

ter, ongoing information and support efforts, sexual problems associated with medical illness can be prevented, or identified early and referred for brief treatment, as described by Kaplan (1983). A third reason for hesitating to discuss sexual issues with patients is the sense that ''the patient is mainly concerned with having cancer.'' This perception has, as previously noted, been contradicted by Vincent and colleagues (1975), who found that 80% of patients receiving cancer treatment desired more information about sex, although 75% said they would not broach the subject themselves. Finally, the staff may be reluctant to raise the topic because they find it embarrassing. With some time, education, patience with oneself, and practice, most health professionals can come to feel that they have something beneficial to offer the confused and often hesitant patient, who has new problems (or exacerbated old ones) with sex, but who does not know to whom to speak about them or what to say. Caregivers can gain assurance in initiating such discussions by realizing that for the patient a simple recognition that a problem exists, is not uncommon, and can be helped with a suitable referral, can provide enormous relief.

Patients may also feel that it is inappropriate or embarrassing to bring up the topic. They may try to be ''the good patient'' and let the doctor determine when, if ever, sex should be discussed, or may assume the staff's silence means that their sex life is thought to be over. In sum, the responsibility for monitoring the impact of cancer treatment on sexual function lies with the oncology team, just as with any other side effect of treatment.

### Whom to Ask: Most Patients Have Sexual Concerns

With very rare exceptions, every patient, adolescent, adult, or elderly, may realistically be considered to have sexual concerns. For this reason, questions evaluating sexual well-being should be a routine part of oncological care. Depending on his or her developmental stage, however, the impact of cancer and treatment may arouse very different concerns in a given individual. Young patients, especially teenagers, who have had less time to develop a stable sense of their own sexuality, may require extra support and attention in this area. Patients in their twenties and older, who may look forward to years of active life after successful cancer treatment, may also have special concerns about their sexual future. Older persons are often assumed to have no interest in sex despite ample documentation of continued sexual desire and sexual activity in this population into the eighties and nineties. Until a particular patient's feelings about sex are

**Table 33-3**  Special issues in sexual rehabilitation by patient characteristics

| Patients | Issues |
|---|---|
| Young | May lack basic information about sexual functioning |
| | Have had less time to develop stable sexual identity |
| | Often in young or unstable relationships or not in a relationship |
| | May have difficulty asking for help |
| Single | Face dating and mate selection issues |
| | Appearance issues important to self-esteem |
| | May want to "try out equipment to see if it still works" after treatment |
| | Low self-esteem after treatment can lead to involvement in poor or unstable relationships |
| | Often confront concerns about sexual functioning well after treatment ends, when contact with staff is minimal |

known, older patients' concerns should be addressed exactly as one would those of someone younger.

Single persons of any age (including those divorced and widowed), who face dating, marriage, or remarriage issues, often feel grave doubts about whether anyone will ever find them desirable, and may require time to work through these issues. They may also wonder when and how to discuss the cancer treatment and its effect on sex (e.g., presence of an ostomy, or absence of a breast) with a new partner. In addition, particular patient characteristics may possibly result in some patients being more vulnerable to sexual problems than others (see Table 33-3). Patients whose treatment directly affects sexual response (including those with gynecological, genitourinary, colorectal, breast, and other cancers) in particular require continuing education, support, and encouragement in dealing with the psychological and sexual aftermath of treatment.

It is important to remember that most patients can be helped to have a comfortable and gratifying sex life after treatment. The first step is for the staff to be consistent and comfortable about bringing it up, maintaining a hopeful and positive stance, above all when it is likely to present a major worry to the patient.

## When to Ask: At Diagnosis, During Treatment, After Treatment

Before starting treatment, at the time of diagnosis, is an ideal time to obtain some baseline information about the patient's sexual history and current sexual status, in order to provide to the patient appropriate support and useful information about the possible impact of treatment on sexual functioning. The first con-

versations about diagnosis, treatment, and side effects should optimally include questions about this area of functioning. This conveys to the patient that sex is an appropriate topic to bring up at any future visits. This is important because at the time of diagnosis the patient may be more concerned about the illness and the risk of dying, but worry about the impact of treatment on one's sex life soon follows, often associated with fears of becoming a burden to one's partner and of abandonment. Offering direct reassurance that when sexual problems occur they can be discussed and treated can be very valuable to the patient and to his or her partner.

Obtaining a sexual history at the time of diagnosis also obviates the risk of giving wrong or inappropriate advice to the patient later, during or after treatment. For example, a woman was reassured after vulvectomy that she would be able to have comfortable intercourse; however, it was unknown to her physician (who never asked) that she was homosexual and had enjoyed clitoral stimulation, rather than intercourse, with her partner of many years. In treatment it came out that she was able to reach orgasm with intravaginal stimulation alone, which contributed to a good outcome.

Before surgery, particularly abdominal or pelvic surgery, fears about the effect of the operation on sexual function are often at a peak, and a discussion then can help the patient prepare for the procedure as calmly as possible.

When sex has not been discussed, whether the patient is undergoing active treatment or it has been months or years since treatment, a discussion of the sexual effects of treatment can be introduced with the simple question, "How are things going sexually?" Again, it is important to obtain a history in order to be able to offer appropriate support and information. For many patients, concern about the impact of treatment on sexual function seems to be less during treatment when the focus is on just getting through it, and greater after treatment is over, when the psychological effects of the cancer treatment experience weigh in. Follow-up visits after treatment ends are therefore a crucial time to assess how the patient is doing emotionally and sexually, and to offer help if needed.

Discussion of sexual issues is appropriately deferred whenever the patient is acutely overwhelmed by a crisis, including treatment setbacks, diagnosis of recurrence, or other problems relating to family or work. Privacy is of premium importance whenever sex is discussed. Therefore, it is inappropriate to introduce the topic on rounds, when several staff members are present, or when a roommate is listening. Doing so only ensures a bland exchange with little real information provided, while conveying the staff's desire not to hear about the patient's true concerns or fears.

**Table 33-4**  Evaluation of sexual problems

- Chief complaint
- Sexual status
- Medical status*
- Psychiatric status
- Family and psychosexual history
- Relationship assessment
- Summary and recommendations

*As adapted here, includes cancer treatment status.
*Source*: From H.S. Kaplan (1983).

## What to Ask About: Evaluating Sexual Function

A useful interview model for the evaluation of sexual problems in healthy and medically ill patients has been offered by Kaplan (1983) (see Table 33-4). With a few adaptations this model is suitable for use with cancer patients as well. The outline of the interview is based on the format for the standard medical history-taking. As with its parent model, its value lies in simplifying the information-gathering process, with the purpose of developing a working diagnosis or differential diagnosis. That diagnosis may, of course, be further refined or changed altogether as a result of additional evaluative measures. Some components of this interview sequence may already be known in detail to the oncology clinician, for example the patient's medical status.

In oncology settings the time to spend on evaluation may be very limited. The briefest sexual history should include current sexual status, current relationship assessment, and past sexual history, each of which will be discussed further. When a more thorough evaluation is possible, family background, attitudes toward sex, and cancer myths relating to sexual function should be explored as well. The order in which the patient's current sexual status, relationship status, and past sexual history are covered is not as important as creating a comfortable atmosphere in which the patient can talk openly about sex, something that most people are embarrassed or reserved about mentioning. It can be helpful to open the topic clearly, as in, "Now I would like to ask you some questions about sex." If this is done in a gentle and straightforward manner, the patient soon understands that the purpose of the questions is to help him or her get through treatment (or recovery) with the fewest possible problems in this area.

While learning how to evaluate sexual functioning quickly and accurately, it may be helpful to cover this material in the sequence given. Each part of the interview will be discussed briefly in turn.

1. *Chief complaint.* As has been discussed, the oncology professional is often in the situation of asking whether there are any sexual problems, rather than being told outright that one exists. In order to determine whether there is a sexual complaint, a basic understanding of the nomenclature of sexual dysfunction is needed.

When assessing sexual function, it is helpful to use the simple triphasic model on which current psychiatric and sexual medicine nomenclature is based. Prior to the introduction of this model, sexual problems in men were grouped together and called impotence and in women they were called frigidity. Treatment for both problems was long-term psychoanalysis, which was too often ineffective. With the careful study of human physiological sexual response of Masters and Johnson (1966) and the treatment refinements of Kaplan (1974), sexual response is now understood as occurring in both sexes in the three phases of desire, excitement, and orgasm. Problems in sexual functioning can occur in any phase, and are diagnosed based on the phase affected. Treatment in turn is tailored to the specific problem, with different treatment approaches being used for problems of sexual desire, of excitement (i.e., impotence or difficulty attaining or maintaining an erection, lack of vaginal lubrication and swelling), and of orgasm (i.e., anorgasmia, premature ejaculation, and retarded ejaculation).

Thus, for purposes of sexual evaluation, the health professional should ask the patient about his or her experience with respect to each of these phases. This does not need to be either coldly clinical or inappropriately personal. A few simple questions usually suffice. Has the patient been able to experience desire lately; for example, has he or she had sexy thoughts sometimes, or sexual fantasies or daydreams, or responded to an attractive person? Loss of desire is not uncommon in cancer patients, because of the anxiety about diagnosis, or the physical and psychological stress of treatment. After treatment, sexual desire should gradually be regained.

When in a sexual situation, is the patient able to become sexually excited? Does he develop and maintain an erection, given enough stimulation? Does she feel "excited," and experience swelling and lubrication in her vagina? Excitement phase problems can occur as a result of stress and anxiety, or as a result of treatment (pelvic surgery or irradiation, or chemotherapy resulting in gonadal failure). Excitement phase problems include inability to get an erection (impotence), changes in erectile response (needing more time or more direct stimulation, partial erection, etc.), or insufficient lubrication. This latter problem will result in painful intercourse that often leads to sexual avoidance.

Finally, during sex does he or she have an orgasm? Inability to have an orgasm (anorgasmia) or changes in orgasm can result from the psychological or physical effects of cancer treatment. It is important to ask about frequency of sexual experiences, not forgetting to include masturbation, particularly if the patient is not in a relationship.

Even experienced clinicians need time to become accustomed to questioning patients in such detail about their sex lives. It is important to remember that expressing professional concern about the impact of chemotherapy, irradiation, or major surgery on your patient's relationship and sex life is just as appropriate as inquiring about appetite and bowel function, and may have far greater value to the patient, whose motivation to comply with or continue treatment is based partly on a vision of a full future when treatment is completed.

If all is well sexually, the evaluation is complete. If, however, problems are reported, the clinician should continue the interview, covering the material in the remaining sections.

2. *Sexual status.* Ascertaining the patient's sexual status means inquiring in detail about the current state of the patient's sexual functioning. This is most straightforwardly addressed by asking, ''What happened the last time you made love?'' This part of the evaluation seems the hardest for the oncology professional to do, for many reasons, including simple embarrassment. However, the information derived from it is often essential to an accurate sexual diagnosis.

The goal of the sexual status is a clear, chronological description from the patient of the thoughts, feelings, and behaviors that made up his or her most recent sexual experience, even if months ago, covering the desire, excitement, and orgasm phases. Appropriate questions include: Who initiated sex? What setting were you in? What kind of foreplay did you have? For how long? Did you have intercourse? For how long? Did you have an orgasm? Was it pleasurable? Were there any problems with pain at any point? How did you feel later? What was said? How do you think your partner felt about it?

The true picture of the couple's sexual interaction often becomes clear in these details. One also learns at this point what remains healthy and untroubled about the sexuality of the patient and partner. In sum, it is essential that the clinician have a clear mental image of what the patient's recent sexual experiences have been like in order to tailor the treatment precisely to this patient's needs.

3. *Medical and cancer status.* In most clinical situations the patient's current medical status, past medical history, and current use of medications are well understood and may be reviewed before taking a sexual history. Special note should be taken of the presence of diabetes or hypertension, and the use of antihypertensive or antiadrenergic medication, both of which conditions can independently cause sexual dysfunction. Medications affecting sexual response will receive further attention later.

The patient's cancer history of site, stage, and the treatment until the present time is also often known to the clinician in detail. If not, it should be discussed. Reviewing the treatment process that the patient has undergone can be very helpful in clarifying for both clinician and patient what have been the major possible sources of sexual difficulty. Asking the patient what part of treatment was hardest and what part he or she feels may have affected his or her sexual response the most is valuable, in part because it is sometimes not what one might expect (for example, hair loss secondary to chemotherapy may have decreased the patient's sexual self-esteem more than a major surgery). It is important to know how long the patient has been out of treatment. It may take months, a year, or longer after the treatment for the patient to recuperate sufficiently to begin to focus on sexual concerns.

The medical aspects of sexual dysfunction in cancer patients are discussed in greater detail in the treatment section.

4. *Psychiatric status.* The oncology clinician should be aware of a history of depression or other psychiatric illness, previous psychotherapy, hospitalization, and previous treatment with any psychotropic medication. Any significant current symptoms of depression, anxiety, or stress response syndrome may need to be addressed, and perhaps treated, prior to sexual counseling. Current use of antidepressants, anxiolytics, or antipsychotic drugs may impair sexual functioning in all three phases. Any sexual counseling endeavor should be undertaken with caution, if at all, when major psychiatric syndromes are present.

If it has not already, the psychological impact of the cancer treatment should also be assessed. The patient's level of functioning, coping style, and current supports (family, friends, work, etc.) should be known. Serious problems in any of these areas may need attention before sexual issues may be addressed.

5. *Family and psychosexual history.* Whereas family issues may be deferable, some knowledge of the patient's past sexual functioning is very helpful in assessing sexual problems arising during the course of treatment. In this area, a useful guideline is to make no assumptions regarding the patient's previous sexual experience; let the patient tell you. Depending on the time available for this part of the evaluation, appropriate questions might include some or all of the following: How old were you when you first noticed sexual feelings? First masturbated? Did you date in high school? Have a boyfriend or girlfriend? How old were

you when you first had intercourse? It is helpful to know what the patient's relationship history has been since high school: a series of short-term relationships? A single long-running monogamy? Marriage? Was there a good sexual relationship in the marriage? Questions about pregnancy, childbearing, miscarriage, abortion, and divorce should also be asked. A question about whether the patient has ever experienced any difficulty with sex before is very important. What kind of problem and under what life circumstances? What happened to the problem? With older patients it is important to know what aging-related changes in sexual response there may have been before starting treatment.

The purpose of the past sexual history is to clarify what risk to the patient the cancer treatment presents. Tying in information from the current situation and the recent past also serves to establish a "best and worst" baseline for comparison purposes. A history of having had a healthy, comfortable sexual adjustment before treatment, and of being in a stable ongoing relationship, augurs well for posttreatment sexual outcome. A history of previous sexual difficulty, which is identified before treatment, will suggest to the cancer clinician that special attention be paid to sexual issues during and after treatment, so that treatment stresses do not serve to magnify sexual problems, or, worse still, cause the patient's sex life to end. For example, a married middle-aged man with a history of occasional impotence (related to age or stress), who faces abdominal or pelvic surgery, may benefit from special counseling to help prevent loss of sexual functioning and sexual avoidance after treatment, which would needlessly magnify the toll of cancer treatment on his marriage and well-being.

When it is possible to do a more complete evaluation, the attitudes of the patient's family toward sex and the influence of religious teachings on the patient's feelings about sex may both be explored. Patients raised in families with strongly puritanical, conservative, or judgmental attitudes toward sex may have more trouble talking about sexual matters initially and voicing their worries. Concerns that sexual difficulties (pain and impotence) represent a "punishment" of some sort are not uncommon. The presence of cancer myths may also require some reeducation of the patient. It is still not unusual for patients to worry that all cancer is contagious, or that radiotherapy has made them radioactive. Cultural influences play a role that should not be overlooked. In some cultures, for example, a woman who has had a hysterectomy is perceived as valueless as a sexual partner, and a man who sleeps with her is viewed questioningly. Offering support and clarification while patients struggle with these issues may be a most important aspect of aftercare.

6. *Relationship assessment.* In oncology settings it is often easier to begin a discussion of sexual issues with questions about the patient's current relationship status, because both patient and staff members may feel more comfortable if the dialogue proceeds from a general discussion of the relationship (if any) and moves to a more specific focus on sex. The health professional will need to know the patient's age, sex, and whether he or she is single, married, separated, divorced, widowed, or remarried; whether he or she is heterosexual or homosexual; whether he or she has children; finally, if single, whether he or she is dating, or if there is an ongoing relationship of some duration.

It is expected that patients will reveal themselves only gradually over time. With greater trust, the health professional may learn of homosexuality or bisexuality that has been concealed, an extramarital liaison, or a history of child abuse, rape, or incest. These are not uncommon experiences and have obvious significance for sexual functioning. The course of any sexual counseling may appropriately be modified when they are revealed. Direct questioning about these issues is also appropriate, particularly so with regard to the experience of child abuse or any sexual violence, as a child or as an adult. Patients who have been the victim of a sexual assault may be more vulnerable to anxiety, depression and sexual dysfunction in the aftermath of cancer treatment.

When there exists an ongoing sexual relationship, the health professional needs from the patient a clear picture of the relationship, its quality, duration, and stability. Is it a "good" relationship? How has the partner responded to the current illness? The patient's concerns about the impact of the illness on the partner should be explored. Open discussion of these issues creates a natural context in which to ask about sexual activity.

7. *Summary and recommendations.* Kaplan (1983) reminds us that anyone who has mastered his or her anxiety enough to discuss sexual matters with a stranger, even a professional, deserves a few supportive words acknowledging the difficulty of doing this. (The fledgling oncologist–sex therapist too may feel he or she deserves a mite of praise for embarking on this endeavor.) At the end of the interview, it is helpful to summarize what has been covered and what is recommended at this point (no treatment, further discussion, specific suggestions, or referral), always with the reassurance that sexual problems are not uncommon and are treatable. While realism in the face of serious illness should never be compromised, and true losses should be sympathetically acknowledged, placing the final emphasis squarely on what is well and good in the situation, what can be expected to improve, and what is treatable does much to lift the patient's anxiety. This in turn eases the return of normal sexual functioning.

## How to Ask: The Stance to Take

The cancer clinician who learns how to discuss and evaluate basic sexual concerns with patients soon finds that simply asking about sexual function is reassuring to many patients. It conveys that the topic is acceptable, that concerns can freely by raised with the staff, and that problems can be discussed and treated. Creating the awareness that sexual concerns can be discussed and that problems in this area can be treated is therapeutic; it constitutes "an ounce of prevention" in dealing with sexual dysfunction.

Sexual response can be disrupted as much by anxiety and depression as by somatic cancer treatment. Cancer patients who complain of sexual difficulties often suffer from a combination of anxieties, relationship issues, and treatment-related physical problems that even the most helpful and optimistic clinician might find daunting. The first step in the treatment of any sexual problem is to begin alleviating some of the patient's anxiety and restoring a measure of hope. This is done by taking a supportive stance and conveying clearly that treatment is available. The importance of starting by alleviating some of the patient's anxiety is crucial for several reasons.

First, unless the patient feels some hope, there will be no treatment. The patient who feels anxious, isolated, and hopeless, whose sexual concerns have been long ignored or dealt with in a passing or "clinical" manner, cannot instantly cooperate in his or her own recovery. Anxiety initially prevails and impedes the treatment effort. When the patient begins to feel less anxious and more hopeful, sometimes after a series of discussions with a clinician, or after a depression has been treated, he or she can begin to participate in the treatment of the sexual problem, by providing information to the clinician, asking questions about areas of concern, involving the partner, and trying offered therapeutic suggestions instead of despondently shrugging them off.

Second, decreased anxiety itself can foster the return of sexual function. The anxious cancer patient with a sexual complaint often has both psychological and medical influences contributing to the problem. While the medical problems are evaluated, the psychological issues must also be addressed to clarify the extent of their contribution to the situation. Sometimes successful medical treatment is not enough. The anxious woman with vaginal stenosis secondary to radiation therapy for cervical cancer can be treated medically with dilators and lubricants, but even so, persisting anxiety can effectively disrupt her sexual response and lead to a poor outcome of pain, discomfort, and continued sexual avoidance. Treating her anxiety and its cause (e.g., fear of pain, fear of rejec-tion, and misinformation) along with her medical problem can lead to the resumption of a comfortable sex life, with or without intercourse. Sometimes when anxiety is alleviated with support and information, medical conditions turn out to be much less of a problem than originally expected.

Third, it is very likely that someone who has gone through a cancer treatment has heightened anxiety about many issues impinging on sexual response. Concerns about being sick and possibly dying can eradicate sexual interest, but they are only the "tip of the iceberg." Concerns about changed appearance, hair loss, weight gain or loss, skin changes, wounds and scars, prostheses and appliances, disfigurement either temporary or permanent, cause greater distress than many patients will admit and directly affect the patient's sexual response. Fear of the impact of the illness on the relationship and on the partner, of estrangement, loss, abandonment, rejection, being a burden, of the partner straying or seeking sexual relief elsewhere are all common, and reflect the damage to self-esteem that typically accompanies a cancer diagnosis and treatment. They can also impair sexual expression. Financial concerns can also weaken self-esteem and cause people to feel less strong, less capable, and less sexy. Fears of being poorer, losing major assets such as a house or savings, placing a whole family under a financial strain, being unable to work to provide for oneself or others, becoming dependent on family or on governmental assistance are likely to be more prevalent than is often assumed, and are associated with feeling powerless, worthless, and undesirable. Concern about the impact of the illness on children or parents, or other loved ones, can lead to preoccupation with the damage caused by the disease and lead to loss of sexual interest. Any of these concerns can lead to increased use of drugs or alcohol, which further diminishes sexual function.

Because the patient is saddled with these anxieties and concerns, it is crucial for the staff when they introduce issues of sexuality into discussions during and after the treatment, to convey a reasonable and positive attitude about sexual expression and about treatment for any sexual problems that may arise. A cool, extremely "professional" stance does little to help the patient or to allay his or her concern; an overly familiar or joking stance is equally inappropriate and may be anxiety-provoking as well. What is required is a warm, intelligent, professional concern about problems that are acknowledged as particularly "personal" in nature and perhaps difficult to discuss. For staff members, developing an individual style of discussing sexual matters that combines concern, warmth, and a relaxed professional demeanor may take some time, but is a worthwhile investment, because being able to talk about sex in a comfortable manner makes it possible to prevent some sexual problems and vastly facilitates the identification and treatment of others. Most cancer clinicians will feel some trepidation about learning to discuss sexual problems with patients, and some will never choose to or be able to have such discussions. But for many, with a little time and practice, the initial fears related to learning to work with sexual issues will subside, and the reward of being able to help one's patients with these very personal problems will be felt.

Even without specialized training, cancer treatment professionals can convey important messages about sex to patients. These might be summarized as follows:

*Everyone has a sex life.* This may sound obvious on the one hand or misleadingly Pollyanna-ish on the other. However, a common concern of people who have been sexually active is that cancer treatment will end their sex lives; a concern of people who have not been sexually active (single patients and teenagers) is that cancer treatment will make it impossible to resume sexual activity ever again, or even begin a sexual life. Patients in active treatment who have temporarily lost sexual desire, older patients who have had less active sex lives, and patients with metastatic disease are all concerned about their attractiveness and desirability, and about the emotional relationships in which sex has been an important part of the tie. Many have sexual thoughts or daydreams, which sometimes take on a wistful and wishful quality, and with these patients particularly, the wish to be perceived as masculine or feminine is often responded to intuitively by the staff. It is important to understand that the patient's view of himself or herself as sexually alive in some way, with fantasies and hopefulness temporarily replacing actual sexual experience (i.e., during or after treatment), constitutes the central component in his or her sex life, and can and should be supported as such.

For example, a man in his middle forties, who was depressed while receiving a lengthy chemotherapy for advanced lymphoma at a hospital far from his wife and family home, flirted gallantly during every visit from his female consulting psychiatrist. The beneficial effect on his mood from this verbal swashbuckling, which was flowery rather than offensive or demeaning, was obvious. With male house officers he talked vigorously about sports and cigars in a "hail fellow well met" way. His need for psychological compensation for this injured masculinity was clear, and staff members responded appropriately by playing along with his overdone macho demeanor in a relaxed, accepting way. This helped enable him to tolerate months of treatment and separation from his family.

For younger patients, sexually active patients, former patients now free of disease, the concerns about attractiveness and sexual functioning may be even greater. It is important that staff not underestimate the anxiety aroused by sexual impairment or the threat of it, and begin by reassuring patients that during and especially after treatment, sex and the affectional relationships around it continue to be part of life, sometimes with some changes, but still enjoyable. This message will bear repeating in different ways for different patients.

*Everyone can keep a partner sexually happy.* For many cancer patients the chief concern regarding sex is not the potential loss of personal gratification, but concern that a troubled sex life will cause a partner to seek sexual company elsewhere, or eventually to abandon the relationship altogether. At some point it is often helpful to remind the patient that even if desire is less or absent, or if it is not possible to have sex in the accustomed way, it is still possible to keep one's partner sexually gratified, to be a good lover to someone. In simple terms this means reminding the patient that touching, caressing, and closeness are always possible and that oral or manual stimulation can lead to orgasms if more active sex or vaginal intercourse is not possible (i.e., for reasons of fatigue, debility, impotence, vaginal stenosis, discomfort). It is appropriate also to reinforce the idea that people make adaptations in their sex practices as situations evolve, in order to continue to have an active sex life. People too often find their preferred mode of sexual expression disrupted by the illness or treatment and, rather than talk together or try something new, they become embarrassed or avoidant of sex altogether, leading to greater distress in the relationship than might otherwise occur.

*Problems with sex are not uncommon in connection with cancer treatment.* Because most patients will not raise the topic of sex with their oncologist and most cancer treatment professionals avoid the topic as well, many patients wonder if they are alone in having problems coping sexually during chemotherapy, after surgery, or after radiation therapy. Letting the patient know that sexual problems are not uncommon during or after cancer treatment is not only consonant with what the literature suggests, but also helps to diminish the isolation many feel. "It's good to know I'm not the only one," is an often-voiced sentiment among patients who learn it is not unusual to lose desire or have an excitement problem after cancer treatment. Again, when anxiety is less, patients are more receptive to learning; sexual functioning often begins to improve spontaneously as well.

*Problems with sex in the context of cancer treatment are treatable.* Patients with sexual problems after cancer treatment often believe there is no treatment for these problems. Unfortunately, staff members are also frequently unaware of treatment possibilities to recommend. Men with impotence after bladder surgery may be told they will have no sex life; women with pain on intercourse may be told a certain amount of discomfort is to be expected, and appropriate treatment options remain unexplored.

It greatly reassures patients who have not yet begun treatment or who are in treatment to know that if problems arise, help is available. For patients who have encountered problems, or who have problems of long standing after treatment, and who may have been told no help was available, such information is crucial. The staff must be able to follow through with a referral to an appropriate professional as indicated. Above all, adopting the stance that a sexual problem is another, different type of medical side effect that can be prevented or treated successfully, serves to make it less frightening to patients and more readily discussed.

In summary, even without special training in sex therapy, staff can and should play an active role in sexual rehabilitation. The oncology professional should be able to assess sexual functioning, identify problems in the sexual area, provide reassurance and education about sexual function, offer simple, practical suggestions for treatment, and provide referral for more serious or long-standing sexual complaints. These principles are outlined in Table 33-5. In the following section more specific information is given regarding the treatment of sexual dysfunction in cancer patients.

## TREATMENT: WORKUP AND MANAGEMENT GUIDELINES

Treatment of sexual dysfunction in cancer patients can range from simple reassurance and education that is accomplished in one visit, to longer combined medical and psychological treatments, that is done by different staff working together, to an extended couples therapy that is carried out by a specialist in sexual medicine in weekly sessions with a couple over a year's time. Different staff will play different roles in treatment at different points. However, at any point some basic principles governing treatment of sexual problems are helpful to bear in mind. The following section covers some treatment guidelines that should be familiar to any clinician working with sexual dysfunction.

Treatment of any sexual dysfunction in a cancer patient should be tailored to the presenting problem or sexual diagnosis, and tailored to the patient. As mentioned earlier in the section on evaluation, sexual diagnosis is based on the triphasic model of sexual response (desire, excitement, and orgasm). Cancer treatment affects each phase of sexual response, both medically and psychologically (see Table 33-6).

Feelings of sexual desire can take the form of thoughts, fantasies, dreams, or daydreams, as well as

**Table 33-5** Guidelines for sexual rehabilitation after cancer treatment

1. Ask about sex. Avoidance—by staff and patients—is the chief obstacle to sexual rehabilitation
2. Include the partner whenever possible. The partner's attitudes are crucially important to the patient, and a supportive partner makes rehabilitation quicker and easier.
3. Take a positive stance with the patient. Some form of sexual expression is always possible for the patient, and helping the patient to feel less anxious will help foster a better sexual response.
4. Take a good sexual history. Evaluate sexual response (desire, excitement, orgasm phases), and ask about pain, fatigue, alcohol, and depression. Consider both medical and psychological aspects.
5. Be prepared to offer:
   - Basic information about human sexual response, and sexual side effects of treatment and medication.
   - Reassurance where there is no true sexual problem.
   - Support and hope where a sexual problem exists.
   - Diagnosis and workup of associated medical or treatment-related conditions, including medication change where indicated.
   - Treatment of medical causes of sexual dysfunction.
6. When counseling patients on sexual issues, after evaluating the problem and offering information (and workup where indicated), try simple suggestions first, and follow up on these in later visits.
7. Be able to refer patients with persisting sexual problems to a colleague with training and/or experience in human sexuality and sex therapy.

of body sensations. These signify a state of sexual aliveness or responsiveness that many healthy people take for granted, but that is diminished or absent during or after treatment for many cancer patients and/or their partners. Normal desire is governed by physical and psychological influences, both of which can be affected by cancer treatment. In both sexes baseline desire is maintained by and influenced by circulating androgens, and to a lesser extent by other hormones. The presence of an attractive, interested partner enhances sexual desire. With any illness, sexual desire is often diminished or lost early, returning as health is regained; cancer is no exception. Cancer treatment may disrupt the hormonal support for desire, and may cause both partners to lose interest. Prolonged loss of sexual desire is often associated with avoidance of sexual situations, a pattern that can become entrenched over time.

In a normal sexual situation, sexual desire leads to a state of sexual excitement, involving the development of an erection in a man and of vaginal engorgement and lubrication in a woman. With continued and sufficient sexual stimulation, sexual excitement in both sexes leads to orgasm. As with desire, impairment of the

**Table 33-6** Application of the triphasic model to assessment of sexual dysfunction in cancer

| Phase | Sexual dysfunction | Relevance to cancer patients and survivors |
|---|---|---|
| *Desire* | Inhibited sexual desire | Not unusual when patient is in active treatment |
| Sexual thoughts, fantasies, daydreaming; finding potential partner attractive | Loss of interest in sex:<br>Few or no thoughts about sex<br>Negative ("antisexual") attitudes about sex<br>Anxious, panicky feeling about sex<br>Avoidance of sexual situations | After treatment, loss of desire may be related to the cancer itself, treatment side effects, psychological factors (depression, anxiety), and partner issues<br>Often requires longer treatment of couple by sex therapist because of prominent psychological component |
| *Excitement* | Inhibited sexual excitement | Requires thorough medical evaluation, including medication |
| Penile erection in men | Erectile impotence in men: difficulty attaining or maintaining an erection | Common after bladder, prostate, colorectal surgery, and radiation therapy<br>May have psychological component even when physical cause is present<br>Supportive partner is essential<br>Treatment depends on cause—counseling to decrease anxiety, decrease focus on performance<br>For complete organic impotence, consider penile prosthesis |
| Vaginal lubrication and engorgement in women | Impaired vaginal lubrication and engorgement in women | Common after surgery, irradiation to pelvis, or any treatment that causes ovarian loss or failure<br>Patient may complain of dry, sore vagina or painful intercourse<br>Treatment: with estrogens (local or systemic), lubricant, taking more time for foreplay, communication issues |
| *Orgasm* | Inhibited female orgasm: anorgasmia | May be related to fatigue, depression, stress, medication, anxiety |
| Reflex muscle contractions, associated with pleasure, ejaculation, and emission in men, pleasurable sensation in women | | Need for longer or more direct stimulation of clitoris<br>Address need for time and relaxation, communication issues with partner |
| | Inhibited male orgasm: retarded ejaculation | May be related to fatigue, depression, stress, medication, anxiety |
| | Premature ejaculation: inability to control timing of orgasm | Rare complaint in cancer patients, unless preexisting<br>Easily treated by sex therapist—good prognosis with brief therapy<br>Retrograde ejaculation and anejaculatory orgasm occur after some abdominal or pelvic cancer surgeries |
| *Other* | Dyspareunia: pain with intercourse | Leads to sexual avoidance unless treated promptly<br>Requires thorough gynecological evaluation and treatment of cause (surgical change in vagina, irradiation changes, estrogen lack)<br>Practice "no painful sex" rule (i.e., no intercourse unless medical cause is adequately treated) |
| | Vaginismus: vaginal muscle spasm, making penetration painful or impossible | Response to pain or fear of pain with penetration<br>Good prognosis with combined relaxation and sequenced penetration treatment, done by patient herself, then with partner |

excitement and orgasm phases of sexual response can occur in cancer patients as a result of treatment or in response to the psychological impact of the illness. Two brief examples serve to illustrate the diagnostic process. In the first case, a man who has been treated for bladder cancer with radical cystectomy reports being physically unable after surgery to develop or maintain an erection, while still remaining desirous of sex (excitement phase problem: erectile impotence). If medical workup confirms organic impotence, the treatment is to work with the couple on sexual alternatives to intercourse, and to consider a penile prosthesis. In the second case, a woman receiving chemotherapy for breast cancer reports that she is unable to achieve orgasm, despite her interest in sex and full excitement by her husband's caresses (orgasm phase problem: anorgasmia). The treatment should include a review of her medications, discussion of the impact of the breast cancer treatment on her sexual self-esteem, clarification of her physical needs in order to reach orgasm (type and duration of stimulation, fantasies, etc.), and review of whether and how she is communicating her needs to her partner, with support for this communication process as needed.

As can be seen, for cancer patients as well as healthy persons, sexual problems can arise in the *desire, excitement* or *orgasm* phase of sexual response, and can have medical or psychological roots. However, with cancer patients, the medical influences and psychological response to treatment are often the cause of the problem.

It is important to note that if a problem in the orgasm or excitement phase persists over time, it is likely to create problems in the preceding phases of response. In other words, orgasm phase problems lead to excitement phase problems and these to desire problems. For example, if a woman has painful intercourse after pelvic irradiation, her ability to become excited will rapidly disappear (excitement phase problem), and she may lose all desire for sexual contact out of fear of pain (desire phase problem).

It is the observation of Kaplan and others with extensive clinical experience treating healthy persons and those with noncancer medical problems that orgasm phase disorders are often easiest to treat, excitement phase problems more difficult, and desire phase problems the most difficult. In essence, an orgasm phase problem usually signifies a normal desire and healthy excitement response; the orgasm is impaired either from physical or psychological causes, typically of no great magnitude. In contrast, a desire phase problem more likely signifies either a greater psychological barrier to sexual response, or a more serious physical problem, or both, and will require a different, more intensive, and longer treatment for optimal results.

Whether this holds true for cancer patients remains to be seen, but it offers a useful clinical guidepost.

Sometimes, while working with cancer patients, it is difficult or impossible to distinguish clearly among desire, excitement, and orgasm phase sexual problems, and the best treatment approach is not always self-evident. Furthermore, even a careful medical evaluation may fail to determine how much of the problem is physical and how much is psychological. This is particularly true when the patient is only tenuously motivated to pursue a medical workup. More doctor visits, tests, and expense are often the last thing in which a cancer patient or survivor wants to be involved. When this happens, one option is a trial of sexual counseling. If no progress is made, it is much clearer that workup is needed; if some progress is achieved, the patient may be more motivated to comply with workup if it is still indicated. Of course, the special problems cancer patients have with pain, fatigue, medications, drug use, and communication all affect sexuality and require the special attention of trained oncology staff. Here the cancer professional can provide the information, reassurance, support, and practical suggestions that enable the patient to have a better sexual experience.

## Desire Phase Problems: Loss of Desire In Cancer Patients

The frequency of the loss of sexual desire during or after treatment for cancer has not been established. However, clinical experience indicates that sexual desire is diminished or lost during active treatment in many patients as a result of the direct effects of the cancer, the side effects of the treatment, and the emotional stress involved. The patient who experiences loss of desire during treatment requires reassurance that this is normal, that when treatment is over sexual response gradually returns as health is regained, and that any persisting problem with sexual response can be addressed and treated after the cancer treatment itself is over. Many patients are most concerned about the effect of the lack of sex on their spouse or partner and on the future of the relationship. Some patients worry that the spouse will wander, but more often patients feel that the sexual deprivation is yet another burden that the cancer treatment places on their partner, and they feel saddened and worried about how the spouse must feel. If it seems that the couple need to discuss this more straightforwardly, bringing the spouse in to talk can help. It is not unusual for the spouse also to lose desire during the patient's treatment and to be relatively unconcerned about sex during that time, despite the patient's fears. If the spouse would like more sex, the couple may be encouraged to have more "one-way" sex, offering sexual relief for the spouse and holding and caressing for the patient, which may be just what each would like.

Other nonsexual issues may turn out to be of greater concern to the couple, for example, the fear that treatment may not work. For some people it is easier to use a sexual concern as a "ticket into treatment" (or into the psychiatrist's office) when the real issue is hard to face (e.g., fear of death, or a painful marital conflict).

During the months and years of follow-up after treatment, the patient may at some point reveal that he or she has never renewed sex. Again the incidence of this problem is not ascertained for most cancers, although for some radical surgeries for gynecological cancer a complete abstention from sex after treatment is apparently the norm. Clinical experience indicates that posttreatment loss of desire and sexual avoidance is probably not rare even among young, previously sexually active persons treated for cancer. In some cases a couple may not have sex for months while one of them is being treated, and then may have difficulty simply getting "back into the habit" again after treatment is over. One man treated for testicular cancer revealed to his physician 3 years after treatment ended that he had had sex only twice a year since treatment. In a couples therapy that lasted a year, issues of feeling like "half a man" turned out to be central for this patient, compounded by sexual difficulties predating the cancer diagnosis that started during a lengthy, highly stressful infertility workup. His wife had always preferred to let him initiate sex and was especially reluctant to "make a pass" at him after treatment, for fear of "pressuring" him. With time, significant improvement was made in all areas and the couple was able to resume lovemaking two to three times a week.

Loss of desire at times may be related to changes in appearance caused by treatment, such as hair loss, weight loss or gain, skin changes, surgical scars, loss of a breast, loss of a limb, and presence of prostheses, special appliances, or equipment. Either patient or partner may react initially to changes in appearance with anxiety, avoidance, or depression. Mastectomy and ostomy patients may require special counseling in this area. With counseling, both parties can learn to accept the change without either ignoring or obsessing about it. A more difficult problem is raised when the partner alone loses interest, in part because of changes in the patient's appearance of which the patient chooses to be "unaware." One young woman sought help when her boyfriend of several years was treated for a brain tumor with irradiation and chemotherapy. His regimen included steroids, and as a result he gained 30 pounds, and developed moon facies and severe acne on his face and back. Seemingly uncon-

cerned about his altered appearance, he remained interested in sex, while she, though very attached, was not. In consultation she decided not to discuss her complete loss of interest with him, but to continue to have sex occasionally to bolster his spirits, using a vaginal lubricant as needed to keep sex comfortable for her.

Absence of sexual desire may continue during psychological recuperation from cancer treatment. Single patients who are recovering after treatment may defer resuming a sexual life until they have successfully resolved other issues facing them, such as returning to work full time, regaining a healthier appearance, and figuring out when and how to discuss the cancer treatment with a potential partner. This may take as long as 1 or 2 years, or longer. Sexual avoidance can also occur when a couple has had preexisting sexual difficulties that are exacerbated by the cancer treatment, or when a particularly preferred, long-standing pattern of lovemaking is disrupted in some way by the cancer treatment or its aftermath. Older couples may have more difficulty making adjustments in their sexual repertory to accommodate a changed physical reality after treatment, and so may need extra support and counseling in this area.

In all sexual problems in cancer patients, the relative contribution of the patient's medical problems must be evaluated and worked up. In cases of the loss of desire, serum prolactin and hormone assays may be useful. Serum prolactin is elevated in prolactinoma and is associated with loss of sexual desire, which may be the earliest symptom of this pituitary tumor. Serum testosterone may be diminished after treatment for some cancers in men, and is also associated with loss of sexual desire. If low serum testosterone is documented, testosterone replacement should be considered. Testosterone replacement has variable effectiveness and should be carried out only in consultation with an endocrinologist. A young man in his early thirties was treated for lymphoma with abdominal irradiation. He appeared 3 years after treatment with a complaint of loss of sexual desire and partially impaired erectile capacity. He was found to have a low serum testosterone, and testosterone replacement was started by an endocrinologist. This resulted in complete and continuing resolution of his sexual difficulty.

While androgens govern sexual desire in both sexes, testosterone replacement for women who complain of the loss of desire after treatment-related ovarian loss or failure requires careful consideration. While desire may improve with testosterone therapy, masculinizing side effects such as increased facial hair and deepening of the voice will be unacceptable to most patients and require close monitoring in all.

Other possible causes of loss of desire include underlying noncancer medical illness and medications. Hepatic and renal impairment, low thyroid function, and diabetes are of particular concern. As common causes of sexual dysfunction in the cancer-free population, these medical conditions can also affect the cancer patient population. Evaluation of loss of desire in the healthy patient is discussed in detail in Kaplan (1983). Medications associated with sexual dysfunction are discussed further in the next section.

With desire problems, treatment decisions will parallel closely psychological influences first gleaned from the evaluation. The cancer patient who complains of loss of desire should be interviewed with the partner present. As with any sexual problem, the goal of the interview is to provide a clear picture of the current situation, a brief overview of the couple's previous sexual functioning, and a decision about further counseling, evaluation, or referral. Particularly with desire problems, the patient or couple may initially be vague or embarrassed. Reassurance and simple direct questions ease the transition to talking about sex. The magnitude of the problem must be clarified; it is not uncommon for patients with loss of desire to report having sex twice a year, or not at all in 2 or 3 years, despite feeling very lovingly connected. Obtaining a clear picture of what happened the last time the couple made love, even if months ago, is most helpful in determining what direction treatment should take. As described earlier, this requires asking who initiated sex; what kind of foreplay there was, and for how long; what the response was; whether intercourse was attempted, and for how long; whether either partner reached orgasm; and whether sex is pleasurable. It takes time and practice to become comfortable with these questions. However, the answers clarify a great deal. In the course of one interview, a man in his middle thirties who was treated for testicular cancer and complained of the loss of desire described as his most recent sexual experience a brief sexual encounter a year before while on vacation, which was initiated by him with no foreplay and intercourse for 2–3 minutes, resulting in a pleasureless orgasm for him and no pleasure or orgasm for his wife. The picture of anxiety, haste, and poor communication could not have been clearer. Given that his erectile functioning was normal, it was clear that treatment must focus first on reassurance, slowing down, and better communication, with the couple coming for consultation together. Single patients may also describe loss of desire and sexual avoidance. They may need support and encouragement in order to reengage in the usual social patterns of dating and mate seeking, and to confront the rational and irrational fears that perpetuate the cycle of avoidance and isolation.

Treatment of desire problems can be difficult and lengthy. Couples with desire problems persisting over a year or more should probably be referred to a colleague with training and experience in treating sexual dysfunctions. The focus of treatment is on encouraging the gradual return of sexual feeling, or "resexualizing" the relationship. To that end, therapy may include prearranged dates or time alone together, bath or shower together, light touch or massage, the use of erotic books, films, and fantasy, and helping the couple to communicate preferences simply and clearly in sexual situations. A good outcome is represented by the gradual diminution of anxiety and resumption of sexual relations in a more relaxed, comfortable manner with a focus on pleasure rather than on performance.

## Excitement Phase Problems In Men Treated for Cancer

Excitement phase sexual response in men includes the development and maintenance of an erection. Erectile difficulties occurring during a course of irradiation or chemotherapy may appropriately be ascribed to stress, fatigue, and the physical drain of treatment. Erectile problems arising or persisting after treatment require a careful medical evaluation, as well as review of possible psychological variables.

In the general population, erectile dysfunction is more common in men over 40. Normal aging changes in the erection response include decreased penile sensitivity, slowing of the rate of erection response (how quickly an erection is developed), and longer refractory period (time after orgasm before an erection can be developed again). An older man in good health may need more direct stimulation of his penis for a longer time to get an erection. Because the incidence of cancer is higher in the older age groups, many older men may go into a cancer treatment with already diminished erectile response and are therefore at greater risk for difficulty after treatment than younger men.

The erection response depends on the finely tuned functioning of the neurological, vascular, and endocrine interconnecting systems. The neural structures governing the erection response include the central (brain), spinal column, and lower motor neuron components. Interruption of these at any level by surgery or irradiation can disrupt the erection response. The arterial and venous pathways of the pelvis that support the erection response can also be interrupted or destroyed by surgery or irradiation for abdominal or pelvic tumors including bladder, prostate, or colorectal lesions. The encodrine component of the erection response consists primarily of testosterone and other androgenic compounds that are secreted by testes and adrenals, and secondarily, of other hormones such as luteinizing hormone-releasing hormone (LHRH),

**Table 33-7** Medications that may affect sexual response

Anticancer drugs
Endocrine drugs, including hormones
Antihypertensive agents
Adrenergic-receptor blockers (β blockers)
Thiazide diuretics
Antipsychotic drugs
Tricyclic antidepressants
Sedatives and hypnotics
Antianxiety drugs
Narcotics
Alcohol
Amphetamines
Cocaine
Cannabis
Hallucinogens

whose role remains controversial. Reasons contributing to low testosterone after cancer treatment include testicular surgery, abdominal or pelvic irradiation, and chemotherapy known to affect fertility and testosterone secretion.

In addition, many medications can affect erectile capacity. It is crucial in evaluating cancer patients with impotence to ask about all medications in addition to those related to the cancer treatment (see Table 33-7). Antihypertensive agents are frequently associated with sexual difficulties including loss of desire and erectile dysfunction. The use of these drugs (including adrenergic-receptor blockers such as propranol, and thiazide diuretics) may predate the cancer treatment. Antipsychotic drugs frequently are used in cancer patients in low doses to treat nausea (prochlorperazine, compazine, and chlorpromazine), delirium (haloperidol), and anxiety (thioridazine), to produce anesthesia, and for sedation; in higher doses they are used to treat psychotic symptoms arising during treatment. The clinician should be aware, however, that the use of these neuroleptic drugs may be associated with increased serum prolactin and the loss of desire; neurological side effects such as low blood pressure may influence erectile response, and orgasm may be slowed. Tricyclic antidepressants, used in cancer patients for depression, anxiety states, and pain management, similarly may impair desire and excitement phase responses. Monoamine oxidase inhibitor antidepressants (MAOI), less frequently used in the cancer population, may also delay or inhibit the orgasm response.

Any CNS depressant may affect all phases of sexual response, and these are widely used in cancer treatment. Sedative-hypnotic agents, including benzodiazepines, barbiturates, and antihistamines, are widely prescribed for sleep during and after treatment. Anxiolytic drugs such as benzodiazepines are used for tran-

sient anxiety states, and for more enduring anxiety conditions such as phobias or panic attacks that can arise in chemotherapy settings. Opioids and synthetic narcotics are used during and after treatment for pain management. Cannabis may be used by some patients to control nausea during chemotherapy. Alcohol is used by patients and partners in many ways during and after treatment, often to relax, but also to treat depression, anxiety, pain, or insomnia, in amounts that may or may not contribute to difficulties in sexual functioning.

Endocrine drugs such as testosterone or estrogen may improve or impair sexual function. The use of estrogens in men with prostate cancer is often associated with lessened sexual desire. Amphetamines may be used in low doses in cases of depression refractory to antidepressant treatment. Finally, for the relief of pain, stress, or for other reasons, besides alcohol and cannabis, patients may self-treat with a host of other drugs, which include cocaine, barbiturates, anxiolytics, sedative-hypnotics, hallucinogens, narcotics and other analgesics, and megavitamins. Only with a good rapport and a careful recording of the patient history is there the possibility of understanding all drugs being used and their potential impact, singly or in concert, on sexual function. Not uncommonly a patient may be taking two, three, or more drugs that adversely affect sexual function (e.g., a sleeping pill, an antianxiety medication, and a pain medication). Weeding out (or weaning off) medications that are optional or superfluous then becomes the first step in improving sexual function. Making appropriate changes in medication, or cutting down on the dose when possible, can offer benefit.

Furthermore, what may have been a tolerable medication regimen to the patient before treatment in terms of sexual function may not be so after treatment. For example, a man whose erection response was perhaps minimally organically impaired before cancer treatment and whose use of medication or alcohol was moderate may go through a cancer treatment and experience a significant change in sexual function later simply because one too many conditions has been altered. The effects of the aging process, initial medication, and occasional alcohol use when combined with cancer treatment aftereffects (including stress, fatigue, and the use of further medication for anxiety, pain, and sleep) can turn minimally compromised but still adequate sexual function into a case of complete, if temporary, organic impotence. In situations in which there are multiple external etiologies, treatment should focus on identifying each of the influences involved, and addressing each in turn. If one or more can be alleviated, sexual response may begin to return.

Men who have been treated for cancer can also develop difficulty with erections for psychological reasons. Anxiety and depression can impair potency. Worry about illness, dying, being weak and dependent, effects on the spouse and family, work and financial concerns may all adversely effect erectile function. Cancer myths and misinformation can also contribute to loss of erections (e.g., impotence may result if a man fears he might give his wife cancer by having intercourse). Similarly, if a man fears that his sex life has been ended by surgery or irradiation, he may interpret posttreatment erectile failures as confirmation of his fears, and may anxiously avoid sex thereafter in order to escape humiliation. In doing so he perpetuates a cycle of anxiety, impotence, and avoidance.

Evaluation of erectile difficulty in men after cancer treatment should emphasize a careful history and medical assessment. The contribution of a partner, in terms of both emotional support and factual information, can be invaluable. The duration of the problem, and the nature of the circumstances at the onset, should be determined. It is most important to learn whether the impotence is situational, whether there are any circumstances under which full erections occur (e.g., in the morning, during masturbation, or with another partner); this suggests a psychological cause for the erectile problem. To overcome vagueness on the subject, it is helpful to ask the patient to rate his recent erections on a scale from 0 to 10, with 0 equaling no erection and 10 equaling the hardest erection he ever had. On this scale a 5 or thereabouts is an erection firm enough to permit penetration. Although it may sound too "clinical," in practice this scale is often readily accepted by patients who are relieved to have a simple way to describe their state and see the clinician as experienced and understanding for suggesting it. The scale is also useful for keeping track of progress as treatment evolves.

As with desire problems, it is very helpful to obtain a clear mental picture of what happened the last time the couple made love, including the reaction of the partner, whose caring response is crucial; a critical or anxious partner contributes to any erectile dysfunction. It is also important to get a detailed sense of the patient's thoughts and fears in sexual situations. A man in the peak of health can lose an erection when he worries that he might lose it; a man who has been treated for cancer carries, if anything, a greater burden of anxiety.

The medical evaluation of erectile dysfunction begins with a physical examination, an endocrine screen, and possibly penile blood pressure and a nocturnal penile tumescence study or NPT. The NPT involves the use of a small, light, circular gauge that is worn on the penis during sleep, and that measures the number, duration, and fullness of erections that occur normally during rapid-eye-movement (REM) phase sleep several times a night. A partial or complete organic impotence can be diagnosed this way, and the patient, who is often relieved that "it's not all in my mind," can then proceed to treatment. Further medical evaluation, including neurological or vascular assessment of erectile function, should be undertaken conjointly with a urologist.

Treatment for impotence depends directly on the cause. In the case of complete organic impotence caused by surgery or irradiation to the pelvis, the couple may want to explore other, nonintercourse approaches to sexual gratification, including oral and manual stimulation. Many men who are unable to have erections are still able to have orgasm, and once the couple understand the physical basis for the problem, they may decide to keep things as they are. It is important that the wife understand that her husband's impotence does not reflect a loss of desire for her but has an organic basis. Under these circumstances, it is often easier for the woman than for the man to accept the loss of the erections, and to explore other nonintercourse sexual possibilities. When either or both partners continue to want erections or intercourse, a penile prosthesis should be considered, and a referral to a urologist (if not already done) should be made so that the couple can pursue this option.

Treatment for partial organic impotence focuses on decreasing anxiety, clarifying what is needed by way of direct stimulation to the penis to maximize the erection response, and focusing not on performance but on pleasure for both partners. Manual or oral stimulation are often more exciting and effective for erection than intercourse, and the sexual practices of the couple will need to be adapted to take this altered physical response into consideration. Some partners have difficulty accepting oral sex practices and may require time and support in order to become familiar with them; others may never be comfortable with this practice and may use only manual stimulation.

When either medical evaluation including NPT or a clear history of situational impotence suggests that impotence is psychogenic in origin, a referral to a colleague experienced in treating sexual problems should be considered. In sex therapy for psychogenic impotence, the couple is seen together. Weekly session time is spent gradually clarifying the psychodynamics of the situation, while specific "homework" assignments for the couple are given, to be done in private at home. These may start with gentle touching and lead over time to increasing sexual stimulation in a context free of any requirement for sexual performance, including erections or intercourse. Often it is suggested initially that the couple abstain completely from intercourse. As anxiety decreases, the erection response usually improves. The underlying personal or marital conflicts that maintain the pattern of impotence are carefully explored, and the couple learns to respond to each other in a more adaptable, supportive way that fosters pleasure rather than performance. The duration of therapy is variable. The work can extend in weekly sessions over weeks to months and may require persistence and dexterity on the part of the therapist.

## Excitement Phase Problems in Women Treated for Cancer

The excitement phase of sexual response in women includes vaginal engorgement and lubrication and is mediated by neurological and vascular structures and by hormonal activity. Among healthy women the excitement response is considered to be less sensitive to transient physical stresses than is the erectile response in men. The latter is felt to represent a more complex interaction among neurological and other systems and is thus more vulnerable to intermittent dysfunction. As a consequence, loss of the excitement response per se is a rare complaint among healthy women.

During cancer treatment, a woman's excitement response may be diminished by stress, fatigue, anxiety, and medications. After treatment, however, it should gradually return, unless treatment itself has affected the structures involved. Surgery and irradiation to the pelvis may interrupt the neural and vascular pathways governing engorgement and lubrication. A loss of adrenal or ovarian function can occur surgically (oophorectomy or adrenalectomy) or as a result of chemotherapy or irradiation to the pelvis. When this occurs, women often experience lack of lubrication and vaginal dryness, which makes intercourse uncomfortable or painful. With time, estrogen insufficiency causes a degree of atrophy of the vaginal mucosa, which may feel raw or irritated and be too sore to permit intercourse. Local or systemic estrogen replacement offers significant relief for this problem, but may be contraindicated for the breast or gynecological cancer survivor. Anatomical changes after surgery to the pelvis may present sexual difficulty (shortening or narrowing of the vagina). Radical gynecological procedures may entail loss of internal or external structures connected with sexual response (labia majora and minora, clitoris, vagina, uterus, or ovaries). Painful intercourse may result from any of these conditions; if untreated, this symptom leads rapidly to complete sexual avoidance.

The evaluation of complaints related to excitement phase dysfunction in women, such as diminished lubrication, requires careful history and a thorough gynecological examination. History should cover the nature of the cancer treatment, whether surgery (pelvic or genital excision, oophorectomy, adrenalectomy, or pituitary surgery performed?), radiation therapy (to pelvis, brain, breast, or other?), or chemotherapy (did chemotherapy cause amenorrhea?). In addition to clarifying what pelvic organs, vascular and neurological structures may have been affected by treatment, the history should often give some indication of the current hormonal and menopausal status of the patient. Medications taken by the patient should be reviewed, including any of the medications listed previously as impairing sexual function (see Table 33-7), as well as replacement hormones, and antiestrogenic or antiandrogenic compounds. Antihistamines and other anticholinergic drugs, including antidepressants, may diminish lubrication. Testosterone provides hormonal support for sexual response in women as well as in men, and women who have had oophorectomy, adrenalectomy, or pituitary surgery may have impaired desire or excitement partially in response to lower circulating levels of this hormone. Thyroid deficiency, not uncommon in the cancer-free population, may also contribute to lowered sexual desire and excitement in the cancer treatment population, especially in postlymphoma and postleukemia treatment groups.

The woman who complains of inability to become excited or lack of lubrication should also be questioned about changes in her lovemaking patterns since treatment, especially regarding the time spent on foreplay. The anxious couple after cancer treatment often spend less rather than more time on foreplay, and the woman's sexual response is not given the extra time needed for it to develop fully. She then often finds intercourse mildly or moderately uncomfortable, but does not communicate this to her partner for fear of burdening him or of appearing still to be sick or damaged. He often senses the change but has no idea how to fix things for her even though he may wish he could; his solution is often to speed up further, in order to spare her any discomfort. In time both may lose desire and become avoidant of sex altogether.

A careful hormonal assessment with serum assays will help determine whether hormone replacement is indicated. A good gynecological examination will provide invaluable data on hormonal status and status of the vaginal mucosa, as well as information about vaginal patency, surgical anatomical changes (if any), degree of irradiation fibrosis or stenosis (if any), and presence of vaginismus during the pelvic examination (if any). Vaginismus is a spasm of the muscles of the vagina that occurs involuntarily, and may make intercourse difficult, painful, or impossible. It often occurs after an experience of painful vaginal penetration, or may be a response to fear of pain alone. It can persist for years after it has developed as a learned reflex, but has an excellent prognosis when treated by a competent sex therapist, assuming any underlying physical cause of discomfort is also treated. Treatment consists of education, reassurance, relaxation exercises, Kegel exercises, and gradual, sequenced vaginal penetration either digitally or using vaginal dilators.

Treatment of women with excitement phase difficulties begins with the consideration of estrogen replacement, either systemic (using oral maintenance doses) or local (using an estrogen cream). After cancer treatments for lymphomas or leukemias in which chemical menopause may have been induced, estrogen replacement may be appropriate and may provide relief of both local and systemic symptoms.

Where estrogen replacement is contraindicated, as after many breast or gynecological cancer treatments (and even when it is possible), sexual counseling should address the need for adjusting sexual activities. Emphasis is given to the need for taking extra time for foreplay and providing whatever stimulation is needed so that the woman's slowed excitement response is given ample opportunity to emerge and develop. Counseling will often involve a discussion of communication issues, so that the woman, single or married, feels able to tell her partner what she needs in order to have enjoyable, comfortable sex. The generous use of a lubricant is also encouraged. The problem of anxiety leading to hurried sex and possibly to sexual avoidance has been described. The result is pleasureless, uncomfortable sex, or no sex, and the treatment requires reassurance, slowing down, decreasing the anxiety by clarifying the issues at hand, and giving the troubled response a chance to heal in a supportive, nondemanding atmosphere.

Irradiation to the pelvis causes fibrosis not only of the nerves and blood vessels supporting excitement but also of the vagina itself. This gradual process can be prevented or reversed to a significant degree by regular use of a lubricant and vaginal dilators (stents). Because this mode of treatment may sound unusual to some patients, they may need to talk over what a plastic vaginal dilator is, looks like, and how it is used before trying it. Because dilators must be used regularly for a period of time before results are seen, patients need continued support and encouragement to use them until there is a significant improvement in vaginal patency. With regular use, which should be comfortable and not problematic, considerable improvement in vaginal circumference and length can be obtained, making intercourse or partial penetration a possibility again.

When the complaint is of painful intercourse, both evaluation and treatment are more urgent. The nature and onset of the pain should be ascertained, as well as its location (upon penetration, in mid-vagina, or with deep thrusting) and whether it persists or goes away during intercourse. A careful gynecological examination is mandatory. When the vagina is irritated from irradiation or estrogen insufficiency and no specific medical treatment is indicated, or surgical change in the vagina is present that will persist, then sexual counseling must address the woman's fears of pain. Left unaddressed, these fears can rapidly destroy sexual desire and lead to complete sexual avoidance, a much harder problem to treat and one with far more implications for the relationship.

The first step in treatment is for the couple to practice the "no painful sex" rule, which means that the patient and her partner may enjoy touching, kissing, caressing, and gradually any form of sexual stimulation that is pain-free; intercourse, however, is absolutely forbidden on the grounds that further association of sex and pain will work against the treatment. This serves to keep sexuality alive and pleasurable in the relationship (often a relief to both partners), while separating only intercourse out for treatment. After pleasurable sex (without intercourse) has been attained (which may take time), a stepwise exploration of very gradual penetration may be considered if the results of the gynecological examination indicate this is feasible and appropriate. The woman may use her fingers or vaginal dilators; as a next step her partner uses his fingers while she controls the timing and degree of penetration by placing her hand on top of his. A good lubricant used plentifully is essential. Finally, for penile penetration, the woman-on-top position is used so that the woman again controls the degree and rate of thrusting. If at any point she feels pain, the woman withdraws partially until the pain disappears. With support and time, gradually increased degrees of penetration can become possible, and eventually pleasurable intercourse may be resumed.

This treatment approach resembles the treatment for vaginismus and can extend for similar periods of time, that is, over several weeks when psychological adaptation is rapid and physical constraints are few, or over several months when anxiety is great or there is a greater physical problem to resolve. One 28-year-old woman who was engaged to be married appeared after vaginal surgery and irradiation for adenocarcinoma of the vagina with a complaint of painful intercourse. A gynecological examination had revealed a mild postirradiation irritation from a course of radiotherapy that had recently been completed. The patient and her fiance began by practicing the "no painful sex" rule, and went on, over a period of 6 weeks, to try gradual penetration of the vagina, using a lubricant and the woman-on-top position. Pain-free intercourse was gradually resumed over 3 months. Over a year later, recurrent pain with intercourse, caused by late irradiation-induced changes in the vagina, responded well to using an estrogen cream.

Sex without intercourse is an appropriate recommendation in a number of situations, such as where the vagina has been surgically removed (i.e., following exenteration, and some bladder and colorectal cancer surgeries) or is too short for pleasurable intercourse, or when strictures or fibrosis or other postsurgery or postirradiation changes are resistant to therapy. Intramammary, intrathigh, or anal intercourse, as well as oral and manual stimulation, are all possible sources of gratification that can be considered in the effort to help the couple maintain the pleasure and intimacy of sexual relations.

Some radical gynecological procedures raise special issues. Women treated for cancer of the vulva with radical vulvectomy experience significant changes in excitement. They will need to mourn the loss of the clitoris and external genitalia, then will need to find what kinds of stimulation feel best for them. Some areas not previously experienced as sexual may become so, and others may become more sensitive. Vaginal stimulation and stimulation of other erogenous zones, as well as the area where the clitoris was, may all become ways to attain orgasm. After pelvic exenteration, the same process of mourning followed by reexploration of the body may be followed. Any ostomy may become erotized, and other erogenous places may develop. A caring partner is an essential ingredient in this healing process.

The value of reconstructive procedures is less clear for gynecological than for breast cancer patients. Construction of a neovagina after vaginectomy remains an imperfect art; some patients who have undergone vaginal reconstruction are pleased with the outcome, while others, in retrospect, feel they would not do it again. The procedure and recovery can be too arduous and draining, the results much less than expected. As different approaches to vaginal reconstruction are explored, it is hoped more widely satisfactory methods will become available. Until then, counseling efforts must continue to focus on finding ways to adapt that offer comfort, gratification, and intimacy.

## Orgasm Phase Problems

Although premature ejaculation in men and anorgasmia in women occur commonly in the healthy population, problems with orgasm alone do not at present appear to constitute a frequent clinical complaint of cancer patients. However, the neurological, vascular, and endocrine structures that govern orgasm are unquestionably influenced by cancer treatment, and orgasm may therefore be directly affected. Surgery, irradiation, and preexisting underlying disease affect both the blood vessels and the central and peripheral nerves that govern orgasm. Diabetes, hepatic and renal impairment, and lowered testosterone and thyroid hormone levels may also be associated with cancer treatment and may impair the orgasm response. Many of the drugs used in conjunction with cancer treatment may also impede orgasm (see Table 33-7). Little is known of the effect of particular chemotherapy agents on the orgasm response, but one, procarbazine, has a structure like MAO inhibitors and may be associated with difficulty reaching orgasm.

In assessing a woman's complaint of difficulty in reaching orgasm, the patient is questioned about her previous orgasmic capability: under what circumstances, with what stimulation was she able to have orgasm before treatment? The type and duration of stimulation that worked best for her, when and how, must be clearly defined. Stress, fatigue, and anxiety at any point in recovery may cause delayed orgasm, and the woman may need longer or more direct stimulation of the clitoris in order to come to orgasm. These and other psychological causes, more than physical conditions, are probably responsible for orgasmic dysfunction in women. Any fears or anxieties the woman experiences during sex may distract her and make orgasms difficult or impossible. These include concerns about mortality, desirability, relationships, family issues, work and finances, and fear of pain. Any significant physical discomfort also usually eradicates the possibility of orgasm.

When these influences seem to be at work in causing anorgasmia, it is not enough to focus on increased stimulation during sex. Even more important is planning ahead so that there is enough time to create a relaxed, private atmosphere. Spending time on foreplay (including baths and touching) so that an excitement response, dampened by cancer treatment and its psychological aftermath, has more time to bloom, becomes even more important. Many couples initially feel a little ridiculous about planning time alone together, something they may last have done when they were dating each other. However, if they can cross this initial obstacle, the rewards of a few special, private, cozy interludes begin to become clear. The couple that is motivated to "heal up" their sex life after cancer treatment will not find it too hard or burdensome to plan time, protecting themselves from distractions for a while and making foreplay special again, essentially restoring to their lovemaking some of the circumstances and practices enjoyed by couples who are courting at any age. Many couples continue to plan time alone together after their sexual counseling is ended.

Anxious or negative distracting thoughts during sex ("He's looking at my scar," "My erection isn't as hard as I'd hoped") can derail sexual excitement and contribute to excitement and orgasm problems. Women or men who are distracted during sex by such "anti-sexual" thoughts may benefit from learning how to use sexual fantasies as an aid or boost to sexual response. Most people are aware of having one or more sexual images, daydreams, or fantasies, often gleaned from movies, books, or magazines, which are particularly exciting for them. The patient need not confide the content of the fantasy to his or her sexual counselor, but can practice focusing mentally on that particular image during sex. While initially the distracting worrying thoughts will "break through," with time the patient becomes more adept at maintaining a sexy picture in his or her mind, and the anxious thoughts are blocked out while sexual feelings are increasingly disinhibited. This approach may be very helpful for women with orgasm problems, and can help other cancer patients to feel more sexual after treatment. In summary, if depression and anxiety are alleviated with time, talk, and medication (if needed), if fatigue is well managed, if drugs and alcohol are kept to a minimum, and if enough time and consideration are given to improving the quality of the couple's sexual experience, many problems with excitement and difficulty in reaching orgasm will be resolved and disappear.

Orgasmic dysfunction in men is more complex, and referral for medical evaluation should always be considered. Premature ejaculation presents rarely in cancer patients as a sole complaint, but may be present as a preexisting condition that is then complicated by a cancer treatment. This condition occurs when a man reaches orgasm more quickly than he wishes, often after brief but intense stimulation. Premature ejaculation has an excellent prognosis with treatment, which focuses on learning how to moderate the amount of stimulation and pleasure being experienced and how to recognize the premonitory sensations of orgasm, so that control is gradually gained over the timing of orgasm.

Retarded ejaculation occurs when, after prolonged and sufficient stimulation, a man is unable or rarely able to achieve orgasm. This is a less common complaint in the healthy population and may be difficult to treat, as it frequently has a significant psychological component. In a man who has been treated for cancer, however, retarded ejaculation requires careful medical evaluation. During and after treatment, fatigue, malaise, pain conditions, medications, and depression may all serve to lower both drive and responsiveness to sexual situations and stimuli in men. Each of these potential contributors to dysfunction should be addressed and treated specifically where appropriate in order to ease and enhance sexual responsiveness. Some men may need to devote special attention to rest, setting, and type of foreplay, and may need longer or more direct stimulation of the penis in order to reach orgasm. Manual stimulation, often using a lubricant, and oral stimulation may be more effective and erotic here than intercourse. Medications such as opioid narcotics, barbiturates, and some psychotropic drugs may slow the orgasm response. Psychological influences may also delay the orgasm response, including cancer myths and misinformation.

Retrograde ejaculation occurs when the sympathetic nerves responsible for reflex closure of the bladder neck are surgically transected. Semen then passes into the bladder rather than down the urethra, and the result is a "dry" orgasm. This is not harmful; the semen passes out of the bladder with the next voiding. Anejaculatory orgasm occurs when the nerves governing emission of the components of seminal fluid from vasa, seminal vesicles, and prostate are transected. Again, no semen is released, and therefore the orgasm, while otherwise unchanged, is dry. Among surgical procedures for cancer, the most common ones producing these latter outcomes are abdominoperineal resection, low anterior resection of sigmoid colon, lymph node dissections done in association with radical nephrectomy for cancer of the kidney, operations for bladder or prostate cancer, staging procedures for lymphoma, and treatment of testicular cancer. Drugs can also produce retrograde ejaculation or anejaculatory orgasm via effects on the sympathetic nervous system. Antipsychotics, ganglion blockers, antidepressants, and antihypertensive agents all have sympatholytic effects. When the probable outcome of surgery is retrograde ejaculation or, less often, anejaculatory orgasm, this should be discussed with the patient and sperm banking accomplished before the procedure is done.

A man who is having surgery that may impair his orgasm response should know that the surgery may cause a change in his experience of orgasm; that he will still have orgasms, as well as erections and sexual desire (assuming this is expectable); what the specific change is likely to be (retrograde ejaculation or anejaculatory orgasm), as best can be determined; finally, that this change will not be dangerous to his or his partner's health. With a good presurgical explanation, the anxiety of the patient and partner is diminished, and postsurgical adaptation should be easier. When patients face testicular, bladder, prostate, or rectal surgery for cancer, anxiety is great about many issues and this reassurance can be very helpful.

## Other Influences in Sexual Response

The role of stress, fatigue, pain, or depression in the etiology of sexual dysfunction cannot be overemphasized. It is normal for mammals, including humans, to lose sexual desire while undergoing a physical or psychological stress; cancer treatment constitutes a major life stress in both domains.

## FATIGUE

Fatigue is a common consequence of cancer treatment regardless of treatment modality and can by itself dampen or eradicate sexual desire. In response to treatment-related fatigue, many patients must learn to manage their lives with a constant eye toward conserving energy. Planning time alone together, at a time when the patient is likely to be feeling stronger, to talk, cuddle, perhaps make love, is one way to help sustain each other through the difficult and sometimes divisive experience of a major illness.

However, there are many times in a cancer treatment when sex may seem or simply be out of the question. Even when physical symptoms are in abeyance, discouragement, resentment, anger, disappointment in oneself or others, a desire to withdraw and pull away, and other negative feelings are an expectable part of the cancer treatment experience. At those times simple talking, touching, or being silent together can be unifying and restoring (Leiber et al., 1976). Sometimes being alone, to sleep, putter, or think, can be what's needed. The goal of the oncology professional is to help people find a way to fit sex into their lives during treatment that works for them, is comfortable, and takes into consideration the realities of their circumstances and personalities.

## PAIN

Patients who complain of pain interfering with sexual response require careful medical assessment first. The pain complaint should be evaluated, diagnosed, and managed with analgesics, behavioral relaxation, and other approaches as indicated (see Chapter 32 on pain). Pain arising only during sex also requires medical evaluation. Possible causes of painful sex in women have been discussed previously, as well as treatment with estrogens, dilators, and counseling. It should be kept in mind that pain during sex may herald a recurrence of a pelvic tumor. The complaint of local pain in the penis, testes, or groin during sexual excitement or orgasm is infrequent outside the cancer population, and probably within this group as well. A thorough urological evaluation is indicated. If no medical cause for the discomfort is found, sexual counseling may be undertaken in an effort to decrease anxiety, find ways to avoid discomfort, and determine what the psychological component of the problem may be.

## DEPRESSION

Patients who have sexual problems are often depressed. A difficult clinical decision that arises early is whether the depression must be treated separately before any sexual counseling begins. Careful evaluation of this dimension is important because if the patient's depression is too great, any sexual counseling effort is doomed. When this happens, the patient responds to every question or suggestion regarding sexual function with a hopeless, despairing, or hostile attitude: ''It probably won't do any good,'' ''This sounds pointless to me,'' and so on. Missed appointments and failure to act on suggestions made in previous sessions are signals that the patient is too depressed to comply with any sequenced sexual counseling. The appropriate decision then is to stop focusing on sexual feeling and address the patient's depression. The symptoms and treatment of depression in cancer patients are covered in detail in Chapter 23.

Once the patient's depression is treated and has lessened or disappeared, sexual counseling can be undertaken or reintroduced. If it is necessary for the patient to remain on antidepressants or other psychotropic medications during counseling, the treating professional should bear in mind that these medications sometimes dampen desire or response, though rarely not to the extent they would be affected by an untreated major depression. The patient should be helped to focus on what his or her mind and body can do; the net effect of antidepressant medication on sexual response is usually not great.

When the patient's depressed feelings do not appear to be so severe as to mandate a delay in sexual counseling, the treating professional should take a gentle but firm stance, move ahead with education and counseling suggestions, and observe the patient's response. If the patient is able to retain some of what is said, follow through on suggestions, keep follow-up appointments, and work with the treating professional, and if the depressed feelings have been related to sexual concerns, then over several weeks the depression should gradually be alleviated, and the patient should appear more relaxed and hopeful. When this does not occur, attention should be returned to persisting depressive symptoms. Some resistance is an expected part of any sexual counseling endeavor; too great a resistance indicates a need for a different approach. If at some point, the patient may benefit from referral for further psychological counseling around illness or other life issues.

### Finding a Referral

Because the field of sexual rehabilitation is new, in many parts of the country simply finding a colleague who is interested in the area of sexual recovery after cancer treatment, to whom one could refer patients, represents a challenge. A useful first step is to contact a local medical school or hospital department of psychiatry, gynecology, or urology and ask who on the staff works in the area of human sexuality or sexual medicine. Departments of psychology, nursing, or social work may also be good sources for local referrals. Health professionals from diverse training backgrounds who work in the area of human sexuality and medical illness can soon develop some expertise in working with cancer patients if they are willing to accept the first few referrals; oncology professionals may need to assist by offering clinical backup, teaching, and support for the cancer treatment-related aspects of the situation. A national organization that may be helpful in locating health professionals trained in human sexuality is the American Association of Sex Educators, Counselors and Therapists (AASECT). Researchers in the field may also be able to provide referral to experienced therapists in their geographic vicinity.

Many patients express interest in reading material on this subject. The American Cancer Society has published two booklets written by Leslie Schover, Ph.D., titled *Sexuality and Cancer,* for men and women patients. Well-written, clear, complete and concise, these constitute an excellent resource for patients; they are available through the ACS.

## SUMMARY

As cancer treatments become more rigorous and more effective, and our ability to provide medical support to people through treatment improves, a population of cancer survivors is developing of whom an undetermined proportion have acquired a sexual dysfunction as a result of or in association with their cancer treatment. Research interest in this area is rapidly increasing. Research data regarding prevalence of sexual dysfunction, risk factors predisposing to development of sexual dysfunction, and intervention methods will hopefully soon become available. The course of these treatment-related sexual dysfunctions over time is also of interest, specifically how many cancer survivors return gradually to normal sexual function over time without need of counseling? While the outcome of current and future research efforts is awaited with interest, it is possible to begin to address these issues with patients in the clinical setting where cancer treatments are carried out. Oncology professionals should be able to identify and evaluate problems with sexual function that arise during or after treatment, to provide accurate information and support about sexual issues to patients, and to refer to a competent colleague with interest, training, and experience in treating sexual dysfunctions when appropriate. In this chapter a brief literature review and some guidelines regarding evaluation and treatment are offered as a beginning step toward improving the quality of care available to pa-

tients in this area. With more time, continuing research, and increasing willingness on the part of oncology professionals to undertake this responsibility, it is hoped that problems with sexual function will be identified and successfully treated more often, so that people who come through the lonely trial of a cancer treatment may look forward with realistic hope to restoration of the full measure of rich human interrelationships that any patient treated for cancer so deeply values and has so clearly earned.

## REFERENCES

Abitbol, W.M. and J.H. Davenport (1974). Sexual dysfunction after therapy for cervical cancer. *Am. J. Obstet. Gynecol.* 119:181–89.

Abt, V., M.C. Mc Gurrin, and A.A. Heintz (1978). The impact of mastectomy on sexual self-image, attitudes, and behavior. *J. Sex Educ. Ther.* 4:43–46.

Andersen, B.L. (1985). Sexual functioning morbidity among cancer survivors. *Cancer* 55:1835–42.

Andersen, B.L. (1987). Conceptualization, assessment, and research design: a study of sexual functioning among cancer survivors. *Proc. of the Workshop on Psychosexual and Reproductive Issues Affecting Patients with Cancer—1987.* A Service and Rehabilitation Education Publication, American Cancer Society, Atlanta 2–12.

Andersen, B.L. (ed.) (1986). *Women with Cancer: Psychological Perspectives.* New York: Springer-Verlag.

Andersen, B.L. and N.F. Hacker (1983a). Psychosexual adjustment following pelvic exenteration. *Obstet. Gynecol.* 61:331–38.

Andersen, B.L. and N.F. Hacker (1983b). Psychosexual adjustment after vulvar surgery. *Obstet. Gynecol.* 62:457–62.

Andersen, B.L. and N.F. Hacker (1983c). Psychosexual adjustment of gynecologic oncology patients: A proposed model for future investigation. *Gynecol. Oncol.* 15:214–23.

Annon, J.S. (1976). *Behavioral Treatment of Sexual Problems,* Vol. 1. *Brief Therapy.* Honolulu: Enabling Systems.

Battersby, C., J. Armstrong, and M. Abrahams (1978). Mastectomy in a large public hospital. *Aust. N.Z. J. Surg.* 48:401–4.

Bernstein, W.C. (1972). Sexual dysfunction following radical surgery for cancer of rectum and sigmoid colon. *Med. Aspects Hum. Sexuality* 6(3):156–63.

Bernstein, W.C. and E.F. Bernstein (1966). Sexual dysfunction following radical surgery for cancer of the rectum. *Dis. Colon Rectum* 9:328–32.

Blake, D.J., C. McCartney, F.A. Fried, and L.G. Fehrenbaker (1983). Psychiatric assessment of penile implant recipient. *Urology* 21:252–56.

Bracken, R.B. and D.E. Johnson (1976). Sexual function and fecundity after treatment for testicular tumors. *Urology* 7:35–38.

Bransfield, D.D. (1983). Breast cancer and sexual functioning: A review of the literature and implications for future research. *Int. J. Psychiatry Med.* 12:197–211.

Brown, R.S., V. Haddox, A. Posado, and A. Rubio (1972). Social and psychological adjustment following pelvic exenteration. *Am. J. Obstet. Gynecol.* 114:162–71.

Bullard, D.G., G.G. Causey, A.B. Newman, R. Orloff, K. Schanche, and D.H. Wallace (1980). Sexual health care and cancer: A needs assessment. *Front. Radiat. Ther. Oncol.* 14:55–58.

Capone, M.A., K.S. Westie, and R.S. Good (1980). Sexual rehabilitation of the gynecologic cancer patient: An effective counseling model. *Front. Radiat. Ther. Oncol.* 14:123–29.

Chapman, R.M., S.B. Sutcliffe, and J.S. Malpas (1979). Cytotoxic-induced ovarian failure in Hodgkin's disease: II. Effects on sexual function. *J.A.M.A.* 242:1882–84.

Cobliner, W.G. (1977). Psychosocial factors in gynecologic or breast malignancies. *Hosp. Physician* 13:38–40.

Decker, W.H. and E. Schwartzman (1962). Sexual function following treatment for carcinoma of the cervix. *Am. J. Obstet. Gynecol.* 83:401–5.

Dempsey, G.M., H.J. Buchsbaum, and J. Morrison (1975). Psychosocial adjustment to pelvic exenteration. *Gynecol. Oncol.* 3:325–34.

Derogatis, L.R. (1980). Breast and gynecologic cancers: Their unique impact on body image and sexual identity in women. *Front. Radiat. Ther. Oncol.* 14:1–11.

Derogatis, L.R. and S.M. Kourlesis (1981). An approach to evaluation of sexual problems in the cancer patient. *CA* 31:46–50.

Di Saia, P.J., W.T. Creasman, and W.M. Rich (1979). An alternate approach to early cancer of the vulva. *Am. J. Obstet. Gynecol.* 133:825–32.

Dlin, B.M., A. Perlman, and E. Ringold (1969). Psychosexual response to ileostomy and colostomy. *Am. J. Psychiatry* 126:374–81.

Donahue, V.C. and R.C. Knapp (1977). Sexual rehabilitation of gynecologic cancer patients. *Obstet. Gynecol.* 49:118–21.

Druss, R.G., J.F. O'Connor, and L.O. Stern (1969). Psychologic response to colectomy: II. Adjustment to a permanent colostomy. *Arch. Gen. Psychiatry* 20:419–27.

Fisher, S.G. (1979). Psychosexual adjustment following total pelvic exenteration. *Cancer Nurs.* 2:219–25.

Frank, D., R.L. Dornbush, S.K. Webster, and R.C. Kolodny (1978). Mastectomy and sexual behavior: A pilot study. *Sexuality Disabil.* 1:16–26.

Frank, E., C. Anderson, and D. Rubinstein (1978). Frequency of sexual dysfunction in "normal" couples. *N. Engl. J. Med.* 299:111–15.

Goldstein, I., M. Feldman, P.J. Deckers, R.K. Babayan, and R.J. Krane (1984). Radiation-associated impotence: A clinical study of its mechanism. *J.A.M.A.* 251:903–10.

Good, R.S. and M. Capone (1980). Emotional considerations in the care of the gynecologic cancer patient. In D.D. Youngs and A.A. Erhardt (eds.), *Psychosomatic Obstetrics and Gynecology.* East Norwalk, Conn.: Appleton-Century-Crofts, pp. 117–25.

Herr, H. (1979). Preservation of sexual potency in prostatic cancer patients after [125]I implantation. *J. Am. Geriatr. Soc.* 27(1):17–19.

Hurny, C. and J.C. Holland (1985). Psychosocial sequelae of ostomies in cancer patients. *CA* 36:170–83.

Jamison, K.R., D.K. Wellisch, and R.O. Pasnau (1978). Psychosocial aspects of mastectomy: I. The women's perspective. *Am. J. Psychiatry* 135:432–36.

Kaplan, H.S. (1974). *The New Sex Therapy: Active Treatment of Sexual Dysfunctions.* New York: Brunner/Mazel.

Kaplan, H.S. (1979). *Problems of Sexual Desire.* New York: Brunner/Mazel.

Kaplan, H.S. (1983). *The Evaluation of Sexual Disorders.* New York: Brunner/Mazel.

Knorr, N.J. (1967). A depressive syndrome following pelvic exenteration and ileostomy. *Arch. Surg.* 94:258–60.

Lamb, M.A. and N.F. Woods (1981). Sexuality and the cancer patient. *Cancer Nurs.* 4:137–44.

Lamont, J.A., A.D. DePetrillo, and E.S. Sargent (1978). Psychosexual rehabilitation and exenterative surgery. *Gynecol. Oncol.* 6:236–42.

Leiber, L., M. Plumb, M.L. Gerstenzang, and J.C.B. Holland (1976). The communication of affection between cancer patients and their spouses. *Psychosom. Med.* 38(6):379–89.

Lewis, F.M. and J.R. Bloom (1978–1979). Psychological adjustment to breast cancer: A review of selected literature. *Int. J. Psychiatry Med.* 9:1–17.

Maguire, G.P., E.G. Lee, D.J. Bevington, C.S. Kuchemann, R.J. Crabtree, and C.E. Cornell (1978). Psychiatric problems in the first year after mastectomy. *Br. Med. J.* 1:963–65.

Masters, W.H. and V. Johnson (1966). *Human Sexual Response.* Boston: Little, Brown & Co.

Masters, W. and V. Johnson (1970). *Human Sexual Inadequacy.* Boston: Little, Brown & Co.

Metcalfe, M.C. and S.H. Fischman (1985). Factors affecting the sexuality of patients with head and neck cancer. *Oncol. Nurs. Forum* 12(2):21–25.

Meyerowitz, B.E. (1980). Psychosocial correlates of breast cancer and its treatment. *Psychol. Bull.* 87:108–31.

Morley, G.W. (1981). Cancer of the vulva: A review. *Cancer* 48:597–601.

Morley, G.W., S.M. Lindenauer, and D. Youngs (1973). Vaginal reconstruction following pelvic exenteration: Surgical and psychological considerations. *Am. J. Obstet. Gynecol.* 116:996–1002.

Narayan, P., P.H. Lange, and E.E. Fraley (1982). Ejaculation and fertility after extended retroperitoneal lymph node dissection for testicular cancer. *J. Urol.* 127:685–87.

*Proceedings of the Workshop on Psychosexual and Reproductive Issues Affecting Patients with Cancer*—1987. A Service and Rehabilitation Education Publication, American Cancer Society, Atlanta.

Rowland, J.H., J.D. Holland, E.R. Jacobs, T. Chaglassian, N. Geller, and G. Petroni (1984). Psychological response to breast reconstruction. Paper presented at the 137th Annu. Mtgs. Am. Psychiatric Assoc., Los Angeles, May.

Schain, W.S. (1980). Sexual functioning, self-esteem and cancer care. *Front. Radiat. Ther. Oncol.* 14:12–19.

Schain, W.S. and S.S. Howards (1985). Sexual problems of patients with cancer. In V. DeVita, Jr., S. Heilman, and S.A. Rosenberg (eds.), *Cancer Principles and Practice of Oncology,* 2nd ed. Philadelphia: Lippincott, pp. 2066–82.

Schain, W.S., D.K. Wellisch, R.O. Pasnau, and J. Landsverk (1985). The sooner the better: A study of psychologic factors in women undergoing immediate versus delayed breast reconstruction. *Am. J. Psychiatry* 142:40–46.

Schover, L.R. and M. Fife (1985). Sexual counseling of patients undergoing radical surgery for pelvic or genital cancer. *J. Psychosoc. Oncol.* 3:21–41.

Schover, L.R., and A.C. von Eschenbach (1984). Sexual and marital counseling with men treated for testicular cancer. *J. Sex Marital Ther.* 10:29–40.

Schover, L.R., A.C. von Eschenbach, D.R. Smith, and J. Gonzalez (1984). Sexual rehabilitation of urologic cancer patients: A practical approach. *CA* 34:3–11.

Schover, L.R. (1987). Sexuality and fertility in urologic cancer patients. *Cancer* 60:553–558.

Schover, L.R. (1988). *Sexuality and Cancer for the Woman Who Has Cancer, and Her Partner* and *Sexuality and Cancer for the Man Who Has Cancer and His Partner.* New York: American Cancer Society.

Seibel, M.M., M.G. Freeman, W.L. Graves (1980). Carcinoma of the cervix and sexual function. *Obstet. Gynecol.* 55:484–87.

Sewell, H.H. and D.W. Edwards (1980). Pelvic genital cancer: Body image and sexuality. *Front. Radiat. Ther. Oncol.* 14:35–41.

Shipes, E. and S. Lehr (1982). Sexuality and the male cancer patient. *Cancer Nurs.* 5:375–81.

Stellman, R.E., J.M. Goodwin, J. Robinson, D. Dansak, and R.D. Hilgers (1984). Psychological effects of vulvectomy. *Psychosomatics* 25:779–83.

Stoudemire, A., T. Techman, and S. Graham (1985). Sexual assessment of the urologic oncology patient. *Psychosomatics* 26:405–10.

Sutherland, A.M., C.E. Orbach, R.B. Dyk, and M. Bard (1952). The psychological impact of cancer and cancer surgery: I. Adaptation to the dry colostomy: Preliminary report and summary of findings. *Cancer* 5:857–72.

Sutcliffe, S.B. (1987). Clinical Problems and Their Management. Female Patients—Lymphoma Proc. of the Workshop on Psychosexual and Reproductive Issues Affecting Patients with Cancer. A Service and Rehabilitation 72–73. Education Publication Atlanta American Cancer Society 72–74.

Vaeth, J.M. (ed.). (1986). *Body Image, Self-Esteem, and Sexuality in Cancer Patients,* 2nd ed. Basel: Karger.

Vera, M.I. (1981). Quality of life following pelvic exenteration. *Gynecol. Oncol.* 12:355–66.

Vincent, C.E., B. Vincent, F.C. Greiss, and E.B. Linton (1975). Some marital-sexual concomitants of carcinoma of the cervix. *South. Med. J.* 68:552–58.

von Eschenbach, A.C. and L.R. Schover (1984). The role of sexual rehabilitation in the treatment of patients with cancer. *Cancer* 54:2662–67.

Walbroehl, G.S. (1985). Sexuality in cancer patients. *Am. Fam. Physician* 31:153–58.

Schultz, W.C.M., K. Wijma, H.B.M. Van De Wiel, J. Bouma, and J. Janssens (1986). Sexual rehabilitation of radical vulvectomy patients: A pilot study. *J. Psychosom. Obstet. Gynecol.* 5:119–26.

Weinberg, P.C. (1974). Psychosexual impact of treatment in female genital cancer. *J. Sex Marital Ther.* 1:155–57.

Wellisch, D.K., K.R. Jamison, and R.O. Pasnau (1978). Psychosocial aspects of mastectomy: II. The man's perspective. *Am. J. Psychiatry* 135:543–46.

Wise, T.N. (1978). Effects of cancer on sexual activity. *Psychosomatics* 19:769–75.

Wise, T.N. (1983). Sexual dysfunction in the medically ill. *Psychosomatics* 24:787–805.

Witkin, M.H. and H.S. Kaplan (1982). Sex therapy and penectomy. *J. Sex Marital Ther.* 8:209–21.

Yeager, E.S. and J.A. van Heerden (1980). Sexual dysfunction following proctocolectomy and abdominoperineal resection. *Ann. Surg.* 191:169–70.

# 34

# Nausea and Vomiting: Physiology and Pharmacological Management

Lynna M. Lesko

Nausea and vomiting constitute a frequent, and sometimes profoundly distressing, side effect of cancer and chemotherapy (Laszlo and Lucas, 1981). If untreated, vomiting leads to dehydration, disturbances in serum electrolytes, malnutrition, metabolic imbalance, aspiration pneumonia, and occasionally esophageal tears (Mallory–Weiss syndrome). Physicians sometimes are forced to reduce the optimal dose of a chemotherapeutic regimen because of nausea or vomiting. If these side effects remain severe and are left untreated, the intolerable quality of life will lead some patients to abandon traditional treatment and seek out unproven remedies that may result in shortened survival. Considerable effort in medical oncology has gone into finding safe and effective antiemetics to ensure patients' ability to tolerate curative treatment regimens. This area has emerged as a critical component of supportive care and research.

The physiology of vomiting is well known. Controlled by the vomiting center in the medullary reticular formation, the response is influenced by receptors in the cerebral cortex, the chemoreceptor trigger zone (CRTZ), and in the periphery. This vomiting center coordinates the intricate act of emesis, including salivation, diaphragmatic contraction, breath holding, contraction of the abdominal muscles, and the retching reflex. The nausea and vomiting experienced secondary to chemotherapeutic treatment, however, are complex; the mechanisms are described here.

## PHYSIOLOGICAL MECHANISMS OF NAUSEA AND VOMITING

The physiological mechanism of the ''vomiting reflex'' has been thoroughly documented in the physiology literature (Borison and Wong, 1953; Harris, 1978; Laszlo, 1983). It begins with the sensation of nausea (salivation, cold sweat, gastric relaxation, ta-

chycardia, diarrhea, and swallowing). Nausea always precedes vomiting, except in the unusual circumstance of explosive vomiting. Physiological, behavioral, and psychological input contribute to its development.

Emesis, or vomiting–retching, is controlled by the vomiting center located in the dorsolateral reticular region of the medulla, and is triggered by afferent input to this center that converge from the several areas listed here.

*Viscera.* The upper GI tract sends afferent impulses to the CNS via sympathetic and vagal stimulation. Clinical situations that stimulate that route are myocardial infarction, certain drugs, bacterial toxins, irradiation, chemotherapy drugs (in particular nitrogen mustard and cisplatin), and metastatic disease to certain sites in the GI tract.

*Chemoreceptor trigger zone (CRTZ).* Bacterial toxins, metabolic products (e.g., uremia or diabetic acidosis), and most important, chemotherapeutic agents and irradiation, produce emesis by stimulating the CRTZ located in the area postrema of the fourth ventricle. The CRTZ in turn activates the ''vomiting center,'' and emesis follows. This is the classic pathway of the apomorphine-induced vomiting paradigm. Emesis mediated by the CRTZ may involve dopaminergic pathways. This fact has been the basis for the major class of drugs used in pharmacological management of vomiting (i.e., those drugs causing dopamine receptor blockade).

*Other areas.* The limbic system, diencephalon, and areas of higher cortical function also play an important role in the vomiting reflex. Tastes, smell, increased intracranial pressure, and psychogenic stimuli can each contribute to and evoke the vomiting response. Anticipatory nausea and vomiting develop through this last pathway and are described in greater detail by Redd in Chapter 35.

In summary, stimuli from a number of different

**Table 34-1** Common causes of nausea and vomiting in the cancer patient

| Cause | Examples |
|---|---|
| Physiological-metabolic | Bowel obstruction |
| | Uremia |
| | Hepatic dysfunction |
| | CNS disorders (tumor, metastases, increased intracranial pressure) |
| | Fluid and electrolyte imbalance |
| | High fever |
| | Endocrine abnormalities |
| Treatment-related | Chemotherapeutic agents |
| | Radiation |
| | Analgesics |
| | Antibiotics |
| Psychological (?physiological) | Anticipatory nausea and vomiting |
| | Anxiety |
| | Anorexia nervosa, bulimia |

**Table 34-2** Chemotherapy agents causing nausea and vomiting

| Agents | Degree of nausea and vomiting |
|---|---|
| Cisplatin | Severe |
| Dacarbazine (DTIC) | |
| Actinomycin-D | |
| Intravenous alkylating agents | |
| Nitrosureas | |
| Anthracyclines | |
|   Doxorubicin | |
|   Daunorubicin | |
| Cyclophosphamide | Moderate |
| Procarbazine | |
| Mitomycin-C | |
| Cytosine arabinoside | |
| Etoposide | |
| Methotrexate | Mild |
| 5-FU | |
| Vinca alkaloids | |
| Bleomycin | |
| 6-Mercaptopurine | |

*Source*: Modified after Gralla (1983).

areas can initiate nausea and emesis via the physiological routes outlined.

## ETIOLOGY OF NAUSEA AND VOMITING IN THE CANCER PATIENT

The common causes of nausea and vomiting in the oncological patient are physiological metabolic, treatment-related, and psychological (Frytak, 1981, 1983) (see Table 34-1).

Metabolic and physiological causes of vomiting are usually clear-cut and easily identified but perplexing to treat. They include bowel obstruction due to tumor, metastasis, or mechanical, drug-related ileus (as seen with use of anticholinergic agents), metabolic abnormalities (e.g., uremia, hepatic dysfunction, fluid and electrolyte imbalance, high fever, and ketoacidosis), endocrine dysfunction (e.g., adrenocortical insufficiency and hypercalcemia), and CNS complications related to primary brain tumor, metastasis, or increased intracranial pressure. Cancer patients are also susceptible to the usual causes of vomiting unrelated to cancer; these should never be overlooked. They include gastritis, gastric ulcers, pancreatitis, renal or biliary colic, and myocardial infarction.

Treatment-related nausea or vomiting is one of the most common problems faced by the cancer patient. Chemotherapeutic agents, radiation, analgesics and intravenous antibiotics elicit mild to severe nausea or vomiting. Table 34-2 lists cytoreductive agents commonly used in cancer patients by their relative potential for producing emesis (Gralla, 1983; Laszlo, 1983). The route of administration, dosage, and individual

variation among patients and treatment cycles also affect the incidence and severity of emesis. Emesis usually occurs 1–3 hours after chemotherapy, although there are exceptions to this general pattern; emesis from cyclophosphamide may be delayed 12 or more hours after administration. Chemotherapeutic agents also vary in their route of emetic action. For example, cisplatin, a highly emetic chemotherapeutic agent, acts primarily on the GI tract, producing vomiting via transmission from the vagus nerve to the CRTZ, while 5-fluorouracil (5-FU) elicits vomiting by direct stimulation of the CRTZ. Pharmacological agents offer the primary means of control of chemotherapy-related emesis (see Tables 34-3 and 34-4); behavioral interventions are rapidly finding an adjunctive but important role in management.

Psychological and behavioral causes of nausea or vomiting are also common and frustrating to treat. Nausea and vomiting in anticipation of chemotherapy (following a classical behavioral conditioning paradigm), discussed more extensively in the next chapter, are far more common than is often appreciated (Morrow, 1982; Pratt et al., 1984). Anticipatory nausea and vomiting can occur hours before a patient actually receives chemotherapy and are frequently encountered by patients who receive repeated cycles of a chemotherapy regimen, usually developing after three to four treatments that have been accompanied by vomiting. Patients most likely to develop anticipatory symptoms are those who receive a highly emetogenic cytoreduc-

**Table 34-3**  Management of treatment-induced emesis in cancer patients

| Management | Examples |
|---|---|
| Pharmacological | Dopamine antagonists (chlorpromazine, prochlorperazine, metoclopramide, haloperidol) |
| | Anticholinergic agents and antihistamines (hydroxyzine, diphenhydramine) |
| | Adrenergic stimulants (dextroamphetamine, ephedrine) |
| | Cannabinoids (THC) |
| | Benzodiazepines (lorazepam) |
| | Steroids (dexamethasone, methylprednisolone) |
| Behavioral treatment | Relaxation |
| | Desensitization |
| | Distraction |

**Table 34-4**  Frequently used antiemetic agents

| Agent class | Examples |
|---|---|
| Dopamine antagonists | Chlorpromazine (Thorazine) |
| | Prochlorperazine (Compazine) |
| | Metoclopramide (Reglan) |
| | Haloperidol (Haldol) |
| Adjuvant | |
| Anticholinergic and/or antihistaminic | Hydroxyzine pamoate (Vistaril) |
| | Diphenhydramine (Benedryl) |
| Adrenergic stimulants | Dextroamphetamine (Dexedrine) |
| | Ephedrine |
| Cannabinoids | $\Delta^9$-Tetrahydrocannabinol (THC) |
| Benzodiazepines | Lorazepam (Ativan) |
| Steroids | Dexamethasone (Decadron) |
| | Methylprednisolone (Solumedrol) |

tive regimen, those who experience severe posttreatment nausea and vomiting, and those who have high levels of anxiety and/or who develop alterations of taste and smell associated with the chemotherapy infusion. Studies at Memorial Sloan-Kettering Cancer Center of long-term survivors of Hodgkin's disease reveal that anticipatory nausea and vomiting is experienced not only during active treatment, but similar sensations of nausea and anxiety can be elicited as long as 10 years after treatment has been completed in response to smells and sights that remind the individual of the clinic and the chemotherapy (Cella et al., 1986). Present treatment approaches to this phenomenon include use of agents with antiemetic properties (butyrophenones and phenothiazines), and the use of anxiolytics. Alprazolam appears to be quite effective given 12–24 hours before treatment. Some have found the simultaneous infusion of lorazepam during chemotherapy helpful. While serving as a sedative, this drug also produces retrograde amnesia for the experience, thus eliminating recall of the treatment-related stimulus and avoiding the conditioned response. Behavior therapy has been introduced more recently to control anticipatory responses (see Chapter 35 by Redd for a detailed review of research and techniques in this area).

Nausea and vomiting may result from a number of other psychological causes. Anxiety related to unfamiliar treatments (e.g., radiation equipment, intravenous infusions, and new procedures) can be extreme enough to produce nausea. It is well managed by anxiolytics such as alprazolam, lorazepam, or diazepam.

There will, of course, be an occasional patient who develops cancer in the context of a preexisting psychiatric eating disorder in which one of the symptoms is

vomiting, such as anorexia nervosa or bulimia. Secondary eating disorders and anorexia nervosa develop rarely in young adult cancer patients. We have reported two cases. One was a young woman with acute nonlymphocytic leukemia treated by bone marrow transplantation (BMT). She developed severe secondary anorexia nervosa 6 months after BMT; symptoms continued for 2 years until she died of opportunistic infections. The second case was a Hodgkin's disease survivor who, though healthy and considered "cured," developed symptoms of anorexia nervosa several months after completion of her treatment regimen.

Because early satiety is a feature of advanced cancer, large meals can contribute to anorexia and nausea. Concern about weight loss and concerns about adequate intake can also produce anxiety and related nausea. Frequent, small, and visually appealing meals may result in less nausea and higher caloric intake.

The remainder of this chapter focuses on the psychopharmacological management of nausea and vomiting.

## PHARMACOLOGICAL MANAGEMENT

There are several classes of pharmacological agents with proven efficacy in the management of chemotherapy-related nausea and vomiting. They are phenothiazines, butyrophenones, cannabinoids, steroids, antihistamines, and anxiolytics. Table 34-5 gives the dosage, route, side effects, and site of action of the commonly used drugs. Each requires proper schedule and dosage to be effective. In addition, patients vary in their response so that no one drug or dosage can be assumed to be best for all patients.

The choice of antiemetic agent depends on the etiology of the symptoms, the emetogenic potential of the chemotherapy agent and its method of action (in the case of chemotherapy-related emesis), route of administration and side effects of the antiemetic agent, and concurrent medical problems.

Emesis and nausea secondary to physiological or metabolic causes is best treated by correcting the underlying cause, for example treating a fluid or electrolyte imbalance, hepatic dysfunction, uremia, or bowel obstruction. Often in these circumstances physicians are reluctant to use pharmacological agents to reduce nausea and vomiting, because the symptoms are used to monitor progression of the disease process, and side effects of drugs can confuse the clinical picture. In this situation, antihistamines are the safest agents for temporary control.

The most commonly used chemotherapy agents can be ranked in order of their relative emetogenicity (Table 34-2). The agents that produce the most severe nausea and vomiting (cisplatin, dacarbazine, actinomycin-D, doxorubicin) require a strong antiemetic regimen composed of several agents that are usually begun before the administration of the chemotherapeutic drugs for the most effective control of the nausea and vomiting.

Certain patients, because of their concurrent medical problems, need special attention to the route of administration of drugs to control nausea and vomiting. Many patients receive their chemotherapy through a Broviac or Hickman catheter or heparin lock, making the intravenous route easily available. This route is indicated in patients with severe nausea and vomiting or in those whose hematological picture prohibits subcutaneous or intramuscular administration. When an oral route is impossible and intravenous or intramuscular administration is impractical, rectal suppositories are useful (see Table 34-5).

## Dopamine Antagonists

Phenothiazines have been the most widely employed antiemetic agents among the dopamine antagonists that have been most effective in emesis control. In fact, prochlorperazine has been the gold standard against which new agents have been tested in clinical trials. Phenothiazines produce their antiemetic effects by partial inhibition of the CRTZ via their antidopaminergic properties. They are effective for patients receiving nitrosureas and methotrexate, but they are usually ineffective when used alone in patients receiving the most highly emetogenic chemotherapeutic agent, cisplatin. To utilize the antiemetic properties of the phenothiazines, the higher dose range also produces extrapyramidal side effects of muscle rigidity, acute dystonia, akathesia, cogwheeling, and akinesia. Table 34-5 outlines the use of neuroleptics as antiemetics and their side effects. They are administered in oral (po, tablet and elixir), parenteral (im or iv) and rectal sup-

pository forms. Each is useful in specific clinical situations. The parenteral (iv) route is utilized in hospitalized patients who are under close supervision, especially those with low platelet counts who always require intravenous administration. The most practical route is oral (e.g., pills, capsules, or elixir) for long-term and outpatient treatment.

Rectal administration of phenothiazines should be reserved for patients in whom emesis or physiological conditions prohibits oral administration and when parenteral routes are impractical. The efficacy of most rectal preparations is variable and unreliable and should be limited to terminal patients at home with very low platelet counts or to other patients in the hospital in whom there is no intravenous or oral route available. In summary, the oral route is the most practical and economical for long-term antiemetic control. It should be noted, however, that expensive, slow-release forms of oral dosage add no special advantage in symptom relief.

Metoclopramide, a procainamide derivative and CNS dopamine antagonist with peripheral GI cholinergic effects, was used for years in low dosage in diabetic patients to increase the tone of the lower esophageal sphincter, promote gastric emptying, and stimulate motility of the upper GI tract. It has been found in high-dose intravenous use to be highly effective in controlling chemotherapy-related emesis (Albibi and McCallum, 1983). Metoclopramide exerts its antiemetic effects by blocking dopamine receptors in the CRTZ of the medulla. Given over 15 minutes at a dosage of 2 mg/kg iv 30 minutes prior to chemotherapy and repeated every 2 hours for two to five doses (a level 10 times higher than previously used), it is effective in control of vomiting with the highly emetogenic agent, cisplatin. It was significantly more effective when compared to chlorpromazine (3.0 mg/kg) or haloperidol (1.0 mg/kg) in clinical trials (Gralla et al., 1981; Strum et al., 1984).

Of diagnostic concern to the psychiatric consultant are the common extrapyramidal system (EPS) side effects of high-dose metoclopramide. The earliest signs are anxiety, restlessness, pacing, and agitation that may initially be assumed to be functional in origin. Later signs of acute dystonia, akathesia, and muscle rigidity may also develop. Tardive dyskinesia has been observed by our group and others in patients following oral and intravenous metoclopramide administration during cyclic chemotherapy (Breitbart, 1986; Lazzara et al., 1986). The EPS (dystonia) can usually be controlled by antiparkinsonian or antihistamine drugs, but it may be necessary to lower dosages or switch to another antiemetic.

Butyrophenones, especially haloperidol, whose primary use has been as an antipsychotic, are potent in-

**Table 34-5** Characteristics of antiemetic drugs

| Drug | Dosage and route | | | | Side effects | Site of action |
|---|---|---|---|---|---|---|
| | po | im | iv | pr* | | |
| *Dopamine antagonists* | | | | | Sedation EPS‡ symptoms, agitation, hypotension | *CRTZ*: block dopamine receptors |
| Chlorpromazine (Thorazine)† | 10 mg q6h | 25 mg | | | | |
| Prochlorperazine (Compazine)† | 10 mg | 20 mg | 10 mg | 25 mg bid | | |
| Haloperidol (Haldol)† | 1–3 mg q3h | 1–2 mg q3h | 1–2 mg q3h | | | |
| Droperidol (Inapsine) | | 0.5–2.5 mg before chemotherapy | 0.5–2.5 mg before chemotherapy | | | |
| Metoclopramide (Reglan) | | 1–2 mg/kg 30 minutes before and 10 minutes after chemotherapy | | | | *Periphery*: ↓ Abdominal distension; ↑ gastric emptying; ↑ GI motility; ↓ gastroesophageal sphincter tone; *CRTZ*: block dopamine receptors |
| *Adjuvant* | | | | | | |
| Anticholinergic and antihistaminic | | | | | Sedation | *Vomiting center*: ↓ Activation |

| Drug | | | | Side effects | Mechanism |
|---|---|---|---|---|---|
| Hydroxyzine pamoate (Vistaril) | 25 mg q3h | 25 mg q3h | 25 mg q3h | | |
| Diphenhydramine (Benadryl)† | 50–75 mg q3h | 25–50 mg q3h | 25–50 mg q3h | Patch | *Periphery:* ↑ gastroesophageal sphincter tone; ↓ retrograde motility. *CRTZ to vomiting center:* Block |
| Adrenergic | | | | | |
| Dextroamphetamine (Dexedrine)† | 5 mg | | | Agitation | Stabilization of vomiting center. *Pathways from CRTZ to vomiting center:* adrenergic tone |
| Cannabinoids | | | | | |
| Δ⁹-Tetrahydrocannabinol (THC) | 7.5–15 mg (5–10 mg/m²) 2 h before and q3–4 h for 24–48 | | | Sedation, dry mouth, agitation, ataxia, depersonalization | ↑ Threshold of vomiting center |
| Benzodiazepines | | | | | |
| Lorazepam (Ativan) | 1–8 mg × 2 | 4–5 mg × 1 (0.05–1 mg/kg) 30 minutes before chemotherapy | | Sedation | *CNS:* Sedation, amnesia |
| Steroids | | | | | |
| Dexamethasone (Decadron) | 3–10 mg × 2 | 10–20 mg before and 10–20 mg q6h × 4 | | Agitation, mood changes | Prostaglandin synthesis |
| Methylprednisolone (Solumedrol) | | 200–500 mg q6h × 4 | | | |

*Rectal suppository
†Elixir form available.
‡Extrapyramidal system.

hibitors of the CRTZ. Haloperidol at 1–3 mg/day has shown significant postoperative antiemetic activity. However, its effect against the highly emetogenic drugs such as doxorubicin and cisplatin has not been substantiated in controlled studies, although it is used in some combination drug regimens. Droperidol at 0.5–2.5 mg 30 minutes to 1 hour before and 4–6 hours after the administration of chemotherapy agents has been used with some success as an antiemetic. They also cause EPS side effects.

## Adjuvant Antiemetics

Antihistamines (diphenhydramine) or anticholinergics (hydroxyzine), commonly used in labyrinthine-induced vomiting or motion sickness, have a minor role in the management of oncological patients with treatment-induced emesis. They are inferior to the more commonly used phenothiazines, but are widely used in control of metabolically related symptoms of nausea and vomiting. They are most valued for their relative safety in seriously ill patients.

The cannabinoids, $\Delta^9$-tetrahydrocannabinol (THC) and synthetic cannabinols such as nabilone, have proved to have superior antiemetic efficacy for use with several chemotherapeutic agents (e.g., high-dose methotrexate) when compared to placebo. However, their efficacy is selective, with poorer patient response to cisplatin, doxorubicin, and cyclophosphamide (Carey et al., 1983; Lucas and Laszlo, 1980; Sallen et al., 1980). It is felt that the cannabinoids act centrally to raise the nausea–vomiting threshold of the emetic center. The average oral THC dose is 5–10 mg/m$^2$ (7.5–15 mg) taken 2 hours before chemotherapy and also repeated every 3–4 hours for 24–48 hours. Side effects are considerable for many patients, especially older ones who complain of dysphoria and confusion. Some authors feel that smoking marijuana is more effective and reliable in that intestinal absorption of the pill is incomplete and drug delivery via inhalation is more efficient.

Other antiemetic agents are adrenergic steroids, stimulants, and benzodiazepines. Steroids have proved to be an effective antiemetic when used in conjunction with other agents, appearing to enhance the antiemetic effects of the other drugs given at the same time. Dexamethasone at 3–10 mg im or iv or methylprednisolone at 200–500 mg iv has some antiemetic activity alone. As noted earlier, parenteral (iv) lorazepam used prior to or concurrently with the infusion of chemotherapy, and in combination with other antiemetics, reduces vomiting and produces a mild amnesia for the noxious episodes, and thus offers a way to inhibit the development of anticipatory nausea and vomiting (Bishop et al., 1984).

## Combination Regimens

The most effective regimens for emesis control currently combine several agents (Gralla, 1983; Fiore et al., 1985). Designed for highly emetogenic chemotherapy protocols, usually containing cisplatin, these regimens generally involve a combination of a dopamine antagonist, a steroid, and an anxiolytic. The combination of metoclopramide, dexamethasone, and lorazepam has been found to be highly effective for the more toxic chemotherapy regimens (Strum et al., 1984; Gagen et al., 1984). As illustrated in Fig. 34-1, the medications in the combination regimens are begun orally a few hours before chemotherapy, continued by intravenous iv infusion just prior to and during treatment, then continued orally 24–36 hours after completion of the chemotherapy infusion. In the protocol developed by Gagen and colleagues (1984), the dexamethasone may be given orally as early as the night before (see in Fig. 34-1B). Researchers are actively exploring new analogs and new combinations of presently used antiemetics.

One of the advances in research in this area is the development of several standardized methods for measuring nausea and vomiting. The new instrumentation has added to the quality and sophistication of the research in this supportive care area. Clinical trials of antiemetic agents have benefited by the incorporation of standardized scales that permit more valid comparison of study results. These scales are described in articles by Rhodes and colleagues (1984), Morrow and Morrell (1982), and Redd and Andrykowski (1982).

## Side Effects of Antiemetic Medication

There are two major side effects of antiemetic agents. An anticholinergic crisis can be seen with diphenhydramine. It is most often seen in the elderly patient or the cancer patient who is receiving other medications with anticholinergic properties in whom an additive effect occurs. The second major side effect is extrapyramidal (EPS) movement disorders seen with the dopamine antagonist drugs, the phenothiazines, butyrophenones, and metoclopramide. Sedation, EPS signs of acute dystonias (oculogyric crisis, trismus, opisthotonos, or respiratory stridor), tardive dyskinesia, parkinsonian symptoms (cogwheeling rigidity), and akathesia are similar to those seen with neuroleptic use in schizophrenia. The higher potency neuroleptics such as haloperidol and metoclopramide produce more EPS side effects. All of these neurological side effects occur more often in the very young or very old patient and disappear after the antiemetic is stopped. Acute symptoms of dystonia and sometimes akathesia are relived within minutes by di-

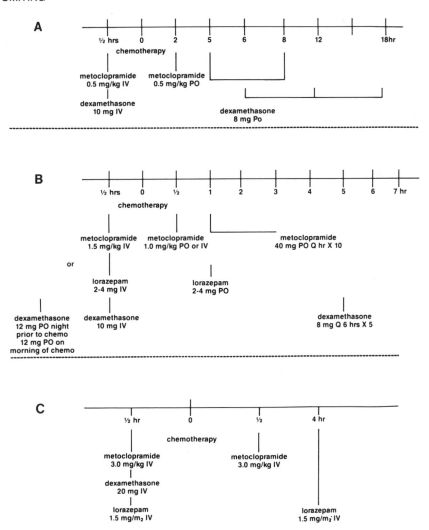

**Figure 34-1.** Combination antiemetic regimens. (A) From Strum et al. (1984); (B) from Gagen et al. (1984); (C) from Fiore et al. (1985).

phenhydramine (Benadryl) 25–50 mg iv or im, or ben-zotropine mesylate (Cogentin) 1–2 mg po. With pro-longed use of the dopamine antagonist antiemetic agents, tardive dyskinesia may develop. These invol-untary movements usually involve the tongue, lips, and face and improve after patients have stopped the drug (Breitbart, 1986).

Phenothiazines that have a piperazine moiety, (i.e. prochlorperazine (Compazine) and perphenazine (Tri-lafon)), are usually associated with less hypotensive side effects and more potential for antiemetic qualities. Those phenothiazines with an alkyl chain, however, such as chlorpromazine (Thorazine) and promethazine (Phenergan), produce more hypotensive sequelae.

THC should not be considered a first-line antiemetic medication because it has a few undesirable psycho-logical side effects in dosage sufficient to control emesis. However, cannabinoids may be an appropriate option in some younger patients who may prefer to smoke marijuana or in those who can tolerate the side effects of ataxia, dry mouth, and sedation produced by THC. Depersonalization, agitation, and psychotic symptoms of paranoia and hallucinations are a few of the side effects usually seen in patients requiring high-er dosage to control emesis, in the elderly, or in pa-tients with preexisting psychiatric disorders.

## SUMMARY

In summary, chemotherapy-related nausea and vomit-ing remain major but increasingly effectively con-trolled side effects of cancer therapy. Treatment of this problem has proved to be an important new application of psychotropic drugs in oncology and continues to be an exciting research area. However, for some patients, aversion to drugs that control nausea and vomiting makes behavioral intervention, especially for the anticipatory symptoms of nausea, of considerable interest. Research in this area is described in the following chapter (chapter 35).

## REFERENCES

Albibi, R. and R.W. McCallum (1983). Metoclopramide: Pharmacology and clinical application. *Ann. Intern. Med.* 98:86–95.

Bishop, J.F., I.N. Oliver, M.M. Wolf, J.P. Matthews, M. Long, J. Bingham, B.L. Hillcoat, and I.A. Cooper (1984). Lorazepam: A randomized, double-blind, crossover study of a new antiemetic in patients receiving cytotoxic chemotherapy and prochlorperazine. *J. Clin. Oncol.* 2:691–95.

Borison, H.L. and S.C. Wong (1953). Physiology and pharmacology of vomiting. *Pharmacol. Rev.* 5:193–230.

Breitbart, W. (1986). Tardive dyskinesia associated with high-dose intravenous metoclopramide. *N. Engl. J. Med.* 315:518.

Carey, M.P., T. Burish, and D. Brenner (1983). Delta-9-Tetrahydrocannabinol in cancer chemotherapy: Research problems and issues. *Ann. Intern. Med.* 99:106–14.

Cella, D.F., A. Pratt, and J.C. Holland (1986). Persistent anticipatory nausea, vomiting and anxiety in cured Hodgkin's disease patients after completion of chemotherapy. *Am. J. Psychiatry* 143:641–43.

Fiore, J.J., R.J. Gralla, M.G. Kris, R.A. Clark, L.B. Tyson, and P. Hetzel (1985). The effects of adding lorazepam to metroclopramide plus dexamethasone in patients receiving cisplatin. *Proc. Twenty-First Annu. Mtg. Am. Soc. Clin. Oncol.* 4:266 (Abstract No. C1036).

Frytak, S. (1981). Management of nausea and vomiting in the cancer patient. *J.A.M.A.* 245:393–96.

Frytak, S. (1983). Management of nausea and vomiting in the cancer patient. In R.J. Gralla (ed.), *Supportive Care of the Cancer Patient*. Proceedings from a symposium sponsored by Memorial Sloan-Kettering Cancer Center, New York, February 25, 1983. New York: Biomedical Information, pp. 18–21.

Gagen, M., D. Gochnour, D. Young, T. Gaginella, and J. Neidhart (1984). A randomized trial of metoclopramide and combination of dexamethasone and lorazepam for prevention of chemotherapy-induced vomiting. *J. Clin. Oncol.* 2:696–701.

Gralla, R.J. (1983). Metoclopramide as an antiemetic agent.

In R.J. Gralla (ed.), *Supportive Care of the Cancer Patient*. Proceedings from a symposium sponsored by Memorial Sloan-Kettering Cancer Center, New York, February 25, 1983. New York: Biomedical Information, pp. 25–32.

Gralla, R.J., L.M. Itri, S.E. Pisko, A.E. Squillante, D.P. Kelsen, D.W. Braun, L.A. Bordin, T.J. Braun, and C.W. Young (1981). Antimetic efficacy of high-dose metoclopramide: Randomized trials with placebo and prochlorperazine in patients with chemotherapy-induced nausea and vomiting. *N. Engl. J. Med.* 305:905–9.

Harris, J.G. (1978). Nausea, vomiting and cancer treatment. *CA* 4:194–201.

Laszlo, J. (ed.). (1983). *Antiemetics and Cancer Chemotherapy*. Baltimore: Williams & Wilkins.

Laszlo, J. and V.S. Lucas (1981). Emesis as a critical problem in chemotherapy. *N. Engl. J. Med.* 305:948–49.

Lazzara, R.R., A. Stoudemire, D. Manning, and K.C. Prewitt (1986). Metoclopramide-induced tardive dyskinesia: A case report. *Gen. Hosp. Psychiatry* 8:107–9.

Lucas, V.S. and J. Laszlo (1980). Delta-9-Tetrahydrocannabinol for refractory vomiting induced by cancer chemotherapy. *J.A.M.A.* 243:1241–43.

Morrow, G.R. (1982). Prevalence and correlates of anticipatory nausea and vomiting in chemotherapy patients. *J.N.C.I.* 60:585–88.

Morrow, G.R. and C. Morrell (1982). Behavioral treatment for the anticipatory nausea and vomiting induced by cancer chemotherapy. *N. Engl. J. Med.* 307:1476–80.

Pratt, A., R. Lazar, D. Penman, and J. Holland (1984). Psychological parameters of chemotherapy-induced conditioned nausea and vomiting: A review. *Cancer Nurs.* 1:483–90.

Redd, W.H. and M.A. Andrykowski (1982). Behavioral intervention in cancer treatment: Controlling aversion reactions to chemotherapy. *J. Consult. Clin. Psychol.* 50:1018–29.

Rhodes, V.A., P.M. Watson, and M.H. Johnson (1984). Development of reliable and valid measurements of nausea and vomiting. *Cancer Nurs.* 7:33–41.

Sallen, S.E., C. Cronin, M. Zelen, and N.E. Zinberg (1980). Antiemetics in patients receiving chemotherapy for cancer: A randomized comparison of Delta-9-Tetrahydrocannabinol and prochlorperazine. *N. Engl. J. Med.* 302:135–38.

Strum, S.B., J.E. McDermed, B.R. Steng, and N.M. McDermott (1984). Combination metoclopramide and dexamethasone: An effective antiemetic regimen in outpatients receiving non-cisplatin chemotherapy. *J. Clin. Oncol.* 2:1057–63.

# 35

# Management of Anticipatory Nausea and Vomiting

William H. Redd

During the protracted course of chemotherapy, between 25 and 65% of patients become sensitized to treatment and develop phobiclike reactions. They report being nauseated in anticipation of treatment. There are patients who begin vomiting as they enter the oncology clinic or as the nurse cleans their skin with alcohol in preparation for the infusion. In some instances the mere thought of treatment makes them nauseated. These reactions represent learned aversions and result from automatic conditioning processes.

In this chapter we examine anticipatory side effects of chemotherapy and describe nonpharmacological behavioral methods of controlling them. The discussion begins with a brief description of the development of anticipatory side effects and then shifts to prevalence and the variables that influence it. Attention is also given to the mechanisms underlying the development of these side effects. Five behavioral procedures (passive relaxation with imagery, active relaxation with imagery, biofeedback with imagery, systematic desensitization, and cognitive-attentional distraction) used to control anticipatory side effects are presented and evaluated. The chapter ends with an examination of clinical issues encountered in the implementation of behavioral procedures to control aversive side effects of cancer treatment.

## ANTICIPATION REACTIONS

Patients beginning chemotherapy are typically apprehensive; most have heard stories about the horrors of ''chemo'' (a term now well known to many nonmedical people). Their fears are only heightened as a clinic nurse or oncologist lists the possible side effects of treatment. Some clinicians maintain that many patients are ''primed'' for problems, starting the first course of treatment with the clear expectation that treatment is going to be tough. This hypothesis is supported by empirical evidence indicating that patient expectations at the beginning of treatment are predictive of the severity of both anticipatory and posttreatment side effects later in the course of treatment (Jacobsen, et al., 1988; Andrykowski, et al., 1988), that is to say, patients who expect to experience nausea and vomiting with treatment are more likely to do so than patients who do not believe that treatment will be difficult. For most patients the first infusion is actually easier to tolerate than they had expected. Except with the most toxic protocols, patients typically experience only mild posttreatment nausea and vomiting following their first infusion. But, as the course of treatment continues with weekly or bimonthly infusions, patients begin to notice side effects (e.g., hair loss, and nausea and vomiting). Unfortunately with subsequent infusions these side effects generally become more severe.

For some patients the situation becomes worse, such that any event or stimulus that is repeatedly associated with posttreatment side effects becomes an elicitor of anticipatory reactions. The likelihood that a particular stimulus will require nausea-eliciting properties depends on how closely it is associated with treatment. Clearly the most potent stimulus for the chemotherapy patient is the smell of the rubbing alcohol used to clean the skin in preparation for an infusion. After four or five infusions, the nurse's perfume, the handsoap the doctor uses, and the odor of coffee may elicit it. Visual and auditory stimuli (e.g., the sight of clinic staff, the name of the hospital printed on a road sign, the sound of the nurse's voice, and the music played in the waiting room) can also become powerful cues eliciting anticipatory reactions.

As indicated in the introduction, cognitively generated images and thoughts of treatment can also elicit nausea and vomiting. For example, during patient interviews conducted by a research assistant who is not directly associated with treatment, it is not uncommon for a patient to ask that the conversation be terminated because talking about treatment brings on nausea. In many cases the mere mention of chemotherapy, cancer, or hospitalization elicits significant nausea.

Researchers in the area have concluded that there are two different "types" of anticipatory nausea and vomiting (ANV). In some patients anticipatory side effects occur only in response to physical stimuli directly associated with the treatment setting. This "clinic-specific" ANV are primarily elicited by the smell and the sight of the drugs. Other patients' anticipatory reactions are "pervasive," experienced during a period of time prior to clinic visits (e.g., the entire day before treatment). ANV in these patients would therefore not be limited to clinic stimuli only. Some patients do, however, display ANV of both types.

Many patients also experience insomnia and other anxiety-mediated problems during the week immediately preceding treatment. Patients often report being preoccupied by thoughts of chemotherapy and find themselves thinking about upcoming events in terms of their proximity to treatment. In research reported by Andrykowski and colleagues (1985) on the development of anticipatory side effects, patients were interviewed before and after each chemotherapy infusion, beginning with the first. A steady increase in anxiety and depression is observed in those patients who develop anticipatory side effects. The pattern is quite striking. The patient who appears cheerful and optimistic after the first treatment may become withdrawn and fearful if side effects become more severe later in the course. Such reactions are quite understandable, considering that many patients must continue treatment for a year or longer and dread repeated bouts of nausea and vomiting.

It is not uncommon for patients and staff members to think that their reactions represent psychological weakness and, thus, to be reluctant to admit that they have the problem or to seek help. A patient was once overheard ridiculing another, saying: "Why are you throwing up before you even get the drugs? That's silly, it's all in your head." Unfortunately, such patient and staff misunderstanding only compound the patient's distress and result in classic victim blaming. As the subsequent discussion shows, anticipatory aversion reactions are the result of normal learning processes and do not represent psychopathology. Indeed, the vast majority of patients who experience anticipatory aversion reactions are psychologically healthy and well adjusted.

## PREVALENCE OF ANTICIPATORY SIDE EFFECTS

Exactly how common are anticipatory side effects? Do all patients receiving chemotherapy experience nausea and vomiting before their regularly scheduled infusions? Can we tell a patient beginning chemotherapy the likelihood that he or she will develop aversion reactions? Although there exists considerable interest among clinicians and researchers regarding the prevalence of anticipatory side effects and at least 20 (see Jacobsen and Redd, 1988; Redd and Andrykowski, 1982) separate studies have addressed the issue, precise data are difficult to obtain.

The likelihood that a particular patient will develop anticipatory reactions depends on a number of influences, some of which are only partially understood. Indeed, it has been suggested that current research on chemotherapy-induced nausea and vomiting should focus on the identification of specific patient and situational variables that can be used to predict which patients are at risk.

Research has revealed a strong association between the intensity, duration, and frequency of posttreatment nausea and vomiting and the development of pretreatment reactions among patients receiving the same chemotherapy protocol. Those patients who report either longer, more frequent, or more severe bouts of nausea and vomiting following each treatment are more likely to develop anticipatory reactions. Two correlates follow from this relationship. First, patients receiving highly emetic drugs are at great risk for developing anticipatory reactions. For example, patients treated with cisplatin, the chemotherapeutic agent that produces the most severe posttreatment side effects, are at greatest risk. Second, patients entered on protocols that incorporate relatively large numbers of different chemotherapeutic agents that cause nausea and vomiting are at greater risk, because such protocols are generally associated with more severe posttreatment side effects. Thus, it appears that any variable that increases the pharmacological effect also increases the likelihood that patients will experience nonpharmacological side effects (Redd and Andrykowski, 1982).

Research has failed to identify a personality "type" or set of attitudes that characterize the patient who is most likely to experience anticipatory reactions. However, there does appear to be a strong association between the appearance of anticipatory side effects and patient anxiety. First, patients who are characteristically anxious and are preoccupied by worry (e.g., high trait anxiety) are more likely to develop anticipatory side effects (van Komen and Redd, 1985). Moreover, these patients with high trait anxiety are also more likely to experience chemotherapy infusions as unpleasant and depressing. A second example of the role of anxiety is the relationship between anxiety experienced during chemotherapy infusions and the development of anticipatory side effects. Patients who report feeling highly anxious during initial treatments are most likely to experience ANV during subsequent treatments.

There are several "external" influences that also appear to have a mediating role in the development of anticipatory reactions. One of these is the physical setting in which treatments are administered. Patients treated in large clinic wards with other patients present are more likely to have anticipatory reactions than are patients treated in small, private cubicles (van Komen and Redd, 1985). It has been suggested that observing others vomiting might increase the patient's anxiety as well as directly evoke emesis.

Because of the large number of factors influencing the development of anticipatory reactions and the complexity of their interaction(s), it is not possible to specify the exact prevalence of such aversions. Different protocols are associated with different prevalence rates. For example, Andrykowski and colleagues (1985) found that only 20% of patients receiving weekly infusions of 5-fluorouracil (5-FU) developed anticipatory reactions during the course of treatment, whereas 80% of patients receiving a combination of cyclophosphamide, doxorubicin, vincristine, and prednisone developed such reactions. Prevalence rates shown in Table 35-1 also demonstrate this problem. For this reason it is impossible to specify an overall prevalence rate. A conservative estimate would be that at least 33% of chemotherapy patients eventually acquire aversions to their treatment. Research by Dolgin and colleagues (1985) suggests that this estimate holds for pediatric patients on chemotherapy as well.

## MECHANISMS UNDERLYING THE DEVELOPMENT OF ANV

Our understanding of the process by which patients develop anticipatory side effects is based on indirect clinical evidence, extrapolation from basic laboratory research on animal learning, and theoretical speculation. Because of ethical and practical concerns, direct experimental research on the development of aversions in humans has not been conducted. At least four hypotheses have been offered to explain ANV: underlying psychological readjustment problems associated with life-threatening illness, severe anxiety experienced immediately before treatment, physiological changes associated with advanced disease, conditioned learning. However, the first three hypotheses have been rejected by the majority of those working on the problem. Indeed, research to date has failed to identify any pattern of psychopathology or psychological maladjustment in patients who experience anticipatory side effects. Moreover, these side effects occur independent of physiological complications of the disease. As the following argument attests, the development of ANV in patients receiving chemotherapy rep-

**Table 35-1** Prevalence of anticipatory nausea and vomiting

| Reference | Protocol* | Prevalence (%) |
|---|---|---|
| Morrow et al. (1982) | Range of chemotherapy regimens at three hospitals | 24 |
| Nerenz et al. (1982) | Cisplatin | 65 |
| | Cytoxan, MTX, 5-FU | 15 |

*MTX, Methotrexate.

resents an automatic, normal, and quite common type of learning. The process is referred to as respondent or Pavlovian conditioning. In laboratory research with dogs, Pavlov repeatedly paired a tone or some other neutral external stimulus with the presentation of a naturally potent stimulus (e.g., food powder to the tongue or injections of small doses of highly emetic apomorphine). After several pairings, presentation of the tone alone elicited a response that reliably mimicked that produced by the potent stimulus. Depending on the experiment, the dogs came either to salivate or to vomit at the sound of the tone. This respondent-conditioning process, as Pavlov called it, was automatic and robust. Applying this respondent-conditioning conceptualization to chemotherapy, the patient becomes conditioned to respond to previously neutral clinic cues with nausea and vomiting because of the cues' association with posttreatment side effects. It was interesting that Pavlov reported the inadvertent development of anticipatory vomiting to "laboratory" cues. After 5 or 6 days of daily pairings of the tone with injections of apomorphine, activities preliminary to the injection (e.g., opening the box containing the syringe, and cleaning the skin with alcohol) elicited vomiting. In some cases the dogs began vomiting in response to the mere sight of the investigator.

Evidence supporting the respondent-conditioning explanation of the development of anticipatory side effects is drawn from three other sources: Garcia's research on the acquisition of taste aversions in laboratory animals, Bernstein's investigation of experimentally induced taste aversion in chemotherapy patients, and a series of clinical reports of inadvertent aversion conditioning following chemotherapy treatment.

Garcia and his colleagues (1955) allowed laboratory rats to consume a saccharin solution (for which they had previously demonstrated a strong preference) while being exposed to $\gamma$ radiation. Shortly after the radiation exposure they became ill. On subsequent presentations of the saccharin solution they showed strong aversion to the taste of saccharin. When given a choice between drinking water and saccharin, the rats chose water whereas before they chose saccharin.

Since this initial work, an extensive experimental

literature has arisen demonstrating that a variety of experimental animals will develop strong aversions to the taste of food that has been associated with illness. It is assumed, though not proven, that the animals would display "illness reactions" (e.g., retching and gagging) if they were not allowed to avoid the stimulus and were forced to ingest the food. The development of such taste aversions has conventionally been accounted for in terms of a respondent-conditioning paradigm, with the taste of the food ingested viewed as the conditioned stimulus and the illness as the unconditioned response.

Although ethical considerations have prevented the replication of Garcia's research with humans instead of animal subjects, Bernstein and Webster (Bernstein, 1978; Bernstein and Webster, 1980) have experimentally established taste aversions in both adult and pediatric cancer chemotherapy patients. In both studies, patients ate a novel flavor of ice cream (Mapletoff—maple and black walnut) 15–60 minutes before receiving regularly scheduled chemotherapy infusions. When patients' ice cream preferences (and aversions) were assessed 2–16 weeks later, patients avoided Mapletoff ice cream. When compared to control patients who were not presented Mapletoff ice cream before chemotherapy, patients who had the flavor paired with chemotherapy ate significantly less Mapletoff. The patients' understanding that the ice cream played no role in their posttreatment nausea and vomiting did not affect their preference; they still avoided the flavor. This fact is noteworthy in that it shows that aversive conditioning is automatic and that "intellect" and cognitive awareness cannot override or prevent the development of taste aversions in humans.

Perhaps the clearest examples of classically conditioned nausea in humans (and certainly the most relevant to the present discussion) come from clinical reports of patients' responses to stimuli (e.g., THC used as an antiemetic) repeatedly paired with their postchemotherapy nausea and emesis. Kutz and colleagues (1980) found that patients initially reported that marijuana helped reduce postchemotherapy nausea–emesis; however, subsequent to repeated use of marijuana following chemotherapy treatments, patients began to notice that the odor of marijuana cigarettes in social settings made them slightly nauseated. For some patients, the taste or smell of marijuana became extremely aversive, eliciting nausea and vomiting. Regardless of how it was presented (in a cookie, brownie, or cigarette), marijuana began to produce the aversive side effects it was intended to control. Morrow and colleagues (1982) observed an even more dramatic example of inadvertent aversive conditioning. Some of his patients actually became nauseated in an-

ticipation of consuming the THC tablet that had originally been prescribed to reduce chemotherapy side effects.

Redd and Andresen (1981) observed a similar phenomenon when taped relaxation inductions were used to control nausea and vomiting caused by cisplatin. Patients in that research were initially trained by a therapist in the use of passive relaxation (self-hypnosis) and then given an audiotape recording of one of their training sessions to use for practice and during subsequent posttreatment periods. The response was uniform, in that patients reported that relaxation training made them more comfortable and less nauseated, and they said they preferred using the relaxation tape. However, an interesting pattern of responding emerged as patients continued to use the audiotapes immediately following chemotherapy infusions. The patients began complaining that the sound of the therapist's voice made them nauseated. Although none of the patients actually vomited in response to the therapist's voice, they reported that when they heard his voice on the tape they felt nauseated. Even talking to the therapist on the phone made them slightly nauseated. All six of our subjects had the same experience. Of course, the patients were free to stop using the audiotape, and four of the six did so. Those four reported, interestingly, that they planned to continue using passive relaxation, but without the audiotape. These responses suggest that the strong effect of the drug outweighed the effect of the hypnosis and the audiotape, similar to what Kutz, Morrow, and their colleagues observed with THC associated with chemotherapy. The therapist's voice became a conditioned stimulus, eliciting nausea.

Based on the published data and clinical observations available, it appears most useful to view the nausea and vomiting experienced by many patients in anticipation of chemotherapy infusions within the framework provided by the respondent-conditioning paradigm. This conditioning process is considered to be automatic and to occur without the individual's awareness.

## BEHAVIORAL CONTROL OF ANTICIPATORY SIDE EFFECTS

In response to the failure of sedative and antiemetic drugs to control anticipatory nausea and vomiting and the research on the role of respondent conditioning in the development of these side effects, researchers have investigated the application of behavioral methods of control. Five procedures have been studied, specifically hypnosis used with guided imagery (i.e., passive relaxation), progressive muscle relaxation training with imagery (i.e., active relaxation), electromyo-

**Table 35-2** Behavioral control of anticipatory side effects (nausea and vomiting) of cancer chemotherapy

| Reference | Behavioral method | Outcome |
|---|---|---|
| Burish et al. (1981) | EMG biofeedback with guided imagery | Reduction in nausea and anxiety |
| Lyles et al. (1982) | Progressive relaxation with guided imagery | Reduction in nausea and anxiety |
| Morrow and Morrell (1982) | Systematic desensitization | Reduction in nausea and vomiting |
| Redd et al. (1982) | Passive relaxation (hypnosis) with guided imagery | Reduction in nausea; elimination of anticipatory vomiting |
| Redd et al. (1987) | Cognitive and attentional distraction (via videogames) | Reduction in nausea and anxiety |

graphic (EMG) biofeedback combined with relaxation training and imagery, systematic desensitiza tion, and cognitive-attentional distraction. Each of these procedures has been studied by independent groups of investigators, using different research designs. Table 35-2 summarizes these studies; in all instances nausea and vomiting were controlled through behavioral intervention. Because no direct comparison of the four procedures has been conducted, the following discussion focuses on each procedure separately.

## Hypnosis with Imagery (Passive Relaxation)

A major focus of initial research on behavioral techniques for the control of ANV has centered on the use of hypnosis in conjunction with pleasant, relaxing imagery. Early clinical reports consistently indicated that this technique reduced nausea and vomiting as well as distress both before and after chemotherapy (Dash, 1980; LeBaron et al., 1975). Unfortunately no quantifiable data were collected.

The research conducted by Redd, Andresen, and Minagawa (1982) sought to determine if the use of hypnosis could result in objectively observable and clinically significant reductions (i.e., eliminations) of ANV. Six women treated with chemotherapy at an outpatient oncology clinic participated in the study. Each subject had been observed vomiting before the actual chemotherapy injection, and none of the antiemetic drugs that were prescribed proved successful in reducing their anticipatory side effects.

Hypnotic induction was achieved in three steps. First, the patient was asked to focus on a fixed point on the wall or ceiling and to concentrate on the psychol-

ogist's voice and suggestions. Second, deep-muscle relaxation was induced by suggesting comfortable sensations in different muscle groups, while progressing from the feet to the head and back two times. Third, relaxing imagery was introduced through the therapist's descriptions of various pleasant scenes. Interwoven with the imagery were suggestions of comfort. After 30 minutes the patient was aroused by the technique of the therapist counting from 1 to 20. This training session was recorded on audiotape and the patient was instructed to listen to the audiotape daily in order to increase her responsiveness to hypnosis.

On the day of the chemotherapy treatment the patient met with the psychologist in his office. Hypnosis was then induced and the patient was taken by wheelchair to the treatment room for the chemotherapy injection. After the treatment the patient was taken back to the psychologist's office to be awakened from hypnosis. This procedure was repeated each chemotherapy treatment session until the patient had completed her prescribed chemotherapy protocol.

Hypnosis eliminated anticipatory vomiting in all patients regardless of when it was introduced during the course of chemotherapy. This ranged from the eighth to the fifteenth session. The effectiveness of hypnosis was also not related to the total number of chemotherapy sessions in which patients had experienced anticipatory vomiting. During those treatments in which hypnosis was not used, anticipatory vomiting reappeared. When hypnosis was reintroduced during subsequent chemotherapy sessions, anticipatory vomiting was again eliminated.

During the actual day that chemotherapy was scheduled, patients initially experienced increased nausea as the time of treatment neared. This trend drastically reversed when hypnosis was introduced. This effect was replicated across all patients on the 21 days when chemotherapy injections were administered with the aid of hypnosis. The patients' ratings of nausea also indicated they experienced little nausea when they were aroused immediately following chemotherapy.

These preliminary results have been replicated in subsequent research as well as in clinical practice. The technique has since been streamlined; patients now receive only one training session, and greater emphasis is placed on the patient working independently. Rather than having a therapist ''guide'' the patient through the infusion by directing relaxation and providing distracting imagery, patients now use audiotapes during treatment. The usual procedure is for the patient to sit quietly and listen to the audiotape (via headphones) for 5 or 10 mintues before the infusion. Once the patient appears comfortable and relaxed, the nurse begins treatment, administering the drugs as the patient listens to the audiotape. This ''automated'' method is effective and requires considerably less professional time and input. We have also taught nurses and other health care providers how to train patients, because they are immediately available in the chemotherapy setting. The goal of our current clinical research is to devise effective and relatively inexpensive methods of intervention.

## Progressive Muscle Relaxation Training with Imagery (Active Relaxation)

Progressive muscle relaxation training is a widely used general relaxation procedure that has been shown to be effective in reducing a number of symptoms, including hypertension, migraine headaches, tension headaches, and preoperative distress. Relaxation training can reduce muscle tension (EMG) levels throughout the body, reduce autonomic arousal, and lead to sensations of deep relaxation. In order to deepen the effects of these briefer versions of relaxation training and to promote cognitive relaxation as well as somatic relaxation, the relaxation exercises are followed by several minutes of guided relaxation imagery in which tranquil scenes are described to the patient.

Burish and colleagues (Burish and Lyles, 1979; Burish et al., 1981; Lyles et al., 1982) have conducted a series of studies assessing the effectiveness of progressive muscle relaxation training used with imagery to control anticipatory side effects. Their procedures are similar to ours, the major difference being the way in which relaxation is brought about. Whereas Redd and colleagues ask the patient to focus on sensations in different muscle groups and provide suggestions of warmth, heaviness, and relaxation, Burish uses a series of tensing and releasing exercises. Once Burish's patients have learned "how to relax," a therapist then directs them through the relaxation and guided imagery during subsequent chemotherapy infusions. In this research patients with anticipatory nausea were studied across 5–10 consecutive chemotherapy treatments divided into baseline, treatment, and follow-up phases. Measures of pulse rate, blood pressure, anxiety, and depression were obtained during chemotherapy infusions, as well as nurses' observations of vomiting. After no-treatment baseline conditions, the therapist directed patients in progressive muscle relaxation and guided-relaxation imagery both before and during chemotherapy injections. During the follow-up phase, the therapist withdrew and patients were instructed to use the relaxation and imagery intervention on their own before and during chemotherapy. In their group comparison research, no-treatment and therapist contact-only control groups were added to assess better the contribution of nonspecific influences.

Results have been consistent across their research. Therapist-directed progressive muscle relaxation with

guided imagery resulted in reductions in pulse rate and blood pressure as well as in self-reported anxiety and nausea. Patients in control conditions did not show these reductions. Follow-up results have been less impressive, however. When the therapist was no longer present, patients in the treatment groups did not display as large a reduction in nausea and physiological arousal.

## Biofeedback with Imagery

Multiple-muscle site EMG biofeedback in conjunction with relaxation training and imagery has been used in one case study by Burish and colleagues (Burish et al., 1981). Both their intervention strategy and assessment methods closely followed those of Burish's previous research cited earlier. Biofeedback was used to augment the relaxation training during drug infusions. Once the patient could effectively reduce his or her physiological arousal (as measured by EMG) and maintain that quiet state, relaxing images were presented during drug infusions. Results replicated their earlier findings; both patient distress and nausea were reduced.

## Systematic Desensitization

Systematic desensitization is a counterconditioning procedure developed for treatment of phobias and related anxiety disorders. It involves having a deeply relaxed individual confront, in imagination, each of a series of increasingly potent anxiety-eliciting stimuli. The aim is to eliminate the anxiety-eliciting value of the feared stimuli by systematically associating those stimuli with relaxation. The procedure involves three general steps. First, the patient is instructed in the use of a relaxation technique, usually progressive muscle relaxation training. Second, the patient and therapist construct a hierarchy of stimuli relevant to the feared situation, ranging from the least to the most anxiety-provoking. For example, in the chemotherapy experience the training sequence might start with an image of driving to the clinic and work up to one in which the patient imagines feeling the needle prick. Third, the patient practices relaxation training while visualizing the increasingly aversive scenes or stimuli within the hierarchy. Although the most commonly used training technique is the muscle tensing–releasing procedure previously described, other methods for inducing relaxation (such as more hypnotic relaxation induction methods and biofeedback) are equally effective. It is hypothesized that, by pairing stimuli that elicit fear with sensations of relaxation, the fear stimuli would lose their aversive properties (their fear-eliciting value). That is, because clinic stimuli acquired their nausea-eliciting strength through conditioning, then presumably they could be counterconditioned in the same way.

In a study on the use of systematic desensitization, Morrow and Morrell (1982) randomly assigned 60 cancer patients to one of three conditions: (1) systematic desensitization, in which patients were taught an abbreviated form of relaxation training and while relaxed were asked to imagine chemotherapy-related stimuli (e.g., seeing the drugs and feeling the needle stick), (2) supportive counseling, intended to control for therapist attention, expectancy effects, and other nonspecific influences, and (3) no treatment control. Patients were asked to rate the frequency, severity, and duration of their prechemotherapy nausea and vomiting during two baseline and two follow-up chemotherapy treatments. Between chemotherapy treatments, patients assigned to treatment groups received two sessions of either the systematic desensitization or the counseling procedure. The results showed that during the two follow-up chemotherapy treatments, desensitized patients reported significantly less severe ANV, and a significantly shorter duration of anticipatory nausea than patients in the other two conditions, who did not differ significantly from each other.

The results of the desensitization studies, particularly those of Morrow and Morrell (1982), suggest two conclusions regarding this technique. First, systematic desensitization can be effective in reducing ANV. Moreover, these effects occur even though the desensitization procedure is administered at a time and place removed from the actual chemotherapy treatment. This point is important because it suggests that a therapist need not be present during actual chemotherapy treatments in order to teach patients to overcome their conditioned responses. Second, the benefits of systematic desensitization are not due solely to patient expectancy or therapist support, since patients in the counseling control condition did not show similar effects.

## Cognitive or Attentional Distraction

Researchers have speculated at length about the mechanism(s) that may underlie the effectiveness of behavioral interventions in controlling anticipatory reactions to chemotherapy (e.g., Redd and Andrykowski, 1982). A major controversy concerns whether behavioral techniques yield reductions in ANV by inducing relaxation, by distracting attention away from nausea sensations or nausea-eliciting stimuli, or by a combination of both processes. Studies employing hypnosis, progressive muscle relaxation, and systematic desensitization have not been able to answer this question because each of these techniques combines distraction with relaxation. During these procedures patients are typically presented with distracting visual imagery only after relaxation has been induced.

Are there techniques that permit an examination of the effects of distraction alone? Redd and colleagues (1987) recently tested whether the behavioral application of videogame-playing could be used for this purpose. They studied 15 pediatric cancer patients with ANV. After a no-videogame baseline assessment, all participants played commercially available videogames at bedside for 10 minutes, followed immediately by a 10-minute no-videogame period, and then by a second 10-minute videogame period. Results indicated that the introduction and withdrawal of the opportunity to play videogames resulted in significant changes (reductions and exacerbations, respectively) in the intensity of anticipatory nausea. The effects of videogame-playing on anxiety were less clear-cut. Although changes in self-reported anxiety mirrored changes in anticipatory nausea, no comparisons of changes in anxiety between adjacent periods reached significance. Pulse rate and systolic/diastolic blood pressure were not consistently altered by the presentation or withdrawal of videogames; in the one instance in which a physiological measure did change significantly, videogame-playing was associated with an increase in systolic blood pressure. These results suggest that reductions in anticipatory nausea can be achieved independently of physiological relaxation and anxiety reduction.

## Preliminary Conclusion

The consistency of the positive results obtained in the group of studies just reviewed is remarkable, because clinically significant reductions in ANV were achieved despite wide variations in type of cancer, stage of the disease, and chemotherapy protocol (Table 35-2). This fact is especially noteworthy when one considers that the research was conducted by separate groups of investigators using different research methods and working independently at three medical centers. Moreover, because most patients in these studies had been receiving antiemetic medication before the behavioral treatment was initiated, the results of these studies suggest that the effects achieved with behavioral interventions extend beyond those that could be obtained by medication alone. Thus, behavioral techniques clearly appear to have a place as an adjunctive treatment in the care of many chemotherapy patients.

## BEHAVIORAL CONTROL OF POSTCHEMOTHERAPY NAUSEA AND VOMITING

Although early clinical case studies of hypnosis with cancer patients reported reductions in postchemotherapy vomiting in patients trained in self-hypnosis, with few exceptions (see Scott et al., 1983), behavioral research has not focused on the treatment of postchemotherapy side effects. Rather, the research has almost exclusively dealt with anticipatory reactions. This bias in focus reflects the presumption that behavioral intervention is more effective in cases of nonpharmacological reactions (i.e., anticipatory) than with vomiting directly related to the presence of toxic drugs (e.g., posttreatment vomiting). The notion is that because anticipatory side effects are the result of conditioning and are not biochemically mediated, then counterconditioning procedures are more likely to work. Indeed, our own experience is consistent with this hypothesis. In cases of severe posttreatment side effects (e.g., vomiting following cisplatin therapy), patients initially report being helped by self-relaxation audiotapes, yet after continued use they say that the audiotapes are unpleasant. Posttreatment reactions appear to outweigh the effects of the tapes and result in the tapes themselves becoming conditioned aversive stimuli. As pointed out earlier in this discussion, this same conditioning process can occur with antiemetic drugs taken to control vomiting secondary to cisplatin therapy, because the drugs themselves become aversive and elicit nausea and vomiting. However, this is not necessarily the case for patients in less toxic protocols. Burish and colleagues consistently report reductions in posttreatment reactions when their patients use self-relaxation and distraction with protocols that do not incorporate cisplatin. Although posttreatment nausea is not eliminated, statistically significant reductions are observed.

## Clinical Issues

Although the behavioral procedures outlined in this chapter are straightforward, lend themselves to empirical quantification and evaluation, and can be easily learned, a number of clinical issues must be considered before implementing a comprehensive behavioral program. There are two broad areas of concern. The first is how to implement these procedures successfully in the context of a busy clinic setting. The second involves the role of rapport, trust, and nonspecific issues in behavioral intervention. Each of these topics introduces certain questions that have yet to be systematically studied. For this reason the following discussion will be largely speculative.

A critical issue is how to make behavioral intervention practical. In most outpatient oncology clinics a psychologist is not available to treat patients. For this reason we have explored the training of nurses, social workers, and patients's spouses or close friends in the use of behavioral techniques. Because the nurse has easy access to patients, he or she is able to identify the first occurrence of anticipatory reaction and intervene

rapidly. Also, nurses trained in behavioral intervention are able to reduce patient anxiety by correctly explaining the cause of anticipatory symptoms when they first appear. Intervention by a family member is a more complex matter. There is the issue of staff time required to train each new patient. Nevertheless, such training requires less staff time than direct professional intervention. There can also be control issues between family members. On the other hand, spouses are often glad to have the opportunity to be meaningfully involved in the care of the patient and prefer "doing something" to sitting and watching. Also, some patients prefer to work with their spouses. For these reasons it is necessary that these issues be assessed and appropriate alternatives be explored before family members are enlisted.

Another way to make behavioral intervention most cost effective is to use audiotaped relaxation training. A set of two 25-minute audiotapes are available that provide a male voice directing either active or passive (hypnotic) relaxation induction. The audiotapes begin with the muscle tension and muscle relaxation induction described earlier. After 10 minutes the focus shifts to descriptions of tranquil scenes such as a still mountain lake or a calm ocean tide washing back and forth. The patient is instructed to practice with the audiotape at home until he or she is able to become relaxed quickly and with little effort. If a patient is apprehensive regarding the procedures, he or she can merely listen to the audiotape without trying to become relaxed, "just to know what the procedure is like." This usually helps the patient overcome any fear of losing control or of becoming hypnotized. After the patient is able to follow the audiotape and achieve a deep state of relaxation, he or she is given a second tape. This "maintenance" audiotape is similar to the training tape, but with a shorter relaxation induction (less than 5 minutes) and a longer period of guided imagery. This audiotape is intended to be used during actual infusions. The patient typically begins the tape, and after 10 minutes the nurse starts the infusion. If the infusion extends longer than 25 minutes, the patient can simply flip the audiotape and listen to the opposite side, which presents the same recording. This allows the patient to play the audiotape repeatedly, with minimal interruption. Although patients often say that they would prefer a "live" therapist, they understand the reasons for using the audiotape and report that the audiotape helps them control their nausea.

An obvious concern with the use of audiotapes is that the relaxation induction and guided imagery cannot be individualized. Regardless of how well the patient is doing, the audiotape continues. It is interesting that this rarely poses a problem. Once patients have learned how to induce a state of relaxation, they are able to attend selectively to the material on the audiotape. That is, patients are able to individualize their experience on their own.

After listening to the audiotape five or six times, many patients report that they can become relaxed without the audiotape. They remark that they can do this while waiting for an appointment or while riding a bus. However, they continue to use the audiotapes during infusions. Many patients state that the audiotape is a crutch that they like to have. The decision as to when to use the tapes is left to the individual patient.

Although the large majority of our patients appreciate the benefits they receive from the behavioral procedures and actually enjoy them, some are reluctant to devote the time and effort to practicing the techniques. Listening to the audiotapes at home can serve as an additional reminder that they have cancer and must undergo further chemotherapy. We are sensitive to this issue and usually discuss it with patients at the onset of our intervention, because patients are often unwilling to admit that they did not practice. These patients may require additional support and the opportunity to practice. In some cases we ask the nurse to help the patient begin listening to the audiotape. Even those patients who do not consistently practice at home interestingly benefit from listening to the audiotapes during their infusions.

Many of our patients state that they find the audiotapes helpful with other problems such as insomnia, headaches, and pain. It is also not unusual for patients to play the audiotapes during blood tests and other procedures requiring intravenous injections. Because of peripheral vascular dilation associated with relaxation, it is easier for the nurse to locate a vein. Patients typically report that procedures seem much quicker when they use the relaxation–imagery tapes.

Some patients appear to have a mild form of amnesia following the use of these procedures. Their first response when regaining attentiveness after listening to the audiotape during an infusion is often with the question: "Is it over? Have I already had chemotherapy?" This reaction is quite similar to the time distortion many individuals experience during hypnosis.

Perhaps our most interesting clinical finding is that patients feel a greater sense of personal control and competence when they receive behavioral intervention. They understand their role in controlling their aversion reactions and enjoy being able to master their behavior in a situation that they generally experience as overwhelming.

For the clinician working with these patients, which procedure to use is a difficult question. As noted, a direct comparison of the available techniques has not yet been conducted. And, as pointed out earlier, it is

generally held that the techniques of hypnosis with imagery and that of progressive muscle relaxation with imagery differ only in respect to the manner in which relaxation is initially induced. Hypnotic relaxation incorporates direct suggestion of warmth, comfort, heaviness, and so forth, whereas active relaxation involves sequentially tensing and relaxing various muscle groups.

We have encountered real fear among many patients regarding hypnosis. Both the popular literature and entertainment industry have done a great disservice by characterizing the procedure as a method of mind control. Those patients who have ever observed hypnosis have typically witnessed hypnotic subjects behaving in an embarrassing manner (one patient asked if he would act like a chicken). These portrayals have led patients to refuse to participate in our treatment procedure and opt to continue to suffer from the side effects of chemotherapy or actually to refuse continued drug treatment. Fortunately, such notions are malleable through straightforward discussion of the patient's beliefs and expectations regarding the behavioral intervention.

More sophisticated knowledge regarding the theoretical foundations of hypnosis has led to confusion as to how best to understand the processes involved in behavioral method of nausea control. Is it hypnosis or relaxation training? Moreover, what do the procedures have in common? There are two major areas of concern, involving how investigators conceptualize the hypnotic process and how patients conceptualize what they will experience. Those doing research procedures on the topic have adopted a behavioral perspective. Many procedures commonly associated with hypnosis (e.g., age regression and posthypnotic suggestion) are not employed. Moreover, the procedures do not induce an altered state of consciousness or tap unconscious processes. Nevertheless, the passive-relaxation induction procedures are identical to those frequently used by many professionals who identify their procedures as hypnosis. For these reasons it seems prudent to identify the procedures operationally (i.e., by describing what is done) rather than by using a term based on presumed processes underlying the methods. That is, the procedures might be best called "passive- and active-relaxation training with guided imagery" and identified as such to patients.

Finally, behavioral intervention is an interpersonal event; both the clinician and patient are active participants. The importance of the development of rapport and trust cannot be overemphasized. With adequate training and supervision, most health care personnel can be effective. Indeed, the intervention work of both Burish and Redd has employed various health care workers as interventionists, including psychologists, nurses, and social workers. In addition, behavioral intervention often results in a positive snowball effect. Rapport between the clinician and patient is enhanced through the use of relaxation–distraction techniques. In turn, patients often feel more comfortable disclosing emotional concerns and seeking help from a clinician they come to know in a nonthreatening context, such as what exists in the behavioral intervention.

## SUMMARY

Many cancer patients display chemotherapy side effects that appear to be behavioral responses to a pharmacological treatment: they experience severe nausea and/or vomiting occurring *before* the drugs are infused. Of the several hypotheses that have been proposed to explain the etiology of anticipatory side effects, the one that appears the most viable is that based on respondent conditioning. Through repeated association with postchemotherapy side effects, the sights, smells, tastes, and even thoughts associated with the treatment come to elicit nausea and vomiting. At least five influences may be important in the development of anticipatory side effects, and they include the emeticity of the drugs used, severity of nausea and vomiting following previous treatments, number of chemotherapy treatment cycles completed, presence of anxiety during initial chemotherapy infusions, and treatment setting.

The first interventions used to reduce chemotherapy nausea and vomiting were antiemetic and antianxiety medications. (A review of these is given by Lesko in chapter 34). These drugs have little to moderate effect on anticipatory side effects, although it should be noted that they are usually not administered until the chemotherapy treatment has begun. Therefore, their potential effect on anticipatory symptoms has not been adequately assessed. Within the last few years three separate groups have studied the effectiveness of behavioral relaxation procedures in reducing the conditioned side effects of cancer chemotherapy. Results from this research indicate that behavioral techniques can reduce the distress of cancer chemotherapy. This conclusion is remarkably robust considering that it has been generated by independent research teams, using uncontrolled as well as controlled experimental designs, and assessing outcome with a wide variety of self-reported, observational, and physiological measures.

## REFERENCES

Andrykowski, M.A., W.H. Redd, and A.K. Hatfield (1985). The development of anticipatory nausea: A prospective analysis. *J. Consult. Clin. Psychol.* 4:447–54.

Andrykowski, M.A., W.H. Redd, P.B. Jacobsen, E. Marks, K. Gorfinkle, T.B. Hakes, R.J. Kaufman, V.E. Currie, and J.C. Holland (1988). Prevalence, predictors, and course of anticipatory nausea in women receiving adjuvant chemotherapy for breast cancer. *Cancer*. 62:2607–2613.

Baxley, N. (producer) (1984). *Relaxation Procedures in Cancer Treatment* (Videotape). Urbana, Il.: Carle Medical Communications.

Bernstein, I.L. (1978). Learned taste aversions in children receiving chemotherapy. *Science* 200:1302–3.

Bernstein, I.L. and M.M. Webster (1980). Learned taste aversions in humans. *Physiol. Behav.* 25:363–66.

Burish, T.G. and J.N. Lyles (1979). Effectiveness of relaxation training in reducing the aversiveness of chemotherapy in the treatment of cancer. *Behav. Ther. Exp. Psychiatry* 10:357–61.

Burish, T.G., C.D. Shartner, and J.N. Lyles (1981). Effectiveness of multiple-site EMG biofeedback and relaxation in reducing the aversiveness of cancer chemotherapy. *Biofeedback Self-Regulation* 6:523–35.

Dash, J. (1980). Hypnosis for symptom amelioration. In J. Kellerman (ed.), *Psychosocial Aspects of Childhood Cancer*. Springfield, Il: Charles C Thomas, pp. 215–30.

Dempster, C.R., P. Balson, and B.T. Whalen (1976). Supportive hypnotherapy during the radical treatment of malignancies. *Int. J. Clin. Exp. Hypn.* 24:1–9.

Dolgin, M.J., E.R. Katz, K. McGinty, and S.E. Siegel (1985). Anticipatory nausea and vomiting in pediatric cancer patients. *Pediatrics* 75:547–52.

Fetting, J.H., P.M. Wilcox, B.A. Iwata, E.L. Criswell, L.S. Bosmajian, and V.R. Sheidler (1983). Anticipatory nausea and vomiting in an ambulatory oncology population. *Cancer Treat. Rep.* 67:1093–98.

Garcia, J., D.J. Kimeldorf, and R.A. Koelling (1955). Conditioned aversion to saccharin resulting from exposure to gamma radiation. *Science* 122:157–58.

Jacobsen, P.B., and W.H. Redd (1988). The development and management of chemotherapy-related anticipatory nausea and vomiting. *Cancer Invest.* 6:327–34.

Jacobsen, P.B., M.A. Andrykowski, W.H. Redd, M. Die-Trill, T.B. Hakes, R.J. Kaufman, V.E. Currie, and J.C. Holland (1988). Nonpharmacologic factors in the development of post-treatment nausea with adjuvant chemotherapy. *Cancer* 61:379–85.

Katz, E.R. (1982). Behavioral conditioning in the development and maintenance of vomiting in cancer patients. *Psychosomatics* 23:650–51.

Kutz, I., J.Z. Borysenko, S.E. Come, and H. Benson (1980). Paradoxical emetic response to antiemetic treatment in cancer patients. *N. Engl. J. Med.* 303:1480.

LeBaron, W., C. Holton, K. Tewell, and D. Eccles (1975). The use of self-hypnosis by children with cancer. *Am. J. Clin. Hypn.* 17(4):233–38.

Lyles, J.N., T.G. Burish, M.G. Krozely, and R.K. Oldham (1982). Efficacy of relaxation training and guided imagery in reducing the aversiveness of cancer chemotherapy. *J. Consult. Clin. Psychol.* 50:509–24.

Morrow, G.R. (1982). Prevalence and correlates of anticipatory nausea and vomiting in chemotherapy patients. *J.N.C.I.* 68:484–88.

Morrow, G.R. and B.S. Morrell (1982). Behavioral treatment for the anticipatory nausea and vomiting induced by cancer chemotherapy. *N. Engl. J. Med.* 307:1476–80.

Morrow, G.R., J.C. Arseneau, R.F. Asbury, J.M. Bennmet, and L. Boros (1982). Anticipatory nausea and vomiting with chemotherapy. *N. Engl. J. Med.* 306:431–32.

Nerenz, D.R., H. Leventhal, and R.R. Love (1982). Factors contributing to emotional distress during cancer chemotherapy. *Cancer* 50:1020–27.

Nesse, R.M., T. Carli, G.C. Curtis, and P.D. Kleinman (1980). Pre-treatment nausea in cancer chemotherapy: A conditioned response? *Psychosom. Med.* 42:33–36.

Nesse, R.M., T. Carli, G.C. Curtis, and P.D. Kleinman (1983). Pseudohallucinations in cancer chemotherapy patients. *Am. J. Psychiatry* 140:483–85.

Nicholas, D.R. (1982). Prevalence of anticipatory nausea and emesis in cancer chemotherapy patients. *J. Behav. Med.* 5:461–63.

Pavlov, I.P. (1927). *Conditioned Reflexes: An Investigation of Physiological Activity of the Cerebral Cortex (Lecture III)*. Oxford: Oxford University Press.

Redd, W.H. and G.V. Andresen (1981). Conditioned aversion in cancer patients. *Behavior Therapist* 4:3–4.

Redd, W.H., and M.A. Andrykowski (1982). Behavioral intervention in cancer treatment: Controlling aversion re-actions to chemotherapy. *J. Consult. Clin. Psychol.* 50:595–600.

Redd, W.H., G.V. Andresen, and R.Y. Minagawa (1982). Hypnotic control of anticipatory emesis in patients receiving cancer chemotherapy. *J. Consult. Clin. Psychol.* 50:14–19.

Redd, W.H., P.B. Jacobsen, M. Die-Trill, H. Dermatis, M. McEvoy, and J.C. Holland (1987). Cognitive/attentional distraction in the control of conditioned nausea in pediatric cancer patients receiving chemotherapy, *J. Consult. Clin. Psychol.* 55:391–95.

Redd, W.H., P. Rosenberger, and C. Hendler (1982). Hypnosis as a behavior procedure in cancer treatment. *Am. J. Clin. Hypn.* 25:161–72.

Redd, W.H., A.L. Porterfield, and B.A. Andresen (1979). *Behavior Modification: Behavioral Approaches to Human Problems*. New York: Random House.

Scott, D.W., D.C. Donahue, R.C. Mastrovito, and T.B. Hakes (1983). The antiemetic effect of clinical relaxation: Report of an exploratory pilot study. *J. Psychosoc. Oncol.* 1:71–84.

van Komen, R. and W.H. Redd (1985). Personality factors associated with anticipatory nausea/vomiting in patients receiving cancer chemotherapy. *Health Psychol.* 4:189–202.

# 36

## Anorexia

Lynna M. Lesko

The cachexia seen in adults and children with advanced cancer of certain sites has been carefully studied. Characterized by extensive weight loss and muscle wasting, this process is due to altered carbohydrate and protein metabolism and an associated negative energy balance (Kisner and De Wys, 1981; De Wys, 1982). The precise pathophysiological mechanism, however, remains poorly understood. Much cancer research has gone into studying the effects of undernutrition on organ and host cell function (Good et al., 1982) and the effect of nutritional status on response to cancer therapy (Van Eys, 1982). Patients with cachexia usually have anorexia, especially with an aversion for meat, leading to speculation about the contribution of appetite, metabolism, and psychological influences in the development of this cardinal sign of progressive illness. Within this complex picture of anorexia and cachexia of cancer, psychological determinants and their management are explored here, following a brief review of the common physiological causes.

## ANOREXIA–CACHEXIA SYNDROME

In both animals and humans with cancer, reduced appetite and oral intake with weight loss are common. This occurs at the same time that energy needs increase to support tumor growth. Speculation about the role of the tumor in producing altered central or peripheral metabolic responses in the host that result in this syndrome of anorexia–cachexia has been lively.

Despite the role that the ventromedial hypothalamus and the lateral nucleus of the hypothalamus play in satiety and appetite, studies of hypothalamic lesions in tumor-bearing animals have not revealed a likely etiological role in those centers in the anorexia of cancer (Bernstein, 1982). Likewise, the role of noradrenergic, dopaminergic, serotoninergic, and other endorphinergic neurotransmitters in control and modulation of food intake has not been proven in cancer anorexia models. Elevation of tryptophan, 5-hydroxyindoleacetic acid (5-HIAA, a serotonin metabolite), and depletion of endorphin resources has been explored in relation to anorexia in tumor-bearing rats without conclusive evidence (Krause et al., 1979; Lowry and Yim, 1980). With respect to protein loss, some studies suggest that the presence of a tumor accelerates muscle wasting and protein loss independently of food intake (Norton et al., 1981).

Cachectin, also called tumor necrosis factor (TNF), a multipotent protein secreted by macrophages, has emerged as a possibly major influence in cachexia; it has also been implicated as playing the central mediator role in toxic shock (Beutler and Cerami, 1987; Old, 1985). Cachectin produces a picture of weight loss, poor food intake, and apathy, as well as fever in animals. Elucidation of this important protein's mode of action may enhance our understanding of this problem in cancer.

## DISEASE- AND TREATMENT-RELATED ANOREXIA

Anorexia seen in patients with oncological disease has both physiological and psychological causes. The contribution of each of these causes will be discussed separately. Early review articles by Holland and colleagues (1977), Ohnuma and Holland (1977), Shils (1979), and the more recent volume edited by Burish and colleagues (1985), provide a concise background for this discussion.

Table 36-1 provide a comprehensive list of the physiological or disease-related and treatment-related causes of anorexia. Anorexia and weight loss occur early in the course of several tumors of the GI tract, specifically stomach, colon, rectum, and pancreas. In

**Table 36-1** Disease and treatment-related causes of anorexia

| Types of anorexia | Examples |
| --- | --- |
| Disease-related | Anorexia–cachexia syndrome |
| | Early symptoms of GI or pancreatic cancer |
| | Fever, anemia, chronic illness |
| | Obstruction by the tumor |
| | Protein-losing enteropathy (gastric cancer) |
| | Ectopic hormone production by tumors (lung) |
| | Uremia and hepatic dysfunction |
| | Pain and discomfort |
| Treatment-related | Surgery |
| |   Oropharyngeal resection: loss of dentition, chewing and swallowing difficulties, tube feeding |
| |   Esophagectomy and reconstruction: ↓ gastric acid secondary to vagotomy, fibrosis, tube feeding |
| |   Gastrectomy: lack of gastric acid, malabsorption, "dumping" syndrome |
| |   Pancreatectomy: diabetes, malabsorption |
| |   Bowel resection: malabsorption, diarrhea secondary to bile salt loss, malnutrition |
| |   Ileostomy/colostomy: fluid electrolyte imbalance |
| | Drugs |
| |   Chemotherapeutic agents: nausea, vomiting, fluid and electrolyte imbalance, stomatitis of alimentary canal, abdominal pain, constipation, intestinal ulceration, diarrhea, neuropathy, CNS complications of confusion |
| |   Pain medication: somnolence, constipation |
| |   Antifungal, antibacterial agents |
| | Radiation therapy |
| |   Oropharyngeal area: ↓ taste and smell; stomatitis |
| |   Neck and mediastinal area: dysphagia, esophagitis, esophageal fibrosis |
| |   Abdominopelvic area: nausea, vomiting, diarrhea, malabsorption, obstruction, stenosis, fistula |
| | Other |
| |   GvHD (BMT): diarrhea, electrolyte imbalance, ileus, malabsorption |

carcinoma of the pancreas, nonspecific anorexia and weight loss may antedate any diagnostic signs of disease. Fever, pain, anemia, uremia, mechanical obstructions, hepatic dysfunction, a protein-losing enteropathy, and malabsorption can each produce anorexia when they occur. Several tumors, primarily in the lung, produce ectopic hormones including kinins, steroids, and polypeptides that alter appetite.

Loss of appetite can occur secondary to all three major treatment modalities, specifically, surgery, chemotherapy, and radiation (see Table 36-1). Surgical procedures on the mouth, pharynx, esophagus, stomach, and lower GI tract result in poor food intake related to loss of taste, nasogastric tubes, and malabsorption. Psychological state, sense of well-being, and appetite are seriously impaired when normal eating is impossible, or when bowel function is altered or impaired.

Chemotherapeutic agents may produce anorexia through a variety of mechanisms. A number of chemotherapeutic agents, in particular, cyclophosphamide, nitrogen mustards, and cisplatin, produce anorexia as a consequence of the associated experience of nausea and vomiting (for a more detailed explanation of this association see Chapter 35 on nausea and vomiting). Only a few agents such as some alkylating agents (chlorambucils and busulfan), vincristine, and steroids are not associated with nausea, vomiting, and subsequent anorexia. Vincristine may cause anorexia as a result of constipation and ileus. Stomatitis, glossitis, pharyngitis, and esophagitis are extremely common side effects of several chemotherapeutic agents, especially methotrexate, 5-fluorouracil, and high-dose adriamycin. The rapid turnover of the mucosal epithelial cells of the alimentary canal renders the GI tract extremely vulnerable to ulcerations; pain and difficulty in eating ensue. Other drugs also produce transient anorexia, including antibiotics, analgesics, and oral antifungal agents. In the case of analgesics, excessive sedation may result in inability to take food at mealtimes, leading to weight loss.

Radiation therapy causes impairment of taste and appetite when certain sites are involved, that is, head and neck, chest, and abdomen. Eating problems are usually related to cumulative dose effect, appearing after several treatments. The course of these changes may reflect transient or permanent sequelae of treatment. Transient effects include stomatitis, mucositis, pharyngitis, esophagitis, nausea and vomiting, and diarrhea. Permanent changes result from radiation effects on taste and smell, with altered or diminished taste, decreased saliva production, dysphagia secondary to pharyngeal or esophageal fibrosis, and GI obstruction secondary to stenosis or fistulas. The sense of taste and appetite are acutely sensitive to changes in the GI system. The emotional response to loss of appetite as a basic pleasure may be significant and produce secondary depression in someone for whom sharing of food is a source of major social interaction, such as a mother, who cooks for a family.

Finally, the effect on appetite of one treatment modality may be complicated by the added effects of a second or third treatment modality. For example, the effects of ablative surgery for cancer on taste and nutrition can often be profound, complicating the later chemotherapy and radiation-induced anorexia. This is particularly the case for cancers that involve the head and neck, upper GI tract, and bowel.

A serious consequence of the rigorous treatment of leukemia by high-dose chemotherapy, irradiation, and bone marrow transplantation (BMT) is graft-versus-host disease (GvHD). Despite the matching of donor and recipient, 70% of patients developing GvHD with major effects on GI tract, skin, and liver. Diarrhea, abdominal pain, ileus, and anorexia are common, as well as impaired liver function. Chronic GvHD, usually seen 150 days or more after BMT, is characterized by a less severe, but distressing picture of anorexia, weight loss, malabsorption, and failure to thrive.

## PSYCHOLOGICAL CAUSES OF ANOREXIA

In addition to its multiple physical etiologies, cancer anorexia may also have multiple psychological causes. Some may result in primary anorexia or may be secondary effects of the physical causes leading to anorexia (see Table 36-2).

### Anxiety

At the time of diagnosis, appetite is exquisitely sensitive to mood, especially anxiety. Upon learning the diagnosis of cancer, many patients note that along with signs of distress such as insomnia and poor concentration, they lose their appetite. The loss of a few pounds is enough to frighten them even more, because their first assumption is that the recently diagnosed cancer is causing the weight loss. Reassurance that the emotional turmoil they are feeling may have an impact on appetite and on eating is often sufficient to reduce the anxiety and encourage return to normal intake.

### Fears of Recurrence

The fear of relapse and recurrence is greatest immediately after treatment, but it does not ever fully disappear. Concerns about eating and weight loss can become a focus of control for some anxious individuals, and at times their families. A concerned and anxious family member, alarmed by the signs of poor eating, may attempt to force food on the patient, making eating the source of a conflict. Concerns on the part of patient and family are greatest in individuals who have had a tumor of the GI tract and in whom initial symptoms may have been difficulty in eating and weight loss. Surgical procedures are often followed by minor transitory difficulties with discomfort or regurgitation. For these patients, fear of recurrence can reach panic proportions, making eating very difficult.

CASE REPORT

A middle-aged woman had had a gastrectomy for an early gastric carcinoma with negative nodes at surgery. Previously

**Table 36-2**  Psychological causes of anorexia

| Cause | Explanation |
|---|---|
| Anxiety | Fears related to meaning of weight loss, which is assumed to be associated with tumor progression, concerns about inability to eat and loss of normal appetite |
| Depression | Inability to eat, no appetite, progressive weight loss, sense of hopelessness |
| Unrelated psychiatric disorders | Anorexia nervosa<br>Affective disorders<br>Schizophrenic disorders<br>Personality disorders<br>Paranoia (suspicious of poisoning and refusal to eat) |
| Food aversion | Specific food aversion (dislike of meat, protein; often treatment-related) |

anxious and with a history of several phobias, this woman had a postoperative course complicated by anxiety attacks, chronic fears, and difficulty eating and maintaining weight. This required psychotherapy, medication with antianxiety drugs, and repeated visits to the surgeon for reassurance that the symptoms were not physical in origin.

In some individuals the fear of weight loss and its potential significance as a sign of tumor progression leads to compulsive behavior and overeating. This is of equal concern, as forced eating in the absence of hunger, as a compulsive habit, can result in obesity. This appears most often in women with breast cancer during chemotherapy. The reasons are unclear, but compulsive eating and the use of food as a means to reduce anxiety appear to be influences (see Chapter 14 on breast cancer).

### Depression

Anorexia is a cardinal symptom of depression; it is also a major symptom of the anorexia–cachexia syndrome of advanced cancer. It is in the advanced stages that both are more common, and the differential diagnosis between major depression and physical origin of anorexia becomes a difficult problem. Thus, the anorexia may be a consequence of the medical situation that results in secondary depression about the inability to eat, or the depression may be a prime contributor to the anorexia.

Patients begin to feel helpless in the face of continuing anorexia and weight loss, and the picture of despair and hopelessness are painful emotional states requiring intervention. It is important to make an accurate assessment of possible physical etiologies and to treat the psychological component by counseling and by pharmacological intervention (see later) that is directed at improving appetite and at treating the major depressive symptoms. Often a therapeutic trial of an antidepressant is worth attempting when the diagnostic issue cannot be resolved.

CASE REPORT

A 58-year-old man with pancreatic cancer was treated with chemotherapy but experienced profound anorexia, weight loss, abdominal pain, depression, and withdrawal. He wished to be treated at home and was kept comfortable by family and home care nursing, using analgesics, antidepressants (those with minimal sedating effects), amphetamines in low dosage, and frequent psychotherapeutic visits with him and his wife during a course of the 3 months in which the disease progressed.

## Unrelated Psychiatric Disorders

A range of psychiatric disorders that preexist in individuals who develop cancer can complicate their care and contribute to anorexia. In particular, anorexia nervosa, affective disorders, schizophrenic disorders, and personality disorders result in altered intake and weight loss in cancer. Such patients present complicated treatment issues. Anorexia nervosa, common in young women, has constituted a particularly difficult problem in these individuals if they are later treated for leukemia and lymphomas. Weight loss, unusual difficulty with taste, and relentless preoccupation with food may not be illness-related, but evidence of a concurrent and complicating psychiatric disorder, as illustrated here.

CASE REPORT

Ms. M. was diagnosed at 21 as having acute nonlymphocytic leukemia. The fourth of eight children, she had come to the United States with her parents from Greece. Her leukemia treatment was uneventful until, during a second relapse, she began to "fake" taking drugs at home to avoid the nausea and vomiting, even injecting saline to fool the family. Following a second relapse she was hospitalized for a bone marrow transplantation. Her hospital course was complicated by a longer than normal weaning period from total parenteral nutrition (TPN) and disinterest in follow-up. Over 3 years, she had anorexia, difficulty swallowing, and inability to take food except iced tea, and she did not take oral medications regularly at home. She was evaluated by several psychiatrists, who felt she had had early symptoms of anorexia nervosa prior to leukemia and that this was exacerbated by the transplantation. She was hospitalized for infections, dehydration, failure to thrive, and weight loss. The complaints of anorexia and difficulty swallowing continued, with the patient finally refusing to eat because it would "make me feel ugly." Her family, who could barely speak English, focused their attention on the patient's cachexia, interpreting the symptoms as due to the leukemia. The patient's noncompliance and passivity in the face of efforts to maintain her oral intake necessitated placement of a percutaneous feeding tube. She complained of bloating, abdominal pain, and diarrhea. Eventually this young woman become immunologically compromised and died of generalized sepsis.

## Food Aversions

Another appetite change noted in cancer is that of an aversion to a specific food or foods, or tastes. As noted earlier, this may develop secondary to metabolic changes produced by the disease or its treatment, particularly radiation therapy to the head and neck regions, and reflect an alteration in physiological taste thresholds. More recently attention has focused on the role of learned food aversions. Research by Bernstein and Webster (1985) has shown that learned food aversions develop as a result of the association between a given food or foods and an unpleasant symptom such as nausea and vomiting. Studied extensively in animals and referred to as the "Garcia effect," this phenomenon is one in which animals learn, in a classical conditioning paradigm, to avoid a taste with which they associate a prior unpleasant symptom. So strong is their association in some cases that it is possible to introduce a delay of many hours between the taste (conditioned stimulus) and the subsequent discomfort (unconditioned stimulus) and, after only a single trial, still produce the effect.

Bernstein and colleagues (Bernstein, 1978, 1982, 1986; Bernstein and Sigundi, 1980; Bernstein and Webster, 1985; Bernstein et al., 1979), in an attempt to examine this response in humans, examined learned food aversions in children receiving chemotherapy for cancer. In their elegant series of studies, children receiving chemotherapy were randomized to a control or experimental group who were offered a novel food (Mapletoff ice cream) shortly before their scheduled chemotherapy treatment. Control patients received no novel food but were occupied with a toy; other control groups consisted of patients receiving chemotherapy with no GI distress or no chemotherapy treatment. All patients were offered several ice cream flavors and tested for food aversions 1–4 weeks later. Those exposed to the Mapletoff were three times more likely to show significant food aversion than other control groups. These studies were later expanded to evaluate responses to common, preferred, and familiar foods. The conclusion of these researchers was that whether novel or part of a regular diet, foods eaten shortly before a treatment with an agent that produces GI discomfort, may likely be avoided later by the individuals. They suggest that neutral foods might be offered before chemotherapy to avoid association with foods that may be important for nutrition. In fact, they demonstrate in an animal model that it is possible to increase caloric intake by presenting a novel diet.

Eating itself may occasionally result in biochemical changes and altered metabolism that in turn may precipitate a learned food aversion. De Wys (1982) noted that patients with cancer produce elevated levels of lactate, a metabolite known to cause nausea if infused into normal volunteers. He suggested that cancer patients eating even a normal-sized meal or a high-carbohydrate diet may develop nausea that then in turn becomes a learned response. Thus, there is possibly a biochemical contribution to learned food aversions that should be explored.

### CASE REPORT

Mr. H. was a 45-year-old traveling salesman with acute lymphocytic leukemia, who was treated with a chemotherapy regimen of induction and consolidation that resulted in acute but transient episodes of nausea, vomiting, anorexia, and change in taste. Mr. H. was then quickly admitted to a sterile room for an allogeneic BMT. Over 3 months he received hyperalimentation that was necessary secondary to stomatitis. Weaning from TPN was stormy. Anorexia was severe despite the absence of any physical problem. However, following struggles with his physician to eat more, he was discharged with continued anorexia and nausea. After a week at home on a bland diet, he became dehydrated and was started on TPN. He became depressed and developed nausea first to solids, then to semisolids; finally, the smell of food or sight of his menu resulted in anxiety and nausea. Antiemetics in adequate doses produced side effects, and he was finally successfully treated by desensitization and relaxation.

This case illustrates the interplay of psychological (anxiety, conflict around weaning from TPN, and subsequent discharge), organic (liver damage, change in taste secondary to inradiation and chemotherapy), and behavioral (learned food aversions) etiologies of anorexia. Psychological intervention was multimodal, including behavioral and pharmacological management. The patient's liver dysfunction slowly resolved without any physiological treatment.

## Psychological Issues in Nutrition Therapy

During the last two decades, artificial feeding techniques have been improved and are being more widely applied. These are now used during chemotherapy, BMT, and after head and neck surgery, in contrast to their earlier more limited use in instances of bowel obstruction and terminal illness. Feedings by hyperalimentation are given by either enteral or parenteral routes (Miller et al., 1986). Enteral feeding includes use of vasogastric, gastrostomy, or jejunostomy routes, each of which serves to bypass the dysfunctional part by employing a flexible thin tube to deliver appropriate nutrients to the functional part. On a short-term basis, the nasoenteral route is used; often patients can insert these very small-diameter catheters daily at home for nutritional support. When it is required on a longer basis, gastrostomy or jejunostomy feeding tubes are inserted by endoscopically guided per-

cutaneous placement. Patients usually begin enteral feedings at half-strength concentrations of polymeric or elemental formulas using continuous or cyclic infusion schedules, and gradually increase infusion rates and concentrations to achieve the desired caloric and volumetric intake (Miller et al., 1986). The polymeric formula consists of fat, protein, and carbohydrate in high molecular weight and is used in patients with normal proteolytic and lipolytic GI capacity. Elemental or monomeric formulas contain nonessential and essential amino acids, little or no triglycerides in the form of medium-chain triglycerides that do not require bile salts or pancreatic enzymes for metabolism, and carbohydrates in the form of monosaccharides and oligosaccharides. Unlike the polymeric formulas, those that are elemental are employed in patients with little proteolytic or lipolytic GI capacity. These formulas are high in osmolality and can result in diarrhea.

Another form of artificial feeding is total parenteral nutrition (TPN). This approach is used for patients who are unable to ingest, digest, or metabolize sufficient nutrients or who have increased caloric or protein needs because of malignancy or infection (Brennan, 1981). Central TPN access allows administration of formulas with high osmolarity that contain high concentrations of dextrose plus vitamins, trace metals, and electrolytes (Shike, 1984). TPN has gained wide success because it involves access via a percutaneous central catheter in the subclavian vein. These silastic catheters with Dacron cuffs, Broviac and Hickman lines, can be cared for by the patient and can remain in place anywhere from months to a few years, allowing home administration of medications as well as alimentation. In addition to Broviac and Hickman lines, a totally subcutaneous central venous access (Port-A-Cath) system is also available (Strum et al., 1986). The Port-A-Cath consists of a silastic central venous system catheter connected to a small-volume subcutaneous injection port. These access systems are advantageous not only for TPN but also for administration of drugs and blood products, alleviating the discomfort of repeated venous punctures. The Port-A-Cath has fewer problems with infection and is less distressing to patients.

Parenteral nutrients can also be administered through peripheral-vein catheters (PTPN) on a temporary basis, using lipid emulsions (soybean or safflower oil) as a nonprotein calorie source to prevent venous sclerosis. Amino acids and carbohydrates constitute the calories; however, the dextrose concentration must be lower than 10% to prevent damage to the vein.

Although patients generally tolerate well the artificial feeding used for short periods of time during hospitalization, feedings are associated with common psychological concerns that can be problematic during prolonged use of this therapy. The patient's initial concerns often involve fears about the meaning that artificial feeding has in terms of their illness, and concern about the impact on their ability to eat normally both immediately and in the future. Patients often equate placement of a tube or catheter as a poor prognostic sign. When such therapy is required, a careful explanation about why it is being placed and for how long needs to be given. The freedom from repeated venipunctures afforded by placement of a line is readily appreciated as a gain. Hyperalimentation during the first 2 weeks after BMT when mouth sores, stomatitis, and esophagitis are common, is well understood. However, weaning off feedings can be problematic. Long-term nutritional treatment results at times in a psychological dependence. In addition, the high caloric content of the feedings increases satiety, reducing physiological hunger and appetite. Weaning is often initiated when patients are still receiving intravenous antibiotics, anorectic in themselves. Because discharge often depends on adequate caloric intake, a conflict can develop between the patient and the physician over eating behavior. Patients feel helpless and need to be encouraged to eat small meals and foods that have appeal.

Table 36-3 summarizes studies of the psychological sequelae of parenteral and enteral artificial feeding. Taken overall, the major psychological issues reported with parenteral access are responses of anxiety and depression to loss of normal appetite and eating, and the impact the feeding equipment has on body image and interpersonal—including sexual—function. In comparison, enteral feedings cause less psychological distress and more distress with the tube or problems with the mechanical aspects of such feeding (Padilla and Grant, 1985). From our clinical experience, patients adjust well if they accept a Broviac or Hickman catheter, which is used for nutritional supplement, for administration of chemotherapy and blood products, and to obtain blood samples. The relative comfort and convenience usually compensate for the psychological problems they experience.

## MANAGEMENT OF ANOREXIA

### Psychotherapeutic, Educational, and Behavioral Interventions

In caring for the patient with anorexia, a full assessment of the causes of appetite change and establishment of a treatment plan is required. The reassurance gained by the patient from an understanding of the cause of the anorexia and a plan to treat it is critically important. Weekly psychotherapy sessions will often begin with a review of appetite changes as a sign of progress toward feeling better. Careful assessment and treatment of underlying anxiety or depression or poten-

tial personal personality problems contributing to anorexia must be undertaken. Referral for behavioral or concrete education about diet may be helpful and critical to management. Books and information on high-calorie foods, ways to serve them, and recipes for small, frequent meals are useful.

Simple behavioral techniques are quite often overlooked by the distraught patient and family. For example, attention to the ambience around meals can have a significant effect. Having a family member share a meal with the hospitalized patient, and/or serving a favorite wine or beer, with candles and special table settings, add to the ''normality'' of eating, despite illness. Patients receiving chemotherapy or irradiation may manage better if they avoid strongly flavored foods like barbecued meats or fish, selecting instead bland foods such as cottage cheese. Special problems, such as reduced saliva secondary to head and neck surgery, chemotherapy, irradiation, or GvHD, mandate a nutritionist's consultation.

A variety of more sophisticated behavioral techniques have been applied to eating disorders in cancer, especially among children. Because anorexia may be accompanied by anxiety or worry concerning food intake and anticipatory anxiety or nausea before a meal, the symptoms of fear, anxiety, worry, and anorexia may become behaviorally coupled to one another. In these situations, behavioral techniques such as relaxation or self-hypnosis can lower anxiety, ameliorate the anticipatory phenomena around eating, and improve fluid and caloric intake. Conflicts with staff and with family members around eating develop easily and quickly, and need to be assessed. Attention to situations that create problems and are associated with refusal to eat is important. A behavioral consultation and intervention may be beneficial. When anxiety is at the center of the problem, relaxation exercises before meals in an effort to reduce the focus on eating and diminish anticipatory distress symptoms, coupled with the use of an antianxiety medication, can improve the anorexia. Sometimes the symptom the patient complains of is ''nausea at the thought or sight of food.'' The same treatments apply as those when it is an anxiety-induced reaction. Symptoms may be experienced as worse in socially embarrassing situations, such as in restaurant where inability to eat or nausea increase self-consciousness and may become a reason to remain at home and not eat with others.

### Pharmacological Interventions

The anorexia seen in cancer, despite its complex causes, often responds to psychological, pharmacological, and behavioral interventions (see Table 36-4). All three may be employed in difficult cases in which a psychological component exists (Holland et al.,

**Table 36-3**  Psychological sequelae of parenteral and enteral feeding

| Reference | Number of patients | Age (years) | Length of feeding (months) | Disease | Findings |
|---|---|---|---|---|---|
| *Parenteral (intravenous or catheter)* | | | | | |
| MacRitchie (1978) | 9 | 18–64 | 3–58 | Noncancerous | Stages of adjustment: (1) Immediate: disbelief, hopelessness, grief, fear of death (2) Intermediate: overdependence on staff (3) Long term: depression, ↓ sexual activity, sleep disturbances secondary to polyuria, loss of vital functions, loss of control, equipment-related ambivalence |
| Price and Levine (1979) | 19 | 17–60 | 1–6 | Unknown | Series of stages: Early: anxiety, disbelief, anger, grief, ↓ body image, feelings of loss Adaptation: loss of control, love–hate relation, depression, some hope for future Long term: ↓ sexual function, ↓ sleep |
| Gulledge et al. (1980) | 50 | 21–63 | 1.5–42.5 | Inflammatory bowel syndrome | Based on first 4 weeks: depression, grief reactions, drug dependency, change in body image, equipment-related anxiety, ↓ sexuality and relationship strains |
| Hughes et al. (1980) | 10 | 15–66 | 3–54 | 9 Crohn's disease 1 Short bowel syndrome | Compliance measures: ↑ Compliance in males with no children and with wives who participated ↓ Compliance in long-term users |
| Malcolm et al. (1980) | 59 | | 1–12 | Noncancerous | Depends on medical diagnosis and length of time on TPN: Acute: transient delirium, depression, hypomania, organic brain syndrome Intermediate: 1–12 weeks depression, ↓ body image, loss of control, dependency, equipment-related fears Long term: ↓ sexual activity, family stress, manipulation of caregivers |
| Perl et al. (1980, 1981) | 10 | 24–66 | 7–48 | 4 Crohn's disease 2 Gardner's syndrome 1 Carcinoid 1 Stab wound 1 Anorexia nervosa 1 Bowel inflammation | Stages: Early: equipment-related fear, loss of control, depression Later: dysphoric mood, crying, insomnia, hopeless body image, ↓ sexual function, mental stress |
| Hall et al. (1981) | 100 | | | Mixed population | Short term (<8 weeks): ↑ organic brain syndrome, confusional states Long term (>8 weeks): transient depression Control (no TPN): no physical differences |

**Table 36-3**  (*Continued*)

| Reference | Number of patients | Age (years) | Length of feeding (months) | Disease | Findings |
|---|---|---|---|---|---|
| Hall et al. (1981) | 30 | | | | More extensively examined: relationship disturbances, equipment-related anxiety |
| | | | | | Chronic versus acute illness: Acute: ↑ symptoms, noncompliance, no severe change in body image, embarrassment, self-consciousness |
| Ladefoged (1981) | 13 | 24–62 | 2–43 | 7 Crohn's disease<br>4 Mesenteric infarction<br>2 Other GI noncancerous illnesses | Low physical effort, fatigue, inertia, loss of eating, equipment-related anxiety, ↓ sexual activity in patients over 55 |
| *Enteral nutrition* | | | | | |
| Padilla et al. (1979) | 30 | >40 | 2 days–2 weeks | Head and neck cancer, trauma | Irritation of pharynx: physical adjustment to texture, smell of food, equipment, dry mouth and soreness in throat and nose |
| | | | | | Absence of swallowing: limited mobility, helplessness, dependence |
| Rains (1981) | 10 | 52–80 | 10 days–5 years | Head and neck cancer | Deprivation of swallowing: social engagement, activity, adjustment with control of GI symptoms |
| Padilla and Grant (1985) | 35 | 15–71 | 24–72 hours | Head and neck cancer, trauma | Deprived of swallowing food: thirst, dry mouth |
| | | | | | Tube-related distress or soreness of nose, throat, secretions, ↓ anxiety with ↑ information on sensory experiences and procedures |

1977). Among the pharmacological agents known to be useful in promoting appetite and weight gain are the antihistamines with anticholinergic effects (cyproheptadine), steroids (prednisone, dexamethasone), and megestrol—(a progestational agent), THC, and amphetamine-like agents (dextroamphetamine). Antihistamines and low doses of tricyclic antidepressants with anticholinergic and antihistaminic properties also promote weight gain and improve appetite. It is often difficult to identify whether appetite loss is due to the tumor or represents an early symptom of depression in the cancer patient; often both contribute. Consequently, a trial of low-dose antidepressants can be extremely helpful to the patient in regaining appropriate food intake. Steroids produce euphoria and an enhanced sense of well-being, which initially improves appetite. Over time, however, increased appetite can result in obesity and severe problems in controlling weight. Amphetamine and amphetamine-like agents also stimulate appetite. Small morning doses of dextroamphetamine or methylphenidate reduce the withdrawal and apathy experienced by patients with advanced disease

and also reduce somnolence caused by analgesics. Excessive doses, however, reduce appetite, and if given toward evening can inhibit sleep. Consequently, these medications must be given before noon and with careful attention to effect (see also Chapter 39 on psychopharmacology). Dizziness, somnolence, depersonalization, and dysphoria can occur with cannabinoids at sufficient dosage to improve appetite, resulting in limitations to their usefulness as well.

## SUMMARY

Anorexia, with its associated decreased food intake and weight loss, is a common and important symptom in cancer, and one that has at times a psychological as well as a physical component. When it is physical in origin, it may be caused directly or indirectly by the disease process of treatment. Most poorly understood is the anorexia–cachexia syndrome of advanced disease. Psychological causes often reflect anxiety about cancer, its possible progression, and depression. Preexisting psychiatric disorders, especially anorexia ner-

**Table 36-4**   Management of anorexia

| Types of management | Interventions |
|---|---|
| Psychotherapeutic and educational counseling | Supportive psychotherapy for fears and depression related to weight loss |
| | Advice about meals with high caloric and protein content, appetizing recipes, visually appealing presentation |
| | Ambiance of mealtime, novel ways of preparing favorite foods |
| | Special consultation for medically related problems of head and neck tumors, stomatitis, artificial feeding |
| Behavioral | Operant-conditioning methods in regard to weight gain |
| | Relaxation techniques before meals |
| | Interventions to reduce learned food aversions |
| Pharmacological | Antihistamines |
| |    Cyproheptadine (Periactin), 4 mg po tid (tablet or elixir) |
| | Steroids |
| |    Dexamethasone (Decadron), variable dosage |
| |    Prednisone, variable dosage |
| | Amphetamines* |
| |    Dextroamphetamine (Dexedrine, Eskatol), 10 mg bid |
| |    Methylphenidate (Ritalin), 2.5–5 mg bid |
| | Antidepressants |
| |    Tricyclic antidepressants, 25–100 mg/day |
| | Cannabinoids |
| |    $\Delta^9$-Tetrahydrocannabinol (THC), 15 mg/day po or inhalation |

*Should be taken in morning or early afternoon to prevent insomnia.

vosa or paranoid states, can substantially complicate cancer treatment.

Regardless of etiology, psychological management of the psychological effects of the anorexia is often helpful. Optimal management often involves the use of a combination of modalities, including psychotherapeutic, behavioral, and/or pharmacological, supplemented by education, counseling, and support. Artificial feeding, used for poor intake, poses a special set of psychological problems for patient and family, depending on whether it is accomplished by tubes (enteral) or by catheters (parenteral). These need to be carefully monitored and addressed. Learned food aversions, which can further restrict limited intake, have been demonstrated in children receiving chemotherapy and may also contribute to aversions to specific foods seen among adult patients after chemotherapy or irra-

diation. Behavioral techniques such as relaxation exercises are useful tools to alter this response as well as to relieve the anxiety precipitated by patient concerns about anorexia and weight loss. Environmental interventions and nutritional advice can also be of considerable value in reversing the negative effects of this distressing symptom in cancer.

# REFERENCES

Bernstein, I.L. (1978). Learned taste aversion in children receiving chemotherapy. *Science* 200(4347):1302–3.

Bernstein, I.L., M.J. Wallace, I.D. Berstein, W.A. Bleyer, R.L. Chard, and J.R. Hartman (1979). Learned food aversions as a consequence of cancer treatment. In J. Van Eys, M.S. Seelig, and B.L. Nichols (eds.), *Nutrition and Cancer*. New York: S P Medical & Scientific Books, pp. 159–64.

Bernstein, I.L. and R.A. Sigundi (1980). Tumor anorexia: A learned food aversion? *Science* 209(4454):416–18.

Bernstein, I. (1982). Physiological and psychological mechanisms of cancer anorexia. *Cancer Res.* 42(Suppl.):715s–20s.

Bernstein, I.L. and M.M. Webster (1985). Learned food aversions: A consequence of cancer chemotherapy. In T.G. Burish, S.M. Levy, and B.E. Meyerowitz (eds.), *Cancer, Nutrition and Eating Behavior*. Hillsdale, N.J.: Erlbaum.

Bernstein, I. (1986). Etiology of anorexia in cancer. *Cancer* 581:1881–86.

Beutler, B. and A. Cerami (1987). Cachectin: More than a tumor necrosis factor. *N. Engl. J. Med.* 316:379–85.

Brennan, M.F. (1981). Total parenteral nutrition in the cancer patient. *N. Engl. J. Med.* 305:375–81.

Burish, T.G., S.M. Levy, and B.E. Meyerowitz (eds.). (1985). *Cancer, Nutrition and Eating Behavior*. N.J.: Erlbaum.

De Wys, W.D. (1982). Pathophysiology of cancer cachexia: Current understanding and areas for future research. *Cancer Res.* 42(Suppl.):721s–26s.

Frymus, M.M. and T.H. Lyons (1986). Prolonged venous access in cancer patients: A review of currently used modalities. *Conn. Med.* 50:225–27.

Good, R.A., A. West, N.K. Day, Z-W. Dong, and G. Fernandes (1982). Effects of undernutrition on host cell and organ function. *Cancer Res.* 42(Suppl.):737s–46s.

Gulledge, A.D., W.T. Gipson, E. Steiger, R. Hooley, and F. Srp (1980). Home parenteral nutrition for the short bowel syndrome: Psychological issues. *Gen. Hosp. Psychiatry* 2:271–81.

Hall, R.C., S.K. Stickney, E.R. Gardner, and M.K. Popkin (1981). Psychiatric reactions to long-term intravenous hyperalimentation. *Psychosomatics* 22:428–43.

Holland, J.C., H.J. Rowland, and M. Plumb (1977). Psychological aspects of anorexia in cancer patients. *Cancer Res.* 37:2425–28.

Hughes, B.A., C.R. Fleming, S. Berkner, and R. Gaffron (1980). Patient compliance with a home parenteral nutrition program. *J. Parent. Ent. Nutr.* 4:12–14.

Kisner, D.L. and W.D. De Wys (1981). Anorexia and cachexia in malignant disease. In G.R. Newell and N.M. Ellison (eds.), *Nutrition and Cancer: Etiology and Treatment*. New York: Raven Press, pp. 355–65.

Krause, R., J.H. James, V. Ziparo, and J.E. Fischer (1979). Brain tryptophan and the neoplastic anorexia–cachexia syndrome. *Cancer* 44:1003–8.

Ladefoged, K. (1981). Quality of life in patients on permanent home parenteral nutrition. *J. Parent. Ent. Nutr.* 5:132–37.

Lowry, M.T. and G.K.W. Yim (1980). Similar feeding profiles in tumor-bearing and dexamethasone-treated rats suggest endorphin depletion in cancer cachexia. *Neurosci. Abst.* 6:518.

MacRitchie, K.J. (1978). Life without eating or drinking: Total parenteral nutrition outside the hospital. *Can. Psychiatr. Assoc. J.* 23:373–79.

Malcolm, R., J.R.K. Robson, T.W. Vanderveen, and P.M. O'Neal (1980). Psychosocial aspects of total parenteral nutrition. *Psychosomatics* 21:115–25.

Miller, L.S., G.D. Pinchcofsky-Devin, R.E. Yen, and M.V. Kaminski, Jr. (1986). Enteral and parenteral nutrition in the critically ill patient. *Hosp. Form.* 21:672–82.

Norton, J.A., R. Shamberger, T.P. Stein, G.W.A. Milne, and M.F. Brennan (1981). The influence of tumor-bearing on protein metabolism in the rat. *J. Surg. Res.* 30:456–62.

Ohnuma, T. and J.F. Holland (1977). Nutritional consequences of cancer chemotherapy and immunotherapy. *Cancer Res.* 37:2395–2406.

Old, L.J. (1985). Tumor necrosis factor (TNF). *Science* 230(4726):630–32.

Padilla, G.V. and M.M. Grant (1985). Psychosocial aspects of artificial feeding. *Cancer* 55:301–4.

Padilla, G.V., M. Grant, H. Wong, B.W. Hansen, R.L. Hanson, N. Bergstrom, and W.R. Kubo (1979). Subjective distresses of nasograstric fluid tube feeding. *J. Parent. Ent. Nutr.* 3:53–57.

Perl, M., R.C. Hall, S.J. Dudrick, D.M. Englert, S.K. Stickney, and E.R. Gardner (1980). Psychological aspects of long-term home hyperalimentation. *J. Parent. Ent. Nutr.* 4:554–60.

Perl, M., L.G. Peterson, S.J. Dudrick, and D.M. Benson (1981). Psychiatric effects of long-term home hyperalimentation. *Psychosomatics* 22:1047–63

Peteet, J.R., C. Medeiros, L. Slavin, and K. Walsh-Burke (1981). Psychological aspects of artificial feeding in cancer patients. *J. Parent. Ent. Nutr.* 5:138–40.

Price, B.S. and E.L. Levine (1979). Permanent total parenteral nutrition. *J. Parent. Ent. Nutr.* 3:48–52.

Rains, B.L. (1981). The non-hospitalized tube-fed patient. *Oncol. Nurs. Forum* 8(2):8–13.

Shike, M. (1984). Trace metals in parenteral and enteral nutrition. *Curr. Concepts Perspect. Nutr.* 3(1):1–10. (Available from The Nutrition Information Center, 515 East 71 Street, S 904, New York, N.Y. 10021 [The New York Hospital–Cornell University Medical Center and Memorial Sloan-Kettering Cancer Center]).

Shils, M.E. (1979). Nutritional problems induced by cancer. *Med. Clin. North Am.* 63:1009–25.

Strum, S., J. McDermed, A. Korn, and C. Joseph (1986). Improved methods for venous access: The Port-A-Cath, a totally implanted catheter system. *J. Clin. Oncol.* 4:596–603.

Van Eys, J. (1982). Effects of nutritional status on response to therapy. *Cancer Res.* 42(Suppl.):747s–753s.

# 37

# The Older Patient with Cancer

Mary Jane Massie and Jimmie C. Holland

The risk of developing cancer increases rapidly with advancing age. Approximately 50% of all cancers occur in people over 65 years of age (Cutler and Young, 1975). Because the nation's number of older individuals is increasing rapidly as well, cancer can be expected to become an even greater public health problem by the next century. Despite the magnitude of the problem of cancer in the aged, little systematic work has focused on the epidemiology, diagnosis, and treatment of cancer in this group. In fact, clinical studies excluded the elderly patient from entry in most clinical investigations until a change was instituted in NIH policy in the early 1980s (Kennedy, 1985). Cancer was not as vigorously treated in the elderly, on the assumption that tolerance of treatment side effects would be poor. However, these concerns were reappraised when Begg and Carbone (1983), as part of the Eastern Cooperative Oncology Group, reviewed 19 studies of older individuals' responses to therapeutic regimens for eight common tumors. They found that toxicity rates were nearly identical for older and younger groups, with the exception of higher incidence in the older patients of leukopenia and hematological toxicity in those regimens containing methotrexate and methyl-CCNU, due to diminished creatinine clearance in older individuals.

Whereas the biological significance of increased cancer in the older individual is unclear, cell-mediated immunity is known to decline with aging and may represent a principal influence in increased cancer incidence. Additionally, some tumors behave differently in the aged in contrast to the young, underscoring additional biological differences and suggesting a need for further research on cancer in this age group. There are equally compelling reasons to study the psychological adaptation of older versus younger individuals.

The older individual who develops cancer in our society faces the dual social stigma of being old and of

having cancer. This occurs at a time when these individuals are also facing the additional burdens commonly associated with aging, such as loss of spouse, siblings, and friends, reduced physical strength and mobility, diminution of sight and hearing, and restricted social and financial resources. These developmental issues, which are relevant to care of the older adult, are reviewed by Rowland in Chapter 4. This chapter is concerned with the special psychosocial problems facing the older patient in the context of the common cancers, their treatment, and the psychosocial and psychiatric complications that occur in older age groups.

## COMMON NEOPLASMS AND THEIR TREATMENT

The common sites of tumors in older individuals are skin, prostate, lung, GI system (esophagus, stomach, colon–rectum, pancreas), and (in women) breast and gynecological (ovaries, uterus) cancer. The common hematological malignancies are leukemia and lymphoma.

Skin cancers, when diagnosed and treated early, are responsive to treatment, but basal-cell carcinomas on the face can be extensive and recurrent. Treatment may require repeated wide excision, occasionally with significant facial disfigurement and associated emotional distress.

Prostatic cancer, a common tumor of older men, is often advanced when diagnosed. Surgical removal, radiotherapy, or both are used for local control. Advanced prostate cancer is responsive to hormonal management by bilateral orchiectomy or estrogen administration. Such treatment promotes survival over several years, even when there has been metastatic spread. Side effects are limited largely to diminished sexual function and feminization of body fat distribution, and risk of cardiovascular complications. Cytotoxic chemotherapy may be useful (Kennedy, 1985).

The peak appearance of lung cancer is in the sixth decade. Previously confined to men, the incidence of lung cancer in women is regrettably rapidly reaching that of men and has already surpassed breast cancer in mortality rates. The increase in lung cancer in U.S. women lags about 20 years behind the onset of cigarette smoking, which began in the 1920s. Unresected lung cancer is associated with a short survival. Pneumonectomy or lobectomy carry a higher operative mortality in patients over 65, but when the lesion is resectable, survival is improved by a few years. Radiotherapy may be used for limited disease or for palliation. Chemotherapy has achieved some success in treating small-cell lung carcinoma, producing cure in a few patients. However, this has not been true for non-small-cell carcinoma, which responds poorly to chemotherapy.

Colorectal carcinoma is one of the most common neoplasms in older individuals and is by far the most common GI tumor in both older men and women. Unfortunately, these tumors have often spread at time of diagnosis in older patients. They respond poorly to chemotherapy when they recur after surgical excision. Pancreatic cancer is increasing without a clear reason in both sexes and, with its survival rate of less than 1% at 5 years, has the poorest prognosis not only among GI tumors, but all tumors generally. The prevalence of stomach cancer, on the other hand, is decreasing in both sexes for reasons that are also not well understood. Esophageal tumors, treated by surgical excision, are often found to have spread locally at time of diagnosis, and therefore often have a more limited prognosis.

The prevalence of breast cancer in women increases with age; in fact, it is estimated that 50% of all breast cancers occurs in women over 65. However, it is a slower growing tumor and metastatic disease takes a more indolent course (Kennedy, 1985). The incidence of estrogen-positive tumors increases with age, which may contribute to favorable response. Hormonal management of metastatic disease is highly effective in older women.

Ovarian and uterine cancers are the most common gynecological neoplasms in the older woman, although uterine cancer is decreasing in prevalence and, because of earlier diagnosis, mortality as well. Women who have been previously treated for breast or endometrial cancer are more likely to develop cancer of the ovary as a second primary cancer (Griffiths, 1982).

The lymphomas seen in older patients are primarily the non-Hodgkin's lymphomas. Acute nonlymphocytic leukemia (ANLL) and chronic lymphocytic leukemia (CLL) are the common leukemias seen at middle and older ages, with CLL being the most common type of leukemia after age 60 (Gunz, 1982). ANLL in the elderly carries a poor prognosis, while CLL may continue many years in an indolent state, but is rapidly fatal when transformed into a blastic phase. Chemotherapeutic regimens are the primary means of treatment for these hematological tumors; bone marrow transplant (BMT) has not been successful in older adults.

## PSYCHOLOGICAL COMPLICATIONS

The best prognosis for cancer in older individuals is associated with early diagnosis and treatment. Unfortunately, older individuals may neglect an early symptom of cancer for a longer period than would a younger individual, leading to delay in diagnosis as a cause for poor outcome. Pain, blood in stools, coughing of blood, weakness, and fatigue may be ignored initially. A number of causes can contribute to procrastination, including worry about the cost of doctor visits and treatment in those with poor financial resources, lack of knowledge, less education, and/or language barriers to information and care, social isolation, and pessimistic and fatalistic attitudes about disease and treatment outcome. "If I have cancer, I'll die of it anyway, so why bother to be treated?" is an attitude more common in older than younger patients. A study by Wilson and colleagues (1984) on attitudes about cancer in 267 older individuals found that they believed that cancer treatments are worse than the disease, and that doctors cause patients to worry more by not explaining things. These strongly held negative beliefs can encourage delay in consultation. Moreover, not having a personal physician or being unable to identify community facilities can contribute to delay in the older person as well (Snider, 1980).

The psychological complications encountered in the older patient during treatment for cancer can be seen as falling into the three broad areas of those occurring during active treatment (adjustment disorders, depression, and delirium), those associated with palliative and terminal care, and those faced by survivors of active treatment who may or may not be cured but who must take up their usual life. The description and management of problems within these three major treatment phases are outlined here.

### Psychological Problems During Active Treatment

The special psychological and rehabilitative problems of older patients have been inadequately addressed. However, the few available studies suggest that older patients adapt better to illness than younger. A study of

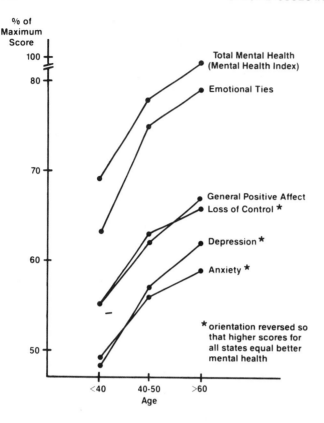

**Figure 37-1.** Psychological status according to age category for six patient groups combined (*n* = 758). *Source:* Reprinted with permission from B. R. Cassileth, E.J. Lusk, T.B. Strouse, D.S. Miller, L.L. Brown, P.A. Cross, and A.N. Tenaglia (1984). Psychosocial status in chronic illness: A comparative analysis of six diagnostic groups. *N. Engl. J. Med.* 311:506–11.

758 patients who had one of six different chronic illnesses was carried out by Cassileth and colleagues (1984), who examined their scores on the Mental Health Index. The five groups of physically ill patients did not differ significantly from each other or the general population, but all had significantly higher psychological status scores than the physically healthy but psychiatrically depressed group. Additionally, when grouped across three age categories (<40, 40–60, and >60), the mental health scores for older groups were found to be higher than younger, irrespective of the chronic illness (arthritis, diabetes, cancer, renal disease, dermatological disorder, or depression). Figure 37-1 illustrates these results, showing the total mental health score and the five component scores increasing as a function of better mental health in the older ages, despite presence of chronic illness. In interpreting their findings, Cassileth and colleagues postulate that older patients may have developed more effective skills to manage stress; illness in the older patient may also result in increased attention and involvement from others. Plumb and Holland (1981) also found better adjustment and less distress in older versus younger patients with advanced cancer. Examining psychological adjustment, using a semistructured interview schedule of current and past adjustment, these researchers found that psychological distress was greater in each decreasing decade in age, from the oldest group to the youngest in their twenties.

Maisiak and colleagues (1983) reported data from a large sample (230) of elderly patients with cancer. Those patients aged 60–97, despite lower income and education, had a somewhat better overall psychosocial status, were less likely to be depressed, and managed work and leisure better than younger patients aged 21–58. The older group missed appointments more often than the younger groups, however, because of lack of faith in the treatments and dislike of the confusing clinic atmosphere.

Ganz, Schag, and Heinrich (1985) used the self-administered Cancer Inventory of Problem Situations (CIPS) to assess psychosocial and rehabilitative issues in a sample of 240 men with cancer. They used an age cutoff of 65 to distinguish between older and younger patients and matched the older and younger for cancer site and Karnofsky level of performance. Despite a higher rate of cardiac and other chronic diseases in the older group (mean age 72) as compared to the younger (mean age 53), there were surprisingly few differences between groups in marital and sexual functioning, or in reported problems of daily living. In terms of ability to deal with the medical setting, the older men communicated better with the team and tended to report less psychological and social distress than younger, per-

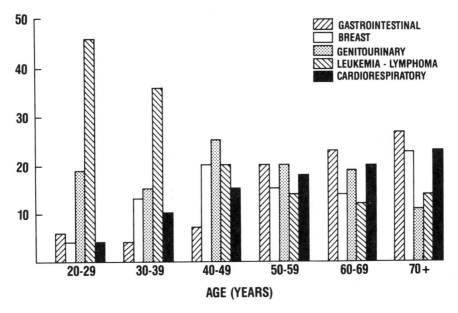

**Figure 37-2.** Average percentage of psychiatric consultations by age (per decade) by cancer diagnosis ($n = 546$).

haps because of more experience with illness and prior hospitalizations.

Although overall adaptation to illness in older patients may be as good as or better than that seen in younger ones, older patients may be at greater risk for developing specific types of problems necessitating psychiatric consultation during active treatment periods.

Whereas Popkin, MacKenzie, and Callies (1984) have reported a review of psychiatric consultations on elderly medically ill patients, most attention has been given to the prevalence and problems of confusional states and dementia in the elderly (Liston, 1984; Seymour et al., 1980). A monograph on psychiatric disorders in the elderly, and their pharmacological management by Salzman (1984) provides an extensive review of these issues. Few studies have focused on the particular psychiatric problems of older patients with cancer. A review of the psychiatric consultations performed during an 18-month period (1980–1981) by the Psychiatry Service at Memorial Sloan-Kettering Cancer Center (MSKCC) has provided helpful information in this regard (Holland and Massie, 1987). Of the 546 patients for whom a consultation was requested, 294 (54%) were 50 years of age or older. Diagnostic information for these patients was compared to that for those aged 49 and younger. Of patients in the sample, most (975) were white, 60% were married, and 70% lived with their family.

With respect to the older group, the sites of cancer represented the common tumor types seen in this age group, namely colorectal, lung, prostate, ovarian,

uterus, breast, leukemia, and lymphoma. Figure 37-2 shows the diagnoses by decade for the whole sample and reflects the rising proportion of patients with cardiorespiratory (largely lung) and GI tumors in the older age groups. The distribution of psychiatric (DSM-III) diagnoses for the two groups of patients is shown in Table 37-1. Prevalence data of these disorders reported in the PSYCOG study of cancer patients (Derogatis et al., 1983) are included for comparative purposes. Figure 37-3 shows the distribution of these psychiatric diagnoses by decade from age 20 through 70 and older for the MSKCC sample. The most marked differences between older versus younger groups are the increased frequency of organic mental disorders in patients 60 and over and the decrease in the frequency of adjustment disorder diagnosed in these older age groups. There was, however, an increase in major depression in the group over 70.

## ADJUSTMENT DISORDERS AND MAJOR DEPRESSION

The most common psychiatric diagnosis in the older patients, as in the younger, is adjustment disorder (with depressed, mixed, or anxious mood). However, older patients particularly at risk may be those with meager social supports or another concurrent medical illness. Financial worries, other recent losses, and bereavement contribute to greater stress and may result in more anxiety and depressive symptoms.

When an older individual faces cancer, the reaction is highly variable. All patients fear becoming "a bur-

**Table 37-1**  Comparison of DSM-III diagnoses in psychiatric consultations in younger and older patients, total and PSYCOG prevalence study

| DSM-III diagnosis | MSKCC Consultation data (%) | | | PSYCOG prevalence data* |
| --- | --- | --- | --- | --- |
| | Age <50 yr (n = 252) | Age >50 yr (n = 294) | Total (n = 546) | |
| Adjustment disorder | 59 | 50 | 54 | 32 |
| Organic mental disorder | 12 | 26 | 20 | 4 |
| Depression | 14 | 10 | 9 | 6 |
| Major psychiatric disorder | 7 | 5 | 5 | — |
| Anxiety disorders | 4 | 3 | 4 | 2 |
| Other | 4 | 4 | 4 | 3 |
| None | 4 | 3 | 4 | 53 |

*Source*: From Derogatis et al. (for PSYCOG) (1983).

den'' on children or others; many often must face loss of independence that might otherwise have been maintained. However, older individuals, perhaps by virtue of facing life stresses before, as noted earlier, show less acute response to the crisis of diagnosis, feeling less surprise and anger at illness than younger individuals.

Differentiating between adjustment disorder with depressed mood and a major depression can be a diagnostic challenge in the older cancer patient, in whom the presenting features can reflect the continuum of depressive symptoms. This is especially true in the more disabled patient, who may have weight loss in addition to other vegetative symptoms related to the cancer. However, the presence of a sad mood, with pessimism, hopelessness, worthlessness, guilt, and suicidal ideation are important diagnostic signs (Mas-

sie and Holland, 1984). The older patient may initially resist referral for psychiatric consultation, even when quite distressed, because of the implied suggestion of ''mental illness'' or the fear that others will suspect or assume that he or she is unable to manage the problems of illness. The usual reluctance of older individuals to utilize mental health facilities is even greater in those who have cancer (Butler, 1975).

The depressed older cancer patient should first be assessed for medications that frequently produce depressive symptoms, including cimetidine, diazepam, guanethidine, narcotic analgesics, propranolol, methyldopa, L-dopa, and reserpine. Older patients also take nonprescription drugs in efforts at self-medication. The physician should inquire about the use of these drugs and about alcohol use. Accuracy of dosages of prescribed medications should additionally be

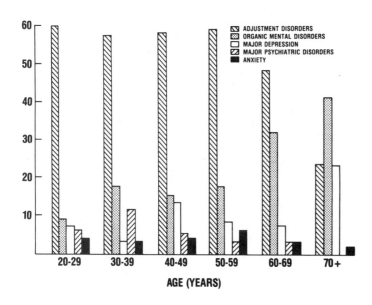

**Figure 37-3.** Average percentage of psychiatric consultations by age (per decade) by DSM-III diagnosis (n = 546).

reviewed; faulty vision, or poor memory can result in medications being taken in excessive amounts. Commonly used cancer chemotherapeutic agents that cause depression include prednisone, dexamethasone, procarbazine, vincristine, and vinblastine (Young, 1982). Evaluation of possible drug-induced depression should be completed before any pharmacotherapy is considered.

In cases in which the predominant symptom is cognitive impairment, it is essential to make a distinction in the elderly, between physiological dementia and pseudodementia caused by depression. This differential diagnosis does not arise often in patients with cancer. However, older patients may have a mild dementia that, when cancer develops, may become complicated by depression or a superimposed, transient delirium occurring secondary to drugs or complications of disease (see Chapter 30).

Treatment of the depressed older patient should combine short-term supportive psychotherapy that explores underlying psychological or concurrent social problems with, when appropriate, pharmacotherapy to control symptoms. The treatment of depression in the elderly by antidepressants has been reviewed elsewhere (Salzman, 1984; Gerner, 1984). Tricyclic antidepressants have been the class of medications most commonly used. Nortriptyline and desipramine are usually better tolerated by the elderly because they are less likely to produce orthostatic hypotension at therapeutically equivalent doses than other tricyclics (e.g., amitriptyline and imipramine). Treatment is usually started at low dosage, which is titrated slowly upward as tolerated.

A therapeutic daily dose of nortriptyline for elderly cancer patients may be as low as 30–40 mg. The tricyclics have a long half-life, and hence the total daily dose is often taken at bedtime. The sedating effects are useful in the depressed patient with insomnia. The clinician should monitor blood levels of both nortriptyline and desipramine. Before starting antidepressants in the elderly, an electrocardiogram (ECG) should be obtained.

Orthostatic hypotension is one of the most troublesome anticholinergic side effects of tricyclics in the elderly. Other anticholinergic side effects that may limit dosage are delirium and cardiac arrhythmias (Friedel, 1983; Meyers and Mei-tal, 1983). The elderly male with prostatic hypertrophy and urinary retention and patients of both sexes with constipation often have difficulty tolerating strongly anticholinergic drugs, as does the cancer patient who has obstructive symptoms associated with GI or genitourinary surgery. Patients with stomatitis secondary to chemotherapy or radiotherapy likewise will benefit

from the least anticholinergic drugs or from the short-acting benzodiazepine, alprazolam (see later). Doxepin, amitriptyline, and imipramine are tricyclics that are useful in reducing pain and potentiating the effect of narcotic analgesics (Massie and Holland, 1984).

The new, short-acting benzodiazepine, alprazolam, is of interest in older cancer patients. It has both anxiolytic and antidepressant properties and is proving to be useful in the clinical treatment of depression among elderly patients (Pitts et al., 1983; Ayd, 1984; Rickels et al., 1985). Because of its short half-life and absence of anticholinergic effects, it is well tolerated.

## DELIRIUM

Delirium, the second most common psychiatric diagnosis among older cancer patients (and especially frequent in hospitalized patients 70 and older in the MSKCC series reported here), arises from the direct effects of cancer consequent to structural damage caused by invasion or extension of the disease into the CNS as well as—more commonly—nonmetastatic involvement or metabolic encephalopathy related to organ failure (liver, kidney, lung, thyroid, or adrenal gland), electrolyte imbalance (hypercalcemia, hyponatremia), vitamin deficiencies (vitamin $B_1$); drug effects (narcotic analgesics, chemotherapeutic agents, sedatives, hypnotics, and cumulative effects of medications with anticholinergic properties), sepsis, intravascular coagulation (often associated with lung cancer), or hormone-producing tumors (Posner, 1979; Lipowski, 1983).

Failure of an organ system is common in terminal states, and often causes mental confusion. Prompt recognition and treatment of delirium in the older cancer patient can reduce distress for patient and family during terminal stages. Having on record a "baseline" mental status examination makes it easier to identify the early symptoms of delirium, including restlessness, irritability, mood lability, suspiciousness or confusion with mild disorientation, recent memory loss, and poor judgment.

Early symptoms of delirium are often misdiagnosed as depression by referring physicians (Levine et al., 1978; Trzepacz et al., 1984; Massie et al., 1983). The erroneous assumption is that "the impact of the disease has finally caught up with him." Because elderly cancer patients are often reluctant to report mild mood disturbances or mild changes in thinking to physicians, delirium often progresses to late or more severe stages with symptoms of agitation, paranoid delusions, or hallucinations, before etiological workup is started or treatment is instituted.

Careful evaluation of CNS dysfunction must be included in the medical and psychiatric evaluation of the elderly cancer patient. Several points should be kept in mind during the evaluation and treatment of delirium (Massie et al., 1983).

1. It is often necessary to treat a patient's agitation or disturbed behavior while simultaneously trying to determine its cause.
2. Careful serial review of mental status and medical and laboratory data must be undertaken; neurological consultation should be obtained when focal signs are present.
3. Patients with delirium benefit from short, frequent contacts with a supportive person, preferably a family member who speaks quietly and reassuringly about the environment, correcting misinterpretations and assisting in the patient's orientation to objects and people around him or her. Continuity in nursing staffing from shift to shift can help allay the patient's anxiety about surroundings.
4. When agitation is severe or the patient is delusional or hallucinating, constant nursing observation is indicated. Suicidal ideation or acts may occur in response to frightening hallucinations or delusions or awareness of change in mental functioning. When this occurs in the presence of impaired impulse control resulting from mild delirium, there is serious suicidal risk (see Chapter 24 on suicide).
5. A psychopharmacological approach should be used with patients exhibiting agitation or disruptive behavior as a part of their delirium. In those cases haloperidol is the most effective drug, orally or by intramuscular injection of 0.25–1.0 mg. This reduces agitation without causing oversedation or hypotension in the elderly. Doses, repeated at intervals of 30 to 60 minutes, are titrated against behavior. Extrapyramidal system (EPS) effects of haloperidol are more frequent in older patients, and they can be controlled with benztropine (see chapter 39 on psychopharmacology).

## COMPLIANCE WITH ACTIVE TREATMENT

It is essential that patients adhere to cancer treatment for best results. Older patients surprisingly have been found to be more likely to comply with therapeutic regimens than younger (Haug, 1979). An important consideration in helping older patients comply is the presence of supportive people who encourage utilization of available services (Lewis et al., 1983). Social isolation has been related to poorer resistance to illness in general (Berkman, 1982). There is a great need for attention to the psychosocial care of older patients who must receive lengthy and arduous regimens of either chemotherapy or radiotherapy.

## Psychological Issues Associated with Palliative Care

For those older patients in whom curative treatment is ineffective, the role of the oncologist and psychiatrist is to assure maximal comfort during the advanced stages of disease. It is during this period that the psychiatrist can provide crucial interventions by managing behavior related to delirium, evaluating and treating pain, depression, and anxiety, evaluating suicidal statements (which may be secondary to delirium, depression, and/or pain), helping staff reduce conflicts regarding patient care, evaluating both patient and family conflicts that can arise from a prolonged and uncertain course of illness, and counseling the bereaved.

In the terminal stages of cancer, a decision to respect the patient's comfort by not drawing blood or doing invasive procedures may preclude establishing a cause of delirium. The delirium seen in end-stage disease usually has more than one cause. Likely irreversible, management is predicated on providing maximal psychological support and pharmacological management. Delirium, pain, and anxiety should be controlled while attempting to avoid excessive sedation. A survey by Jaeger and colleagues (1985) showed that, in advanced disease stages, older patients are prescribed fewer psychotropic drugs, particularly antidepressant and antianxiety drugs, than younger (see Fig. 37-4).

The psychiatric consultant may be needed to assist the family with the stress of long or repeated hospitalizations. Awaiting and anticipating how and when death will occur becomes a major preoccupation. If the decision is made for the elderly patient to die at home, the family must be informed about available home care programs and nursing support, and a plan for home care instituted (see also Chapters 48 and 49).

Anticipatory bereavement and bereavement counseling for elderly widows and widowers provides important support for the survivors of cancer patients, and may reduce the frequency and morbidity of a range of illnesses that occur more frequently in settings of loss and grief (Helsing and Szklo, 1981). In their study of the incidence of mortality following loss of a spouse, Helsing and Szklo found that widowers between the ages of 55 and 75 are at increased risk. The psychiatrist who has seen the patient before he or she dies is ideally situated to provide ongoing counseling to the bereaved relative.

## Psychological Issues Related to Long Survival and Cure

Today's oncologists are increasingly concerned with issues related to the cured patient and the survivor who

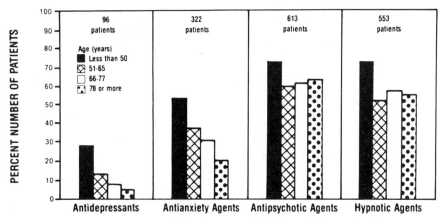

**Figure 37-4.** Age-related utilization of psychotropic drugs in advanced-cancer patients. Collapsed across drug classes, the difference between age groups is statistically significant ($p < .005$). Those patients 50 years of age or less were prescribed on the average significantly more psychotropic medications than any of the other age groups. *Source:* Reprinted with permission from H. Jaeger, G.R. Morrow, P.J. Carpenter, and F. Brescia (1985). A survey of psychotropic drug utilization by patients with advanced neoplastic disease. *Gen. Hosp. Psychiatry* 7:353–60.

finishes treatment and returns to normal activities. This is a stressful period, irrespective of age, when long-term outcome is unclear. The older patient may have many worries about his or her ability to pursue plans for retirement or an independent living situation. Counseling may be critical at this time. As increasing numbers of older patients are surviving with their disease, physicians and mental health professionals are turning their attention to their special rehabilitative needs. For example, the patient treated for head and neck cancer requires special attention to assure appropriate prostheses are obtained and to promote cooperation with care. Complications of treatment must be watched for, in addition to monitoring for and controlling the effects of other chronic diseases. The patient, especially the older woman with breast cancer, may fear for herself and her daughter.

## SUMMARY

Cancer in the older individual has been subjected to increasing scrutiny, with the result that several commonly held myths have been rejected. Not only do older patients tolerate and comply with most treatment for cancer as well as younger individuals, but they also cope better psychologically and maintain better mental health than younger patients. Several psychological risks, however, must be recognized in this group, including a tendency to delay in seeking consultation for early symptoms, a greater tendency toward development of delirium, response to psychotropic medications requiring cautious use, tendency for preexisting psychiatric problems (alcohol abuse and depression) to complicate care, and increased need for support of the surviving spouse. Management during active treat-

ment, palliative and terminal care, and a successful treatment completion poses challenging problems for the psychiatric consultant who seeks to help the older patient with cancer. Work with this group of cancer patients, however, is equally rewarding.

## REFERENCES

Ayd, F.J., Jr. (1984). Psychopharmacology update: Alprazolam—anxiolytic and antidepressant. *Psychiatr. Ann.* 14:393–95.

Ban, T.A. (1980). *Psychopharmacology for the Aged.* New York: Karger.

Ban, T.A. (1984). Chronic disease and depression in the geriatric population. *J. Clin. Psychiatry* 45:18–23.

Begg, C.B. and P.P. Carbone (1983). Clinical trials and drug toxicity in the elderly: The experience of the Eastern Cooperative Oncology Group. *Cancer* 52:1986–92.

Berkman, D. (1982). Social support and mortality in an elderly community population. *Am. J. Epidemiol.* 115:684–94.

Butler, R.N. (1975). Psychiatry and the elderly: An overview. *Am. J. Psychiatry* 132:893–900.

Casslieth, B.R., E.J. Lusk, T.B. Strouse, D.S. Miller, L.L. Brown, P.A. Cross, and A.N. Tenaglia (1984). Psychosocial status in chronic illness: A comparative analysis of six diagnostic groups. *N. Engl. J. Med.* 311:506–11.

Cutler, S.J. and J.L. Young (1975). *Third National Cancer Survey: Incidence Data.* DHEW Publ. No. (NIH)75-787) (National Cancer Institute Monograph No. 41). Bethesda, Md.: National Cancer Institute.

Derogatis, L.R., G.R. Morrow, J. Fetting, D. Penman, S. Piasetsky, A.M. Schmale, M. Henrichs, and C.M. Carnicke (1983). The prevalence of psychiatric disorders among cancer patients. *J.A.M.A.* 249:751–57.

Friedel, R.O. (1983). Affective disorders in the geriatric patient. In L. Grinspoon (ed.), *Psychiatry Update*, Vol.

II. Washington, D.C.: American Psychiatric Association, pp. 118–30.

Ganz, P.A., C.C. Schag, and R.L. Heinrich (1985). The psychosocial impact of cancer on the elderly: A comparison with younger patients. *J. Am. Geriatr. Soc.* 33:429–35.

Gerner, R.H. (1984). Antidepressant selection in the elderly. *Psychosomatics* 25:528–35.

Griffiths, C.T. (1982). Carcinoma of the ovary and fallopian tube. In J.F. Holland and E. Frei, III (eds.), *Cancer Medicine,* 2nd ed. Philadelphia: Lea & Febiger, pp. 1958–71; 2391.

Gunz, F.W. (1982). Chronic lymphocytic leukemia. In J.F. Holland and E. Frei III (eds.), *Cancer Medicine,* 2nd ed. Philadelphia: Lea & Febiger, pp. 1460–77; 2357–59.

Haug, M. (1979). Doctor–patient relations and the older patients. *J. Gerontol.* 34:852–60.

Helsing, K.J. and M. Szklo (1981). Mortality after bereavement. *Am. J. Epidemiol.* 114:41–52.

Holland, J.C. (1982). Psychologic aspects of cancer. In J.F. Holland and E. Frei III (eds.), *Cancer Medicine,* 2nd ed. Philadelphia: Lea & Febiger, pp. 1175–1203; 2325–31.

Holland, J.C. and M.J. Massie (1987). Psychosocial aspects of cancer in the elderly. *Clin. Geriatr. Med.* 3:533–39.

Jaeger, H., G.R. Morrow, P.J. Carpenter, and F. Brescia (1985). A survey of psychotropic drug utilization by patients with advanced neoplastic disease. *Gen. Hosp. Psychiatry* 7:353–60.

Kennedy, B.J. (1985). Specific considerations for the geriatric patient with cancer. In P. Calabresi, P.S. Schein, and S.A. Rosenberg (eds.), *Medical Oncology: Basic Principles and Clinical Management of Cancer.* New York: Macmillan, pp. 1433–45.

Levine, P.M., P.M. Silberfarb, and Z.J. Lipowski (1978). Mental disorders in cancer patients: A study of 100 psychiatric referrals. *Cancer* 42:1385–91.

Lewis, C., M. Linet, and M. Abeloff (1983). Compliance with cancer therapy by patients and physicians. *Am. J. Intern. Med.* 74:673–78.

Lipowski, Z.J. (1983). Transient cognitive disorders (delirium, acute confusional states in the elderly. *Am. J. Psychiatry* 140:1426–36.

Liston, E.H. (1984). Diagnosis and management of delirium in the elderly patient. *Psychiatr. Ann.* 14:109–18.

Luchins, D.J. (1983). Review of clinical and animal studies comparing the cardiovascular effects of doxepin and other tricyclic antidepressants. *Am. J. Psychiatry* 140:1006–9.

Maisiak, R., R. Gams, E. Lee, and B. Jones (1983). The psychosocial support status of elderly cancer outpatients. *Prog. Clin. Biol. Res.* 120:395–403.

Massie, M.J. and J.C. Holland (1984). Psychiatry and oncology. In L. Grinspoon (ed.), *Psychiatry Update, Vol. III* Washington, D.C.: American Psychiatric Association, pp. 239–56.

Massie, M.J., J.C. Holland, and E. Glass (1983). Delirium in terminally ill cancer patients. *Am. J. Psychiatry* 140:1048–50.

Meyers, B.S. and V. Mei-tal (1983). Psychiatric reactions during tricyclic treatment of the elderly reconsidered. *J. Clin. Psychopharmacol.* 3:2–6.

Pitts, W.M., W.E. Fann, C. Sajadi, and S. Snyder (1983). Alprazolam in older depressed inpatients. *J. Clin. Psychiatry* 44:213–15.

Plumb, M. and J.C. Holland (1981). Comparative studies of psychological function in patients with advanced cancer: II. Interview-rated current and past psychological symptoms. *Psychosom. Med.* 43:243–54.

Popkin, M.J., T.B. MacKenzie, and A.L. Callies (1984). Psychiatric consultation to geriatric medically ill inpatients in a university hospital. *Arch. Gen. Psychiatry* 41:703–7.

Posner, J.B. (1979). Neurological complications of systemic cancer. *Med. Clin. North Am.* 63:783–800.

Rickels, K., J.P. Feighner, and W.T. Smith (1985). Alprazolam, amitriptyline, doxepin, and placebo in the treatment of depression. *Arch. Gen. Psychiatry* 42:134–41.

Salzman, C. (1984). *Clinical Geriatric Psychopharmacology.* New York: McGraw-Hill.

Seymour, D.G., P.J. Henschke, R.D. Cape, and A.J. Campbell (1980). Acute Confusional states and dementia in the elderly: The role of dehydration/volume depletion, physical illness and age. *Age Ageing* 9:137–46.

Snider, E.L. (1980). Awareness and use of health services by the elderly: A Canadian study. *Med. Care* 28:1177–82.

Trzepacz, P.T., G.B. Teague, and Z.J. Lipowski (1984). Organic mental disorders in a general hospital (Abstract). *Psychosom. Med.* 46:83.

Young, D.F. (1982). Neurological complications of cancer chemotherapy. In A. Silverstein (ed.), *Neurological Complications of Therapy: Selected Topics.* New York: Futura Publishing, pp. 57–113.

Weinberger, D.R. (1977). Tricyclic choice for elder patients (Letter to the Editor). *Am. J. Psychiatry* 134:1048.

Wilson, C.M., B.K. Rimer, D.J. Bennett, P.F. Engstrom, E. Kane-Williams, and J. White (1984). Educating the older cancer patient: Obstacles and opportunities. *Health Educ. Q.* 10(Spec. Suppl.):76–87.

# PART VII

## Therapeutic Interventions

# 38

## Psychotherapeutic Interventions

Mary Jane Massie, Jimmie C. Holland, and Norman Straker

## HISTORICAL PERSPECTIVE

Psychological interventions for patients with cancer were slow to develop. Since the 1950s, efforts to develop interventions have grown steadily out of the greater emphasis on quality of life of patients with cancer. Individuals who had adjusted to illness or to a particular treatment such as colostomy or laryngectomy came to be seen as sources of support for new patients. These individuals formed self-help groups that were viewed initially with some suspicion by the medical profession but eventually became a remarkably important resource not only for individual patients and families, but also as advocates at a national level (see Chapter 41 on self-help and mutual help). Social workers, the first professionals to give support and assistance to patient groups, began to play a greater role in both describing the problems of patients and intervening to provide emotional support. Psychiatrists began to take greater interest in the emotional problems of the medically ill patient at about the same time (Bard, 1959). These historical issues were reviewed in Chapter 1 and elsewhere (Holland and Rowland, 1981).

## TYPES OF PSYCHOSOCIAL INTERVENTIONS

Psychosocial interventions have developed from several directions, and this has contributed to the forms in which support is given today. They may be best described as the two models of individual counseling and group counseling. Both may be provided by health professionals or by fellow or veteran patients through visitor programs and through mutual support groups. Table 38-1 indicates the types of interventions each model employs.

Spiritual counseling is another important source of psychosocial support. Especially for those who have religious ties, it provides a philosophical and spiritual context for the understanding and expression of painful emotions associated with illness by a trusted representative of the individual's own faith. Chapter 57 outlines the role of clergy.

This chapter describes the psychosocial interventions available to health professionals working with cancer patients, outlines the application and efficacy of both individual and group methods, and discusses the special skills required of persons who undertake these interventions.

## STUDIES OF PSYCHOSOCIAL INTERVENTIONS

It has been assumed that a wide range of psychosocial interventions are beneficial to cancer patients, and personal and clinical accounts have supported this view (Bard, 1959; Creech, 1975; Cunningham, et al., 1978). It has been difficult, however, to carry out studies that test interventions in a standardized way because psychosocial support and psychotherapy are usually individualized. However, advances have been made in the research methods used in psychosocial and psychotherapeutic studies of patients with cancer (Conte and Plutchek, 1986). Giving more careful attention to the homogeneity of samples in patient studies, in regard to medical aspects of site and stage of disease, has been important in enhancing the researchers' ability to arrive at valid conclusions. Psychotherapy research in general has become more sophisticated; models for testing medically ill patients have been developed. To provide the reader with a background of research in the area, several major studies that used both individual and group counseling methods are described in the following paragraphs.

Watson (1983) provided the first extensive review

**Table 38-1**  Models of psychosocial interventions in cancer

| Providers | Intervention type | |
| --- | --- | --- |
| | Individual | Group |
| Health professionals | Education | Education |
| | Supportive psycho- | Psychotherapy |
| | therapy | Cognitive-behavioral |
| | Crisis intervention | |
| | Supportive inter- | |
| | vention | |
| | Psychodynamic | |
| | Combinations of | |
| | above | |
| Fellow and veteran | Hospital visits and | Education, practical |
| patients (see | education | advice |
| Chapter 41) | Practical advice | Mutual support |
| | from personal | Advocacy |
| | knowledge | Coping models |
| | Coping models | |

of studies of psychosocial interventions that she viewed as generally methodologically sound. Her critique of available studies described several common flaws, including the absence of a control or comparison group, absence of an objective psychological evaluation, potential for biased findings when assessment and intervention were often done by the same individuals, lack of uniformly applied intervention, and absence of a description of statistical methods. However, several studies permitted valid analysis for efficacy of a particular intervention. Table 38-2 outlines the studies reviewed by Watson that had a control or comparison group and describes the methods, intervention, and outcome. Later studies are included in chronological order.

In the five studies done in the late 1970s, patients received an intervention by either group or individual counseling, and showed some benefits on one or more outcome measures (Golonka, 1977; Bloom et al., 1978; Baum and Jones, 1979; Farash, 1979; Ferlic et al., 1979). Most were studies of interventions for women with breast cancer, and showed that counseling resulted in less preoperative anxiety (Baum and Jones, 1979), better sense of control (Bloom et al., 1978), and better response to body image change and greater satisfaction with care (Farash, 1979; Ferlic, 1979).

Capone and colleagues (1980) used crisis intervention counseling for newly diagnosed patients with gynecological neoplasms and found that counseled patients had better self-image and faster return to work and prior level of sexual function. Gordon and colleagues (1980) showed individual counseling given by a team for patients with newly diagnosed cancer of three sites had more rapid decrease in negative affect.

Maguire and co-workers (1980), using a nurse-counselor with mastectomy patients, showed increased anxiety at 4 months but decreased anxiety at 12 and 18 months in the group who were counseled. The impact of the nurse intervention and the high rate of referral to psychiatrists was felt to account for the long-term improvement. Blake (1983) failed to find any differences in women with breast cancer who received psychotherapy versus relaxation and information. Linn and colleagues (1982), using individual counseling in men with stage IV cancer, showed reduced distress and enhanced self-esteem in those who received an intervention. No effect was seen on the length of survival.

The studies by Spiegel, Bloom, and Yalom (1981) and Spiegel and Bloom (1983) demonstrated the effect of group counseling sessions for women with advanced breast cancer. The latter study used group therapy and hypnosis to reduce emotional distress and to control pain in 54 women with metastatic breast carcinoma. Patients were randomized as they entered the program, which was a 90-minute weekly outpatient group meeting attended by 6–10 patients. Two therapists, a psychiatrist or social worker, and a woman who had breast cancer conducted the sessions that covered a range of common issues, including family problems, illness and treatment, and death. The sessions ended with a hypnosis exercise lasting 5–10 minutes to assist in pain control. The support group plus hypnosis contributed to both better pain control and a sense of well-being. Spiegel and Glafkides (1983) reported similar findings in women with advanced breast cancer. Using group supportive psychotherapy, they enhanced patients' ability to discuss death, while maintaining a more positive affect.

Worden and Weisman (1984) compared a patient-centered individual psychotherapeutic model, focused on handling of specific problems, with a cognitive didactic model for patients who were identified as being at high risk of poor adjustment. The therapist's role over four sessions of psychotherapy was to facilitate identification of problems, to encourage expression of affect, and to engage the patient in exploring ways of problem solving. The other intervention emphasized training in use of cognitive skills, using behavior therapy methods, progressive relaxation, and supporting a stepwise approach to solving problems commonly encountered by cancer patients. Those who received either intervention showed lower distress and had better problem resolution than those in the control group. They concluded that both these techniques were cost-effective means to improve low morale and poor self-esteem.

A study by Forester and colleagues (1985) used weekly psychotherapy visits during 6 weeks of radiotherapy for a group of patients who were compared

**Table 38-2**  Studies of psychosocial interventions

| Reference | Intervention(s) | Study design | Outcome |
|---|---|---|---|
| Golonka (1977) | Group: counseling approach | 45 women with breast cancer receiving chemotherapy; half received group counseling | There was minimal effect on anxiety. |
| Bloom et al. (1978) | Individual and group: team approach | 39 women with breast cancer, after mastectomy; half received team approach; half none | At 1 week after surgery, the therapy group was significantly more tense, less vigorous and more confused. At 2 months, there was significantly higher health locus of control. There was no difference in mood. |
| Baum and Jones (1979) | Individual: nurse-counselor; preoperative and postoperative counseling | Women before and after mastectomy; some women were in control group | Counseled patients had lower preoperative anxiety levels. There were no postoperative differences. |
| Farash (1979) | Individual and group: individual crisis counseling versus a self-help group | 80 women with newly diagnosed breast cancer; one-third designated control without intervention | There were no differences between the two interventions in effectiveness; with depression, however, both intervention groups were more likely to have body-image disturbances. |
| Ferlic et al. (1979) | Group: team approach with nurse, physician, chaplain, occupational therapist, and dietitian; crisis intervention | Newly diagnosed metastatic cancer ($n = 60$); control group matched for age, sex, and education | Counseled patients were more satisfied with care and had greater confidence in the doctor. There was no outcome measure of anxiety or depression used. |
| Capone et al. (1980) | Individual: female psychologists; crisis intervention technique | 97 women with newly diagnosed gynecological cancer; half received intervention | Counseled patients had a better self-image and more had returned to work and prior sexual function at 12 months. |
| Gordon et al. (1980) | Individual: team of oncology counselors | 308 women with newly diagnosed breast cancer, lung cancer or melanoma; half received intervention | Negative affect declined more rapidly among patients who received counseling. |
| Maguire et al. (1980) | Individual: nurse-counselor; sessions weekly for 12–18 months | Breast cancer after mastectomy ($n = 75$); 35 women with breast cancer following mastectomy; 75 received interventions; 77 did not; randomized | At 4 months, counseled showed more anxiety but at 12–18 months significantly less. |
| Spiegel et al. (1981) | Group: weekly sessions using team approach with psychiatrist, social worker, or patient-counselor; supportive | 58 women with metastatic breast cancer; 34 received intervention; 24, none | Intervention group showed significant decrease in distress, but no difference in self-esteem, denial of illness, or health locus of control. |
| Spiegel and Bloom (1983) | Group: sessions as above plus hypnosis for pain control | 54 women with advanced breast cancer randomized to group or group plus hypnosis | Women receiving group plus hypnosis had better sense of well-being and better pain control. |
| Blake (1983) | Group: two nurse-counselors; compared psychotherapy with relaxation and information | 16 patients with early-stage breast cancer, not in active treatment; half received intervention | No differences between groups on measures of depression, anxiety, and health locus of control. |
| Linn et al. (1982) | Individual: counselor, using crisis intervention | Men with stage IV cancers, estimated life expectancy of >3 months; part of group received no intervention | Individual counseling improved perceived quality of life, internal control, and self-esteem; length of survival was the same. |

*(continued)*

**Table 38-2**   (*Continued*)

| Reference | Intervention(s) | Study design | Outcome |
|---|---|---|---|
| Spiegel and Glafkides (1983) | Group: led by psychiatrist and patient-counselor; supportive | 34 women with metastatic breast carcinoma; 23 received no intervention as control | Patients were better able to discuss dying; negative effect was reduced. |
| Worden and Weisman (1984) | Individual: comparison of two approaches, a psychotherapeutic model and a didactic model for relaxation | Patients with five sites of cancer with prognosis >3 months; half received interventions; half, none | Both interventions were cost-effective, resulting in improved self-esteem, morale, and problem resolution. |
| Forester et al. (1985) | Individual: psychiatrist; supportive therapy with educational, and dynamic components | 102 patients (half men, half women) with neoplasms of multiple sites; all receiving radiotherapy | Individually counseled group had fewer emotional and physical symptoms during radiotherapy and persisting 4 weeks later. |
| Goldberg and Wool (1985) | Individual: social support counseling with spouses | 20 lung cancer patients; 23 spouses | Intervention produced no differences in patients or spouses. |
| Cain et al. (1986) | Individual or group: patients randomized to one of three interventions composed of eight sessions: (1) structured thematic model (covering common themes over sessions), individual sessions; (2) structured thematic in group sessions; (3) standard counseling | 80 women with gynecological cancer randomized to one of three groups | Women who received the thematic model, group or individual sessions, were less depressed and anxious, had fewer sexual problems, better knowledge of illness, and better relationship to caregivers than those with standard counseling. |
| Holland et al. (1987) | Patients with elevated levels of anxiety or depression (Covi and Raskin scores >6) randomized to progressive relaxation exercises three times a day or alprazolam 5 mg tid for 10 days | 147 ambulatory patients with neoplasms of multiple sites | Both groups showed significant drop in Hamilton Anxiety and Depression scores between 1 and 10 days; drug group showed slight advantage in depression and overall level of symptoms at 10 days. |

*Source*: Adapted from M. Watson (1983). Psychosocial intervention with cancer patients: A review. *Psychol. Med.* 13:839–46.

with a similar group who served as controls. The supportive psychotherapy utilized educational and psychodynamic methods. Using items from the Schedule of Affective Disorders Scale, depression, pessimism, hopelessness, somatic preoccupation and worry, social isolation, insomnia, and anxiety were significantly lower in those who received counseling. Anorexia, fatigue, and nausea and vomiting were also less, suggesting that a simple intervention during radiotherapy may contribute to better quality of life.

Goldberg and Wool (1985), in providing social support counseling for spouses of men with advanced lung cancer, found no impact on either the spouse or the patients. However, because samples were small and outcome measures limited, an effect might have been missed.

Cain and colleagues (1986) carried out a randomized trial of an eight-session intervention for women with gynecological cancer. Patients were randomized into the three groups of eight standard counseling sessions led by a social worker, or eight sessions geared to providing information related to common themes (diet, exercise, illness, emotional, and sexual reactions) given as group sessions or individual sessions. The cognitive approach was termed structured thematic counseling. Patients' level of depression, anxiety, and sexual and social functioning was evaluated. Those who received the information-structured approach, either in the individual or group model, were better adjusted at both 6 months and 1 year later than were those who received standard counseling. The value of a problem-solving approach appeared to be supported.

A study reported by Holland and co-workers (1987)

for the Psychosocial Collaborative Oncology Group (PSYCOG) identified patients undergoing radiotherapy or chemotherapy as having high level of distress, if they had an observer-rated score on the Covi Anxiety or Raskin Depression Scale of 6 or greater. To reduce the confounding problems of illness-related changes in mood, the time period studied was limited to 10 days. Patients were randomized to groups. Patients in one group had a single session with a counselor who taught progressive relaxation. During the session, instructions were taped, and the patient was asked to practice relaxation three times daily at home. Patients in the other group received alprazolam, a benzodiazepine effective in relieving symptoms of both anxiety and depression. Using changes on the Hamilton Anxiety and Depression Scale, scores on the Hamilton scales were significantly lower at 10 days for both groups, with a slight advantage for drug over relaxation for depression and overall scores. Most patients received a diagnosis of reactive anxiety and/or depression. Benefit was expressed by 75% of the patients, suggesting that simple cost-effective techniques employed during outpatient treatment are effective, and that their use should be encouraged by the oncologist when he or she identifies a patient with high level of distress.

These studies provide support for the usefulness of psychotherapeutic interventions utilizing a range of methods in individual and group models. However, carefully designed intervention studies that test a large number of patients randomized to receive various treatment models are still needed. Also needed are studies of patients with cancer that are similar to the one carried out by Schlesinger and colleagues (1983). This study showed a reduced number of medical visits by those patients who had received a limited number of outpatient mental health visits. Similar to Schlesinger's findings, results might be found in cancer patients that would support not only reduced emotional distress but fewer medical visits for control of symptoms.

## WHO SHOULD RECEIVE INTERVENTIONS?

As attention to psychological aspects of cancer has grown, and studies such as those outlined earlier have shown the efficacy of psychosocial interventions, the issue has repeatedly been raised of which patients should receive psychosocial interventions. Some enthusiasts have advocated offering counseling to all patients on the assumption that they need help, and, of course, want it. Several studies, which were outlined earlier, showed improvement in patients who uniformly received intervention, irrespective of the level of their distress, on the assumption that all would bene-

fit. In fact, however, Worden and Weisman (1980) found that many patients rejected the offer of help. Investigative efforts were then directed toward finding ways to identify those cancer patients who were most distressed and who were at greatest risk of making a poor adaptation to cancer. One could then intervene early in those for whom counseling would be expected to produce the greatest benefit.

Worden and Weisman (1984) used this approach with 372 patients with newly diagnosed cancer in the aforementioned study. Utilizing their Index of Vulnerability as a screen for risk of poor adjustment, they identified high-risk patients (Weisman and Worden, 1976). Only about two-thirds of the patients identified as being at high risk accepted counseling. Those who refused had a positive outlook, minimized the implications of their diagnosis, and viewed the offer of therapy as a threat to their emotional equilibrium by opening the possibility of increasing their distress by unleashing emotions. Patients who accepted were less able to deny the diagnosis and its implications; they were less hopeful and were more apt to experience their situation in religious or existential terms. Among those who accepted counseling, an improvement in their psychological state was seen, supporting the concept that early identification of those at risk allows for helpful intervention. One might speculate that among those who refused counseling initially, some might have accepted it later, if their positive stance was seriously threatened. At any rate, those who were identified as vulnerable and accepted help did benefit from it.

In Canada, Stam and colleagues (1986) found that 20% of 449 ambulatory cancer patients seen in a single cancer center, which received most cancer patients within the geographic area, were referred and seen for psychosocial counseling over a 1-year period. This may be an underestimate of actual need for help, because according to the three-center study by Derogatis and colleagues (1983), 50% of the patients had sufficient distress to receive a psychiatric diagnosis and, it might be assumed, would benefit from intervention. Family and personal problems were the most common reasons for seeking help. Interventions were either psychotherapeutic or educational in type. Irrespective of the exact number, there is a significant subset of patients with cancer who have greater distress and for whom intervention is likely quite beneficial.

## PSYCHOSOCIAL INTERVENTIONS: DEFINITION, GOALS, AND VARIOUS MODELS

Psychosocial interventions for cancer patients are systematic efforts applied to influence coping behavior through educational or psychotherapeutic means. In

**Table 38-3**  Psychosocial interventions

*Definition*:  Systematic efforts applied to influence coping behavior through educational or psychotherapeutic means

*Aims*:

- ↑  Morale
- ↑  Coping ability
- ↑  Self-esteem
- ↑  Sense of control
- ↑  Resolution of problems
- ↓  Emotional distress

*Source*: Adapted from J.W. Worden and A.D. Weisman (1984). Preventive psychosocial intervention with newly diagnosed cancer patients. *Gen. Hosp. Psychiatry*, 6:243–49.

**Table 38-4**  Educational psychosocial interventions

| Recipient | Interventions |
|---|---|
| Patient | Clarifying information about the medical condition (tests, diagnosis); treatment side effects (and control of side effects); medical system (costs, access) |
|  | Reinforcing information from staff |
|  | Identifying community resources |
|  | Explaining expected emotional reactions |
| Family | Encouraging asking questions as needed (ways to cope) |
|  | Preparing for common problems encountered at home and at work |
|  | Facilitating their communication about illness with others (doctor, family, friends, employer) |
|  | Enhancing their understanding of the patient's illness, treatment, and emotional responses and making recommendations for management facilitating communication with the medical staff |
|  | Enhancing their understanding of the patient's reactions to illness and making recommendations for management facilitating communication |
| Staff | Clarifying reasons for behavior of patient, explaining management principles |
| Employer or school | Clarifying absences, physical problems, work load, and emotional responses with consent of patient |

general, the aims are to increase morale, self-esteem, and coping ability, while simultaneously decreasing distress. Interventions also seek to enhance the individual's sense of personal control during the struggle with illness and help bring about a better resolution of the practical problems being faced (Worden and Weisman, 1984) (Table 38-3). Recognizing these broad goals, one can examine the two types of psychosocial interventions, educational (Table 38-4) and psychotherapeutic (Table 38-5), using the concept of Gordon and colleagues (1980). The educational approach is directive, utilizing problem-solving and cognitive methods. The other approach utilizes psychodynamic and exploratory methods to understand emotional responses. Clinical work with an individual patient will use both of these approaches, interweaving them as needed.

## Educational Interventions

Educational interventions are critically important, especially for patients who are timorous and who fear "bothering the staff" by asking questions (Table 38-4). Clarifying information that has not fully been understood because of anxiety, correcting misinformation, and giving reassurance about the situation are all helpful interventions. Reinforcing information given, explaining and preparing patients for tests and procedures that sound frightening, and sometimes reviewing the rights of patients when negotiating access to the medical system, all become important interventions. Extending the doctor's explanations about chemotherapy and radiotherapy side effects and their control is helpful for all patients. Identifying and arranging for the use of community resources is also a useful intervention, as is anticipating problems likely to be encountered on return to home, school, or work.

Another educational role is explaining common emotional reactions to cancer, why they occur, why they are normal, and why they are not cause for alarm. These explanations often include interpretation and explanation of psychological mechanisms as a way to encourage more effective ways of coping. Patients or their families often express fear that recently experienced depression or anxiety may have caused the cancer or will cause it to return. Feeling anxious or depressed is viewed as a "weakness" to be overcome. Explanation that these symptoms are expected, normal at certain times during cancer, and do not adversely affect treatment is important. Educational interventions may also need to be extended to the patient's social environment, including the family, the treating doctor and staff, and the employer or school (Wellisch et al., 1978). The family may need more extensive discussion of their concerns than was possible with the doctor, or they may have special concerns about the patient's troubling emotional response. Clarification of and suggestions for management enable family members to cope more effectively with the patient; this, in turn, enhances the patient's sense of support (Wellisch et al., 1978).

**Table 38-5** Psychotherapeutic psychosocial interventions

| Recipient | Interventions |
| --- | --- |
| Patient | Encouraging expression of feelings about illness |
| | Offering verbal support and reassurance about illness |
| | Exploring present situation in relation to prior situations influencing response to it (e.g., prior death in family by cancer) |
| | Clarifying and interpreting feelings, behaviors, and defenses in psychodynamic terms |
| | Examining ways of coping with uncertainty about the future and existential concerns |
| | Exploring related areas of concurrent stress (recent divorce, job loss) |
| Family | Exploring impact of illness on family members and their response |
| | Identifying psychopathological reactions preexisting or concurrent, which influence the situation |
| | Reviewing decisions required about treatment (desired place, expense, feasibility) |
| | Encouraging sharing of concerns and feeling about illness with patient |
| | Meeting with patient and family together to encourage sharing of emotions about illness |
| | Identifying children who may be vulnerable and need intervention |

The doctor and nurse may be similarly puzzled or annoyed by a particular patient's attitude or behavior. When an explanation of the attitude or behavior is provided and ways of managing it are outlined, negative reactions disappear and support follows because the health care workers understand the cause of the behavior. Particularly with the hospitalized patient, the psychiatrist or psychotherapist may become an advocate for the patient, clarifying information for both the staff and the patient, and assisting in obtaining modifications of hospital procedures to accommodate a particular patient's needs. An example is the patient awaiting surgery who has agoraphobia and cannot tolerate spending the night alone before surgery (see Chapter 8 for case history). Although this problem occurs infrequently, the psychiatrist may recommend that a relative be permitted to sleep in the patient's room. Refusal to modify hospital policy could preclude the patient's ability to tolerate admission and surgery. The therapist makes the patient "human" to medical and nursing staff by explaining reasons for behaviors; the staff then can often become more supportive of modifications in routine.

The psychotherapist may need to serve as intermediary between a child's teacher and the hospital, explaining the emotional and cognitive problems that are anticipated as a result of treatments. School absences,

plans for tutoring, and the level of work that the child can be expected to accomplish need to be discussed and arranged. The same plans often need to be made for high school and college students. Discussion by the therapist with an employer or health nurse (with the patient's permission), regarding physical strength and emotional responses may alleviate potential misunderstandings.

The following two examples show the importance of education in understanding of illness and treatment side effects.

### CASE REPORTS

A middle-aged woman who had been treated with chemotherapy and radiotherapy for Hodgkin's disease in the neck and mediastinum was found at the time of a hysterectomy to have had disease spread to the abdominal lymph nodes. She misunderstood her situation and believed that she now had two cancers, lymphoma and "stomach cancer." She felt that two cancers were "unbeatable." She was demoralized and felt hopeless, and chose to refuse treatment. Upon fuller explanation that she had an extension of Hodgkin's disease and that the treatment recommended by the oncologist was effective, she became more optimistic and accepted treatment.

A hardworking 60-year-old professional businesswoman vowed that she would not "cave in to cancer" during chemotherapy and radiotherapy for stage II breast cancer. She was determined to continue her 60-hour workweek and her busy family and social life. She became enraged at herself and depressed as she felt her "determination was failing her," because she became progressively more fatigued and had to reduce her work load. She was relieved to learn that fatigue was a side effect of her treatment, not a manifestation of a "bad attitude." Recognizing that her depressed feelings were transient and normal, and would not cause poor tumor response to treatment (a fear acquired from a magazine), she began to cope more effectively and reduced her activities in such a way that her limited energy was directed toward the most important activities.

Helping the patient deal with the return to work is a role for educational intervention.

### CASE REPORT

A recently married 37-year-old accomplished professional woman adjusted to mastectomy and adjuvant chemotherapy. However, she was fearful about returning to work because she felt she would be "pitied, shunned, or devalued as being half a worker." The social worker whom she saw initially in the hospital encouraged her to anticipate the reactions she might experience and to plan how she might respond without being caught unprepared. She realized that absence of questions about her illness or a tactless remark might reflect a friend's self-consciousness. She decided to approach coworkers first, offering the level of information that she wanted each to know, thus avoiding uncomfortable interactions on initial meetings with colleagues.

## WHO SHOULD RECEIVE EDUCATIONAL INTERVENTIONS?

The educational interventions just outlined are clearly the purview of no single professional group; in fact they are given routinely by all members of the health care team as part of routine care (see Chapter 6). The doctor and nurse, who are primary to care, are substantially assisted in the task by the social worker, rehabilitation counselors, and mental health professionals. Oncology units and centers currently place far more emphasis than before on patient education, developing written materials, videotapes, and verbal instruction packages that help patients anticipate surgical procedures, chemotherapy, and radiation side effects. The materials have all served to make the patient feel more an active rather than a passive participant in treatment. In addition, the affinity of one who has been through a difficult experience with another places the veteran and fellow cancer patient as central figures in giving this type of advice and information from a credible witness who has been there (see Chapter 41 on self-help).

### Psychotherapeutic Interventions

## WHO SHOULD GIVE THEM?

Whereas educational interventions are given by many who work in oncology, psychotherapeutic interventions should be given by health professionals who have been trained in mental health or who have developed skills through special training, added to their own professional training. For example, there are some graduate programs for nurses to learn psychotherapeutic interventions with cancer patients. Social workers, psychiatric nurse-clinicians, psychologists, and psychiatrists have training that equips them well to work effectively with patients with cancer. Each, however, is ineffectual without acquiring a familiarity with oncology in order to know about the types of neoplasms, treatments available, and general prognosis.

The term therapist is used throughout this chapter to indicate such mental health professionals who, irrespective of background, undertake the difficult psychotherapeutic task of working with those individuals who have a life-threatening illness. The precise mental health training of the therapist may be unimportant in assuming an effective role with a large number of patients who will be treated equally well by any individual from one of the disciplines. However, some patients require special skills of the therapist to achieve a desired goal. Each mental health professional should therefore be aware of his or her own strengths and limitations, and should be able to recognize when the special skills of another mental health discipline might

be better applied. Cognitive or behavioral therapy is most often in the domain of psychologists, whereas diagnostic and management problems that have medical implications are probably in the psychiatrist's purview. A willingness on the part of the professional to obtain consultation for specialized skills is important.

In many settings, however, a single mental health professional assumes all these responsibilities simultaneously and must function truly as a generalist without opportunity for consultation. In larger centers, where several mental health professionals may be present and where the role of each is new and evolving, the potential for nonproductive professional jealousies to develop is great. The issues arise because neither the staff nor the newly assigned mental health professional has a clear picture of expected role or function in a setting in which these roles are new and ill-defined. Conflicts can be avoided by mutual respect for the contributions of each discipline, and by maintaining a constant review of the nature and quality of management of all psychosocial aspects of care given within a unit or center, making changes in staff members and disciplinary background as needed. Some models have developed that provide these services in single integrated units or collaborative teams that encourage constructive and full use of all resources.

## WHAT ARE PSYCHOTHERAPEUTIC GOALS?

Psychotherapy with a patient who has cancer has several goals that include maintaining a primary focus on the illness and its implications, while exploring only those issues from the past and present that affect the adjustment to illness (Gordon et al., 1980; Holland and Rowland, 1981). Using a brief therapy crisis intervention model, focus is kept on the illness and present concerns. The therapist first encourages expression of feelings and fears about the illness and its outcome; fears are often considered by the patient to be too painful and too burdensome to reveal to family and friends, and hence the therapy plays a useful role in exploring and exposing the feelings. Support is offered by the therapist, who usually can help the patient see that most concerns are universal.

Reassurance is given always in the context of reality; blanket reassurances that are not realistic are never offered. The therapist's reassurance should be related to providing a sense of security that he or she and the medical staff are reliable. Often recall of a situation from the past makes the adjustment to illness much more difficult, as is demonstrated in several case histories in this book in which a death by cancer in the family, a traumatic loss in childhood, combat experience, or memories of the holocaust are triggered when confrontation with death is posed by a cancer diagnosis. Sourkes (1982) suggests always obtaining a "loss history" from the individual facing serious illness, which will ensure a review of these important issues. A series of vague, poorly understood recollections of how the death of the relative occurred are activated by a personal illness, especially when the loss occurred during childhood.

## CASE REPORT

An example of the impact of past experience on coping was seen in a 49-year-old firefighter who developed esophageal cancer. On the way to the operating room for an esophagogastrectomy, he became panic-stricken and could not go through with the surgery. He was discharged home later in the day after agreeing to return to see the psychiatrist. Over several visits, he remembered that when he was 6 his mother had gone to the hospital to have an operation. She had never returned home, having died on the operating table. He had always feared having an operation. After reliving these memories and reexamining his fears of hospitals and operations, he successfully managed admission 10 days later.

Old defenses and methods of coping come to the fore with the crisis of illness and the uncertainty of the future. At times a clarification of the origin of counterproductive defenses, and exploring their impact on behavior in relation to illness provides helpful insight. Existential issues of life and death that patients commonly put aside "for the future" will be explored. At times, cancer is felt to be a punishment by God for some real or imagined prior act. Because mystical and irrational beliefs are associated with cancer, and guilt may be an associated emotion, psychotherapy may help to clarify the sources of distress, especially in some teenagers who sense that illness may be retribution for sexual experimentation.

Cancer is always viewed as having occurred at the worst possible time (although there is no good one), and a recent divorce, concurrent loss of job, or other loss must be reviewed for the painful impact of dealing with more than one loss at the same time.

Because cancer involves not only the patient but the whole family, the family must often be included in a psychotherapeutic intervention. Sometimes this is achieved best by arranging one or more sessions with the patient and family together when issues that affect the resources of the family require clarification or when decisions about where the patient will be treated must be made. The impact of the patient's illness on the family member(s) can be observed in a family meeting. It may indicate a need for a separate meeting with a family member whose own problems need attention because of the presence of a psychiatric disorder or a special problem created by the illness. The impact of a family member's illness on the children in the family is particularly important. They may need

attention to explore their reactions and to give them an opportunity to express their fears and concerns. When the illness of the relative, especially mother or father, is life-threatening and likely fatal, psychotherapeutic intervention to deal with anticipatory grief may contribute to a far better immediate and long-term outcome (see Chapter 50).

## SPECIAL ISSUES OF PSYCHOTHERAPY WITH THE ONCOLOGY PATIENT

Several issues complicate psychotherapy with cancer patients, requiring a modified approach from the way in which treatments would commonly be carried out with physically healthy patients. The therapist may initially feel as if he or she is "breaking the rules" learned in supervision doing psychotherapy with healthy individuals. Some of the problems are discussed here.

### Frequency of Visits

The supportive psychotherapy model, the most widely employed, utilizes visits once or twice a week for the ambulatory patient over 4–6 weeks. This usually adequately addresses most transient crises that occur in cancer. This allows time to explore, clarify, and interpret psychodynamic issues that are relevant to the immediate situation. In contrast to the traditional psychotherapy model that is set up as a contract with a fixed schedule and responsibility for missed hours, modifications in scheduling appointments are frequently necessary with the cancer patient. Appointments often need to be rescheduled, the number of weekly or monthly sessions may have to be increased or decreased, and the length of visits altered depending on the physical status of the patient. When the crisis passes, visits may be tapered or discontinued, but with a clear message that they can be resumed if or when another crisis occurs.

Sourkes (1982, p. 14) notes the difference imposed by illness on the therapeutic process and content.

A hallmark of traditional psychotherapy is the unstructured flow of content and process. Past, present and future interweave in the unfolding themes. Letting a process emerge at its own pace and time is a luxury precluded by the very nature of the life-threatening illness. Its immediacy demands a focus on the present, framed by the themes of separation and loss.

A sense of "time-limited" therapy results in a feeling of urgency, which is transmitted to the therapist from the patient. This is a countertransference issue that must be recognized by the therapist.

If the person's illness requires hospitalization for

THERAPEUTIC INTERVENTIONS

medical reasons during therapy, the therapist should be available by phone and make visits to the hospital when possible. This sense of continuity, irrespective of the level of illness, and whether visits are in the office or hospital is often what patients find most reassuring and helpful. Visits with the hospitalized patient should be as short as 15–20 minutes in length; the therapist should be responsive to the level of the patient's fatigue and discomfort. The hospital room with more than one bed offers little privacy for an interview; taking the patient in a wheelchair to a private place is desirable, but illness may preclude this. Quiet conversations, recognizing the absence of full confidentiality, can still be highly meaningful. Talk is usually focused on immediate concerns, although at times important events unrelated to the illness may require attention.

## Shifting from Supportive to Exploratory Psychotherapy

When patients experience a remission and health becomes more normal, the confrontation with cancer and death sometimes is an impetus to explore problems that might otherwise have been tolerated, such as a troubled marriage or a delayed separation from the family of origin for a young adult. Such chronic unpleasant situations become less tolerable for one who has had to examine life and mortality directly. Patients often have the need to prioritize life concerns. Psychotherapy, begun during cancer treatment, may be the proper place to consider priorities. The format of this therapy should revert to the more usual contract of regular visits in which the therapist takes a less active stance. It is preferable to move closer to the traditional model during any period of remission or when the patient is well enough to benefit from a more exploratory model of psychotherapy. It may be wisest to refer the patient to a therapist away from a cancer center, signaling that illness is no longer the focus.

### CASE REPORT

A 22-year-old single man recovered from treatment for testicular cancer and returned to his job at the family business and his room in the family home. Attempts to break away in the past had been circumvented by parental pressure. Increasing depression, despite good health, led him to call the psychiatrist with whom he had had brief contact in the hospital a year earlier. He recognized his distress in dealing with issues from childhood and requested referral to a psychiatrist near his home.

If a recurrence develops, a more supportive psychotherapeutic approach is resumed temporarily, but this need not be seen as excluding the possibility of renewing a traditional approach when the patient improves and can again benefit from it. Concepts developed by

Horowitz and others for brief therapy for stress response syndromes are helpful in dealing with cancer patients (Horowitz, 1973; Horowitz et al., 1984; Malan, 1976; Mann, 1973).

## Dealing with Medical Treatment Options

There are times when a distressed patient who must make an important decision about treatment may benefit from a therapist who serves as an impartial observer and who assists the patient in considering the options for a course of action. This is seen often in women who become overwhelmed by making a decision about the treatment options between mastectomy and segmental resection and irradiation for primary breast cancer (see Chapter 14).

It is helpful to review the steps involved in both courses of action and encourage the patient to imagine her feelings, assuming one treatment, then the other, thereby coming to a conclusion about her own wishes.

At times, the highly personal reasons for indecision or reluctance to accept a treatment can be explored with a therapist when the individual feels they are too trivial or embarrassing to discuss with the doctor. This situation arises more often as patients are encouraged to participate in decisions about treatment (Bukberg and Straker, 1982).

## Defenses as They Relate to Illness

It is important to evaluate the defenses of the patient that, contrary to being a barrier to understanding the past in traditional psychotherapy, become the vehicle whereby constructive coping with illness is accomplished. Because the coping mechanisms employed are those that have been used in prior crises, the therapist is searching for ways to bolster, not weaken, the usual adaptive defensive patterns. Sometimes, however, maladaptive coping may interfere with treatment. Two examples using denial and regression are offered. Patient A with multiple myeloma continues about his usual course of business and family activity while undergoing chemotherapy. He has a positive attitude and focuses on the expected benefits of the treatment while denying the risks of side effects or recurrence. Patient B with multiple myeloma denies his risk of pathological fracture and joins a health club to "strengthen his leg." It is the task of the therapist to encourage Patient B to examine his actions, helping him see that he may be too frightened to consider his diagnosis. Similarly, the therapist may actively attempt to limit regression in a patient who is not overtly ill and to encourage functioning at full capacity. In contrast, the therapist should recognize and allow regression when it is adaptive to the comfort of the terminal patient. A previously independent adult may, in the course of terminal illness, be cared for by a parent again. Both assume earlier patterns of behavior, reminiscent of the patient's childhood. For the terminally ill patient, this may be adaptive.

## Psychotherapy Combined with Other Modalities

Patients who have cancer often have insomnia, depression, and anxiety. These nonspecific symptoms may be secondary to the underlying disease. When the patient is in psychotherapy, there is an opportunity to explore psychological reasons for heightened distress, while also assessing the contribution of underlying disease or side effects of treatment. The exploration of the underlying problem and the development of a positive transference may reduce symptoms and obviate the need for medication. However, if the symptoms are severe and do not abate, medication may be appropriate as an adjunct to psychotherapy. The overzealous use of medication initially for target symptoms may limit the exploration of psychological issues; however, it is equally important to protect the patient from excessively painful affects, and if indicated, to explore patient reluctance to using medication. This latter situation is common in cancer patients who resist the thought of adding another "medicine in my body. I already take so much." Abuse of drugs by cancer patients is extremely rare (see Chapter 39).

Similarly, some patients may need the addition of a behavioral intervention for control of a specific symptom like pain or conditioned nausea and vomiting. As shown by the study of Spiegel and Bloom (1983), supportive psychotherapy and instruction in hypnosis in group sessions led to the most effective control of symptoms.

## The Therapist: Personal and Countertransference Issues

The therapist working with cancer issues must be knowledgeable in psychotherapeutic techniques and oncology (Klagsbrun, 1983). He or she must know the principles of crisis intervention, supportive psychotherapy, and family intervention. In addition, the constant confrontation with threat to life, dying, and death makes it essential that the therapist have insight into his or her personal views of death and the ability to deal with losses (Eissler, 1955). Sourkes (1982) suggests that just as one needs to take into account the loss history of patients, so too, should one take into account the personal loss history of therapists as well. Psychotherapeutic work in cancer demands a far more active stance and use of the self than is true of traditional psychotherapy, making the need for self-reflection more important. Introspection about one's own vulnerability from prior losses, and acknowledgment of

it, help to reduce the errors made out of personalized responses. Sourkes suggests that the test of objectivity is always a reflection on whether the patient's needs are being served, not one's own. Therapy in these situations that are characterized by uncertainty and loss require a high level of commitment as a "characteristic of the therapist. The richness and depth of this commitment are intensified by the omnipresence of separation and loss" (Sourkes, 1982, p. 122).

The therapist should have expert knowledge of psychological techniques, as well as a working knowledge of treatment options for major cancer sites, of the usual side effects and their management, of complications and particularly those that occur in the CNS (e.g., vincristine-related peripheral neuropathy, interferon "flulike symptoms," and depression). The therapist can assist the patient in anticipating side effects and thereby control response, only when he or she has a good understanding of these problems.

In the oncology setting, psychotherapeutic and counseling interventions are utilized with patients or their families at all stages of illness, often within the context of a complex and changing medical situation with multiple specialists involved. The therapist must be able to adapt treatment to the patient's needs and illness changes, and to adapt interventions with physicians and nurses on the patient's behalf. The therapist's role is often ambiguous in the setting of acute illness, and personal responses to these anxiety-provoking situations must be frequently examined. Accurate information about the individual patient's diagnosis, treatment, and prognosis must be obtained from the referring physician before undertaking psychotherapy. Sometimes individuals coming from mental health disciplines lack knowledge of treatment for each cancer site and, like the general public, may assume a worse prognosis for a patient than is appropriate. One cannot deal with a patient's fears or give realistic reassurance without some knowledge of the effectiveness of treatment and survival statistics.

Therapists encourage patients to express openly their thoughts and feelings about illness and death; their impact on the therapist results in a repetitive dealing with loss. Because empathic concern results in attachment (albeit at a professional level), working with patients with life-threatening illness carries with it problems for the therapist that may result in common personal countertransference reactions that are employed as self-protective devices. These reactions can be detrimental to patient care, and the common ones should be so well known to therapists in this work that they can recognize them in themselves and colleagues.

The first is the psychological need to try to "save" patients from their illness. The therapist may wish to rescue patients from their plight or may sense that patients are asking him or her to do so. These feelings are often poignant when dealing with patients whose cancer is in an advanced or terminal stage. "What can I do? What do I have to offer?" are the inner questions that arise and create a sense of futility and discouragement for the therapist. Feelings of helplessness and impotence to change the situation result, especially in the therapist who is doing this work for the first time. Low self-esteem and depression may occur, and resentment may be felt toward the patient for creating the conflict. In an attempt to deal with these feelings, the therapist may encourage or demand inappropriate or unrealistic efforts on the patient's behalf that may deny the reality of the situation. This is seen most often in a cancer center at the time that active treatment that has been directed toward cure or control must be changed to palliative and comfort care. Staff members, including the psychiatrist, go through the painful transition of accepting altered treatment goals, with varying degrees of difficulty in accepting reality and relinquishing the idea of survival of a special patient (Spikes and Holland, 1975). The opposite response is to choose premature withdrawal from the patient based on unrecognized angry feelings that reflect the frustration in dealing with a patient with inexorably advancing illness. This reaction, like the former, alters clinical judgment about patient care.

The other common problem is the concern about causing the patient additional emotional distress associated with confronting the patient with evidence of maladaptive defenses. There may be an unwillingness to bring up a painful topic for discussion, even when appropriate, because it may cause additional discomfort. This is similar to the medical staff's reluctance to carry out a needed procedure because of the pain or side effects it will cause. It is important for the therapist to confront maladaptive defenses that are harmful to the patient by the use of a tactful question, confrontation, or interpretation. This problem is often encountered when the patient is denying some aspect of his or her situation to ward off depression or anxiety, and in doing so is engaging in an activity that may be detrimental to the treatment of the illness or personal situation.

We, as well as others, have found that the therapist requires support, self-awareness, and opportunity to reflect on "problem" cases with another, to minimize maladaptive ways of dealing with countertransference feelings.

## Group Counseling

The group model of psychological support in cancer has rapidly developed since the early 1970s (Berger, 1984; Blacher, 1984). As outlined at the beginning of the chapter, two general types of groups are used, that is, groups run by professionals for patients and/or families using educational, psychotherapeutic, or cognitive behavioral methods; or self-help or mutual support groups, often composed of patients with the same tumor site or treatment, focusing on education, practical advice, modeling, coping, and serving as a source of mutual support and advocacy (Cordoba et al., 1984) (Table 38-1). Self-help groups are often independent of medical care; nevertheless they provide an important link between health care and the outside world (see Chapter 41). Groups run by health professionals are outlined here.

There was initial resistance to the use of therapy groups in cancer because of the concern about a potentially negative effect on members if one member in the group died. This concern proved to be ill-founded. In fact, patients found early groups helpful in dealing with anxiety about their own possible death through confronting the loss of others (Yalom and Greaves, 1977). The extensive experience of Yalom and associates is reported earlier in the chapter. Using a group mode for ambulatory patients with advanced cancer (Spiegel et al., 1981; Spiegel and Bloom, 1983; Spiegel and Glafkides, 1983), they found that the optimal number of persons in a group was seven; new patients were allowed to enter as places became available. The unique philosophy of "living to the fullest in the context of dying" appeared to be accomplished by the group members who experienced more depth and meaning to life as a consequence of the group experience. Members' feelings of alienation were lessened by talking with others who were "in the same boat"; belonging to a group supported identification with others who were successfully coping with similar problems. The sense of personal psychological growth that was fostered countered the uncomfortable feelings of being victimized and feeling powerless. Participants felt less sad, lonely, and isolated. They also experienced heightened self-esteem and viewed their communication with their physician and family as improved. They had less need to deny cancer.

Studies such as that by Cain and colleagues (1986), showing efficacy of both individual and group therapy and using a structured thematic model, supports the American Cancer Society model of eight semistructured sessions, called "I Can Cope." Psychological problems that arise in the course of daily living and adapting to illness are particularly amenable to the group setting. Group work with larygectomy patients in the immediate postoperative period and with patients who have had recent surgery for head and neck cancer is helpful to encourage early return to socialization and easier confrontation with the common feelings of self-consciousness faced by these individuals after surgery (Holley, 1983).

Parents of children with cancer who participate in groups have reported feeling more supported during crises and having a greater sense of the understanding of their own and their children's responses, gained particularly by sharing and identifying with other parents (see Chapter 41 and 45). Most pediatric oncology units have regular meetings for parents, which vary from a purely educational to a dynamic group therapy model.

The use of groups for hospitalized patients has proved more difficult, in part because of the acute nature and severity of illness of hospitalized patients, which preclude regular and full participation (Cunningham et al., 1978). Inpatient groups have been found useful, however, when organized as discussion groups coordinated by the staff, which most often includes a social worker, a nurse, or psychiatrist working as a team. The groups may be structured for patients alone, patients and their families, or families alone. At Memorial Sloan-Kettering Cancer Center, groups geared toward considering practical problems and psychological responses of relatives are held weekly on all floors.

Groups for women who have had a mastectomy have been particularly successful and have been a part of support at our hospital for well over a decade. Group sessions are held on a daily basis; leadership is rotated regularly among the nurse, physiotherapist, and social worker. Patients learn exercises from the physiotherapist, ask a nurse questions about medical problems, and are encouraged by the social worker to participate in discussions about the emotional impact of mastectomy. A Reach-to-Recovery volunteer attends sessions and provides an opportunity for patients to meet someone who has successfully dealt with this loss and who can field queries about the practical aspects of adaptation. A useful adjunct to the multimodality rehabilitation group for mastectomy patients is a separate optional session for patients interested in learning about breast reconstruction. Postsurgery groups for patients who have had limited resections for breast cancer are best held separately from postmastectomy groups; these two subsets of patients perceive their cancer adjustment tasks to be very different.

Pretreatment groups for radiotherapy patients demonstrate the usefulness of a highly specific, task-centered intervention. Centered around an orientation to the clinic, its routines, equipment, and technicians, group leaders (usually members of the clinic staff) generate discussions that are used to diminish the anxiety associated with referral for and commencement of a treatment often seen as strange and frightening. The group leader must be comfortable with existential issues, medical illness, radiation side effects, and group dynamics.

## Models: Open Versus Closed

Another question raised is whether groups should be open or closed with a more traditional psychotherapeutic model. In general, the open model is used with changing membership, using a strong informational and directive approach, usually encouraging an individual to attend a "series" that covers the basic information and provides support as well. Patient's ties to other group members usually persist for ongoing support.

## Cognitive Behavioral Therapy

This model of psychotherapy is increasingly applied to patients with psychiatric disorders and medical illnesses, including cancer (Rush, 1984; Childress and Burns, 198). Because it can be developed with a repeatable intervention (even using a manual of interventions for the therapist), it has been more widely studied than supportive models. Cognitive behavioral therapy has been of particular interest in cancer because it is short-term and is aimed at control of target symptoms. Clinicians have found it to be effective for pain management, anxiety, some eating disorders, and depression in cancer; however, few controlled studies have been conducted in medical illness (see Chapter 40).

This approach has appeal to many patients with cancer who have little interest in a psychological inquiry into their problems, and who prefer to learn to control troublesome, identified symptoms. Symptoms are viewed as clues to mental cognitions and assumptions that play a key role in the development or sustaining of a psychopathological state, such as increased perception of pain. Thus, the patient learns to recognize the cognitions, to modify assumptions, and to understand their impact on symptom development. In this model the therapist serves as a guide and teacher; homework is required.

Beck (1976) has used this method in managing depressed patients. Efficacy has not yet been shown in cancer, but in certain chronic situations when disease is stable and depression persists, it may be a useful technique to consider, especially if chronic pain is present (Fishman and Loscalzo, 1987).

## SUMMARY

Studies have increasingly supported the value of a range of psychosocial interventions to provide emotional support in cancer patients. The actual percentage who need help or would benefit remains unclear, but it is likely that at least 25% of patients and their families need additional psychological support. Psychosocial interventions, by both health professionals and veteran patients, in both group and individual sessions appear in controlled trials to be efficacious. They utilize educational and psychotherapeutic methods. Any utilized psychotherapy model must be flexibly applied, having frequency, duration, and the type of approach altered to accommodate to the level of illness. Cognitive behavioral therapies geared to problem solving have proved useful.

Therapists who offer these services should know techniques of individual and group therapy, be familiar with oncological diagnosis, prognosis, and treatment, and be aware of personal responses to work with patients who have a life-threatening illness. Finally, psychotherapeutic work with cancer is challenging and requires commitment to do it effectively; it is also highly personally rewarding.

# REFERENCES

Bard, M. (1959). Implications of analytic psychotherapy with the physically ill. *Am. J. Psychother.* 13:860–71.

Baum, M. and E.M. Jones (1979). Counseling removes patients' fear. *Nurs. Mirror* 8(3):38–40.

Beck, A.T. (1976). *Cognitive Therapy and the Emotional Disorders*. New York: International Universities Press.

Berger, J.M. (1984). Crisis intervention: A drop-in support group for cancer patients and their families. *Soc. Work Health Care* 10:81–92.

Blacher, R.S. (1984). The briefest encounter: Psychotherapy for medical and surgical patients. *Gen. Hosp. Psychiatry* 6:226–32.

Blake, S.M. (1983). *Group Therapy with Breast Cancer: A Controlled Trial.* Unpublished master's thesis, University of Manchester, Department of Psychiatry.

Bloom, J.R., R.D. Ross, and G. Burnell (1978). The effect of social support on patient adjustment after breast surgery. *Patient Counsel. Health Educ.* 1:50–59.

Bukberg, J.B. and N. Straker (1982). Psychiatric consultation for the ambivalent cancer surgery candidate. *Psychosomatics* 23:1043–50.

Cain, E.N., E.I. Kohorn, D.M. Quinlan, K. Latimer, and P.E. Schwartz (1986). Psychosocial benefits of a cancer support group. *Cancer* 57:183–89.

Capone, M.A., R.S. Good, S. Westie, and A.F. Jacobsen (1980). Psychosocial rehabilitation in gynecologic oncology patients. *Arch. Phys. Med. Rehabil.* 61:128–32.

Childress, A.R. and D.D. Burns (1981). The basics of cognitive therapy. *Psychosomatics* 22:1017–27.

Conte, H.R. and R. Plutchek (1986). Controlled research in supportive psychotherapy. *Psychiatr. Ann.* 16:530–33.

Cordoba, C., M.B. Shear, P. Fobair, and J. Hall (1984). *Cancer Support Groups Practice Handbook.* Oakland, Calif.: American Cancer Society.

Creech, R.H. (1975). The psychologic support of the cancer patient: A medical oncologist's viewpoint. *Semin. Oncol.* 2:285–92.

Cunningham, J., D. Strassberg, and H. Roback (1978). Group psychotherapy for medical patients. *Compr. Psychiatry* 19:135–40.

Derogatis, L.R., G.R. Morrow, J. Fetting, D. Penman, S. Piasetsky, A.M. Schmale, M. Hendricks, and C.L. Carnicke (1983). The prevalence of psychiatric disorders among cancer patients. *J.A.M.A.* 249:751–57.

Eissler, K.R. (1955). *The Psychiatrist and the Dying Patient.* New York: International Universities Press.

Farash, J.L. (1979). Effects of counseling on resolution of loss and body image disturbance following a mastectomy. *Diss. Abstr. Int.* 39:4027.

Ferlic, M., A. Goldman, and B.J. Kennedy (1979). Group counseling in adult patients with advanced cancer. *Cancer* 44:760–66.

Fishman, B. and M. Loscalzo (1987). Cognitive-behavioral interventions in management of cancer pain: Principles and applications. *Med. Clin. North Am.* 71:271–87.

Forester, B., D.S. Kornfeld, and J.L. Fleiss (1985). Psychotherapy during radiotherapy: Effects on emotional and physical distress. *Am. J. Psychiatry* 142:22–27.

Goldberg, R.J. and M.S. Wool (1985). Psychotherapy for the spouses of lung cancer patients: Assessment of an intervention. *Psychother. Psychosom.* 43:141–50.

Golonka, L.M. (1977). The use of group counseling with breast cancer patients receiving chemotherapy. *Diss. Abstr. Int.* 37:6362–63.

Gordon, W.A., I. Freidenbergs, L. Diller, M. Hibbard, C. Wolf, L. Levine, R. Lipkins, O. Ezrachi, and D. Lucido (1980). Efficacy of psychosocial intervention with cancer patients. *J. Consult. Clin. Psychol.* 48:743–59.

Holland, J.C. and J. Rowland (1981). Psychiatric, psychosocial and behavioral interventions in the treatment of cancer: An historical review. In S.M. Weiss, J.A. Herd, and B.H. Fox (eds.), *Perspectives on Behavioral Medicine* New York: Academic Press, pp. 235–260.

Holland, J.C., G. Morrow, A. Schmale, L. Derogatis, M. Spefanek, S. Berenson, P. Carpenter, W. Breitbart and M. Feldstein (1987). Reduction of anxiety and depression in cancer patients by alprazolam or by a behavioral technique. *Proc. Twenty-third Annu. Mtg. Am. Soc. Clin. Oncol.* 6:258. (Abstract No. 1015).

Holley, B. (1983). Counseling the head and neck cancer patient: Laryngectomy. *Prog. Clin. Biol. Res.* 121:215–25.

Horowitz, M.J. (1973). Phase-oriented treatment of stress response syndromes. *Am. J. Psychother.* 27:506–15.

Horowitz, M.J., C. Marmar, D.S. Weiss, K.N. DeWitt, and R. Rosenbaum (1984). Brief psychotherapy of bereavement reactions. *Arch. Gen. Psychiatry* 41:438–48.

Klagsbrun, S. (1983). The making of a cancer psychotherapist. *J. Psychosoc. Oncol.* 1:55–60.

Linn, M.W., B.S. Linn, and R. Harris (1982). Effects of counseling for late-stage cancer patients. *Cancer* 49:1048–55.

Maguire, G.P., A. Tait, M. Brooke, C. Thomas, and R. Sellwood (1980). The effects of counseling on the psychiatric morbidity associated with mastectomy. *Br. Med. J.* 28:1454–56.

Malan, D.H. (1976). *A Study of Brief Psychotherapy.* New York: Plenum.

Mann, J. (1973). *Time-Limited Psychotherapy.* Cambridge, Mass.: Harvard University Press.

Rush, A.J. (1984). Cognitive therapy. In T.B. Karasu (ed.),

*The Psychiatric Therapies,* Vol. 2. *The Psychosocial Therapies.* Washington, D.C.: American Psychiatric Association, pp. 397–414.

Schlesinger, H.J., E. Mumford, G.V. Glass, C. Patrick, and S. Sharfstein (1983). Mental health treatment and medical care utilization in fee-for-service system: Outpatient mental health treatment following the onset of a chronic disease. *Am. J. Public Health* 73:422–29.

Sourkes, B.M. (1982). *The Deepening Shade: Psychological Aspects of Life-Threatening Illness.* Pittsburgh: University of Pittsburgh Press.

Spiegel, D. and J.R. Bloom (1983). Group therapy and hypnosis reduce metastatic breast carcinoma pain. *Psychosom. Med.* 45:333–39.

Spiegel, D. and M.C. Glafkides (1983). Effects of group confrontation with death and dying. *Int. J. Group Psychother.* 33:433–74.

Spiegel, D., J. Bloom, and I. Yalom (1981). Group support for patients with metastatic cancer. *Arch. Gen. Psychiatry* 38:527–33.

Spikes, J. and J.C. Holland (1975). The physician's response to the dying patient. In J. Strain and S. Grossman (eds.), *Psychological Care of the Medically Ill.* East Norwalk, Conn.: Appleton-Century Crofts.

Stam, H.J., B.D. Bultz, and C.A. Pittman (1986). Psychosocial problems and interventions in a referred sample of cancer patients. *Psychosom. Med.* 48:539–47.

Watson, M. (1983). Psychosocial intervention with cancer patients: A review. *Psychol. Med.* 13:839–46.

Weisman, A.D. and J.W. Worden (1976). The existential plight in cancer: Significance of the first 100 days. *Psychiatr. Med.* 7:1–15.

Wellisch, D.K., M.G. Mosher, and C. Van Scoy (1978). Management of family emotion stress: Family group therapy in a private oncology practice. *Int. J. Group Psychother.* 28:225–31.

Worden, J.W. and A.D. Weisman (1980). Do cancer patients really want counseling? *Gen. Hosp. Psychiatry* 2:100–103.

Worden, J.W. and A.D. Weisman (1984). Preventive psychosocial intervention with newly diagnosed cancer patients. *Gen. Hosp. Psychiatry* 6:243–49.

Yalom, I.D. and C. Greaves (1977). Group therapy with the terminally ill. *Am. J. Psychiatry* 134:396–400.

# 39

# Psychopharmacological Management

Mary Jane Massie and Lynna M. Lesko

Effective pharmacological management of psychological distress, psychiatric syndromes (depression, delirium, and anxiety), and insomnia in cancer patients often presents a challenge to psychiatrist and oncologist. The challenge is often greatest for physicians attempting to control distressing psychological symptoms in patients whose treatment is palliative and in whom comfort is the major goal. Distress at certain times in cancer illness is normal. When distress becomes intolerable or when it impairs the patient's ability to adjust to the demands of illness and treatment, then the use of psychotropic medications should be considered to increase comfort and reduce distress.

In the past, psychopharmacological agents have been underutilized in oncology. Several issues appear to have contributed to this underuse.

1. Physicians lacked familiarity with psychotropic medications, and few psychiatrists served as consultants on oncology wards or in clinics.
2. Relatively less importance was given to changes in mood, behavior, and quality of life, because the major concern was directed to the life-threatening aspects of cancer.
3. Oncology staff lacked information about the common psychiatric syndromes seen in cancer patients and the efficacy of psychotropic drugs.
4. There was concern that seriously ill cancer patients could not tolerate the potential side effects of psychoactive medications.
5. It was feared that psychotropic drug interactions and metabolism might adversely alter patient response to cancer treatment.
6. There was concern about the addictive potential of some psychoactive medications (e.g., benzodiazepines).
7. Many patients were reluctant to accept a psycho-

tropic drug that they associated with the treatment of ''mental illness'' or ''weakness of character.''

This chapter is intended to provide oncology staff with the indications for the use of psychotropic medications in cancer patients, the specific agents available, and the special considerations in the use of psychotropic medications. The chapter also directs the reader to pertinent references for further study. We have chosen to discuss the most frequent disorders and symptoms seen in cancer patients for which a psychotropic drug may be indicated, that is, depression, anxiety, insomnia, delirium, and the functional psychoses. For each disorder or symptom, we describe the indications for drug use, the classes of drugs to be considered, and recommended clinical use (choice of drug, dosage, side effects, pattern of response, and special considerations in regard to the effects of patient age and tumor site on psychotropic drug metabolism.)

## PSYCHOTROPIC DRUG USE

The first survey of prescribing practices of psychotropic medications by oncologists was carried out by the Psychosocial Collaborative Oncology Group (PSYCOG) in primarily inpatients admitted to five oncology centers over a 6-month period (Derogatis et al., 1979). Of the 1579 patients, 51% received a psychotropic drug, of which 48% were hypnotics ordered for insomnia. The next most common drug class prescribed was antipsychotics (26%), which were ordered for control of nausea and vomiting. Anxiolytics accounted for 25% of medications and were prescribed for preoperative or preprocedural anxiety. Antidepressants accounted for only 1% of prescriptions, even though depressive symptoms are commonly seen in patients with cancer. Rationales for the psychotropic medications ordered were sleep (44%), nausea and vomiting (25%), psychological distress (17%), and anxiety associated with medical procedures (12%). Three drugs accounted for 72% of all prescriptions—namely, flurazepam, prochlorperazine, and diazepam—suggesting that oncologists chose a limited number of the total of 49 psychotropic drugs available in the formularies.

The PSYCOG group repeated the survey in three of the five cancer centers initially studied (Holland et al., 1986). Of the 82 psychotropic drugs available in the three hospital formularies, only 30 were prescribed. Of the 602 patients reviewed, 87% received one or more psychotropic drugs from five drug classes: anxiolytics, antipsychotics, antidepressants, hypnotics, and stimulants. Hypnotics (43.9%) were most widely used; antipsychotics (30.2%), anxiolytics (23.4%), and antidepressants (2.5%) followed. The most common reasons for prescribing a psychotropic drug were sleep (29.8%), medical procedures (26.2%), nausea and vomiting (26.1%), psychological distress (11.0%), pain (5.4%), seizures (0.1%), and other (1.4%). The drugs most often used were diazepam, hydroxyzine, prochlorperazine, metoclopramide, triazolam, flurazepam, and pentobarbital. Data from these two studies show that more psychotropic drugs are available now in hospital formularies than were available at the time of the survey. More patients (51% in 1979 versus almost 90% in 1986) are receiving prescriptions for psychotropics to control a range of physical and psychological symptoms. Oncologists are now more familiar with the use of a wider range of drugs, which often have several indications for the cancer patient (e.g., amitriptyline prescribed for pain as well as depression). However, the majority of psychotropic drugs are still prescribed for insomnia, discomfort of medical procedures, and nausea and vomiting.

In 1985 Jaeger and colleagues reported the psychotropic drugs used in management of 1000 hospitalized patients with advanced and terminal cancer. At least one psychotropic agent was prescribed to 82% of the patients. Hypnotics were prescribed to 56% of the patients, 61% received antipsychotics, 32% received antianxiety drugs, and 10% received antidepressants. Anxiolytics comprised 20% of all psychotropics given and antidepressants 5%. Another study by Goldberg and Mor (1985) similarly reviewed the utilization patterns of psychotropics in terminal cancer patients. They reported that 3–5% of patients received antidepressants within the last 6 weeks of life. Clearly, psychotropics (particularly antidepressants) are prescribed more widely for symptom control in patients receiving palliative care and in whom symptoms of pain, nausea, vomiting, and psychological distress, especially depression, are greater.

The following sections outline the guidelines for use of psychoactive drugs.

## BASIC PRINCIPLES FOR PSYCHOACTIVE DRUG ADMINISTRATION

Several principles should be kept in mind when considering the use of any psychoactive drug in any patient with cancer. Although there have been virtually no studies of psychotropic drug trials in cancer patients, our clinical experience suggests these four important rules:

1. Start with a lower dose than ordinarily indicated in a physically healthy patient.
2. Increase drug dose more slowly than in a physically healthy patient.
3. Therapeutic maintenance dose may be significantly lower in a cancer patient than in a physically healthy patient.
4. Know the major side effects of the drug being considered, which could have a deleterious effect on organ dysfunction related to tumor site or treatment (e.g., anticholinergic effects in a patient with bowel obstruction, orthostatic hypotension in a debilitated patient, delirium in an elderly patient).

These rules will be described in relation to specific drug groups discussed here, as they are used in relation to management of the major psychiatric disorders, namely, depression, anxiety, insomnia, delirium, and major psychotic disorders (e.g., schizophrenia and bipolar affective disorder).

## DEPRESSION

Depression in cancer patients can result from the stress of cancer diagnosis and treatment, medications (steroids, interferon, or other chemotherapeutic agents, a biologically determined (endogenous) depression that is not related to a precipitating event, or bipolar affective disorder (manic-depressive illness) (see Chapter 23).

### Classes of Antidepressants used in the Oncology Setting

The antidepressant agents used most frequently in the oncology setting are the tricyclic antidepressants, second-generation antidepressants, monoamine oxidase inhibitor (MAOI), lithium carbonate, sympathomimetic stimulants, and the triazolobenzodiazepine, alprazolam. Table 39-1 shows the drugs, starting doses, and therapeutic range of these drugs. Each class is discussed in the following paragraphs.

**Table 39-1**  Antidepressant medications used in cancer patients

| Generic name | Trade name | Starting daily oral dosage (mg) | Usual therapeutic daily oral dosage (mg) | Therapeutic plasma level (mg/ml) |
|---|---|---|---|---|
| *Tricyclic antidepressants* | | | | |
| Amitriptyline | Endep, Elavil,* Amitid | 25 | 75–150 | 100–200 |
| Doxepin | Adapin, Sinequan† | 50 | 75–150 | 75–200 |
| Imipramine | Janimine, SK-Pramine, Tofranil* | 25 | 75–150 | 200 |
| Desipramine | Norpramin | 25 | 75–150 | 40–160 |
| Nortriptyline | Aventyl, Pamelor† | 50 | 75–150 | 50–150 |
| *Second-generation antidepressants* | | | | |
| Trazodone | Desyrel | 50 | 150–250 | |
| Maprotiline | Ludiomil | 25 | 50–75 | |
| Amoxapine | Asendin | 25 | 100–150 | |
| Fluoxetine | Prozac | 20 | 20–60 | |
| *Monoamine oxidase inhibitors* | | | | |
| Phenelzine | Nardil | 15 bid | 30–60 | |
| Tranylcypromine | Parnate | 10 bid | 20–40 | |
| Isocarboxazid | Marplan | 10 bid | 20–40 | |
| *Lithium carbonate* | | | | |
| Lithium | Eskalith,† Lithane, Lithobid, Lithotabs | 300 bid | 600–1200 | |
| *Sympathomimetic stimulants* | | | | |
| Dextroamphetamine | Dexedrine, Obetrol | 2.5–5.0 in morning | | |
| Methylphenidate | Ritalin | 5–10 mg (8 A.M. and noon) | | |
| *Benzodiazepines* | | | | |
| Alprazolam | Xanax | 0.25–1.00 qd | 0.75–6 | |
| *Experimental antidepressants* | | | | |
| Carbamazepine | Tegretol | 200 bid | 200 tid–qid | |

*Available for intramuscular injection.
†Available in elixir

## TRICYCLIC ANTIDEPRESSANTS

The tricyclic antidepressants are safely and effectively prescribed for depressed physically ill patients. Raskind and colleagues (1982) and Glassman and colleagues (1983) have reported effective use of imipramine in depressed patients with ischemic heart disease and congestive heart failure. Orthostatic hypotension was the most serious side effect of imipramine, and was the most important limitation on its use. Both of these authors encouraged consideration of the use of nortriptyline in the physically ill. Lipsey et al. (1984) have reported results of a double-blind comparison of nortriptyline versus placebo in patients after stroke or intracerebral hemorrhage. Patients treated with nortriptyline showed greater improvement in depressive symptoms than those treated with placebo. Similarly,

Rifkin and colleagues (1985) have reported results of a double-blind comparison of trimipramine versus placebo in 42 physically ill outpatients with endogenous major depression (including some patients with cancer). Trimipramine was superior to placebo on some measures of depression, with improvement in depressive symptoms occurring without concomitant improvement in the physical disorder.

Purohit and colleagues (1978) reported the efficacy of low-dose (25 mg tid) imipramine in a study of a small number of cancer patients. Popkin and colleagues (1985) retrospectively reviewed the outcome of antidepressant (desipramine, imipramine, amitriptyline, doxepin, and nortriptyline) use in 50 hospitalized physically ill depressed patients (including 15 patients with cancer). Of the patients studied, 40% had a positive response to antidepressants, a response rate lower than that normally achieved in psychiatric patients with primary affective disorder. Of the antidepressant trials, 32% were discontinued because of unacceptable drug side effects (e.g., delirium, nausea and vomiting, and urinary retention).

Costa and colleagues (1988) reported the efficacy and safety of mianserin (an antidepressant not available in the United States) in a randomized placebo-controlled trial of 73 depressed women with cancer. Both groups were matched for cancer site clinical stage, Karnofsky scores, duration of depression, baseline values on standard depression rating scales and types of depression.

There is a need for more systematic studies of antidepressants in cancer patients, although such studies are difficult to conduct because of the difficulty of establishing the diagnosis of depression, the lack of accurate standardized screening instruments to measure depression, and multiple confounding variables related to cancer and cancer treatment. However, as Rifkin et al. (1985) state, "the clinician must act in the present" and psychiatrists and oncologists effectively prescribe antidepressants for seriously ill depressed cancer patients.

## Choice of Tricyclic Antidepressant

The tricyclic antidepressants have been found effective in patients of all ages. Before starting to administer an antidepressant, the patient's blood count should be obtained and history of cardiovascular disease reviewed. If the patient has an abnormal electrocardiogram (ECG) or history of a prior cardiac problem, these should be reviewed with a cardiologist before an antidepressant is started. These considerations, along with several others to be discussed, influence the tricyclic chosen.

The choice of the tricyclic in a particular patient depends on the nature of the depressive symptoms, the medical problems present that would be adversely affected by drug side effects, and the side effects of the individual tricyclics. Within these three areas, several questions often arise in cancer patients, and influence the choice of a tricyclic.

*Is sedation desired?* The depressed cancer patient who is restless or agitated and has insomnia will respond best to a tricyclic with sedative properties such as amitriptyline or doxepine. The patient who has psychomotor slowing will benefit from a less sedating tricyclic, such as desipramine or protriptyline. Table 39-2 indicates the degree of sedative and anticholinergic side effects of the tricyclics, the second-generation antidepressants, and the triazolobenzodiazepine alprazolam.

*Does the patient have problems that will be wors-*

**Table 39-2**  Drug characteristics of antidepressant medication*

| Drug | Sedative effect | Anticholinergic effect |
|---|---|---|
| *Tricyclic antidepressants* | | |
| Amitriptyline | + + + + | + + + + |
| Doxepin | + + + + | + + + |
| Imipramine | + + | + + |
| Desipramine | + | + |
| Nortriptyline | + + | + + |
| Protriptyline | + | |
| *Second–generation antidepressants* | | |
| Maprotiline | + + | + + |
| Trazodone | + + + + | 0 |
| Amoxapine | + + | + |
| Fluoxetine | 0 | 0 |
| *Benzodiazepines* | | |
| Alprazolam | + + | 0 |

*Least effect, +; greatest effect, + + + +.

*ened by anticholinergic effects?* The depressed patient who has stomatitis secondary to chemotherapy or radiotherapy, or who is recovering from gastrointestinal or genitourinary surgery and has slowed intestinal motility or urinary flow, or who has graft-versus-host disease (GvHD) secondary to bone marrow transplantation (BMT) should have prescribed a tricyclic with the least anticholinergic effects, such as desipramine or nortriptyline. Strong anticholinergic effects and sedative effects (antihistaminic effects) usually occur together (Table 39-2).

*Is the patient unable to take medication orally?* Depressed patients who are unable to take medications by mouth because of oral, pharyngeal, or esophageal surgery, restricted oral intake, or severe esophagitis or stomatitis can be given the tricyclic antidepressants amitriptyline and imipramine intramuscularly. Patients should be switched to the oral form as early as possible. Currently, tricyclic antidepressants are not approved for intravenous use in the United States; however, several studies from Europe indicate their effectiveness and safety by this route (Carton et al., 1976; Mucha et al., 1970).

*Does the patient have a seizure disorder?* Although reports in the literature differ, desipramine and doxepin probably lower the seizure threshold less than other tricyclics, and hence are the preferred tricyclics for patients with seizure disorders (Richardson and Richelson, 1984; Markowitz and Brown, 1987).

## Dosage

Common starting dosage and range of usual daily therapeutic dosages of the tricyclic antidepressants for cancer patients are shown in Table 39-1. Treatment is started with a low dose range of 10 to 25 mg, usually given at bedtime. The dose is increased by 25 mg every 1–3 days until a therapeutic effect is seen. Maximum recommended dosages for physically healthy patients are up to 300 mg daily; maximum effective dosages for cancer patients are often in the range of 75–150 mg daily.

To ensure an adequate therapeutic trial of a tricyclic, a patient should be maintained on a therapeutic dosage of the tricyclic for 2–3 weeks. If a patient shows a therapeutic response, he or she should be maintained on the dosage producing that response for at least 4 months *after* he or she is free of significant symptoms, before treatment is discontinued (Prien and Kupfer, 1986). Tricyclic antidepressants are never abruptly discontinued; the dosage is lowered to 50% of the therapeutic dosage for 2 months and then tapered and discontinued.

## Pattern of Response

The pattern of symptomatic response to tricyclic antidepressants usually proceeds in phases consisting of improvement in sleep and appetite noted within 2–7 days, and mood improvement seen in 2–3 weeks. Depressed cancer patients often show response to doses of 25–150 mg/day, far lower than those required for therapeutic response in physically healthy depressed patients. Why a lower dosage is both effective and more rapidly achieved is unclear, but tumor or treatment effects may alter drug metabolism and drug absorption (Sokol et al., 1978).

## Changing to a Different Medication

If a patient has not benefited from an adequate therapeutic trial of a tricyclic, a different tricyclic or a second-generation antidepressant (e.g., amoxapine, trazodone, maprotiline or fluoxetine) should be tried. Like the tricyclic compounds, the second-generation antidepressants vary in their antihistaminic and anticholinergic effects. Trazodone is more sedating and some patients report fewer anticholinergic effects; maprotiline is reportedly less cardiotoxic. Fluoxetine, a selective serotonin reuptake inhibitor has no anticholinergic activity and few adverse cardiovascular effects.

Most depressed cancer patients will respond to either a tricyclic or a second-generation compound. In presence of an unresponsive and unremitting major depression, MAOI can be tried. They are safer than often assumed, even in medically ill patients, but patients must avoid eating tyramine-containing foods (see later).

## Monitoring Plasma Concentrations

Plasma concentrations for nortriptyline, amitriptyline, imipramine, and desipramine can be determined in many laboratories (Table 39-1). We consider it unnecessary to obtain plasma concentrations routinely; however, plasma level determination may be helpful in special situations such as the following.

1. In the event that a patient fails to respond to a presumed adequate dosage, if the plasma concentration is low, the patient may either not be taking the prescribed dose or the drug is not being metabolized normally. A higher dosage is warranted as a trial (Hollister, 1983).
2. When the tumor or treatment is suspected to enhance metabolism and degree of protein binding of the antidepressant, this can result in excessively high blood levels.
3. When a tricyclic antidepressant (e.g., nortriptyline) that has a therapeutic "window" is used, a blood level determination will establish whether the plasma concentration is within the therapeutic range, and hence whether the dosage must be increased or decreased.

## Antidepressants in Combination with Other Psychoactive Drugs

One does not regularly prescribe combinations of tricyclic antidepressants or the "second-generation" antidepressants in the cancer patient. The combined use of tricyclics and the "second-generation" antidepressants does not increase antidepressant effect. De'Montigny and co-workers (1981) have reported that adding lithium carbonate (900 mg qd) as an adjunct to tricyclic antidepressants for patients with unipolar major depression who are nonresponders to tricyclic antidepressants alone can produce good antidepressant effect. Tricyclic antidepressants and an antipsychotic are usually prescribed for patients whose depression has psychotic features. Procarbazine is a mild MAOI, and patients receiving it should be monitored when a tricyclic is given. However, the risk of hypertensive crisis resulting from combined use of tricyclic antidepressants and MAOI appears to be lower than previously believed. Occasionally tricyclics and MAOI are given in combination to depressed patients who are refractory to single agents (White and Simpson, 1981). Feighner and co-workers (1985) have reported that some patients with major depression who have failed to respond to tricyclics alone have been treated safely with tricyclic, MAOI, and stimulant (dextroamphetamine or methylphenidate) combinations. These authors suggest that imipramine be avoided when combining tricyclics and

MAOI. Combinations of antidepressants should always be administered carefully.

## Age Restrictions

In depressed children and adolescents, individual psychotherapy is the primary treatment modality. Antidepressants should be prescribed as an adjunct treatment (Ambrosini, 1987). Several authors have described prescribing principles for antidepressants for children and adolescents (Rancurello, 1985; Pfefferbaum-Levine et al., 1983; Geller et al., 1986) (see Chapter 44). Caution must be used when prescribing tricyclics for the elderly because of the increased risk of orthostatic hypertension and delirium, which are caused by anticholinergic effects.

## Tricyclics in the Treatment of Pain

Tricyclic antidepressants (amitriptyline, doxepin, and imipramine) are increasingly used as adjuvant analgesic drugs in the management of cancer pain (Foley, 1985). Walsh (1986) reported results of a randomized double-blind trial of placebo versus imipramine for chronic pain in patients receiving palliative cancer care. A lower dose of morphine was required in patients who received imipramine in addition to morphine. This effect was seen in 7 days, and there was no change in mood. The efficacy of antidepressants has been proven in the treatment of migraine headache, postherpetic neuralgia, diabetic neuropathy, and neuropathy related to total parenteral nutrition (TPN). Suggested starting dosage is 10 mg for elderly patients or 25 mg for the average patient at bedtime. Whereas the initial assumption was that the analgesic effect resulted indirectly from the tricyclics' effect on depression, it is now clear that tricyclics have a separate analgesic effect mediated by enhancing serotonin activity within the CNS. Clifford (1985) cites evidence that the presence of depression is not necessary for an analgesic response, the antidepressant effect on pain is more rapid (days) than its effect on depression (weeks), and serum levels that are effective for pain relief are much lower than those needed for an antidepressant action (see Chapter 23).

## Side Effects

Physicians may underprescribe tricyclics because of concern about side effects (Table 39-3). Our discussion of the adverse effects is not meant to discourage their use, but rather to alert the clinician to the spectrum of common to rare side effects.

The common side effects of the tricyclics are drowsiness, sedation, orthostatic hypotension, dry mouth,

**Table 39-3** Side effects of tricyclic antidepressant medications

|  | Side effects | |
|---|---|---|
|  | Common | Uncommon |
| Anticholinergic | Dry mouth, constipation, ↓ intestinal motility, urinary hesitancy or retention | Blurred vision, worsening of glaucoma, confusion or delirium |
| Cardiovascular | Orthostatic hypotension | ECG changes (arrhythmias, delayed cardiac conduction) |
| Endocrine and/or metabolic | Weight gain | Amenorrhea, impotence |
| Neurological | Sedation | EEG abnormalities, paresthesias, neuropathy, confusion |
| Sexual | — | Anorgasmia, ↓ enjoyment, impaired ejaculation |
| Sympathomimetic | — | Tremor, sweating, tachycardia, insomnia |
| Toxic | — | Agranulocytosis, cholestatic jaundice |

constipation, urinary hesitancy, and weight gain. Patients usually become tolerant to the unpleasant sedating effects, which often diminish after the first few days. Severe orthostatic hypotension is more apt to occur in older patients and may limit dosage, although some patients can tolerate this effect if the dosage is increased gradually. Nortriptyline has been shown to be less likely to cause orthostatic hypotension than imipramine (Glassman et al., 1983; Roose et al., 1987). The discomfort of dry mouth can be diminished by frequent sips of water or use of a synthetic saliva (Remick, 1988). Constipation is common and particularly difficult to control in patients receiving other constipating medications such as narcotics. Constipation often is relieved by adding fiber to the diet, use of bulk-forming laxatives (psyllium or methylcellulose), or lubricants (mineral oil).

Intramuscular use of the tricyclics seems to cause fewer anticholinergic effects; however, it is impractical to administer antidepressants by injection for a prolonged period of time. Although weight gain is a common side effect of antidepressants in healthy individuals, it is rarely a problem and may be a beneficial side effect in the debilitated cancer patient.

Less common side effects of the tricyclic antidepressants are shown in Table 39-3. Delirium resulting from anticholinergic effects occurs more frequently in medically ill patients and in the elderly. The potential cardiotoxic effects of the tricyclics (e.g., arrhythmias and delayed cardiac conduction) should be considered when prescribing for the cancer patient who has cardiac disease.

Harrison and colleagues (1986) have reported results of a double-blind randomized study of imipramine, phenelzine, and placebo on sexual function. Both drugs were associated with adverse effects on sexual function in terms of interest in and enjoyment of sex, impaired ejaculation, and anorgasmia. Of the two drugs, phenelzine was more frequently associated with altered function.

Other rare adverse effects are a central anticholinergic syndrome, allergic reactions, neurotoxicity (tremor), and endocrine disorders.

## SECOND-GENERATION ANTIDEPRESSANTS

The second-generation compounds (e.g., trazodone, maprotiline, and amoxapine) are usually prescribed after a therapeutic trial of the tricyclic compounds has proved nonbeneficial. Initially these compounds were described as having few cardiovascular side effects, which made them appear particularly useful for medically ill patients. However, experience has shown they have many of the same side effects as tricyclics (Glassman, 1984).

Common starting dosage and range of daily therapeutic doses for these compounds are seen in Table 39-1. The daily dosage of trazodone needed to produce antidepressant effects in cancer patients is usually higher (e.g., 250 mg) than the usual daily dosage of tricyclics (e.g., 75–150 mg). Amoxapine has a chemical structure similar to the antipsychotics and may be selected for use because of its combined antipsychotic and antidepressant action (Cohen et al., 1982).

The common side effects of the second-generation compounds are drowsiness, dizziness, fatigue, and orthostatic hypotension. There are reports of priapism (Scher et al., 1983) and aggravation of preexisting ventricular arrhythmias with trazodone (Janowsky et al., 1983).

Fluoxetine, a selective serotonin reuptake inhibitor, may be useful for some cancer patients because of its lack of anticholinergic activity. Starting dose is 5 mg qid; side effects include insomnia, anorexia, anxiety, and nausea.

## MONOAMINE OXIDASE INHIBITORS

MAOI are usually prescribed for depressed patients who have not benefited from therapeutic trials of either the tricyclic or second-generation antidepressants or who have had unacceptable side effects from these drugs. If a cancer patient has a history of a previous response to MAOI, their use should be considered if depression appears during cancer treatment. Patients taking MAOI must be cautioned about eating tyramine-containing foods (e.g., aged cheese, red wine, beef extract) to avoid hypertensive crisis.

The starting daily dosage and daily therapeutic dose range of the MAOI (phenelzine, tranylcypromine, isocarboxazid) are listed in Table 39-1. Phenelzine and tranylcypromine are the most commonly prescribed in the United States. MAOI are started in much lower dosage (10 mg bid) than are tricyclics; antidepressant effect is often achieved with doses of 20–60 mg daily. Combined use of tricyclics and MAOI, should be cautiously approached in physically ill patients. Anesthesiologists often discontinue MAOI 24–48 hours prior to surgery (or 1–2 weeks prior to elective surgery) if monoamine compounds are to be used during anesthesia. The analgesic meperidine should never be prescribed to patients taking MAOI, because of potential fatal reactions.

The undesirable effects of phenelzine are anorgasmia, impotence, hypomania, and syncope (Rabkin et al., 1984).

## LITHIUM CARBONATE

Lithium carbonate's specific usefulness is for the treatment of bipolar affective disorder. It is the drug of choice for the treatment of mania and is effective in the prevention of depression in some patients with recurrent depressive disorder. Lithium carbonate has been prescribed experimentally to stimulate granulocytopoiesis in neutropenic cancer patients and to prevent mood changes and psychosis associated with steroid administration. Neither of these uses has proved highly effective, and both are discussed here.

### Initiation of Lithium Therapy

Before starting lithium therapy, the patient's history of renal or thyroid disease should be reviewed. ECG, thyroid function tests (serum thyroid-stimulating hormone or TSH), blood urea nitrogen (BUN), and creatine and creatinine clearance should be obtained.

### Dosage

The usual starting dosage of lithium for the treatment of depression is 300 mg bid. The daily dose is adjusted to achieve plasma levels of 0.8–1.2 mEg/L, measured 12 hours after the last dose. There is wide variability in the dosage of lithium needed to maintain therapeutic blood levels; the dosage may range from 300 to 1200 mg daily. Once therapeutic levels are reached, they should be monitored frequently in the patient whose medical situation is unstable. Maintenance dosage may have to be lowered as the patient's metabolic status changes. Lithium is available in concentrate form for patients unable to swallow pills.

## Lithium in the Periods Before and After Surgery

Patients who are well stabilized on lithium are often reluctant to discontinue its use preoperatively because of fear of recurrence of depression. Lithium can be continued in usual doses until the patient is ordered to have nothing orally and can be restarted postoperatively as soon as the patient is permitted to have fluids. It is useful to request psychiatric consultation for assistance in monitoring lithium dose and salt and fluid intake during periods before and after the operation to avoid lithium toxicity.

## Side Effects

The side effects of lithium include lithium poisoning, dehydration, and sodium deficiency. The early signs of lithium poisoning are fine tremor and muscle weakness. Muscle twitching, ataxia, nausea, diarrhea, difficulty concentrating, somnolence, and dysarthria appear later. Because some of these signs and symptoms can result from cancer or cancer treatment, the physician must be particularly alert to signs of lithium toxicity in the cancer patient. If a patient taking lithium has fever, or diarrhea, is sweating or vomiting, or is being treated with diuretics and low-salt diet, the danger of dehydration or sodium deficiency is more severe.

Nephropathy induced by lithium, characterized by reduction in urine-concentrating capacity (DePaulo et al., 1986), is of concern in cancer patients who are receiving potentially nephrotoxic chemotherapeutic agents (e.g., cisplatin). Lithium decreases thyroid function in most patients, however, few patients develop thyroid enlargement or symptoms of hypothyroidism (Hollister, 1983). Cardiac effects of lithium include T-wave changes, sinus node dysfunction, and ventricular arrhythmias.

## Experimental Uses of Lithium in the Oncology Setting

Lithium carbonate, in doses similar to those used to treat manic-depressive illness, has been shown to cause neutrophilic leukocytosis due to mobilization of polymorphonuclear (PMN) leukocytes from bone marrow reserves (Scala and Visconti, 1985). Several authors have reported possible beneficial effects from the use of lithium in neutropenic cancer patients (Cantane et al., 1977; Lyman et al., 1980; Stein et al., 1979;

Turner et al., 1979); however, the functional capabilities of these leukocytes have not been determined.

## Other Pharmacological Uses of Lithium

The corticosteroids predisone and dexamethasone, commonly used in cancer treatments, can cause a range of psychiatric symptoms including affective changes with manic and depressive symptoms. There are several reports in the literature regarding the potential usefulness of lithium carbonate for the prevention of steroid-induced mood changes (Falk et al., 1979; Goggans et al., 1983). We have not found this use of lithium helpful in preventing steroid psychosis and prefer to use antidepressants or neuroleptics if symptoms appear.

## SYMPATHOMIMETIC STIMULANTS

The use of sympathomimetic stimulants (e.g., dextroamphetamine and methylphenidate) for the treatment of depression has been controversial (Chiarello and Cole, 1987). In the oncology setting, dextroamphetamine has been found to improve both mood and appetite in patients who are in terminal stages of illness (Hackett, 1978). A controlled trial of methylphenidate in patients with advanced cancer showed reduced narcotic consumption and improved activity and interest. The major negative side effect was appetite suppression (Bruera et al., 1986). Kaufmann and Murray (1982) reported beneficial antidepressant effects with dextroamphetamine in three patients, two of whom had poor response to tricyclics and one depressed cancer patient who had severe pain that was poorly controlled with morphine. Amphetamines are useful to counter sedating effects of narcotics in patients who require large amounts of analgesics. A retrospective review of the use of psychostimulants in 66 medically ill patients showed that psychostimulants can safely produce rapid and continuing relief of depressive symptoms in medically ill patients in whom tricyclic antidepressants are contraindicated (Woods et al., 1986). Starting dosage of dextroamphetamine in medically ill patients is 2.5–5.0 mg qd, and starting dosage of methylphenidate if 5–10 mg at 8 A.M. and noon (see Table 39-1).

## BENZODIAZEPINES IN DEPRESSION

Alprazolam, a triazolobenzodiazepine, has sparked considerable interest in cancer settings, because of its antidepressant and anxiolytic effects. Alprazolam has been tested against the tricyclic imipramine and has been found to be equally efficacious (Feighner et al.,

1983; Rickels et al., 1985,1987). Holland and colleagues (1987) have reported results of a study carried out in several cancer settings testing the efficacy of alprazolam versus relaxation techniques for patients with mixed symptoms of anxiety and depression. Although both treatments were found to be effective, patients receiving alprazolam showed a more rapid decrease in anxiety and showed greater reduction in depressive symptoms. The drug also reduces nausea and vomiting, especially anticipatory distress prior to chemotherapy. Table 39-1 shows the starting dosage and approximate therapeutic dose range for alprazolam. Studies indicate the dosage of alprazolam needed for treatment of depression may be higher (2.0–8.0 mg/day) than that required for treatment of anxiety (0.5–1.5 mg/day).

## ANXIETY

The types of anxiety seen in the oncology setting are episodes of acute anxiety related to problems associated with cancer and its treatment and chronic anxiety disorders that antedate cancer diagnosis, but are exacerbated during cancer treatment.

Patients are especially apt to experience acute anxiety at several points, specifically, while waiting to hear about their diagnosis or test results, before procedures (e.g., bone marrow aspiration, start of chemotherapy, wound debridement, and lumbar puncture), and before surgery or major diagnostic tests. Physical problems, especially pain or hypoxia, also produce acute anxiety; medications (e.g., steroids and neuroleptic drugs) may cause symptoms of anxiety and restlessness. Anxiety symptoms can be encountered in cancer with hyperthyroidism, hyperparathyroidism, depression, delirium, and drug withdrawal (e.g., alcohol, barbiturates, and narcotics).

The most common chronic anxiety states that antedate the cancer diagnosis are phobias (e.g., claustrophobia or fear of needles) and panic disorder (see Chapter 25 for discussion of anxiety disorders). Anxious patients often benefit from an antianxiety drug to reduce fear, distress, and panic irrespective of the cause, and to assist the patient in reasserting control over his or her emotions. Specific indications for anxiolytics are outlined here.

## Classes of Antianxiety Medications Used in the Oncology Setting

The classes of drugs used for the treatment of anxiety are the benzodiazepines, antipsychotics, antihistamines, antidepressants, adrenergic blocking agents, and buspirone (Table 39-4).

Barbiturates and meprobamate, a glycerol deriva-

**Table 39-4**  Antianxiety medications used in cancer patients

| Generic name | Trade name |
| --- | --- |
| *Benzodiazepines* | |
| Alprazolam | Xanax |
| Oxazepam | Serax |
| Lorazepam | Ativan |
| Triazolam | Halcion |
| Diazepam | Valium |
| Chlordiazepoxide | Librium |
| Flurazepam | Dalmane |
| Clorazepate dipotassium | Tranxene |
| *Antipsychotics* | |
| Thioridazine | Mellaril |
| Trifluoperazine | Stelazine |
| Haloperidol | Haldol |
| Perphenazine | Trilafon |
| *Antihistamines* | |
| Diphenhydramine | Benadryl |
| Hydroxyzine | Atarax, Vistaril |
| *Antidepressants* | |
| Imipramine | Tofranil |
| Phenelzine | Nardil |
| *Adrenergic blocking agents* | |
| Propranolol | Inderal |
| *Others* | |
| Buspirone | Buspar |

tive, were once the mainstay of treatment of anxiety, but because they are highly addictive and lethal in overdose, the benzodiazepines have largely replaced them for the treatment of acute and chronic anxiety. The barbiturates are occasionally used for preoperative sedation and insomnia. Intravenously administered amobarbital sodium is used diagnostically to help distinguish between a neurological disorder and a conversion reaction. Antipsychotic medications are occasionally prescribed for acute anxiety when the maximal therapeutic dose of a benzodiazepine is not effective; however, concern about tardive dyskinesia limits their usefulness for treatment of anxious states. The low efficacy of the antihistamines for anxiety limits their general application; however, they can be used for patients who have respiratory impairment and for those in whom physicians have concern about suppression of central respiratory mechanisms by the benzodiazepines. Antihistamines also relieve the akathesia associated with phenothiazines. The β blockers (e.g., propranolol), tricyclic antidepressants (e.g., imipramine), the MAOI (e.g., phenelzine), triazolobenzodiazepines (e.g., alprazolam), and clonazepam are all useful in the treatment of panic disorder. Benzodiazepines (e.g., alprazolam) are prescribed for panic disorder and agoraphobia with panic attacks (Ballenger et al., 1988; Noyes et al., 1988; Lesser et al., 1988). Imipramine is the drug of choice for maintenance treatment of panic disorders. Kahn and colleagues (1986) have reported results of a double-blind placebo-controlled comparison of imipramine and chlordiazepoxide in outpatients with anxiety disorders. Imipramine was found to be a more effective antianxiety agent than chlordiazepoxide. Although this study requires replication, the results support the independence of the antianxiety and antidepressant actions of imipramine.

Buspirone, a nonbenzodiazepine anxiolytic, has been found not only to be effective in treating anxiety (Feighner et al., 1982), but also to produce relatively little psychomotor or cognitive impairment with no addiction liability.

## Choice of Anxiolytic Medication

Although there are a large number of anxiolytic drugs from which to choose, it is best to be fully familiar with

the use of a selected number of these compounds in regard to their metabolism, half-life, side effects, and efficacy.

The antianxiety drug selected in a specific situation depends on the acuteness or chronicity of the anxious state, the drug's absorption rate (distribution and duration of action), the desirable and/or available route of drug administration, concurrent medical problems that affect drug metabolism, and drug side effects.

The drugs of choice for specific anxiety syndromes commonly encountered in a cancer population are outlined here (see Fig. 39-1).

## ACUTE ANXIETY

For patients with acute anxiety, diazepam or clorazepate, which have a rapid absorption and quick onset of action, are useful (Greenblatt et al., 1983a). Diazepam given orally has its onset of action in 30 minutes, with peak plasma levels in 60 minutes. Oral administration of diazepam produces more rapid and complete ab-

**Figure 39-1.** Decision tree for selection of antianxiety agent.

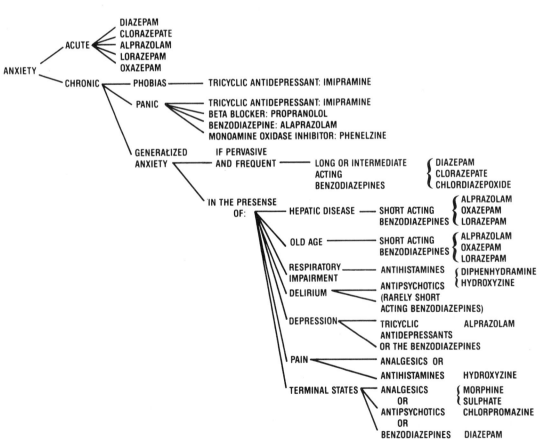

sorption than does parenteral administration. The acutely anxious patient who is unable to take medication orally can be given some benzodiazepines (e.g., diazepam, chlordiazepoxide, and lorazepam) parenterally. If diazepam must be administered parenterally, intravenous administration is preferred over intramuscular, because substantially higher plasma concentrations are achieved by the intravenous route and intramuscular dosages have an unpredictable absorption rate. Intramuscular administration is, of course, contraindicated in patients with thrombocytopenia.

## CHRONIC ANXIETY

Patients with chronic anxiety states are usually best treated with long-acting benzodiazepines such as diazepam, chlordiazepoxide, or clorazepate, which usually require administration only twice a day. These three anxiolytics are all metabolized by oxidation to desmethyldiazepam, an active metabolite, and hence have a long half-life.

## ANXIETY IN PATIENTS WITH HEPATIC DISEASE

Patients who need an antianxiety medication, but who have impaired hepatic function due to tumor or cholestatic jaundice, should be treated with the short-acting compounds (e.g., oxazepam and lorazepam) that are metabolized by conjugation and excreted rapidly by the kidney.

## ANXIETY IN PATIENTS WITH SEVERE RESPIRATORY IMPAIRMENT

All benzodiazepines cause some central respiratory depression. Anxious patients with chronic obstructive pulmonary disease or lung metastasis may get moderate relief of anxiety symptoms from antihistamines such as hydroxyzine or diphenhydramine (Jenike, 1983).

## ANXIETY IN THE ELDERLY

Elderly patients often have slowed metabolism of drugs; consequently, if benzodiazepines are to be given to anxious elderly patients, short-acting drugs such as alprazolam, oxazepam, and lorazepam are the drugs of choice (Jenike, 1983).

## ANXIETY ASSOCIATED WITH PAINFUL PROCEDURES

Anxiety is a feature of acute pain; patients undergoing painful procedures such as bone marrow aspiration or

lumbar puncture often need medications. The sedative effects of analgesics combined with the sedative effects of antihistamines (e.g., hydroxyzine), commonly used to potentiate analgesics, often effectively reduce anxiety symptoms. Intravenous anesthetics such as fentanyl and ketamine have been used effectively in children undergoing bone marrow aspiration or biopsy. They produce both anesthetic and tranquilizing effect within minutes of intravenous administration. Ketamine is usually given 1–2 mg/kg body weight and will produce 5–10 minutes of surgical anesthesia. Ketamine can produce unpleasant dreamlike states and visual hallucinations, which are reduced by adding intravenous diazepam or lowering the dose of ketamine. Fentanyl is also useful for anxiety arising from minor painful surgical procedures, and will provide some pain relief during the postoperative period. Dosage is 0.05–0.1 mg (or 0.002 mg/kg) iv or im given slowly over 1–2 minutes, approximately 30 minutes prior to the procedure. Drug effect can be reversed by naloxone.

## ANXIETY AS A FEATURE OF DELIRIUM

Anxiety symptoms are often early symptoms of delirium; if delirium goes untreated, severe agitation may ensue. Often anxiety or agitation must be controlled to enable a workup to determine the etiology of the delirium. The use of benzodiazepines should be avoided in the delirious patient, because they often worsen confusion. Low dosage of a high-potency antipsychotic, such as haloperidol, is the treatment of choice (see Chapter 30 and delirium and dementia sections in this chapter).

## MIXED ANXIETY AND DEPRESSIVE SYMPTOMS

Patients with cancer often have symptoms of both anxiety and depression as a response to stresses during cancer (see Chapter 22). Often these symptoms of distress resolve with psychological support alone. However, if the symptoms are manifestations of a depressive disorder, pharmacological management is best achieved with antidepressant medication with sedative properties (e.g., amitriptyline, doxepin) (see Chapter 23). Alprazolam, with demonstrated antidepressant effect, is useful for many patients with these mixed symptoms (Feighner et al., 1983; Rickels et al., 1985).

## ANXIETY IN TERMINAL ILLNESS

Often dying patients are anxious (or agitated) because of pain, hypoxia, or delirium resulting from multiple

**Table 39-5** Benzodiazepines commonly prescribed for cancer patients

| Drug (trade name) | Approximate dose equivalent | Initial oral dosage (mg) | Absorption | Half-life | Active metabolites | Metabolic pathway |
|---|---|---|---|---|---|---|
| Alprazolam (Xanax) | 0.5 | 0.25–0.5 tid | Intermediate | Intermediate | Yes | Oxidation |
| Oxazepam (Serax) | 10 | 10–15 tid | Slow–intermediate | Intermediate | No | Conjugation |
| Lorazepam (Ativan) | 1 | 0.5–2.0 tid | Intermediate | Intermediate | No | Conjugation |
| Chlordiazepoxide (Librium) | 10 | 10–25 tid | Intermediate | Long | Yes | Oxidation |
| Diazepam* (Valium) | 5 | 5–10 bid | Fast | Long | Yes | Oxidation |
| Clorazepate (Tranxene) | 7.5 | 7.5–15 bid | Fast | Long | Yes | Oxidation |

*Available in intramuscular and intravenous forms.

metabolic abnormalities (Massie et al., 1983). Although the use of benzodiazepines is usually avoided in delirious patients because of their tendency to exacerbate confusion, nonconfused anxious or agitated dying patients can benefit from a combined use of intravenous morphine sulfate and benzodiazepines (diazepam or lorazepam). Recommended starting dosage of morphine sulfate is highly variable (0.5–100 mg/qh) as are maximum dosages (4–480 mg/qh). Guidelines for appropriate continuous morphine use are comprehensively summarized by Portenoy and colleagues (1986) and in Chapter 32 by Portenoy and Foley.

## Dosage

The initial dosage, as well as frequency and length of administration of antianxiety agents depends on the nature and cause of the anxious state, the desired effect, the patient's physical condition, and the concomitant use of other medications (e.g., antidepressants, analgesics, and antiemetics). Table 39-5 lists an approximate dose equivalent, the commonly used starting dosage of benzodiazepines, absorption, half-life, presence of active metabolites, and metabolic pathway.

For effective treatment of anxiety, an adequate dose of medication must be given. Physicians often err on the side of undertreating anxious states because of their fear of using too high a dosage or causing addiction. Both worries are exaggerated. It is important to reduce distress by giving enough anxiolytic on a 24-hour schedule. An ''upon request'' order places the burden to ask for medication on an already anxious patient. Anxiety increases if drugs are administered late or in insufficient amounts.

The dosage schedule depends on the patient's tolerance and the duration of action of the anxiolytic. Because of their long half-life, chlordiazepoxide, clorazepate, and diazepam are useful for chronic generalized anxiety and can be given twice a day. Although timed-release forms of diazepam are available, it is best to avoid the use of these preparations when drug metabolism is impaired because of hepatic dysfunction. The shorter-acting benzodiazepines are given three to four times a day because of their short half-life and absence of active metabolites.

If a patient's anxious state does not respond to the initial dose of benzodiazepine, it is best to increase the dose to the maximal recommended dose before switching to another drug in the same class or to another class of anxiolytics. If a patient is refractory to maximal recommended dose of antianxiety agents (e.g., diazepam 40 mg/day), then it may be useful to switch to a different class of anxiolytic for treatment, or low dosage of an antipsychotic (e.g., thioridazine or perphenazine).

Length of maintenance on antianxiety agents depends on the nature of the problem being treated. Patients who have anxiety before a procedure (e.g., anxiety before chemotherapy) often take an antianxiety agent only on the day of chemotherapy, before coming to the clinic. Patients with chronic anxiety often need to take an antianxiety agent for months or years. In our experience, most cancer patients do not take more benzodiazepines than they absolutely need to control symptoms; patients appropriately discontinue medication as soon as symptoms remit. Physicians and patients are often concerned about the risk of creating a physical dependence on benzodiazepines and occurrence of a withdrawal syndrome. Busto and colleagues (1986) have reported that symptoms of withdrawal from long-term use of therapeutic doses of benzodiazepines occur, but are usually mild and can be managed by gradual reduction in the dose of benzodiazepines.

## Age Limitations on the Use of Benzodiazepines

There are no age limitations on the use of benzodiazepines. Pfefferbaum (Chapter 44) has reported the safe use of benzodiazepines in children with cancer. Benzodiazepines should be used with caution in the elderly because they can produce a confusional state (see later discussion of pharmacological management of the elderly patient with cancer).

## Side Effects

The most common side effects of the benzodiazepines are sedation, somnolence, confusion, and motor incoordination. These dose-dependent effects disappear when the dosage is lowered, uncomfortable sedation often disappears while the antianxiety effects continue. Sedation is common and can be severe in patients with impaired liver function. Patients should be cautioned regarding the additive sedative effects of the benzodiazepines when used with other medications with CNS-depressant properties (e.g., analgesics and alcohol).

The short-acting benzodiazepine lorazepam produces anterograde amnesia after both oral and intravenous administration (Healey et al., 1983). This effect is clinically useful in the cancer setting, where it is given intravenously to control nausea and vomiting associated with chemotherapeutic agents (e.g., *cis*-platinum) with high emetic potential. When administered as the sole antiemetic agent in doses of 2–4 mg, lorazepam does not decrease the number or frequency of emetic events; however, patients remember little of their vomiting episodes (Laszlo et al., 1985). Lorazepam given with metoclopramide reduces the motor restlessness caused by metoclopramide and, because of the amnestic effect, reduces patients' tendency to develop anticipatory nausea and vomiting.

Physicians should be mindful of two important drug interactions involving anxiolytics:

1. Cimetidine, a histamine $H_2$ receptor antagonist, inhibits hepatic enzymes that metabolize diazepam, chlordiazepoxide, and alprazolam (Klotz and Reimann, 1980). Combined administration of cimetidine with these benzodiazepines can lead to as much as a threefold reduction in plasma clearance of the benzodiazepine. Because lorazepam and oxazepam are excreted by the kidney, they are not affected by this interaction.
2. Long-term use of estrogen contraceptives impairs the plasma clearance of diazepam and greatly increases its plasma half-life (Abernethy et al., 1982).

## INSOMNIA

Patients with cancer often have difficulty falling asleep and/or maintaining a restful sleep cycle in the hospital and at home. A disruption of sleep can be the result of

**Table 39-6**  Causes of insomnia in cancer patients

Physical illness (hypoxia, urinary frequency, fever, pruritus, endocrine disorders)
Pain
Psychiatric syndromes (depression, mania, delirium)
Anxiety
Medication/drugs (prolonged use and withdrawal)
Disturbing hospital and/or home environment

pain, fever, respiratory difficulty, pruritus, medications, interference from the environment, anxiety, or depression (see Tables 39-6 and 39-7). Chronic usage of hypnotic agents may cause or perpetuate sleep disturbances. Rebound insomnia, a withdrawal phenomenon, may be caused by short-acting benzodiazepines. Long-acting benzodiazepines such as flurazepam can have a cumulative effect, especially in older patients.

The treatment of insomnia in the cancer setting involves management of the underlying physical and emotional causes. Treatment approaches are psychological support and reassurance, patient education, relaxation training, and the use of pharmacological agents. This section outlines pharmacological management (Table 39-8).

The "ideal" bedtime hypnotic should have a half-life equal to an average night's sleep, no active metabolites, immediate effectiveness, little possibility for disruption of the sleep cycle, and no abuse potential (Hollister, 1983). Of course the "ideal" hypnotic is nonexistent. Active metabolites cause desired sedation as well as undesirable "hangover" and cumulative sedative effects.

When selecting a hypnotic for a cancer patient, the

**Table 39-7**  Agents that cause insomnia in cancer patients

| Application | Agents |
| --- | --- |
| Prolonged usage | CNS stimulants (caffeine, amphetamines, aminophylline) |
| | Steroids |
| | Antidepressants (MAOIs) |
| | Chemotherapy agents, antimetabolites |
| | Thyroid preparations |
| | Antihypertensive agents (α-methyldopa, propranolol) |
| | Alcohol |
| | Hypnotic sedatives |
| Withdrawal | CNS depressants and hypnotics |
| | Anxiolytics (benzodiazepines) |
| | Antidepressants (tricyclics, MAOIs) |
| | Antipsychotics |
| | Recreational drugs |
| Regular usage | Diuretics |

**Table 39-8**　Management of insomnia in hospitalized cancer patients

- Rule out and manage underlying pain or medical illness.
- Relieve environmentally induced sleep disruptions.
- Provide psychological intervention: behavioral (relaxation training); education; psychological support by staff.
- Institute pharmacological management.

physician should consider the patient's medical problems that affect drug metabolism and elimination, and the hypnotic's side effects.

The class of hypnotic agents most commonly used for the patient with cancer are the benzodiazepines; less commonly prescribed are chloral derivatives and antidepressants. Barbiturates, antihistamines, and the amino acid tryptophan are less often prescribed (Table 39-9).

## Classes of Hypnotic Agents

### BENZODIAZEPINES

The safe and effective benzodiazepines are the most commonly prescribed medications for many cancer patients. They include triazolam, diazepam, flurazepam,

and temazepam. Diazepam and flurazepam rarely cause "rebound" insomnia or early-morning awakening. However, because of their long half-life (50–100 hours) and active metabolites, they can produce morning hangover and grogginess. Temazepam, which has an intermediate half-life of 8–10 hours and no active metabolites, is a useful hypnotic because it has less potential for drug accumulation and can be used in patients with hepatic disease. Unlike diazepam clearance, that of temazepam is not affected by cimetidine administration. Triazolam, with a short half-life of 2–3 hours and no active metabolites, is also useful for patients with hepatic dysfunction. The advantage of triazolam—that it produces virtually no morning hangover—must be weighed against the disadvantage of rebound insomnia, early-morning awakening, and daytime anxiety Greenblatt et al., 1983b). We recommend a starting dosage of triazolam of 0.125 mg for debilitated or elderly cancer patients, because some develop irritability, confusion, delirium, and agitation at a higher dose (see Table 39-9 for dosage guidelines). Scavone and co-workers (1986) have reported that the bioavailability of triazolam after sublingual administration is increased by an average of 28% compared with oral administration of the same dose, possibly because first-pass hepatic extraction is bypassed.

**Table 39-9**　Sedatives and hypnotics commonly used for cancer patients

| Drug | Trade name | Initial oral dosage (mg) | Oral dosage range (mg) | Half-life (hours) | Active metabolites |
|---|---|---|---|---|---|
| *Benzodiazepines* | | | | | |
| Triazolam* | Halcion | 0.25 | 0.25–0.50 | 2–3 | No |
| Temazepam* | Restoril | 15 | 15–30 | 8–10 | No |
| Flurazepam[†] | Dalmane | 15 | 15–30 | 50–100 | Yes |
| Diazepam[†,‡] | Valium | 5 | 5–10 | 20–100 | Yes |
| *Antihistamines* | | | | | |
| Diphenhydramine[‡,§] | Benadryl | 50 | 50–75 | | |
| *Chloral derivatives* | | | | | |
| Chloral hydrate[§] | Noctec, SK-Chloral Hydrate | 500 | 500–1000 | 8–10 | |
| *Short-acting barbiturates* | | | | | |
| Phenobarbital[‡,§,‖] | Nembutal | 100 | 100–200 | | |
| Secobarbital[‡,‖] | Seconal | 100 | 100–200 | | |
| *Intermediate-acting barbiturates* | | | | | |
| Amobarbital sodium | Amytal sodium | | | | |
| *Amino acid* | | | | | |
| L-Tryptophan | Trofan, Tryptacin | 1000–5000 | | | |

*Metabolism by conjugation.
[†]Metabolism by oxidation.
[‡]Available for intramuscular or intravenous injection.
[§]Available in elixir.
[‖]Available in suppository.

## ANTIHISTAMINES

Antihistamines (e.g., hydroxyzine and diphenhydramine) have low efficacy as hypnotics; however, they are useful for patients with respiratory impairment and in whom hypnotics, which cause central respiratory depression, must be avoided. If prescribed in large doses, they may precipitate an anticholinergic crisis with symptoms of disorientation, confusion, urinary retention, and tachycardia.

## CHLORAL DERIVATIVES

Chloral hydrate is an effective bedtime hypnotic in doses of 500–1000 mg. It can be used with relative safety in most patients, including the elderly. It has the advantage of producing little respiratory depression; however, it should be used judiciously in cancer patients with gastritis and peptic ulcer disease, because it can cause gastric irritation. The chloral derivatives are contraindicated for patients with severe liver dysfunction and those patients taking anticoagulants detoxified in the liver. Chloral hydrate potentiates the effects of anticoagulants.

## BARBITURATES

Barbiturates are indicated for cancer patients who have severe chronic sleep disturbances that are refractory to benzodiazepines, antihistamines, or chloral derivatives. Barbiturates should be used with caution because of addictive potential and withdrawal effects. These agents stimulate hepatic enzymes involved in the degradation and detoxification of many other drugs, and hence they decrease the clinical efficacy of anticoagulants, quinidine, digoxin, hydantoins, antipsychotics, and tricyclic antidepressants.

## TRYPTOPHAN

Berlin (1984) reported that when the amino acid L-tryptophan is given in doses of 1–5 g, sleep latency is shortened. However, other investigators cite the necessity for further research regarding the usefulness of L-tryptophan as a hypnotic (Adam and Oswald, 1979; Hartmann, 1977; Weilburg and Donaldson, 1988).

### Sleep Disorders in the Elderly

Older patients may be especially sensitive to the sleep disturbances associated with cancer. Depression, anxiety, or a mild organic brain syndrome may also contribute to sleep disorders in the elderly, who normally experience age-related decrease in total sleep time, frequent awakenings, and lighter sleep. The pharma-

cokinetics of lipophilic drugs such as the barbiturates and benzodiazepines are affected by age. With advancing age, there is a decrease in muscle and liver mass, a decrease in total body water, and an increase in body fat. Because drug half-life is proportional to volume of distribution, and drug elimination is proportional to hepatic blood flow and enzymatic metabolism, the elderly metabolize drugs more slowly. All hypnotic agents should be prescribed cautiously for elderly cancer patients, usually at 25–50% the dosage for younger patients. Benzodiazepines are usually the drug of choice. Chloral hydrate is usually safe; diphenhydramine is effective in some patients, but can cause paradoxical excitement in the elderly (and children). Depressed geriatric patients with sleep disturbances may benefit from low dosage of tricyclic antidepressants at bedtime.

Sleep disturbance is often associated with delirium, which is found in 15–20% of hospitalized cancer patients (Posner, 1978) and (see Chapter 30). If bedtime sedation is needed for delirious patients, an antipsychotic is the drug of choice, because both barbiturates and benzodiazepines may worsen the underlying delirium.

## THE MAJOR PSYCHOTIC DISORDERS: SCHIZOPHRENIA AND BIPOLAR AFFECTIVE DISORDER

The functional psychotic disorders (schizophrenia and the manic phase of bipolar affective disorder) are seen in a relatively small number of patients with cancer. The symptoms of a major psychotic disorder can include anxiety, agitation, irritability, hallucinations, and delusions, and often require pharmacological management. A patient who has symptoms of disorganized or illogical thinking or suspiciousness may require psychiatric treatment before cancer therapy, which requires a high level of cooperation. (see Chapter 28).

*Antipsychotics*[1] are the treatment of choice for both acute and chronic schizophrenia and the acute manic phase of bipolar affective disorder. Lithium carbonate and carbamazepine are used for maintenance treatment of bipolar affective disorder. Antipsychotics and antidepressants (usually tricyclic) are used in combination for the treatment of depression with psychotic features. Antipsychotics are discussed here (see the earlier sections on lithium carbonate).

The antipsychotic compounds commonly pre-

---

1. Antipsychotics are often referred to as neuroleptics (producing signs of neurological disorders; however, the general term antipsychotic is preferable given the discovery of antipsychotic agents without neurological effects (Baldessarini, 1984).

**Table 39-10** Approximate equivalent doses of commonly used antipsychotic agents in the oncology setting

| Generic name | Trade name | Approximate equivalent dose | Relative potency |
|---|---|---|---|
| *Phenothiazines* | | | |
| Aliphatic | | | |
| Chlorpromazine | Thorazine | 100 | Low |
| Piperidines | | | |
| Mesoridazine | Serentil | 50 | Low |
| Thioridazine | Mellaril | 90–100 | Low |
| Piperazines | | | |
| Perphenazine | Trilafon | 8–10 | Intermediate |
| Trifluoperazine | Stelazine | 3–5 | Intermediate |
| Fluphenazine | Prolixin | 2 | High |
| *Thioxanthenes* | | | |
| Thiothixene | Navane | 3–5 | High |
| *Dibenzoxazepines* | | | |
| Loxapine | Loxitane, Daxolin | 10–15 | |
| Butyrophenones | | | |
| Haloperidol | Haldol | 2–3 | High |
| *Indolones* | | | |
| Molindone | Moban, Lidone | 8–10 | Intermediate |

*Source*: Adapted from R.J. Baldessarini (1984). Antipsychotic agents. In T.B. Karasu (ed.), *The Psychiatric Therapies: Part I. The Somatic Therapies*. Washington, D.C.: American Psychiatric Association, pp. 119–70, with permission.

scribed in the oncology setting are the butyrophenones (haloperidol) and phenothiazines (chlorpromazine, mesoridazine, thioridazine, perphenazine, and trifluoperazine). Far less frequently used are thioxanthenes (thiothixene), dihydroindolones (molindone), and dibenzoxazepines (loxapine). Table 39-10 gives the names and approximate equivalent doses. Most antipsychotics are remarkably similar in their main actions and overall antipsychotic efficacy (Baldessarini, 1984).

Schizophrenic patients who have been well stabilized on antipsychotics prior to treatment for cancer should be maintained on their usual medication. Adjustments in drug, dosage, or route of administration may have to be made if psychiatric symptoms worsen or complications of cancer or chemotherapy alter drug metabolism. Occasionally the diagnosis of schizophrenia is first made in the oncology setting. A psychiatric consultation is required to establish the diagnosis and to determine pharmacological management of these patients.

The selection of an antipsychotic depends on the nature of presenting symptoms, concurrent medical problems (e.g., seizure disorder, hepatic dysfunction,

thrombocytopenia, or restriction of oral medication), past history of a response to an antipsychotic, and side effects of the antipsychotic.

Patients who have an acute psychosis with agitation need a psychotropic drug that is rapidly effective and easily administered. Presenting symptoms may determine the route of administration. If the presenting symptoms include suspiciousness with refusal to take medications orally, agitation, or poor compliance, then an antipsychotic such as haloperidol should be administered in parenteral form. The patient should be switched to oral medication as soon as he or she can and will take medication by mouth. Clinicians often initiate treatment with ''high-potency'' compounds (i.e., more potent on a milligram-for-milligram basis as compared with chlorpromazine) such as butyrophenones or thioxanthenes.

Antipsychotic drugs vary in their sedating properties and likelihood of producing orthostatic hypotension, neurological side effects (e.g., acute dystonia or extrapyramidal symptoms), and anticholinergic effects. The acutely agitated cancer patient requires a sedating medication; the patient with hypotension requires a drug with the least effect on blood pressure (e.g., haloperidol or perphenazine). The delirious postoperative patient who has mechanical ileus or urinary retention and who requires treatment with medications with anticholinergic properties (such as narcotics) should receive an antipsychotic with the least anticholinergic effects (e.g., haloperidol). Patients with hepatic dysfunction should be treated with *low* doses of antipsychotic agents, because all are metabolized in the liver. Those with a seizure disorder should be treated with compounds that lower seizure threshold least (haloperidol, molindone or the piperazines) (Baldessarini, 1984).

The special features of useful medications from various classes are discussed here.

## Classes of Antipsychotic Drugs

### BUTYROPHENONES

Haloperidol, a high-potency antipsychotic, is most commonly prescribed in our setting for patients with schizophrenia because of its effectiveness, availability in multiple forms, and low incidence of cardiovascular and anticholinergic effects. Haloperidol can be given orally (tablet or concentrate) or by intramuscular or intravenous injection. The latter are useful routes of administration for the agitated patient or the patient who initially will not take medication by mouth. Peak plasma concentrations of haloperidol are achieved in 2–4 hours after an oral dose, and measurable plasma concentrations occur in 15–30 minutes after intramuscular administration. Although not yet approved by the FDA for intravenous use, haloperidol is commonly and safely administered by this route for the agitated patient (see organic mental disorder in a later section).

Haloperidol causes less hypotension and has fewer anticholinergic effects than the low-potency compounds (e.g., chlorpromazine and thioridazine). It can produce significant extrapyramidal system effects (EPS), which usually are controlled by the use of antiparkinsonian medications.

## THIOXANTHENES, DIBENZOXAZEPINES, AND INDOLONES

If a schizophrenic patient does not respond to haloperidol, a different class of high-potency antipsychotics should be tried (e.g., thiothixene, loxapine, or molindone). These high-potency compounds all have a potential for causing EPS side effects; however, they have fewer anticholinergic effects than the low-potency phenothiazines.

## PHENOTHIAZINES

Although they are effective antipsychotics, low-potency phenothiazines such as chlorpromazine and mesoridazine are often avoided with cancer patients, especially the elderly, because of the risk of postural hypotension. Thioridazine may have some antidepressant effects in addition to having sedating and antipsychotic properties. Perphenazine and trifluoperazine are often well tolerated by the ambulatory patient. Chlorpromazine is useful for sedation of the terminally ill and for patients with intractable hiccups and nausea.

## Dosage

The initial dose and effective daily dose of antipsychotics vary widely because of the wide range of potency of these medications (see Table 39-10). In cancer patients, it is best to start treatment with a low dosage of a high-potency drug (e.g., haloperidol 0.5–1.0 mg po). Treatment is usually started using divided daily doses. Often patients are switched to a single nighttime dose when the effective 24-hour dosage has been determined. Target symptoms that improve with antipsychotics are hallucinations, acute delusions, combativeness, agitation, and insomnia. Length of maintenance treatment should be individualized; treatment is discontinued with gradual reduction of dose. Some authors (Adams, 1984) advocate the use of extremely high-dose haloperidol (or haloperidol and lorazepam combination) for the management of confusional states in cancer patients. High doses increase the risk of toxicity and effective results can be achieved with lower doses of haloperidol (Baldessarini, 1984). If antipsychotics are started by intravenous or intramuscular administration, a switch to an oral form should be made as soon as possible.

## Common Side Effects

The common side effects of the antipsychotic medications are neurological and anticholinergic in nature. Neurological effects are acute dystonia, akathesia, and a parkinsonian syndrome. Acute dystonia and akathesia usually appear within hours to days after the start of antipsychotic drug treatment. Drug-induced parkinsonism (tremor and rigidity) usually has its onset within the first week to month of treatment. These EPS effects rarely necessitate termination of treatment in the cancer patient, because the use of intramuscular, intravenous, or oral diphenhydramine or benztropine is effective for acute dystonic reactions and other EPS side effects. High-potency antipsychotics more readily induce dystonic reactions and parkinsonian symptoms than do the low-potency agents.

In cancer patients, these neurological side effects are frequently seen in patients receiving the neuroleptics prochlorperazine and metoclopramide to reduce distress of chemotherapy-induced nausea and vomiting. Motor restlessness, agitation, or akathesia related to drug effect may be incorrectly diagnosed as anxiety; if the drug is continued the patient experiences a worsening of symptoms (Fleishman et al., 1988). Patients with these symptoms secondary to metoclopramide or prochlorperazine are often more comfortable by giving a low dosage of a short-acting benzodiazepine. Sometimes these neurological symptoms necessitate discontinuation of the neuroleptic antiemetic.

Tardive dyskinesia (TD) is an EPS syndrome that consists of involuntary choreiform movements of the tongue, face, and neck muscles, as well as muscles of the extremities and chest wall. Orolingual-masticatory movements are the most common presentation. TD usually occurs after many weeks of treatment with an antipsychotic mediation or after discontinuation of the drug. The repetitive short-term high-dosage use of metoclopramide as an antiemetic in cancer patients has been reported to produce this disorder (Breitbart, 1986). Prevalence of these symptoms in patients chronically treated with antipsychotics may reach 50% (Baldessarini, 1984). The symptoms of TD usually become temporarily worse when the antipsychotic is withdrawn (rebound phenomenon), and symptoms may improve with readministration of the antipsychotic. Although the cause of TD is unknown, the traditional view that TD reflects supersensitivity of dopamine receptors caused by neuroleptic-induced dopamine receptor blockade is most likely inaccurate, because receptor supersensitivity is probably a ubiquitous consequence of neuroleptic administration (Jeste and Wyatt, 1981). It is felt that noradrenergic mechanisms may be involved in modulating symptoms (Jeste et al., 1982). All neuroleptics can cause TD, although those with higher affinity for niagrostriatal dopamine receptors carry a higher risk for delayed sequelae (Kane and Smith, 1982). The risk of TD increases with dosage and with duration of treatment, although it can occur at low dosages, and after treatment for only months or even weeks.

Treatment of TD involves suspending the administration of the drug, if possible, or lowering the dosage. Anticholinergic medications tend to exacerbate the choreiform movements. Most cases of TD that occur in younger patients who have been on a low dosage of antipsychotics for a short period of time will improve spontaneously if the antipsychotic is discontinued (Glazer et al., 1984). Indications for chronic administration of antipsychotic medication should be compelling because of the risk of TD.

The common anticholinergic effects of the antipsychotics vary from mild to severe and can contribute to patient noncompliance or necessitate change to a drug with fewer anticholinergic properties. Caution is suggested when using antipsychotic drugs with the strongest anticholinergic effects in particular types of cancer patients:

1. Those in the immediate postoperative period who are susceptible to urinary retention (after genitourinary surgery) or mechanical ileus (after abdominal surgery)
2. Those who are receiving several drugs with anticholinergic properties (atropine, tricyclic antidepressants, antiemetics, and analgesics)
3. Those who have stomatitis secondary to chemotherapy or radiotherapy
4. Those who are elderly and hence are more sensitive to anticholinergic effects
5. Those who are susceptible to developing a delirium secondary to toxic cause

## Rare Side Effects

The rare adverse reactions to antipsychotics are cardiovascular toxicity, cholestatic jaundice, agranulocytosis, neuroleptic malignant syndrome, and lowered seizure threshold. The risk of severe cardiovascular toxicity due to antipsychotics is low (Baldessarini, 1984); it most often involves the development of orthostatic hypotension and, infrequently, ventricular arrhythmias. Orthostatic hypotension is more commonly seen with the low-potency antipsychotics and

can be a problem in elderly or very physically ill patients. Because hypotensive effects are not related to dosage, the practice of administering test doses of antipsychotics is unnecessary (Baldessarini, 1984). The risk of ventricular arrhythmias is greatest with thioridazine; high-potency phenothiazines, haloperidol, and molindone have the least risk for cardiac patients. Transient cholestatic jaundice, now a relatively rarely reported side effect, was seen more often with the early use of chlorpromazine and was felt to be due to problems related to pharmaceutical formulation. Agranulocytosis, if it occurs, is seen in the first several weeks of drug treatment. This rare idiosyncratic side effect has an incidence of less than 0.01%, although it can be potentially serious in cancer patients with hematological malignancies.

Neuroleptic malignant syndrome (NMS) is characterized by altered levels of consciousness, severe EPS symptoms, autonomic dysfunction, and fever (Caroff, 1980; Kurlan et al., 1984; Levenson, 1985; Guze and Baxter, 1985; Pope et al., 1986). This disorder, which occurs in 1.4% of patients (Pope et al., 1986) treated with neuroleptics, is thought to be caused by dopaminergic blockade. Pearlman (1986) has reviewed 330 cases and reports that with wider recognition, the mortality rate has decreased from 22% of cases reported through 1980 to 4% of the last 50 cases he reviewed. Patients die of respiratory or renal failure, arrhythmias, and/or cardiovascular failure. Patients at higher risk for developing NMS are those who have prior muscular damage and/or are debilitated. This life-threatening syndrome should be considered in the differential diagnosis of any cancer patient receiving a phenothiazine who has fever and rigidity without clear basis. The presence of an elevated serum creatine kinase helps to make the diagnosis. Treatment involves discontinuation of the antipsychotic drug, and supportive care that includes hydration. Several authors report success with the use of dantrolene sodium (0.8–10 mg/kg per day) or bromocriptine mesylate, a dopamine antagonist 2.5–10 mg tid) (Guze and Baxter, 1985). NMS resembles malignant hyperthermia, a skeletal muscle syndrome that occurs in 1 in 50,000 patients exposed to inhalation anesthesia (e.g., halothane). Kurlan and co-workers (1984) reviewed both syndromes and risks of anesthesia in patients with NMS. It appears that the concern that anesthesia may precipitate NMS in a patient with a history of previous NMS is unwarranted. Levinson and Simpson (1986) have reviewed reports of NMS and question the assumption of a unitary NMS. They suggest that attention must be directed toward identification of medical complications in patients with severe EPS symptoms. Diagnosing coincidental occurrence of fever (which can result from multiple causes in the cancer patient) and severe EPS symptoms as "NMS" can inappropriately lead to the decision never to prescribe neuroleptics to patients who may need them in the future.

Antipsychotics can produce transient diffuse slow electroencephalograph (EEG) activity; however, the incidence of seizures associated with the use of low doses of antipsychotics is less than 1%. Seizure activity is more common in patients taking large doses of antipsychotics or in patients who have brain injury or a history of epilepsy (Remick and Fine, 1979; Itil and Soldatos, 1980). The relevance of this drug-induced lowered seizure threshold becomes important for the cancer patient when one uses a psychotropic medication in an epileptic patient, in a patient with a primary or metastatic brain lesion, or in a patient receiving intrathecal chemotherapy. Antipsychotic medications that produce less sedation or more EPS side effects have lower epileptic potential [i.e., the aliphatic phenothiazines (chlorpromazine) are more epileptogenic than those in the piperazine class (trifluoperazine, perphenazine, and fluphenazine) or the indolone (molindone)].

## Clinical Use of Lithium Carbonate

Lithium carbonate is the drug of choice for the treatment of mania. Because there is a "lag" time between the initiation of lithium therapy and clinical effect, patients often are started on an antipsychotic (haloperidol or chlorpromazine) in addition to lithium for initial treatment of mania with psychosis. Antipsychotics are gradually discontinued when the acute mania is improved, and lithium is continued as maintenance treatment for protection from further manic episodes. Starting dosage of lithium for acute mania in cancer patients is 300 mg bid–qid.

## ORGANIC MENTAL DISORDERS: DELIRIUM, DEMENTIA, AND STEROID PSYCHOSIS

The organic mental disorders that are frequently seen in the oncology setting are acute confusional states, namely delirium, dementia, and organic affective disorders (steroid psychosis) (see Chapter 30). The symptoms of these disorders vary in degree of severity but may include agitation, confusion, disorientation, memory impairment, suspiciousness, hallucinations, delusions, irritability, and inability to attend to a conversation or to sustain an activity due to distractibility. The acute brain syndromes sometimes require treatment with antipsychotics to reduce symptoms of agitation and suspiciousness to permit the physician to carry out a workup to determine the etiology of the disorder.

The class of medications most useful for the management of symptoms seen in delirium and dementia are the antipsychotic agents. The choice of specific drug is outlined here.

## Choice of Medication

The hospitalized cancer patient who is confused and disoriented, or who has hallucinations or delusions, should be started on a low dose of an antipsychotic medication, because confusion and psychotic symptoms may worsen and progress to agitation. An antipsychotic (e.g., haloperidol, perphenazine, or trifluoperazine) should be given orally if the patient can take them by this route. It is best to start with a low dosage of haloperidol (0.25–0.5 mg) in the elderly or debilitated patients, or 1–2 mg in the patient with good physical condition. Maintenance doses always need to be titrated against clinical signs of agitation, confusion, and irritability.

The acutely agitated delirious patient presents a special management problem that requires safe yet effective use of antipsychotic drugs. Because the agitated patient is often unable to cooperate with taking medications orally, we start treatment with intravenous or intramuscular administration of haloperidol at a dose of 0.5–2.0 mg. Administration by the intravenous route is 1 mg/min. Doses can be repeated at 15-minute intervals for 1 hour and should be titrated against observable clinical signs of agitation and irritability as well as side effects. Intravenous haloperidol can cause EPS signs that often can be controlled by benztropine (0.5–1.0 mg bid). If a patient appears to be increasingly agitated with haloperidol administration, the clinician must consider akathesia as a side effect of haloperidol in his or her differential diagnosis. There is a wide variability in the amount of haloperidol needed in any one patient to reduce symptoms to a level that is comfortable for the patient. Dubin and colleagues (1986) have reviewed the comparative efficacy of several drug regimens for rapid tranquilization in an emergency situation. They suggest that approximately 50% of the recommended dosage be used for debilitated patients.

When acute symptoms of agitation resolve, often within 24 hours, the patient should be switched to oral haloperidol at a dose of 75–150% of the parenteral dose given over the previous 24 hours. Conversion from parenteral to oral equivalents depends on the patient's ability to metabolize the drug and the overall well-being.

## SUMMARY

In this chapter, we have reviewed the psychotropic medications that are used for the treatment of depression, anxiety, insomnia, and major psychotic disorders that are commonly seen in the patient with cancer. In the past, psychotropic medications were underutilized in the oncology setting; however, clinicians are gaining familiarity with their beneficial effects of reducing the discomfort of emotional symptoms of cancer and its treatment.

## ACKNOWLEDGMENTS

We thank Dr. S. Fleishman and Dr. S. Roth for providing additional information and references.

## REFERENCES

Abernethy, D. R., D. J. Greenblatt, M. Divoll, R. Arendt, H. R. Ochs, and R. I. Shader (1982). Impairment of diazepam metabolism by low dosage estrogen-containing oral-contraceptive steroids. *N. Engl. J. Med.* 306:791–92.

Adam, K. and I. Oswald (1979). One gram of L-tryptophan fails to alter the time taken to fall asleep. *Neuropharmacology* 18:1025–27.

Adams, F. (1984). Neuropsychiatric evaluation and treatment of delirium in the critically ill cancer patients. *Cancer Bull. Univ. Texas M.D. Anderson Hosp. Tumor Inst. (Houston)* 36:156–60.

Ambrosini, P. J. (1987). Pharmacotherapy in child and adolescent major depressive disorder. In H. Y. Meltzer (ed.), *Psychopharmacology,* The Third Generation of Progress. New York: Raven (pp. 1247–54).

Baldessarini, R. J. (1984). Antipsychotic agents. In T. B. Karasu (ed.), *The Psychiatric Therapies: Part I. The Somatic Therapies.* Washington, D.C.: American Psychiatric Association, pp. 119–70.

Baldessarini, R. J. and J. O. Cole (1988). Chemotherapy. In A. M. Nicholi (ed.), *The New Harvard Guide to Psychiatry.* Cambridge, Massachusetts: Harvard University Press (pp. 481–533).

Ballenger, J. C., G. D. Burrows, R. L. DuPont, I. M. Lesser, R. Noyes, J. C. Pecknold, A. Rifkin, and R. P. Swinson (1988). Alprazolam in panic disorder and agoraphobia: results from a multicenter trial. *Arch. Gen. Psychiatry* 45:413–22.

Ballenger, J. C. (1988). The clinical use of carbamazepine in affective disorders. *J. Clin. Psychiatry* 49:13–19.

Berlin, R. M. (1984). Management of insomnia in hospitalized patients. *Ann. Intern. Med.* 100:398–404.

Breitbart, W. (1986). Tardive dyskinesia associated with high-dose intravenous metoclopramide. *N. Engl. J. Med.* 315:518.

Bruera, E., N. MacDonald, S. Chadwick, and C. Brenneis (1986). Double-blind cross-over study of methylphenidate with narcotics for the treatment of cancer pain. *Proc. Am. Soc. Clin. Oncol.* 989:253.

Busto, U., E. M. Sellers, C. A. Naranjo, H. Cappell, M. Sanchez-Craig, and K. Sykora (1986). Withdrawal reaction after long-term therapeutic use of benzodiazepines. *N. Engl. J. Med.* 315:854–59.

Caroff, S. N. (1980). The neuroleptic malignant syndrome. *J. Clin. Psychiatry* 41:79–83.

Carton, M., E. Cabarrot and C. Lafforgue (1976). Interet de l'amitriptyline utilisee comme antalgigue en cancerologie (The value of amitriptyline as an analgesic in cancer). *Gaz. Med. France* 83:2375–78.

Catane, R. L., J. Kaufman, A. Mittelman, and G. P. Murphy (1977). Attenuation of myelosuppression with lithium. *N. Engl. J. Med.* 297:452–53.

Chiarello, R. J. and J. O. Cole (1987). The use of psychostimulants in general psychiatry: A reconsideration. *Arch. Gen. Psychiatry* 44:286–95.

Clifford, D. B. (1985). Treatment of pain with antidepressants. *Am. Fam. Physician* 31:181–85.

Cohen, B. M., P. Q. Harris, R. I. Altesman, and J. O. Cole (1982). Amoxapine: Neuroleptic as well as antidepressant? *Am. J. Psychiatry* 139:1165–67.

Costa, D., I. Mogos, and T. Toma (1985). Efficacy and safety of mianserin in the treatment of depression of women with cancer. *Acta. Psychiatr. Scand.* 72 (Suppl. 320): 85–92.

De'Montigny, C., F. Grunberg, A. Mayer, and J. P. Deschenes (1981). Lithium induces rapid relief of depression in tricyclic antidepressant drug non-responders. *Br. J. Psychiatry* 138:252–56.

DePaulo, J. R., E. I. Correa, and D. G. Sapir (1986). Renal function and lithium: A longitudinal study. *Am. J. Psychiatry* 143:892–95.

Derogatis, L. R., M. Feldstein, G. Morrow, H. Schmale, M. Schmitt, C. Gates, B. Murawski, J. Holland, D. Penman, N. Melisaratos, A. J. Enelow, and L. M. Adler (1979). A survey of psychotropic drug prescriptions in an oncology population. *Cancer* 44:1919–29.

Dubin, W. R., K. J. Weiss, and J. M. Dorn (1986). Pharmacotherapy of psychiatric emergencies. *J. Clin. Psychopharmacol.* 6:210–22.

Falk, W. E., M. W. Mahnke, and D. C. Poskanzer (1979). Lithium prophylaxis of corticotropin-induced psychosis. *J.A.M.A.* 241:1011–12.

Feighner, J. P., G. C. Aden, L. F. Fabre, K. Rickels, and W. T. Smith (1983). Comparison of alprazolam, imipramine and placebo in the treatment of depression. *J.A.M.A.* 249:3057–64.

Feighner, J. P., J. Herbstein, and N. Damlouji (1985). Combined MAOI, TCA, and direct stimulant therapy of treatment-resistant depression. *J. Clin. Psychiatry* 46:206–9.

Feighner, J. P., C. H. Merideth, and G. A. Hendrickson (1982). A double-blind comparison of buspirone and diazepam in outpatients with generalized anxiety. *J. Clin. Psychiatry* 43:103–7.

Fleishman, S. F., M. Satler, H. Szarka, and M. Walczak (1988). Incidence of subjective motor restlessness from prochloperazine and metoclopramide: observations of cancer patients receiving chemotherapy. *Proc. ASCO* 7:282 (abstract # 1093).

Foley, K. (1985). The treatment of cancer pain. *N. Engl. J. Med.* 313:84–95.

Geller, B., T. B. Cooper, E. C. Chestnut, J. A. Anker, and M. D. Schluchter (1986). Preliminary data on the relationship between nortriptyline plasma level and response in depressed children. *Am. J. Psychiatry* 143:1283–86.

Glassman, A. H. (1984). The newer antidepressant drugs and their cardiovascular effects. *Psychopharmacol. Bull.* 20:272–79.

Glassman, A. H., L. L. Johnson, E. V. Giardina, B. T. Walsh, S. P. Roose, T. B. Cooper, and J. T. Bigger (1983). The use of imipramine in depressed patients with congestive heart failure. *J.A.M.A.* 250:1997–2001.

Glazer, W. M., D. C. Moore, N. R. Schooler, L. M. Brenner, and H. Morgenstern (1984). Tardive dyskinesia: A discontinuation study. *Arch. Gen. Psychiatry* 41:623–27.

Goggans, F. C., L. J. Weisberg, and L. M. Koran (1983). Lithium prophylaxis of prednisone psychosis: A case report. *J. Clin. Psychiatry* 44:111–12.

Goldberg, R. J. and V. Mor (1985). A survey of psychotropic drug use in terminal cancer patients. *Psychosomatics* 26:745–51.

Greenblatt, D. J., R. I. Shader, and D. R. Abernethy (1983a). Drug therapy: Current status of benzodiazepines (Part 1). *N. Engl. J. Med.* 309:354–58.

Greenblatt, D. J., R. I. Shader, and D. R. Abernethy (1983b). Drug therapy: Current status of benzodiazepines (Part 2). *N. Engl. J. Med.* 309:410–16.

Guze, B. H. and L. R. Baxter, Jr. (1985). Neuroleptic malignant syndrome. *N. Engl. J. Med.* 313:163–66.

Hackett, T. P. (1978). *The Use of Stimulant Drugs in Medicine.* Paper presented at the annual meeting of the American Psychiatric Association, Atlanta, Ga., May.

Harrison, W. M., J. G. Rabkin, A. A. Ehrhardt, J. W. Stewart, P. J. McGrath, D. Ross, and F. M. Quitkin (1986). Effects of antidepressant medication on sexual function: A controlled study. *J. Clin. Psychopharmacol.* 6:144–49.

Hartmann, E. (1977). L-Tryptophan: A rational hypnotic with clinical potential. *Am. J. Psychiatry* 134:366–70.

Healey, M., R. Pickens, R. Meisch, and T. McKenna (1983). Effects of clorazepate, diazepam, lorazepam, and placebo on human memory. *J. Clin. Psychiatry* 44:436–39.

Holland, J. C., S. Cohen, G. Morrow, A. Schmale, L. R. Derogatis, J. Fetting, R. Cherry, and P. Carpenter (1986). The pattern of psychotropic drugs prescribed for patients in 3 cancer centers: A survey. *Proc. Am. Soc. Clin. Oncol.* 27:239.

Holland, J. C., G. Morrow, A. Schmale, L. Derogatis, M. Spefanek, S. Berenson, P. Carpenter, W. Breitbart, and M. Feldstein (1987). Reduction of anxiety and depression in cancer patients by alprazolam or by a behavioral technique. *Proc. Am. Soc. Clin. Oncol.* 6:258 (Abstract No. 1015).

Hollister, L. E. (1983). *Clinical Pharmacology of Psychotherapeutic Drugs,* 2nd ed. New York: Churchill-Livingstone.

Itil, T. M., and C. Soldatos (1980). Epileptogenic side effects of psychotropic drugs. *J.A.M.A.* 244:1460–63.

Jaeger, H., G. R. Morrow, P. J. Carpenter, and F. Brescia (1985). A survey of psychotropic drug utilization by patients with advanced neoplastic disease. *Gen. Hosp. Psychiatry* 7:353–60.

Janowksy, D., G. Curtis, S. Zisook, K. Kuhn, K. Resovsky, and M. Le Winter (1983). Ventricular arrhythmias possibly aggravated by Trazodone. *Am. J. Psychiatry* 140:796–97.

Jenike, M. A. (1983). Treating anxiety in elderly patients. *Geriatrics* 38(10):115–19.

Jeste, D. V. and R. J. Wyatt (1981). Dogma disputed: Is tardive dyskinesia due to postsynaptic dopamine receptor supersensitivity? *J. Clin. Psychiatry* 42:455–57.

Jeste, D. V., M. Linnoila, C. M. Fordis, B. H. Phelps, R. L. Wagner, and R. J. Wyatt (1982). Enzyme studies in tardive dyskinesia. III. Noradrenergic hyperactivity in a subgroup of dyskinetic patients. *J. Clin. Psychopharmacol.* 2:318–20.

Kahn, R. J., D. M. McNair, R. S. Lipman, L. Covi, K. Rickels, R. Downing, S. Fisher, and L. M. Frankenthaler (1986). Imipramine and chlordiazepoxide in depressive and anxiety disorders. *Arch. Gen. Psychiatry* 43:79–85.

Kane, J. M. and J. Smith (1982). Tardive dyskinesia: Prevalence and risk factors, 1959 to 1979. *Arch. Gen. Psychiatry* 39:473–81.

Kaufmann, M. W. and G. B. Murray, (1982). The use of d-amphetamine in medically ill depressed patients. *J. Clin. Psychiatry* 43:463–64.

Klotz, U. and I. Reimann (1980). Delayed clearance of diazepam due to cimetidine. *N. Engl. J. Med.* 302:1012–14.

Kurlan, R., R. Hamill, and I. Shoulson (1984). Neuroleptic malignant syndrome. *Clin. Neuropharmacol.* 7:109–20.

Laszlo, J., R. A. Clark, D. C. Hanson, L. Tyson, L. Crumpler, and R. Gralla (1985). Lorazepam in cancer patients treated with cisplatin: A drug having antiemetic, amnesic and anxiolytic effects. *J. Clin. Oncol.* 3:864–69.

Lesser, I. M., R. T. Rubin, J. C. Pecknold, A. Rifkin, P. Swinson, R. B. Lydiard, G. D. Burrows, R. Noyes, and R. L. DuPont (1988). Secondary depression in panic disorder and agoraphobia. *Arch. Gen. Psychiatry* 45:437–43.

Levenson, J. L. (1985). Neuroleptic malignant syndrome. *Am. J. Psychiatry* 142:1137–45.

Levinson, D. F. and G. M. Simpson (1986). Neuroleptic-induced extrapyramidal symptoms with fever. *Arch. Gen. Psychiatry* 43:839–48.

Lipsey, J. R., R. G. Robinson, G. D. Pearlson, K. Rao, and T. R. Price (1984). Nortriptyline treatment of post-stroke depression: A double-blind study. *Lancet* 1:297–300.

Lyman, G. H., C. C. Williams, and D. Preston (1980). The use of lithium carbonate to reduce infection and leukopenia during systemic chemotherapy. *N. Engl. J. Med.* 302:257–60.

Markowitz, J. C. and R. P. Brown (1987). Seizures with neuroleptics and antidepressants. *Gen. Hosp. Psychiatry* 9:135–41.

Massie, M. J., J. C. Holland, and E. Glass (1983). Delirium in terminally ill cancer patients. *Am. J. Psychiatry* 140:1048–50.

Mucha, H., E. Lange, and G. Bonitz (1970). Amitriptylin in der psychiatrischen Therapie [Amitriptyline in psychiatric therapy]. *Psychiatr. Neurol. Med. Psychol.* 22:116–20.

Noyes, R., R. L. DuPont, J. C. Pecknold, A. Rifkin, R. T. Rubin, R. P. Swinson, J. C. Ballenger, and G. D. Burrows (1988). Alprazolam in panic disorder and agoraphobia: results from a multicenter trial. *Arch. Gen. Psychiatry* 45:423–28.

Pearlman, C. A. (1986). Neuroleptic malignant syndrome: A review of the literature. *J. Clin. Psychopharmacol.* 6:257–73.

Pfefferbaum-Levine, B., K. Kumor, A. Cangir, M. Choroszy, and E. A. Roseberry (1983). Tricyclic antidepressants for children with cancer. *Am. J. Psychiatry* 140:1074–76.

Pope, H. G., P. E. Keck, and S. L. McElroy (1986). Frequency and presentation of neuroleptic malignant syndrome in a large psychiatric hospital. *Am. J. Psychiatry* 143:1227–33.

Popkin, M. K., A. L. Callies, and T. B. MacKenzie (1985). The outcome of antidepressant use in the medically ill. *Arch. Gen. Psychiatry* 42:1160–63.

Portenoy, R. K., D. E. Moulin, A. Rogers, C. E. Inturrisi, and K. M. Foley (1986). Intravenous infusion of opioids in cancer pain: Clinical review and guidelines for use. *Cancer Treat. Rep.* 70:575–81.

Posner, J. B. (1978). Neurologic complications of systemic cancer. *Disease-a-Month* 2:7–60.

Prien, R. F. and D. J. Kupfer (1986). Continuation drug therapy for major depressive episodes: How long should it be maintained? *Am. J. Psychiatry* 143:1823.

Purohit, D. R., P. L. Navlakha, R. S. Modi, and R. Eshpumiyani (1978). The role of antidepressants in hospitalized cancer patients. *J. Assoc. Physicians India* 26: 245–48.

Rabkin, J., F. Quitkin, W. Harrison, E. Tricamo, and P. McGrath (1984). Adverse reactions to monoamine oxidase inhibitors: Part I. A comparative study. *J. Clin. Psychopharmacol.* 4:270–78.

Rancurello, M. D. (1985). Clinical applications of antidepressant drugs in childhood behavioral and emotional disorders. *Psychiatr. Ann.* 2:88–100.

Raskind, M., R. Veith, R. Barnes, and G. Gumbrecht (1982). Cardiovascular and antidepressant effects of imipramine in the treatment of secondary depression in patients with ischemic heart disease. *Am. J. Psychiatry* 139:1114–17.

Ray, W. A., M. R. Griffin, W. Schaffner, D. K. Baugh, and L. J. Melton (1987). Psychotropic drug use and the risk of hip fracture *J.A.M.A.* 316:363–69.

Remick, R. A. (1988). Anticholinergic side effects of tricyclic antidepressants and their management. *Prog. Neuropsychopharmacol. Biol. Psychiatr.* 12:225–31.

Remick, R. A. and S. H. Fine (1979). Antipsychotic drugs and seizures. *J. Clin. Psychiatry* 40:78–80.

Richardson, J. W. and E. Richelson (1984). Antidepressants: A clinical update for medical practitioners. *Mayo Clin. Proc.* 59:330–37.

Rickels, K., H. R. Chung, I. B. Casnalosi, A. M. Hurowitz,

J. London, K. Wiseman, M. Kaplan, and J. D. Amsterdam (1987). Alprazolam, diazepam, imipramine, and placebo in outpatients with major depression. *Arch. Gen. Psychiatry* 44:862–66.

Rickels, K., J. P. Feighner, and W. T. Smith (1985). Alprazolam, amitriptyline, doxepin, and placebo in the treatment of depression. *Arch. Gen. Psychiatry* 42:134–41.

Rifkin, A., G. Reardon, S. Siris, B. Karagji, Y. Kim, L. Hackstaff, and N. Endicott (1985). Trimipramine in physical illness with depression. *J. Clin. Psychiatry* 46:4–8.

Roose, S. P., A. H. Glassman, E. G. V. Giardina, B. T. Walsh, S. Woodring, and J. T. Bigger (1987). Tricyclic antidepressants in depressed patients with cardiac conduction disease. *Arch. Gen. Psychiatry* 44:273–75.

Scala, S. M. and J. A. Visconti (1985). Lithium in the treatment of leukopenia. *Hosp. Form.* 20:613–28.

Scavone, J. M., D. J. Greenblatt, H. Friedman, and R. I. Shader (1986). Enhanced bioavailability of triazolam following sublingual vs. oral administration. *J. Clin. Pharmacol.* 26:208–10.

Scher, M., J. N. Krieger, and S. Jeurgens (1983). Trazodone and priapism. *Am. J. Psychiatry* 140:1362–63.

Sokol, G. H., D. J. Greenblatt, B. L. Lloyd, A. Georgotas, M. D. Allen, J. S. Harmatz, T. W. Smith, and R. I. Shader (1978). Effect of abdominal radiation therapy on drug absorption in humans. *J. Clin. Pharmacol.* 18:388–96.

Stein, R. S., J. M. Flexner, and S. E. Graber (1979). Lithium and granulocytopenia during induction therapy of acute myelogenous leukemia. *Blood* 54:636–41.

Turner, A. R., R. N. MacDonald, and T. A. McPherson (1979). Reduction of chemotherapy-induced neuropenic complications with a short course of lithium carbonate. *Clin. Invest. Med.* 2:51–53.

Walsh, T. D. (1986). Controlled study of imipramine (Im) and morphine (M) in chronic pain due to advanced cancer. *Proc. Am. Study Clin. Oncol.* 5:237.

Weilburg, J. B., and S. R. Donaldson (1988). L-Tryptophan for sleep. Massachusetts General Hosp. Newsletter Biological Therapies in Psychiatry 11:13,16.

White, K. and G. Simpson (1981). Combined MAOI–tricyclic antidepressant treatment: A reevaluation. *J. Clin. Psychopharmacol.* 1:264–82.

Woods, S. W., G. E. Tesar, G. B. Murray, and N. H. Cassem (1986). Psychostimulant treatment of depressive disorders secondary to medical illness. *J. Clin. Psychiatry* 47:12–15.

# 40

# Behavioral Techniques: Progressive Relaxation and Self-Regulatory Therapies

## Rene Mastrovito

The last two decades have seen a dramatic rise in the use of behavioral therapies for control of symptoms in medical settings. Particularly in cancer, they are now extensively applied to control psychological distress and pain. Contributing to this change are an increased interest in Eastern religions and philosophies with their emphasis on self-control through meditation, an increasing emphasis on the individual's role in maintaining personal health and in actively participating in treatment and care during illness, a generally greater "antiestablishment" and "antimedical" climate, the search for "naturalistic" and "holistic" approaches to treatment of disease, new evidence demonstrating that meditation and biofeedback can alter physiological function, and the emergence of the discipline of behavioral medicine with its focus on the clinical application within medical settings of cognitive-behavioral approaches developed by behavioral psychologists.

Behavioral methods of coping with cancer offer patients not only the possibility of stress management but also a sense of enhanced self-control. Lerner (1985), who has studied the use of some of these methods and alternative therapies in cancer, prefers to call them "integrative therapies," suggesting a desirable union of traditional and alternative therapies. These methods, however, are used at present largely as distinct ancillary techniques in traditional medical settings.

The behavioral techniques, encompassing hypnosis, meditation, autogenic training, progressive relaxation, and biofeedback, are also called by some cognitive-behavioral, holistic, and alternative modes of therapy. All are forms of self-regulating therapies (Stoyva, 1976), a more comprehensive and appropriate term. Such therapeutic interventions generally are characterized by two basic stages in which the patient is first guided through a primarily cognitive activity

that creates the second stage, an altered state of awareness (Ludwig, 1966; Hilgard, 1969).

This chapter reviews the development of these therapies as adjunctive methods in the general medical setting, and in cancer in particular, where they are for the most part primarily used for the purposes of reducing anxiety and pain, controlling anticipatory and post-treatment nausea and vomiting associated with chemotherapy, and assisting in the management of eating and sleep disorders. By far the most widely used technique in cancer is relaxation therapy, which promotes an altered state of awareness through reducing distressing emotions and producing a physiologically quiescent state in which there is selective awareness of specific sensory stimuli to the exclusion of others (Hilgard, 1969; Walsh, 1980). The historical antecedents of the different techniques are discussed to place these therapies into perspective. Their origins, which have been associated historically with religious, "magical," and sometimes charlatan practice, are important to explore because they affect current attitudes about the use of such interventions and patients' willingness to employ them. Their use is traced historically by the major techniques of hypnosis, autogenic training, meditation and relaxation, and biofeedback (see Table 40-1).

## HISTORICAL BACKGROUND OF BEHAVIORAL INTERVENTIONS IN MEDICINE

### Hypnosis

Of the several major techniques used to produce an "altered state," hypnosis has the longest history and provides a generic model as well as a perspective from which to view other methods in use today. The hypnotic state constitutes a classical model of altered

**Table 40-1** Historical influences on the development of behavioral interventions

| Date | Person/event | Impact on techniques |
|------|--------------|----------------------|
| *Hypnosis* | | |
| 1734–1815 | Mesmer | Father of modern hypnosis; "animal magnetism," "mesmerism" |
| 1840s | Braid | Introduced term "hypnosis"; determined induction of trance enhanced by focusing on one subject or idea, "monoideism" |
| 1846 | Esdaile | Recorded use of mesmerism in cases of major as well as minor surgery in India |
| 1860s | Quimby | Cured a bedridden invalid, Mary Baker Eddy (later founder of Christian Science), with mesmerism |
| 1880–1890s | Charcot | Used hypnosis to treat hysterical patients in France; but associated it with illness |
| 1880–1890s | Freud | Used hypnosis to discover the unconscious but then abandoned it in favor of free association |
| 1889 | First International Congress for Experimental and Therapeutic Hypnosis | Reflected a peak of interest in hypnosis and served to validate practice of hypnosis as acceptable |
| 1940 | Hilgard, Erickson, Spiegel | Modern applications to medicine. |
| *Autogenic Training* | | |
| 1920 | Schultz and Luthe | Development of autogenic training focusing on awareness of natural feelings associated with state relaxation |
| 1950 | Sargent, Walters & Green | Self-suggestion to induce relaxation and alter physiologic function (e.g. temperature, migraine) |
| | | Practice of meditation and yoga in a religious context, particularly eastern cultures, brought west. |
| *Progressive relaxation and meditation* | | |
| 1938 | Jacobson | Publishes book of progressive relaxation technique |
| 1958 | Wolpe | Modifies and repopularizes Jacobson's technique |
| 1974 | Benson | Application of Transendental Meditation (TM) and a simple relaxation response to situations and diseases associated with increased sympathetic activity (e.g., anxiety, hypertension, headache) |
| *Biofeedback* | | |
| 1969 | Miller | Publishes "Learning of Visceral and Glandular Responses in Animal Studies: Human Application in Clinical States and Pain" |
| 1970s | Schwartz | Widely applied in clinical medicine to migraine, Reynaud's disease and hypertension |
| 1975 | Weiss and Engel | Operant Conditioning in premature ventricular contractions |

awareness. During the hypnotic state, perceptions, beliefs, emotions, and behavior are drastically altered so that the subject responds to the reality suggested by the hypnotist and reality becomes temporarily suspended from the usual perception of the "real" world.

Both hypnosis and hypnoidal states were well known among ancient civilizations, where they were linked to religious rites and magic. The priest–physicians of ancient Egypt produced trance states by these means in the temples of Isis, goddess of the Nile.

Hypnosis was used in the sleep temples of ancient Greece, and in the British Isles by the Celts who produced a "Druidic" or "magic" sleep that cured patients of complaints, worries and grief. Trancelike states were also recorded in China in the eighteenth century B.C. (Zilboorg and Henry, 1941). There appears to be no one special observable behavior indicative of the hypnotic trance state. Hypnotic behaviors reported by Ambrose and Newbold (1968) in a historical review varied from the tranquil "Druidic sleep" to frenzied states of hyperactivity. Induction methods similar to those of ancient times, in which rhythmic repetitive sounds and movements accompanied by music and dance were used to induce trancelike states in groups of people, are still in use today.

The modern era of these therapies was introduced by Mesmer who, during the latter half of the eighteenth century, engaged in the practice of passing magnets over the body of patients to restore normal magnetic fields. The technology involved in producing artificial magnets (as opposed to the naturally magnetic lodestone) had been recently discovered, and magnets were not only great playthings but also the subject of scientific investigation. Mesmer's approach was based on a complex theory that held that health depended on maintaining a correct relationship with the planets and that magnets could restore imbalances in this relationship. He produced trances, and often cured symptoms by means of what was referred to as "animal magnetism." He soon found that he could produce the same trances by performing "magnetic passes" over the body of his patients with his hands alone, which he assumed had become magnetized. Forced by the traditional medical establishment to leave Vienna, he started group treatments in Paris in 1778 using large tubs or "baguets" filled with water and iron filings and out of which projected iron rods. Grasping the rods permitted the "magnetism" to flow into the patients being treated; a hysterical frenzy resulted that passed from one to the other. When attempts by distinguished scientists to duplicate his methods failed, it was determined that "animal" magnetism was worthless unless both the doctor and patient strongly believed in it.

Although "animal magnetism" was largely discredited, many had learned from Mesmer and continued their own investigations of hypnotism. Of particular note, was the work of the Marquis de Puysequr, who demonstrated the phenomenon of hypnotic somnambulism and proved that a state analogous to sleep could be induced by suggestion in an awake individual. As a technique, however, mesmerism languished until James Braid, a Manchester surgeon, revived interest in it in the nineteenth century. In experiments aimed at getting away from the still-used "magnetic passes," he found that induction of a hypnotic state could also be achieved by having the individual stare at a flickering candlelight. When the eyes tired, the lids closed, and the patient fell into a sleep or a "hypnotized" state (Fromm and Schor, 1972). Eye fixation subsequently became the classical induction technique. As he progressed in his research, Braid leaned more toward a psychological explanation of the phenomenon, noting that the attainment of a trancelike state depended more on the beliefs of the subject rather than those of the physician. He observed further that

induction of the trance state was enhanced by encouraging the patient to concentrate on one subject or idea. Braid is also credited with introducing the term "hypnotism."

At about the same time, James Esdaile, a Scottish doctor reported in 1846 that while working in India he had used mesmerism as anesthesia for 345 cases of major surgery and for thousands of minor procedures. In the United States, Phineas Quimbey cured a bedridden invalid, Mary Baker Eddy, by mesmerism. She later founded the Christian Science Church, which has been an advocate of self-healing concepts, coupled with strong religious faith.

In France, Charcot began to use hypnosis for hysteria in the late nineteenth century. Freud also became interested in its use and, while using the trance state in treatment, made the startling discovery of an unconscious level of awareness that could influence behavior. It is upon this history that the present use of suggestion and hypnosis is based. In the modern era, medical applications have been explored by Hilgard (1969) and Sacerdote (1966).

## Autogenic Training

A derivative of hypnosis, autogenic training, was developed by Schultz in 1920 (Schultz and Luthe, 1969). In this technique for stress reduction, attention is directed toward internal functions, resulting in changes in states of awareness and consciousness. Schultz noted that while individuals were being induced using eye fixation, other subjective phenomena occurred spontaneously, such as a warming of the hands and feelings of heaviness in the limbs, presumably mediated through parasympathetic pathways. He used these as self-suggestions to enhance relaxation, asking patients to focus on these effects, and followed them by meditation exercises and "passive concentration." He found that patients preferred the use of sensory awareness for induction over the classical eye fixation. The method was developed further by the middle of the twentieth century by others who applied the technique particularly to treat disorders of temperature control (e.g., Reynaud's disease) and migraine (Sargent et al., 1972).

## Meditation

Meditation, with its roots in Buddhism and Hinduism, has received much attention in the Western world in the past 25 years, enhancing interest in altered states of awareness and a deepened appreciation of "inner" consciousness (Walsh, 1980). Some aspects of meditation undoubtedly predate the rudimentary and fragmentary historical evidence for hypnotic states. The potential applications to medicine have more recently been widely explored. Benson (1975) in particular has contributed to the use of meditation in medicine. He has used transcendental meditation (TM) in medical settings, developing a noncultic, simple form of what he termed "the relaxation response" to produce a quiescent state. Meditation is often used with other self-regulatory therapies, making it difficult at times to determine which method has been most effective (Shapiro, 1982).

The goal of a meditative state is to reach a state of detached self-observation. This is accomplished by two widely recognized methods of meditation, namely, concentration meditation, of which TM is the most popular, and mindfulness meditation, which encourages the mind's attention to focus on spontaneously occurring mental images. The practice of TM involves focusing attention on a repetitive body function, such as breathing, while simultaneously repeating a sound or word (mantra) in rhythm with the breathing (Benson et al., 1974). The meditative state is best attained in a relaxed posture with the eyes closed in a quiet environment without distraction (Benson, 1977). The subject is taught to push away distracting thoughts (Kutz et al., 1985; Kabat-Zinn, 1982). On the other hand, mindfulness meditation, while similar to concentration meditation in its initiation by attention to breathing and repeating a mantra, encourages the subject to allow his or her mind to wander, with the goal of achieving a detached sense of self-observation. Thus, concentration meditation focuses on a specific object (the mantra); mindful concentration places less importance on the content and more on the process of allowing thoughts to come and go (Goldman and Schwartz, 1976; Kraines, 1963).

The meditative state produces physiologically, a hypometabolic state, with decreased oxygen consumption, decreased blood lactate, increased skin resistance, and increased $\alpha$-wave production. The degree of $\alpha$-wave production observed in masters of meditation is quite striking. Kasamatsu and Hirai (1969) showed that $\alpha$-wave production in Zen Buddhist masters was greater than in novices and monks who did not practice meditation. While considerable emphasis has been given in the popular press to $\alpha$-wave production, it is increased only in meditation. No change in $\alpha$ waves occurs in hypnotic trance states, autogenic training, and progressive relaxation. What is important is that while each of these self-regulatory therapies is different in method, they each achieve similar results.

Although Shapiro (1982) warned that we should not equate meditation with autogenic training or hypnosis, the therapeutic effectiveness in control of anxiety and pain is frequently indistinguishable.

## Progressive Relaxation

Progressive relaxation, progressive muscle relaxation, and Jacobson's modified progressive relaxation are all terms for the simplest and most popular of the self-regulatory therapies today. Jacobson originated the technique and popularized it in 1938 as a treatment for insomnia, tension, nervousness, and psychophysiological disorders (Jacobson, 1938). He based his therapeutic approach on the thesis that relaxation and anxiety are mutually exclusive states. Modified by Wolpe (1958), progressive relaxation was also used with systematic desensitization for treatment of phobias.

Progressive relaxation is a method in which the patient is instructed to close his or her eyes and concentrate on relaxing sequentially one body part at a time, beginning with one area such as the feet and focusing progressively on legs, knees, thighs, hips, arms, shoulders, neck, jaws, and tongue, consciously allowing each part to become as relaxed as possible. The specific body areas covered are not critical; practitioners generally vary the areas suggested depending on the desired result and their personal style. The "passive" procedure is used by some in contrast to others who use an "active" method in which the subject is asked to tense each body part before relaxing it, thus increasing awareness of the sense of relaxed versus tense muscles. The intended goal of both passive and active approaches is the same, that is, the attainment of a state of muscle relaxation as profound as is possible (Ferguson et al., 1977). The degree of success generally depends on the extent of motivation, discipline, and perseverance necessary to carry out frequent, regular practice.

Whereas it is not clear how muscle relaxation training serves to reduce anxiety, it does in most instances seem to do so (Davidson and Schwartz, 1976). Some studies have shown that diminished anxiety is not a given consequence of relaxation under all circumstances, and that relaxation training alone is not always an effective procedure for anxiety reduction (Cooke, 1968; Davison, 1968; Heide and Borkovea, 1983). However, the weight of clinical evidence supports the value of this technique for control of psychological distress (Goldfried and Trier, 1974; Goldfried, 1973; Jacobson, 1938), and for physiological relaxation of muscles and decreased skin resistance (Paul, 1969).

## Biofeedback

Since its introduction by Miller in 1969, biofeedback, with its clinical application to treatment of migraine, hypertension, Reynaud's disease, and other psychosomatic disorders, has proved an important tool in the repertoire of behavioral therapists (Miller, 1980). In this technique, the patient is instructed to exert conscious control over selected physiological functions (e.g., heart rate and muscle tension) by use of feedback from continuous displays of an index of the selected activity (e.g., ECG or EMG monitor) and is given instruction in behaviors to alter physiological activity. The application of biofeedback can serve three important purposes. First, it can provide an observable measure of a physical correlate to a problem (e.g., previously unrecognized areas of tension). Second, it can assist in sensitizing the individual to that phenomenon. Third, and that which is perhaps most important, it can help the individual learn that control of this event is within his or her power, diminishing a sense of helplessness that often accompanies illness.

Although the impact of biofeedback on significant long-term control of blood pressure, temperature, and pain has been questioned, the technique has been of value in short-term control of a range of symptoms, including motion sickness. Its application in cancer patients has been more limited. Pain control can be enhanced by demonstration to the patient that he or she can alter responses. In such cases, demonstrating this effect with individual biofeedback data is useful. Exploration of the technique to prevent conditioned nausea and vomiting is also of interest. Research among astronaut candidates has shown that when subjects are given early signs of temperature or vascular changes associated with initial signs of nausea, they can be taught behavioral exercises to prevent or delay symptom progression to the full retching reflex. Underutilized in cancer, further exploration of biofeedback's clinical usefulness in these settings is desirable.

### Guided Imagery

Though not an independent behavioral therapy in its own right, guided imagery is a technique commonly used in conjunction with the aforementioned techniques and deserves brief mention. Guided imagery describes a process whereby the practitioner instructs patients to imagine a fantasized scene or body process. Patients may be asked, for instance, to imagine walking on a beach, or lying in the sun, or to imagine their body growing stronger. There are many images that can be suggested. The use of guided imagery is typically embedded within one of the behavioral therapies, usually to enhance the altered state being sought.

### COMBINED BEHAVIORAL THERAPIES

In the clinical setting, the most common practice today is the combined use of several of the cognitive-behavioral strategies described. This is particularly true of progressive relaxation, which is sometimes used as an induction for hypnosis and meditation, followed by visual imagery of a pleasant memory (French and Tupin, 1974), or of guided imagery suggested by the therapist, usually involving a tranquil, pleasant setting (Donovan, 1980). In the former, the patient starts with instructions in relaxation, progressively engaging a focus on each body part. Following this exercise, the person is asked to think of a pleasant memory, dwell on it, and become immersed in it, returning to it if thoughts drift. This serves a function somewhat similar to the mantra in meditation in excluding other extraneous stimuli. The patient is allowed to remain in this state for about a minute. It is characterized by a relaxed state with flickering eyelids and lateral eye scanning movements. The person is then asked to open his or her eyes and repeat the procedure. This simple technique can be used at will for insomnia, pain, or anxiety.

Progressive relaxation is also often combined with guided imagery suggested or imposed by the clinician. The patient is told to think of a pleasant, restful scene, such as being on a beach by the ocean, in a forest, or by a brook. With children, imagery is chosen that will engage them in places or fantasies they like. The choice of a setting can be determined through discussion with the patient about his or her likes and dislikes or recall of ''happy'' places.

### USE OF BEHAVIORAL THERAPIES IN CANCER

The interest in the application of behavioral interventions in cancer is not just a reflection of a change in social mores. The movement also reflects the usefulness, and frequently dramatic success, of these techniques in managing special problems in patient care that are often resistant to conventional treatment alone. Specifically, these are control of pain, chemotherapy-induced anticipatory nausea and vomiting, anxiety, eating and sleep disorders, and enhancement of a sense of self-control and well-being.

In keeping with its primarily medical origins and application, hypnosis has a long history of use among cancer patients (Kroger, 1976, 1979; Sacerdote, 1966). The easy suggestibility and readiness to engage in imaginative ventures of children has made hypnosis a particularly viable adjunct to care in pediatric oncology, especially for control of pain and anxiety, associated with painful procedures (Hilgard and Hilgard, 1983; Lebaw et al., 1975; Olness and Gardner, 1978; Hilgard and Lebaron, 1984). In a review by Jay and colleagues (1986), they note the lack of attention paid to pediatric pain and especially cancer pain. Beyond the sensory stimulus, the meaning of the pain to a child is highly variable and can enhance (or diminish) the pain level. Most research on behavioral interventions has focused on management of the acute pain of medical procedures; of these studies, most have utilized hypnosis (Jay et al., 1985). Kellerman and colleagues (1983), in their work with adolescents, found that the use of relaxation and hypnosis during painful procedures reduced anxiety and discomfort. Hilgard and LeBaron (1984) used hypnosis effectively in children undergoing bone marrow aspiration, whereas Zeltzer and LeBaron (1982) showed that hypnosis using imagery and fantasy was more effective than distraction in 6- to 17-year-olds during these procedures. The 1986 review of Jay and colleagues draws attention to the dearth of studies on pain control in children under age 6 (see also Chapter 46 by Redd on behavioral interventions in pediatric oncology).

In adults hypnosis is useful as an adjunct in the management of cancer pain. Orne and Dinges (1984) discuss the advantage of psychological control over the debilitating pain related to terminal illness afforded by use of hypnosis. The technique permits the patient to gain some control over the pain (even though the disease does not abate), thus dealing with the psychological significance of the pain and disease to the person. Spiegel (1985) provided an excellent review of the use of hypnosis in cancer, both alone and combined with group therapy. In a study by Spiegel and Bloom (1983) among terminally ill patients, they found that those who participated in a group that received group sessions and a regular self-hypnosis exercise had no increase in pain over a 1-year period, despite a 30% mortality rate in the sample. They felt that group support and hypnosis influenced those aspects of the pain experience attributed to the psychological reaction of the sensation of pain and the associated suffering it caused.

It should be noted, however, that benign pain and pain with a strong psychological component respond less well to this treatment modality. Hypnosis or other behavioral approaches should be tried early in the course of managing cancer pain, especially in patients who are reluctant or fearful to take medication and who have a strong need to remain in control. Paradoxically, because it may also be perceived as frightening to those who see in the technique a mechanism for possible "loss of control," it can have limitations as an approach in these same individuals. In other instances, the patient may simply be a poor candidate for hypnosis. It is estimated that approximately 10% of the population is refractory or nonsusceptible to hypnosis (Hilgard and Hilgard, 1983). This is a relatively enduring trait and, if hypnosis has not been previously successful, further attempts are likely unwarranted. Finally, hypnosis should only be used by well-trained clinicians, especially in seriously ill patients. Availability of trained staff to carry out hypnosis and to follow

patients is essential and may be a limitation in its broader applicability in cancer settings. Although autogenic training alleviates some of these problems, hypnosis per se requires more patient–therapist interaction than the other modalities.

Less information has been published on the use of meditation with cancer patients (Balon, 1974). Patients who have used meditation prior to becoming ill find these skills helpful in coping with their illness-related distress. Lack of prior exposure to meditation, however, should not be a reason for exclusion. Again, the sense of calm produced and control over emotions may be extremely reassuring and can contribute to well-being.

Progressive relaxation, combined with other behavioral techniques, is being used increasingly for control of pain, anxiety, and nausea and vomiting (Cob, 1984; Cotanch, 1983; Grzesiak, 1977; Keefe et al., 1981; Arnoff et al., 1981). A series of studies has shown that the use of progressive relaxation, usually in combination with other techniques, immediately before and/or during chemotherapy with patients who had developed a negative conditioned response to chemotherapy lessened the nausea and emotional distress of patients in comparison to those who received no such training or interventions (Burish and Lyles, 1981; Lyles et al., 1982; Cotanch, 1983). Redd (1982), using passive relaxation, demonstrated the same finding in reducing anticipatory nausea and vomiting. Morrow and Morrell (1982), addressing the same problem, used progressive relaxation as part of a desensitization technique with significantly positive results. Scott and colleagues (1983), using slow-stroke back massage and progressive relaxation with guided imagery, reduced the frequency, intensity, and volume of vomiting during and following chemotherapy infusions in women being treated for gynecological cancer. (For greater elaboration on the use of these behavioral techniques in the control of nausea and vomiting, see Redd's Chapter 35 on nausea and vomiting and Chapter 46 on behavioral interventions in pediatrics.)

Relaxation has been utilized in combination with guided imagery in cancer patients by Simonton and others (1980) in which the imagery used encourages the patient to visualize ways by which the natural body defenses are fighting the neoplastic cells in the body. These techniques are aimed not only at promoting a sense of self-control but also at controlling tumor progression. The latter goal remains controversial in the field with respect to the validity of the claims made by its practitioners and the weighing of the salutary versus potentially adverse consequences of the methods to patients. (Some of the controversies arising out of this approach are reviewed in Chapter 42 in which alternative therapies are discussed.)

Because of its practicality and safety, the use of relaxation in cancer patients is receiving increasing attention. Progressive relaxation, with or without the use of imagery, is a useful, versatile tool because it can be applied readily by any oncology staff member who has been trained in its use. This training must however include awareness of the limitations of the method. Patients experiencing severe distress or behavior that suggests significant psychiatric disturbance, or those who have a history of psychiatric illness, should be carefully evaluated before beginning relaxation. Although there is little inherent risk in the procedure per se, there may be significant risks in missing the diagnosis of serious psychiatric problems that require assessment and treatment. The severely depressed patient, or the one who has mild confusion related to pain medication or delirium from CNS effects of disease or treatment, should not be managed by relaxation. It is important that a psychiatric consultant be available for such cases in which initiation of relaxation is questionable, or in which an unexpected negative response suggests an underlying serious disturbance not amenable to relaxation techniques.

In oncology units and clinics, progressive relaxation is particularly helpful in situations that provoke fear and apprehension, such as painful diagnostic and treatment procedures (e.g., bone marrow aspiration, lumbar puncture, and chemotherapy infusions). As a therapeutic technique, progressive relaxation has several unique assets. First, it can be applied in almost any setting that provides a small, quiet spot and, ideally, a comfortable reclining chair or one with a headrest. For the bedridden patient, the head of the bed should be cranked up partway. Second, progressive relaxation has widespread patient acceptance, and almost any cooperative patient will achieve some degree of positive results. Negative or adverse effects are rare; their occurrence is likely due to an unrecognized psychiatric disorder. Third, it is not time-consuming, and the cost–benefit ratio is positive. Fourth, progressive relaxation can be applied readily in many situations, even on an "emergency" basis. For example, in the patient who is highly fearful while anticipating bone marrow aspiration, the clinician can start the relaxation procedure while the patient is being prepared on the table for the procedure, talking to the patient, and encouraging muscle relaxation and control of anxiety while the aspiration is being performed. If the distress is substantially reduced, the patient may wish to master the technique to use at other times. Several sessions are often needed to ensure that the patient can utilize the technique on his or her own.

It is important to be aware of the risks associated with progressive relaxation, although they are few.

Application of progressive-relaxation training may occasionally *increase* rather than diminish a patient's anxiety. This can occur in a patient whose expectation was too high for success, in the patient who has a personality disorder that results in anger and negative response to most efforts to help, in the patient who has severe cancer pain (e.g., plexopathy pain) that requires analgesic or nerve block intervention for control, in the self-critical patient who blames himself or herself for being a failure and not "trying hard enough," and in the patient for whom complete relaxation is equated with losing control, which may be equated with fears of death.

Another response, seen in some patients, is that in which a relaxed state progresses to a hypnotic trance. This is unusual and is not necessarily a drawback unless it arouses anxiety and concern in the patient, family member, or medical staff. The clinician needs to know how to manage trance states if they occur. These caveats to the effective use of progressive relaxation are few. However, they can become critical to both patient and practitioner in the absence of adequate training and experience on the part of the therapist.

## TRAINING

The training of the clinician in progressive relaxation must address the appropriate selection of patients, the procedural steps involved, the impact of the technique on psychological and physiological processes, potential risks and benefits, limitations of the technique, and recognition of the necessity of having a psychiatric backup. For example, emergency intervention for the patient with a severe panic attack is apt to fail; psychiatric evaluation and intervention should be recommended instead.

The simplicity and ease of application of progressive relaxation tends to engender an inappropriately casual approach to the use of this technique. Progressive relaxation should be viewed as a measured, planned intervention requiring adequate time for preparation of the practitioner, as well as the patient.

Thus, the clinician who wishes to become proficient in progressive relaxation must involve himself or herself in a full teaching program given by a tutor who is fully grounded in the use of all behavioral techniques, including progressive relaxation, hypnosis, and meditation.

A minimum of 6 hours is recommended to train a clinician adequately in progressive relaxation. The student should learn the concepts of stress and the mental and physiological responses to it. The history of progressive relaxation and the rationale for its use should be reviewed, as well as that for hypnosis, trance states, and meditation. Problems that can arise in the use of these techniques need also to be thoroughly discussed. The student should be put through several progressive relaxation sessions acting as the patient, with practice sessions outlined to carry out at home. During the last half of the training sessions, students should pair off and carry out the procedure with each other. The subject (recipient) functions as a critic of the operator's delivery. Students can practice on willing subjects among family and friends. The last part of training occurs in the hospital or clinic among referred patients with the teacher as observer. A return consultation for all students 1–2 months later for a formal review of methods and problems should be built into the training program.

## USE OF TAPES

It is a common practice in the current application of progressive relaxation to make an audiotape an initial session with a patient for his or her use at home or in other situations. The patient can practice at home with the tape, following the recorded procedure as frequently as recommended or needed; it serves as a reminder of what to do and how to do it. Although benefits are clearly present, some feel that there are disadvantages to fostering dependence on the use of tapes. First, the patient is more likely to develop his or her own timing and cadence for relaxation if given the chance, and practice while alone may help motivate a patient to "tailor" the technique to achieve optimal relaxation. Second, unaided practice avoids the problem faced by a patient who may need to evoke his or her self-regulation in settings in which the use of a tape player is awkward (e.g., waiting in the clinic area). Third, patients more quickly establish confidence in their own ability to accomplish a relaxed state. Finally, the greatest drawback is that an audiotape quickly loses its impact. It becomes boring and is reduced to a neutral, or sometimes annoying, or even anxiety-arousing stimulus. When the use of a tape at home is deemed important, it is a far better tactic to lend the patient a cassette with instructions to return it in a short time (e.g., after a week of practice). An alternative to the use of a tape is to provide the patient with a typewritten list of short "reminders" of the key points in the process.

## PATIENT SELECTION

The following broad criteria are useful in determining who is an appropriate candidate for progressive-relaxation training. Patients with cancer who should be considered include the following:

1. A patient who has anxiety, pain, or a conditioned response to chemotherapy that is not controlled by usual methods
2. A patient who has a great need for self-control and who is afraid to use medication (e.g., hypnotics and sedatives) to control pain or distress (such individuals often say "I never even take an aspirin")
3. A patient who has heard of benefits and knows that such intervention is available and asks about it

Patients who are poor candidates for relaxation are the following:

1. A patient who has a CNS complication of cancer (delirium or dementia)
2. A patient who has a history of serious mental illness and in whom cooperation would be marginal
3. A patient who is not motivated to try and who is disinterested and unenthusiastic after initial exposure to the technique (included are the patient who professes real interest in the procedure but who does not "find the time" to practice diligently at home, and also the patient who reports that his or her mind wanders and that it is impossible to "stick with it")

## NEW DIRECTIONS

A recent development in cancer pain control is the application of cognitive-behavioral techniques in clinical management. This approach is based on the premise that behavioral and emotional responses to physical sensations of pain are determined in part by cognitions and appraisals of the sensations, and by coping ability. Because pain is often equated with disease progression in patients' minds, the element of "suffering" (i.e., the meaning of the pain) may intensify it (Meichenbaum and Turk, 1979). In the technique designed by Turk and Rennert (1981), pain is addressed early in the course of disease by teaching patients specific coping skills to manage pain from both the sensory and the emotional side. This is accomplished through the use of rational restructuring, coping skills training, and problem-solving training. These authors have proposed a preventive pain control intervention that, while not yet systematically tested, appears useful. This method has also been applied and tested in children by Jay and colleagues (1985) in a multicomponent package designed to reduce distress during bone marrow aspirations and spinal taps. It has five parts consisting of filmed modeling, reinforcement, breathing exercises, imagery, and rehearsal, and appears to be effective in reducing pain, distress, and arousal. Other applications in children have also been helpful (LeBaw et al., 1975; Redd, 1982; Spiegel,

1985; Spiegel and Bloom, 1985; Stacher et al., 1975; Stewart, 1976).

## SUMMARY

Although in some cases they have a long history of use in medicine, behavioral interventions represent the most recent approach to management of distress in cancer, following psychotherapeutic and psychopharmacological interventions. Resurgence of interest in these modalities has been spurred by social pressure toward greater patient participation in care, as well as the publication of research detailing the unique efficacy of self-regulatory techniques in helping patients manage a variety of highly specific situations, such as conditioned nausea and vomiting, which are often refractory to more conventional intervention.

The self-regulatory therapies offer a potentially powerful adjunct to maximizing quality of life for patients. The relative ease with which they can be applied also makes them an appealing therapeutic approach. Of the approaches discussed, progressive relaxation is a particularly good model. Much research still needs to be conducted, however. Premature or misapplication of new behavioral interventions is particularly apt to occur in a society that adheres less to spiritual values and has unrealistic expectations of psychology.

## REFERENCES

Ambrose, G., and G. Newbold (1968). *The Handbook of Medical Hypnosis*. Baltimore: Williams & Wilkins.

Arnoff, G. M., R. Kamen, and W. O. Evans (1981). The relaxation response: a behavioral answer for chronic pain patients. *Behavioral Medicine* 8:20–25.

Balon, J. J. (1974). Meditation—psychotherapy in the treatment of cancer. *Psychiatry* 6:19–22.

Benson, H. (1975). *The relaxation response*. New York: William Morrow.

———— (1977). Systemic hypertension and the relaxation response. *N. Engl. J. Med.* 296:1152–56.

————, J. C. Beary, and M. P. Carol (1974). The relaxation response. *Psychiatry* 37:37–46.

Burish, T. G., and J. N. Lyles (1981). Effectiveness of relaxation training in reducing adverse reactions to cancer chemotherapy. *J. Behav. Med.* 4:65–78.

Cobb, S. C. (1984). Teaching relaxation techniques to cancer patients. *Can. Nursing* 7:157–61.

Cooke, G. (1968). Evaluation of the efficacy of the components of reciprocal inhibition psychotherapy. *J. Abnorm. Psychol.* 73:464–67.

Cotanch, P. H. (1983). Relaxation training for control of nausea and vomiting in patients receiving chemotherapy. *Can. Nursing* 6:277–83.

Davidson, R. J., and G. E. Schwartz (1976). The psycho-

biology of relaxation and related states: A multi-process theory. In D. Mostofsky (ed.), *Behavior Control and Modification of Physiological Activity*. Englewood Cliffs, NJ: Prentice Hall, pp.399–442.

Davison, G.C. (1968). Systematic densitization as a counter-conditioning process. *J. Abnorm. Psychol.* 73:91–99.

Donovan, M. (1980). Relaxation with guided imagery: a useful technique. *Can. Nursing* 3:27–32.

Enskine-Milliss, J., and M. Schonell (1981). Relaxation therapy in asthma: a critical review. *Psychosom. Med.* 43:365–72.

Ferguson, J. M., J. N. Marquis, and C. Barr Taylor (1977). A script for deep muscle relaxation. *Dis. Nerv. Sys.* 38:282–87.

French, A. P., & Tupin, J. P. (1974). Therapeutic application of a simple relaxation method. *Am. J. Psychother.* 28:282–87.

Fromm, E., and R. C. Shor (1972). *Hypnosis: Research Developments and Perspectives*. Chicago: Aldini-Atherton.

Goldeman, D. J., and G. E. Schwartz (1976). Meditation as an intervention in stress reactivity. *J. Consult. Clin. Psychol.* 44:456–66.

Goldfried, M. R. (1973). Reduction of generalized anxiety through a variant of systematic desensitization. In M. R. Goldfried and M. Merbaum (eds.), *Behavior Change Through Self-Control*. New York: Holt, Rinehart & Winston.

————, and C. S. Trier (1974). Effectiveness of relaxation as an active coping skill. *J. Abnorm. Psychol.* 83:348–55.

Grzesiak, R. C. (1977). Relaxation techniques in treatment of chronic pain. *Arch. Phys. Med. Rehab.* 58:270–72.

Heide, F. J., and T. D. Borkovec (1983). Relaxation-induced anxiety: paradoxical anxiety enhancement due to relaxation training. *Journal of Consult. Clin. Psychol.* 51:171–82.

Hilgard, E. R. (1969). Altered states of awareness. *J. Nerv. Men. Dis.* 149:68–79.

————, and J. R. Hilgard (1983). *Hypnosis in the Relief of Pain*. Los Altos, CA: William Kaufmann.

Hilgard, J. R., and S. LeBaron (1984). *Hypnotherapy of Pain in Children With Cancer*. Los Altos, CA: William Kaufmann.

Jacobson, E. (1938). *Progressive Relaxation*. Chicago: University of Chicago Press.

Jay, S. M., C. M. Elliott, M. Ozolins, R. Olson, and S. Pruitt, (1985). Behavioral management of children's distress during painful medical procedures. *Behav. Res. Ther.* 23:513–20.

————, C. M. Elliott, and J. W. Varni (1986). Acute and chronic pain in adults and children with cancer. *J. Consult. Clin. Psychol.* 54(5):601–7.

Kabat-Zin, J. (1982). An outpatient program in behavioral medicine for chronic pain patients based on the practice of mindfulness meditations: theoretical considerations and preliminary results. *Gen. Hosp. Psychiatry* 4:33–47.

Kasamatsu, A. and I. Hira (1969). An encephalographic study of the Zen meditation (Zazen). In C. Tart (ed.), *Altered States of Consciousness* New York: Wiley and Sons, pp. 489–501.

Keefe, F. J., A. R., Block, R. B. Williams, and R. S. Surwit (1981). Behavioral treatment of chronic low back pain: clinical outcome and individual differences in pain relief. *Pain* 11:221–31.

Kellerman, J., L. Zeltzer, L. Ellenberg, and J. Dash (1983). Adolescents with cancer: hypnosis for the reduction of acute pain and anxiety associated with medical procedures. *J. Adol. Health Care* 4:85–90.

Kraines, S. H. (1963). Emotions: a physiologic process. *Psychosomatics* 4:313–24.

Kroger, W. S. (1976). *Hypnosis and Behavior Modification: Imagery Conditioning*. Philadelphia: Lippincott.

———— (1979). *Clinical Experimental Hypnosis*. Philadelphia: Lippincott.

Kutz, I., J. Z. Borysenko, and H. Benson (1985). Meditation and psychotherapy: A rationale for the integration of dynamic psychotherapy, the relaxation response, and mindfulness meditation. *Am. J. Psychiatry* 142:1–8.

LaBaw, W., C. Holton, K. Tewell, and D. Eccles (1975). The use of self-hypnosis of children with cancer. *Hypnosis* 17:233–38.

Lerner, M., and N. Remen (1985). Varieties of integral cancer therapies. *Advances* 2:14–33.

Ludwig, A. (1966). Altered states of consciousness. *Arch. Gen. Psychiatry* 15:225–34.

Lyles, J. N., T. G. Burish, M. G. Krozely, and R. K. Oldham (1982). Efficacy of relaxation training and guided imagery in reducing the aversiveness of cancer chemotherapy. *J. Consult. Clin. Psychol.* 50:509–24.

Meichenbaum, D., and D. Turk (1976). The cognitive behavioral management of anxiety, anger and pain. In P. O. Davidson (ed.), *The Behavioral Management of Anxiety, Depression and Pain* New York: Bruner-Mazel, pp. 1–34.

Miller, N. E. (1980): Effects of learning on physical symptoms produced by stress. In H. Selye (ed.), *Selye's Guide to Stress Research* New York: Van Nostrands Reinhold, pp. 131–67.

Morrow, G. R., and C. Morrell (1982). Behavioral treatment for the anticipatory nausea and vomiting induced by cancer chemotherapy. *N. Engl. J. Med.* 307:1476–80.

Olness, K., and G. G. Gardner (1978). Some guidelines for use of hypnotherapy in pediatrics. *Pediatrics* 62:228–33.

Orne, M. T., and D. F. Dinges (1984). Hypnosis. In P. D. Wall and R. Melzack, (eds.), *Textbook of Pain* New York: Churchill Livingstone, pp. 806–16.

Paul, G. L. (1969). Physiological effects of relaxation training and hypnotic suggestion. *J. Abnorm. Psychol.* 74:425–37.

Redd, W., and M. A. Andrykowski (1982). Behavioral intervention in cancer treatment: Controlling aversion reactions to chemotherapy. *J. Counsel. Clin. Psychol.* 50: 1018–29.

Sacerdote, P. (1966). Hypnosis in cancer patients. *Am. J. Clin. Hypnosis* 9:100–8.

Sargent, J. D., E. E. Green, and E. D. Walters (1972). The use of autogenic feedback training in a study of migraine and tension headaches. *Headache* 12:120–24.

Schultz, J. H., and W. Luthe (1969). In W. Luthe (ed.), *Autogenic Methods: Vol. 1. Autogenic Therapy*. New York: Grune and Stratton.

Scott, D. W., D. C. Donahue, R. C. Mastrovito, and T. B. Hakes (1983). The antiemetic effect of clinical relaxation: Report of an exploratory pilot study. *J. Psychosoc. Oncol.* 1(1):71–84.

Shapiro, D. H., Jr. (1982). Overview: clinical and physiological comparison of meditation with other self-control strategies. *Am. J. Psychiatry* 139:267–74.

Simonton, O. C., S. Matthews-Simonton, and T. F. Sparks (1980). Psychological intervention in the treatment of cancer. *Psychosomatics* 21:226–27, 231–33.

Spiegel, D. (1985). The use of hypnosis in controlling cancer pain. *Ca - A J. Clin.* 36:221–31.

————, and J. R. Bloom (1983). Group therapy and hypnosis reduce metastatic breast carcinoma pain. *Psychosom. Med.* 45:333–39.

Spiegel, H., and D. Spiegel (1978). *Trance and Treatment: Clinical Uses of Hypnosis*. New York: Basic Books.

Stacher, G., P. Schuster, P. Bauer, R. Lahoda, and D. Schulze (1975). Effects of suggestion of relaxation or analgesia on pain threshold and pain tolerance in the waking and in the hypnotic state. *J. Psychosom. Res.* 19:259–65.

Stewart, E. (1976). To lessen pain: relaxation and rhythmic breathing. *Am. J. Nursing,* 76:958–59.

Stoyva, J. (1976). Self-regulation and the stress-related disorders: A perspective on biofeedback. In D. Mostofsky (ed.), *Behavior control and modification of physiological activity* Englewood Cliffs, NJ: Prentice-Hall, pp. 366–98.

Turk, D. C., and D. Rennert (1981). Pain and the terminally ill cancer patient: a cognitive social learning perspective. In H. J. Sobel (ed.), *Behavior Therapy in Terminal Care* Cambridge, MA: Ballinger Publishing, pp. 95–123.

Walsh, R. (1980). The consciousness disciplines and the behavioral sciences: questions of comparison and assessment. *Am. J. Psychiatry* 137:663–73.

Weiss, T., and B. T. Engel (1975). Evaluation of intracardiac limit of learned heart rate control. *Psychophysiology* 12:310–12.

Wolpe, J. (1958). *Psychotherapy by Reciprocal Intuition*. Stanford, CA: Stanford University Press.

Zelzer, L., and S. LeBaron (1982). Hypnosis and nonhypnotic techniques for reduction of pain and anxiety during painful procedures in children and adolescents with cancer. *J. Pediatr.* 101:1032–35.

Zilboorg, G., and G. Henry (1941). *A History of Medical Psychology*. New York: Norton.

# Self-Help and Mutual Support Programs

Rene Mastrovito, Rosemary Moynihan, and Lissa Parsonnet

"Sometimes fear is so engulfing it precludes the ability to call for help. It is this fear that those of us called patients understand and can help to diminish for one another"

Robert Fisher, founding member,
Patient-to-Patient volunteer program

Sol Weiss vividly remembers when he first learned about Memorial Sloan-Kettering's Patient-to-Patient volunteers. It was the day before his colon cancer surgery, 4 years ago. "The nurses told me I had one of the best rooms in the house," he recalled at the program's regular monthly meeting this May. "A volunteer brought me flowers. Another asked if I wanted a book, I didn't care about anything. I was trying my best to think about anything but cancer—when another volunteer walked into my room. He said, 'I had cancer. And I had many complications.'

He went on talking about his experiences while I just stared. I never knew anybody could have had a disease like this and look as healthy as he did. Finally I asked how he'd got here. I meant, how had it happened. He said, 'I bicycled here, 68 blocks.'

"I don't think anyone who hasn't been a patient could possibly know what our talk meant to me. That night, I was offered a sedative, but I didn't need it. I slept like a baby."

These vignettes express the distinctive meaning of help to a cancer patient from another who had "been through it" (MSKCC *Center News,* 1986). They reflect the instant bond that forms between two individuals who truly "understand" what it is like to have cancer. Life crises, particularly separation, loss, and crippling or life-threatening illness, cause individuals to seek emotional support from others. While they may receive loving help from family and friends, often no one may seem quite to understand "what it is like to have my problem" except someone who has "been there."

In relation to cancer and most other diseases, physicians used to discourage this kind of dialogue because of the fear that patients would upset each other by comparing medicines and doctors. Despite the concerns, the natural desire of one individual with cancer to help another with the same problem, has resulted in patient-to-patient self-help programs that have slowly been accepted and encouraged (Barish, 1971; Gartner and Reissman, 1982). Like Alcoholics Anonymous and widow-to-widow groups, the value of patient-to-patient support in cancer is that it is a powerful source of support for patients with cancer and their families (Guggenheim and O'Hara, 1976). This chapter outlines the development of self-help support programs and our own experience with such a program at Memorial Sloan-Kettering. The origin of the program is described by the founding volunteer, Robert Fisher, whose energy, commitment, and efforts led to the evolution of our highly effective Patient-to-Patient volunteer program.

An understanding of the value of self-help support in physical illness in general, and in cancer in particular, derives from three sources, namely, studies of crisis theory, coping strategies, and social support systems theory (Killilea, 1982). Crisis theory has evolved from the information showing the value of intervention during acute crises (such as at the time of a catastrophic event), during transitional periods (such as bereavement and divorce), and during chronic crises in which restitution to the prior state will not be attained (such as with chronic or fatal illness). Also relevant for the studies of coping strategies, which are utilized by individuals in stressful circumstances such as illness. They have been studied by Hamburg and others in terms of the tasks that must be accomplished in a crisis, that is, containing distress, maintaining self-esteem, remaining a valued member of a group, and meeting the demands of the present while preparing for the future (Hamburg and Adams, 1967).

Evidence derived from social support systems theory has shown that social support can modify the deleterious effects of stress on behavior and health, either by buffering the impact of stress or by enhancing coping strategies. The purpose served by social networks appears to be to maintain social identity, and to provide emotional support, material aid, and services, access to information, new social contacts, and maintenance of social roles (Walker et al., 1977). Programs have arisen out of the gap perceived in available supports from traditional medical care, the decrease in extended family support due to geographic dispersion, and the needs engendered by a chronic illness with its associated burden of physical care and rehabilitation (Tracey and Gussow, 1976).

Understanding the existential plight of the patient with cancer and the adaptation demanded in order to cope effectively makes the need for social support readily apparent, for the cancer survivor who benefits from the shared support to meet the social stigma. It is also beneficial for patients with advanced stages of cancer and their families who face the problems of adapting to advancing illness.

## HISTORICAL PERSPECTIVE

By examining the first mutual-help effort in the medical care field, we can gain some insights into the current proliferation of mutual-help groups. In 1905, Joseph Pratt organized a program for poor tuberculosis patients in Boston who took their bed rest at home on porches and the roofs of tenements (Killelea, 1982). They had a "friendly visitor," usually a nurse, or another patient who offered encouragement and guidance. The patients came weekly to Dr. Pratt's office at the Massachusetts General Hospital, where they held classes in which he reviewed the diaries they had kept and discussed their health problems. The concept of a partnership in which the patient provided important expertise from having been through the experience was a critical principle.

The self-help and mutual-support programs for cancer patients date to the 1940s after World War II when the American Cancer Society (ACS) began its visitor programs, which offered practical help for patients at home. These programs offered by volunteers, and the programs that followed, developed support needed to cope with the consequences of the radical surgical procedures, which offered the only hope of cure at that time (see Table 41-1). The International Laryngectomy Association was founded in 1942, as laryngectomy became a common surgical procedure. Reach-to-Recovery was taken over by the ACS in 1952 to meet the emotional needs of women after mastectomy and has served as a model for patient-to-patient support programs. Around this time, ostomy clubs formed as colostomy became a common procedure from which

**Table 41-1** Some national self-help groups for cancer patients

| Group | Related to |
|---|---|
| American Cancer Society (ACS)* | |
| Visitor programs | General |
| CanSurmount | General |
| Reach-to-Recovery | Breast |
| Candlelighters | Childhood cancer |
| International Laryngectomy Society | Laryngectomy |
| Ostomy Clubs | Colostomy |
| Make Today Count | Chronic disease |
| S.H.A.R.E. | Breast reconstruction |
| Living with Cancer | General |
| Compassionate Friends | Loss of child with cancer |
| Can-Do | General |
| Coalition of Cancer Survivorship | Survivors and their relatives |

*The ACS partially supports several of these organizations.

patients survived, developing into an international society. A Cured Cancer Club was developed in the 1950s to help cancer patients meet the social stigma faced by these early survivors. Self-help groups have tended to develop as grassroots efforts to meet special needs perceived by patients, families, and concerned staff. The Leukemia Society of America is a major nonprofit organization that is exploring not only professional but self-support methods.

Although programs vary in the way they meet sociomedical needs, these mutual-help groups make possible "person-to-person" exchanges that provide identification, reciprocity, and access to a body of specialized information. An opportunity to share coping techniques based on realistic expectations is helpful. An increased sense of worth develops when members can see and hear about how similar their feelings and experiences are to those of others in the same situation. Reinforcement for change, maintenance of effort, and feedback on performance are given. The group serves also as a focus for advocacy and social change. The group activities provide powerful methods for confronting the adverse effects of stigma of cancer (Killilea, 1976).

### Self-Help Models in Cancer

Most of the self-help support groups in cancer work in close proximity to professional medical services, thus offering social supports as an adjunct to traditional care (Toseland and Hacker, 1982). This interface requires physician approval, especially for "visitation programs" in which the patient with cancer can meet a "veteran" who has been through the experience and who can serve as a model for the new patient. The goal is to help patients and their families adapt to the illness and the changes it brings (Chesler et al., 1984; Gussow and Tracey, 1976; Mantell, 1983). The access to patients by these visitors is often facilitated by physicians, social workers, psychiatrists, nurses, and clergy, who readily recognize their value (Vattano, 1972; Mantell et al., 1976; Mantell, 1983; Mastrovito et al., 1980).

Patient-visitors can offer a dimension of help beyond the scope of professional practitioners, namely, that of experiential empathy (Katz, 1965, 1970; Davies et al., 1973; Levy, 1976). The uniquely special knowledge and sensitivity that come from having had the same experience, and the willingness to share it, assist the new patient in coping more effectively. Mantell and colleagues (1976) stressed the importance of this dimension, because cancer patients often have difficulty in communicating their distressed feelings to others, leading to a sense of isolation and alienation. Without attention to this tendency in cancer patients, a wall of silence can arise between a patient and those with whom he or she has previously shared fears and concerns. The patient may attempt to protect others with a facade of cheerfulness. The distressed relative or friend often may not understand the experience, and may allow the patient to withdraw. Evidence shows that patients who lack confidence become apathetic and withdrawn. Absence of social support has been correlated with poorer outcome of disease (Adams, 1979; Mantell, 1983).

The veteran-patient volunteer who visits the new patient facilitates coping by providing a source of credible information based on description of their past "patient" experiences, by demonstrating constructive alternative ways of living and managing despite illness, providing motivation for rehabilitation and enhancing a sense of self-worth, by providing protection from alienation and isolation, by encouraging the new patient's participation in their own treatment, by functioning as a "surrogate patient" of whom families can ask questions and express feelings concealed from the patient, and by serving to educate professionals and the public about the needs of people with cancer. In carrying out these functions successfully for another person, the patient-visitor benefits as well, according to the "helper therapy" principle (Reissman, 1965, 1982).

### Formation of the Memorial Sloan-Kettering Hospital Group

At our hospital a patient-visitor program has flourished through the efforts of individuals, all of whom have or have had cancer and who have successfully adapted to it. Known as the Patient-to-Patient Volunteers, these individuals see newly admitted cancer patients who have the same or a similar cancer diagnosis. Because they have firsthand knowledge of the disease, they are able to provide expertise possessed by few medical and ancillary medical personnel. This experiential expertise provides a powerful core experience that binds the volunteers and the new patients together.

The concept of a patient-volunteer program in our cancer research hospital began in 1977 when Robert Fisher, a patient with chronic myelocytic leukemia, was asked by his physician to visit a particularly anxious, newly diagnosed leukemia patient. This first patient-to-patient encounter led to further similar requests from the physician. As time passed, requests for patient visits sprang from other sources, specifically, from floor nurses, other physicians, and patients themselves. A hospital psychiatrist (coauthor Mastrovito) occasionally consulted informally with the patient-volunteer. The positive rapport established between the newly hospitalized patients and the patient-volunteers was impressive. It became apparent that this phenomenon was based mainly on two conditions. The first was the ready identification of the volunteer as a fellow patient with leukemia. This established an immediate empathic relationship with an individual who had survived the rigors of hospitalization and treatment for the same illness. The veteran could be trusted with certain revelations (thoughts, fears, and concerns) that could not easily be discussed with the family and often not revealed to the professional staff. Second, the veteran was a person outside the medical fraternity who was at the same time approved by the institution and thus was an adjunct to formal care by the medical staff. He or she was thus a nonprofessional who, nevertheless, knew a great deal about the disease and treatment experience from the patient's point of view and who had mastered many aspects of the situation.

Bard and Sutherland noted 30 years ago that, in some measure, every patient wishes to be a "model" patient (1955). The individual does not want to challenge or question the medical system too greatly because his or her life and well-being depend on it (Bard and Sutherland, 1955). The need to believe in and trust the medical establishment and its members is great. Thus many feelings, concerns about illness, and apprehensions about treatment are viewed by patients as too threatening to the relationship to be voiced to the nurse or physician. For instance, patients may perceive, correctly or not, that their doctors will view their feelings of despair or fear as evidence that they are lacking moral fiber. They also fear that their questions may not be answered honestly. The veteran patient is a natural consultant in these matters, for he or she is one who has felt the fears, apprehensions, and concerns. He or she listens and understands the concerns, without surprise or dismay.

**Table 41-2**  Volunteers by site of illness* in MSKCC program

| | |
|---|---|
| Amputation | Leukemia |
| Bone | Lung |
| Bone marrow transplant | Lymphoma |
| Breast | Lymphosarcoma |
| Cervix | Melanoma |
| Colon | Ovary |
| Hodgkin's disease | Spinal cord |
| Kidney | Testicle |

*Laryngectomy and ostomy patients are handled by special programs.

**Table 41-3**  Criteria for selection of patient volunteers

- Personal experience with cancer ("experiential expertise")
- Committment to the program—willingness to work in conjunction with medical staff
- Good communication skills, sensitivity, empathy, good listening skills
- Emotional stability
- Ability to present a good model of coping in which the patient has returned to normal life activities and interests
- Education not important

On the basis of the experience of Robert Fisher, the first patient-volunteer, and a few others found to be doing similar patient visits at Memorial Sloan-Kettering Hospital, the viability of utilizing peer-patient referrals was accepted, at least in great part, by the medical staff. In 1979, the status of patient-volunteers was formalized, and they became part of a special group. Formed within the Department of Volunteer Services, the Psychiatry Service and the Department of Social Work participated in the administration of the program. Two social workers and a psychiatrist have served as links between the professional staff and this nonprofessional group. The core group, having begun with 10 volunteers, has since expanded to 25. The membership changes periodically with the addition of new volunteers and loss of others due to medical reasons and evolving life choices. In order that patient concerns associated with specific tumor types, sites, and treatments can be better addressed, participating volunteers are individuals who have had a spectrum of types of cancer namely, lymphoma, melanoma, Hodgkin's disease, leukemia, as well as tumors of the testicles, spinal cord, colon, breast, kidney, and bone (sarcoma with amputation) (see Table 41-2).

The selection and screening of new volunteers is an important function of the professional staff. Candidates, usually self-referred, are interviewed by at least two members of the professional staff. They are admitted if their concept of the role of patient volunteer is generally consistent with the goals and philosophy of the group. The basic credential is a personal experience with cancer. In addition, individuals are chosen who are sensitive and empathic, who are good listeners, and who are able to discuss their personal experiences in such a way as to provide constructive support for another person. They must represent an example of good coping and adaptation to the cancer experience (see Table 41-3). The occasional individual who is profoundly dissatisfied with his or her prior medical treatment is not a good candidate. This is true because such individuals sometimes intend to "right the wrongs" of the entire medical system. Such individuals are discouraged from joining. Similarly, indi-

viduals who advocate unproven medical treatments are also discouraged from joining. Those who profess such beliefs are not accepted by the medical establishment. Candidates who seem psychologically fragile and who are covertly seeking support from similarly affected individuals within the group are referred to other resources.

Before undertaking his or her duties, the new volunteer attends two 2-hour teaching and orientation sessions in which the staff assists volunteers in understanding their role. The volunteers also learn listening skills, and discuss the limits of what they should expect of themselves. Monthly meetings serve to monitor the activities of each volunteer, to assess the quality of their interaction with patients, and to provide emotional support for them. One concern of those overseeing the program has been that a training too extensive or a supervision too intense might lead to regimentation with a loss of spontaneity in interactions.

Supportive supervision places little emphasis on skill development. It is pointed out that the volunteer's role is not to offer therapy and that treatment is not their responsibility. Rather, focus is placed on orientation to the hospital system, patient needs, new developments in cancer care, and visiting skills such as limit setting. The patient-visitor role is explored, and information and techniques are reviewed in order to increase volunteers' confidence and their ability to tolerate the demands of their role.

There is no minimum amount of time that each person must devote as a volunteer. Most volunteers are active in their business and family life, and may be able to devote only a few hours a month. Others who are retired or who have few outside responsibilities devote much more time.

Each member of the group functions independently, relating to one of the supervisors. Activity is, except for very unusual circumstances, carried on within the hospital, although visits may be made at home and telephone contact maintained. Most often patients are visited at the bedside several times. The exact number of visits depends on the patient's needs and on the volunteer's availability. Ideally the patient is always seen when anxiety or fear may be greatest, for example, shortly after admission and/or before undergoing a new treatment. Assignments are monitored to check for situations in which the volunteer becomes overly responsible for a patient, or becomes overidentified. Participants are encouraged to ask another volunteer to take a particular patient when they feel overly burdened or distressed.

The problem of linking the patient and the volunteer is difficult in the Patient-Volunteer Program. When the group was first formed, volunteers were already receiving referrals, usually from their own physician. As the group enlarged and stabilized, an attempt was made to institute a formal referral process. A memorandum went out to physicians and staff that announced the existence of the group, described its function, and provided a telephone extension at which services could be reached. This formal referral system has since been abandoned in favor of the original, more effective informal contact system. Referrals are usually made by word of mouth.

Some physicians absolutely rejected the concept of patient-volunteers and wished none of their patients to be seen without a formal request. Others embraced the program and requested that patient-volunteers see as many of their patients as possible. Many physicians delegated the decision whether or not to refer to the floor nurse or the social worker assigned to the unit. The patient-volunteers are encouraged to strengthen their own informal system, because these contact represent a rapport and trust between the professional and the volunteer. Usually a volunteer works closely with one or two doctors and the related floor staff.

A major issue that patient-volunteer programs raise is that of the emotional burden on the volunteer who has had cancer. Visiting distressed patients who have the same diagnosis, and may be near the same age, is painful to any volunteer. It may be difficult to handle, even with good defenses (Mastrovito et al., 1980; May et al., 1979). Because of this, those who wish to become volunteers when they may be motivated out of an effort to understand their own experience rather than to help others are discouraged (Manell et al., 1976; Rogers and Bauman, 1984). The overall monitoring of the program is managed by frequent telephone contact between volunteers, patients, and medical staff. Monthly meetings are held with the full group, and the morale of the volunteers and staff is monitored (Koocher, 1979) (Table 41-4).

The effectiveness of patient-visitor programs is difficult to evaluate for two reasons. First, models vary, making empirical research difficult, and second, such interventions usually address only one part of a detailed, multifaceted coping process at different illness stages (Lieberman and Bond, 1979). It is difficult to

**Table 41-4** MSKCC program review

- Frequent telephone contact between volunteers and professional staff
- Monthly meeting of volunteers and professional staff
- Meeting between individual volunteers and assigned professional staff (minimum of once every 3 months)
- Participation of volunteers and professional staff in training of new volunteers

show objective changes in levels of distress such as anxiety and depression as a function of visitor efforts (Spiegel et al., 1981; Killilea, 1976). Irrespective of these considerations, patients and families report great benefit from this program. The ACS, which has the most extensive visitors program, has found evaluation difficult because the work depends on volunteers who have considerable autonomy and who work loosely within broad guidelines.

Empirical research is needed to document the effectiveness of visitor programs. Prospects for their utilization and further implementation by the health care system must be explored. A clearer definition of the training and supervision needed for such programs must be established. Pertinent issues to be addressed in greater depth include determination of the optimal times for the use of patient volunteers and evaluation of the psychosocial needs of each patient visitor.

## REFERENCES

Adams, J. (1979). Mutual-help groups: Enhancing the coping ability of oncology clients. *Cancer Nurs.* 2:95–98.

Bard, M. and A. M. Sutherland (1955). Psychological impact of cancer and its treatment. *Cancer* 8:656.

Barish, H. (1971). Self-help groups. In R. Morris (chief ed.), *Encyclopedia of Social Work*, 16th issue, Vol. 2. Washington, D.C.: National Association of Social Workers, pp. 1163–68.

Chesler, M., O. Barbarin, and J. Lebo-Stein (1984). Patterns of participation in a self-help group for parents of children with cancer. *J. Psychosoc. Oncol.* 2(3/4):41–64.

Davies, R. K., D. M. Quinlan, P. McKegney, and C. P. Kimball (1973). Organic factors and psychological adjustment in advanced cancer patients. *Psychosom. Med.* 35:464–71.

Gartner, A. and F. Reissman (1982). The self-help revolution. New York: Human Services Press.

Guggenheim, F. G. and S. O'Hara (1976). Peer counseling in a general hospital. *Am. J. Psychiatry* 133:1197–99.

Gussow, Z. and G. S. Tracey (1976). The role of self-help clubs in adaptation to chronic illness and disability. *Soc. Sci. Med.* 10:407–14.

Hamburg, D. A. and J. E. Adams (1967). A perspective on coping behavior. *Arch. Gen. Psychiatry* 17:277–84.

Katz, A. H. (1965). Application of self-help concepts in current social welfare. *Soc. Work* 10:68–74.

Katz, A. H. (1970). Self-help organizations and volunteer participation in social welfare. *Soc. Work* 15:51–60.

Killilea, M. (1976). Mutual help organizations: Interpretations in the literature. In G. Caplan and M. Killilea (eds.), *Support Systems and Mutual Help.* New York: Grune & Stratton, pp. 37–93.

Killilea, M. (1982). Interaction of crisis theory, coping strategies and social support systems. In H. C. Schulberg and M. Killilea (eds.), *The Modern Practice of Community Mental Health.* San Francisco: Jossey-Bass, pp. 163–214.

Koocher, G. P. (1979). Adjustment and coping strategies among the caretakers of cancer patients. *Soc. Work Health Care* 5:145–50.

Levy, L. H. (1976). Self-help groups: Types and psychological processes. *J. Appl. Behav. Sci.* 12:310–22.

Lieberman, M. A. and G. R. Bond (1979). Self-help groups: Problems of measuring outcome. *Small Group Behav.* 9:221–41.

Mantell, J. E. (1983). Cancer patient visitor programs: A case for accountability. *J. Psychosoc. Oncol.* 1(1):45–58.

Mantell, J. E., E. S. Alexander and M. A. Kleiman (1976). Social work and self-help groups. *Health Soc. Work* 1:86–100.

Mastrovito, R., R. Moynihan, J. F. Lee, and R. Fisher (1980). The veteran patient program at Memorial Hospital. *Proc. Natl. Forum Compr. Cancer Rehabil. Vocat. Implications,* Williamsburg, VA., pp. 211–15.

May, C. H., M. C. McPhee, and D. J. Pritchard (1979). An amputee visitor program as an adjunct to rehabilitation of the lower limb amputee. *Mayo Clin. Proc.* 54:774–78.

Memorial Sloan-Kettering Cancer Center (MSKCC) Department of Public Affairs (1986). Patient-to-patient volunteer program: Experts in hope. *Center News,* June 7, p. 7.

Reissman, F. (1965). The "helper-therapy" principle. *Soc. Work* 10:27–32.

Reissman, F. (1982). The self-help ethos. *Soc. Policy* 13:42–43.

Rogers, T. F. and L. J. Bauman (1984). Effects of peer support: Reach-to-Recovery and the mastectomy patient. *Advances in Cancer Control: Epidemiology and Research.* New York: Alan R. Liss, pp. 335–51.

Spiegel, D., J. R. Bloom, and I. Yalom (1981). Group support for patients with metastatic cancer. *Arch. Gen. Psychiatry* 38:527–33.

Toseland, R. W. and L. Hacker (1982). Self-help groups and professional involvement. *Soc. Work* 27:341–47.

Tracey, G. S. and Z. Gussow (1976). Self-help health groups: A grass-roots response to a need for services. *J. Appl. Behav. Sci.* 12:381–96.

Vattano, A. J. (1972). Power to the people: Self-help groups. *Soc. Work* 17:7–15.

Walker, K. N., A. MacBride, and M. L. S. Vachon (1977). Social support networks: The crisis of bereavement. *Soc. Sci. Med.* 11:35–42.

# 42

## Alternative Cancer Therapies

Jimmie C. Holland, Natalie Geary, and Alice Furman

Alternative cancer therapies raise perplexing questions for patients, their families, and oncology staff. The extent of their use is evident from the economic impact, estimated at $4 billion per year (Cassileth et al., 1984). The "alternatives" range from treatments that are outright frauds and dangerous to health, to others that are aimed at improving well-being and thereby are assumed to enhance the body's ability to fight the cancer. The latter offer individuals a participatory role in their own care and reflect the increased popularity of more naturalistic approaches among the public. They also reflect a negative view of the cancer treatment and research effort as part of a negative view of medicine in general. Tension between the alleged cancer establishment and a cancer counterculture, however, reached its peak in the 1970s with the debates over the use of laetrile. Presently the issues remain in an era in which individuals assume more responsibility for their own health, hold more holistic health beliefs, and are interested in treatments of cancer that are built on assisting the body in its fight against cancer.

These alternative therapies pose problems for psychooncology because the same behavioral, psychosocial, and psychological intervention methods used in cancer for the management of emotional distress and symptoms control are presented by some alternative therapists as ways to both control tumor growth and to cure it. Combined with simple explanations for the cause of cancer, including response to stress, and drawing upon data from the new field of psychoneuroimmunology, naturalistic treatments appear not only rational but lacking in negative side effects. Patients are confused, searching for hope, yearning for an antidote to feelings of helplessness caused by a tumor whose uncontrolled growth in their body threatens life (Holland, 1982). They have legitimate questions to ask oncology staff members about these alternative methods. In the past, their questions were often stifled for

fear of an angry reaction from the doctor that sometimes amounted to, "If you do that, I won't treat you anymore." This response is growing less common, and oncologists are providing more information about alternative therapies, discussing them more readily and offering advice about use of the specific alternative treatments presented for consideration (ASCO, 1983). Physicians have an obligation to be well informed about these treatments because patients are bombarded with information about them. They may learn of them from the network of individuals who are committed to holistic medical concepts, health food, and the use of alternative therapies. Visits to health food stores reveal an array of cancer therapies supported by testimonials of their efficacy. Questions about these treatments are appropriately brought to oncology staff members. This chapter provides guidelines for responding to such questions and advising patients about the highly emotional issues posed by alternative therapies.

The field of psychological oncology has a particular obligation to serve as a source of information to both patients and staff. As an informed resource, psychooncologists should be able to understand and discuss the psychological appeal of these treatments, know the range of available alternative therapies, their risks and benefits, and be able to assess the likely economic impact with patient and family.

### HISTORICAL CONTEXT

"Cancer cures" by folk remedies have been available for centuries, representing the natural need for people to find the means of treating an otherwise incurable disease (Geary, 1985). In the nineteenth century, cancer quackery, as it was called until the middle of this century, consisted of quasi-medical remedies. Cassileth and others have provided a picture of cancer remedies over the past 150 years (Cassileth, 1986;

**Table 42-1** Popular unorthodox treatments used for cancer in the United States

| Time period | Treatments |
|---|---|
| 1800–1850 | Thomsonianism: stimulation of "vital heat" by steam baths, emetics, enemas (with cayenne pepper) |
| 1850–1900 | Homeopathy: founded by Hahnemann, treatment was based on highly diluted "homeopathic" doses of drugs |
| 1890s | Naturopathy: "natural" approaches by diet, massage, colonic irrigation |
| | Osteopathy and chiropracty: manipulative therapy of bones and spine |
| 1900s | Pills, ointments, tonics, some specific for cancer |
| 1920s | Energy cures: "cosmic energy," "psychic" diagnoses, and "tumor removal" by bloodless surgery |
| 1940s | Koch's glyoxylide |
| 1950s | Hoxsey's cancer cure |
| 1960s | Krebiozen |
| 1970s | Laetrile |
| 1980s | Metabolic therapies, diet treatments, megavitamins, mental imagery applied for antitumor affect, spiritual or faith healing, "immune" therapies |

*Source*: Adapted from B. Cassileth (1986). Unorthodox cancer medicine. *Cancer Invest.* 4:591–98.

Whorton, 1987; Gevitz, 1987) (Table 42-1). Thomsonianism was a popular faith-healing method in this country from 1800 to the 1850s. Thomson, a New Hampshire farmer, felt that he was a gifted healer. He applied the ancient philosophy of treating disease by stimulating the body's "vital heat." His rigorous treatments included enemas containing cayenne pepper, emetics, and steam baths. Whorton (1987) points out that in the mid-1800s people found Thomsonianism appealed to their common sense, which was extolled as a virtue of the common man. There was a prevalent distrust of the medical profession at that time also.

It is interesting that around the same time, the concepts of health maintained through vegetarianism and "natural" foods were popular, similar to the current emphasis on diet. Graham, and later Kellogg, were health authorities who felt that protein resulted in autointoxication, which caused many ailments. The treatment was based on cereals, bran, and laxatives (Whorton, 1987). Many of these concepts persist today in cancer autointoxication remedies that "purify" and cleanse the body through vegetarian diets and colonic irrigations.

Homeopathy, naturopathy, osteopathy, and chiropracty appeared in the latter half of the last century. Hahnemann, the founder of homeopathy, purported to cure disease by employing extremely dilute doses of medicinals. The naturopathic movement of the 1890s—which stated that diseases arose, not from bacteria, but rather from the violation of the natural laws of living—utilized diets, massage, and colonic irrigation for detoxification and purification. Prevention of disease as recommended by Graham and by Kellogg had similar concepts to those applied to treatment of disease. Still founded a school of osteopathy in Missouri and took a far different approach based on manipulation of the spine and limbs to cure disease. "Tonics," pills, and ointments, which were promoted for a variety of ailments, were popular in the early part of this century. Those identified specifically for cancer differed largely in their description of cause and the method of cure. Dr. Chamlee's "Cancer-Specific Purifies the Blood" remedy, for instance, was designed to remove cancer viruses from the blood. In the first half of this century, cosmic-wave and "energy"-wave cures were popular, perhaps mirroring the first medical uses of radiation for cancer.

Beginning with the 1940s, each decade has been dominated by a single widely popular cancer cure. Koch's glyoxylide, popular in the 1940s, was found to be no more than distilled water, representing a fraudulent product promoted solely for economic gain. In the 1950s, Hoxsey's herbal tonic gained national attention. It was composed of "ten herbs said to have been learned from Hoxsey's great-grandfather, whose horse was said to have been cured of leg cancer after grazing in a field where such plants were growing" (ASCO, 1983). Calling himself a naturopath, Harry Hoxsey had no medical degrees. He maintained that cancer was the result of a "major chemical imbalance in the body" that caused "normal cells to mutate into cancerous form," and his tonic restored the "original chemical environment, checking and killing the cancerous cells." He offered no scientific evidence for either his claims about the cause of cancer or its cure, stating that he was "kept too busy to spare time, personnel and facilities for objective study." When challenged on scientific grounds, Hoxsey identified the medical establishment as "the real cancer quacks." Hoxsey realized large profits from the exclusive sale of his tonic. Despite lack of evidence of efficacy and criticism from the medical community, the case against him was in court for 10 years before a federal court injunction made sale of his tonic illegal. The Hoxsey treatment, still available in Mexico, is composed of lactated pepsin, potassium iodide, and herbal balms.

Krebiozen followed a similar course in the 1960s. However, the major sponsor was a distinguished physiologist who became involved in what turned out to be a hoax. No valid evidence of the efficacy of the substance against cancer was ever provided. Said to have been derived from the blood of 2000 horses inoculated with a fungus that causes ''lumpy jaw'' in cattle, it was claimed to stimulate the body's inherent anticancer substances. Again, nothing but anecdotal evidence was offered and the promoters attacked the medical establishment and the FDA for suppressing the use of the drug they claimed saved lives. The popularity of Krebiozen declined after the FDA revealed that on chemical analysis, it was nothing but mineral oil containing creatinine monohydrate, an amino acid present in all animal tissue. No clinical trial was felt warranted by the National Cancer Institute's (NCI) division responsible for screening all potential anticancer agents reported from anyplace in the world (Holland, 1967).

Laetrile, an extract of apricot pits, was the primary alternative treatment of the 1970s. It is still used as part of some unorthodox treatments, despite clearly waning popularity in the 1980s. Developed by Ernst Krebs, laetrile was also called vitamin $B_{17}$ and amygdalin, which placed it beyond the limits of FDA regulation. The laetrile phenomenon is perhaps most notable for the political issues it raised. The concept of a remedy for cancer being suppressed by a ''conspiracy'' of drug companies, medical specialists, researchers, and the FDA was appealing at the time to both ultraconservatives who opposed government regulation as interference with the rights of the individual and to antiestablishment liberals who believed the actions of these agencies were based solely on the profit motive. These otherwise strange bedfellows joined forces as a powerful lobby to obtain passage of a ''Medical Freedom of Choice'' bill to assure that patients with cancer could obtain laetrile (Cassileth, 1982).

In fact from 1957 to 1977, the NCI had carried out drug trials of laetrile in animals. Even though the drug had no evidence of efficacy against cancer, political support was strong and public pressure mounted for a clinical trial. The NCI ran its first clinical trial of an alternative therapy without preclinical proven efficacy in 1977. In 1982 results were published, showing that ''no substantive benefit was observed in terms of cure, improvement, or stabilization of cancer, improvement of symptoms related to cancer, or extension of life span'' (Moertel et al., 1982). In fact, laetrile can produce cyanide toxicity when combined with certain foods (Miller and Howard-Ruben, 1983).

The most accurate and continuous record of the numerous unorthodox cancer treatments has been kept by the American Cancer Society (ACS). All reported remedies since the 1940s have been reviewed by a formal committee of the ACS. The committee has provided thorough reports on major claims over the decades and has made its reports available to physicians and to the public. The Unproven Methods Committee continues to keep a record not only of current alter-

native therapies but also of those that have become inactive in this country (although they may persist elsewhere, especially in Mexico). In 1986, they identified 51 therapies that were placed on the inactive list, including Carcin and Neo-Carcin, Grape Diet, Hett ''Cancer Serum,'' Organic Energy Devices, and Koch's ''antitoxins.'' It is interesting that many of these recycle every few years, making the total registry of treatment identified throughout the last 50 years an important resource. Olsen (1977) noted that 57 cancer cures were widely used in the country between 1893 and 1971, although hundreds were in use regionally.

The term ''unorthodox'' and ''unproven methods'' began to emerge as umbrella terms in the 1970s, replacing the term quackery, which became less acceptable.

## CURRENT ALTERNATIVE THERAPIES

The 1980s have seen a departure from alternative therapies that rely on a single substance such as laetrile (I. J. Lerner, 1984). Our society has come to value personal responsibility for maintaining a healthy state. A holistic approach to health and illness is popular, which includes the concept of the unity of mind and body. When combined with a disaffection with medicine's highly technological and less personalized health care delivery, it is not surprising that the present alternative therapies reflect these social views. The ''cancer establishment,'' consisting of researchers, clinicians, and the organized cancer societies, are targeted for the most severe criticism. As a sign of resistance to the medical establishment, the current alternative therapies (like naturopathy) rely on a holistic approach that recommends purification of the body, detoxification through internal cleansing, and attention to nutritional needs and emotional well-being through life-style changes (Cassileth, 1986). They depend for implementation on the individual's extensive attention to daily routine, food preparation, psychological state, and physical exercise. Participation of family members is often encouraged as well. Perhaps of equal importance, they offer understandable explanations for how cancer developed and why it is potentially controllable by these means. Data are used that show scientific support for the role of diet in cancer risk and evidence of the effect of stress and emotional states on the immune system and hence on the immune system's surveillance of cancer. The oncologist, who offers no such simple or logical explanations for why cancer develops, also uses treatments that have unpleasant and toxic side effects. Their efficacy is discussed with the patient in terms of the potential benefits to be expected and the risk of side effects. Informed consent requires that these be fully and accurately described as an ethical obligation. Some alternative cancer therapists promise cure of cancer, disregarding the moral obligation for informing the patient as honestly as possible. When these facts are coupled with the debate in the public and professional press as to whether the "battle against cancer" is being won or lost, the climate encourages some individuals to explore alternatives.

An added consideration today is the testimonials given by an increasing number of individuals who have survived cancer and who, even though they had traditional medical treatments, often attribute cure to their own attitude or to a particular alternative treatment utilized. In earlier days, the numbers of cured patients were small and those who survived did not reveal that they had had cancer. Such individuals today are articulate and express their beliefs and experiences in detail, giving added support for the use of alternative treatments.

These therapies are now called alternative, adjunctive, complementary, and integrated, which all suggest that they may be used alone or in conjunction with established medical treatments (I. J. Lerner, 1984). Most of the information about this new genre of nontraditional cancer therapies was hearsay until Cassileth and colleagues (1984) reported the first systematic study of contemporary alternative treatments, which explored the attitudes of patients, their practitioners, and the treatments given. Their data, now extended to over 1000 patients, challenged a great many widely held assumptions about alternative therapies. The patients who used unconventional therapies initially used them in conjunction with conventional therapy. Eventually, however, 40% of these patients abandoned standard medical treatment in favor of alternative therapy. The patients were highly educated individuals who were not "grasping at straws" and had often just been diagnosed or were in the early stages of illness. Very few patients (4%) had refused conventional treatment, and 42% perceived that their physicians had been supportive (30%) or neutral (12%) about the pursuit of alternative therapy.

They noted that 60% of the 138 alternative practitioners interviewed had M.D. degrees; 18% of these were board-certified, although none were oncologists. "Although some unorthodox practitioners may well fit the characteristic portrait of quacks and charlatans, many are well-trained, few charge high fees, and most, on the basis of patients' views and their own observations, sincerely believe in the efficacy and rationality of their work" (Cassileth et al., 1984, p. 112). Similarly, 58% of alternative practitioners were either supportive (22%) or neutral (36%) about the patients' continuing conventional treatment.

The following year, M. Lerner provided a journalistic investigation of complementary cancer therapies based on visits to over 30 well-known centers offering these treatments around the world, using his background in social theory and psychology, and his commitment to complementary medicine to examine them. He made observations that confirmed some of those made by Cassileth, despite their approaches from different perspectives (M. Lerner, 1985; M. Lerner and N. Remin, 1985). His observations are helpful to reduce the gulf between the worlds of alternative therapies and conventional medicine. He noted that he found no decisively successful cure for cancer among the complementary therapies he explored. He felt that there was little scientific evidence with which to evaluate the modest contributions to the quality of the patients' lives or to extending their lives. Anecdotal evidence suggested an improved quality of life for some and a small (but significant) number who experienced improvement, which might or might not have been due to the complementary therapy. He noted that there was an increased use of psychological, nutritional, and spiritual approaches by many resourceful patients who attempted to integrate conventional and complementary therapies to make a personalized treatment program that made sense to them (M. Lerner, 1985).

Most alternative treatments studied by Cassileth shared a common view of the cause of cancer and involved a corrective or preventive approach; that is, cancer was seen as symptomatic of an underlying systemic disorder, dysfunction, or "toxicity," which could only be improved by the use of the patient's own biological or psychological abilities. They provided simple, commonsense illness attributions based on eating, elimination, and stressful events. The cause translated directly into a treatment lacking in unpleasant side effects. It appears that treatments that can be clearly explained, make sense, and are consonant with the patient's spiritual or philosophical belief system are most appealing. Some patients comply with established treatment but find emotional support from alternative therapies.

In their national survey, Cassileth and colleagues found six alternative therapies most widely used today, namely, metabolic therapy, diet treatments, megavitamins, mental imagery approaches, mental imagery applied for antitumor effect, spiritual or faith healing, and immunotherapy. Actually, most of the alternative cancer centers use combinations of these treatments. Most include psychological and nutritional components even when more "biological" treatments are given.

## Metabolic Approaches

Metabolic therapy, received by 45% of patients in Cassileth's study, attributes the cause of cancer to toxins and waste materials that interfere with the metabolism, causing liver and pancreatic failure and a degeneration in the immune and "oxygenation" systems. Treatment claiming to reverse this process is based on cleansing the body by dietary manipulations, vitamins, minerals, and enzymes. Treatment consists of "detoxification" of cells by means of colonic irrigations (often using coffee or wheat grass enemas), high doses of vitamins and minerals, and diets that are largely vegetarian.

No scientific evidence exists to demonstrate a positive correlation between metabolic therapy and cancer prevention or cure. In fact, studies have shown that metabolic therapy can be life-threatening, as a result of electrolyte imbalance, bowel necrosis and perforation, amebiasis, toxic colitis, and vitamin deficiency (Cassileth, 1986). Of the metabolic practitioners, 65% had medical degrees, a substantially higher percentage than with any other type of alternative therapy. Several of these metabolic therapies are also claimed to enhance immune function.

## Nutritional Approaches

Dietary change along with psychological approaches are present in most alternative cancer therapy programs and were used by 37% of those seen in Cassileth's study, varying from a grape cure popular several years ago to the present emphasis on two major diets, the wheat grass diet of the Hippocrates Health Institute and the macrobiotic diet of the East–West Foundation.

In the macrobiotic approach, cancer is attributed to body dysfunction resulting from an imbalance, in this case, of Yin and Yang. Tumors are designated as either Yin (hollow tumors of the stomach and bladder) or Yang (compact tumors in organs such as the pancreas or liver). Like many Eastern and Asian medical theories, health is based on maintaining a balance between opposing forces, and treatment recommends consumption of whichever force the patient lacks. Combined with a way of life that emphasizes self-reflection and restoration of universal balance are 10 levels of macrobiotic diets (Howard-Ruben and Miller, 1984).

There is no available scientific evidence to support the effectiveness of macrobiotic diets in cancer management (ACS, 1983). The support, thus far, as with many alternative therapies, has been anecdotal reports from a small number of patients who may have been utilizing a plurality of treatments, including conventional therapy, vitamin D, and ascorbic acid. Iron deficiencies and weight loss are severely detrimental side effects of these diets for the cancer patient (ACS, 1983).

Although macrobiotic therapy is the most common nutritional approach to cancer therapy, megavitamin therapy represents a significant alternative nutritional

therapy. Of the patients in Cassileth's study, 20% consumed large quantities of high-dose vitamins as part of the protocol. Practitioners claim that high-dose vitamins enhance the body's capacity to destroy malignant cells, despite the data suggesting that excessive vitamin intake can be toxic. It has been difficult for the public to distinguish between diets that are measures to reduce cancer risk and those that promote cure. In 1982, The National Research Council published a report on diet, nutrition, and cancer that recommended minimizing carcinogenic substances and fat intake in the diet, and increasing whole-grain, fruit, and vegetable consumption. These preventive guidelines were immediately incorporated by alternative therapists into treatment strategies that have gained widespread popularity (M. Lerner, 1985).

## Psychological-Spiritual Approaches

A more clearly psychological approach widely practiced in the United States is that of the Simonton method, developed by Carl Simonton, M.D. in 1973, and widely promoted through the book, *Getting Well Again* (Simonton et al., 1980). Cancer is said to develop because of a complex interaction between negative personality traits and stressful events, suggesting personal responsibility for illness. The personality traits common to cancer patients described include poor self-image, limited capacity for trust, tendency toward self-pity, and inability to develop long-term relationships. Therapy at the Simonton Center Counseling and Research Center consists of psychosocial assessment and analysis of the patient's previously unhealthy behavior, and visual imagery and relaxation techniques. While the Simontons have softened their approach, which was noted to have the potential of producing guilt in some patients whose disease progressed despite treatment, the therapy still places major responsibility for improvement on the individual's role. A similar approach by Bernard Siegel, a surgeon, places emphasis on a positive attitude to survive by becoming an "exceptional" patient (1986). There is a similarity to the "blame the victim" philosophies, common in our culture in relationship to crime and other misfortunes, suggesting that those who do not survive somehow did not have a sufficiently strong will or attitude. A debate over the ethical implications of these positions is needed.

Visual imagery, central to the Simonton therapeutic approach, is assumed to assist the immune system to fight the cancer. Patients are asked to visualize their cancer cells as weak, and healthy cells as strong, using an acceptable model for visual destruction of cancer cells. This imagery assists in the destruction of the patient's cancer cells, and relaxation reduces stress, thereby enhancing immune function in order to fight the cancer. Although the relationship between stress, the immune system, and cancer progression in humans is thus far inconclusive, data are used by some alternative cancer therapists to promote simplistic explanations of benefit. In 1983, because of the popularity of the psychosocial and behavioral approaches to cancer treatment, the ACS evaluated the effectiveness of unproven psychological methods; they reported that "there is not enough evidence to support the theory that the use of techniques for reducing stress (such as visual imagery, hypnosis, relaxation) can change the risk of developing cancer or the length of survival. While these therapies may substantially reduce patient distress during treatment, there is no evidence to support their use except as adjuvant, not alternative therapies (ACS, November, 1984).

Finally, there is an array of alternative therapies that fall into the category of life-style and health promotion therapies, which include spiritual and philosophical theories about how to achieve harmony between the patient and nature. The promotion of spiritual and mystical approaches to healing is an integral component of the macrobiotic diet, the Hippocrates program, the Lukas Klinik, Rudolf Steiner anthroposophical approach, and the Bristol Cancer Help Center in England, which uses spiritual healers. Cancer is commonly attributed to an external evil that must be exorcised in order to control the disease (Cassileth et al., 1984). Unlike other alternative healers, faith healers do not publish any results but promote their treatments on the basis of patients' faith, hope, and belief in the method. Hence, patients become proponents of the therapy and make pilgrimages to the treatment centers. One of the most popular faith healers was Tony Agpoa, whose followers continue to practice in the Philippines. Through massage, prayer, and "psychic" surgery, they remove the patient's cancer from the body. Analyses of samples from the tumors "removed" by "bloodless" surgery have revealed animal tissue.

## Immunotherapy

Hans Nieper's clinic in Hannover, Burton in the Bahamas, and Levingston in California are well-known examples of alternative immunotherapies. Immunoaugmentative cancer therapy (IAT), developed by L. Burton, Ph.D., and practiced exclusively at the Immunology Research Center in the Bahamas, is among the most popular. Cancer is attributed to a defective immune system, and treatment attempts to restore protein balance through the injection of human serum protein fractions, to restore the immune system and destroy tumor tissues (ASCO, 1983; Miller and Howard-Ruben, 1983). In 1974, the research center

was denied FDA approval of an investigational drug application, noting insufficient evidence of antitumor effects. The clinic closed in July 1985 but reopened in early 1986 because of public pressure. Analysis at that time by the NCI found the injections to be contaminated with the HIV and hepatitis-B viruses (Curt et al., 1986).

Finally, these alternative cancer treatments represent those that have gained national or international popularity. Folk medicines for cancer peculiar to one culture or another are continuously used. When they are brought to its attention, the NCI subjects all of them to a screening test for possible efficacy. "Cures" continue to appear, whether new or recycled from the past, but until cancer is more generally seen as a curable disease, these alternatives will continue to flourish and be touted as potential cures (M. Lerner, 1985).

## ONCOLOGY STAFF AND ALTERNATIVE THERAPIES

Those who work in oncology can gain useful insights about the importance of addressing emotional needs during cancer treatment by examination of some of the psychologically oriented alternative methods that largely provide hope, control by self-help, and a sense of concern for the whole person. These issues have been raised as criticisms of our conventional cancer treatment settings in which, despite best efforts, patients sometimes perceive that our emphasis is on the biological aspects of the therapy, without the equal emphasis on the person and his or her participation in treatment. The laetrile trial provided an interesting insight into why some patients chose to participate in treatment by this unproven method. A common answer was "The doctor said there was nothing more he could do for me. What did I have to lose?" (Redding et al., 1981). The sense of failure of traditional therapy, the loss of hope, and the perceived lack of the physician's commitment to continued care with altered treatment goals resulted in their leaving the doctor at a time that they most needed emotional support from the same physician and staff. Indeed, there is never a time that *nothing* can be done; comfort care in the face of advancing illness is an integral part of continuity of care. Clearly, part of the onus is on the oncology community to provide maximal emotional support in the context of conventional treatment. The more patients' needs are met, the less their likelihood of seeking alternative care.

Several guidelines should be used in approaching the issues of alternative treatments with patients and families (Table 42-2).

1. When patients indicate an interest in an alternative treatment, evaluate the reason they appear to be

**Table 42-2**  Oncology staff and alternative therapies

- Evaluate the reason for the patient's wish for an alternative therapy. Does it reflect emotional needs that are not being addressed during conventional therapy?
- Be well informed about current alternative therapies.
- Provide accurate information about them to patients.
- Encourage questions, take all questions seriously.
- Discuss risks and benefits.
- Avoid moral judgments.
- Advise pro and con based on therapy presented, its potential to interfere or not with conventional therapy and its possible adjunctive versus alternative use.
- Follow up with questions after a few weeks to monitor for any negative emotional or physical signs.

pursuing it. Sometimes it may reflect that their emotional needs are not being met.

2. Health professionals working in oncology should be well informed about current alternative therapies, including their potential physical or emotional risks, as well as their benefits. Because they change all the time, one must maintain information about those that are popular with patients in a specific geographic area.

3. The oncology office or clinic should have information available to patients on alternative treatments; the guide to laypersons prepared by the American Society of Clinical Oncology is excellent (ASCO, 1983). A new program has developed which provides a data base to store this information and to make a summary of a given remedy available, which can be accessed quickly on the doctor's computer terminal and by patients and families (Monaco, 1986). It might be a good idea for regional cancer centers to appoint one individual to keep abreast of information on unproven methods in order to serve as a resource to others.

4. The doctor or oncology staff member should have a relationship to the patient that indicates to the patient that a question about an alternative therapy will be taken seriously without anger or ridicule and certainly without the threat of withdrawing conventional treatment if it is pursued.

5. Patients may be referred to a psychiatrist if the staffperson has trouble understanding the reasons for requesting information and to help patients assess it more objectively. A psychiatric consultant may feel more familiar with the emotional process that leads patients to seek unproven methods.

6. In honestly discussing unproven remedies with the patient, the health care professional must be careful to avoid moral judgments. The "theory" behind many methods may seem ridiculous, but it may be quite plausible to others. For the cancer patient whose education has not been in the physical sciences, whose understanding of body mechanisms is not sophisti-

cated, and who is facing a devastating illness, simple remedies that make sense are appealing.

The discussion of an alternative treatment may bring to light misconceptions about the cause of cancer and the rationale for treatment. It provides an opportunity to extend the explanations for the medical treatment plan, its rationale, and expected benefits. Optimism in the doctor and staff conveys a spirit of "working together" for a common outcome and makes the patient a "team player" and not a passive recipient of treatment.

7. The pros and cons of the particular therapy should be discussed in a dispassionate manner, asking the patient for details of what has been proposed. If there are contraindications, especially caloric reduction, debilitating enemas, or hazardous immunotherapy, the treatment should be advised against, citing medical risks. When there appear to be no medical contraindications to pursuing a given treatment while simultaneously continuing conventional therapy, this should be pointed out. The treatments, used as adjuncts to medical treatments, can contribute to psychological well-being.

8. When potentially psychologically negative aspects appear with a particular treatment, benefits and risks should be discussed. The benefits of self-participation in treatment and the sense of hope and control can be recognized. However, the negative aspects of personal responsibility for having developed cancer and the responsibility for disease progression should it occur, should also be discussed. The person should be assured that transient depression or discouragement does not contribute to tumor growth, as patients sometimes believe.

9. The physician or oncology staff member should follow up in a few weeks with a question about how the alternative treatment is going. Should there be obvious negative physical or emotional consequences, discontinuance should be recommended. Monitoring progress and showing concern about the alternative therapy confirms concern for the person as a whole and reflects absence of criticism about the decision.

## SUMMARY

Alternative cancer therapies over this and the past centuries are reflections of the culture's views of medicine and health. Contemporary alternative cancer treatments incorporate a naturalistic, holistic appeal that parallels the health-conscious culture with its strong emphasis on mind–body relationships. Present alternative therapies are utilized by educated, resourceful individuals seeking to use all means at their disposal to fight cancer. Such approaches reduce the sense of helplessness and reestablish hope. Most alternative cancer centers use combined approaches, which include metabolic therapies aimed at body purification and cleansing (by colonic irrigation, diets, and megavitamins) and immune enhancement, psychological approaches to mind–body and spiritual healing, and dietary regimes. Some, particularly the metabolic and rigid dietary regimes, may carry hazardous risks to cancer patients. Psychological approaches, while more benign, have negative effects when accepted to the extent of establishing guilt for disease or disease progression.

The staff must discuss alternative therapies with patients, encouraging their questions, and offering advice about risks and benefits. Alternative cancer therapies, while constantly changing, are apt to continue until cancer is more generally successfully treated. This suggests a strong need for those working in oncology centers to understand the appeal of alternative treatments to patients and the need for staff to deal sympathetically and thoughtfully with patients' questions about them.

## REFERENCES

American Cancer Society (1984). Statement on the effects of emotions on cancer. Internal communication. New York: American Cancer Society, June.

American Cancer Society (1983). *Unproven Methods of Cancer Management: Macrobiotic Diets*. New York: American Cancer Society.

American Society of Clinical Oncology (ASCO), Subcommittee on Unorthodox Therapies (1983). Ineffective cancer therapy: A guide for the layperson. *J. Clin. Oncol.* 1:154–63.

Cassileth, B. (1982). After laetrile, what? *N. Engl. J. Med.* 306(24):1482–84.

Cassileth, B. (1986). Unorthodox cancer medicine. *Cancer Invest.* 4:591–98.

Cassileth, B., E. J. Lusk, B. A. Strouse, and B. J. Bodenheimer (1984). Contemporary unorthodox treatments in cancer medicine. *Ann. Intern. Med.* 101:105–12.

Curt, G., A. Katterhagen, and G. Mahoney (1986). Immunoaugmentative therapy: A primer on the perils of unproved treatments. *J.A.M.A.* 255:505–7.

Gavitz, N. (1987). Sectarian medicine. *J.A.M.A.* 257:1636–40.

Geary, N. (1985). *Indian Explanatory Models of Illness and Cancer*. Unpublished honors thesis, Harvard University, Boston.

Holland, J. C. (1982). Why patients seek unproven cancer remedies: A psychological perspective. *CA* 32:10–14.

Holland, J. F. (1967). The Krebiozen story: Is cancer quackery dead? *J.A.M.A.* 200:213–18.

Holleb, A. (ed.). (1982). *Unproven Methods of Cancer Management*. New York: American Cancer Society.

Howard-Ruben, J. and N. J. Miller (1984). Unproven methods of cancer management: II. Current trends and implications for patient care. *Oncol. Nurs. Forum* 11(1):67–73.

Janssen, W. F. (1979). Cancer quackery: The past in the present. *Semin. Oncol.* 6:526–35.

Lerner, M. (1985). A report on complementary cancer therapies. *Advances: J. Inst. Advancement Health* 2(1):31–43.

Lerner, M. and N. Remin (1985). A variety of integral cancer therapies. *Advances: J. Inst. Advancement Health* 2(3):14–33.

Miller, J. and J. Howard-Ruben (1983). Unproven methods of cancer management: I. Background and historical perspectives. *Oncol. Nurs. Forum* 10(4):46–52.

Moertel, C. A., T. R. Fleming, J. Rubin, L. K. Kvols, G. Sarna, R. Koch, V. E. Currie, C. N. Young, S. E. Jones, and J. P. Davignon (1982). A clinical trial of amygdalin in the treatment of human cancer. *N. Engl. J. Med.* 306(4):201–6.

Monaco, G. P. (1986). The primary care physician: The first line of defense in the battle against health fraud. *Med. Times* 114(5):43–48.

Olsen, K. B. (1977). Drugs, cancer and charlatans. In J. Horton and G. Hill (eds.), *Clinical Oncology*. Philadelphia: W. B. Saunders, pp. 182–91.

Redding, K., L. Beutler, S. Jones, F. Meyskins, and T. Moon (1981). Psychosocial attitudes of cancer patients treated with laetrile or other phase II agents. *Proc. Seventy-Second Annu. Mtg. Am. Assoc. Cancer Res. and Seventeenth Annu. Mtg. Am. Soc. Clin. Oncol.* 22:394 (Abstract No. C-243).

Siegel, B. (1986). *Love, medicine and miracles*. New York: Harper and Row.

Simonton, O. C., S. Matthews-Simonton, and J. L. Creighton (1980). *Getting Well Again: A Step-by-Step, Self-Help Guide to Overcoming Cancer for Patients and Their Families*. New York: Bantam Books.

Whorton, J. C. (1987). Traditions of folk medicine in America. *J.A.M.A.* 257:1632–35.

# PART VIII

# Childhood Cancer: Psychological Issues and Their Management

# 43

# Developmental Stage and Adaptation: Child and Adolescent Model

## Julia H. Rowland

In caring for the young patient, health care professionals necessarily bring with them a broad model of age-related milestones and tasks against which to measure the individual child's growth and development. These include an awareness of the relative timing and progression of changes in physical maturation and coordination, acquisition of language and cognitive skills, and expression of affective and social behavior. It is these sets of criteria that permit evaluation of healthy development and that also serve, at times, to define pathology. Although there is a natural emphasis on a developmental perspective in providing and tailoring medical care for children and adolescents, two important changes have led to a greater need to look closely at the role developmental issues play in the management of cancer patients.

The first of these is the dramatic progress over the past two decades in developing effective treatments for the common childhood tumors (see Fig. 1-1). Overall mortality from cancer in children has been almost halved since 1950 (ACS, 1987). In the 1960s acute lymphocytic leukemia (ALL), the most common form of childhood cancer, was almost uniformly fatal. All but 4% of children diagnosed were dead in 6 months. Today 65% of children treated for ALL can expect to be cured of their disease. Depending on biological indicators and place of treatment, this figure may increase to 75–80%. Although 5-year survival rates vary widely depending on site of the tumor (Table 43-1), more and more children can now expect to be cured or experience long periods in which their illness is controlled and they can resume routine activities. The growing number of survivors and children whose disease is chronic has raised concerns about the delayed effects on psychological and social as well as physical functioning, of the more aggressive multimodal therapies that have made cure possible (Meadows and Silber, 1985; Lansky et al., 1986; Teta et al., 1986;

Maguire, 1983; see also Chapter 7, this volume). Additionally, as research within the population of treated patients has grown, it has become apparent that age at the time of treatment may be an important mediating variable in subsequent adjustment. A number of studies have shown that younger children (<6 years) who receive cranial irradiation as part of their therapy for leukemia are at greater risk of subsequent cognitive deficits than older ones (Eiser and Lansdown, 1977; Goff et al., 1980; Moss et al., 1981; Meadows et al., 1981). On a more general level, Koocher and colleagues (1979) found that treatment produces less persistent and severe developmental disruptions in infants and young children than in school-aged children or adolescents. The improved prospect for cure makes imperative closer attention to what normal tasks of development may be affected transiently or permanently by treatment.

The second change fostering renewed emphasis on developmental concerns has been the greater participation of psychologists in all aspects of medical care (Stone, 1983; Roberts et al., 1984). Although the roots of this movement are varied, there has been a general uniformity of purpose, namely, to provide a coherent integration between biomedical and behavioral knowledge with the goal of using information generated from these efforts to promote health and improve disease prevention, diagnosis, therapy, and rehabilitation (Miller, 1981). As interest in the field of behavioral medicine has grown, so too has the contribution of developmental psychologists to these efforts. Contrary to what one might expect given the roots of this field in early childhood development, the emphasis on incorporating developmental issues in medicine has been most strongly evidenced in the area of geriatric care (Bellak and Tokso, 1976; Birren and Schaie, 1977; Kart et al., 1978; Solomon et al., 1982). The research toward establishing a synthesis between child develop-

**Table 43-1**   Incidence, peak age at onset, and survival estimates for the major pediatric tumors

| Disease | Annual incidence* | Peak age | Relative 5-year disease-free survival rate (%) |
|---|---|---|---|
| Leukemia | 42.1 | | |
|   ALL | | 4–10 Years | 75 |
|   AML | | Even distribution | 30 |
| Brain tumors | 23.9 | | |
|   Medulloblastoma | | <5 Years | 40 |
|   High-grade astrocytoma | | Even distribution | 20 |
|   Brain stem glioma | | Even distribution | 10 |
| Lymphoma | 13 | | |
|   Hodgkin's disease | | Adolescence | 90 |
|   Non-Hodgkin's lymphoma | | Adolescence | 70 |
| Neuroblastoma | 9 | <2 Years | 5 (stage IV) |
| Soft-tissue sarcoma | 8 | <5 Years and adolescence | 50 |
| Wilms' tumor | 8 | 1–3 Years | 90 |
| Bone tumors | 6 | | |
|   Osteosarcoma | | Adolescence | 70 |
|   Ewing's sarcoma | | Adolescence | 60 |
| Retinoblastoma | 3 | Infancy | 90 |

*Source*: Courtesy of Dr. Paul A. Meyers, Department of Pediatrics, Memorial Sloan-Kettering Cancer Center, New York.
*Given as per million population. Overall incidence of childhood cancer is estimated at 6600 cases per year, making it a rare disease. However, with estimated 1800 deaths in 1988, it remains the chief cause of death by disease in children aged 3–14 (*Cancer Facts and Figures*: ACS, 1988).

ment theory and behavioral and psychiatric disorders represents a more recent effort (Achenbach, 1978, 1982; Bowlby, 1988). As Maddux and colleagues (1986) point out, application of a developmental perspective in pediatric health care is only in its infancy.

This movement has extended most recently into the field of pediatric oncology. While there is beginning to be an extensive literature on the psychological impact of life-threatening illness in childhood (Adams and Deveau, 1984; Hall, 1982; Koocher, 1986b; Spinetta, 1982; Spinetta and Lansky, 1982; see also the excellent review by Van Dongen-Melman and Sanders-Woudstra, 1986), researchers are also beginning to turn their attention to determining what impact cancer or life-threatening illness has on specific age groups within childhood (Spinetta, 1974; Geist, 1979; Bibace and Walsh, 1980; Blum, 1984; Burbach and Peterson, 1986; Dinkfelt et al., 1986; Rait and Holland, 1986; Bush, 1987). One consequence is greater sensitivity in medical education to the role of psychosocial issues in management of pediatric malignancies (Hays et al., 1985).

This chapter reviews briefly the developmental tasks of childhood and how the physical, cognitive, emotional, and social changes that occur as the child grows are both affected by and determine, to a large extent, the psychological impact of life-threatening illness. Because of its importance to our patients, particular attention is given to understanding children's con-

cepts of illness and death at different ages. Using this information, stage-specific interventions are presented that address the different needs of the growing child and suggest ways to minimize the most common acute and chronic disruptions associated with pediatric malignancies and their treatment.

This chapter does not present a theoretical model; rather, it attempts to synthesize the findings of existing research on child development as they relate to response to illness. The emphasis is on adopting a developmental perspective from which one can evaluate the psychological impact of cancer on a child.

While it is recognized that age is not synonymous with stage or development, some divisions must be imposed to provide a structure within which to organize the information available. This chronological structure consists of infancy to toddler (birth to 2 years), preschool age (3–5), school-aged child (6–11), and adolescence (12–18). For each of the periods delineated, the age-related developmental tasks are reviewed. These include the physical, cognitive, affective, social, and psychosexual changes associated with each period. The ways in which childrens' concepts of illness and death evolve are also covered. The well-known life cycle models of stage development formulated by Erik Erikson and Sigmund and Anna Freud are also presented to provide a framework of reference.

While the common tumors and the periods with which they are associated are summarized in Table

**Table 43-2** Common psychosocial concerns of illness ("the five D's")

| Five D's | Nature of concern |
|---|---|
| Distance | Altered interpersonal relationships, dislocation |
| Dependence | Versus independence |
| Disability | Achievement disruptions |
| Disfigurement | Body–sexual image and integrity |
| Death | Existential concerns: painful death |

43-1, the disruptions caused by illness and treatment specific to each period are covered in detail. In reviewing adaptation to illness across the life span, Rowland and Holland identified five common sources of problems, referred to as the "five D's." They are *distance* in interpersonal relations, issues related to *dependence* and independence, *disability* in social or school achievement, *disfigurement* or physical impairment, and fears or anxieties about *death* (see Table 43-2). Although the primacy of each problem area may vary in a given period or with respect to a specific person, these common areas of stress appear across the life span. When analyzed with respect to its source, almost any specific problem in adjustment can be seen as falling into one of these basic categories. The content of each, however, varies across age periods. For example, in considering alterations in interpersonal relations secondary to illness, separation from one or both parents during hospitalization causes acute distress for the 2-year-old, whereas absence from peers may be more stressful for the hospitalized adolescent. While both responses reflect a disruption in interpersonal relationships, the roles of the individuals involved and meaning attached to the changes may be very different depending on the child's developmental needs. Finally, interventions that address each of these five areas of disruption and that are specific to each period are presented. (A brief summary of all this information is contained in the full developmental chart that appears in the appendices at the back of this volume.)

Before proceeding to each of the sections, however, several caveats are needed about the interpretation and use of such information. First, this chapter is only a beginning effort to describe the needs of sick children and to foster an appreciation for the utility of embracing a developmental perspective in anticipating and managing these needs. The rapidity and complexity of changes during childhood make their full elaboration impossible. Still, it is possible to summarize the essential changes in each period and how they affect psychological response during illness. This leaves to the reader the job of elaborating, from personal experience and broader research or reading, the finer details of growth

and development in the population with which he or she works.

Second, individuals progress at their own rate. While all children are expected to accomplish the developmental milestones described, the age brackets for doing so vary. In some cases, achievement of a specific milestone occurs within a very narrow period. In other instances, such as in the onset of puberty, the range may span several years, and even several developmental periods. Some children may be precocious in their acquisition of one skill and average or slow in others. This is particularly true for children who are ill. Frequently in school-aged children who are ill, motor skills are compromised while verbal and reasoning ability, because of the significant time spent among adults in medical settings, may be advanced.

Third, the developmental and much of the illness-related information provided reflects norms and responses reported within study samples of predominantly white, middle-class children. While there is a whole body of literature detailing cross-cultural studies of development, we cannot hope to begin to address the results of this research here. It is important to be aware, however, that the value placed on achievement of specific milestones varies across cultures as well as across economic class. The emphasis on education seen in highly industrialized countries may be second to that of meeting obligations to family or community in more rural or agrarian settings. Hence, while illness causes concern for absence from school in the young child in our culture, failure to carry on social or family roles may be the more acute concern for the child from a third-world country who is ill. Similarly, while inability to hold a job during illness may not be important for the adolescent from a middle-class background, it may be critically important to the welfare of the family of the adolescent from a blue-collar background.

In a similar vein, rates at which milestones are achieved and their nature may also vary by individual and social background. In an interesting study of concepts of cancer, black schoolchildren reported that they felt significantly more vulnerable to the disease than did their white peers (Michielutte and Diseker, 1982). Thus, in applying a developmental perspective, the clinician must be sensitive to differences in cultural and social mores as well as to individual differences.

## INFANCY TO TODDLER: BIRTH–2

Of the four periods of childhood, the developmental changes that occur in the first 3 years of life are probably the most dramatic. At the beginning of the period, a wholly dependent, immature (though physically highly complex) child progresses through a rapid and systematic series of maturational processes that enable him or her by the end of the period to walk, talk, feed himself or herself, engage in reasonably coordinated purposive behavior, and in the case of most children by 36 months, exert control over bowel and bladder functioning. Maturation of the CNS is principal among the forces driving these changes. Infants were once thought to be helpless at birth. Greater sophistication in research techniques has permitted researchers to discover that infants come with more sophisticated "hard wiring" than earlier recognized. We now know that babies have visual acuity and show recognition of and preference for humanlike facial patterns (Cohen, 1979); at only several hours of age they also manifest distinct taste preferences. Finally, as any parent will attest, infants, just in the way they cry and coo, exert enormous control over the behavior of their adult caretakers. It is of interest to note, however, that babies born more than 4 weeks premature have difficulty molding to the cuddle of their caretaker, because of the immaturity of the frontal and parietal brain regions; this consequence may have import for early bonding processes.

Two key requirements for normal development are the presence of a primary caretaker, usually the mother, and consistency in caretaking. The importance of the mother–infant bond has been a historical focus of attention (Stern, 1985). The assumption has always been that initially infants do not experience themselves as separate from their mother, a state referred to as normal autism. Anna Freud (1963, 1965) described the work of infancy as the task of separating the self from this symbiotic relationship, thus permitting the child to begin to develop a sense of self as an individual (separation to individuation) (see also the work of Margaret Mahler and Sybil Escalona). Erik Erikson (1963) emphasized that the child's basic sense of trust and hope in the world grows out of a recognition of a consistent pattern in the response of providers as well as of internal stimuli.

This early appreciation that people will respond to him or her in a certain fashion and that he or she will be able to meet their expectations leads to a sense of rudimentary ego identity. Trust enables the child to let the mother go because her return is reliable. The converse, however, is also true. Inconsistency in caretaking, by undermining the child's belief that his or her needs will be met and providing mixed cues as to how the world views him or her, results in withdrawal or clinging overdependency. This latter behavior is distinct from the natural "clinginess" seen at 6–9 months when children exhibit stranger anxiety, or at 24–36 months as their motor skills enable them to dash off in different directions resulting in bouts of separation anxiety when they find themselves in unfamiliar territory.

Consistency is also a fundamental element in cog-

nitive development. Dependent at the start on reflexive activity, development proceeds in what Piaget refers to as the sensorimotor period (ages birth–2), through repetition of movements and imitation of goal-oriented actions (reaching, grasping, and moving toward objects or persons). The growth of these behaviors is facilitated by the maturing nervous system, and importantly, the sensory pleasure the activities initially bring (e.g., sucking and feeding, crying and being cuddled), and later because they are met with a supportive response (e.g., getting a desired object, the applause of a parent, a hug). It is hard to imagine an infant being able to make sense of a world in which the same action brought a different response every day. It is equally difficult to imagine wanting to interact with a world that was boring or lacked change. Hence stimulation is another critical component of healthy development.

A third critical component is the opportunity to explore or interact with the environment. As Piaget's research (1952) elegantly displayed, children (indeed all humans) learn by doing. Restriction as a consequence of physical limitation, handicap, or environmental deprivation (poverty, protected-environment care) leads to slowing down of the acquisition of or failure to develop essential skills in infancy and early childhood.

As infants increase their field of exploration, learn to walk, and move into toddlerhood, the developmental emphasis shifts away from that of establishing trust to one of achieving autonomy. Mastery of bladder and bowel control, completed by the end of this or the beginning of the next period (age 2–3), has long been viewed as a critical milestone because of its importance in socialization. Its power to produce pleasure and displeasure from internal (physical) as well as from external (social) sources makes control of these functions the unique metaphor for the fundamental struggle of the toddler period, that is, mastery and control of the internal and external environment. Efforts at self-control and control over objects in the environment increase, as do stubbornness, negativism, and tantrums. Erikson (1963) stresses that during this period failure to gain a sense of control without the loss of self-esteem results in shame and self-doubt.

The parallel to individuation in the terms of Piaget is the cognitive achievement of object concept, or the ability of a child to see himself or herself as separate from the objects in the environment (For a lucid review of Piaget's developmental stages see Ginsburg and Opper, 1969). The attainment of this seemingly simple yet profound ability is manifest by the child who, when an object is hidden under a blanket in front of him or her, searches for it rather than acting as though it had ceased to exist. This occurs around 4–10 months. Object constancy, the capacity to represent objects or persons mentally in their absence, is achieved much later than object permanence and marks the end of the sensorimotor period.

The acquisition of language heralds the beginning of preoperational thought, which characterizes the child from 2 to 7 years. During this stage, the child's growing vocabulary enables him or her to talk about and imagine objects and events not present, and to express feelings. Because it is hard to know what the preverbal child is thinking, it is difficult to know what children under the age of 2 think of illness and death. Maurer (1961) has suggested that perception of the differences between the physiological states of sleeping and waking may represent early development of appreciation of being and nonbeing. Death is most commonly thought to be understood as separation from parents at this stage, that is, loss of parental comfort. (Table 43-3 summarizes the developmental changes in concepts of death over the life span.) Before age 2 there is probably little understanding of illness. Rather, the child likely interprets and responds to perceived fear, anxiety, anger, and sadness in the parent. Once children begin to acquire a vocabulary, however, we can begin to explore their feelings. Bibace and Walsh (1980) describe the child of 2 as beginning to have a phenomenistic view of illness. Children at this age conceptualize illness in terms of a single external symptom, often a sensory phenomenon, at one time in the child's experience associated with an illness (e.g., "A heart attack is from the sun"). Burbach and Peterson (1986) provide an excellent review of the developmental literature on children's thinking about illness and health. Their summary of the relevant findings by age is provided in Table 43-4. It is important to note at the onset that illness concepts tend to lag behind overall cognitive development (Perrin and Gerrity, 1981), and that siblings of ill children often have a less developed concept of disease than their unaffected peers (Caradang et al., 1979).

## Disruptions of Illness: Birth–2

### ALTERED INTERPERSONAL RELATIONS

Although interpersonal relationships may be dramatically altered when illness and treatment occur during other periods in the life span, disruption of these important ties, particularly parental ties, probably has no more profound effect than in the earliest years of life. Evidence for the dramatic effect of parental separation in childhood comes from early studies of hospitalized infants (Spitz, 1945) as well as from the literature on animals (Harlow and Zimmerman, 1959; Harlow and Harlow, 1962) and human babies who lack or lose a parent (Bowlby, 1960; Mahler et al., 1975).

**Table 43-3**  Developmental stages in the concept of death and life

| Age or period | Understanding and response |
|---|---|
| 0–2 Years | (<18 months) No formal concept of death. Perception of differences between sleeping and waking may represent early development of appreciation of being and nonbeing. In addition, infants do react emotionally to loss of a significant person, especially the mother. At the latter end of this period, death is thought to be understood as separation from parents, loss of parents' comfort, resulting in anger, worry, withdrawal. |
| 3–5 Years | Expansion of death concept to include loss of loving and protective object. Death is seen as temporary departure or absence, hence reversible. Child sometimes exhibits thoughts that indicate that he or she believes it is possible to come back to life—magical thinking. At the latter end of this period, there is an appreciation of removal from one kind of physical existence to another (e.g., angels in heaven). |
| 6–11 Years | During the early school years, the concept of death is incomplete and concrete, and death is often personified (e.g., "bogey man"). Death may also be associated with darkness, evil, violence, and sleeping. Death is associated with grief for anticipated (or actual) separation from loved ones, and with fear when seen as punishment for wrong acts (external versus biological process). Latency-age child begins to understand death as permanent, nonreversible, contributing to fears of mutilation and physical injury. |
| Adolescence | Death comes to be recognized as a final and irrevocable biological event, yet it is accompanied by disbelief in the possibility of one's personal death (adolescent egocentricity). |
| Early adulthood | Death is viewed as a universal and natural end point of physical life. |
| Middle adulthood | This stage requires the anticipation of and preparation for parental death and formulation of personal wills. |
| Mature adulthood | Change in the time perspective leads to the individual's awareness of being on the upper half of the age curve with time perceived as "years left" versus "years since birth." It involves the personalization of and mental rehearsing for death: men from heart attacks and women left with widowhood. |
| Late adulthood | This stage is characterized by the realistic assessment of life expectancy with concerns for dying more than for death itself. |

**Table 43-4**   A cognitive-developmental synthesis of important findings concerning children's concepts of physical illness

| Reference | Stage of cognitive development | | |
| --- | --- | --- | --- |
| | Preoperations (approx. 2–6 or 7 years) | Concrete operations (approx. 7–11 or 12 years) | Formal operations (approx. 12 years–adult) |
| Bibace and Walsh (1980) | Phenomenism; contagion | Contamination; internalization | Physiologic; psychophysiologic |
| Blos (1956) | Descriptive stage | Explanatory stage | Causative stage |
| Brewster (1982) | Lack of understanding; egocentricism; finalism | Physicalism; semiphysical reasoning | Physicalism; interaction of illness variables with underlying logic |
| Campbell (1975a,b, 1978) | More likely to accept sick role; less likely to see themselves as stoic in the face of illness | Increasing denial of sick role; more likely to see themselves as stoic in the face of illness, particularly in males | Attention to specific diseases and/or diagnoses; deviations from role behaviors; and use of restrictive illness concepts |
| Gellert (1961) | Self-blame | Self-blame, increasing objectivity | Objectivity |
| Kister and Patterson (1980) | Overextension of contagion concept; illness as a form of immanent justice | More appropriate use of contagion concept; less likely to use immanent justice explanations | |
| Nagy (1951) | Incapable of understanding the real cause of illness; all illness caused by infection | All disease, illnesses, infections caused by one type of germ | Different diseases, illnesses, infections caused by different germs; not all illnesses are caused by germs |
| Neuhauser et al. (1978) | Use external rather than internal cues to determine illness | Use internal rather than external cues to assess illness; increasing control over illness | More control over illness; less vulnerable to illness |
| Perrin and Gerrity (1981) | Global | Concrete rules, internalization | Physiologic; psychophysiologic |

*Source*: Reprinted with permission from D.J. Burbach and L. Peterson (1986). Children's concepts of physical illness: A review and critique of the cognitive-developmental literature. *Health Psychol.* 5:317.

Inconsistency may result from care given by a number of different individuals, or provided by the same person but in an unpredictable way, as in the care given by a psychiatrically disturbed parent or one who is acutely stressed and whose ability to parent effectively is compromised. Inconsistency in caregivers and caregiving may result in a sense of mistrust manifested by exaggerated stranger anxiety in the infant or separation anxiety in the toddler. For their part, parents often feel overwhelmed by helplessness and guilt at their inability to protect and provide for their child.

Critical illness in the young couple's first infant is particularly devastating. With no previous childrearing experience to draw on for strength and confidence, the couple's sense of competence is severely challenged. So too are their new roles as mates with a family. Research by Morrow and colleagues (1981) found that parents over age 30 showed better adjustment than younger parents. If the patient is a toddler, there may be a new baby at home or on the way, making additional demands on the mother's time and energy. If there are older siblings, they often feel guilty, angry, sad, and neglected, all of which affect their demands of their parents as well as color their feelings toward their sick sibling.

## DEPENDENCE–INDEPENDENCE ISSUES

Precisely because trust, the seed from which independence is nourished, is nurtured by consistency, any threat to this also threatens movement toward self-sufficiency. Inconsistent daily routines and unexpected handling (e.g., forced feedings and painful procedures) cause helpless feelings, fears, and mistrust.

## ACHIEVEMENT DISRUPTIONS

In the infant and young child, achievement is measured in terms of the acquisition and rate at which development milestones are attained. At times assessing these is difficult because children, whether sick or well, progress variably with respect to different skills, such as motor, affective, cognitive, linguistic, and social. A child who drops behind the normal limits for acquisition of a skill is a cause for concern. Immobilization due to hospitalization, surgery, fever, or neutropenia can contribute significantly to developmental delay. Inability to explore, utilize, and develop burgeoning skills is a major source of disruption and retardation in development of the very young child. Here the line between regression versus retardation in developing skills is fine. Until illness occurs, a parent may not have noticed any problems in development. Alternately, once their child is diagnosed with cancer, some parents may reflect that their baby exhibited previously a number of unusual characteristics.

For the older infant or early toddler, loss of skills may reflect inability to practice newly acquired skills (e.g., bladder control) because of physical intervention (e.g., catheterization), a stress response, or a combination of both (e.g., inability to ingest food in the context of multiple vomiting episodes secondary to receiving chemotherapy). Finally, the nature of treatment may put the infant at special risk for developmental delay. For example, studies now show that children under age 5 with ALL who receive cranial irradiation in conjunction with intrathecal methotrexate as part of their CNS prophylaxis are at particular risk of cognitive deficits (Meadows et al., 1981).

## BODY–SEXUAL IMAGE AND INTEGRITY

When treatment involves care in special settings (e.g., isolettes, reverse-isolation units, or rooms with high-barred cribs), and experiences with intravenous tubes, catheters, or other physical appliances, the infant or small childs' ability to develop a sense of separateness from external events is compromised. There may be a lack of body image apart from the environment. When treatment results in severely altered appearance or disfigurement (e.g., craniofacial surgery and cushingoid facies), the distress of caregivers in seeing the child may produce early distortions in the child's nascent sense of self-esteem and perceived ability to elicit pleasure in others.

## EXISTENTIAL ISSUES

Finally, in the world of the infant, where separation may be equated with death itself, the disruption produced by the illness may quite literally be worse than the disease itself. Critical in this period, when the small, sick child has so little control, is the response of the parents. Cancer forces the family to deal with the inconceivable, the possible death of a young member. When the outcome is bleak, parents' ability to continue providing support until the end is at times overtaxed. Some families, in an effort to cut short their pain, may emotionally mourn and prematurely bury the child before he or she dies; they emotionally withdraw. The risk of this occurring is greater today because of our ability with sophisticated medical technology to keep a terminally ill child alive through multiple crises.

The opposite response also occurs in which the parents are unable to let a child go. Although families have frequently sought magical cures for their critically ill children (witness the centuries-old pilgrimage to Lourdes), there is a sense that the compelling need to seek alternatives to traditional care has heightened. This is partially because of the increased medical sophistication of the lay public, and the availability of quasi-medical alternative therapies that purport to carry no side effects and "can do no harm" (see Chapter 42). When the focus of such efforts is a young child who cannot say no and may endure pain and suffering for the benefit of the family only, there is great reason for concern.

## Interventions: Birth–2

The primacy of their role in caring for and mediating the response of the infant and very young child with cancer make the parents the major focus of interventions during this life cycle period. Supporting maximal family contact with the ill child is crucial. Recognition of the importance of the mother–infant bond and greater support for parental involvement in the hospitalized child's care have done much to diminish the negative impact of treatment. Practices with respect to parental involvement in care of the young patient have changed significantly over the years, and it is now common for parents to be involved in their child's care over the course of the illness and treatment. This is achieved through encouraging participation in the infant's hospital care by providing flexible visiting privileges, sleep-in arrangements, and homelike housing, such as the Ronald McDonald houses in major cities. Oncology staff must in particular provide new parents with information about how to care for and play with their child in the hospital and at home. Even seasoned parents may feel afraid to do what comes naturally in the sterile and formal environment of a hospital. In providing such support, it is important that the guidance be given in a way that bolsters rather than detracts from self-esteem and a sense of efficacy, while reinforcing and teaching new skills. The emphasis is on maximizing positive parenting behaviors for both parent and child (see also M.A. Adams, 1978; and Chapter 45 by Adams-Greenly).

If parents are to be successful in maintaining their nurturing role during the infant's illness, they may have to shift radically other functions and tasks. The staff needs to evaluate closely the resources available to the family, including financial and material as well as social and emotional. The response of parents and siblings and at times other key family members (e.g., grandparents) needs to be monitored and counseling provided to members who exhibit disturbed responses such as irrational guilt or inappropriate anger.

Supporting the caretaking role of the mother and father, and keeping the number of other caregivers to a minimum—especially during periods of hospitalization—reduces separation anxiety and promotes consistency in caretaking. Attention needs to be given, however, to providing time out for the mother to preserve her own integrity and to replenish energy needed to care for her sick child.

Keeping procedures to a minimum and facilitating play and manipulation of the environment by the child are also central to promoting healthy development. Special efforts at social, physical, and play stimulation may be necessary for children who are confined, or temporarily (e.g., attached to an intravenous tube) or permanently (e.g., because of amputation or the nature of tumor excision) handicapped. Holding, cuddling, and talking are especially important for the sick infant, for whom special focus on using motor and sensory skills may be needed while encouraging emotional interaction.

Finally, the parents' responses need to be monitored and expression of emotions encouraged when there is threatened or actual loss of their small offspring (Easson, 1968). Assistance in anticipating the loss is important. The special issues in bereavement are reviewed in Chapter 50 (see also Krupnick, 1984). Koocher (1986a) provides a thoughtful discussion of the special issues associated with a cancer death.

## EARLY CHILDHOOD: AGES 3–5

The world of the normal 3- to 5-year-old is filled with endless play and self-absorbing activity; children begin to move out of the close family circle to explore the world. Such activity, sometimes referred to as "true socialization," is set into full swing during this period. Greater physical mobility and language skills are key prerequisites to this self-assertion process. The preschooler is growing in size, strength, and coordination. Development of gross and fine motor skills enable the child in this age group to master such skills as riding tricycles or bicycles with training wheels and using roller skates, to writing, buttoning clothes, and tying shoelaces. With each of these accomplishments come a parallel growth in self-esteem and a sense of achievement.

There is also a preoccupation, born of increased skill and recognition of human differences, with the adequacy of the body for its appropriate sex role as well as general functioning. This is accompanied by a greater concern about real and imagined physical injury. Associated in psychoanalytical theory with the phallic period, the years from 3 to 6 are typified by an increased interest in sex differences and a pronounced attachment to the parent of the opposite sex, with accompanying anxiety about potential disruption of the relationship with the same-sex parent (e.g., castration anxiety in boys and penis envy in girls).

While the child continues to be dependent on the parents for care and nurturance, there are incipient stirrings toward autonomy. The child bathes himself or herself, helps a little in household tasks, masters bladder and bowel control, and enters nursery school, leaving parents (and young siblings) at home. Anna Freud (1963) characterizes the period as one in which the focus is on the shift from dependence to independence. The newly found ability to get around and leave home facilitates the growth of initiative. In Erik Erikson's (1963) model, the child at this stage is involved in undertaking, planning, and attacking tasks (*initiative versus guilt*). A sense of primitive morality is manifested in the struggle with a sense of guilt (described by Freud as superego development) over impulsive goals or acts initiated in exuberance. This is also a period of sibling rivalries.

Finally, the transition to symbolic thought that evolves with language development leads to a whole new cognitive world for the child, one that, because of the new vehicle of communication (speech), is understood better than in the preceding period. The ability to talk about and imagine objects or events not present and feelings makes possible fantasy and imaginative play, both of which are important activities of this period. The parallel play seen among children in the preceding stage is replaced by interactive and, toward the end of this period, competitive play. Thinking is, however, egocentric; the child is unable to take another's viewpoint and exerts little effort to adapt communication to the listener's needs. It is also prelogical. This has important influence on the preschool child's understanding of illness-related concepts.

Perhaps the most fundamental keys to interpreting children's responses to medical settings at this age is to recognize that they do not see illness as representing one end on the continuum of well-being; rather, health and illness are seen as two separate states. Additionally, while parents (or God) are generally seen as responsible for health, the child at this age is more likely to feel he or she is responsible for illness. Bibace and Walsh (1980) suggest that the concepts of phenomenism and contagion correspond to the preoperational level of thought. *Phenomenism*, as mentioned in the preceding age period, refers to a conceptualization of illness as a concrete phenomenon that may co-occur with illness but is not necessarily spatially or temporarily proximal (e.g., people get colds from "the sun"). In the *contagion* stage, illness is seen as located in objects or people who are proximate but not touching the child, eliciting a "magical" connection (e.g., people get colds "when someone else gets near them''). In their research, Kister and Patterson (1980) found that less cognitively mature and more anxious children were more likely than more cognitively mature and less anxious children to view illness in moralistic terms and to apply what Piaget referred to as a sense of immanent justice and animism in explaining illness (i.e., "people get what they deserve"). Children in this cognitive period are also more likely to believe that there are rules to follow to stay healthy, thus there may be a heightened sense of guilt when illness occurs. Other researchers have found that preschool children are likely to express less perceived control over the healing process (Bibace and Walsh, 1980), to rely more heavily on external versus internal cues to monitor the recovery process (Neuhauser et al., 1978), to have greater difficulty differentiating the symptoms from the causes of illness and the effects of illness from treatment (e.g., staff actions and medical procedures are often viewed as punishment for past misdeeds, or forbidden, hostile, or erotic impulses directed toward caregivers) (Farley, 1981; Perrin and Gerrity, 1981), and to regard themselves as more vulnerable to contagion than older (concrete operational) children (Potter and Roberts, 1984). Also, because young children sometimes conceptualize internal space as hollow, there appears to be greater emphasis on changes manifest on the body surface. One ramification of this is that it is easier for children who have externally visible symptoms to appreciate that they are getting better than for those with internal symptoms (Neuhauser et al., 1978).

With respect to concepts of death, studies among healthy children in this age group suggest that there is an expansion of the concept from mere separation to loss or absence of a loving and protective object (Nagy, 1948). Death is frequently seen, however, as a temporary departure. When listening to children speak about the death of a grandparent or a pet, one sometimes hears expressed thoughts indicating that they believe the person or animal will come back to life (magical thinking). Later in the period there is a growing appreciation that death represents removal from one kind of existence to another (e.g., person will become an "angel in heaven").

It is important to note at this juncture that the appreciation of death in healthy children as well as siblings of ill patients may differ from that of seriously ill groups (Caradang et al., 1979). A growing body of research indicates that even young children with cancer are aware of the seriousness of their illness and the threat of death (Binger et al., 1969; Schowalter, 1970; Waechter, 1971; Spinetta and Maloney, 1975). Bluebond-Langner (1977, 1978) in her observations goes even further to say that exposure to death of peers and repeated bouts with acute illness accelerate a child's cognitive understanding of death. However, the converse likely also holds true, that a relatively easy course of treatment may protect a child from this premature development of a more sophisticated grasp of the meaning of death. Thus, in caring for children it is important to be aware of the role of illness events and previous exposure to death have on the level of understanding of death.

## Disruptions of Illness: Ages 3–5

### ALTERED INTERPERSONAL RELATIONS

Separation from family and home during hospitalization and during frequent outpatient visits is particularly stressful. While loss of contact with parents is a central concern, children at this age may also express anxiety, sadness, and anger about separation from siblings. The sick child may feel jealous of the good health of a sibling, of the imagined attention he or she is getting at home, or of the possible usurping of his or her (the patient's) role in the family. For their part, healthy siblings often exhibit anger and at times depressed affect in the face of a brother or sister's illness and perceived diversion of parental attention. These feelings create tensions and guilt on both sides. The natural growth of rivalry in this period can cause guilty feelings over such responses to be strongly felt by the sick child.

Parents, whose normal role in this period is to provide behavioral boundaries for and to support efforts toward independence of their young child, find it hard to maintain this stance during illness. The temptation to protect, pamper, and reassert a level of control more appropriate to the earlier period is great, even after the child is no longer acutely ill. Sometimes, though rarely, parents may try to push their child to grow up and handle illness and treatment more maturely. Conflict results when parents diverge in views. The situation is worsened by preexisting marital discord. If the change in role responsibilities necessitated by increased level of care for the ill child is resented by or overburdensome to one or the other parent, further conflict occurs.

Because he or she continues to live in an egocentric world and imagines himself or herself to be responsible for the illness, the 3- to 5-year-old also feels acutely guilty about any changes, tensions, or conflicts at home that he or she perceives to result from the illness and care.

### DEPENDENCE–INDEPENDENCE ISSUES

The emphasis on achieving independence makes the constraints of illness and treatment difficult to tolerate.

When efforts at autonomy are thwarted, anger, depression, and withdrawal may result. The drive to reexert control can lead to increased oppositional behavior (stubbornness) and tantrums.

## ACHIEVEMENT DISRUPTIONS

Occasional loss of recently acquired skills and motor functions (e.g., bowel control) is distressing for the young child who may not be able to see it as caused by illness or treatment but views it rather as a sign of personal failure or inadequacy. Such occurrences serve to magnify the personal sense of loss of control and vulnerability; they can also raise doubts in the child's mind concerning ability to control his or her internal and external environment.

At times, because of frequent contacts with adults and medical settings, the child with cancer will give the appearance of being more mature than might be expected for his or her age. This is often based on the observation among these children of more relaxed adult relationships and greater sophistication in speech patterns than would be seen in healthy age peers. An apparent precocious maturity, however, is often accompanied by much slower development in other spheres (e.g., poorer peer relationships and slowed acquisition of motor skills). If these gaps in proficiency go unacknowledged, the child may be placed in the position of having to be overly responsible for his or her own care, emotions, and development, and be at risk for an inability to seek or receive the critical support, nurturance, and protection he or she needs to develop in these other realms.

## BODY–SEXUAL IMAGE AND INTEGRITY

The growth and awareness of body in the 3- to 5-year-old bring into sharp focus issues of body damage. Although a concern through later periods and adulthood, fears and concerns about real or imagined injury are greatest in these years through latency. Research indicates that children under the age of 7 are significantly more likely than older children to exhibit higher levels of distress during medical procedures; the procedures themselves (e.g., placing of intravenous tubes, finger pricks, and lumbar punctures) are both confusing and frightening, and are likely to be seen as punishment for misdeeds (Jay et al., 1983; Jay and Elliott, 1984). Because children of this age rely on their parents to protect them, parental inability to stop or control pain and painful procedures can produce significant anxiety. Additionally, pain responses are exacerbated by parental communication of anxiety as well as by disinhibition of fear behaviors (Shaw and Routh, 1982). This may be manifested by withdrawal, panic,

obstinacy, tantrums, or agitated behavior. Research has also shown that children in chronic pain who cope inadequately are at risk for developing depression (Masek et al., 1984). A study by Steward and Steward (1981), which looked at what types of stimuli were threatening to different age groups, found that preschool children were more threatened by medical instruments. (For an excellent review of the role of developmental issues in pain in children, see Bush, 1987). Perceived assaults on their body threaten a sense of personal safety and security. Physical alterations produced by disease and treatment (e.g., hair loss, surgical amputation, incisional scarring, and steroid changes) threaten body image and shake the nascent foundations of positive self-esteem and sex role identity.

## EXISTENTIAL ISSUES

Because death may continue to be equated with abandonment, the separation from parents through hospitalization may precipitate acute anxiety and withdrawal. At times during this and in the earlier period, parents may add to this fear by prematurely mourning their dying child, withdrawing care and comfort during the final stage of illness. Also, whether or not the young child has a clear understanding of death, the anxieties of the adults around him or her are inevitably communicated, leaving the child with little chance of escaping a sense of threat (Goggin et al., 1976; Spinetta, 1974; Waechter, 1971).

### Interventions: Ages 3–5

Because of the child's continued dependence on the family, parents continue to be extremely important in the child's response to illness. For any child through the age of 5, having a parent stay over during hospitalization is critically important. However, because of the role it plays in their lives normally and the dramatic results it can produce therapeutically, play becomes the primary form of intervention in this period.

The use of play is important not only because of its link with the activity of normal growth and development, but also because of its powerful role as a means of communication. On the one hand, play serves to reinforce developing motor and social skills critical in this period. Efforts to assure maximal opportunity to engage in peer play behavior both in hospital and at home minimizes achievement disruptions and at the same time diminishes the sense of being different. On the other hand, play provides a unique opportunity to observe how the child sees the world. Although language is rapidly evolving during this period, children are not always able to communicate clearly their fears, pain, or needs. Adults similarly do not always make themselves clear to children. Thus play offers a means of monitoring and sharing information that might otherwise go uncommunicated. Play and therapeutic play have multiple uses and serve as an important intervention on many levels. In undertaking therapeutic play, it is important to be aware that good behavior may be just as important as misbehavior in alerting the staff to child distress. (For a broader review of interventions in this area see also Chapter 45.)

Engaging in play with a child before initiating a procedure permits an accelerated development of trust and the establishment of a therapeutic alliance. Rehearsal of a procedure (e.g., injections, anesthesia, surgery, or radiotherapy) prior to implementation is also helpful to allay the young child's concerns. Such techniques also permit the health care professional to gain a better understanding of what the child thinks is going to happen and how he or she feels about it.

Although it is not always possible in acute situations to prepare the preschool child for what is about to happen, every effort should be made to do so under less pressing circumstances. Research in behavioral medicine shows that such a rehearsal promotes mastery and that providing certain kinds of information is useful in dealing with the preschool-aged child. Information provided should be concrete and nontechnical. The situation should be carefully described and include sensory data (e.g., where, how long, and what it will feel like). Providing the child with exposure to the environment and equipment (e.g., tours and the opportunity to see the equipment to be used) under less stressful conditions, perhaps starting with a favorite doll or animal (e.g., Teddy tries on anesthesia mask, then the child), can be helpful at least on the first hospital visit or encounter with a given procedure. It should be noted, however, that repeating this type of exposure on subsequent visits may increase rather than diminish anxiety. On subsequent visits or repeat procedures, emphasis might be placed instead on how well the child did or how things will be different this time. Filmed modeling is sometimes helpful. Consistency of information is also important, as is the timing of communications. All discussions should be done in the presence of a parent who can "translate" for the child and provide reassurance. Because of their limited grasp of time, information sessions and opportunity for rehearsal should occur within a day, at most two, of the event, and reminders and reviews need to be given. (See also Elkins and Roberts, 1983, for a detailed review of issues related to preparation for hospitalization.)

Despite the importance of parents to the young child in managing the stress of illness, opinions regarding the desirability of their presence during painful procedures are mixed. In one study of 4- to 10-year-olds, researchers found crying was greater for those children whose mothers were present during venipuncture than for those whose mothers stayed in the waiting room (Gross et al., 1983). By contrast, Ross and Ross (1984) found that of 994 children 5–12 years old who were interviewed about pain, 99% reported parental presence as the most helpful influence. What appears to be most important is what the parent actually does while interacting with the frightened or anxious child (Bush and Cockrell, 1987). Teaching parents and staff limit-setting strategies, simple distraction, and coping techniques is very helpful in promoting a sense of mastery for all involved, child, parent, and staff members (Carpenter, 1987; P.B. Jacobsen, personal communication, 1988). For some parents unable to deal with pain in their child, permission to wait outside during an unpleasant medical procedure may be best for all.

Parents also benefit from education and support in other areas. Group meetings with the staff for parents with sick children are an important means of providing both information and support. Use of veteran parents is another increasingly popular intervention in the oncology setting. Parents need to be encouraged to maintain a growing experience as normal as possible for their child. This means controlling the need to overindulge, encouraging social autonomy appropriate to the child's age, and being able to set limits and boundaries.

A number of interventions outlined in the preceding period also apply here. Support needs to be given to enable the family to have maximal contact with the sick child while still meeting family role obligations. Families also need to be assessed for adequacy of social, emotional, and tangible support as well as ongoing functioning. As the decision to care for the dying child at home is being made by an increasing number of families, medical and psychological supports must be provided for those who choose this as an option. Wherever children are treated, they need to be reassured that they will not be abandoned.

## MIDDLE CHILDHOOD AND LATENCY: AGES 6–11

The world of the child aged 6–11 is dominated by entry into and participation in formal school. While not entirely eclipsing the home and family, school is a major socializing environment for children in this period. Many of the skills that come into prominence during this period are reinforced by early formal education, including increased physical and athletic prowess (focus on gross motor skills), acquisition of an enriched vocabulary as well as sophisticated grammar and reading skills, acquisition of elemental logic and principles of reversibility and conservation (ability to understand relationships among observations and to show thought independent of experience), greater conformity to social rules, increased sharing as well as competitiveness, and intensification of peer relationships with friends of the same and opposite sex.

As a consequence of working and playing with contemporaries for most of every day, an overriding developmental theme is comparison of self to peers: who is tallest, strongest, prettiest, who has lost more teeth, who can run fastest, jump rope longest, who got the highest grades, and who has the most friends. Because competence in achievement and performance is such a focus of attention, damage to the body is also a primary focus. Toward the end of this period, entry into puberty begins to push girls into the next developmental period. Paradoxically, in contrast to being best or first in other spheres, it is sometimes easier for a girl to be average in the acquisition of secondary sex characteristics. Developing breasts or beginning to menstruate too early or too late relative to peers can be devastating.

Erikson (1963) described the middle childhood and latency years as the age of industry. Mastery of school life and harnessing earlier exuberance to fit the laws of the impersonal realm (e.g., mastery of the three $R$'s) are goals of this stage. Recognition is gained by producing things. At the same time, cultural and social identity are acquired. In Erikson's model, mastery of this stage can be hindered if the child despairs of the adequacy of his or her personal skills, tools, or status among peers, and leads to a sense of inferiority.

From a psychoanalytical perspective, the successful positive identification with the parent of the same sex and internalizaion of parental values to form a conscience (achieved in the prior period) enable the child to relegate a lesser emphasis to sexual impulses (hence the term latency), and to increase concern with mastery of the external environment (e.g., school, hobbies, peers, and sports). Anna Freud (1965) refers to this as the transition from autonomous play to the work role.

The acquisition of concrete operational thought (ages 7–11) has particular ramifications for how children during these years view illness, pain, and death. Health for the school-aged child is seen as a positive feeling state. This goes beyond the mere association with absence of illness held by younger children. Although much of the control for personal health is still perceived as under the control of others, especially physicians, there is a growing awareness of personal control. In the model proposed by Bibace and Walsh (1980), two stages of illness causality are reflected in the concrete operational period. In the first of these, referred to as the *contamination* stage, the child de-

fines illness in terms of multiple symptoms and views illness as transmitted primarily through physical contact with a source (e.g., germs and dirt). In the second, or *internalization* stage, the child still considers the cause of illness to be external but begins to view illness as the result of internalizing an external contaminant (e.g., people get colds by breathing in bacteria and swallowing germs). The mechanisms most often associated with the process are swallowing or inhaling. It is important from a behavioral perspective that both of these stages increase the likelihood of being able to engage effectively the child in health-promoting activities (e.g., avoiding germs). There is a marked decrease in a moralistic or immanent justice concept of illness causality.

The increased sense of control also extends to healing processes. Because they generally have greater experience than younger children, school-aged children also have a broader repertoire of coping skills. Consequently, they exhibit greater ability for management and sense of control over painful procedures or stressful situations (Brown et al., 1986). Health information provided at school also helps. It should be noted, however, that while treatment is more likely than in the earlier periods to be viewed as a help rather than an assault, children until about age 10 have a limited ability to benefit from empathic efforts of staff. For example, it is not clear if telling a child a procedure is going to hurt a lot decreases screaming or acting out. However *not* telling him or her it is going to hurt when it does, destroys the caregiver's credibility and promotes future anxiety in similar situations.

Children tend to reduce reports of pain as they mature. However, during this period there may be an increased fear of needles more than of the pain itself. A study by Steward and Steward (1981) suggests that in the older school-aged child, fear of medical instruments, seen as a primary concern of younger children, is replaced by concern over the interaction with medical personnel. In addition, learned anxiety from previous medical experience plays an increasingly important role in the older child's response to illness, pain, and hospitalization. The frequency of posttraumatic stress disorder in children with cancer has not been systematically studied, but it is likely high, based on clinical observations (E. Heiligenstein, 1988, personal communication). It should be remembered that while the traits described earlier are characteristic of older children, acutely stressed children who are upset or frightened may regress to the earlier, egocentric reasoning of the younger child, viewing illness and hospitalization as punishment for wrongdoing. Also, research oriented to age distinctions indicates that older boys are more reluctant than girls of the same age or younger children to acknowledge illness and pain, and are more likely to deny or reject the sick role than other children (Campbell, 1975a, 1978).

The latency-aged child begins to understand death as permanent and not reversible, contributing to fears of mutilation and physical injury. Death may at times be personified (e.g., as the "bogeyman"). It is also associated with grief for anticipated separation from loved ones and fear when seen as punishment for wrongful acts or thoughts.

## Disruptions of Illness: Ages 6–11

### ALTERED INTERPERSONAL RELATIONS

All the potential sources of family dysfunction noted in earlier periods occur in the world of the sick school-aged child. There may be concerns about parental conflict over caretaking, presence of other children at home needing or demanding attention, sibling guilt, anger, and depression in the face of a brother or sister's illness and source of diversion of parental attention, exacerbation of preexisting parental marital or family discord, and threatened abandonment or withdrawal of one or both parents from the ill child and/or each other. Also, the school-aged child frequently experiences isolation from peers. Fears of being rejected by parents, especially during hospitalization, and problems of reentry into the social life of contemporaries are common themes (Kagen-Goodheart, 1977). Added to this is the burden of threatened loss of or change in the role of the family, peer group, and school milieu. The impact of this latter concern also has ramifications for dependence–independence issues and achievement disruptions. Change in status within the family can produce profound feelings of displacement and a sense of loss of control. Additionally, restriction of peer group or school standing, through illness changes or absence, can lead the child to despair of his or her competency to meet perceived social and school achievement standards. Because of the high value placed on social acceptance and personal achievement, repeated or extensive separations from peers, school, familiar routines, as well as from family members, may significantly affect developing self-esteem. Signs of distress may include regressive behavior (e.g., clinging, tantrums, and bed-wetting), separation anxiety, depression, and school phobia.

### DEPENDENCE–INDEPENDENCE ISSUES

The thrust toward industry and competency during this particular period places the school-aged child at special risk for fears of inability to cope during illness.

Parental overprotection and the child's reluctance to assert himself or herself may both contribute to overdependency. The loss of autonomy from the restrictions on activities may lead to diminished self-esteem and result in behavioral regression. Looking at it from the child's point of view, illness is seen "in terms of what things he or she can or cannot do: seeing the doctor, going to the hospital, not being able to play with friends all the time, and worrying about being hurt. In an effort to regain control, the child may try to exert control in inappropriate ways, such as refusing to participate in activities that are possible" (Rait and Holland, 1986, pp. 2–3). Loss of self-control (e.g., crying, clinging, and tantrums), tolerated in younger children, is less socially acceptable as the child matures. As a consequence, it is more distressing to both child and parent or caregiver when it occurs.

### ACHIEVEMENT DISRUPTIONS

Because of the importance of the school setting in the normal development of the child of this age group, school disruption, resulting from absence or poor performance, can have a major adverse impact on sense of competence and self-esteem. Multiple absences from school and physical side effects of treatment (e.g., fatigue, diminished attention and concentration, IQ loss secondary to tumors or treatment of the CNS) can compromise academic position. Similarly, physical alterations in appearance (e.g., hair loss, weight gain or loss, and amputation), and associated embarrassment or fear of ridicule—real or imagined—can compromise social position. Fears of inadequacies in either of these spheres can lead to behavior problems (e.g., acting out, overdependency, and "school phobias"). The young child may view the consequences of his or her treatment as stigmatizing and perceive the changes as a threat to reputation. The child's sense of being different and isolated may be exacerbated by teachers who are threatened by having a child with cancer in the classroom or who, believing the child's future to be grim, lower achievement expectations for him or her, thereby missing the opportunity to provide a normalizing experience or to evaluate the child for special needs or placement as appropriate.

### BODY–SEXUAL IMAGE AND INTEGRITY

The natural preoccupation with physical adequacy in this period leads to an increase in mutilation anxiety and fears of being attacked or disfigured when illness occurs (Spinetta, 1974). School-aged children tend to focus on the discomfort associated with a procedure and its potential for physical harm. As a consequence, they are more apt to develop frightening fantasies about intrusive procedures (e.g., EEG will turn me into Frankenstein or chemotherapy will kill me), and may see them as punishment. There may be a particular fear about painful procedures, surgery, and anesthesia. Self-consciousness about the body also leads to increased shyness and embarrassment. When his or her sensitivity about the body goes unacknowledged, as when groups of physicians on rounds look at a child's scar, it may confirm loss of control. For children who are feeling relatively well at the time of diagnosis, their treatment may indeed seem worse than the disease itself.

## EXISTENTIAL ISSUES

Although there is not necessarily a full appreciation of the irreversibility of death yet, children with cancer in this age are aware of the seriousness of their disease. This awareness is associated with increased levels of anxiety (Spinetta, 1974). Boys appear to be at greater risk for anxiety than girls (Goggin et al., 1976). As in the case of the younger child, and despite greater cognitive capacity, the school-aged child may express concern that the illness is a consequence of a misdeed or ''bad'' thought. The child may also fear that his or her actions caused the disease or its recurrence, or will cause death. The school-aged child may experience nightmares of a ''monster'' taking him or her away from the family. Concrete fears of death may also be expressed (e.g., worry about being buried alive). There is also disquiet and at times preoccupation about the family circle in his or her absence.

### Interventions: Ages 6–11

For the school-aged child with cancer, the importance of the social world to growth and development makes the creation of a therapeutic environment of particular use. For that reason the role of milieu and school is emphasized in any planned interventions.

In addition to the interventions proposed to minimize stress on interpersonal relationships for younger children, several are important to this age group. Interaction with peers, both in and out of the hospital, is important to ensure continued development of social skills and competence. Long recognized by others (Langford, 1961), play groups and therapeutic play sessions are particularly beneficial in this age group. Attention should be given to maintaining the sick child's connection with and role in the family. In the hospital this might include sibling visits, visits by pets as permitted, and contact via telephone calls, audio cassettes, and videotapes. Once at home, parents should be encouraged to support the child's return to

normal chores and responsibilities as well-being permits.

Issues of dependency can be addressed by helping parents (and staff) support the child's autonomy while still setting boundaries. The child can decide when to take a medication (e.g., now or in 20 minutes), but not whether to take it or not. As with younger children, establishing trust and describing and rehearsing anticipated procedures and consequences supports a sense of control. School-aged children are particularly receptive to behavioral interventions to reduce pain and distress. Along with sensory data and concrete information, children of this age are also able to respond to metaphor (e.g., going into the CT scan machine is like lying in a big doughnut). Rehearsing new coping skills and setting realistic goals for the patient is helpful. Filmed modeling, use of audiotapes, and use of peer modeling and counselors are also beneficial. Unlike the younger child, for whom immediate information is critical, school-aged children have a better grasp of time frames. Consequently, they benefit from lead time in preparation to allow for the information to ''sink in.'' Coping skills and strategies can then be reinforced at the stress point.

It is important to note that, although children move away from parental dependence as they grow older, illness almost always leads to a greater desire for support. Family responses to illness continue to play a strong role in children's coping well into adolescence. In particular, the ability of the parents to foster family integration, (e.g., building a close relationship with the spouse) and maintain self-stability (e.g., ''keep myself in shape'') during a child's illness can reduce a sense of hopelessness in children (8–16 years old) early in the cancer experience (Blotcky et al., 1985).

In planning any intervention it is particularly important to appreciate the child's understanding of the meaning of illness. Their increased experiential, logical, and reasoning capacity makes it possible to enlist the older child's cooperation through understanding of the reasons for treatment. Parents often serve as valuable interpreters of how their child is coping. Drawing on this expertise, parents can be trained to be alert to specific distress cues and to provide critical coping support, diminishing feelings of helplessness in both child and parent.

Relaxation and meditation, as well as distraction, are powerful intervention techniques (see also Chapter 46). Positive self-talk (i.e., verbally encouraging oneself in mastering a task) and attention diversion are techniques frequently used by healthy children in managing stressful situations (e.g., dental visit, giving a school report) that can be applied in the cancer setting (Brown et al., 1986). For some ''high-tech'' families, the use of videogames or biofeedback training to reduce distress or symptoms may have particular appeal (Spinetta and Lansky, 1982). Contingency contracting (e.g., making a desired toy or a promised outing contingent on meeting a specified goal such as sitting still for a venipuncture) is also useful in promoting behavioral control in this age group. In addition to enabling the child to tolerate a needed procedure, success at achieving a goal (e.g., sitting still) also promotes a feeling of being in control and able to cope. That experience is helpful in going forward to meet the next challenge, although it should be cautioned that staff and parents should not expect generalization of skills. Each new crisis will likely require that concrete guidelines in management be given to the child. The important key in restoring and supporting control is to help the child realize that mastering the situation is within his or her power and that there are people ready to help with a variety of techniques.

The increasing efficacy of treatments for the majority of childhood tumors and emphasis on outpatient care have reversed earlier patterns of school absenteeism. Recognition of the importance of the school experience on all levels of the child's healthy development has led to a growing emphasis on returning the child with cancer to the classroom as quickly as possible (Spinetta and Deasy-Spinetta, 1986). The success of this endeavor depends on addressing the concerns of both the student and the school. Discussions about fears related to the child's reactions to school reentry are needed. Arrangements should be made to find wigs, scarves, or prostheses to minimize changes in appearance. Time is also necessary for rehearsing the young patient in answering peers' questions or reactions. Tutoring should be provided as needed, especially when therapy has involved treatment to the CNS. Evaluation of possible effects of particularly neurotoxic regimens on cognitive and academic functioning is important. Establishing a dialogue between parents and teachers reduces the likelihood that problems will go unnoticed (Eiser, 1980). In a model used at Memorial Sloan-Kettering, teachers of children treated here are invited to attend a 1-day workshop to familiarize them with the special needs of their students (see Chapter 45).

It is important that the returned student have tasks that he or she can master. At times this may mean allowing the student to spend more time on assignments (being flexible), to give verbal instead of written reports (modifying procedures), or to obtain special educational services (providing assistance). Classmates need to be sensitized to the experience of their returned peer. Attention should be given to open discussion of concerns they may have about how to respond to their classmate and friend, and fears about contracting the disease themselves. When a student

with cancer dies, the class needs the opportunity to grieve. Having a commemorative can be helpful. However, it is also important to recognize and facilitate the students' need to go on.

In planning school interventions, it is also important to include issues for healthy school-aged siblings. Teachers can help alert parents to emotional difficulties that may occur for the well child. They can also help normalize routine during stressful periods for the siblings by providing a consistent learning environment and support for their continued emotional as well as physical and academic growth and development (for a discussion of related issues in school attendance, see Chapter 44 on childhood psychopathology and Chapter 45 on psychosocial interventions in children with cancer).

The sick child's concerns about physical damage are lessened by open discussion of illness and treatment in terms the child can understand, and of what is happening or will happen to him or her. It is vital to listen to the child. Having the child relate back what he or she has heard can help the staff and parents find out what has been understood or misunderstood. The need for privacy should be recognized and honored.

Frank discussion about the causes of the child's illness will minimize fantasies and guilt, although specific fears and nightmares need to be individually addressed as they arise. Open discussion of a peer patient's death, with emphasis on how the survivor's situation is different, can lessen fear, guilt, and grieving. Unless the child is seriously mentally compromised, secrets (conspiracy of silence) about diagnosis and death at this age are only harmful. The literature on young patients and survivors of cancer provides convincing evidence that adjustment problems decrease when children have the opportunity to talk about their disease (Karon and Vernik, 1968; Kellerman et al., 1977; Koocher and O'Malley, 1981; Slavin et al., 1982). When the subject of death arises, staff and family need to respond to the child's questions about life after death and concerns about family life without him or her.

## ADOLESCENCE: AGES 12–18

Unlike earlier periods of development in which one could single out particular aspects of growth that seemed to predominate (e.g., birth to 2 years with physical growth and maturation, 3 to 5 with cognitive and affective development, 6 to 11 with the acquisition and elaboration of skills in prosocial and academic spheres), in adolescence major changes are occurring in the physical, cognitive, social, and affectional and sexual spheres simultaneously. Whereas earlier theorists viewed adolescence as a period of *Sturm und*

*Drang* (Blos, 1962), more recent research suggests that passage through this developmental period is for many adolescents more benign (Csikszentmihalyi and Larson, 1984; Offer, Ostrov and Howard, 1981).

Adolescence is sometimes considered to be synonymous with, or at least its onset is defined by, puberty. However, because girls begin puberty approximately 2 years earlier than boys (around age 8–10 years) and reach their maximum velocity in height growth around 12 years (as opposed to 14 years in boys), this leaves a fairly loose boundary for definitional purposes and frank differences in rate of development of puberty between the sexes. The dramatic physical and physiological changes that accompany puberty are both a focus of attention and the catalyst for psychological changes in this period.

The principal developmental tasks of adolescence are fourfold, namely, to achieve a stable identity or self-image, to adjust to an adult sex role and enter into mature relationships with peers of both sexes, to gain independence from the nuclear family unit, and to begin to prepare for the future, often by making an initial vocational or career choice. As summarized by Blumberg and colleagues (1984, p. 133),

If developmental tasks are successfully completed, the adolescent will emerge from this period with adequate self-esteem, a comfortable body image, an established identity, emotional independence, economic independence or the ability to achieve it when the completion of school or training makes it appropriate, a sexual identity, and a realistic, goal-oriented view of the future.

The "physiological revolution" that occurs in adolescence intensifies the concern with the body seen in the preceding period. In contrast to the need to measure and compare as seen in the preceding age group, there is a shift in focus to "fitting in"; an affirmation of sameness becomes central in adolescence. In part, the response is a counterbalance to the feeling of change in the self. Overmaturation or underdevelopment, or development that is accelerated or delayed relative to peers can lead to concern and even behavior problems. As noted earlier, being on schedule relative to a peer group with respect to puberty is important. Studies evaluating the effects of timing of puberty on psychological adjustment have shown that early-maturing boys tend to exhibit fewer behavior problems, to be more secure and self-assured, to excel at sports, to be better accepted by peers, and often to be a better student than late-maturing males (Money and Clopper, 1974). In contrast, it is the late-maturing girl who appears to have an easier time of adolescence and to get along better with peers.

"Who am I" (or "How am I different") is the question of the day. To answer this question the ado-

lescent depends heavily on the feedback from his or her peer group. Erikson sees the need for strong peer connections, the "in-group" feeling, clannishness, and intolerance of differences, as a "necessary defense" against the dangers of self-diffusion that are present until such time as an identity is established (Erikson, 1968).

The advent of puberty, entry into the genital period in Freud's psychoanalytical model, sets the stage for the completion of psychosexual differentiation in courtship, mating, and parenting. (It is also the time at which earlier errors in genetic or psychosexual differentiation become fully appreciated.) Acceptance of sexuality and channeling appropriately the sexual drives experienced are a major task of adaptation (A. Freud, 1958). Sexual experimentation, falling in love, and pursuit of romantic interests are hallmarks of this period.

Because part of the answer to the question "Who am I" is "Where am I going?" and "Whom will I become?" the adolescent must in addition to accepting his or her sexuality, also establish an orientation to the future and develop a commitment to a system of values. Thus, search for vocational and career interests and life goals is a major task.

Finally, the adolescent must also establish independence from parents and family. Often this separation is made complete by the end of the period when the teenager goes off to college or moves away to start a life of his or her own. Pressure for emancipation from previously set limits and for greater privacy increase.

In Erikson's model (1963), the developmental issue of adolescence is the achievement of a sense of personal identity. The search for identity involves the formulation of a meaningful self-concept, one that incorporates and links together past, present, and future. Successful search for identity also requires assessment of assets and liabilities and how the adolescent wants to use them. Erikson saw devotion and fidelity to principle(s) and person(s) as characteristic of this period. Developing new relations with contemporaries of both sexes and preparing for marriage and family life are both part of the tasks of sexual adjustment associated with Freud's genital period. The basic Freudian assertion (that there are somatically rooted social changes) is at least upheld in adolescence.

Levinson et al. (1978) characterizes the years from age 17 to 22 as the early-adult transition. Like Erikson, he sees the period as one of questioning the nature of the world and one's place in it. Key relationships are evaluated in the context of these changes. There is by the end of these years a consolidation of initial adult identity and a testing of some choices for adult living.

Although many children by the end of the preceding period are capable of formal operational thought, this type of thinking blossoms in adolescence. Formal operational thinking is characterized by the mastery of the ability to apply logical rules and reasoning to abstract problems, the use of propositional and combinational operations, and the ability to imagine the many possibilities inherent in a situation. The following example illustrates the differences between preadolescent, concrete reasoning and adolescent reasoning based on verbal propositions.

The 9-year-old can arrange a series of dolls according to their height and can even supply each doll with a stick of corresponding size from a series of different sticks. He can do this even if the sticks are presented in reverse order. But not until formal operations can he solve a similar, but verbal problem: "Edith is fairer than Susan; Edith is darker than Lilly; who is the darkest of the three?" (Muuss, 1975, pp. 192–93)

Unlike the younger child whose thinking is concretely bound, the adolescent is able to transcend the here and now, to think about thinking. "The most distinctive property of formal thought is this reversal of direction between *reality* and *possibility* (Inhelder and Piaget, 1958, p. 251). There tends, however, to be an egocentric quality to the adolescent's thinking. Preoccupation with his or her own thinking at this stage often leads to the assumption that everyone sees things in a like manner, or conversely that no one has ever thought about the world in quite the same way.

The more complex thinking in adolescence is reflected in more sophisticated notions of health. Unlike younger children who tend to view illness as an all-or-none phenomenon (i.e., they are or are not sick), adolescents can be a little sick. They also understand that most illness and treatment has an end point. It should be noted, however, that comprehension of healing can come and go during this developmental period and often relates to how stressed the young person is. In the model of Bibace and Walsh (1980), physiologic and psychophysiologic concepts of illness are thought to be associated with formal operational thought. In the *physiologic* stage the child believes that while the cause of illness may be triggered by external events, the source and nature of illness are understood to be within specific internal structures and functions. The child is able to conceptualize the breakdown of physiologic processes and structures as a step-by-step sequence (e.g., What is cancer? "Cancer is when there's too many cells. They're invisible but I know that they grow"). Important in this concept is the child's perception of having greater control over onset and cure of illness; illness has multiple causes hence multiple cures (Bibace and Walsh, 1980).

The child in the *psychophysiologic* stage of development also regards illness in terms of internal physiologic processes. However, he or she appreciates ad-

ditionally that thoughts and feelings can affect the way the body functions (e.g., people get "heart attacks" by being "nerve wracked"). There is greater awareness of the importance of one's own actions in adolescence on health, but not necessarily the appropriate action. This has implications for compliance with medical recommendations as well as for maintenance of good health practices.

Paralleling the greater understanding of illness during adolescence is a greater sense of control over illness and a different sense of vulnerability. Indeed, the egocentricity in thinking typical of adolescence may lead to the feeling of invulnerability, or the opposite of vulnerability. As a consequence, the adolescent may be shocked by or apt to deny serious illness when it occurs, reacting as if such a circumstance "can't happen to me." A similar pattern is seen in the adolescent's appreciation of death. While adolescents understand both the universal and irrevocable nature of death, this awareness is accompanied by the disbelief in the possibility of their own death. Although capable of grasping the full implications of a diagnosis of cancer, both on present and future life, the adolescent's sense of the invincible self may lead to a denial of death as a possible outcome.

## Disruptions of Illness: Ages 12–18

The very nature and normative tasks of adolescence, with its emphasis on physical and sexual development, intensification of interpersonal bonds, move toward independence from parents and family, and emphasis on personal achievement, make confrontation with the diagnosis and treatment of cancer a serious challenge. Whereas adolescents with a life-threatening illness do not invariably manifest psychopathological symptoms, illness-related life disruptions make it likely that major changes and distress will develop in at least one or more areas of functioning over the course of treatment (Kellerman et al., 1980; Zeltzer et al., 1980, 1984). In 1977, Schowalter reflected on how little had been written regarding the impact of illness and hospitalization in adolescence, despite its recognized importance in development. Since then, there have been a growing number of articles written about the unique issues that face this special group of patients.

### ALTERED INTERPERSONAL RELATIONS

Hospitalization, physical limitations, and the separation from peers necessitated by intensive or prolonged periods of illness and treatment place the adolescent at risk of feeling isolated. Missing out on important social experiences, including the opportunity to develop intimate relationships and to engage in sexual activities, can be felt more strongly than the threat to life (Koocher and O'Malley, 1981). The negative impact of social isolation from a critical reference group is often compounded by the adolescent's need for increased dependence on parents; a situation that threatens the drive toward emancipation, and that may at times be as distressing to parents as it is to the adolescent. Although more commonly associated with younger patients, separation anxiety occurs in ill adolescents as well. The loss of ego con ol and lack of confidence in a new-found sense of self-reliance can lead to more regressive behavior causing acute distress to patient and parent alike.

## DEPENDENCE–INDEPENDENCE ISSUES

Whereas control is a critical issue across developmental periods, its importance is magnified in adolescence. Control is central to establishing self-identity, maintaining identity integration (Erikson, 1963), and harnessing libidinal impulses (Blos, 1962). In their study of the psychological effects of illness in adolescence, Zeltzer and co-workers (1980) found that restriction of freedom was the area of greatest concern. In their study, adolescents with cancer were more likely to view their treatment as highly disruptive. Loss of independence and privacy secondary to illness not only engenders feelings of helplessness, but also produces distrust, alienation, anger, acting out, and uncooperativeness. Such responses may be exacerbated by parental overprotection, as well as staff paternalism.

In their research, Hoffman, Becker, and Gabriel (1976) found that adolescents entering and leaving this period tolerated the restrictions imposed by illness better than those in middle adolescence, who tended to be more confrontational. This likely reflects the transitional nature of middle adolescence; young patients in this stage have already begun to redefine themselves, but have not yet consolidated a new or complete self-conception. Avoiding power struggles and setting limits often become major issues.

## ACHIEVEMENT DISRUPTIONS

Changes in physical and mental ability secondary to illness, even when transient, can lead to a diminished perception of self-value and personal worth. When the changes are permanent, as in loss of a limb or intellectual acumen, serious depression can result. The adolescent may express concern about the ability to fulfill ambitions. Sports and academic standing, often vital status symbols in the valued peer network, are jeopardized or lost. Many children undertake extensive and dedicated efforts to succeed at the same sports and

activities despite the loss, refusing to acknowledge it. As with younger children, fear of failure or being seen as different can result in school phobia and increased somatic complaints.

## BODY–SEXUAL IMAGE AND INTEGRITY

The primary concern in adolescence is with peer relations and fitting in with the crowd. It is not surprising that the greatest stress of illness for adolescent cancer patients is the disruption of body image. In this regard, females report greater impact of illness on physical appearance than males (Zeltzer et al., 1980). Deviation from critical peer conformity can be traumatic. Schowalter (1977) emphasized the negative impact of debilitation on self-esteem and ego-ideal formation. Alopecia, delayed physical growth resulting from chemotherapeutic and radiation treatment, and altered sexual maturation have a major impact on both self-image and emerging sexuality. The adolescent may express fears of being somehow "dirty." Shyness and embarrassment about body exposure during examinations are acutely felt. The greater consciousness about mind–body interactions in illness raises concerns about body disintegration and possible insanity. Finally, illness poses a major threat to adolescent sense of physical invulnerability. (For a discussion of the psychological effects of limb amputation in adolescence, see Chapter 20; see also Earle, 1979.)

## EXISTENTIAL ISSUES

Because of the centrality of the body to adolescent development, illness is intimately tied to identity, and vice versa. Their more philosophical style of thinking makes adolescents become keenly aware of the seriousness of their illness and its meaning for the future. Anxiety, panic, depression, faltering belief in immortality, and anguish at not living to "grow up" may all be evidenced. Greater awareness of the uncertainty of prognosis is associated with more fears of recurrence than is seen in younger children. Research by Goggin and colleagues (1976) found that older boys tend to be more realistic and less anxious than girls. Recurrence when it happens may be seen as punishment, as in younger age groups, but is more commonly associated with guilt for specific actions (versus thoughts), such as masturbation or shoplifting. It may also be viewed as a punishment by God or as a means of punishing others (form of noncompliance). In their struggle to create life roles, the adolescents' confrontation with cancer can precipitate a search for life meaning; survival may be associated with guilt or a special purpose in life.

## Interventions: Ages 12–18

The critical role peer groups play in mediating the adolescent's search for identity makes them a powerful source of intervention in illness. Peer support thus is the theme for interventions in this period. Contrary to what one might expect, however, it is not the adolescent's accustomed social group whose company is sought most during illness. Many ill adolescents complain that their friends and classmates don't understand them, or avoid them. Rather, it is fellow teen patients who serve best as sources of support. The use of peer-support groups to promote self-confidence and bolster self-efficacy, and "veteran patients" to model effective coping strategies, are powerful means of helping the sick adolescent deal with the impact of disease and treatment (see also Chapter 45). Family counseling focusing on excessive passivity and overprotection, as well as on how to manage exaggerated adolescent behavior (e.g., rebellion, overdependency, and regression) is also helpful in minimizing strains in interpersonal relationships at home. As with all age groups, special attention needs to be given to the emotional well-being of healthy siblings.

In addition to providing a new, more appropriate and supportive referent group, it is essential in caring for the adolescent to minimize the sense of loss of control that accompanies physical illness. The need for independence and the adolescent's greater intellectual capacity dictate more open and detailed communication throughout the disease course. Several researchers have shown that this approach not only fosters a greater sense of control, but also promotes better early as well as long-term adjustment to illness (Vernick and Karon, 1965; Nannis et al., 1982). Their more adultlike logic, grasp of internal, invisible effects of illness and treatments, and greater knowledge of biological and physical mechanisms enable the adolescent to benefit from explanations and frank discussion of outcomes, procedures, and medications. Although it is still important to include parents—and parents should still have responsibility for most decisions—they are less important in the communication process. Caregivers need to spend time alone with the adolescent, establish trust, and enlist patient cooperation. Signs of secrecy or dishonesty (and failure to share information is apt to be interpreted as such) are to be avoided. In arranging care it is important to formulate plans with maximal input from the patient, and to adhere to them, or to explain fully deviations when they arise (Nannis et al., 1982). It should be noted, however, that some adolescents may object to participating in the decision-making process. They may not wish to be (or may fear being) responsible for life-and-death decisions. Parents and staff need to be prepared to make those choices.

Encouraging self-care and as much autonomy as possible also lessens a sense of dependency. The adolescent's need for privacy (both physical and emotional) should be respected, with attention given to how he or she is treated during rounds or examinations, and how much time or space is allowed for being alone.

In many ways, the task of providing support for the adolescent who is ill is made easier by his or her greater breadth of experience and more versatile reasoning. The adolescent generally has a larger range of coping strategies available both through prior illness encounters and life events, and through the use of metaphor than the younger child (Brown et al., 1986). However, skills often need to be taught for each new situation. Although success in facing prior stresses boosts a sense of confidence in the ability to tackle new challenges, the often very different demands of new treatments and procedures puts a high premium on developing new skills. For example, whereas the use of videogame distraction may have been helpful in reducing anxiety during chemotherapy infusions, a different strategy will need to be employed to cope with the isolation and enforced immobilization experienced during radiation treatments (e.g., progressive relaxation and audiocassette tapes).

Because control issues are such a common theme in management problems with adolescents, it is important to speak briefly here about issues of non-compliance. Although not uncommon in the preceding age group and adult populations, noncompliance is most commonly associated with adolescence and when it occurs can be very troublesome in this age group, particularly among older adolescents. Research by Blotcky and colleagues (1985) found that non-compliant adolescents exhibited high levels of trait anxiety and religiosity, and exhibited an external locus of control. These youngsters were prone to anxiety and coped with their illness-related distress by maintaining a belief that their lives were determined by fate or religious convictions. These researchers felt that a fear-arousal orientation to increasing compliance would have little effect in such individuals. They advocated an approach that reduced anxiety and fostered a sense of personal mastery. In addition to specific personality traits, a number of other influences also cause noncompliance, including failure of the adolescent to grasp the importance of a treatment or regimen, conflict with the physician or in the parent–child relationship, a regimen of treatment that is too distasteful to patient, parent, or both, and lack of confidence in the likely success of the treatment or failure to see improvements over time. Similarly, other influences increase the likelihood of compliance including a decrease in symptoms associated with institution of treatment, greater illness experience, increasing degree of disability, and positive attitude toward and complete understanding of the regimen by parents. Mutual respect, confidence, and honesty are key elements to optimal communication and compliance.

In addressing adolescent concerns about achievement disruptions consequent to illness, it is important to encourage gradual return to prior activities or, when not possible, to explore new areas of expertise or mastery (e.g., intellectual versus physical pursuits). It is important to recognize the emphasis in this age group on the physician as "ego-ideal" and role model, and to be aware that this can turn to "hate object" or "feared object" as well. The physician's interest in and respect for his or her young patient often provides vital self-esteem building support. In planning treatments, it is important to strive for fullest possible return to prior abilities and normal school attendance. This should include encouragement to take up extracurricular activities as soon as possible. All the recommendations about school and fellow student counseling discussed for the preceding age group should be employed here as well to minimize achievement disruptions and development of school phobias.

Ironically, despite more complex reasoning and abstracting powers, it is often the concrete symptom(s) that is the focus of concern and attention for the adolescent (Plumb and Holland, 1974; Mechanic, 1983). The critical importance of body image makes it especially useful to plan for wigs or prostheses when alopecia or limb loss are anticipated. Counseling about self-image and sexual identity is important and may be facilitated through use of veteran peers. The adolescent also needs to discuss the meaning of any delays in maturation and possible sequelae (for older adolescents) of treatment on sexual function and fertility. Ways to look normal need to be explored, along with fears and anxieties about how to handle feeling and being treated as though they were different. Changes in his or her body image may be as frightening to the teenager as they are frustrating. Although discussions concerning the physical impact on the adolescent are important early in treatment, they should also be repeated after treatment ends.

The dramatic impact that loss of health and body changes have on the adolescent's developing existential view of the self requires special efforts to ensure that these concerns are addressed. New information about treatments, results, and future prospects should be discussed gradually to enable the youth to "dose" anxiety. The adolescent should be encouraged to express fears and concerns, and to discuss means of coping with them. Concerns about illness as a cause for shame or a sign of weakness must be aired, and the adolescent reassured about his or her ability to take control of life and find meaning. At times having been a cancer patient for a prolonged period makes it hard for the adolescent to return to a "normal" life; it is difficult and frightening to abandon one persona, especially if he or she has mastered that one well, to take on a role that was temporarily set aside during illness. This task is often made harder because in the course of treatment, youngsters are so well socialized to adjust and operate in an adult (medical) setting, that they no longer have the skills or confidence to be a child or adolescent.

The adolescent's greater awareness of death makes discussion of likely outcome of care and the future important. Counseling is helpful in dealing with irrational fears of punishment and unresolved conflicts of childhood, and in helping the adolescent develop reasonable expectations of self and a positive, realistic appraisal of achievements.

## FAMILY ISSUES

The impact of the developmental stage of the family and the needs of specific family members in the context of a child's illness care are considered elsewhere (see Chapters 44, 45, 47 and 50). However, several themes regarding the family's role in the care and adaptation of the child who is ill cross all developmental periods and deserve special emphasis.

First, while there may be deemphasis on their centrality in planned interventions outlined for the older child and adolescent, families—in particular, parents—play a key role in the response of children of all ages to illness and treatment. If anything, their involvement in the support of the ill child has become more complex as the complexity of treatment has increased and the burden of care provided at home has grown. At the same time, a number of changes in the social composition of families in the United States suggest that the family with a young child with cancer may be more vulnerable to stress than in an earlier period. Hodgekinson, in his book *All One System,* notes that of children born in 1983, 59% will live with only one parent before reaching the age of 18. Of every 100 children born in 1987, 12 will be born out of wedlock, 40 will be born to parents who will divorce before the child is 18, 2 will be born to parents one of whom will die before the child is 18, and 41 will reach 18 "normally." Thus, whatever programs or efforts are developed to promote a child's adaptation at any age must necessarily include an evaluation of the family, its strengths and weaknesses, and attention to its critical role.

Second, another consistent theme is the crucial role of good communication among patient, family, and staff in the care of children of all ages. There has been a dramatic shift away from what Karon and Vernick (1968) referred to as the "conspiracy of silence" in discussions of illness and death with children. It is significant that the movement toward greater candor and dialogue has paralleled the tremendous advances made toward curing childhood malignancies. The change in approach toward disease-related communication reflects, however, a greater appreciation for what the child knows about illness, health, and dying. Clear understanding by child and parent of what is expected during treatment is often pivotal to successful outcome of an intervention to improve well-being. Follow-up studies of survivors further suggest that open communication has an important positive impact on long-term adaptation (Koocher and O'Malley, 1981; Slavin et al., 1982). While thoughtful guidelines on how to inform parents and children about life-threatening illness already exist (see chapters by Koocher and Spinetta in Kellerman, 1980), more research needs to be done concerning how best to tailor communication throughout illness to address the changes in children's cognitive ability at each age.

Third, careful attention needs to be given to siblings' responses to an ill brother or sister (Sourkes, 1980; Koocher and O'Malley, 1981; Carpenter and Sahler, 1987). Because their reactions affect not only their well-being but also that of the ill child and parents, attention to sibling needs is important. Toward this end it is useful to review the developmental tasks and concerns of a sibling as well as those of the patient. It should be noted, however, that as this group comes under closer scrutiny, patterns of differences between their development and that of children whose siblings are well will likely emerge. For example, it has already been observed that concepts of illness are less well developed in children whose siblings are ill than in children with healthy siblings (Caradang et al., 1979).

Fourth, the importance of the family in a child's adaptation to illness and the greater involvement of its members in the care of the seriously ill child make the family a likely target for psychosocial interventions at all developmental stages. However, interventions that capitalize on the family's role have several other advantages. The use of a family member can be cost effective. For example, a parent can be taught to distract a child during a painful procedure, thus freeing an already overburdened staff. Involving a family member can serve to diminish the sense of helplessness. In the example just given, the parent may not be able to prevent a child from receiving a needle, but can help make the procedure less distressing to the child. Enlisting family support also has the potential for promoting better family communication, especially if all members are given a role.

Finally, in contrast to an earlier period, there now exists both a growing body of lay literature for the family of a child with cancer (cf. Adams and Deveau, 1984; Bracken, 1986; Chesler and Barbarin, 1987; see also the superb annotated bibliography published by the Candlelighters, 1987), and formalized support services (e.g., Candlelighters and Leukemia Society). Health professionals need to be aware of these resources and to use them as appropriate in providing supportive care for every child and family (Monaco, 1986). For their part, families are often grateful to know about material they can read and often derive enormous comfort and support from these very special self-help groups.

## SUMMARY

Cancer in a young person is a devastating experience affecting not only the child but also the family and health care professional. Recent advances in treatment, however, have increased dramatically the prospect for survival from many of these diseases, making this a challenging and rewarding field in which to work. With growing numbers of children going on to live healthy lives, increasing attention has been given to minimizing the negative psychosocial effects of their disease. Although the need to adjust to the regression caused by loss of ego control and to adjust to unknown people, procedures, and machines is experienced by all ill children, specific tasks of development are affected when illness occurs and need to be addressed. Knowledge of ways to address these difficulties will enable health professionals to recognize and anticipate distress in their patients and thereby help both children and families to manage during and to adjust after the clinical course.

## REFERENCES

Achenbach, T.M. (1978). Psychopathology of childhood: Research problems and issues. *J. Consult. Clin. Psychol.* 46:759–76.

Achenbach, T.M. (1982). *Developmental Psychopathology*, 2nd ed. New York: Wiley.

Adams, D.W. and E.J. Deveau (1984). *Coping with Childhood Cancer*. Reston, Va.: Reston Publishing.

Adams, M.A. (1978). Helping the parents of children with malignancy. *J. Pediatrics* 93(5):734–38.

*American Cancer Society (ACS) (1988). Cancer Facts and Figures*. New York: American Cancer Society.

Bellak, L. and B.D. Tokso (eds.). (1976). *Geriatric Psychiatry*. New York: Grune & Stratton.

Bibace, R. and M.E. Walsh (1980). Development of children's concepts of illness. *Pediatrics* 66(6):912–17.

Binger, C.M., A.R. Ablin, R.C. Feuerstein, J.H. Kushner, A. Zoger, and C. Mikkelsen (1969). Childhood leukemia: Emotional impact on patient and family. *N. Engl. J. Med.* 280:414–18.

Birren, J.E. and K.W. Schaie (1977). *Handbook of the Psychology of Aging.* New York: Van Nostrand Reinhold.

Blos, P. (1956). *An Investigation of the Healthy Child's Understanding of the Causes of Disease.* Unpublished doctoral dissertation, Yale University, New Haven, Conn.

Blos, P. (1962). *On Adolescence.* New York: Free Press.

Blotcky, A.D., D.G. Cohen, C. Conatser, and P. Klopovich (1985). Brief report: Psychosocial characteristics of adolescents who refuse cancer treatment. *J. Consult. Clin. Psychol.* 53:729–31.

Blotcky, A.D., J.M. Raczynski, R. Gurwitch, and K. Smith (1985). Family influences on hopelessness among children early in the cancer experience. *J. Pediatr. Psychol.* 10:479–93.

Bluebond-Langner, M. (1977). Meanings of death to children. In H. Feifel (ed.), *New Meanings of Death.* New York: McGraw-Hill, pp. 48–66.

Bluebond-Langner, M. (1978). *The Private Worlds of Dying Children.* Princeton, N.J.: Princeton University Press.

Blum, R.W. (ed.). (1984). *Chronic Illness and Disabilities in Childhood and Adolescence.* New York: Grune & Stratton.

Blumberg, B.D., M.J. Lewis, and E.J. Susman (1984). Adolescence: A time of transition. In M. Eisenberg, L. Sutkin, and M. Jansen (eds.), *Chronic Illness and Disability through the Life Span. Effects on Self and Family.* New York: Springer, pp. 133–49.

Bowlby, J. (1960). Grief and mourning in infancy and early childhood. *Psychoanal. Study Child* 15:9–32.

Bowlby, J. (1988). Developmental psychiatry comes of age. *Am. J. Psychiatry* 145:1–10.

Bracken, J.M. (1986). *Children with Cancer: A Comprehensive Reference Guide for Patients.* New York: Oxford University Press.

Brewster, A. (1982). Chronically ill hospitalized children's concepts of their illness. *Pediatrics* 69:1156–59.

Brown, J.M., J. O'Keeffe, S.H. Sanders, and B. Baker (1986). Developmental changes in children's cognition to stressful and painful situations. *J. Pediatr. Psychol.* 11:343–58.

Burbach, D.J. and L. Peterson (1986). Children's concepts of physical illness: A review and critique of the cognitive-developmental literature. *Health Psychol.* 5:307–25.

Bush, J.P. (1987). Pain in children: A review of the literature from a developmental perspective. *Psychol. Health* 1:215–36.

Bush, J. and C. Cockrell (1987). Maternal factors predicting parenting behaviors in the pediatric clinic. *J. Pediatr. Psychol.* 12:505–18.

Campbell, J.D. (1975a). Attribution of illness: Another double standard. *J. Health Soc. Behav.* 16:114–26.

Campbell, J.D. (1975b). Illness is a point of view: The development of children's concepts of illness. *Child Dev.* 46:92–100.

Campbell, J.D. (1978). The child in the sick role: Contribu-

tions of age, sex, parental status and parental values. *J. Health Soc. Behav.* 19:35–51.

Candlelighters Childhood Cancer Foundation (1987). *Bibliography and Resource Guide,* rev. ed. Washington, D.C.: Candlelighters Childhood Cancer Foundation.

Caradang, M.L., C.H. Folkins, P. Hines, and M.S. Seward (1979). Role of cognitive level and sibling illness in children's conceptualizations of illness. *Am. J. Orthopsychiatry* 49:474–81.

Carpenter, P.J. (1987). Parent involvement in preparing pediatric cancer patients for invasive medical procedures: A cognitive-behavioral approach (Abstract). *Proc. Am. Soc. Clin. Oncol.* 6:256.

Carpenter, P.J. and O.J. Sahler (1987). Siblings' perceptions of the pediatric cancer experience (Abstract). *Proc. Am. Soc. Clin. Oncol.* 6:225.

Chesler, M.A. and O.A. Barbarin (1987). *Childhood Cancer and the Family.* New York: Brunner/Mazel.

Cohen, L.B. (1979). Our developing knowledge of infant perception and cognition. *Am. Psychol.* 34:894–99.

Csikszentmihalyi, M. and R. Larson (1984). *Being Adolescent: Conflict and Growth in the Teenage Years.* New York: Basic Books.

Dinkfelt, P., G. Gilchrist, W. Smithson, E. Burgert, S. Obetz, R. Colligan, and T. Therneau (1986). Development of pediatric patients' conceptions of cancer (Abstract). *Proc. Am. Soc. Clin. Oncol.* 5:238.

Earle, E.M. (1979). The psychological effects of mutilating surgery in children and adolescents. *Psychoanal. Study Child* 34:527–46.

Easson, W.M. (1968). Care of the young patient who is dying. *J.A.M.A.* 205:203–7.

Eiser, C. (1980). How leukemia affects a child's schooling. *Br. J. Soc. Clin. Psychol.* 19:365–68.

Eiser, C. and R. Lansdown (1977). Retrospective study of intellectual development in children treated for acute lymphoblastic leukemia. *Arch. Dis. Child.* 52:525–29.

Elkins, P.D. and M.C. Roberts (1983). Psychological preparation for pediatric hospitalization. *Clin. Psychol. Rev.* 3:275–96.

Erikson, E.H. (1963). *Childhood and Society,* 2nd ed. New York: Norton.

Erikson, E.H. (1968). *Identity: Youth and Crisis.* New York: Norton.

Farley, G. (1985). Cognitive development. In R. Simons (ed.), *Understanding Human Behavior in Health and Illness,* 3rd ed. Baltimore: Williams & Wilkins, pp. 249–54.

Freud, A. (1952). The role of bodily illness in the mental life of children. *Psychoanal. Study Child* 7:69–81.

Freud, A. (1958). Adolescence. *Psychoanal. Study Child* 16:225–78.

Freud, A. (1963). The concept of developmental lines. *Psychoanal. Study Child* 18:245–65.

Freud, A. (1965). *Normality and Pathology in Childhood. Assessment of Development.* New York: International Universities Press.

Freud, S. (1927). *The Ego and the Id.* London: Hogarth Press.

Geist, R.A. (1979). Onset of chronic illness in children and adolescents: Psychotherapeutic and consultative intervention. *Am. J. Orthopsychiatry* 49:4–23.

Gellert, E. (1961). Children's beliefs about bodily illness. Paper presented at the annual meeting of the American Psychological Association, New York, September.

Ginsburg, H. and S. Opper. *Piaget's Theory of Intellectual Development. An Introduction.* Englewood Cliffs, N.J.: Prentice-Hall.

Goff, J.R., H.R. Anderson, and P.F. Cooper (1980). Distractability and memory deficits in long-term survivors of acute leukemia. *J. Dev. Behav. Pediatrics* 1:158–63.

Goggin, E.L., S.B. Lansky, and K. Hassanein (1976). Psychological reactions of children with malignancies. *J. Acad. Child Psychiatry* 15:314–25.

Gross, A., R. Stern, R. Lenn, J. Dale, and D. Wojnilower (1983). The effect of mother–child separation on the behavior of children experiencing a diagnostic medical procedure. *J. Consult. Clin. Psychol.* 51:783–85.

Hall, B.D. (1982). Issues in the psychological care of pediatric oncology patients. *Am. J. Orthopsychiatry* 52:32–44.

Harlow, H.F. and R.R. Zimmerman (1959). Affectional responses in the infant monkey. *Science* 130:421–32.

Harlow, H.F. and M.K. Harlow (1962). Social deprivation in monkeys. *Sci. Am.* 207:136–46.

Hays, D.M., K.I. Hoffman, K.O. Williams, S.E. Siegel, and R. Miller (1985). Medical students' concepts of childhood cancer and its management. *Med. Pediatr. Oncol.* 13:78–82.

Hoffman, A., R. Becker, and H. Gabriel (1976). *The Hospitalized Adolescent: A Guide to Managing Ill and Injured Youth.* New York: Free Press.

Hodgekinson, H.L. (1985). *All One System.* Washington, D.C.: Institute for Educational Leadership.

Inhelder, B. and J. Piaget (1958). *The Growth of Logical Thinking.* New York: Basic Books.

Jay, S.M. and C.H. Elliott (1984). Psychological intervention for pain in pediatric cancer patients. In G.B. Humphrey, L.P. Dehner, G.B. Grindey, and R.T. Acton (eds.), *Pediatric Oncology,* Vol. 3. Boston: Martinus Nijhoff, pp. 123–54.

Jay, S.M., M. Ozolins, C.H. Elliott, and S. Caldwell (1983). Assessment of children's distress during painful medical procedures. *Health Psychol.* 2:133–47.

Kagen-Goodheart, L. (1977). Reentry: Living with childhood cancer. *Am. J. Orthopsychiatry* 47:651–58.

Karon, M. and J. Vernick (1968). An approach to the emotional support of fatally ill children. *Clin. Pediatrics* 7:174–280.

Kart, C.S., E.S. Metress, and J.F. Metress (1978). *Health and Aging: Biological and Social Perspectives.* Menlo Park, Calif.: Addison-Wesley.

Kellerman, J. (ed.). (1980). *Psychological Aspects of Childhood Cancer.* Springfield, Ill.: Charles C. Thomas.

Kellerman, J., D. Rigler, S.E. Siegel, and E.R. Katz (1977). Disease-related communication and depression in pediatric cancer patients. *J. Pediatr. Psychol.* 2:52–53.

Kellerman, J., L. Zeltzer, L. Ellenberg, J. Dash, and D. Rigler (1980). Psychological effects of illness in adolescence. I. Anxiety, self-esteem and perception of control. *J. Pediatrics* 97:126–31.

Kister, M.C. and C.F. Patterson (1980). Children's conception of the causes of illness: Understanding of contagion and use of immanent justice. *Child Dev.* 51:839–46.

Koocher, G.P. (1986a). Coping with a death from cancer. *J. Consult. Clin. Psychol.* 54:623–31.

Koocher, G.P. (1986b). Psychosocial issues during the acute treatment of pediatric cancer. *Cancer* 58:468–72.

Koocher, G.P. and J.E. O'Malley (1981). *The Damocles Syndrome: Psychosocial Consequences of Surviving Childhood Cancer.* New York: McGraw-Hill.

Koocher, G.P., J.E. O'Malley, G.L. Gogan, and D.J. Foster (1979). Psychological adjustment among pediatric cancer survivors. *J. Child Psychol. Psychiatry* 21:163–73.

Krupnick, J.L. (1984). Bereavement during childhood and adolescence. In M. Osterweis, F. Solomon, and M. Green (eds.), *Bereavement: Reactions, Consequences and Care.* Washington, D.C.: National Academy Press, pp. 99–141.

Langford, W.S. (1961). The child in the pediatric hospital: Adaptation to illness and hospitalization. *Am. J. Orthopsychiatry* 31:667–84.

Lansky, S.B. (1985). Management of stressful periods in childhood cancer. *Pediatr. Clin. North Am.* 32:625–32.

Lansky, S.B., M.A. List, and C. Ritter-Sterr (1986). Psychosocial consequences of cure. *Cancer* 58:529–33.

Levinson, D.J., with C.N. Darrow, E.B. Klein, M.H. Levinson, and B. McKee (1978). *The Seasons of a Man's Life.* New York: Knopf.

Maddux, J.E., M.C. Roberts, E.A. Sledden, and L. Wright (1986). Developmental issues in child health psychology. *Am. Psychol.* 41:25–34.

Maguire, G.P. (1983). The psychosocial sequelae of childhood leukemia. In W. Duncan (ed.), *Paediatric Oncology.* Berlin: Springer-Verlag, pp. 47–56.

Mahler, M.S., F. Pine, and A. Bergman (1975). *The Psychological Birth of the Human Infant.* New York: Basic Books.

Masek, B., D. Russo, and J. Varni (1984). Behavioral approaches to the management of chronic pain in children. *Pediatr. Clin. North Am.* 31:1113–31.

Maurer, A. (1961). The child's knowledge of non-existence. *J. Exist. Psychol.* 2:193–212.

Meadows, A.T., J. Gordon, D.J. Massari, P. Littman, J. Fergusson, and K. Moss (1981). Decline in IQ scores and cognitive dysfunctions in children with acute lymphocytic leukemia treated with cranial irradiation. *Lancet* 2:1015–18.

Meadows, A.T. and J. Silber (1985). Delayed consequences of therapy for childhood cancer. *CA* 35:271–86.

Mechanic, D. (1983). Adolescent health and illness behavior: Review of the literature and a new hypothesis for the study of stress. *J. Human Stress* 9:4–13.

Michielutte, R. and R.A. Diseker (1982). Children's perceptions of cancer in comparison to other chronic illnesses. *J. Chron. Dis.* 35:843–52.

Miller, N.E. (1981). An overview of behavioral medicine: Opportunities and dangers. In S.M. Weiss, J.A. Herd, and

B.H. Fox (eds.), *Perspectives on Behavioral Medicine.* New York: Academic Press, pp. 3–22.

Monaco, G.P. (1986). Resources available to the family of the child with cancer. *Cancer* 58:516–21.

Money, J. and R.R. Clopper, Jr. (1974). Psychosocial and psychosexual aspects of errors of pubertal onset and development. *Human Biol.* 46:173–81.

Morrow, G.R., A. Hoagland, and C.L.M. Carnrike, Jr. (1981). Social support and parental adjustment to pediatric cancer. *J. Consult. Clin. Psychol.* 49:763–65.

Moss, H.A., E.D. Nannis, and D.G. Poplack (1981). The effects of prophylactic treatment of the central nervous system on the intellectual functioning of children with acute lymphocytic leukemia. *Am. J. Med.* 71:47–52.

Muuss, R.E. (1975). *Theories of Adolescence,* 3rd ed. New York: Random House.

Nagy, M.H. (1948). The child's theories concerning death. *J. Genet. Psychol.* 73:3–27.

Nagy, M.H. (1951). Children's ideas of the origin of illness. *Health Educ. J.* 9:6–12.

Nannis, E.D., E.J. Susman, B.E. Strope, P.J. Woodruff, S.P. Hersh, A.S. Levine, and P.A. Pizzo (1982). Correlates of control in pediatric cancer patients and their families. *J. Pediatr. Psychol.* 7:75–84.

Neuhauser, C., B. Amsterdam, P. Hines, and M. Steward (1978). Children's concepts of healing: Cognitive development and locus of control factors. *Am. J. Orthopsychiatry* 48:335–41.

Offer, D., E. Ostrov, and K.I. Howard (1981). *The Adolescent: A Psychological Self-Portrait.* New York: Basic Books.

Offer, D., E. Ostrov, and K.I. Howard (1984). Body image, self-perception, and chronic illness in adolescence. In R.W. Blum (ed.), *Chronic Illness and Disabilities in Childhood and Adolescence.* New York: Grune & Stratton, pp. 59–73.

Perrin, E. and P.S. Gerrity (1981). There's a demon in your belly: Children's understanding of illness. *Pediatrics* 64:841–49.

Piaget, J. (1952). *The Origins of Intelligence in Children.* New York: International Universities Press.

Plumb, M.M. and J. Holland (1974). Cancer in adolescents. The symptom is the thing. In B. Schoenberg, A.C. Carr, A.H. Kutscher, D. Peretz, and I.K. Goldberg (eds.), *Anticipatory Grief.* New York: Columbia University Press, pp. 193–209.

Potter, P.C. and M.C. Roberts (1984). Children's perceptions of chronic illness: The roles of disease symptoms, cognitive development, and information. *J. Pediatr. Psychol.* 9:13–27.

Rait, D.S. and J.C. Holland (1986). Pediatric cancer: Psychosocial issues and approaches. *Mediguide Oncol.* 6:1–8.

Roberts, M.C., J.E. Maddux, and L. Wright (1984). Developmental perspectives in behavioral health. In J.D. Matarazzo, N.E. Miller, S.M. Weiss, and J.A. Herd (eds.), *Behavioral Health: A Handbook of Health Promotion and Disease Prevention.* New York: Wiley, pp. 56–68.

Ross, D. and S. Ross (1984). Childhood pain: The school-aged child's viewpoint. *Pain* 20:179–91.

Schowalter, J.E. (1970). The child's reaction to his own terminal illness. In B. Schoenberg, A. Carr, D. Peretz, and A. Kutscher (eds.), *Loss and Grief: Psychological Management in Medical Practice.* New York: Columbia University Press, pp. 51–69.

Schowalter, J.E. (1977). Psychological reactions to physical illness and hospitalization in adolescence. *J. Am. Acad. Child Psychiatry* 16:500–16.

Shaw, E. and D. Routh (1982). Effect of mother presence on children's reactions to aversive procedures. *J. Pediatr. Psychol.* 7:33–42.

Slavin, L.A., J.E. O'Malley, G.P. Koocher, and D.J. Foster (1982). Communication of the cancer diagnosis to pediatric patients: Impact on long term adjustment. *Am. J. Psychiatry* 139:179–83.

Smith, D.W. and E.L. Bierman (eds.) (1973). *The Biologic Ages of Man.* Philadelphia: W.B. Saunders.

Solomon, J.R., M.V. Faletti, and S.S. Yunik (1982). The psychologist as geriatric clinician. In T. Millon, C. Green, and R. Meagher (eds.), *Handbook of Clinical Health Psychology.* New York: Plenum, pp. 227–50.

Sourkes, B.M. (1980). Siblings of the pediatric cancer patient. In J. Kellerman (ed.), *Psychological Aspects of Childhood Cancer.* Springfield, Ill.: Charles C. Thomas, pp. 47–69.

Spinetta, J.J. (1974). The dying child's awareness of death: A review. *Psychol. Bull.* 81:256–60.

Spinetta, J.J. (1981). The sibling of the child with cancer. In J.J. Spinetta and P. Deasy-Spinetta (eds.), *Living with Childhood Cancer.* St. Louis: C.V. Mosby, pp. 133–42.

Spinetta, J.J. (1982). Behavioral and psychological research in childhood cancer: An overview. *Cancer* 50:1939–43.

Spinetta, J.J. and P. Deasy-Spinetta (eds.) (1981). *Living with Childhood Cancer.* St. Louis: C.V. Mosby.

Spinetta, J.J. and P. Deasy-Spinetta (1986). The patient's socialization in the community and school during therapy. *Cancer* 58:512–15.

Spinetta, J.J. and S.B. Lansky (1982). Behavioral and psychosocial research in childhood cancer. *Cancer* 50(Suppl.):1944–45.

Spinetta, J.J. and L.J. Maloney (1975). Death anxiety in the outpatient leukemic child. *Pediatrics* 65:1034–37.

Spitz, R.A. (1945). Hospitalism: An inquiry into the genesis of psychiatric conditions in early childhood. *Psychoanal. Study Child* 1:53–74.

Stern, D.N. (1985). *The Interpersonal World of the Infant.* New York: Basic Books.

Steward, M. and D. Steward (1981). Children's conceptions of medical procedures. In *New Directions for Child Development. Children's Conceptions of Health, Illness and Bodily Functions.* San Francisco: Jossey-Bass, pp. 67–83.

Stone, G.C. (ed.) (1983). Proceedings of the national working conference on education and training in health psychology. *Health Psychol.* 2(Suppl.).

Teta, M.J., M.C. Del Po, S.V. Kasl, J.W. Meigs, M.H. Myers, and J.J. Mulvihill (1986). Psychosocial consequences of childhood and adolescent cancer survival. *J. Chron. Dis.* 39:751–59.

Van Dongen-Melman, J.E.W.M. and J.A.R. Sanders-Woudstra (1986). Psychosocial aspects of childhood cancer: A review of the literature. *J. Child Psychol. Psychiatry* 27:145–80.

Vernick, J. and M. Karon (1965). Who's afraid of death on a leukemia ward? *Am. J. Dis. Child.* 107:393–97.

Waechter, E.H. (1971). Children's awareness of fatal illness. *Am. J. Nurs.* 7:1168–72.

Zeltzer, L., J. Kellerman, L. Ellenberg, J. Dash, and D. Rigler (1980). Psychologic effects of illness in adolescence: II. Impact of illness in adolescents—crucial issues and coping styles. *J. Pediatrics* 97(1):132–38.

Zeltzer, L., S. LeBaron, and P. Zeltzer (1984). The adolescent with cancer. In R.W. Blum (ed.), *Chronic Illness and Disabilities in Childhood and Adolescence*. New York: Grune & Stratton, pp. 375–95.

# 44

# Common Psychiatric Disorders in Childhood Cancer and Their Management

Betty Pfefferbaum

The psychosocial and psychiatric issues associated with childhood cancer have changed markedly as the prognosis for many of the more common malignancies has improved. Childhood cancer today is a model not only for understanding the psychological aspects of terminal illness, but also for studying chronic illness and long survival. The psychological literature has grown rapidly, reflecting these changes and an increasing sophistication in the understanding of related issues. This chapter reviews the indications for psychiatric consultation, common psychiatric disorders, psychiatric interventions, treatment-related issues, stage-specific issues, and special problems related to school, communication, ethical issues, and staff problems.

## NATURE OF THE PSYCHIATRIC CONSULTATION

The treatment of all children with cancer should include careful attention to the mental health of the child and the family. This attention is an integral part of the routine care given by the pediatric oncologist, nurse, and social worker. However, when significant psychiatric problems develop in the patient, parent, or sibling, it is important that a psychiatric consultant be called. For this reason, it is important that the oncologist and the support team know these indications, especially when emergency intervention may be necessary or when the likelihood of psychiatric problems is so great (''at risk'' families) that a consultation is warranted at the time of diagnosis to provide early assessment and intervention. Table 44-1 outlines these problems. Each is discussed in terms of usual symptoms and management principles in the subsequent sections.

The psychiatric consultant must be informed not only about common psychiatric problems encountered in pediatric oncology but also about common childhood malignancies, their prognoses, treatments, and expected treatment or illness-related side effects. Because patients frequently are referred for adjustment problems and may not have primary psychopathology, they may be suspicious of the psychiatrist and may even refuse to cooperate if the consultation is not presented carefully. The psychiatrist should ideally work closely with the oncologists, making clinical rounds, often simply making recommendations for management to the team without formally seeing the child or parent at all. When a child and/or parent are identified for evaluation, they will have met the psychiatrist already during rounds and recognize him or her as a member of the team who manages certain kinds of physical and psychological problems. The psychiatrist can then explain to the child and family that the evaluation was recommended to help with a specific symptom such as pain, sad feelings, or trouble with sleeping or eating. Reassurance can be given that psychiatric consultation is helpful to many patients in the context of coping with the stresses of cancer and its treatment, and that seeing a psychiatrist does not imply that one is ''crazy.''

The psychiatric evaluation consists of first reviewing the chart, assessing any clinical or laboratory data that might be pertinent to the symptom to be evaluated, and obtaining information from the referring physician, staff, patient, and parents. As part of this review, it is very important to ascertain the family and child's understanding of the diagnosis, treatment, and prognosis. The psychiatric history of the child, parents, and siblings should be carefully taken to determine if any member is at risk for psychiatric decompensation and is in need of close monitoring. The family history should include both medical and psychosocial aspects to determine if there is a history of familial problems. Previous life crises should be reviewed to determine

**Table 44-1** Indications for psychiatric consultation in pediatric oncology

| Level for consultation | Indications |
| --- | --- |
| I. Emergency | Suicidal risk: ideation or behavior (child or family member) |
| | Behavior endangering self or others (child or family member) |
| II. At time of diagnosis | Preexisting major mental illness (child or family member) |
| | Mental retardation and autism |
| | History of child abuse or neglect |
| III. Early referral | Anxiety and panic |
| | Depression |
| | Pain |
| | Organic brain syndrome (delirium) with psychosis |
| | Adjustment problems to treatment |
| |     Compliance |
| |     Side effects |
| |     Special treatment situations |
| | Stage-specific adaptation problems |
| |     Long survival and cure |
| |     Terminal illness |
| | Special problems |
| |     Family (especially "at risk" constellation) |
| |     School |
| |     Coping over time |
| |     Communication and staff issues |

the usual response of the child and parents to crises, coping strategies, and availability of support systems among extended-family members or community organizations. It is additionally important to determine the family members' alliances, attitudes, dynamics, and interpersonal relationships.

Evaluation of the child should include assessment of developmental level, understanding of the illness, reactions to the illness and treatment, and intellectual functioning. A complete mental status examination should be done initially. The documented mental status provides an important baseline with which to compare mental changes later. Areas to be assessed are size and general appearance, motility, coordination, speech, thought and perception, emotional state, manner of relating, fantasies and dreams, insight, cognitive functioning (including orientation, attention span, concentration, memory, information, and vocabulary), abstraction ability, and judgment.

One goal of consultation is to clarify the child's understanding of the diagnosis and treatment plan, and to correct misinformation. It is best initially to use the child's own terms in discussions about the illness. The child's words indicate his or her understanding of the illness and its implications and also provide shelter

from frightening realities. For example, one 5-year-old described her illness by saying, "You know how you have bruises on your body when you get hurt? Well, I have bruises inside and out." Labeling the illness as a "bruising" disease provided a readily acceptable term to enhance communication. Providing too much information, or conveying information with words that confuse or frighten the child, should be avoided.

It is important to let the child set the pace of discussion. It is equally important for the psychiatrist to be a supportive listener while the child expresses his or her problems in his or her own words. It should be cautioned that hasty interpretation of the child's thoughts can be both frightening and counterproductive. One teenager, in an early session with a therapist, described a dream in which she was frightened by a "black sheet" that covered her. The therapist, understanding the child's concerns, identified the "black sheet" as representing fears of death. The child responded with intense anger and refused any further sessions.

It is expected and normal that the child with cancer will have psychological distress, as will his or her family. They will be particularly stressed at certain times, such as at time of diagnosis, when there is a sudden adverse change in physical condition, beginning and ending treatment, upon school reentry, and in the event of disease recurrence. While grief, anxiety, and depression are common, most families cope well with the crises. Psychologically healthy families are able to use available resources and find new ones. Most children and families never ask for psychiatric assistance, managing to cope and make a healthy adaptation. However, many suffer more severe psychological disturbance that requires intervention. Outlined in Table 44-1, these are discussed in greater detail in the following section.

## PSYCHIATRIC DISORDERS

Psychiatric disorders that require consultation in the pediatric oncology setting can be classified into three categories: level I consists of life-threatening conditions that necessitate emergency consultation; level II disorders are preexisting or concurrent psychiatric or social conditions that have a high risk of compromising treatment and that should be evaluated at time of diagnosis; level III includes psychological or social adaptational problems that can occur at any point in the course of illness and for which early referral for consultation is warranted. Because some of these conditions warrant psychopharmacological management, specific psychotropic drugs and recommended dosages are specified where appropriate (for review of current concepts in pediatric psychopharmacology, see also Biederman and Jellinek, 1984; Klein et al., 1980; Weiner, 1984).

## Level I: Disorders Requiring Emergency Consultation

### SUICIDAL RISK

This may be a life-threatening complication occurring in the child or parent in the course of cancer treatment. An emergency consultation should be called when suicidal ideation or behavior is observed in either the child or a family member. The parent with a history of severe prior psychiatric disturbance may become suicidal when informed that his or her child's condition is poor. Management of a suicidal parent on a pediatric floor may necessitate removal of the parent or careful monitoring of behavior.

Adolescents who become depressed may talk of suicide as illness progresses. Noncompliance accompanying depressive symptoms may sometimes be considered a suicidal action. When confusion from encephalopathy occurs, suicidal behavior may be observed, reflecting depressed mood and the associated loss of impulse control. Behaviors such as attempting to place an intravenous line around the neck or grabbing scissors have been seen. Suicidal risk requires careful evaluation, observation, and counseling in management principles for staff and parents. Treatment of depression or a confusional state, usually with tricyclic antidepressants or phenothiazines, may be indicated.

### BEHAVIOR ENDANGERING SELF OR OTHERS

This is another indication for an emergency psychiatric consultation, and it may occur in the child or a family member. In the child or adolescent, such behavior can occur in the context of a psychotic reaction or violent behavior associated with delirium related to a drug (e.g., steroids), or to a metabolic encephalopathy from other causes. The child may be hallucinating and may appear hypervigilant. The child may require sedation to prevent exhaustion or possible combative behavior toward others. If the child refuses oral medication, intramuscular or intravenous (when a central line is in place) sedation must be instituted, using physical restraint as needed, combined with efforts to calm and orient the child.

The psychiatrically disturbed parent who has paranoid, suspicious tendencies may decompensate as the child's condition worsens. The need to blame someone for the impending loss may result in hostility toward the doctor and/or staff who are perceived as neglecting or improperly managing the child. Threats against the physician or staff must be taken seriously, and the psychiatrist must have ready access to security guards in such potentially volatile situations.

## Level II: Disorders Requiring Referral at Diagnosis

### PREEXISTING MAJOR MENTAL ILLNESS

A history of a psychiatric disorder in the child or parent is reason for psychiatric consultation or diagnosis because the stress of the illness may result in exacerbation of the primary psychiatric disorder. Children with attention deficit disorder, schizophrenia, or affective disorder should be followed carefully and treated with medication as needed. A retarded or psychotic child with cancer will need special attention to help him or her understand and cope with the disease and undergo treatments that demand cooperation; special attention is also needed in obtaining informed consent. Collaboration between the pediatric oncologist and the child psychiatrist is essential in these situations.

The parent with a psychiatric history must be assessed early to establish a diagnosis and determine how the parental illness may impinge on the child's treatment. Common problems that occur with these parents are inadequate support for the child, conflict with staff, poor compliance with the child's treatment plan, and conflicts with the spouse that complicate treatment decisions.

### MENTAL RETARDATION

The severely retarded or autistic child presents special problems and needs in regard to management. Special efforts are necessary to explain procedures and enlist cooperation, or to sedate when cooperation cannot be attained. Concern for legal aspects of guardianship, assent, and consent are important.

### HISTORY OF CHILD ABUSE OR NEGLECT

A history of child abuse or neglect, not attributable to a mental disorder in the parent, also needs careful evaluation at the time of diagnosis. Such patterns of disturbed parent–child interactions place the patient and siblings at risk for inadequate care and may require legal attention.

Adequate physical, emotional, and nutritional support of the young patient undergoing intensive treatment may be compromised if a responsible, caring adult relationship is lacking. Both parent and child may use compliance as a battleground for long-standing conflicts. A sibling may alternately be singled out as a scapegoat in these families when crises overwhelm the distressed parent. Early identification of a principal caregiver in this situation is important. The adaptation of the child and family should be carefully monitored over the course of treatment; special efforts may be necessary to provide additional social supports to family members, especially parents.

## Level III: Disorders and Problems Requiring Early Referral When Observed

### ANXIETY AND PANIC

Anxiety and depression often coexist in children with cancer. The anxious child may exhibit mild agitation, features of depression, or physical symptoms. Chronic anxiety often underlies some children's marginal adaptation throughout the course of the illness. Anticipatory and acute situational anxiety and panic usually occur in response to painful diagnostic procedures, treatments, or crises during illness.

Surprisingly, little systematic attention has been paid to anxiety in children with cancer, although clinically this is a common problem that requires attention. Two studies, however, examined incidence of the problem. A study of over 100 children undergoing bone marrow aspiration found anxiety to be ubiquitous. Younger children showed more distress than older children, and girls appeared more anxious than boys (Katz et al., 1980). In a second study, some children were found to have anxiety associated with stressful procedures from the outset. Others appeared to do well for a period of time and then developed severe anxiety or other anticipatory symptoms such as a conditioned nausea response during the course of the illness (Redd and Andrykowski, 1982).

Anticipatory and acute situational anxiety and panic are frequently observed in children during painful procedures such as spinal taps and bone marrow aspirations. The distress may lead the child to withdraw and cry, or to become agitated, angry, and combative, requiring physical restraint. This latter behavior is distressing not only to the child but also to the parents and staff, as well as other children and families. Acute situational anxiety may make painful procedures and treatment procedures impossible to perform. Noncompliance with the medical regimen may be a worrisome result. In addition, underlying unresolved anxiety may cause other serious disturbances in psychosocial functioning.

### CASE REPORT

An 8-year-old boy came to the clinic for his last spinal tap in a long series that had spanned several years. The child had not expressed concern during any stressful procedure until the last one. He became severely fearful, cried and screamed, and refused to undergo the procedure. He ran from the treatment room and was found on one of the inpatient units. After a dose of chlorpromazine, the child agreed to undergo the procedure. He played quietly and calmly for about 30 minutes until it was time for the procedure, and then once again became extremely anxious. He was given a second dose of medication, and time was allowed for it to take effect. The child, still frightened and fighting, had to be restrained as he kicked and screamed throughout the entire procedure.

It is important to avoid these extreme behaviors by careful planning *prior* to the procedure. Intervention for particularly painful procedures, often including medication, may reduce anxiety and noncompliance. Because these anticipatory and acute situational anxiety reactions often continue and even increase over time, even during remission, concern must be raised about the long-term effect of the conditioning on anxiety and its role in the development of posttraumatic stress disorder in adulthood. Retrospective studies of adult psychiatric patients with anxiety and panic disorders show that they often had similar symptoms during childhood (Gittleman and Klein, 1984; Raskin et al., 1982). While this may reflect a genetic basis, it may also represent a conditioned response to stressful childhood events (e.g., physical illness), making management of such events early in life important future determinants.

Chronic anxiety may be difficult to diagnose and often coexists with depression. Although one study of chronically ill adolescent outpatients found them to be no more anxious than healthy controls on self-report measures (Kellerman et al., 1980), there still appears to be reason for concern about the long-term impact of repeated procedures associated with pain and anxiety in childhood cancer outpatients.

Management of the anxiety depends on its severity. Often reassurance, guidance, and support are sufficient to help the anxious child through a painful procedure, treatment, or crisis. At times, however, more intensive psychological intervention is required. Rehearsal of a procedure in play therapy is helpful, especially for young children (see Chapter 45). Relaxation techniques and hypnosis are also useful and popular therapeutic modalities with some children (for an elaboration of these techniques, see Chapter 46 on behavioral interventions). The parent's response is crucial and often functions to reduce or increase the child's anxiety, suggesting the need to help the parent who accompanies the child.

When anxiety is severe—of panic proportions, or prolonged—medication should be used. Major and minor tranquilizers have been used for acute episodes. Diphenhydramine is safe and sedating in sufficient amounts. Minor tranquilizers such as diazepam and alprazolam are helpful in some situations. A recent study reported beneficial results with alprazolam in low doses (0.02 mg/kg tid) for anticipatory and acute situational anxiety in children undergoing procedures (Pfefferbaum et al., 1988). Phenothiazines such as chlorpromazine may at times be necessary. Medication in conjunction with relaxation techniques may be desirable in some cases. Once anxiety has reached panic proportions, medication is required in large doses. However, before symptoms escalate, a drug introduced early will be effective, usually in lower doses, and should be used in the child who is known or expected to be anxious. Tricyclic antidepressants such as amitriptyline and imipramine appear to be helpful in the management of chronic anxiety and should be considered when anxiety is long-standing and accompanied by symptoms of depression (Maisami et al., 1985; Pfefferbaum-Levine et al., 1983).

Lansky and Gendel (1978) described a symbiotic regressive behavior pattern in children with cancer in whom family interactions became markedly disturbed. The pattern was characterized by extreme anxiety, panic, and regressive behavior in the child, with an intense, mutually protective, hostile parent–child relationship, and social withdrawal. When observed, this picture of separation problems and poor individuation indicates that the family is at risk for difficulties during treatment and warrants early intervention; unaddressed, the behavior pattern becomes intractable. During episodes of extreme anxiety, panic, or regression in these disturbed relationships, initiation of intensive family therapy is essential. Psychotherapy aimed at separating the close parent and child must be cautious to avoid enhancement of the pathological attachment. Extreme degrees of separation anxiety and pathological attachment are not uncommon in the context of cancer treatment. One robust teenage boy sat in his mother's lap every time he came to the clinic. When he was hospitalized, his mother shared his bed. Another teenager with a long disease-free period following treatment for Ewing's sarcoma developed a school phobia, refusing to return to school for over 6 years. She lived alone with her widowed mother and the two seldom participated in activities without each other. After the child's death, the mother's grief reaction included hallucinating the child's voice.

Identifying and encouraging the adaptive aspects of the parent–child relationship is crucial and should begin at the earliest hint of a disturbance in the relationship. The therapist should insist that the child attend school and participate in age-appropriate activities. The parent should be encouraged to participate in parental activities and spend time alone with the spouse and other children in the family.

## DEPRESSION

Chronic mild depression mixed with anxiety is often present throughout much of the child's treatment. Kashani and Hakami (1982) found that 17% of their childhood cancer patients showed signs of an affective disorder and over 30% experienced separation anxiety and fear during the illness. Reassurance, guidance, and support are often sufficient to control symptoms. Psychological interventions including individual, play, group, and family therapy may also be helpful and should be considered when more persistent depression occurs.

When depression is severe or persistent, or when it interferes with medical treatment or psychosocial functioning, medication should be used. Successful management of depression, anxiety, sleep disturbance, and other symptoms was reported with low doses (1–2 mg/kg/day) of a tricyclic antidepressant. Tricyclics were effective and safe, without hepatic, renal, and cardiac side effects, although these need to be closely monitored until more experience has been gained with the use of these drugs in ill children (Pfefferbaum-Levine et al., 1983). Another study reported that major tranquilizers and tricyclic antidepressants allay anxiety and facilitate psychotherapeutic intervention in terminally ill children (Maisami et al., 1985). While child psychiatrists are cautious in recommending psychotropic drugs, these medications appear to be especially efficacious in children with depression or anxiety associated with cancer.

### CASE REPORT

An 11-year-old girl who had undergone an amputation for osteogenic sarcoma suffered tremendous anxiety at diagnosis but seemed to improve. Later in the treatment course, however, she became severely depressed, with symptoms of anxiety that were worse when she was scheduled to return to the hospital for chemotherapy. On one occasion, her mother found her hiding in a ditch. Another time on the way to the hospital, she tried to jump from the car, which was going 60 miles per hour. Treatment with low-dose (2 mg/kg/day) tricyclic antidepressant medication was successful, and the child was able to begin school on time several weeks after beginning the chemotherapy treatments.

Both tricyclic antidepressants and major tranquilizers have been reported to lower the seizure threshold. Therefore, if a patient requires a high dose of an antidepressant or has suspicious neurological findings, a baseline EEG should be obtained before beginning treatment. Tricyclic antidepressants have also been associated with ECG changes that are dose-related (Klein et al., 1980). When a child is receiving cardiotoxic chemotherapeutic drugs, particularly adriamycin, it is advisable to monitor cardiac function carefully by ECG, even if doses are low (Pfefferbaum-Levine et al., 1984b). When psychoactive medications are considered or used in children with cancer, a child psychiatrist should be consulted and should follow the patient.

Tricyclic antidepressants are beneficial for a number of symptoms in this population, including anxiety, depression, sleep disturbance, withdrawn behavior, and pain. Although careful studies are needed to assess benefit for specific symptoms such as pain in children, clinical experience shows this class of drugs to have particular efficacy. Different clinicians have preference for specific antidepressants, but experience with imipramine and amitriptyline is most extensive (Maisami et al., 1985; Pfefferbaum-Levine et al., 1983).

## PAIN

Pain has a subjective component that is enhanced in the presence of anxiety or depression. Conversely, the presence of uncontrolled pain causes anxiety and depression. There is a strong tendency to underestimate levels of pain in children who have trouble describing it, but careful attention confirms that pain, even phantom limb pain in young children can be very distressing. Difficulty in assessing the level of pain, coupled with fears of addiction, often result in excessive caution in the use of pain medications.

An Australian study of 170 children recovering from surgery in two major teaching hospitals revealed that no analgesic medication was ordered for 16% of patients, and the narcotic medication ordered was not given to 39% of patients. When an order was written for either narcotic or nonnarcotic medication, the nonnarcotic medication was given exclusively. Irrespective of medication, 75% of children reported pain on the day of surgery and only 53% reported no pain on the first postoperative day; 17% had severe pain. The interpretation of ''PRN'' was ''as little as possible.'' Many children became withdrawn as a means of coping with the pain (Mather and Mackie, 1983). In another study comparing 50 children with 50 adults in the prescription rates and administration of analgesics following open-heart surgery, it was found that children were prescribed significantly fewer potent narcotics than adults. No analgesics were prescribed to 6 children during the first 3 postoperative days, and 12 children received no analgesics during the first 3 to 5 days after their operation. Also, fewer prescriptions for children fell within the therapeutic dosage range (Beyer et al., 1983). Reluctance to medicate adequately, or at all, may result in the child's recall of a painful episode as a traumatic experience, making him or her more vulnerable to anxiety in future episodes.

There is a great need for both systematic study of pain control in children and greater emphasis on the education of medical and nursing staff in pain management in children.

Psychological, behavioral, pharmacological, and surgical interventions are all currently used to achieve pain control in children. Psychological and behavioral interventions include psychotherapy, relaxation, hypnosis, and biofeedback. Psychoactive medications used have included minor and major tranquilizers, antidepressants, and stimulants. Benzodiazepines may decrease symptoms such as anxiety and restlessness, thereby minimizing the general sense of distress accompanying pain (Noyes, 1981). Some argue that minor tranquilizers, while indicated for anxiety and agitation associated with pain, do not potentiate analgesics and may produce depressive symptoms and excessive sedation (Newberger and Sallan, 1981). However, a relatively new benzodiazepine (alprazolam), which may have antidepressant and anxiolytic effect, is of interest for use in children (Fawcett and Kravitz, 1982). Chlorpromazine has antianxiety and sedative properties that diminish pain as well as reduce fear and sleep disturbance associated with the child's suffering. Tricyclic antidepressants, which have anxiolytic, sedating, as well as antidepressant properties, also have been used successfully in children (Pfefferbaum-Levine et al., 1983). Stimulants have been used successfully as adjuvant drugs in pain relief in adults (Forrest et al., 1977; Newburger and Sallan, 1981), but have received little attention in this application with children. In some cases it is not clear how a specific agent provides pain relief. Mode of action may involve direct analgesic effect, potentiation of narcotic agents, sedation, or control of psychological symptoms (e.g., improving mood or diminishing anxiety).

## ORGANIC BRAIN SYNDROME (DELIRIUM) WITH PSYCHOSIS

One of the most distressing psychiatric problems among childhood cancer patients is acute delirium with psychotic manifestations resulting from central nervous system (CNS) complication of the disease. The delirium may be caused by direct CNS invasion or by indirect effect or secondary encephalopathy resulting from infection, metabolic disturbance, narcotics, or organ failure. (For an elaboration of the CNS complications associated with cancer, see Chapter 29.) Treatment of this alarming condition is of great concern for parents and staff as well as the child. The clinical picture is one in which the child's behavior changes, often abruptly; the child may become withdrawn or restless and agitated. Auditory, visual, or tactile hallucinations are common and usually frightening. Some patients fight sleep fearing that sleep will lead to death, and sleep deprivation in turn heightens the psychotic symptoms. Mental status examination reveals altered attention, fluctuating levels of consciousness, varying degrees of cognitive impairment, and disorientation, as well as psychotic symptoms such as hallucinations and paranoia.

## CASE REPORTS

A teenage girl in relapse after a bone marrow transplant for acute leukemia developed a psychotic delirium. She refused to sleep, reasoning that if she closed her eyes she would die. She was hypervigilant, turning toward the slightest sound. She denied hallucinations, but was confused, disoriented, and severely agitated. She required large doses of chlorpromazine to enable her to sleep. She died later in a calm state.

A teenage boy who had central nervous system infiltration of leukemia considered jumping from his hospital window to escape the fear aroused by auditory and visual hallucinations of waterfalls rushing into his room and motorcycles crashing through the walls. High doses of chlorpromazine titrated to symptom control level provided sleep and relief of psychotic symptoms. He was comfortable during the remaining weeks of his terminal illness.

The symptoms associated with an organic brain syndrome may require emergency treatment when panic or suicidal risk is involved. Rapid control of symptoms of agitation and hallucinations is required. Any major tranquilizer is potentially effective. However, the oncology staff's familiarity with chlorpromazine as an antiemetic and sedative drug for the child with cancer makes it a good choice. Haloperidol is preferred by others because it is less sedating, but it is more apt to cause extrapyramidal side effects, which are distressing to patient and staff alike. Determining the safe, efficacious dosage of an antipsychotic drug in children may be difficult. Knowledge of a particular drug is probably most important in establishing a margin of safety. Drug doses must be titrated against symptom control, with careful monitoring of vital signs. The lowest effective dosage should not be exceeded.

## ADJUSTMENT PROBLEMS TO TREATMENT

### Noncompliance

Noncompliance is an increasingly serious problem in pediatric cancer patients. It may stem from psychological problems in the child, especially during adolescence, or in the parent of a younger child. Despite the serious nature of pediatric cancer care, nonadherence to treatment is remarkably high. One study found that 33% of pediatric cancer patients were not compliant with outpatient steroid medication; among the adoles-

cents in this group, the noncompliance rate was an alarming 59% (Smith et al., 1979). A study of psychological influences associated with noncompliance found that, while the rates of compliance were equal in boys and girls, psychological correlates of compliance differed between sexes (Lansky et al., 1983). In girls, the child's own level of anxiety was the best predictor of compliance. In boys, on the other hand, parental anxiety, anger, and obsessive-compulsive behavior correlated positively with compliant behavior. It was hypothesized that parents may expect their daughters to be more responsible and acquiescent, while boys are apt to be seen as more vulnerable and in need of supervision. These differences in parental concerns translate into more careful supervision of the treatments and compliance of boys. Another study found adolescents less compliant than younger children and a number of medical and social influences related to compliance (Tebbi et al., 1986). Although more work needs to be done in the assessment and management of compliance, these reports provide important speculations about the influence of medical, social, and family concerns on treatment.

Noncompliance may take many forms. A child with acute anxiety or panic may flatly refuse a procedure or treatment; he or she may fail to keep appointments, or parents may choose an alternative ''unorthodox'' treatment they find more palatable. A parent may bring a reluctant child for treatment, only to have the child refuse treatment. This is particularly likely to occur when parents and children are in conflict about treatment. In such cases, the staff may be in the uncomfortable situation of having simultaneously to encourage treatment and referee a parent–child disagreement.

When a young child or adolescent refuses a procedure or treatment, staff and parents become very distressed. The child may even threaten or attempt suicide to underscore the seriousness of his or her position. These situations arouse feelings of ambivalence, conflict, and helplessness in the oncologist and staff, magnifying the child's own helpless feeling. The psychiatrist, coming in as an objective outsider, may be able to defuse the situation and restore the child's sense of control; willingness to cooperate often returns when the child feels respected and senses he or she is being considered in the decision-making process. Appealing to the healthy side of his or her ambivalence while acknowledging the helpless and angry feelings may help.

Denial may be adaptive but it must be treated when it leads to noncompliance. Some teenagers who refuse a procedure or treatment may benefit from going home to think about the implications of noncompliance. A psychiatrist can be used to review a treatment refusal with the child or teenager, again permitting him or her to have control by "thinking about it," but encouraging compliance. Having restored a sense of autonomy, the child often will return to continue the recommended treatment. Psychotherapy is highly beneficial in such cases to prevent such behavior from becoming a pattern. Underlying anger and frustration, depression and anxiety, and issues of dependency and control must be explored and understood. However, some children, particularly teenagers, are recalcitrant and completely refuse treatment. The distress of parents and staff is great when noncompliance clearly adversely alters prognosis; fortunately, such instances are rare.

The use of alternative treatments may also represent noncompliance. Such treatments are reported as being or having been used by 6–16% of patients. An even higher proportion of families report having received suggestions about specific unorthodox methods for their child's care (Copeland et al., 1983; Faw et al., 1977; Pendergrass and Davis, 1981). Trust in the oncologist, open communication, and sharing in decision making are essential ingredients in the relationship between a family and oncologist and are the elements that best serve to discourage alternative treatment (see also Chapter 42). When families express interest in an unorthodox treatment, they should be given as much information as possible about both the conventional and nonconventional treatment in question. It is important that information be imparted in a nonjudgmental way. If the alternative method is harmless and does not preclude standard treatment, participation in both may be the most reasonable compromise.

## Side Effects

Adjustment to the consequences of cancer treatment is often as painful as the treatment itself. Disfigurement ranges from alopecia and cushingoid appearance to surgical deformities, including limb amputation. One study found that adolescent cancer and rheumatoid arthritis patients showed greater disruption of body image because of their disease and treatment than did teenagers with other chronic illnesses (Zeltzer et al., 1980). However, a study of long-term survivors of childhood cancer found that the level of psychosocial adaptation was not affected by severity of disfigurement or physical impairment (O'Malley et al., 1980).

Alopecia is a common side effect that represents a serious problem for many children who fear being or looking "different." Some adjust by wearing a wig, some wear scarves or hats, and others dare to reveal their baldness. In a society in which sexual identification is largely determined by hairstyle, sexual identity, personal identity, and self-esteem may be seriously affected by hair loss. Preparation for hair loss, allow-

ing anticipation and planning, along with assurance that it is often only transitory, assist adjustment.

Amputation in adolescent cancer patients is often well tolerated, and long-term adjustment is favorable (Boyle et al., 1982; O'Malley et al., 1980). However, each child's reaction is different. Some have serious problems coping with physical impairment as well as disfigurement. Many children do well immediately after amputation and feel relieved that the cancer has been removed. However, the difficult task of walking with crutches or adjusting to a prosthesis, especially after leaving the hospital, may result in disappointment, fatigue, and depression later.

Psychotherapy may be helpful when physical loss or change must be endured. Management approaches emphasize the child's capabilities and promote hope, while acknowledging the realistic implications of and limitations consequent to treatment. Group therapy in which participants are children who are roughly the same age and are dealing with the same issues or treatments, or support form a youngster who has managed the same problem is particularly helpful (May et al., 1979; see also Chapter 41). In some cases work with the family and environmental manipulations may be needed. The use of a psychotropic drug for symptoms of anxiety and depression may help initially until the child resolves some problems through psychotherapy.

## Special Treatment Situations: Protected Environments

Protected environments, used for children during periods of high susceptibility to infections, restrict the child to a small area where touch is limited by gloves and faces are masked. It is rare that psychiatric problems exclude a child from treatment in such an environment. The major exclusion criteria used in most centers are based on the patient's physical status and compliance. Although sensory deprivation, perceptual changes, mood disturbances, and behavioral changes have been described in children remaining in these environments for long periods of time (Kellerman et al., 1980; Pfefferbaum et al., 1978), long-term adverse psychological sequelae appear to be few (Powazek et al., 1978; Susman et al., 1980).

Psychiatric consultation is necessary most often for CNS complications or treatment side effects. Sensory deprivation is not usually a significant clinical problem in children because special efforts are made in these settings to emphasize orientation and stimulation. Major tranquilizers may be required for antipsychotic, antianxiety, and sedative effects if delirium develops. Antidepressant medication for depression, particularly if vegetative symptoms are present, may be needed. At times it is difficult to discern whether symptoms are related to the primary illness or to the child's emotional state. Most children respond to support, guidance, and structure, and do well psychologically despite the restrictions imposed by care in a protected environment. For a review of the issues related to the late adolescent and adult treated in these settings the reader is referred to Chapter 12.

## Special Treatment Situations: Bone Marrow Transplantation (BMT)

An overview of the procedure itself, general patterns of or stages in adaptation, and common problems and their management in BMT settings are provided by Lesko in Chapter 11. A number of special issues may arise during transplantation in the pediatric setting and warrant greater discussion here.

Often members or entire families must temporarily relocate from their home community to accompany the ill child to the referral treatment center. This relocation is an emotional, physical, and financial burden that adds to the stress of making decisions about care. Seeking treatment in a special setting imposes a multitude of changes, including altered support systems, the necessity of forming new alliances with unfamiliar doctors and staff, empty, merely functional living arrangements for the parent who stays, complicated parking, and perhaps unfamiliar language. Even when the family lives within reasonable proximity of the treatment center, numerous shifts occur in family routines as the patient, and at various times some of the family members, move into the hospital for an extended period of time. Support systems must be identified and strengthened early.

The treatment team ascertains, by a psychosocial as well as medical evaluation, whether or not the patient is thought to be able to tolerate the procedure. Consent, obtained from all members involved in the transplant, must be "informed" by use of age-appropriate explanations. When ethical and legal issues arise, some institutions appoint an advocate to represent a young patient or donor in decisions about transplantation. In some situations, a committee reviews and determines transplant policy, and at times, decisions are referred to the courts. Psychological issues for donors are reviewed in Chapter 11.

Bringing some of their "world" to the room helps children tolerate the social isolation and restriction of physical contact imposed by seeing family and team members behind gowns, gloves, masks, and hats; school can continue, and favorite toys, stuffed animals, games, and even athletic equipment that can be sterilized, are allowed into the room. Many visitors—child development specialists, teachers, nurses, parents, and siblings—reduce the sense of isolation.

Younger children appear to have less difficulty with the isolation experience than do older children and adolescents (Pfefferbaum et al., 1978).

Removal from isolation is experienced with ambivalence and fearfulness by the child who has felt protected and "special" in the isolated environment. The child must cope with new worries of no longer being "special" but just "different" and vulnerable to new stresses of reentry to home and school. Reintegration into the home and school may be a monumental task for both the child and the family. Ongoing psychological support begun in the hospital is essential, and ideally should be provided by the same person(s).

## STAGE–SPECIFIC ADAPTATION PROBLEMS

### Long-Term Survival and Cure

A growing number of children today are considered "cured" of childhood cancer. Although the label "survivor" would seem attractive, status in this group is not without psychological difficulties; the issue has become the focus of an increasing number of clinical and research reports. An extensive review of the physical and psychological issues in survivorship is presented by Tross in Chapter 7. The most comprehensive series of studies addressing psychosocial adjustment in the pediatric population involved more than 100 survivors of childhood cancer (Koocher and O'Malley, 1981). These researchers found that normal developmental milestones were achieved; however, although survivors denied having problems, their psychosocial adaptation, as determined by interviews and testing, showed a lingering sense of vulnerability, heightened anxiety and depression, and lowered self-esteem. Of survivors studied, 12% showed severe psychological impairment and over half had mild symptoms. Children who were youngest at the time of illness had adapted better than those whose illness occurred in middle childhood or adolescence. Learning the diagnosis early in the treatment process and having a supportive family were also associated with better adjustment.

To assess long-term adaptation, education, occupation, and marriage were also used as measures of social and psychological outcome. Of the 36 survivors over 21 years old, many were married and had healthy normal children, despite initial concerns about sexual functioning and the possible effects of prior therapy on their progeny. The proportion of the sample who remained single or were divorced was lower than that in the general population (Gogan et al., 1979). Although the cancer diagnosis might have been made many years earlier, discrimination both in employment and in health and life insurance was reported (Koocher et al.,

1981). The range of psychological problems encountered, as well as comments by survivors themselves, suggest that psychosocial intervention may be valuable, especially in those showing severe problems (Koocher et al., 1980). Many survivors may benefit form special counseling following the end of active treatment. Referral problems frequently focus on educational, physical rehabilitation, vocational counseling, employment, and interpersonal issues. When they arise, potential long-term or late problems should be carefully explored with the patient and family, and referrals made for additional intervention as appropriate.

## Terminal Illness

A child's reaction to unremitting illness is influenced by his or her own emotional maturity, experience, surroundings, and level of intellectual development. The responses of the parents, siblings, and extended family will be important as well. The more limited, age-related understanding of death seen in the healthy child may not apply in the cancer setting. The seriously ill child appears to be more aware of death, acquiring an earlier maturity in dealing with the concept and its consequences (Bluebond-Langner, 1977). These children seem precocious in their understanding and discussions of illness and death, likely the outgrowth of their experience with doctors, nurses, illness, and medical terminology, as well as their exposure to deaths among peer patients experienced in the context of unit or clinic care. The severely ill young children studied by Spinetta (1974) showed anxiety about death, an unexpected finding given their cognitive level. These data are in contrast to normative findings showing that preschool children view death as a form of temporary separation or loss.

According to theories of cognitive development, the child's ability to understand death proceeds in stages (Nagy, 1959). Children under 18 months of age are believed to have no formal concept of death, although they react emotionally to the loss of or separation from a significant person. Between the ages of 3 and 5 death is viewed as absence but is considered reversible. During early school years, death may take on personal attributes (e.g., the "boogeyman") and is seen as an external process. Although death gradually becomes viewed as final, the concept is incomplete and concrete. Children who have lost a grandparent or pet exhibit feelings of anxiety and sorrow associated with death. At this stage death is seen as a punishment for misdeeds, making it an important issue to consider in siblings of the ill child. Children approaching and during adolescence are aware that everyone dies and many think about their own death. They view death as bio-

logical and irreversible. They sense their own vulnerability and that of those they love. These stages are reviewed in the developmental charts (Appendices A–D) and in Chapter 43.

Open, honest communication coupled with emotional support are extremely important with the terminally ill child. The atmosphere should encourage questions and expression of fantasies and fears about illness and death. Exploration of these findings must proceed at the child's own pace, requiring great sensitivity on the part of the therapist who chooses this work. The therapist must listen, answer questions honestly, respond to the child's feelings, and offer assurance that he or she will not be alone or be allowed to have pain or severe discomfort. Most children intuitively understand the significance and severity of their illness. A 7-year-old boy, shortly after learning of his relapse, was asked if he would be available for a visit in 2 weeks. He replied, "I don't know. I don't make plans anymore." Reflecting feelings, acknowledging affect, and encouraging the child to elaborate further on his or her concerns are important aspects of support.

Parents sometimes ask how they should respond to their child's questions about death. Often they want to protect the child from knowledge of terminal illness. In such instances the parents must be helped to understand that the child already knows and understands his or her status, and that experience has demonstrated that the child is more frightened if not allowed to discuss it with those he or she trusts. They should be encouraged to listen carefully to the child, to answer questions, to express understanding and acceptance of feelings, and to offer support, reassurance, and hope. With resistant parents, it may be helpful to determine what they think the child already knows and then work with the child and parents at their own pace. Role playing with anxious parents may be helpful, as well as working with them in anticipation of the impending last days of life. The expression that "death is a blessing" often is not comforting. It is better to acknowledge their grief and try to comfort them.

In working through their anticipatory grief, parents sometimes accept the death of their child prematurely, before death actually occurs. In such instances, the family needs help in maintaining nurturing ties with their child while simultaneously anticipating and accepting inevitable death. This is often the most stressful period for parents because it elicits contradictory feelings. Sometimes voicing of this painful ambiguity is helpful. Parents anticipating the death of a child must at the same time participate in the decisions about level of care during terminal illness, such as when to stop active treatment, stop invasive diagnostic procedures, and initiate "comfort care only," as well as whether resuscitation will be done when cardiac or respiratory failure occurs. When parents must make a decision regarding further, often experimental, treatment or use of heroic procedures, it is often helpful to acknowledge their dilemma and recognize that neither option—continuing treatment by experimental means or taking the child home for terminal care—is comfortable. Discussion with the oncologist, who explains clearly medical data supporting each option, is of value to parents who must be helped not to feel guilty about decisions, especially for limiting life supports and resuscitation.

Parents are increasingly taking the option to have their child die at home. Home care programs, run by nurses and social workers, offer critical support to sustain the stressed parents and siblings, by providing home visits and regular consultation with the physician (Martinson et al., 1978; see also Chapter 48). Every effort should be made to support parents in this decision; however, they should also be assured that if the child is too uncomfortable or they reach a point where they cannot manage, readmission to the hospital is always an option.

Not only the child, but also the family suffers greatly in the terminal phase of illness, and supportive intervention is helpful. Although the pediatric oncologist is the key source of information and solace, the social worker, religious counselor, mental health counselor, or a parent who has gone through it, can be very helpful. Parents will usually relate best to one of these supportive workers and that tie should be encouraged. Candlelighters, as a national resource group, can offer much support as well as information about support networks available in a particular community. Individual and family therapy may also be useful. Groups for bereaved parents and parents of children who are dying can provide special support. Follow-up after death on anniversaries and important holidays provides helpful ongoing support, which also acknowledges the staff's memory of the child. Referral to the nearest chapter of Compassionate Friends may provide an additional support source. Staff members also benefit from group discussions when a favorite child is dying. After the child's death, it is helpful for the staff to hold a meeting in which care of the child is reviewed, conflicts about decisions can be rationally discussed, and feelings of loss shared.

## SPECIAL PROBLEMS

### Family

Family dynamics and interactions change markedly when cancer is diagnosed in one of the family's young members. (See Chapter 47 for a review of the developmental tasks and common issues in family adaptation.)

**Table 44-2**  Influences placing families at risk for adaptational problems

- Psychiatric history in a family member
- History of child abuse and/or neglect
- History of parent—child conflicts
- Parental divorce–marital disruption
- Distance from home
- Cultural and/or language barriers
- Multiple family losses or stressors

Although some disruption is expected, there are symptoms that indicate some family members may be at greater risk for maladaptive responses and in need of close monitoring and early intervention. Listed in Table 44-2, some of these have already been discussed in preceding sections. As noted earlier, history of pre-existing mental illness in the parent warrants evaluation at the time of diagnosis of cancer in an offspring. The stress of having a child or sibling in the family with cancer may cause an exacerbation of psychiatric symptoms in any family member. Coexistence of any of the other risk factors listed in Table 44-2 also requires careful monitoring.

Regardless of other problems, it is safe to assume that all cancer families experience problems related to the cancer illness and treatment. Occurring in parents are depression, conversion reactions, psychosomatic illness, increased alcohol and drug use and abuse, marital conflict, and job performance problems. Using marital status as a measure of family conflict, early studies suggested that divorce and serious marital problems were a frequent consequence of the stress of cancer. However, these studies failed to compare the divorce rate in cancer families with the divorce rate in the general population (Binger et al., 1969; Kaplan et al., 1976). A later controlled study found no significant increase in divorce but did report an increase in marital discord attributed to the diagnosis of cancer in these families (Lansky et al., 1978). The "absent father" (Wyse, 1983) is frequently neglected because he is often less available than the mother or siblings for psychosocial prevention or intervention. As a consequence, less is known in general about paternal reactions to the child's illness and the stress of cancer.

Symptoms indicative of problems in siblings include anxiety, depression, lowered self-esteem, enuresis, somatic complaints, deviant behavior, school phobia, and other school difficulties (Binger et al., 1969; Kaplan et al., 1976). The early literature tended to highlight deviant behavior and adjustment problems rather than successful coping in siblings of cancer patients. Early reports relied almost exclusively on parental report of behavior during stressful periods of the cancer illness (Sourkes, 1980), but more recent studies have provided less biased data. One study compared school-aged cancer patients with their healthy siblings on projective and self-report measures. Well siblings were found to have, among other symptoms, significant anxiety, fears about their own health, and social isolation (Cairns et al., 1979). Comparing siblings of patients from various illness groups, another study found siblings of children with hematological disorders, mostly leukemia, to be coping adequately but to be more fearful, inhibited, withdrawn, and irritable than siblings of healthy controls (Lavigne and Ryan, 1979). However, the siblings of cancer patients did not show more behavioral problems such as aggression or learning problems than other sibling control groups. In a prospective study of siblings, Spinetta (1981a) found their adjustment poorest when their ill sibling was doing well. He hypothesized that parents understandably focus attention on the ill child during crises and at other times, when attention might have turned to healthy siblings, they focus on other neglected matters, essentially leaving the siblings emotionally unattended much of the time. While the extent of sibling problems may still be in dispute, most clinicians and researchers would agree that siblings of cancer patients are frequently neglected in both family and treatment situations.

Comprehensive care of the child with cancer includes careful attention to the needs of the family and its individual members. Depending on the nature and severity of the problems, family, couples, and individual therapy are useful. Special therapy or activity groups for healthy siblings of cancer patients can help promote positive adaptation in these family members.

## School

With improved prognosis, childhood cancer is now considered a chronic disease. Most treatment programs and clinicians emphasize the importance of maintaining as normal physical and psychological development as possible. Because many children can now expect to experience long periods free of both illness and treatment-related symptoms, normalization is particularly important for overall psychological and social development. Klopovich and co-workers (1981) noted five reasons why school attendance is important for the child with cancer: (1) to provide social contact, (2) to boost morale, (3) to counter boredom, (4) to maintain dignity, and (5) to normalize life. School, especially when it is a supportive environment, can provide the ideal setting for the child to adapt to the realities of his or her situation and life.

At times, frequent and sometimes long absences from school are inevitable. Fatigue and lack of stamina impede participation in competitive sports and athletic activities. When coupled with fears of "falling behind" in academic performance and the problems of social reentry with peers, return to school may be traumatic. The child may fear being (or be) socially ostracized, ridiculed, and teased because of the illness, appearance, or absences. Anxiety and depression may also interfere with academic and social functioning.

School phobia (Lansky et al., 1975) and absenteeism (Eiser, 1980; Deasy-Spinetta and Spinetta, 1980; Stehbens et al., 1983), once major problems, have diminished in recent years because of improved prognosis and treatment, as well as better psychosocial support for the child and parents and improved education of teachers about management of the child with cancer. Difficulty completing school assignments, trouble in concentrating, and actual learning disabilities have been reported and can result from treatment effects, especially cranial irradiation (Deasy-Spinetta and Spinetta, 1980; Rowland et al., 1984). Problems in academic performance, particularly in the first year following diagnosis, may be expected. School behavior appeared to be at least moderately affected in almost half of the children studied in one report (Stehbens et al., 1983). Despite this, it is important that parents insist on school attendance and refrain from the understandable tendency to overprotect.

School psychologists most often receive referral of these children to help in the management of anxiety associated with changes in appearance (e.g., weight gain and alopecia), school reintegration after prolonged absence, care for newly diagnosed patients to prevent emotional problems, or evaluation for special placement (Katz et al., 1980). Additional influences that put a child at risk for school problems are depression, problems in parent–child separation, and resistance on the part of school personnel (Klopovich et al., 1981). All of these conditions need to be recognized and treated promptly. It is important for the child to learn early how to deal with the school situation. Special instruction of school personnel on appropriate responses to the child and assistance of the child with cancer in the classroom may be needed. (See Adams-Greenly's section on school programs, Chapter 45.) The school can contribute to normalization best when communication with the treatment team occurs regularly. The treatment team provides information regarding the illness and possible social and academic implications; also, school personnel often provide useful information to the doctor.

A number of medical influences can contribute to school difficulties. These include the complexity of the treatment regimen, frequency and nature of routine follow-up, disease status, neutropenia, infection, and chicken pox in the classroom (Klopovich et al., 1981). To this list must also be added the treatments themselves. Problems in academic performance may result as a function of neuropsychological effects of treatment involving the CNS either as primary treatment, as in the case of brain tumors (Deutsch, 1982; Danoff et al., 1982), or as part of prophylactic therapy used in the prevention of CNS disease as seen in childhood leukemia (Eiser, 1978; Eiser and Lansdown, 1977; Meadows et al., 1981; Moss et al., 1981; Pfefferbaum-Levine et al., 1984a; Rowland et al., 1984). In both cases, results suggest that CNS effects are likely global across cognitive functional areas, although some studies among leukemia samples have identified major effect on perceptual motor skills, quantitative ability, and memory (Copeland et al., 1985; Goff et al., 1980; Pfefferbaum-Levine et al., 1984a). Younger children receiving CNS therapy appear to be at greater risk for neuropsychological impairment than older children (Danoff et al., 1982; Meadows et al., 1981; Moss et al., 1981; Eiser and Lansdown, 1977). In the case of leukemia treatments, the deleterious effects appear to be due to the combined effect of intrathecal methotrexate and cranial irradiation rather than intrathecal medications alone (Rowland et al., 1984), and the level of impairment likely does not progress (Copeland et al., 1985). The effect of poor school attendance, physical and psychological symptoms, potential treatment, or disease-related cognitive deficits in these children combine to hamper the child's school performance. When such treatments are to be used, baseline and periodic cognitive assessment should be done to identify deficits early and, when needed, to introduce remediation geared toward minimizing long-term reduction in performance. Careful assessment by both a pediatric neurologist and psychologist should be part of the follow-up of the child at risk for cognitive difficulties, because it may be difficult to separate psychological symptoms from those of neurological origin.

## Coping Over Time

Recent emphasis on family coping has resulted in several longitudinal investigations designed to assess family coping at discrete points during the cancer illness. At the time of diagnosis, reactive anxiety and depression are common in both the child and parents (Kupst and Schulman, 1980; Powazek et al., 1980). Many children in remission and their parents are generally coping well (Kupst et al., 1982) 1 year after diagnosis, although some may suffer lingering anxiety and depression, somatic complaints, and occasionally disturbed thought processes (Powazek et al., 1980). In the study by Powazek and colleagues (1980), mothers reported that their children quickly returned to school and regained their prior level of functioning. Fathers and siblings, however, had more difficulty coping.

Siblings experienced a variety of behavioral difficulties including fear of going to school, fear of being left alone, achievement and behavioral problems at school, anger and jealousy toward the ill child, discipline problems at home and school, and somatic complaints; in many instances siblings had little understanding of the illness of their brother or sister.

Evaluation of a cohort of families studied over time showed that most families were coping well 2 years postdiagnosis (Kupst et al., 1984). Characteristics associated with good adjustment were quality of the marital and family relationships, coping well with the illness, good social support, lack of additional stresses, open communication within the family, and an attitude of living in the present. Whereas psychosocial intervention correlated with good maternal adjustment earlier in the child's illness, it was not significantly related to coping at 2 years, although having someone to talk with during the treatment period was found to be helpful. Continued intervention at the 2-year point did not seem warranted when the child was doing well medically and life had returned to normal.

Adaptation to loss and bereavement was studied by Spinetta (1981b), who evaluated parents after the death of their child. The parents considered best adjusted were those who had a philosophy that allowed the family to accept the diagnosis and cope with its consequences, felt they had shared information with their child and given emotional support during the illness, and had had an adequate support system during the illness. These studies reflect findings similar to those observed in adult cancer patients and their families. (For review of these see Chapter 47.)

Whereas psychiatric or psychosocial intervention is not usually necessary throughout the entire course of cancer treatment, it is important during crisis periods. Specific times of crisis are at diagnosis, during treatment induction, when serious complications of treatment occur, at time of reentry into normal life, at recurrence, when curative treatment fails, when investigational treatment begins, at termination of treatment, during terminal illness, during bereavement, on anniversaries, and at times of recall of the child's expected developmental markers (Christ and Adams, 1982; Koocher, 1982). It is advisable to assess all families initially for characteristics that would predict psychological problems, including strengths and weaknesses of each family member, prior psychiatric history, family coping style, and availability of social supports. Sensitive inquiry during clinic visits by clinic staff who know a family well will alert the treatment team to those needing attention.

At diagnosis, the first crisis reveals how the family responds, reestablishes psychological equilibrium, and likely will cope with further crises. Careful assessment, including psychiatric consultation, should be initiated when "at-risk" characteristics are found.

Terminating treatment when the child is in remission brings the mixed emotions of relief tempered by feelings of anxiety that relapse may occur after treatment, and of loss to the family of a caring source of structured support (Alby, 1980). Psychological preparation should begin well before the last treatment. Assuring parents that they may feel more worried for a while is helpful; they need to know that their anxiety is normal. Realistic concerns about second malignancies, late relapse, or delayed effects are also understandable, and reassurance should be given that the child will still be monitored closely.

## COMMUNICATION AND STAFF ISSUES

### Communication Issues

In the past, communication issues concerning children with cancer dealt chiefly with what (or whether) to tell the child about his or her diagnosis and prognosis, and how to communicate issues related to death and dying. The improved prognosis and long-term survival for many childhood tumors coupled with a greater appreciation for children's understanding of illness and death have changed this picture. Today, straightforward, honest communication with the child and family is recommended, starting at the time of diagnosis. One outcome of this approach is that parents less frequently try to keep the diagnosis from their child, and communication between child and parent is enhanced.

Several studies emphasize that adolescents depend heavily on their oncologist as a primary source of information, although they and their parents agreed that the parent should be included in the discussions (Levenson et al., 1981). This contrasts with adolescents' otherwise strong preference for confidentiality and exclusion of parents in preference to peers. Adolescents interviewed about their relationships with their oncologists indicated that they appreciated it when the oncologist seemed to respect and like them as a person. Many longed for more time with and concern from their oncologist when this positive relationship was lacking (Young and Pfefferbaum-Levine, 1984). As would be expected, younger children depend more on their parents for information (Levenson et al., 1982). Play therapy or drawing may be needed for very young children to provide information at their level and to enable them to express their unverbalized concerns.

The importance of the physician's role in imparting educational information regarding cancer and its treatment cannot be overemphasized. It is not feasible, however, for the physician to shoulder this burden alone. Other team members and peers who have the same diagnosis should be drawn upon to extend initial information. In addition, audio and visual tapes, and reading material are widely available to provide details to patients and families about a specific disease, such as leukemia, and standard treatment protocols. Some institutions have implemented novel communication formats. One center uses a weekly staff conference that is attended by the oncologist and other specialists involved, the treatment team, the child, and the parents to discuss treatment concerns and formulate a plan of action (van Eys and Copeland, 1982). A similar format is used by some centers or units when treatment options for terminal illness must be reviewed. Options of home care versus phase I and II chemotherapy must be fully explored with respect to risks and benefits with both child and parents participating in the final decision (Nitschke et al., 1977). (Other support and educational group models are detailed in Chapter 45.)

Regardless of the mode, the fostering of open, honest, straightforward communication as an essential part of overall care is a central goal. School and community groups that become involved because of a particular child or children serve as outreach resources, providing a focus for much-needed public education about the current improved treatment for childhood cancer and the improved prognosis for many childhood malignancies.

### Staff Issues

Individuals who choose to work in pediatric oncology are self-selected. Nevertheless, rewards for those who work intimately with such ill children are tempered by the frequent sense of loss, grief, and disappointment. These problems are discussed at length by Lederberg in Chapter 51. Informally or formally established mechanisms for dealing with staff distress have been developed in most large pediatric oncology centers. Any unit, however, either hospital or clinic, should provide support groups, psychosocial conferences, and informal opportunities for managing the responses of all staff members, especially nurses, involved in intimate care. (See also Chapter 45 and 47 on support groups in pediatrics and Chapter 54 on nurse-to-nurse counseling.) Pediatric house staff, not accustomed to the level of illness or complex protocols used with hospitalized children, are particularly vulnerable to distress, often unspoken and unacknowledged.

Psychosocial support and psychiatric consultation must be built into treatment programs for the child, family, and staff. Most pediatric oncology units have psychosocial support teams that include a social worker, chaplain, child life worker, psychologist, and psychiatric consultant. Pediatric units, even with only a few oncology patients, must provide at least one support person who can obtain assistance from other specialists. Support teams foster an environment that is sensitive to the psychological, social, educational, and behavioral needs of the child, parents, and siblings. The expertise of their members also assists the oncologist in assessing the psychological response of child and family to the medical crises and determining when intervention is necessary. A knowledge of predictable crises and the commonly manifested types of psychological distress and psychiatric syndromes assures better planning for interventions when necessary.

## Ethical and Legal Issues

Staff members working in pediatric oncology face special ethical and legal concerns that arise in the context of treating minors. The right to informed consent of parents and right of assent of children to treatment decisions, including right to refuse treatment is protected. In the past most laws involved protection of children. More recently legislation has focused on the rights of the child to participate in decisions. Older adolescents—especially those living apart from their families—are viewed as adults under the law in some treatment situations. Even younger children must be given age-appropriate information, especially regarding investigative protocols, which require their assent by presence of their signature. There are times, however, when conflict between child, parents, and/or the medical team creates ethical dilemmas. Treatment decisions become difficult when the child's right of protection is in conflict with his or her right of self-determination, particularly when the decision is to refuse treatment (Lansky et al., 1979b). Legal rulings in cases in which parents have refused treatment for their child are not yet clear enough to provide clear guidelines for staff (Sokolosky, 1982). Most hospitals require consent for both routine and investigative treatment from the child and the parents. These new requirements have assured that the child is engaged positively (and not coercively) early in treatment. This is important for sustained compliance, especially when side effects may be multiple and frequent.

Clinical investigations by controlled trials in pediatric oncology over the past 20 years have resulted in far better informed parents and children. The process of obtaining consent for research results in more questions, greater participation in decision making, and more frequent review of decisions during treatment (Miller and Haupt, 1982). Thus, it can be argued that the benefits of research are not limited to the physical benefits alone, but include enhanced communication

as well. Physicians have tremendous influence over the patients they treat, as well as over their families. Pediatric oncologists, in their dual roles as clinicians and investigators, have an important and sometimes difficult obligation to weigh these two roles in the care of those children who require investigative treatments.

## Future Perspectives

New psychological issues emerge as pediatric cancer treatments change and psychological research in this population becomes more sophisticated. Studies of psychosocial and neurocognitive late effects of treatment will need to be expanded. Problems of the adult who was cured of cancer as a child will need more study in relation to developmental and career achievements, job stability and discrimination, and the potential for intimate relationships and parenting. Research in psychiatric and psychosocial issues will be an increasingly important aspect of pediatric oncology. The group of children born to childhood cancer survivors may become an important population for study not only for genetic predisposition and possible congenital effects of cancer and its treatment, but also for the impact of early life crises and survivorship on overall individual and family adjustment.

The economic consequences of cancer treatment (including the nonmedical costs of psychosocial support, relocation, and job loss) already examined (Lansky et al., 1979a) will need increasing attention. Although investigational treatment has been responsible for the remarkably improved prognosis of childhood cancer, its high costs will, in the present climate of rapidly changing social policies about medical care, likely be reexamined with important repercussions on overall care.

The use of psychotropic medications for symptom control in children with cancer is receiving increasing attention. Altered metabolism and pharmacokinetics in children who have impaired organ function and chemotherapy side effects will need to be studied to establish safe, but efficacious dosage ranges.

Finally, the child with cancer and the stressed parents treated in the pediatric oncology setting provide an unusual opportunity to study the interaction of neuropsychological, endocrine, and immune function. Some fundamental questions in psychiatry may be addressed by clinical investigations addressing the nature of these diseases, the effects of treatment on the CNS, and the psychological and biological consequences of the prolonged, stressful situation of childhood cancer. The complex nature of cause–effect relationships between stress and illness may be also well examined in these settings.

# REFERENCES

Alby, N. (1980). Ending the chemotherapy of acute leukemia: A period of difficult weaning. In J.L. Schulman and M.J. Kupst (eds.), *The Child with Cancer*. Springfield, Ill.: Charles C Thomas, pp. 175–82.

Beyer, J.E., D.E. DeGood, L.C. Ashley, and G.A. Russell (1983). Patterns of postoperative analgesic use with adults and children following cardiac surgery. *Pain* 17:71–81.

Biederman, J. and M.S. Jellinek (1984). Psychopharmacology in children. *N. Engl. J. Med.* 310:968–72.

Binger, C.M., A.R. Albin, R.C. Feuerstein, J. Kushner, S. Zoger, and C. Mikkelsen (1969). Childhood leukemia: Emotional impact on patient and family. *N. Engl. J. Med.* 280:414–18.

Bluebond-Langner, M. (1977). Meanings of death to children. In H. Feifel (ed.), *New Meanings of Death*. New York: McGraw-Hill, pp. 47–66.

Boyle, M., C.K. Tebbi, E.R. Mindell, and C.J. Mettlin (1982). Adolescent adjustment to amputation. *Med. Pediatr. Oncol.* 10:301–12.

Cairns, N.U., G.M. Clark, S.D. Smith, and S.B. Lansky (1979). Adaptation of siblings to childhood malignancy. *J. Pediatr.* 95:484–87.

Christ, G. and M.A. Adams (1982). Therapeutic strategies at psychosocial crisis points in the treatment of childhood cancer. In A.E. Christ and K. Flomenhaft (eds.), *Childhood Cancer Impact on the Family*. New York City: Plenum, pp. 109–28.

Copeland, D.R., J.M. Fletcher, B. Pfefferbaum-Levine, N. Jaffe, H. Ried, and M. Maor (1985). Neuropsychological sequelae of childhood cancer in long-term survivors. *Pediatrics* 75(4):745–53.

Copeland, D.R., Y. Silberberg, and B. Pfefferbaum (1983). Attitudes and practices of families of children in treatment for cancer: A cross-cultural study. *Am. J. Pediatr. Hematol. Oncol.* 5(1):65–71.

Danoff, B.F., F.S. Cowchock, C. Marquette, S. Mulgrew, and S. Kramer (1982). Assessment of the long-term effects of primary radiation therapy for brain tumors in children. *Cancer* 49:1580–86.

Deasy-Spinetta, P. and J. Spinetta (1980). The child with cancer in school: Teacher's appraisal. *Am. J. Pediatr. Hematol. Oncol.* 2:89–96.

Deutsch, M. (1982). Radiotherapy for primary brain tumors in very young children. *Cancer* 50:2785–89.

Eiser, C. (1978). Intellectual abilities among survivors of childhood leukemia as a function of CNS irradiation. *Arch. Dis. Child.* 53:391–95.

Eiser, C. (1980). How leukemia affects a child's schooling. *Br. J. Soc. Clin. Psychol.* 19:365–68.

Eiser, C. and R. Lansdown (1977). Retrospective study of intellectual development in children treated for acute lymphoblastic leukemia. *Arch. Dis. Child.* 52:525–29.

Faw, C., R. Ballentine, L. Ballentine, and J. van Eys (1977). Unproved cancer remedies: A survey of use in pediatric outpatients. *J.A.M.A.* 238:1536–38.

Fawcett, J.A. and H.M. Kravitz (1982). Alprazolam: Pharmacokinetics, clinical efficacy, and mechanism of action. *Pharmacotherapy* 2:243–54.

Forrest, W.H., Jr., B.W. Brown, Jr., C.R. Brown, R. DeFalque, M. Gold, H.E. Gordon, K.E. James, J. Katz, D.L. Mahler, P. Schroff, and G. Teutsch (1977). Dextroamphetamine with morphine for the treatment of postoperative pain. *N. Engl. J. Med.* 296(13): 712–15.

Goff, J.R., H.R. Anderson, Jr., and P.F. Cooper (1980). Distractibility and memory deficits in long-term survivors of acute lymphoblastic leukemia. *Dev. Behav. Pediatr.* 1(4):158–63.

Gogan, J.L., G.P. Koocher, W.E. Fine, D.J. Foster, and J.E. O'Malley (1979). Pediatric cancer survival and marriage; issues affecting adult adjustment. *Am. J. Orthopsychiatry* 49:423–30.

Kaplan, D.M., R. Grobstein, and A. Smith (1976). Predicting the impact of severe illness in families. *Health Soc. Work* 1:72–82.

Kashani, J. and N. Hakami (1982). Depression in children and adolescents with malignancy. *Can. J. Psychiatry* 27:474–77.

Katz, E.R., J. Kellerman, and S.E. Siegel (1980). Behavioral distress in children with cancer undergoing medical procedures: Developmental consideration. *J. Consult. Clin. Psychol.* 48:356–65.

Kellerman, J., S.E. Siegel, and D. Rigler (1980). Special treatment modalities: Laminar airflow rooms. In J. Kellerman (ed.), *Psychological Aspects of Childhood Cancer*. Springfield, Ill.: Charles C Thomas, pp. 128–54.

Kellerman, J., L. Zeltzer, L. Ellenberg, J. Dash, and D. Rigler (1980). Psychological effects of illness in adolescence. I. Anxiety, self-esteem, and perception of control. *J. Pediatr.* 97(1):126–31.

Klein, D.F., R. Gittelman, F. Quitkin, and A. Raskin (1980). *Diagnosis and Drug Treatment of Psychiatric Disorders: Adults and Children,* 2nd ed. Baltimore, MD: Williams & Wilkins

Klopovich, P., T.S. Vats, G. Butterfield, N.U. Cairns, and S.B. Lansky (1981). School phobia. *J. Kans. Med. Soc.* 82:125–27.

Koocher, G.P. (1982). The crisis of survival: Discussion of Mrs. Christ's and Ms. Adams' paper. In A.E. Christ and K. Flomenhaft (eds.), *Childhood Cancer Impact on the Family*. New York: Plenum, pp. 129–31.

Koocher, G.P. and J.E. O'Malley (1981). *The Damocles Syndrome*. New York: McGraw-Hill.

Koocher, G.P., J.E. O'Malley, and D.J. Foster (1981). The special problems of survivors. In G.P. Koocher and J.E. O'Malley (eds.), *The Damocles Syndrome*. New York: McGraw-Hill, pp. 112–29.

Koocher, G.P., J.E. O'Malley, J.L. Gogan, and D.J. Foster (1980). Psychological adjustment among pediatric cancer survivors. *J. Child Psychol. Psychiatry* 21:163–73.

Kupst, M.J. and J.L. Schulman (1980). Family coping with leukemia in a child: Initial reactions. In J.L. Schulman and M.J. Kupst (eds.), *The Child with Cancer*. Springfield, Ill.: Charles C Thomas, pp. 111–28.

Kupst, M.J., J.L. Schulman, G. Honig, H. Maurer, E. Morgan, and D. Fochtman (1982). Family coping with childhood leukemia: One year after diagnosis. *J. Pediatr. Psychol.* 7(2):157–74.

Kupst, M.J., J.L. Schulman, H. Maurer, G. Honig, E. Morgan, and D. Fochtman (1984). Coping with pediatric leukemia: A two-year followup. *J. Pediatr. Psychol.* 9(2):149–63.

Lansky, S.B. and M. Gendel (1978). Symbiotic regressive behavior patterns in childhood malignancy. *Clin. Pediatr.* 17:133–38.

Lansky, S.B., N.U. Cairns, G.M. Clark, L. Lowman, L. Miller, and R. Trueworthy (1979). Childhood cancer: Nonmedical costs of illness. *Cancer* 43:403–8.

Lansky, S.B., N.U. Cairns, R. Hassanein, B.A. Wehr, and J.T. Lowman (1978). Childhood cancer: Parental discord and divorce. *Pediatrics* 62:184–88.

Lansky, S.B., J.T. Lowman, T. Vats, and J. Gyulay (1975). School phobia in children with malignant neoplasms. *Am. J. Dis. Child.* 129:42–46.

Lansky, S.B., S.T. Smith, N.U. Cairns, and G.F. Cairns (1983). Psychological correlates of compliance. *Am. J. Pediatr. Hematol. Oncol.* 5(1):87–92.

Lansky, S.B., T. Vats, and N.U. Cairns (1979b). Refusal of treatment. A new dilemma for oncologists. *Am. J. Pediatr. Hematol. Oncol.* 1:277–82.

Lavigne, J.V. and M. Ryan (1979). Psychologic adjustment of siblings of children with chronic illness. *Pediatrics* 63(4):616–27.

Levenson, P.M., B.J. Pfefferbaum, D.R. Copeland, and Y. Silberg (1982). Information preferences of cancer patients ages 11–20 years. *J. Adolescent Health Care* 3:9–13.

Levenson, P.M., B. Pfefferbaum, Y. Silberberg, and D.R. Copeland (1981). Sources of information about cancer as perceived adolescent patients, parents, and physicians. *Patient Counsel. Health Educ.* 3(2):71–76.

Lewis, S. and J.D. LaBarbera (1983). Terminating chemotherapy: Another stage in coping with childhood leukemia. *Am. J. Pediatr. Hematol. Oncol.* 5(1):33–7.

Maisami, M., B.H. Sohmer, and J.T. Coyle (1985). Combined use of tricyclic antidepressants and neuroleptics in the management of terminally ill children: A report on three cases. *J. Am. Acad. Child Psychiatry* 24:487–89.

Martinson, I.M., G.D. Armstrong, D.P. Geis, M.A. Anglim, E.C. Gronseth, H. MacInnis, J.H. Kersey, and M.E. Nesbit, Jr. (1978). Home care for children dying of cancer. *Pediatrics* 62:106–13.

Mather, L. and J. Mackie (1983). The incidence of postoperative pain in children. *Pain* 15:271–82.

May, C.H., M.C. McPhee, and D.J. Pritchard (1979). An amputee visitor program as an adjunct to rehabilitation of the lower limb amputee. *Mayo Clin. Proc.* 54:774–78.

Meadows, A.T., D.J. Massari, J. Fergusson, J. Gordon, P. Littman, and K. Moss (1981). Declines in IQ scores and cognitive dysfunctions in children with acute lymphocytic leukemia treated with cranial irradiation. *Lancet* 2:1015–18.

Miller, D.R. and E.A. Haupt (1982). Clinical cancer research: Patient, parent, and physician interactions. In A.E. Christ and K. Flomenhaft (eds.), *Childhood Cancer Impact on the Family.* New York: Plenum, pp. 43–81.

Moss, H.A., E.D. Nannis, and D.G. Poplack (1981). The effects of prophylactic treatment of the central nervous system on the intellectual functioning of children with acute lymphocytic leukemia. *J.A.M.A.* 71:47–52.

Nagy, M. (1959). The child's view of death. In H. Feifel (ed.), *The Meaning of Death.* New York: McGraw-Hill, pp. 79–98.

Newburger, P.E. and S.E. Sallan (1981). Chronic pain: Principles of management. *J. Pediatrics* 98(2):180–89.

Nitschke, R., S. Wunder, C.L. Sexauer, and G.B. Humphrey (1977). The final-stage conference: The patient's decision on research drugs in pediatric oncology. *J. Pediatr. Psychol.* 2:58–64.

Noyes, J.R. (1981). Treatment of cancer pain. *Psychosom. Med.* 43:57–70.

O'Malley, J.E., D. Foster, G. Koocher, and L. Slavin (1980). Visible physical impairment and psychological adjustment among pediatric cancer survivors. *Am. J. Psychiatry* 137:94–96.

Pendergrass, T.W. and S. Davis (1981). Knowledge and use of "alternative" cancer therapies in children. *Am. J. Pediatr. Hematol. Oncol.* 3:339–45.

Pfefferbaum, B., M. Lindamood, and F.M. Wiley (1978). Stages in pediatric bone marrow transplantation. *Pediatrics* 60:625–28.

Pfefferbaum, B., J.E. Overall, H.A. Boren, L.S. Frankel, M.P. Sullivan, and K. Johnson (1987). Alprazolam in the treatment of anticipatory and acute situational anxiety in children with cancer. *J. Am. Acad. Child. Adol. Psychiatry* 26:532–35.

Pfefferbaum-Levine, B., D.R. Copeland, J.M. Fletcher, H.L. Ried, N. Jaffe, and W.R. McKinnon (1984a). Neuropsychologic assessment of long-term survivors of childhood leukemia. *Am. J. Pediatr. Hematol. Oncol.* 6:123–28.

Pfefferbaum-Levine, B., R.B. DeTrinis, M.A. Young, and J. van Eys (1984b). The use of psychoactive medications in children with cancer. *J. Psychosoc. Oncol.* 2:65–71.

Pfefferbaum-Levine, B., K. Kumor, A. Cangir, M. Choroszy, and E.A. Roseberry (1983). Tricyclic antidepressants for children with cancer. *Am. J. Psychiatry* 140:1074–76.

Powazek, M., J.R. Goff, J. Schyving, and M.A. Paulson (1978). Emotional reactions of children to isolation in a cancer hospital. *J. Pediatrics* 92(5):834–37.

Powazek, M., J.S. Payne, J.R. Goff, M.A. Paulson, and S. Stagner (1980). Psychosocial ramifications of childhood leukemia: One year post-diagnosis. In J.L. Schulman and M.J. Kupst (eds.), *The Child with Cancer: Clinical Approaches to Psychosocial Care Research in Psychosocial Aspects.* Springfield, Ill.: Charles C Thomas, pp. 143–55.

Raskin, M., H.V.S. Peeke, W. Dickman, and H. Pinsker (1982). Panic and generalized anxiety disorders. *Arch. Gen. Psychiatry* 39:687–89.

Redd, W.H. and M.A. Andrykowski (1982). Behavioral intervention in cancer treatment: Controlling aversion reactions to chemotherapy. *J. Consult. Clin. Psychol.* 50(6):1018–29.

Rowland, J., O. Glidewell, R. Sibley, J.C. Holland, R. Tull, A. Berman, M.L. Brecher, M. Harris, A.S. Glicksman,

E. Forman, B. Jones, M.E. Cohen, P.K. Duffner, and A.I. Freeman (1984). Effects of different forms of central nervous system prophylaxis on neuropsychologic function in childhood leukemia. *J. Clin. Oncol.* 2:1327–35.

Smith, S.D., D. Rosen, R.C. Trueworthy, and J.R. Lowman (1979). A reliable method for evaluating drug compliance in children with cancer. *Cancer* 43:169–73.

Sokolosky, W. (1982). The sick child and the reluctant parent: A framework for judicial intervention. *J. Fam. Law* 20:69–104.

Sourkes, B.M. (1980). Siblings of the pediatric cancer patient. In J. Kellerman (ed.), *Psychological Aspects of Childhood Cancer*. Springfield, Ill.: Charles C Thomas, pp. 47–69.

Spinetta, J.J. (1974). The dying child's awareness of death. A review. *Psychol. Bull.* 81:256–60.

Spinetta, J.J. (1981a). The sibling of the child with cancer. In J.J. Spinetta and P. Deasy-Spinetta (eds.), *Living with Childhood Cancer*. St. Louis: C.V. Mosby, pp. 133–42.

Spinetta, J.J. (1981b). Adjustment and adaptation in children with cancer. In J.J. Spinetta and P. Deasy-Spinetta (eds.), *Living with Childhood Cancer*. St. Louis: C.V. Mosby, pp. 5–26.

Stehbens, J.A., C.T. Kisker, and B.K. Wilson (1983). School behavior and attendance during the first year of treatment for childhood cancer. *Psychol. Schools* 20:223–28.

Susman, E.J., A.R. Hallenbeck, B.E. Strope, S.P. Hersch, A.S. Levine, and P.A. Pizzo (1980). Separation–deprivation and childhood cancer: A conceptual reevaluation. In J. Kellerman (ed.), *Psychological Aspects of Childhood Cancer*. Springfield, Ill.: Charles C Thomas, pp. 155–70.

Tebbi, C.K., K.M. Cummings, M.A. Zevon, L. Smith, M. Richards, and J. Mallon (1986). Compliance of pediatric and adolescent cancer patients. *Cancer* 58:1179–84.

van Eys, J. and D.R. Copeland (1982). The staffing conference in pediatric oncology. In A.E. Christ and K. Flomenhaft (eds.), *Childhood Cancer Impact on the Family*. New York: Plenum, pp. 87–103.

Weiner, J.M. (1984). Psychopharmacology in childhood disorders. *Psychiatr. Clin. North Am.* 7:831–43.

Wyse, R. (1983). The absent father. In D.R. Copeland, B. Pfefferbaum, and A.J. Stovall (eds.), *The Mind of the Child Who Is Said to Be Sick*. Springfield, Ill.: Charles C Thomas, pp. 170–74.

Young, M.A. and B. Pfefferbaum-Levine (1984). Perspectives on illness and treatment in adolescence. *Cancer Bull.* 36:275–79.

Zeltzer, L., J. Kellerman, L. Ellenberg, J. Dash, and D. Rigler (1980). Psychologic effects of illness in adolescence. II. Impact of illness in adolescents—crucial issues and coping styles. *J. Pediatrics* 97(1):132–38.

# 45

## Psychosocial Interventions in Childhood Cancer

Margaret Adams-Greenly ACSW

The many psychosocial stresses of childhood cancer are well documented and well understood by contemporary medical, nursing, and mental health clinicians. Diagnosis and treatment evoke intense but usually appropriate reactions of helplessness, fear, anger, guilt, and depression that may be manifested in areas of medical noncompliance, school adjustment problems, interpersonal conflicts, marital stress, sibling adjustment problems, and financial strains. The focus of this chapter is not on these issues themselves but rather on interventions to alleviate them. The chapter will briefly describe a team approach and apply it as an organized system of psychological supports integrated into the care of pediatric oncology patients and their families and will also address problems of health care staff and community.

### THE TEAM APPROACH

The hospital treatment staff may easily consist of many professionals, including attending pediatricians, surgeons, medical consultants, house staff, nursing staff, intravenous therapy nurses, psychiatrists, social workers, psychologists, chaplains, pharmacists, recreation-play therapy personnel, hospital schoolteachers, physical therapists, and dietitians. Hospitals usually have varying resources available; some manage with a few professionals who assume the range of functions that in other hospitals might be carried out by several individuals. Any and all of the disciplines represented may, if available, be involved in the care of any one child with cancer. Irrespective of team composition, the crucial issue is that cooperation and collaboration among these professionals is paramount to effective psychosocial management. Although the interdisciplinary team approach to psychosocial management is not a new concept in medical care, it has become an

increasingly important adjunct to patient care, particularly in pediatric oncology settings (Lansky, 1978; Craig, 1973; Drotar and Doershuk, 1979).

This approach reflects an awareness of two important concepts of systems theory, namely, that the system (team) is an entity rather than a conglomeration of parts, and that social phenomena are elements of a continuously flowing interaction (Bertalanffy, 1968). Germain (1984) points out that the goal of a well-functioning interdisciplinary team is to integrate, not simply coordinate, the different skills and perspectives of diverse disciplines in order to provide optimal health care. In an integrated system of psychological support, rather than receiving compartmentalized assistance from each professional, patients receive input from the entire system and are actually a part of it as well. The system utilizes a biopsychosocial approach aimed at understanding patients in relation to all aspects of their situation.

In designing a system of psychosocial supports for pediatric oncology patients, the health care team must consider the broad needs of the total patient population, as well as specific needs of subgroups. Different children and their families may utilize different aspects of the system at different times, based on the child's diagnosis, the stage of disease, the age of the child, the geographic availability of the family or center, cultural considerations, family structure, and personal preference. Thus, the support system must be flexible enough to respond not only to the group but also to the individual.

This chapter presents a model of psychosocial interventions that reflects a philosophy that the child and family should maintain as much of their normal life as possible, within the limits of the medical situation. Interventions are thus focused directly on the child, on his or her parents and siblings, on the hospital staff, and on the school and community.

## PSYCHOSOCIAL INTERVENTIONS FOR PATIENTS AND FAMILIES

Whether a child is admitted directly to an inpatient unit or is seen in a clinic or pediatric day hospital, psychosocial support should be initiated immediately. As the patient and his or her parents are typically quite anxious upon arrival, a thorough orientation will help them feel more secure. Parents benefit from written material, including basic information about the hospital or clinic, as well as guidelines on the emotional management of the patient and siblings useful in promoting good adjustment. A visit to the playroom and schoolroom, if these are available, should be included in the orientation, conveying that, although the child has a serious illness, normal development will be fostered. A nurse may prepare the child and family psychologically for tests, procedures, and surgery, emphasizing a philosophy that open communication lessens fear and enhances compliance. The physician who discusses the diagnosis and the plan of treatment with the parents, encourages them to speak honestly with their child and to involve the child as fully as possible in his or her own care.

The first mental health professional to meet a new family is usually a social worker. A useful team model is one in which one social worker works closely with one or more pediatricians and is available to all families being cared for by them. The advantages of such a model are that it provides comprehensive care, maximizes patient–doctor communication, and affords continuity of caregiving. It is additionally important to provide social workers who are fluent in the first language of patients. The goal of such a model is for all families to have access to a readily identified mental health professional and to have at least an initial psychosocial consultation and assessment shortly after coming for or starting treatment. At this time children or family members at "high risk" for psychosocial stress can be identified. In such an assessment risk factors would include those who have excessive anxiety, prior mental illness, a history of previous loss or of previous problems in work or school adjustment, visibly stressed interpersonal relationships, or a family or individual history of multiple social problems with limited resources.

Individual and family counseling is focused around the key issues of arranging for practical concerns such as transportation and housing, communication about the diagnosis and treatment, the needs of siblings, marital stresses, school adjustment, and emotional reactions to the medical situation. The social worker should also recognize, along with the pediatrician, the need for psychiatric consultation and initiate referral. This is indicated when there is a history of psychiatric illness, when the patient or a family member presents psychotic symptoms or suicidal ideation, or when psychiatric symptoms or behavior require psychotropic medication for control (see Chapter 44 by Pfefferbaum). A referral may also be made for behavioral intervention (see Chapter 46 by Redd).

Throughout the course of treatment, which may last several years, a core program of psychosocial support should remain available to the child patient and his or her family. This should provide (1) ongoing or periodic instruction about the disease, treatment, and medical procedures, (2) age-appropriate recreation and education, (3) family-focused supportive counseling, and (4) psychiatric and behavioral consultation as needed. Two further desirable sources of support include a pediatric home support team who can coordinate home care for families of terminally ill children; and a long-term follow-up program for children who have completed treatment. A program of group interventions greatly expands the range of helpful services to families. Some possible models of group intervention are described in the following paragraphs.

### Groups for Patients

Groups for patients may be both unit-specific and age-specific. In planning patient groups, careful consideration should be given to developmental issues and the impact of serious illness on them (see Chapter 43 by Rowland). The groups described here are planned with this in mind and are appropriate to both ambulatory and hospital settings.

## ADOLESCENT GROUPS

While adolescence represents for most young people a challenging developmental period, it is especially stressful when the adolescent has cancer. Diagnosis and treatment limit autonomy, and the adolescent patient often feels weak and debilitated (Kagen-Goodheart, 1977). Conflicts around separation–individuation are exacerbated by forced dependence on parents and the often accompanying regressive pull (Schowalter, 1977). Physical changes caused by surgery or chemotherapy, especially amputation and hair loss, leave the adolescent feeling vulnerable and unattractive (Kagen, 1976). He or she may withdraw from activities and healthy peers (Plumb and Holland, 1974).

Because the peer group is a natural formation in adolescence, the use of group meetings is a natural tool for enhancing coping and decreasing feelings of isolation. Leadership should be planned to encourage attendance by both sexes and to provide male and female role models. Group sessions should focus on the developmentally normal aspects of adolescence and the impact of catastrophic illness on them (Boyers, 1983), including the tremendous impact on body image, sexuality, and feelings about desirability, issues concerning dependence/independence and conflicts with parents and staff, difficulties with the healthy peer group, and concern about the future (including schooling, career plans, worry about marriage and childbearing ability, and the possibility of terminal illness).

An adolescent group provides multiple opportunities for identification, reality testing, and working through of issues. A particularly impressive aspect of such groups is the development of enhanced compassion among the members. As ill as they are, they may be highly sensitive to each other's needs and provide feedback as well as support through the most difficult times, sharing advice about coping strategies, and offering advice on how to talk to friends and teachers. Once rapport is established, teens feel free to discuss their fear of embarrassment over hair loss, and tell anecdotes of their worst, or even funniest, moments. They use the group to develop insight into their parents and siblings, and to appreciate how their illness is affecting family life (Boyers, 1983).

## HOSPITAL PLAY THERAPY GROUPS

The stressful aspects of physical illness and hospitalization on young children are well known (Chapter 43). They include the child's limited knowledge of life outside the home, cognitive limitations, and the disruption of normal peer activities (including school, sports, and social events). Hospitalization may additionally entail sensorimotor restrictions, physical pain, and frightening procedures. Issues related to the child's developing ego capacities affect his or her response to physical illness and its treatment (Freud, 1952). Cooper and Blitz (1985) identify these issues as separation anxiety, egocentrism, conflicts about body integrity, physical change, control of sexual and aggressive impulses, the need for intellectual development, and sense of mastery.

Hospitalization, particularly for cancer treatment, may result in moderate to severe depression, regression, decreased cooperation, aggression, disruptive behavior, and sleep disturbances (Cofer and Nir, 1975). Koocher and O'Malley (1981) pointed out that being able to express negative feelings and to share anxiety-producing experiences enhances coping. They also observed that anticipating a painful or stressful event increases mastery over it. Cofer and Nir (1975) emphasized the importance of careful preparation for the procedure as a way to enhance mastery.

Play is the child's most natural method of self-expression and self-exploration, as well as being a vehicle for learning about life (Adams, 1976). The literature on the value of play stresses the importance of mastery (Peller, 1952), catharsis and education (Petrillo and Sanger, 1972), and the working through of conflicts (Freud, 1946; Axline, 1947).

Although play therapy may be available and appropriate on an individual basis, hospital play therapy groups have many advantages. As Ginnott (1958) pointed out, group play provides multilateral relationships for the child, opportunities for catharsis of feeling, reality testing, pleasure in activities, and insight into emotions. Hospital play therapy groups have the three goals of educating children about their illness and treatment and thus enhancing compliance, addressing the child's perception of the illness through an understanding of the symbolic content of play, and facilitating the child's ability to cope with the anxiety that inevitably accompanies a complex medical treatment (Cooper and Blitz, 1985).

To achieve these goals, such groups are best led cooperatively by a nurse and social worker or other mental health professional. The co-leaders share psychosocial expertise, but each brings a specialized knowledge. The presence of a nurse makes the group accessible to children who otherwise would not be able to attend, such as those receiving blood transfusions or chemotherapy. The nurse's knowledge of the illness and treatment is important to the teaching function of the group. In addition, he or she can inform other nurses about important problems or attitudes that may become apparent in the group setting. The child's care plan can be altered or expanded to incorporate these issues. The social worker brings skill in understanding group and individual dynamics, encouraging expression of feelings and assessing ego development, and encouraging behavior consistent with developmental stage (Cooper and Blitz, 1985).

Hospital play therapy groups are useful with children between the ages of 30 months and 11 years. Thus, considerable flexibility and knowledge of developmental issues, needs, and capabilities are required of the leaders. The primary focus of the group discussion is to elicit feelings about the hospital experience, but children will often address how this affects other areas of their lives, such as family relationships and school.

### Groups for Parents

It has long been recognized that parents of children with cancer rely greatly on support from one another; identification with others in the same situation limits the sense of isolation and helps them learn new coping strategies (Adams, 1978b; Ross, 1979). Support groups for parents may take three forms of structure: unit-specific, disease-specific, and culture-specific.

## UNIT-SPECIFIC PARENTS' GROUP

Unit-specific parents' groups are best organized to meet weekly on inpatient and outpatient units, and are best led cooperatively by a social worker or other mental health professional, and the head nurse of the unit or a nurse familiar with the issues. Goals of these parent groups are to decrease feelings of isolation, provide relevant information, increase a sense of competence, and strengthen the ability to reflect on the broad implications of the disease and the situation, and to consider the emotional needs of the entire family as well as those of the patient (Adams, 1978b).

The use of co-leaders is beneficial. The nurse answers questions about treatment and procedures, and signifies by her or his presence that the nursing staff is concerned about the stresses for parents. The social worker is trained in group dynamics and is able to identify families in need of individual help. The group leaders should invite all parents who are present on the unit to a planned meeting. Those who attend will likely have children who have different diagnoses and are at different stages in their illness. This may create difficulties in that new parents, who are in need of hope, may be overwhelmed by those parents whose child has relapsed or is terminally ill. However, it can be a strength in that the new parents can learn that it *is* possible to cope with the stresses; experienced parents often provide guidance and serve as role models (Adams, 1978b).

Although the content of the meetings is not structured, there are themes that emerge consistently. The first is the parents' need to express their feelings of helplessness, fear, anger, guilt, and sadness (Chodoff et al., 1964; Futterman and Hoffman, 1973). Parents frequently report that family and friends do not understand them and that they feel alone. They are usually relieved to unburden themselves and to discover that their feelings are normal and appropriate. These expressions should be strongly encouraged by the group leaders, thus validating the parents' feelings and recognizing their universal nature. Of greater concern to the leaders will be meetings in which parents' feelings of helplessness and anger are displaced onto hospital staff. It is important that such reactions be accepted without antagonism and be placed in perspective. It is helpful to emphasize that staff and parents are allies in the treatment process and that everyone's goal is the child's optimum physical and mental health.

A second important theme in parents' meetings is the emotional care of the patient and siblings. The need for communication within the family system (Koocher and O'Malley, 1981) deserves particular emphasis; a sense of trust is essential in order for the family to sustain the impact of the illness on their lives. The importance of maintaining normal family life, including school attendance, household responsibilities, and discipline should be consistently stressed (Kagen-Goodheart, 1977). Although concerns about sibling rivalry are frequently a topic in the outpatient parents' group, the issue of separation of siblings from parents may be raised more often in the inpatient group.

School reentry is a third major area of discussion. Parental concern is often voiced about how best to help a child cope with the stresses of returning to school. Practical advice about managing responses to a changed physical appearance, to questions and teasing from peers, and to dealing with frequent absences from class and the side effects of treatment (in particular fatigue and weakness) are often sought. Concern is also frequently raised about the school's ability to accept and support the child with cancer in the normal classroom.

A fourth major issue, especially in a hospital parents' group, is that of terminal illness and death. These parents repeatedly experience the death of other children on the unit and have contact with the parents of those children. They tend to develop close and intense relationships and may be profoundly devastated by these losses, which, of course, raises their concern about their own children. In the meetings, parents wonder aloud how to talk with their children about serious illness and death in a way that is open, yet not frightening (Adams-Greenly, 1984). As with all other issues, the focus of the group leaders should be on identifying coping strategies and emphasizing that, though painful and difficult, open communication enhances trust and family cohesion.

## DISEASE-SPECIFIC PARENTS' GROUPS

Although all parents may attend unit-specific groups, there may be some aspects of a particular disease that raise unique issues. In this situation, parents may benefit from a disease-specific parents' group that will address site- and treatment-specific concerns. An example of such a group is a meeting for parents of children with brain tumors. At Memorial Sloan-Kettering Cancer Center (MSKCC), the social worker and pediatric nurse-practitioner who work with the two pediatric neurologists became aware that parents of these children face unique coping tasks and developed a special group program for them (M. T. Hanna and D. Schaefer, personal communication, January 1984). This group meets on a monthly basis and has a combined focus of education and support. The leaders invite guest speakers, including the neurologists, to address particular topics for the first half of each meeting, which is then followed by an open discussion of any concerns raised by the parents.

Issues raised in this group include all of those in the unit-specific groups as well as others that are unique to these parents. In the group for parents of children with brain tumors, these include the possibility of gradual intellectual decline of the patient as a function of the tumor or the treatment, cognitive impairment following surgery, loss of the ability to speak or to see, side effects of steroids, loss of motor function or paralysis, personality changes, and the need for special education. Because these patients usually require more physical care than other pediatric oncology patients, this may place a greater burden on the parents' caretaking roles and on the needs of siblings.

Parents who attend these meetings are actively involved in recruiting new group members, identifying parents of children with newly diagnosed brain tumors, and planning the agenda of each meeting. Helping others serves to allay some of the helplessness these parents so often experience. This group is relevant to these particular families; other disease-specific groups may also be helpful (e.g., leukemia, Hodgkin's disease).

## CULTURE-SPECIFIC PARENTS' GROUPS

In a complex medical system, the needs of families whose cultural background is different may be overlooked, especially when language is a barrier. Staff may not recognize or understand cultural differences; they may be simply too rushed to attend to them. For example, a tertiary care facility such as MSKCC is apt to have a substantial number of Spanish-speaking pediatric patients. The parents of these children are usually unable to benefit from the other existing group programs because of the language barrier. One of the Spanish-speaking social workers observed that Hispanic families tended to commiserate and share medical information, misinformation, and tips on coping with their sick children only with other Hispanic families, and not with the predominantly non-Hispanic hospital staff. Although all of the normal interventions were available for these families, it was determined that a group program would provide greatly needed mutual support and problem solving (Schaefer, 1983).

In a group conducted especially for this Spanish-speaking subpopulation, members deal with many of the general issues raised in the unit-specific groups. However, additional unique issues for these parents are the language barrier and its effect on their understanding of their children's treatment, cultural values (concerning sex roles, religion, and childrearing), social isolation, and separation from the rest of the family and community supports at home (Schaefer, 1983).

Hispanics place high value on the concept of ''personalismo,'' or the inclination to relate to and place trust in people rather than institutions. They are more likely to relate well to someone who speaks their language, understands the culture, is flexible, easily accessible, and able to advocate for them in the large, complex hospital system (Schaefer, 1983). In addition to group meetings, the Spanish-speaking social worker sees all group members individually and provides continuity of care. She or he is regarded by the parents not only as the leader but also as their liaison and advocate with the rest of the staff. In turn, she or he provides feedback from the parents to the staff. This culture-specific group helps its members perceive the hospital as warm and caring, and minimizes the feeling of isolation and alienation. Such a group is particularly suitable in areas where large, unique cultural groups live, such as Asians, Native Americans, or recent immigrants.

## Siblings

The special needs of siblings of children with cancer have become an increasing concern in recent years. Reports of work with these youngsters describe feelings of anger, resentment, guilt, and low self-esteem. Siblings may show depression, anxiety, daydreaming, social difficulties, withdrawal, and preoccupation with illness (Binger, 1973; Gogan et al., 1977; Kramer, 1984). Sourkes (1981) found that healthy siblings expressed concern about the cause of the illness, the visibility of the disease, guilt and shame, conflicts in the relationship with parents, impaired academic and social functioning, and somatic symptoms.

In studying siblings, Townes and Wold (1977) found that poor adjustment of the sibling was more likely when there was little communication from parents about the ill child's disease. Spinetta and Deasy-Spinetta (1981) also found that the degree to which parents communicated with siblings influenced how well they coped. Kagen-Goodheart (1977) and Lindsay and McCarthy (1974) recommend that siblings have direct information about the illness, coupled with recognition and understanding by the parents of the importance and validity of their feelings. Wiener (1970) pointed out that staff members who showed interest in and concern for siblings had a positive effect on the whole family.

The stresses for siblings may be reduced by interventions that fall into the areas of communication, education, and support. Each has been identified as helpful in facilitating effective coping (Blumberg et al., 1984). One model of intervention developed at MSKCC is a 1-day workshop, held on a Saturday, which includes both educational and supportive components. Letters are mailed to parents of children on treatment, inviting them to register the patient's school-aged siblings to attend the workshop. The program begins with a lecture on normal cell division, the difference between normal cells and cancer cells, forms of cancer therapy, and side effects of therapy. The siblings are then taken on a tour of the hospital, including a visit to the radiation therapy department and the operating rooms. In the afternoon they view a videotape of four siblings discussing their experiences, problems, and coping strategies. A group discussion follows, stimulated by the videotape, with a focus on identifying constructive coping mechanisms. Evaluations by siblings and by parents show the workshop to be successful in its educational and supportive goals, and to have a positive effect on family life (Adams-Greenly et al., 1986).

## PSYCHOSOCIAL SUPPORTS FOR THE SCHOOLS

It is widely agreed that it is important for the child with cancer to return to school as soon as possible after diagnosis, and be treated as normally as the physical and psychological condition permits (Cyphert, 1973; Deasy-Spinetta, 1981; Lansky et al., 1975). School is the workplace of children; it is there that they learn not only academic skills but also the social skills of teamwork, self-control, discipline, respect for authority, and mutually supportive peer relationships. For the child with cancer, successful school reentry is an important aspect of reestablishing normality and enhancing quality of survival.

Reentry to school following diagnosis of cancer and initial treatment presents problems for parents and students. Teachers and administrators are occasionally reluctant to have a seriously ill child in the classroom. There are several possible reasons for such an attitude, including teachers' unresolved feelings about cancer, worries about being unable to address appropriately the needs of the patient as well as those of the other students, and concern about the response of the patient or classes to information about the illness. Because some teachers fear they may not be able to provide adequate care for the student with cancer, they may withdraw emotionally from these students, and, in so doing, unconsciously influence other students to do the same (Cyphert, 1973). These teachers, who isolate the student with cancer in reaction to personal fear of or misconceptions about the disease, lower academic requirements and standards for the child. This overprotection of the patient serves to isolate the child from his or her peers, emphasize the differences due to illness, and increase the child's feelings of hopelessness and helplessness.

Parents can also contribute to this problem by being overprotective of the child with cancer and being hesitant to return the child to school (Cyphert, 1973). Parents may at times be unable to deal realistically with their child's diagnosis, treatment, and prognosis, a response that can prevent them from encouraging the child and making appropriate scholastic demands. Also, some families encounter problems returning the patient to school if the sick child develops school phobia (Lansky et al., 1975; see also Chapter 44).

A useful model to address the concerns of patients, parents, and teachers is a 1-day workshop for school personnel of pediatric patients and their siblings. The format of this particular workshop provides for didactic instruction on medical and psychological issues and an opportunity to view and discuss videotaped interviews with patients and siblings. The videotapes address developmental issues and provide advice from the children themselves to the school personnel on how to foster a good school adjustment. The goal of such a program is for school personnel to know more about childhood cancer and feel more comfortable with patients and their siblings. Evaluations of this type of workshop at MSKCC have consistently shown that school personnel rate the experience very highly. Results of pretest and posttest assessments also indicate clearly that increased knowledge is gained through exposure to this kind of presentation.

## PSYCHOSOCIAL SUPPORTS FOR HOSPITAL STAFF

Caring for children with cancer and their families is extremely stressful for hospital staff (see section of staff problems in Chapter 44 by Pfefferbaum as well as Chapter 47 by Rait and Lederberg and Chapter 51 by Lederberg). Catastrophic illness and the possibility of death confirm our feelings of inadequacy and elicit strong emotions. We may feel angry at ourselves for failing the patient, at the patient for failing us, or at God for failing all of us. We may feel frightened, or even panicked by the indiscriminate, sudden, and ruthless character of catastrophic illness. We may feel sad and mourn the loss of a person whom we knew, cared for, respected, and even loved (Adams, 1978a). Koocher (1979) points out that there are also rewards to be found in this work. These include the knowledge that one has brought physical or psychological comfort, has helped to enhance the ability of the patient and family to cope, and has shared deeply personal moments in the patient's life. Maintaining a reasonable balance between these stressful and positive aspects of caring for children with cancer is indeed a challenge. Staff members need to allay the feeling of helplessness and develop a feeling of control and competence (Adams, 1978a).

Psychological support groups for staff may either

focus directly on the staff and their own feelings, or utilize a focus on the patient and family to strengthen and enhance staff members' feelings of competence through improved case management. In this section, both support formats are discussed, the first in the form of an inpatient nursing support group and the second in the form of inpatient psychosocial rounds.

## Nursing Support Group

Eisendrath (1981) points out that a support group is different from a psychotherapy group. The group's goal is to support staff and improve patient care, not produce intrapsychic change; the focus is on job-related issues, not personal problems (Moynihan and Outlaw, 1984). Wiener, Caldwell, and Tyson (1983) identify six characteristics that lead to a successful support group: the group reflects a response to a perceived need by the staff and is supported by the administration; the members have had previous positive exposure to the leader, whom they regard as both an expert and a real person; the leader is active and uses a structured approach; the focus is on patient-related issues; affect is regulated and each meeting is summarized; and finally, a distinction is made between therapy and support.

The model of a nursing support group presented here has met on a weekly basis for the past 8 years. It was formed at the request of the staff with the support of the head nurse, and is led by the pediatric social work supervisor at the request of the staff nurses. As Wiener and colleagues point out, an active, directed leadership approach with a focus on problem solving, not simply emotional ventilation, is most effective. It is important to help group members regulate and modify affect and to conclude each meeting with a summary that is positive and helps the staff return to their bedside responsibilities.

The goals of such a group are to help staff be more aware of their own emotional reactions, learn new ways of solving problems and coping with stress, and develop a sense of cohesiveness and support among themselves. As with other groups described in the literature, issues may include professional identity and the professional social system (Beardslee and DeMaso, 1982), reactions to pain and suffering (Moynihan and Outlaw, 1984), and countertransference (Koocher, 1979).

## Psychosocial Rounds

In contrast, and in many respects a complement to the nursing- or staff-focused group, is the patient- and family-focused multidisciplinary meeting. Ideally, these meetings, referred to in some settings as psychosocial

rounds, should be attended by the active treating staff, including pediatricians, fellows, house staff, nursing staff, social workers, psychiatrists, psychologists, and chaplains. Playroom and schoolroom staff, and other professionals such as the physiotherapists and the dietitians involved in specific patients' care should attend.

The leader of psychosocial rounds, in consultation with medical and nursing staff, should develop a list of patients for discussion in advance of the meeting. Patients and families appropriate for discussion are those whose behavior indicates maladaptive coping (i.e., those who seem excessively anxious, angry, or depressed), those families with a history of separation and loss, social and financial problems, or psychiatric illness, patients who are terminally ill, and patients who are newly admitted for whom a collaborative plan must be developed. Each case discussion should begin with a brief medical summary by the responsible physician and a statement about why the patient is being discussed and what questions about care should be addressed by the group. Relevant psychosocial information should be reported by other staff who have seen the family, particularly the social worker, psychiatrist, psychologist, or nurse. Input from all other staff should be solicited, key problem areas identified, and a plan of team intervention developed.

Nasson (1981) points out that team interaction provides a structure for the group's professional functioning, and that tensions and disagreements are a normal part of that process. They reflect not only different members' professional goals and perceptions of the patient, but also their empathic awareness of different aspects of the patient's total life experience. Nasson further points out that interprofessional behavior does not require that members of different professions think alike, but rather that they act together.

Psychosocial rounds provide a forum for the sharing and airing of a variety of viewpoints. By working these out together and agreeing on a plan, all team members have the opportunity to hear and be heard by their colleagues. The effective team is one that is able to advance beyond fragmented thinking about the patient from each particular discipline's point of view, to a broader or comprehensive understanding of the patient–environment relationship. In such an atmosphere, proposed interventions tend to be complementary and, when differences occur, they are recognized and resolved (Germain, 1984).

At psychosocial rounds, the plan of intervention should be agreed on by all. Thus, the tendency to act autonomously and perhaps put the patient or family in the middle of a staff or treatment conflict can be avoided. Similarly, because the implementation of the plan will be consistent from one team member to another, the possibility of "splitting" the staff by patient or family will also be avoided.

## INTEGRATION OF PSYCHOSOCIAL SUPPORTS FOR PATIENTS, FAMILIES, HOSPITAL STAFF, AND THE COMMUNITY

Bertalanffy (1968) defines a system as an "organized complexity" or a "wholeness," and says that an open system "maintains itself in a continuous inflow and outflow, a building up and breaking down of components." This section presents examples of the maximum utilization of the system of psychosocial supports.

### Example A

The following case describes the integration of psychiatric and social work intervention, play group therapy, and primary nursing in the management of a disturbed child.

CASE REPORT

Rebecca was 5 years old when admitted for a bone marrow transplant. Psychiatric intervention was requested because of her serious behavioral problems including enuresis, rocking, shrieking, food refusal, and extreme intractability. If frustrated she quickly regressed into impulsive, aggressive behavior. Her mother was noted to be anxious, depressed, inhibited, and unable to set any limits with Rebecca. There were four other children at home; the oldest, age 7, had many responsibilities for the care of the younger three.

Concerned about her ability to tolerate the frustrations and demands of isolation, skin and mouth care, and other aspects of the transplant procedure, the staff felt that Rebecca's behavior problems were in themselves life-threatening. Transplant was postponed until Rebecca became more manageable.

Psychiatric intervention included medication (to lessen anxiety, mitigate the severity of the regression, and enhance integration of coping), intensive individual psychotherapy with Rebecca, supportive contact with the mother, and consultation with staff (Anna Balas, M.D., personal communication, September 1984).

Rebecca also attended a play therapy group, participating in a total of 15 sessions before entering isolation. Though initially impulsive, possessive, and demanding, she emerged as a group leader and "expert," interacting well with other children and with the leaders. The play group nurse worked closely with Rebecca's primary nurse to incorporate play into her care plan, especially after she entered isolation.

Simultaneously, Rebecca's mother was seen by the social worker for supportive counseling focused on helping her set limits with Rebecca, follow the care plan developed by nursing, and reorganize responsibilities for the 7-year-old at home. This child was also seen by the social worker for play

therapy, and because of their intense sibling rivalry, several joint sessions were held with the patient and sibling.

Because of the complexities of the situation, special case conferences were held on a weekly basis to coordinate the efforts of all involved. Rebecca and her mother responded well to these efforts of intensive supportive intervention. Rebecca entered isolation for transplantation and coped satisfactorily with the frustrations of the arduous procedure.

### Example B

The integration of social work, primary nursing, play therapy, parents' group, and psychosocial rounds in the care of a terminally ill child are the subject of the next case.

CASE REPORT

Marty G., age 8, was put on the list for psychosocial rounds by his resident because he had just been readmitted in the third relapse of his leukemia. The resident expressed concern because Marty's parents had seemed inappropriately cheerful upon admission and he wondered if they understood the medical situation.

Social work input revealed that Marty's parents were divorced, but were able to collaborate on the care of their son. However, they did not communicate with each other on an emotional level and, historically, each had maintained a cheerful bravado when visiting at the hospital together. In separate interviews, both had tearfully admitted that they knew Marty was dying. However, both also expressed an interest in trying a research protocol, feeling that neither they nor Marty were ready to "give up."

In the parents' group meeting, Mrs. G., who had been an active member during previous admissions, told the other parents about Marty's condition. She received support and encouragement from her peers to "take one day at a time." A popular mother on the unit, Mrs. G. used the group to be helpful to new parents, giving advice and sharing her warm sense of good humor. She later told her social worker that the group was "a respite" and that "helping others helps me forget about myself for a while." However, although the group had met her need to be helpful and her need for support, she had not felt free to share some of her deeper concerns about her sadness over Marty's grave prognosis. She used individual counseling to talk about this and about her wish to maintain Marty's trust in her.

Marty, upon hearing that he was again in relapse, clearly stated that he wanted "more drugs." However, the research protocol that he was placed on required daily intravenous injections. Marty used play therapy group to ventilate his anger at this situation, sticking needles mercilessly into doctor and nurse puppets, saying, "It's just too bad for you. There's nothing we can do. Ha, ha." The group leaders commented that "it's hard when you feel angry at people you really like," and Marty admitted that he knew the staff did not really enjoy hurting him but said "I'm just sick of being sick."

After 3 weeks, when Marty had shown no response to the

research drug, his case was again raised at psychosocial rounds, this time for a discussion of whether he should be discharged. The medical staff pointed out that, although there were legitimate reasons to keep Marty in the hospital, he probably could be cared for as well at home until his death. Nursing staff felt strongly that, as long as his bed was not needed for someone more acutely ill, Marty should be allowed to stay. They expressed concern that both Marty and his mother might feel abandoned if he was discharged. A lively discussion ensued in which it became clear that different team members had widely disparate views about management of the terminally ill. It was then concluded that, the disparate viewpoints notwithstanding, Marty and his mother should be allowed to exercise control in this situation and make the decision themselves, with our full support.

The home support team met with Mrs. G. and offered their services in arranging visiting nurse service (VNS) and other community supports, as well as home visits from the team. The attending physician assured Mrs. G. that discharge from the hospital did not imply rejection and that she could bring Marty back should his condition worsen. After careful consideration, Mrs. G. decided to keep her son in the hospital. Her decision followed a conversation with Marty in which he had said, "No matter how much I hate the medicine, we have to keep trying."

Throughout the remainder of Marty's life, which was another 3 weeks, Mrs. G. continued to attend parents' meetings, serving as a role model of acceptance and dignity for newer parents. Marty declined further invitations to attend play group, but welcomed bedside visits from the group leaders. Mrs. G. used individual counseling to deal with her grief and to focus on her communication with Marty. When he asked her if he was going to die, she was able to answer him truthfully, discuss his fear, but reassure him that she would be with him and that he would soon be at peace.

## Example C

The third case report focuses on the integration of the nursing support group and psychosocial rounds in planning collaboratively on behalf of newly diagnosed patients.

CASE REPORT

Nurse D. opened discussion at the nursing support group by saying that Mr. P., father of a new patient, was "annoying." She went on to say that Mr. P.'s anxiety about his son and his questioning and requestioning were interfering with her ability to take care of the boy. Nurse D. said that she was "too busy with too much work and too little time." Several other nurses agreed, saying that "the parents we have right now seem very demanding."

Exploration revealed that the nurses were referring specifically to parents of newly diagnosed children. The group leader gently commented that for new parents to be anxious and have many questions did not seem unusual or inappropriate. She wondered why this was so bothersome to the staff right now, when, at other times, they were highly sensitive to these problems and derived satisfaction from educating and guiding parents through the first weeks of diagnosis and treatment. One nurse commented, "Maybe it's because we don't know them yet, so we don't understand them." Another then said, "Maybe we just don't have the energy to get to know them."

Further discussion revealed that, in the last 3 weeks, several children had died whom the staff had known very well and had cared about deeply. The nursing care that had been provided for them as they were dying had been exemplary. Simultaneously, newly diagnosed children had been admitted, immediately taking the beds of the children who had died. That these usually sensitive and empathic nurses experienced these parents as demanding was a clear indication that they had not been able to mourn the previous patients enough to invest in the new ones. Comments were made, such as, "What's the use? We don't really do any good anyway."

The remainder of this meeting was devoted to a discussion of the sad, the poignant, and the funny moments that the staff had shared with the children who had died and their parents. Leadership efforts were directed at identifying ways in which the staff had helped them and had alleviated potential problems. The group was reminded that all of these children had once been new to us, and that, through our intervention, their lives (and ours) had been enriched. Staff were also reminded that more and more children with cancer are becoming long-term survivors. The meeting concluded with a decision to place the names of the newly diagnosed patients on the list for psychosocial rounds that week, as well as to hear updates on children who had been discharged and were doing well.

At psychosocial rounds, each of the new patients was discussed, with a concerted effort by all team members to individualize them and to develop a care plan consisting of education for patient and parents, supportive counseling, and outreach to the schools. At the end of the meeting, social workers reported on their follow-up bereavement contact with families of the children who had died. In every instance, the family had asked the worker to convey to the staff their gratitude for the care they had given. Brief reports were then given on children who were doing well and leading normal, active lives.

## SUMMARY

It is clear that pediatric cancer patients and their families require supportive interventions at different levels and in different areas. No one aspect of the system "treats" the patient and provides total care. Without the complete support of the total system, each intervention is isolated in only one area of the experience of the patient and family. However, taken together, the whole is surely far greater than all of its individual aspects. Close and consistent collaboration bring to the patient the best in care, and to the staff the satisfaction of a job well done.

PSYCHOSOCIAL INTERVENTIONS IN CHILDHOOD CANCER

# REFERENCES

Adams, M.A. (1976). A hospital play program: Helping children with serious illness. *Am. J. Orthopsychiatry* 46:416–24.

Adams, M.A. (1978a). From life to death: A social worker's response. *Soc. Work Health Care* 4:88–92.

Adams, M.A. (1978b). Helping the parents of children with malignancy. *J. Pediatr.* 93:734–38.

Adams-Greenly, M. (1984). Helping children communicate about serious illness and death. *J. Psych. Oncol.* 2:62–72.

Adams-Greenly, M., T. Shiminski-Maher, N. McGowan, and P.A. Meyers (1986). A group program for helping siblings of children with cancer. *J. Psych. Oncol.* 4:55–67.

Axline, V. (1947). *Play Therapy*. New York: Ballantine Books.

Beardslee, W.R. and D.R. DeMaso (1982). Staff groups in a pediatrics hospital: Content and coping. *Am. J. Orthopsychiatry* 52:712–18.

Beardslee, W.R. and D.R. DeMaso (1982). Staff groups in a pediatric hospital: content and coping. *Am. J. Orthopsychiatr.* 52:712–718.

Bertalanffy, L. (1968). *General Systems Theory: Foundation, Development, and Applications*. New York: George Bazillon.

Binger, C.M., A.R. Aldin, R.C. Feuerstein, J.H. Kushner, A. Zoger, and C. Mikkelsen (1969). Childhood leukemia: Emotional impact on patient and family. *N. Engl. J. Med.* 280:414–18.

Binger, C. (1973). Childhood leukemia: emotional impact on siblings. In E.J. Anthony and C. Koupernik (eds.) *The Child in His Family: Impact of Disease and Death*. New York: John Wiley and Sons.

Blumberg, B.D., J.T. Burklow, J.K. Laufer, M. Cosgrove, M. Adams-Greenly, and S.M. Kranstuber (1988). Responding to the informational needs of young people whose parents or siblings have cancer. *J. Assoc. Pediatr. Oncol. Nurses* 5:16–19.

Boyers, R. (1983). *The Adolescent Group in an Oncology Setting*. Paper presented at the meeting of the International Association of Pediatrics Social Workers, Washington, D.C., October.

Chodoff, P., S. Friedman, and D. Hamburg (1964). Stress, defenses, and coping behavior: Observations in parents of children with malignant diseases. *Am. J. Psychiatry* 120:743–47.

Cofer, D.H. and Y. Nir (1975). Theme-focused group therapy on a pediatric ward. *Int. J. Psychiatry Med.* 6:541–50.

Cooper, S. and J. Blitz (1985). A therapeutic play group for hospitalized children with cancer. *J. Psychosoc. Oncol.* 3:23–37.

Craig, T.J. (1973). Psychiatric consultation to the non-physician staff of an outpatient oncology clinic. *Psychiatr. Med.* 4:291–300.

Cyphert, F. (1973). Back to school for the child with cancer. *J. School Health* 43:215–17.

Deasy-Spinetta, P. (1981). The role of the school in the life of the child with cancer. In J.J. Spinetta and P. Deasy-Spinetta (eds.), *Living with Childhood Cancer*. St. Louis: C.V. Mosby.

Drotar, D. and C. Doershuk (1979). The interdisciplinary case conference: An aid to pediatric interventions with the dying adolescent. *Arch. Found. Thanatol.* 74:79–96.

Eisendrath, S.J. (1981). Psychiatric liaison support groups for general hospital staffs. *Psychosomatics* 22:685–94.

Freud, A. (1946). *The Psychoanalytical Treatment of Children*. New York: International Universities Press.

Freud, A. (1952). The role of bodily illness in the mental life of children. *Psychoanal. Study Child* 7:69–81.

Futterman, E. and I. Hoffman (1973). Crisis and adaptation in the families of fatally ill children. In E. Anthony and C. Koupernik (eds.), *The Child in His Family: The Impact of Disease and Death*. New York: Wiley.

Germain, C.B. (1984). *Social Work Practice in Health Care*. New York: Collier MacMillan.

Ginnott, H. (1958). Play group therapy: A theoretical framework. *Int. J. Group Psychother.* 8:160–66.

Gogan, J., G. Koocher, D. Foster, and J. O'Malley (1977). Impact of childhood cancer on siblings. *Health Social Work* 2:1–10.

Kagen, L. (1976). Use of denial in adolescents with bone cancer. *Health Social Work* 1:71–76.

Kagen-Goodheart, L. (1977). Re-entry: Living with childhood cancer. *Am. J. Orthopsychiatry* 47:651–56.

Koocher, G.P. (1979). Adjustment and coping strategies among the caretakers of cancer patients. *Soc. Work Health Care* 5:143–50.

Koocher, G. and J. O'Malley (1981). *The Damocles Syndrome*. New York: McGraw-Hill.

Kramer, R.F. (1984). Living with childhood cancer: Impact on the healthy siblings. *Oncol. Nurs. Forum* 11:44–51.

Lansky, S.B. (1978). One person—one vote. *Proc. Am. Cancer Soc. Second Ntl. Conf. on Human Values in Cancer*. New York: American Cancer Society, pp. 89–94.

Lansky, S.B., J.T. Lowman, T. Vats, and J.E. Gyulay (1975). School phobia in children with malignant neoplasm. *Am. J. Dis. Child.* 129:42–46.

Lindsay, M. and D. MacCarthy (1974). Caring for the brothers and sisters of a dying child. In L. Burton (ed.), *Care of the Child Facing Death*. Boston: Routledge & Kegan Paul.

Moynihan, R.T. and E. Outlaw (1984). Nursing support groups in a cancer center. *J. Psychosoc. Oncol.* 2:33–48.

Nasson, F. (1981). Team tension as a vital sign. *Gen. Hosp. Psychiatry* 3:32–36.

Peller, L. (1952). Models of children's play. *Ment. Hyg.* 36:66–83.

Petrillo, M. and S. Sanger (1972). *Emotional Care of Hospitalized Children*. Philadelphia: Lippincott.

Plumb, M. and J. Holland (1974). Cancer in adolescents: The symptom is the thing. In B. Schoenberg, A. Carr, A. Kutscher, D. Peretz, and D. Goldberg (eds.), *Anticipatory Grief*. New York: Columbia University Press.

Ross, J.W. (1979). Coping with childhood cancer group intervention as an aid to parents in crisis. *Soc. Work Health Care* 1:381–91.

Schaefer, D. (1983). Issues related to psychosocial intervention with Hispanic families in a pediatric cancer center. *J. Psychosoc. Oncol.* 1:39–46.

Schowalter, J. (1977). Psychological reactions to physical illness and hospitalization in adolescents. *J. Am. Acad. Child Psychiatry* 16:500–515.

Sourkes, B. (1981). Siblings of pediatric cancer patients. In J. Kellerman (ed.), *Psychological Impact of Childhood Cancer.* Springfield, Ill.: Charles C Thomas.

Spinetta, J. and F. Deasy-Spinetta (1981). *Living with Childhood Cancer.* St. Louis: C.V. Mosby.

Townes, B. and D. Wold (1977). Childhood leukemia. In E. Patterson (ed.), *The Experience of Dying.* Englewood Cliffs, N.J.: Prentice-Hall.

Wiener, J. (1970). Reactions of the family to the fatal illness of a child. In B. Schoenberg, A. Carr, D. Peretz, and A. Kutscher (eds.), *Loss and Grief: Psychological Management in Medical Practice.* New York: Columbia University Press.

Wiener, M.W., T. Caldwell, and J. Tyson (1983). Stresses and coping in ICU nursing: Why support groups fail. *Gen. Hosp. Psychiatry* 5:179–83.

# 46

# Behavioral Interventions to Reduce Child Distress

William Redd

The treatment of most childhood cancers is extremely aggressive and, for some children, more painful than the disease itself. Many treatment protocols require repeated infusions of highly emetic chemotherapeutic agents, bone marrow aspirations, lumbar punctures, and blood tests. Moreover, in most cases these procedures must be continued long after the child has ceased feeling ''sick'' or has any observable symptoms. Because of the anxiety and pain caused by such invasive treatment and many children's limited understanding of why treatment is protracted, young patients often become noncompliant and actively resist routine medical procedures. The child's distress often interacts with that of the parents and compounds the difficulties of delivering treatment.

Although pharmacological interventions to reduce pain and anxiety in pediatric cancer patients are available, many clinicians try to limit their use because of feared long-term neurological side effects. For this reason there is increased interest in the use of nonpharmacological behavioral methods for reducing distress. The major effort has been toward developing multifaceted interventions involving positive motivation (reinforcement), attentional distraction, emotive imagery, and hypnosis. These applications of behavioral theory represent a major advance in psychosocial oncology as well as a widening of the domain of behavioral medicine.

The purpose of this chapter is to examine the role of behavioral intervention in the treatment of children with cancer (see also Chapter 45). It begins with the identification of problems pediatric patients experience during the protracted course of treatment. Of major interest is how children's fear and distress reactions to specific procedures can develop into phobiclike patterns of behavior. Influences on the intensity of children's distress reactions are discussed, with emphasis on the role of parents. In describing the use of behav-

ioral techniques to reduce anxiety and distress during medical procedures, the discussion centers on specific behavioral procedures (i.e., positive motivation, attentional distraction, emotive imagery, and hypnosis) to reduce distress and increase patient compliance. A comprehensive behavior modification program to control pain and anxiety during bone marrow aspiration and lumbar puncture is presented. The chapter ends with a review of clinical issues that must be considered when applying behavioral procedures. Because the application of behavioral psychology in pediatric oncology is relatively new, much of what is presented here is based on extrapolation from other areas of clinical psychology. Due to this dearth of empirical research, the author must also draw on his experience as a clinical psychologist and behavioral consultant for the Department of Pediatrics at Memorial Sloan-Kettering Cancer Center (MSKCC).

## THE PAIN AND DISTRESS OF TREATMENT

Cancer treatment often causes more distress than the disease itself. Indeed, it is not uncommon for the physician to have to enlist the assistance of two or three nurses to restrain the patient during routine bone marrow aspiration. In a recent case of a 10-year-old autistic girl with osteogenic sarcoma, seven adults had to assist in order to complete a chemotherapy infusion. Koocher and Sallan (1978) aptly observed that ''patients are often uncertain as to whether the aggressor is the disease or the physician.'' Although older children generally show less distress than younger children and appear to have less anticipatory anxiety, patients do not habituate by becoming less distressed with repeated injections. In fact, in many instances the level of distress (as measured by patient self-report and behavioral observation of crying and behavioral resistance) increases with subsequent treatments. Children are often able to "bite the bullet" initially, but they gradually burn out during the long course of treatment. The anxiety that patients experience in anticipation of treatment is often associated with nausea, vomiting, skin rashes, and insomnia days before diagnostic and treatment procedures are scheduled. For some children the dread of treatment becomes severe and their reactions resemble phobias.

In the case of patients receiving chemotherapy, repeated infusions can lead to phobiclike conditioned aversion responses (Redd and Andrykowski, 1982) (see Chapter 35). After three or four infusions these patients begin feeling nauseated in anticipation of treatment. In some cases the patient begins vomiting before the chemotherapy drugs are even administered. These anticipatory side effects do not represent malingering or psychopathological responses. Rather, they are the direct result of respondent conditioning. Through repeated association of environmental stimuli (e.g., the sight of the clinic, sound of the nurse's voice, and the smell of rubbing alcohol) with treatment and its aftereffects, previously neutral environmental stimuli come to elicit symptoms (i.e., nausea and vomiting). For some patients the mere thought of chemotherapy makes them nauseated. Unfortunately, these symptoms do not extinguish or disappear readily; they can last for years. In follow-up interviews with individuals who were cured of leukemia or Hodgkin's disease as children, they often report that they still feel nauseated whenever they enter the hospital or smell rubbing alcohol (Cella and Tross, 1988). One of our Hodgkin's survivors said that he could still vividly recall the chemotherapy infusions he received 12 years earlier and that the thought of them still made him nauseated. A 30-year-old former patient reported an incident that occurred when she was sailing on the river alongside the hospital where she had been treated early in adolescence. She said that as soon as she noticed the entrance to the chemotherapy clinics she felt nauseated and began vomiting. Although the last two cases are textbook examples and do not represent a uniform pattern, they do demonstrate the powerful impact that treatment can have on patients' behavior and attitudes.

Four distinct patterns of treatment-related distress can be identified. The first is the pain and anxiety experienced during immediate treatment (e.g., the pain of the needle and the sensation of the aspiration). The second is the anxiety experienced in anticipation of treatment; this type of anxiety might be appropriately labeled extreme worry. The third pattern of distress is the conditioned anticipatory reaction seen in patients undergoing chemotherapy. These patients' anticipatory reactions are automatic, conditioned responses to treatment. The fourth pattern includes phobic reactions to needles and syringes that are occasionally seen in pediatric patients. Although similar in form to the anticipatory side effects seen in chemotherapy patients, phobic reactions are typically more pervasive and less related to automatic learning processes. Almost all pediatric patients experience the first form of distress (immediate distress of treatment), and many experience the other types as well.

As will be clear in the discussion that follows, different influences contribute to the development of each type of distress. Moreover, specific treatment methods are required depending on the particular combination of treatment distress the individual patient experiences. As will also become clear, a theoretical understanding of the principles underlying a particular behavioral problem and a thorough assessment of the patient's condition are crucial to effective intervention.

## INFLUENCES ON CHILDREN'S REACTIONS TO INVASIVE MEDICAL PROCEDURES

Children's emotional reactions to medical procedures vary widely; some children begin crying loudly as the nurse cleans the skin for routine blood tests, whereas others sit stoically. The influences that determine the nature and intensity of children's reactions are not well understood. Age of the child and invasiveness of the procedure are clearly relevant. Research has shown that the level of distress is 5–10 times greater in children younger than 7 years old (Jay et al., 1983). Not only are younger children generally poorer at impulse control (i.e., depending on the age of the pediatric patient, equivalent levels of aversive stimulation evoke different magnitudes of expressed distress); they may also fail to understand why the procedures are being done. The younger child often thinks that the doctor and nurse are punishing him or her for some wrong deed (Katz et al., 1980). Moreover, many children believe that they can die from the procedures (Jay et al., 1983; Spinetta and Maloney, 1975). These misattributions regarding the cause of illness and the effect of treatment appear to be related to the child's level of cognitive development. Research has shown that children's causal attributions regarding health and illness are consistent with predictions based on Piaget's theory of cognitive development (Perrin and Gerrity, 1981).

In the face of threat and uncertainty, the young child looks to his or her parents for emotional support and for guidance in understanding what is happening. The child is keenly aware of the parents' reactions and quickly responds to any signs of anxiety on the parents' part. Parental tone of voice, posture, and eye gaze are subtle but powerful cues for the child during stressful events (Bloom, 1975). If the parent is calm and relaxed, the child is more likely to believe that the situation is safe. If, on the other hand, the parent is clearly anxious and out of control, the child's anxiety is fueled. Research suggests that a complex feedback loop exists between the parent and child, with each being exquisitely sensitive to the other's emotional reaction (Bloom, 1977). Although in a particular instance one may not be able to identify which member of the dyad initiated the spiral, it is clear that both contribute to its escalation. This observation is supported by research in medical sociology (Mechanic, 1979), psychoanalytical theory (Freud, 1940), and cognitive development (Piaget, 1963, 1969). It has been shown that parents play an important role in modulating children's expressions of emotional distress. Jay and colleagues (1983) found that the presence of parents during invasive procedures (e.g., bone marrow aspiration) can actually make the child more agitated.

There are at least two distinct patterns of parental behavior that are correlated with high levels of child distress. The first pattern is extreme reactivity and appears to involve the parent's inability to suppress his or her own emotional distress and anxiety. Parents may begin to cry, become faint, or express apprehension regarding the skill of the clinician carrying out the procedure. Though clearly contrary to their intentions, such parents are not providing reassurance or giving the message that the procedure is not to be feared. Even if they are able to convey positive expectation verbally, their nonverbal behavior contradicts these attempts to comfort. Holding the shaking hand of a frightened parent does not calm the child or foster the belief that the parent will provide protection. Although the parent tells the child that there "isn't anything to worry about" and that "everything will be fine," the child probably doesn't believe it. Moreover, the parents' emotional behavior provides a clear message to the child that it is also acceptable for the child to lose control; indeed, such parents actually expect the child to lose control. In most instances the child behaves accordingly.

The second pattern of parental behavior associated with high levels of child distress in medical settings is more subtle. It involves the parents' providing "too much" support. In such instances the parents typically comply with every demand of the child and provide immediate physical comfort whenever the child complains. In an attempt to give emotional support, the parents are actually fueling the child's fears and concerns. That is, the child learns to cry and become upset in order to get what he or she wants. In such cases the parents fail to build on the child's own strengths. In fact, one might identify this parental style of interacting as an unintended, yet highly effective, means of encouraging regression. With such overly solicitous parents there is generally little ability to set limits or to encourage the child to try to control his or her fear. These parents often project the attitude that the child,

like themselves, is helpless in controlling his or her own behavior. It is interesting that older children often reject their parents' attitudes and, on occasion, have been observed to ask their parents to remain out of the room during painful procedures. They comment that their parents' behavior "makes it worse." In many instances they are correct.

Unfortunately, writers in this area have not provided discussion of the role parents play in cases in which the child does better during painful procedures than one would otherwise expect. While we have a fairly clear idea of how parents make the child worse, we really do not know how parents make the child better. Researchers have devised a set of behavioral procedures that can be used to reduce effectively child distress during invasive treatment (Jay et al., 1983; Katz et al., 1980). However, their research does not tell us whether parents of "good copers" employ behavior principles on their own, without explicit training. It is not known whether some parents actually interact with their children in a manner consistent with behavioral theory, but are not aware of it. As in other areas of child psychology, our understanding of how best to treat children's distress might be enhanced greatly by an examination of the behavior and attitudes of those patients and families who do well. These parents might be able to provide important recommendations. On theoretical and clinical grounds, despite the paucity of empirical studies, it seems likely that the helpful parent first conveys that there are no options. The procedure must be done. Second, he or she projects a sense of calm control over the situation and an expectation that the child will assume the same stance. Third, the parent acknowledges that the procedure will hurt, but that the level of pain has been managed by other children and the parent knows that the patient can take it and will be brave. Last, the parent expresses pride and pleasure in the child's performance, saying, for example, "I knew you could."

In conferences with parents during initial workups, the clinician might determine if the parent is likely to provide effective support and structure for the child. The parent who does not appear to be able to maintain such a posture and who is overly protective and anxious should be discouraged from being in attendance and reassured that it is quite acceptable for parents to sit and wait. As with any clinical intervention, a primary aim is to reduce parental guilt and to provide a means for them to be effectively involved.

## CONTROLLING DISTRESS AND INCREASING PATIENT COMPLIANCE

Behavioral interventions to alleviate distress during painful medical procedures and encourage compliance with treatment and rehabilitation generally involve a combination of positive motivation, attentional distraction, emotive imagery, and hypnosis. As was pointed out earlier, recommendations for their application in pediatric oncology are drawn from a number of sources outside pediatric medicine, the primary being childhood early education and child clinical psychology. Specific applications in pediatric oncology are relatively new and preliminary in scope.

## Positive Motivation

Perhaps the most widely used behavioral intervention method with children is positive motivation. The guiding principle is the law of effect initially proposed by Edward L. Thorndike in 1898 and subsequently refined by B.F. Skinner in 1938. According to this law, organisms (both human and infrahuman) behave in ways that increase pleasure and reduce pain; behavior that results in either an increase in positive (i.e., pleasurable) consequences or a reduction of aversive conditions will be strengthened. Those behaviors that reduce the positive and/or increase aversive consequences will diminish in frequency. The idea may sound familiar to most readers; it is the simple principle of carrot and stick (reward and punishment). However, its effective application can be complex. Behavioral psychologists have devised a set of procedures that increase the ease and effectiveness with which clinician, teacher, or parent can use rewards to encourage compliance and reduce patient distress.

The most important principle is positive reinforcement. Here the strategy is to motivate the child by presenting pleasurable consequences (and/or removing unpleasant ones) when the child behaves appropriately. The most obvious application with pediatric populations is praising desired behavior and providing tangible rewards. In clinical applications with pediatric dental and medical patients, stars and points redeemable for prizes and toy trinkets have been effectively used to increase cooperation during treatment and to encourage compliance with follow-up care.

A critical, and often overlooked, ingredient in any positive-motivation system concerns the value the child places on the rewards that are given. Tokens, points, and so on will be ineffective motivators if the child does not value them intrinsically or want the things they buy. It is here that the concept of individualized intervention that is central to behavioral psychology arises. If the motivation system is to be effective then it must be tailored to the child. The object, event, or "thing" used as a reward must be seen by the child as fun, interesting, or enjoyable; the child has to "want it" if it is to function as a motivator. For example, if the child is to be motivated to cooperate with a procedure by earning a trip to the movies or a

sailboat ride by being still and helping the nurse and doctor do their jobs, it is crucial that he or she likes the movie or enjoys sailing. It is interesting that one frequently encounters motivational programs in which this issue has been ignored. Stars and points are given lavishly, but are never redeemed; in such instances the "incentives" are worthless and ineffective. Unfortunately, this oversight is probably the worst mistake that could be made in the implementation of behavioral intervention.

Behavioral psychologists are quite unenthusiastic regarding the "other side of the motivation coin"— that is, punishment. Indeed, no word is more taboo in child psychology and behavior modification. Although little research has addressed this issue, most psychologists and behavioral clinicians contend that punishment produces undesirable emotional side effects (e.g., aggression) and is less effective than positive reinforcement. Rather than using punishment, they suggest that the clinician put heavy emphasis on strengthening those positive behaviors that are incompatible with the undesirable problem behaviors. For example, rather than reprimanding a child for failing to take his or her pill or eating junk food, the behavioral clinician recommends rewarding him or her for taking the daily medicine at regular intervals and providing tangible incentives for eating prescribed meals. The strategy is to establish a strong motivational system in which desirable behavior "replaces" (i.e., effectively competes with) the undesirable behavior. When behavioral technicians are forced to use some method of negative sanction, they generally suggest loss of privileges or some other mild negative consequence.

Positive-incentive programs can be used to encourage patient compliance as well as to motivate the patient to practice the technique that will help control pain and distress. In our work at MSKCC, we often give points exchangeable for special treats and privileges to motivate young patients to cooperate with unpleasant treatment procedures. One example is a 6-year-old boy who kicked and cried during routine mouth care; he was so disruptive that three nurses were required to complete the daily procedure. A simple contingency system was initiated in which, if he did not kick or hit the nurses during mouth care and was generally cooperative, his mother would read him a favorite story. If he actively resisted, two more nurses would be called and he would miss the storybook time with his mother. After 3 days of behavioral intervention his resistance to mouth care was no longer a problem, and he was cooperative and proud of his accomplishment. Similar positive-incentive programs have been used with pediatric patients to increase compliance with radiation treatment (i.e., special privileges given for holding still) and routine blood tests.

## Attentional Distraction

The role of anxiety and physiological arousal in pain and somatic symptom perception has been well documented, and clinical research with adults has repeatedly demonstrated that anxiety reduction results in a decrease in pain intensity. Moreover, research with adult cancer patients has shown that patients can be trained in specific relaxation techniques to control their own anxiety and thereby reduce pain and distress during invasive medical procedures (Redd et al., 1982; Reeves et al., 1983). Although it appears clear that anxiety plays equally important roles with adults and children, the relaxation techniques used with adults are, for the most part, inapplicable with children. The problem is that young children simply cannot sit still, focus their attention on states of muscle relaxation, and go through the muscle exercises that are required.

A more effective strategy has been to distract the child's attention. Through storytelling, fantasy play, and active involvement in an intellectual task (e.g., games) during painful procedures, the child's attention is diverted toward positive activities. Once the child is "cognitively" engaged, the clinician or therapist can complete the procedure. These strategies are quite similar to hypnosis and rely on the child's ability to engage in fantasy. Central to this process is the therapist's skill at engaging the child. Fortunately, the therapist's task can be relatively easy, as children are generally less reality-bound and more open to fantasy than adults.

Techniques involving fantasy and attentional distraction are often used to reduce the pain of invasive procedures and the nausea and vomiting associated with chemotherapy. Our behavioral research team at MSKCC is now investigating the use of distraction via videogames to control anticipatory nausea and anxiety in children receiving chemotherapy. Intervention is really quite simple; it involves children playing videogames during infusions. The goal is to present the child with games of sufficient difficulty to challenge and to require full attention to the visual display. The notion is that the more involved the child is in the game, the less aware he or she will be of the infusion and of the sensations of nausea. This strategy has been effective also in controlling anticipatory nausea and anxiety in children prior to initiation of the chemotherapy infusion. Children's ratings of nausea are at least 50% lower when they are playing the games than when they are passively sitting and focusing on the intravenous infusion.

## Emotive Imagery

In cases of extreme, phobiclike anxiety, a more structured desensitization intervention is often required. The most popular is emotive imagery. Similar to distraction and hypnosis, it takes advantage of the child's openness to fantasy. The therapist begins working with the child in his or her office, away from the medical treatment area. After establishing a rapport with the child, the therapist determines the child's favorite storybook hero and the things the child likes to do. The therapist then tells the child a series of stories involving the child and his or her hero. Each subsequent story brings the child closer to the feared setting, while the hero helps the child master the situation. This procedure is similar to systematic-desensitization procedures used to treat phobias in adults. The rationale is that if strong anxiety-inhibiting emotive images are elicited in the context of feared stimuli, the anxiety reaction to those stimuli will be reduced. By being told a story that involves favorite storybook heroes interacting with the phobic stimulus, the child comes to associate these stimuli with positive feelings of self-assertion, pride, and affection. As the therapist relates the story, the feared stimuli are introduced in a hierarchical fashion, from least to most distressing.

The following description shows how emotive imagery can be used to reduce a young child's fear of needles. In such cases the patient is usually referred because his or her level of agitation and resistance has increased with repeated treatments. At the time of referral this 7-year-old boy's level of noncompliance was high; when his name was called for chemotherapy his father would literally have to carry him into the treatment room. He would often hide behind a chair and begin kicking when anyone came near. In other situations the child was quite pleasant and cooperative; he was well liked by staff and fellow patients.

The therapist began by asking the patient to describe what treatment was like and to try to explain what frightened him. Although many young patients find it difficult to identify the problem, they often state that they wish it wasn't so scary and that they could be braver. The therapist then explained that she wanted to teach him how to get his mind off the needle and how to learn how to keep calm. She also explained to the patient that she would be telling a story and that the child could help by filling in missing parts. She then asked the patient to close his eyes and she began:

David, you know about Batman and Robin, right? You know that they have special powers and can help children do lots of things. They can help us be strong and brave and they can even help take away pain. Let me tell you one way they do this. On one of their trips to a faraway planet they found a special invisible glove. It was in a box with other treasures from long ago. Beside the glove was a note. It told them about the glove's special powers. The glove would protect them whenever they wore it. To test it out Batman put it on and was able to lift the Batmobile with one hand. One day

Robin was going to the doctor and asked Batman if he could use it. Batman knew how much Robin hated going to the doctor's: He doesn't like getting shots. So Batman gave it to Robin and Robin wore it proudly. As Robin got ready to go into the doctor's office he felt scared, but remembered that he had the magic invisible glove for protection. He went into the office for his shot, put out his arm, and, to his great surprise, he didn't feel a thing. It was magic. Robin was so happy. Would you like to try on the glove? Oh, good. Hold out your hand and let me help you put it on. How does it feel? Does it fit? Pull it up high, all the way to your shoulder. Good. Let's go into the treatment room and try on the glove there. It will be fun, okay? Good . . . .

If the child displays any anxiety, the therapist slows the story and approaches the feared object (task) less directly. Throughout the intervention the therapist is careful to be sensitive to the child's emotional reaction and is ready to pace the story according to the child's needs.

In a case reported by Diener (1984) involving a 7-year-old boy who was afraid of needles, the child was quite excited about the possibility of using the imaginary glove and complied with the therapist's instructions. During subsequent treatments the child's parents learned how to help and the therapist reduced her involvement. As the patient's mother stated, "It was amazing. David put on the magic glove and went through chemotherapy without any problem." His mother also recounted an interesting incident. One day David and his parents were waiting to see the doctor when they noticed another child crying and fighting, obviously afraid of the treatment he was about to receive. David leaned over and whispered to his mother "Mom, should I lend him my magic glove? Of course, he'll have to give it back so I can use it later."

Arnold Lazarus, the originator of emotive imagery, reported a case of an 8-year-old boy who was afraid of the dentist and showed reactions quite similar to those observed in pediatric oncology patients undergoing painful medical procedures (Lazarus and Abramowitz, 1962). Using Batman and Robin as heroes, the therapist asked the child first to imagine his heroes visiting the dentist while he watched them. As the therapist elaborated the story, he asked the child to imagine himself in the dentist's chair as Batman and Robin stood beside, watching. After engaging in such fantasies daily for 1 week, the child was able to visit the dentist's office without resisting.

Our clinical experience is that emotive imagery can help reduce anxiety in pediatric oncology patients. However, it is important to point out that such desensitization is best used with fears that are irrational and not directly linked to aversive treatment (e.g., fears of the dark and being alone). In the case of fears of procedures that actually cause significant pain (e.g., bone marrow aspiration), one would not expect emotive imagery used alone to be effective. The problem is that, after the child was desensitized, he or she would again experience the pain and aversive stimulation caused by the procedure and his or her fear would return. That is, the child would be reconditioned. Rather than using a desensitization procedure such as emotive imagery, one would be advised to use relaxation and distraction techniques. That is, rather than trying to remove the fear and later having it reestablished, the therapist should block the patient's perception of the pain during the actual treatment. Such a strategy would help reduce the subjective adversiveness of treatment as well as foster the reduction of anticipatory anxiety.

## Hypnosis

Although the use of hypnosis to relieve acute pain has a long history, many practicing clinicians and most laypersons do not understand it. Many actually fear it. This is quite unfortunate because research has demonstrated the effectiveness of hypnosis with particular pediatric patients (Hilgard and LeBaron, 1984; Zelter et al., 1984). Hypnosis involves a relatively simple dissociation process in which the patient learns to focus his or her attention on stimuli, images, and/or thoughts that are unrelated to the source of pain. Hilgard and LeBaron (1984) have coined the term "imaginative involvement" to refer to the process by which the individual becomes "hypnotized." They maintain that this process involves the individual in becoming cognitively engaged in a task such that other stimuli are blocked or reduced in intensity. This dissociation is common in everyday life, for example, reading a good book and being unaware of what's happening around you, or playing a game of tennis and not being aware of a cut finger until after the match is over. In clinical settings, hypnosis requires the therapist to gain the patient's cooperation and then direct the patient's attention to images that are distinct from those associated with the treatment setting. As with other procedures, the aim is to distract the patient. Although all individuals are capable of this type of cognitive dissociation, some individuals are more skilled than others. Various scales of hypnotizability have been developed to assess this capability. The essential characteristic appears to be an ability to engage in fantasy; individuals who score high on hypnotizability scales also report being able to become deeply involved in reading, dreams, and in the aesthetic appreciation of nature. Research has shown that children are as a group more hypnotizable than adults (Hilgard and LeBaron, 1984). They appear to be less reality-bound and easily become absorbed in fantasy.

## COMPREHENSIVE BEHAVIOR MODIFICATION

Jay and colleagues (1982) have devised a comprehensive behavioral intervention for children undergoing painful cancer treatment. This "package," as Jay has called it, integrates the techniques outlined earlier as well as pain and anxiety reduction procedures devised for pediatric dental patients. The reason for offering a multifaceted program is to ensure that the program is maximally flexible and is able to meet the particular needs of each child. With individual children, emphasis can be placed on particular components, or the components can be adjusted to permit better tailoring of the intervention to the child's individual needs. Treatment components include breathing exercises, reinforcement, imagery, behavioral rehearsal, and filmed modeling. Although a large-scale evaluation of the package has not been conducted, preliminary work with individual cases confirmed the utility of comprehensive behavioral intervention.

Although the actual intervention is carried out during regularly scheduled medical procedures, the therapist or nurse meets with the patient and his or her parent during specially scheduled training sessions. The intervention represents a combination of patient education and direct behavioral treatment.

### Breathing Exercises

In order to help reduce physiological arousal (i.e., anxiety) and to facilitate attentional distraction, deep-breathing exercises are taught during training sessions and then carried out during scheduled treatments. The child might be asked to imagine blowing up a plastic bubble, taking deep breaths and then slowly letting the air out. The therapist might explicitly pace the child's breathing by counting and squeezing the child's hand in rhythm with slow breathing. If the child shows signs of "losing it," the therapist might tell the child to "Keep it up. Slow, easy, soft breathing." "You can do it, slow. Easy, . . . one, two, . . . slow, . . . three . . ." In many ways the therapist functions as a coach. Here the therapist uses all of his or her clinical skill; the therapist must be sensitive to subtle signs of mounting anxiety in the child and, at the same time, be able to engage the child and maintain the child's attention.

### Reinforcement

Before each treatment the child and therapist decide on a toy or prize that the child will "work for." Jay gives the patient a trophy for doing well. To obtain the trophy the child's job is to lie still and do the breathing exercises. We use coloring books, small puzzles, and special outings with parents as rewards. We try to individualize the reinforcement system as much as possible. It is important to point out that the criterion for winning is not mastery of the procedure without crying or getting upset; rather, cooperation and using the skills that have been taught are all that is required. It is our experience that setting standards at realistic levels often helps "turn things around for the child." By earning the prize the child starts to identify himself or herself with winning, with being brave and strong. It also helps the child approach the next treatment with a more positive expectation. It is also our experience that most children want to do well and are ashamed when they resist or fight. By offering techniques that help the child tolerate procedures, the therapist provides a structure that makes treatment less aversive and helps the child feel better about himself or herself.

### Imagery

To help distract the child's attention, the therapist uses emotive imagery during separate training sessions as well as during scheduled treatments. The following quotation is taken from a case report provided by Jay and colleagues involving a young girl undergoing bone marrow aspiration.

Pretend that Wonderwoman has come to your house and told you that she wants you to be the newest member of her Superpower Team. Wonderwoman has given you special powers. These special powers make you very strong and tough so that you can stand almost anything. She asks you to take some tests to try out these superpowers. The tests are called bone marrow aspirations and spinal taps. These tests hurt, but with your new superpowers, you can take deep breaths and lie very still. Wonderwoman will be very proud when she finds out that your superpowers work and you will be the newest member of her Superpower Team.

During the medical procedure, children were reminded of the imagery scenario which had been developed and were coached to use the imagery (e.g., "Remember Wonderwoman—what would she do right now?"). The emotive images presumably transform the meaning of the pain for the child and elicit motivations related to mastery over pain rather than avoidance. (Jay et al., 1982, pp. 9–10)

### Behavioral Rehearsal

In order to teach the child how to cooperate and to reduce anxiety due to fear of the unknown, the patient is taken through all phases of the procedure during the training sessions. During these practice sessions the child assumes each role, namely, playing the doctor, nurse, and patient. The child carries out with a doll each aspect of the medical treatment that the oncologist uses during treatment. The child also practices giving proper instructions, breathing exercises, and emotive imagery material. Finally, the child takes on the role as patient and is coached to lie still and complete breathing exercises.

## Filmed Modeling

Jay has made two films to help train a patient in the completion of bone marrow aspiration (one for children under 8 years of age, the other for children over 8). In these films a child of approximately the same age as a patient viewing the film narrates scenes showing him going through the procedure. The patient describes his anxieties and concerns as the nurse prepares him. He also explains how he copes. The child's description is realistic; he readily admits that he is afraid and that it is not easy. In her accounts of the behavioral intervention she and her colleagues have devised, Jay has stressed that the film is based on a "coping" rather than a mastery model. That is, the film facilitates the child's identifying with the model and is more effective in reducing anxiety. Although the child depicted in the film is successful and cooperates without resistance, his anxiety is acknowledged and his hardiness is reinforced.

## CLINICAL ISSUES

Behavioral intervention in pediatric oncology is typically offered as an adjunct to more traditional methods of psychosocial intervention. Indeed, at Memorial Sloan-Kettering children who are seen because of behavioral problems are also followed throughout their treatment by a clinical social worker, and their parents frequently attend parent group meetings. During the course of behavioral intervention, it is also often the case that the behavioral clinician addresses nonbehavioral issues. Patients typically want to discuss emotional/existential concerns with the clinician because he or she (the patient) has learned to trust that person. Some writers have even argued that behavioral intervention is one of the most effective ways of building rapport and that it serves to facilitate work in other areas. Behavioral intervention is straightforward and does not question more sensitive issues (that the patient and his or her family might wish to keep private). Thus, the patient/family is able to get to know the clinician in a nonthreatening context. Other issues naturally arise and the patient is free to pursue them as he or she wishes.

Behavioral intervention is directed by three general guidelines. The first is a detailed, on-going assessment. Before beginning behavioral intervention, it is important that the clinician determine the strengths and weaknesses (the assets and deficits) that the child

brings to treatment. The clinician must first know "where the child is": What is the child capable of doing? It is also important to determine at the outset the factors that contribute to the behavioral problems. Although this may be difficult and the clinician can never be sure that the assessment is complete, it is essential that the clinician understand the context in which the problem occurs. Questions the clinician might ask include: Does the child have difficulties in other areas of life? If so, what are they? When did the problems first occur and in what situation? The goal is to determine the factors that might be changed in order of alleviate the problem. This assessment and careful monitoring of the child's behavior continues throughout treatment. In essence, this assessment is the clinician's primary source of feedback as to how the intervention is affecting the child's behavior.

Central to behavioral assessment is clinical sensitivity. This is when behavioral intervention resembles "art." The clinician must be sensitive to subtle changes in the patient's behavior in order to ascertain whether the patient understands, agrees, and is affected by what is being done. For example, when using imagery, distraction, and relaxation procedures, it is crucial that the clinician be aware of the patient's level of anxiety. This information allows the clinician to pace his or her work appropriately and to provide appropriate supports and prompts. In the role of coach, the skilled clinician must be exquisitely sensitive to nonverbal cues from the patient. It is important that the clinician is able to perceive subtle signs of anxiety in the patient's facial expression, voice, and posture. When trying to control a child's distress during a painful procedure, the therapist uses such cues to know how to pace the patient's breathing, how quickly to present distracting imagery, and whether to change to another vehicle of distraction. In this regard it is important to note that, although much has been written about patients' relative hypnotizability and it is true that highly hypnotizable patients are easier to work with, a skilled clinician can help even the more reality-bound, difficult to hypnotize patients. Although it may be difficult and require additional time and patience, it is not impossible. Indeed, the clinician should look on such a patient as a challenge.

A second guideline is that intervention relies on the use of positive motivation and incentives, and is designed so that progress is associated with success rather than failure and frustration. In all cases intervention proceeds through small steps. The change from one step to another is, in the ideal instance, not even perceived by the patient. The clinician begins at the patient's baseline level to help assure success. Subsequent steps build on former steps. Prompts, aids, and gentle directions are used so that the child can successfully complete each new task. As the child becomes more skilled, the therapist increases the difficulty of the task so that the child is "stretched" but not frustrated. In all instances the therapist makes lavish use of praise, positive attention, and support.

The third rule of behavioral intervention is that its effectiveness is evaluated in terms of immediate behavior change in the child. If the intervention is appropriate and of real value, then it should have an immediate positive impact on the child's behavior. For example, if a procedure is intended to reduce patient distress, then one would expect the child's anxiety, pain, and discomfort to diminish as soon as the intervention is implemented. If an intervention is designed to control nausea and vomiting, then there should be an immediate reduction in both. In all cases criteria are clear and straightforward.

For many working in the area of psychosocial oncology, this standard represents a welcome change from more traditional psychological and psychiatric practice in which the impact of treatment is measured in subtle changes in attitudes, often over days or weeks. In this regard, the objective criteria of treatment efficacy used by behavioral clinicians is similar to that used in clinical medicine.

## SUMMARY

Behavioral intervention is a critical component to comprehensive psychosocial care of pediatric cancer patients. Although it does not presume to address all, or even the majority, of psychosocial problems facing the young cancer patient and his or her family, it does help control the severe pain, anxiety, and nausea associated with cancer and its treatment. Perhaps because its impact is immediate and often profound, those interested in providing such services can expect to be welcomed by medical staff, patients, and their families.

## REFERENCES

Bloom, K. (1975). Social elicitation of infant vocal behavior. *J. Exp. Child Psychol.* 20:51–58.

Bloom, K. (1977). Patterning of infant vocal behavior. *J. Exp. Child Psychol.* 23:367–77.

Cella, D.F. and S. Tross (1988). Psychological adjustment to survival from Hodgkin's disease. *J. Consult. Clin. Psychol.* In press.

Diener, C. (1984). *Controlling the Behavioral Side Effects of Cancer Treatment.* Urbana, Ill.: Norman Baxley & Assoc.

Freud, S. (1940). *An Outline of Psychoanalysis.* New York: Norton.

Hilgard, J.R. and S. LeBaron (1984). *Hypnotherapy of Pain in Children with Cancer.* Los Altos, Calif.: William Kaufmann.

Jay, S.M., C.H. Elliott, M. Ozolins, and R.A. Olson (1982). *Behavioral Management of Children's Distress during Painful Medical Procedures.* Paper presented at the American Psychological Association Convention, Washington, D.C., August.

Jay, S.M., M. Ozolins, C. Elliot, and S. Caldwell (1983). Assessment of children's distress during painful medical procedures. *Health Psychol.* 2:133–47.

Katz, E.R., H. Kellerman, and S.E. Siegel (1980). Behavioral distress in children with cancer undergoing medical procedures: Developmental considerations. *J. Consult. Clin. Psychol.* 43:356–65.

Koocher, G.P. and S.E. Sallan (1978). Pediatric oncology. In P. Magrab (ed.), *Psychological Management of Pediatric Problems,* Vol. 1. Baltimore: University Park Press, pp. 283–307.

Lazarus, A.A. and A. Abramowitz (1962). The use of "emotive imagery" in the treatment of children's phobias. *J. Ment. Sci.* 108:191–95.

Mechanic, D.K. (1979). Development of psychological distress among young adults. *Arch. Gen. Psychiatry* 36:1233–39.

Perrin, E. and S. Gerrity (1981). There's a demon in your belly: Children's understanding of illness. *Pediatrics* 67:841–49.

Piaget, J. (1963). *The Origins of Intelligence in Children.* New York: Norton.

Piaget, J. (1969). *The Psychology of the Child.* New York: Basic Books.

Redd, W.H., G.V. Andresen, and K.Y. Minagawa (1982). Control of anticipatory nausea in patients undergoing cancer chemotherapy. *J. Consult. Clin. Psychol.* 50:14–19.

Redd, W.H. and M.A. Andrykowski (1982). Behavioral intervention in cancer treatment: Controlling aversion reactions to chemotherapy. *J. Consult. Clin. Psychol.* 50:1018–29.

Reeves, J.L., W.H. Redd, F.K. Storm, and R.Y. Minagawa (1983). Hypnosis in the control of pain during hyperthermia treatment of cancer. In J.J. Bonica, V. Lindbland, and A. Iggo (eds.), *Advances in Pain Research and Therapy.* New York: Raven Press, pp. 857–61.

Skinner, B.F. (1938). *The Behavior of Organisms.* New York: Appleton-Century-Crofts.

Spinetta, J.J. and J. Maloney (1975). Death anxiety in the outpatient leukemic child. *Pediatrics* 56:1034–37.

Thorndike, E.L. (1898). Animal intelligence: An experimental study of the associative processes in animals. *Psychol. Rev.* 2:28–31.

Zelter, L., S. LeBaron, and P.M. Zelter (1984). The effectiveness of behavioral intervention for reduction of nausea and vomiting in children and adolescents receiving chemotherapy. *J. Clin. Oncol.* 2:683–90.

# PART IX

## Family Adaptation

# 47

## The Family of the Cancer Patient

Douglas Rait and Marguerite Lederberg

The importance of close loving relationships to every person's well-being is a truism that may be overlooked, just because it is so universal. The interdependence of family members in both health and disease, until the recent burst of interest in family process and family therapy, was possibly such an unexamined assumption. It was simply taken for granted that the family would be available as an extended agent of patient care. And indeed the family has performed remarkably well, and continues to do so, even as the increasing complexity of medical care has made the demands more onerous.

During the last two decades, in ways that not surprisingly parallel the development of psychooncology, it has become obvious that this view is simplistic and incomplete. Attention has been drawn to the family members, who are deeply and painfully affected by severe illness in one of their members. In effect, they must be viewed as second-order patients in their own right.

A still later development, one that is very new in its applications to psychooncology, addresses the family itself as a dynamic organism and studies the ways in which illness in a member alters and is altered by family process.

This chapter will address these three aspects of family involvement, reviewing some of the available literature and synthesizing it with a view to developing a comprehensive approach to family evaluation and intervention.

## THE FAMILY AS A PROVIDER OF PATIENT CARE

The period spanning the middle of the twentieth century during which patients in Western cultures have been routinely cared for in hospitals may turn out to be a brief aberration in social and medical history. Before this time, patients were cared for at home. Today, currents of social change are conspiring to remove them from the hospital and return them to their home again. Outside the Western world, they had never left their homes.

The ways in which the family cares directly for the patient can be roughly divided into five categories, as described in the following paragraphs.

### Provision of Emotional Support

Providing emotional support is the most abstract, yet the most immediate and compelling of the family's roles. Although family members themselves may be shattered by the diagnosis of cancer in a loved one, they are expected by others—medical staff especially—and by themselves to be able to contain their feelings and function supportively toward the patient.

There are many assumptions about cancer's effect on the family. One is that cancer brings families together, another that it promotes stress and distance. The reality seems more complex and elusive. Kaplan, Grobstein, and Smith (1976) described an increased incidence of divorce in families of leukemic children; experienced workers in the field have all seen marriages flounder during the course of a child's illness, yet Lansky and colleagues (1978) were not able to document these findings.

Tebbi and co-workers (1985) queried adolescents about their best source of support. In descending order they named mothers, fathers, medical staff, and siblings. The peer group, that vaunted source of adolescent intimacy and support, was viewed as distant and disappointing. Yet one does see previously alienated adolescents whose family distance is even increased during their illness and who endure their cancer essentially alone.

There are marked cultural differences in the ways in

which support is mediated. Copeland, Silberberg, and Pfefferbaum (1983) observed that Hispanics expected and desired more family involvement than non-Hispanics when cancer was being discussed. Lons and Lois (1982) observed that Japanese families do not discuss a diagnosis of cancer or a poor prognosis even when death is imminent, but manifest their feeling by "immersing themselves in proper role behavior."

## Shared Responsibility for Decision-Making

It has been noted that a diagnosis of cancer makes immediate complex decision-making demands on the patient at a time when he or she is perhaps least able to meet them. Family members routinely step into this breach, providing tireless involvement and often performing the lion's share of the work needed to explore, learn, and evaluate a sea of new and difficult information. Often a patient gratefully abdicates the decision-making role altogether. Occasionally there is overt conflict, creating a delicate and difficult situation for medical staff. It has been repeatedly observed that family members are not just willing but have a deep need to receive information and share in the decision-making. Derdiarian (1986) found a great deal of invariance and universality in families' informational needs, suggesting that these needs could be more routinely met. Chesler and Barbarin (1984) have observed that one of the most crucial elements of family satisfaction with medical treatment is their sense of involvement in the decision-making; another is the sense of caring and respect on the part of the staff.

## Concrete Care-Taking

Even in the days when women stayed in the home and presented an available pool of caretakers, the demands of nursing a sick patient could be quite disruptive to the household. Today several trends make the situation even more difficult.

First, that female supply of free nursing care no longer exists because a rapidly increasing number of women are in the labor force making key contributions to the family income.

Second, sicker patients are living longer with increasingly complex medical regimens. It is possible for the family of today's cancer patients to be administering tube feedings, multiple regimens of oral, intramuscular, subcutaneous, and even intrathecal medication (Smith, 1986). Increasing numbers of patients go home with intravenous lines in place receiving antibiotics and chemotherapy (Butler, 1984). Some AIDS patients have been receiving maintenance DHPG and other experimental drugs, under the new rules allowing their use in special cases. Long-term home parent-

eral nutrition (HPN) is now frequent enough that Perl (1987) has described the special problems that families encounter with it.

Finally, political and social trends are throwing a growing part of the burden back onto the family, in a backlash against the increase in medical care costs. Faced with necessity and driven by love and/or obligation, families strive to meet the need, but the human costs are enormous.

## Financial and Social Costs

Murinen (1986) has found that 25% of primary caretakers gave up or lost their job. This increased with age, was more frequent and permanent in women, and was most often observed in families with lower income—namely, those that could afford it the least. Of the remainder of caretakers, 60% registered a significant loss in income due to absenteeism or a shift to lesser paid work. The author concluded that the financial savings associated with home care are not really a savings at all but represent a shift from the formal medical sector to the informal one, that is, from third-party payers to individual families. Lansky and colleagues (1979), Bodkin, Pisott, and Mann (1982), and Bloom, Knorr, and Evans (1985) all document the staggering financial burden on families, even where medical expenses are largely paid for, as in Great Britain.

However, no one has quantified the lifetime losses associated with permanent career disruption and overall loss of social mobility, a burden that may in fact be comparable to that described for some surviving patients. McCubbin and Figley (1983b) discuss the issue, and McKeever (1983) reviews it and extends it to siblings.

## Maintenance of Stability in the Midst of Change

Throughout all of these vicissitudes, the family must somehow endure. It must maintain itself in many ways and at many different levels. The tasks include filling in for the lost role and contribution of the sick member, coping with the demands, losses, and drains described earlier, meeting the increased emotional needs generated in all members by the crisis, and finally, continuing to perform the multitudinous functions (feeding, education, nurture, financial maintenance, etc.) for which it was previously responsible. Although these tasks cannot be called direct patient care, they are nevertheless essential to patient well-being. Stam, Bultz, and Pittman (1986) have found that many patients stated that their concern about the burden of illness on their families was even greater than their concern about themselves. Therefore, they benefit directly if the family maintains its integrity and self-sufficiency, and may be willing to undergo considerable personal sacrifice to this end. Lonely hospitalized patients may say that they have refused to let family members visit, so as to spare them fatigue or disruption.

Paradoxically, the maintenance of stability requires a capacity for change because the tasks just-mentioned require major adaptation. In fact, it has been said that change is the family's only constant, because the natural course of cancer presents both patient and family with continually changing demands.

The needs of the diagnostic period are different from those of ongoing treatment. Remission, relapse, deterioration, and long-term survival all present the family with special requirements for patient care and support. Hospitalization versus home care presents a particularly important distinction. Different types of cancer create very different emotional climates; compare the "roller coaster" course of acute leukemia with the slow progression of some colon or lung cancers. Brain tumors make unique demands on family members, with the poignant loss of self that precedes physical deterioration. In reviewing the impact of cancer on the family, Northouse (1984) divided the subject according to three major phases: initial, adaptive, and terminal. The current state of the art would require adding survivorship as a fourth major phase. Perhaps a more flexible and accurate terminology would be acute, chronic, and resolution states.

## FAMILY MEMBERS AS SECOND-ORDER PATIENTS

There is a large body of literature on the emotional stresses and psychopathology generated in families of severely ill patients in general, and a smaller one on cancer patients in particular.

Some authors address the psychological state of all family members. Other authors have focused on special relationships such as spouses, parents, children, and siblings of patients. The bulk of the work focuses on (1) the families of pediatric cancer patients, because the central role of the family has always been obvious in pediatrics, and (2) the problems of bereavement, because death creates a well-defined crisis around which to organize observations. However, many issues overlap. Family dynamics are found to extend across the life cycle, and the understanding of bereavement has inevitably required an examination of pre-bereavement processes. Therefore, one can cautiously expand some of the observations to families of older patients and to the prebereavement period.

## Stresses on the Family as a Whole

Anthony (1969) and Litman (1974), among others, wrote detailed, thoughtful reviews that introduced many of the family process issues that have been developed by later workers. There is a current emphasis on viewing the family not merely as reacting to stress, but also as actively adapting to it (McCubbin and Figley, 1983a; Minuchin and Minuchin, 1987). We can characterize the family's adaptation to stress as occurring in three phases.

### ACUTE PHASE

As documented by Schuler and colleagues (1985), Koocher (1986a,b), and Spinetta (1984a,b), among others, the diagnosis of cancer in a family member presents the whole family with a frightening crisis to which all members react in their characteristic ways. These are variable, and may be more or less compatible with each other and with the needs of the moment. Some family members may be even more acutely distressed than the patient. However, this is also a time of rallying and mobilization. There is much willingness to give active help and support including that from extended family and friends. The availability of accurate information at this time is critical in helping the family move from an affective to an effective response (Sargent, 1985).

In trying to protect themselves and the patient, many families reduce the communication process and create a "conspiracy of silence," which has well-documented and far-reaching negative effects on family relationships and individual well-being (Bluebond-Langner, 1978). This process manifests itself early in the course and may crystallize permanently if it is not addressed directly.

The mechanisms of the "acute" period also extend to initial treatment, relapse, and unexpected complications.

### CHRONIC PHASE

Different mechanisms characterize "chronic" or consolidation periods such as return to the home, lengthy courses of treatment, lengthy hospitalizations, and periods of remission. During consolidation times, the family must juggle the needs of the patient with the needs of other family members and must focus on resumption of normal developmental tasks for all. This is difficult to achieve. Different family members may disagree on goals and process; for example, a primary caretaker may remain overly protective while other family members want the patient to move along. As more time passes, an increasing number of family members may experience and may manifest their anger, jealousy, and neediness, leading to a paradoxical increase in psychological symptoms during these periods. This is worsened by the often decreased support of the extended family, friends, and co-workers, which parallels the emotional process described in the family. Thus the family finds itself more isolated at a time when it most needs help. It has been noted that it may further isolate itself for reasons related to shame, fear, anger, and depression in its members. Hinds (1985) found that only a third of families actually made use of available community supports about which they knew, even at a time when they felt a great need for them.

During this time, the family tends to remain in a holding pattern, to be illness-oriented despite itself, to delay major decisions, and to cope on a day-to-day basis—often at the expense of long-term developmental tasks (Sourkes, 1977). Sometimes this is a direct reaction to ongoing stress, but sometimes it is a "habit"—a resetting of family homeostasis that was changed during a dramatic period and now remains at the new setting. The stressfulness of the ongoing experience is borne out by finding a positive correlation between length and severity of illness and several measures of dysfunction in family members (Cancer Care, Inc. and National Cancer Foundation, 1977; Koocher and O'Malley, 1981). However, it is important to point out that dysfunction is not inevitable and that some families respond adaptively with new roles and new goals that maximize opportunities for all members in the new era.

## RESOLUTION

The bereavement and survivor experiences of the family are covered in Chapters 47 and 50.

The term synchrony has been used to address the issue of the "timeliness" of fatal illness. A family can better tolerate cancer in a grandparent than in a child because it is more "synchronous" with family developmental expectations. This apparently extends to the patient, because Ganz, Schas, and Heinrich (1985) found that older patients were less distressed than younger ones. This, however, refers to emotional response. The loss of a child is the most tragic, but in terms of actual disruption among family members the loss of a generative and nurturing adult member is probably the most disruptive.

### Spouses of Cancer Patients

Spouses are deeply involved and live through the patient's experience vicariously with great intensity. They also play a major role in patient adjustment. It is not unusual to see a sicker patient feeling better because of an upswing in the marital relationship. In

studies of spouses of mastectomy patients (Sabo et al., 1986), men were found to be deeply emotionally engaged but hiding it, and playing a protective, reassuring, minimizing role. They assumed this was the most supportive role, but their wives interpreted it as rejecting and insensitive. It led routinely to increased distance and mistrust in the relationship. This type of interaction is found with many other diagnoses.

Increased involvement of spouses in decision making leads to better adjustment of both patient and spouse (Wellisch et al., 1978; Hinton, 1981). There are contradictory findings about overall marital adjustment and response, but these may be due to the studies' focus on small, highly disparate patient groups across a broad time period. Retroactively, a group of widows of cancer patients described feeling more upset and more helpless about their husbands' death from cancer than did the group of widows of cardiovascular patients (Vachon et al., 1977). Helplessness is a theme that recurs frequently in the vocabulary of cancer families.

### Parents of Cancer Patients

The anguish of parents losing a child to cancer and the impact of parental coping on the child patient are well known and well described (Adams, 1978; Farrell and Hutter, 1984; Koocher, 1986a,b; Lansky et al., 1978; Spinetta, 1981; see also Chapter 50 in this volume). The early studies of the Sutherland group at Memorial Sloan-Kettering Cancer Center (Bozeman et al., 1955) and the 1963 study of parents of leukemic children by Friedman and colleagues still make for instructive reading. There are contradictory findings about the severity of the overall impact on marital stability and other measures of parental functioning such as the incidence of psychiatric syndromes, alcohol and drug use, somatic disorders, and work problems. Some of these may be explained by methodology and patient selection issues. Others relate to stage-of-disease issues. For example, marital stability is strained during the acute phase, consolidated during the chronic phase, and then is strained again during the postmortem period.

In one of the few studies addressing the parents of adult cancer patients, Shanfield, Benjamin, and Swain (1984) found a surprising level of postbereavement "acceptance" and "growth." Poor outcomes were associated with long-standing ambivalence in the relationship, a finding with clear implications for antemortem evaluation and management.

### Children of Cancer Patients

Adams-Greenly and Moynihan (1983) and the 1977 study sponsored by Cancer Care, Inc. and the National Cancer Foundation have extensively described young children of adult cancer patients. They represent a hidden, high-risk group whose problems are minimized by overwhelmed parents and unknown to the medical staff who seldom see them. They experience an increased incidence of vegetative disturbances, psychological symptoms, acting-out behaviors, and school problems. They may have long-term changes in cognitive performance and in personality attributes such as self-esteem.

All children experience guilt about their possible causative role, grief and yearning for lost parenting from both parents, fear for themselves, and anger and resentment about being abandoned or shunted aside. This latter reaction can be quite realistic, as young children are often sent away and are almost always bypassed in the illness communication network. Therefore, fantasies replace fact, and, as child therapists have long known, these are more tormenting than even a grim reality.

Consistent with this is that the younger the children the more serious the problem. Nir, Pynoos, and Holland (1981) have described a case of a 4-year-old child who was attempting to take care of her mother in a role reversal that is frequently found at all ages, if one thinks to look for it. This speaks powerfully to the need to include children as much as possible in the family evaluation and support system. Rosenheim and Reicher (1985) have found that children who were told about a parent's terminal illness showed less anxiety than children who were not.

Rosenfeld and associates (1983), studying adolescent daughters of mastectomy patients, found no increased acting out but increased psychosomatic problems. The daughters felt resentful at being ''left out''; they took on increased maternal duties with resentment in some cases and increased self-esteem in others. Wellisch (1979) reported on four male and one female adolescents, who all acted out in the context of a poor parental marriage and a weak or absent healthy parent. Intervention usually focused on the parents.

Adult children of cancer patients must often take on a caretaker role for which they are variably equipped. Some overshoot into a rigid overprotective role that deprives the patients of a chance to use their strengths and lowers their self-esteem. Others regress or refuse and can make demands for continued parenting even from a very ill patient. Looking back on this period, the children almost universally view it as profoundly stressful and sometimes leaving permanent scars.

## Siblings of Cancer Patients

Like the youngsters just described, siblings have been a neglected group of troubled children. They show a similar range of problems reviewed by Sourkes (1980) and McKeever (1983), but added to them are acute and painful disturbances in the sibling relationship that, given the potential for strong identification and severe rivalry, cuts very deeply indeed. Comparison between patients, siblings, and controls has shown siblings to fare as badly or worse than the patients on selected measures such as self-esteem, social isolation, and fear of confronting family members (Cairns et al., 1979; Spinetta and Deasy-Spinetta, 1981). However, Koocher and O'Malley (1981) described a more positive outcome, namely a lower incidence of problems and a higher number of siblings reporting normal self-esteem, enhanced closeness, and resolution of anger toward the affected child. Significantly, they were addressing families of long-term survivors. On the other hand, Bank and Kahn (1982), Cain, Fast, and Erickson (1964), Pettle Michael and Lansdown (1986), and Fox-Sutherland (1985), in studying sibling bereavement, have all documented poor outcomes, many of which are clearly a continuation of antemortem patterns.

## THE FAMILY-CENTERED APPROACH

Starting in the late 1970s and through the 1980s, the focus in family and illness studies has changed to define the family itself as the treatment unit, not the patient, the disease, or the individual members. The emphasis is no longer on the impact of cancer on the family. It is on studying ways in which the family manages the cancer. This is a direct outgrowth of the family therapy field, itself a complex one with different schools within it. These are well reviewed and summarized by Walsh (1983) and Turk and Kerns (1985). However, there is a growing use of certain major concepts:

1. The family life cycle approach described by Carter and McGoldrick (1980)
2. The structural family approach, pioneered by Minuchin (1974), and applied to families of the medically ill by Munson (1978) and Sargent (1985), among others
3. The importance of history and family beliefs, as emphasized by the Ackerman Chronic Illness Project (Penn, 1983)
4. The importance of the dynamic interface between the family and the treatment setting as described by Imber-Coppersmith (1985)

Practical issues in these areas will be developed later. Family role theory (Bell, 1966) and family stress theory (McCubbin, 1979) are integrated into the overall approach but will not be separately discussed. Turk and Kerns (1985), though not focused exclusively on cancer, provide broad in-depth review of the family-centered approach to illness.

## Family Developmental Stages

Families, like individuals, go through a life cycle with different stages that present their characteristic tasks. Eisenberg, Sutkin, and Jansen (1984) present an extensive survey and discussion of the effect of chronic illness on the family, organized along these lines.

### THE YOUNGEST FAMILY

The newly married couple must create a strong, enduring new system, often while still dealing with issues of separation from the family of origin. Cancer in one of the pair may shatter the union, propelling the patient back into dependency and intimacy with parents and siblings, while excluding the spouse. This is seldom equally acceptable to both spouses and is often associated with friction between the family and spouse. It can lead to acute problems in terminal-care situations, when the family wishes to assume decision-making prerogatives that legally belong to the spouse.

### THE YOUNG FAMILY

The parents of young children are deeply involved in childrearing duties that must be juggled with the needs of the marriage and the individual needs of each partner, while negotiating a workable interface with families of origin, friends, and the larger community. Cancer in any member decreases the available energy for all these tasks and disrupts the balance of relationships usually in the direction of least resistance, which is often not the most constructive one. For example, in a shaky marriage in which the mother tended to turn to one of the children for consolation, the stress of the cancer may well increase the marital distance and the mother's dependency on the child. It may also shatter appropriate boundaries between nuclear and extended families while paradoxically increasing overall family isolation.

### THE FAMILY WITH ADOLESCENTS AND YOUNG ADULTS

The main task of this stage is for parents to promote gradual yet definite separation of the children, a brittle task given the recrudescence of powerful emotional issues adolescents arouse in the family. The younger generation must be moving toward intimacy with peers, as well as toward definition and consolidation of identity and goals. Cancer in any member may disrupt these processes easily. Cancer in a child may arrest his or her normal development abruptly, force regression, and create severe dependence–autonomy conflicts; cancer in a parent may place demands on adolescents

that slow down or arrest their separation process, whether they react with overt engagement and acquiescence or withdrawal and acting out. Parental tasks are equally disrupted.

### THE AGING FAMILY

Parents in the aging family must profoundly refocus their personal and interpersonal concerns and goals in the direction of old age. They must let children consolidate their own adult role and face a probable role reversal in relation to their parents. Often the generations live apart, and there may not be any obvious willing and nurturing adult in any household. This creates a caretaking vacuum that is very stressful.

## Family Organization

All families, even those that appear chaotic, have a complex structure. Each is a system made up of functionally defined subsystems, such as spouses or siblings, who maintain dynamic boundaries and who relate to each other along hierarchical lines. A stable organization that promotes predictability, security, and cohesiveness is highly valued by family members, who will often go to great lengths to protect it.

The cancer crisis is a major destabilizer. Many families try to deny this, as a way of denying the impact of the cancer (Sourkes, 1977). They respond by clinging rigidly to their previous structure, forcing inefficient, even destructive behaviors on the members. Others dissolve under the impact, leaving members needlessly disoriented and bereft of structure. Even flexible families may show signs of stress. They often change their patterns in ways that are not optimal, "overshooting in the direction of their dominant style," namely putting too much reliance on patterns that worked previously because that is the easiest, most natural thing to do (Minuchin and Minuchin, 1987).

The ideal response is that of appropriate flexibility. Families often achieve this remarkably well under very taxing circumstances, but the process is seldom smooth. As the family undergoes transformation, it experiments with new patterns, some of which result in transient signs of strain. These are not necessarily permanent or pathological but must be observed and evaluated. Minuchin (1974) has stated that, from a family process point of view, the pathology lies not so much in the actual pattern of behavior of any given family, but in whether or not the family shows any capacity to change and adapt under stress. Thus a family may appear quite strange to staff members but may be structurally "healthy" if it is changing appropriately to meet the needs of the situation.

## Family History and Family Beliefs

Besides a structure, each family has a unique, cumulative history of its experiences with important events, and a rich body of family myths and traditions that grow up around the emotional impact of that history.

Much of this relates to illness and loss, and provides the blueprints for their present responses to the cancer experience (Penn, 1983; Walker, 1983; Adams, 1978). Past behavior can guide present appraisals and definitions of the crisis, the means by which resources are called on and managed, the roles that different members are expected to assume, and the extent to which success can be expected.

Family histories also provide important clues about the etiology of particular assumptions held by family members about cancer and the prognosis. Miller, Bernstein, and Sharkey (1973) have commented that, in seeking professional help, families are almost purely seeking "corroboration and continuation of existing family values." This latter point can help staff members clarify patient and family behaviors that, on the face of it, appear irrational and counterproductive. Such behaviors can cause severe intrafamilial conflict, because individual members' beliefs are related to their own families of origin and are not necessarily compatible with each other in the current family.

Once implicit assumptions are made explicit and the difference between past and present is pointed out, tensions decrease and behaviors become more appropriate.

## Family–Treatment Interface

The family system viewpoint has also helped to highlight the important relationships that develop between family members and the health care team. This has important implications for patient compliance, case management, and staff morale, and will be discussed in some detail.

## INTENSITY OF THE RELATIONSHIP

It is difficult to overestimate the intensity of the relationship that families develop toward the treatment staff and the institution in which a member is receiving extended care for cancer. As Cassileth (1979) put it, illness-related issues become the "prime referent" for the family's thinking, and medical caregivers become endowed with enormous significance. Their words are repeated and overinterpreted, while their behaviors are scrutinized for covert messages about the patient's condition. A more subtle process occurs in which the family adopts complex, unspoken beliefs and rules from the treatment team. Therefore, families and pa-

tients are powerfully socialized to the medical system. The resulting "good fit" between team and family has obvious advantages, but the pressure to conform may be to the family's detriment if their family's style is too foreign, or if the team philosophy is not optimal for a particular patient's case. In the case of "bad fits" between the family and the team, the treatment is fraught with recurrent problems and complications, and the family may become a scapegoat by frustrated caretakers.

## STAFF BEHAVIORS

Besides an unintentional amount of "socializing," families may be realistically intimidated by the large number of highly trained and specialized professionals who play a role in modern cancer treatment (Imber-Coppersmith, 1985). It makes them feel less capable, and when they receive—as often happens—conflicting reports from different people, they may feel intellectually paralyzed, very anxious, and very angry.

On today's large treatment teams, it is difficult to achieve the right level of communication with families, that is, to give a great deal of current information without being confusing or inconsistent. Small groups and private practitioners have an advantage with this problem. But even there it is easy to underestimate the family's capacity, to become overcontrolling, and to make the family more passive than it needs to be.

At the level of concrete caretaking, the treatment team may not accurately gauge the family's capacity. They may underestimate the family's ability to make a meaningful contribution to care, or they may overestimate them and casually expect the family to perform tasks for which they are emotionally or practically unprepared. When the problems are explicit, they can be dealt with. When they are not, they cause ongoing stress in the family and difficulties with case management.

## FAMILY REACTION TO STAFF BEHAVIORS

What families lack in medical knowledge and decision-making power, they compensate for in intensity and commitment; hence, they wield considerable influence on the treatment team and on the course of the treatment.

When faced with some of the staff behaviors just described, families react in many ways. Some are acquiescent and identify deeply with the treatment team. These are the "good" families from the staff's point of view. Some acquiesce on the surface but remain ambivalent. Their feelings can easily turn into disappointment, anger, and blame—emotions often exaggerated, unrealistic, and not amenable to discussion. This shift is less likely to occur when there is a previously established base of open communication and trust, but has been known to take even seasoned doctors by surprise.

Some families never acquiesce to anything, arguing and negotiating at every step. These are the "exhausting" families. Some families find the experience so painful that they avoid it altogether, either abandoning the patient or taking the patient out of treatment. They may compromise by doctor shopping or seeking alternative treatments. If family dissatisfaction is too great, they may convince even a well-motivated patient to stop treatment. When the staff does not understand the anguish that drives them, these are viewed as "irresponsible" or "impossible" families.

## FAMILY DYNAMICS IN THE TREATMENT SETTING

Even with an ideal treatment team and a very supportive setting, the family brings its own dynamics into the situation in ways that can be quite powerful. Families can subtly manipulate and co-opt staff members into playing a role in preexisting family conflicts. Witness the power struggles on the ward regarding the management of a child whose parents have always disagreed on discipline. Families that are overenmeshed and have poor boundaries will induce staff members to become overinvolved with them. Families that are closed and suspicious will induce a distant, guarded stance from their caretakers, thus confirming the family in their belief about the lack of support to be received from outsiders.

## CONCLUSION

The family–treatment setting is intense and complex, a web of complementarities in which the medical system and the family system join to form a new "ad hoc" system. During acute periods, the shape of the old family system may be almost submerged. During chronic periods it reassumes primacy. But once cancer has occurred in a family, the system is never the same again.

## EVALUATION

### Referral Issues

The occurrence of cancer in a family is catastrophic enough that every family could ideally benefit from a family evaluation early in the treatment course, when patterns of communication and coping are set that tend to solidify during the course and may result in major and permanent alterations in family structure. However, this is not a practical option; nor does it do full justice to the strength, the resiliency, and the generosity that many families demonstrate. Nevertheless, it argues strongly for educating medical staff to look for problems in all family members, and to refer promptly before the situation becomes chaotic. It argues further that all mental health professionals working in this field should learn to "think family" even though they are not trained family therapists.

There are three major ways in which a family usually comes to the medical staff's attention. The earliest and most compelling is when the family fails significantly in its patient care function. This rapidly produces a referral to psychosocial services if they are available, or some concerned discussion, if they are not. Second, obvious psychiatric dysfunction or breakdown in a visible family member also requires a referral. Other common precipitants include a history of psychiatric illness, the presence of drug or alcohol abuse, signs of severe anxiety or depression, suicidal statements, severe somatic complaints, inappropriate or bizarre behavior, and sudden changes in mental state. The same problems may be occurring in unseen family members, such as children sent to their grandparents or a spouse who works long hours, and are then ignored by medical staff. Stepfamilies and families with single parents are at special risk. A third source of referrals is noncompliance and frictions between patient, family, and staff in all combinations, that are severe enough to interfere with case management.

From a family systems perspective, all these presenting complaints are not only problems in their own right, but are also clear markers of family dysfunction. Looking only at the presenting problem may be ineffective because it is fueled by deeper family dynamics. Adding a systems approach to the standard psychiatric evaluation of all family members may allow the designing of an intervention that will address the systems issues and will enable the family as a whole to move into a more constructive adaptation.

The other major advantage of the family-centered evaluation is that it can pick up dysfunctional patterns before they reach the point of acute breakdown and allow much earlier, possibly more effective interventions. For example, the overcompliant "parentified" child-patient will protect his or her parents as long as possible, but will ultimately break down as time progresses, causing major disruption in family and treatment setting. This perspective also addresses the problem of the time lag in response. A family may mobilize so well for a hospital crisis that it cannot demobilize and shift gears for a period of remission or outpatient care. These two types of dysfunction may be missed by medical staff but can ultimately be quite disruptive.

## Components of the Family Evaluation

In the setting of cancer illness a family orientation does not replace traditional evaluations but extends them. Purists in the field might argue this, but they have usually never spent much time on a ward or in a clinic, and underestimate the extent to which the reality of the illness and its relentless demands have become a central focus of family concerns and to which the medical system has literally ''invaded'' the family system, endowing doctors and staff with enormous emotional meaning.

A complete evaluation must therefore give the consultant the following information:

1. A reliable understanding of the patient's disease, the treatment, and the prognosis in order to know what the family must endure
2. Rapid individual screening of the patient and all family members to identify acute psychological symptoms and psychiatric diagnoses that may require immediate treatment
3. A family systems evaluation so as to delineate the way in which the family is functioning as a system of support for the patient and all its members
4. A careful evaluation of the family–treatment setting interface, so as to delineate the medical contribution to family dysfunction as well as the family's ability to hinder delivery of care

## Treatment Decisions

Given these data, the consultant is in the delicate position of weighing many different approaches, some of which may be incompatible. For example, a focus on improving direct patient care and support may as a consequence, further deprive remaining family members of attention. On the other hand, supporting an overextended family member's disengagement may further destabilize the family unless it is coupled with ways of replacing that member's contribution. However, taking family dynamics into account will allow one to select treatment goals more thoughtfully and design interventions that are less likely to flounder or backfire. The overall purpose is not to find the right solution but to approximate the best fit between complex and conflicting requirements.

## INTERVENTIONS

The goals of family intervention can be divided into three broad areas, namely, the provision of immediate emotional comfort, the creation of an extended system of support, and the challenging of dysfunctional patterns.

## Provision of Immediate Emotional Comfort

The direct support of family members is in some ways comparable both in method and intent to direct support of patients themselves. In fact, support of one results in improvement of both. However, a few special points can be made. It is important to legitimize the family's feelings. Members often feel they have no right to their feelings because they are ''healthy.'' They also feel their family customs may have no standing. They may believe that the stress and disruption they are experiencing is unique and shameful. Finally, they keep many thoughts and feelings unstated not only to staff but among themselves. It provides immediate relief for the implicit to be made explicit and for family members to hear that disruption and ambivalence are commonplace, that they as individuals have a right to complex needs at this time, and that, as a family, they are acknowledged and respected.

An important focus at this time should be identifying the family's distinctiveness and strengths, with a purpose to acknowledging and reinforcing them. An added benefit of this type of intervention is that it models open accepting ways of behaving and feeling that the members can carry over to each other and to the patient.

## Creation of an Extended System of Support

Families will have to support themselves emotionally and practically over the course of the illness. Five major areas of intervention that have been shown to be helpful to families will be described in the following paragraphs.

## EDUCATION

Cassileth and associates (1982) found lower anxiety levels in parents who had audiovisual teaching materials. Rudolph and colleagues (1981) received an enthusiastic response to an extensive didactic program. A teaching component is often built into other modalities such as support groups (Berger, 1984; Adams, 1978; Knapp and Hansen, 1975; Wellisch et al., 1978; Sabo et al., 1986; Ringler et al., 1981; Kartha and Ertel, 1976; Gilder et al., 1978), home care training programs (Edstrom and Miller, 1981; Mulhern et al., 1983), and home visitation programs (Michielutte et al., 1981). The nursing profession has played an increasing role in these programs and they are always well received. Conatser (1986) has reviewed the educational requirements for families of children with cancer.

## IMPROVING FAMILY COMMUNICATION

The value of improving communications in the family has been well demonstrated. It is fruitful to open channels of frank discussion between family members (Worby and Babineau, 1974). Adams-Greenley and Moynihan (1983) described this for children of cancer patients at age-appropriate levels, Adams (1978) for parents of cancer patients through the group modality, and Adams-Greenley, Beldoch, and Moynihan (1986) for adolescents. Two particularly important axes of communication to be bolstered are the marital axis (for which the problems have already been described) and the parent–child axis, because children's ways of reacting are often misinterpreted negatively by parents, with destructive consequences that are easily avoidable. Support groups as just described are also very useful for this kind of intervention.

## SMOOTHING THE FAMILY–TREATMENT TEAM INTERFACE

Just as it is helpful to explain children's behaviors to parents, it can be very helpful to explain distraught families' behavior to staff members, after which the latter usually treat them less defensively and with more sensitivity. Consultants can serve as role models for staff or act as an adjunct on the health care team, attending staff–family meetings and ensuring that the full range of issues is discussed adequately (Sourkes, 1977).

Sometimes the ward climate is destructive. It is important to be aware of informal coalitions of families meeting in the hall and visitors' lounge, and upsetting each other rather than performing their more usual function of support (Kartha and Ertel, 1976). Usually one or more troubled families can be identified and their effect defused through personal intervention. Gilder and colleagues (1978) report on a long-established group for parents of leukemic children, in which there was an unusual emphasis on improving the family–treatment interface due to active participation from staff members.

## PROVISION OF SERVICES

Even while the patient's needs are being fully met in the hospital, families may be burdened by many of their own new needs and benefit from instruction and guidance to available resources. Adams-Greenley (1986) has published a detailed method of staging fam-

ilies according to their needs at different stages of the disease process along with a wide range of associated psychosocial interventions. Monaco (1986) has reviewed the range of available resources.

## MOBILIZING OF SOCIAL SUPPORTS

While some of the just-mentioned interventions relate to periods of acute illness, this last area is important throughout the course and becomes especially so during chronic and recovery phases. Families must be encouraged to reopen their connections to the broadest number of community institutions so as to counteract subtle trends toward increasingly entrenched isolation. If it is not friends, clubs, churches, or other preexisting social institutions, it should be cancer-related groups or societies, which exist to meet the needs of people dealing with all diagnoses. The useful effects of these connections are well recognized.

### Challenging Dysfunctional Patterns

Challenging dysfunctional patterns addresses the structure of the family and the ways in which it is being altered by the illness. If what is occurring is a crystallization of preexisting difficulties, it may be difficult to effect any change without the help of long-term family therapy. However, a cancer crisis creates a time of acute change—an "access point," as it were—during which new patterns are being tried and may be in the process of being solidified. If recently formed, these patterns may be easily altered even without the use of special family therapy techniques. In fact they are often altered as an accidental benefit of the interventions just described.

Until now interventions have been discussed as if they were performed in discrete, nonoverlapping ways, but the reality is more fluid. The process of gathering enough information to make a careful evaluation is in itself loaded with inevitable potential for promoting change. Often the family meetings organized to inquire into problems or to gather knowledge turn out to have a mutative impact that comes as a great surprise to the staff and sometimes even to the consultant. Zarit and Zarit (1984) have commented on "the impressiveness of family meetings" to promote change. This is probably because well-run family meetings do, in fact, challenge dysfunctional family patterns even when they may have another overt agenda.

For example, family meetings are often called by the staff to solve a problem in case management even when they are unaware of the family conflicts that are fueling it. Addressing the management problem means, de facto, dealing with the conflictual family area, and resolving the one is tantamount to defusing the other.

Staff members are often present at family meetings and play an important role in the resolution of family problems associated with the course of the illness. During acute crises, one must recognize and act on the reality that members of the health team have become powerful and integral actors in the family drama. On the other hand, during chronic and survivorship periods it may be important to honor the privacy of the family and encourage intimacy and cohesiveness. Individual decisions are required to decide when and whom to include in family interventions during this period.

In the rare cases in which family therapy is indicated, Minuchin and Minuchin (1987) emphasize the importance of understanding the problem as a transitional issue related to the trauma of the illness. ''Access points'' are not only danger points; they are also times of unusual opportunity.

## SUMMARY

This chapter has reviewed the important role of the family in providing care for the cancer patient, as well as the enormous impact on the family of a cancer patient. The short-term and long-term human cost to all members has been emphasized and documented. A family systems approach has been described that highlights the active and adaptive role of the family. Along with traditional methods of needs assessment, it takes into account developmental stages, family structure, family myths, and the family–treatment interface in trying to understand and optimize the family's response.

A tripartite intervention model is outlined. It begins with the immediate provision of emotional comfort, which can occur during the evaluation process as well as later. It moves to the long-range development of the family's capacity to grow and sustain itself, and ends with the option of challenging dysfunctional patterns when they are identified.

To do justice to the family, one must be able to entertain complex and sometimes contradictory hypotheses. One must support both change and stability; one must label and encourage strengths, reframe symptoms in a constructive mode, and yet be unflinching in recognizing and addressing conflicts and dysfunctions. One must make hard choices between conflicting needs without being co-opted by, or arousing guilt in, any part of the system.

The effort is eminently worthwhile, given the level of distress of the human beings involved and given the remarkable benefit that can ensue from even brief interventions.

## REFERENCES

Adams, M. (1978). Helping the parents of children with malignancy. *J. Pediatrics* 93(5):734–38.

Adams-Greenly, M. (1986). Psychological staging of pediatric cancer patients and their families. *Cancer* 58:449–53.

Adams-Greenly, M. and R. Moynihan (1983). Helping the children of fatally ill parents. *Am. J. Orthopsychiatry* 53:219–29.

Adams-Greenly, M., A. Beldoch, and R. Moynihan (1986). Helping adolescents whose parents have cancer. *Semin. Oncol. Nurs.* 2:133–38.

Anthony, J.E. (1969). *The Mutative Impact on Family Life of Serious Mental and Physical Illness in a Parent*. Paper presented at the annual meeting of the Canadian Psychiatric Association, Toronto, Ontario, June.

Bank, S.P. and M.D. Kahn (1982). Siblings as survivors: Bond beyond the grave. In S.P. Bank and M.D. Kahn (eds.), *The Sibling Bond*. New York: Basic Books, pp. 271–95.

Bell, R.R. (1966). The impact of illness on family roles. In J.R. Folta and E.S. Deck (eds.), *A Sociological Framework for Patient Care*. New York: Wiley, pp. 177–90.

Berger, J.M. (1984). Crisis intervention: A drop-in support group for cancer patients and their families. *Soc. Work Health Care* 10(2):81–92.

Bloom, B.S., R.S. Knorr, and A.E. Evans (1985). The epidemiology of disease expenses: The costs of caring for children with cancer. *J.A.M.A.* 253:2393–97.

Bluebond-Langner, M. (1978). *The Private Worlds of Dying Children*. Princeton, N.J.: Princeton University Press.

Bodkin, C.M., T.J. Pisott, and J.R. Mann (1982). Financial burden of childhood cancer. *Br. Med. J.* 284:1542–44.

Bozeman, M.F., C.E. Orbach, and A.M. Sutherland (1955). Psychological impact of cancer and its treatment: Part I. The adaptation of mothers to the threatened loss of their children through leukemia. *Cancer* 8:1–19.

Butler, M.C. (1984). Families' responses to chemotherapy by an ambulatory infusion pump. *Nurs. Clin. North Am.* 19:139–44.

Cain, A.C., I. Fast, and M. Erickson (1964). Children's disturbed reactions to the death of a sibling. *Am. J. Orthopsychiatry* 34:741–52.

Cairns, N.V., G.M. Clark, S.D. Smith, and S.B. Lansky (1979). Adaptation of siblings to childhood malignancy. *J. Pediatrics* 95(3):484–87.

Cancer Care, Inc. and National Cancer Foundation (1977). *Listen to the Children: A Study of the Impact on the Mental Health of Children of a Parent's Catastrophic Illness*. New York: Cancer Care, Inc. and National Cancer Foundation.

Carter, E.A. and M. McGoldrick (eds.). (1980). *The Family Life Cycle: A Framework for Family Therapy*. New York: Gardner Press.

Cassileth, B.R. (ed.). (1979). *The Cancer Patient: Social and Medical Aspects of Care*. Philadelphia: Lea & Febiger.

Cassileth, B.R., R.M. Heiberger, V. March, and K. Sutton-

Smith (1982). Effect of audiovisual cancer programs on patients and families. *J. Med. Educ.* 57:54–59.

Chesler, M.A. and O.A. Barbarin (1984). Relating to the medical staff: How parents of children with cancer see the issues. *Health Soc. Work* 9:49–65.

Conatser, C. (1986). Preparing the family for their responsibilities during treatment. *Cancer* 58:508–11.

Copeland, D.R., Y. Silberberg, and B. Pfefferbaum (1983). Attitudes and practices of families of children in treatment for cancer: A cross-cultural study. *Am. J. Pediatr. Hematol. Oncol.* 5:65–71.

Derdiarian, A.K. (1986). Informational needs of recently diagnosed cancer patients. *Nurs. Res.* 35:276–81.

Eisenberg, M.G., L.C. Sutkin, and M.A. Jansen (eds.). (1984). *Chronic Illness and Disability through the Life Span: Effects on Self and Family.* Vol. 4. In T.E. Backer (ed.), *Springer Series on Rehabilitation.* New York: Springer.

Farrell, F.Z. and J.J. Hutter, Jr. (1984). The family of the adolescent: A time of challenge. In M.G. Eisenberg, L.C. Sutkin, and M.A. Jansen (eds.), *Chronic Illness and Disability through the Life Span: Effects on Self and Family.* Vol. 4. In T.E. Backer (ed.), *Springer Series on Rehabilitation.* New York: Springer, pp. 150–66.

Fox-Sutherland, S. (1985). Children's anniversary reactions to the death of a family member. *Omega—J. Death Dying* 15:291–305.

Friedman, S.B., P. Chadoff, J.W. Mason and D.A. Hamburg (1963). Behavioral observations on parents anticipating the death of a child. *Pediatrics* 32(4):610–25.

Ganz, P.A., C.C. Schas, and R.L. Heinrich (1985). The psychosocial impact of cancer on the elderly: A comparison with younger patients. *J. Am. Geriatr. Soc.* 33:429–35.

Gilder, R., P. Buschman, A. Sitarz, and J. Wolff (1978). Group therapy with parents of children with leukemia. *Am. J. Psychother.* 32:276–87.

Hinds, C. (1985). The needs of families who care for patients with cancer at home: Are we meeting them? *J. Adv. Nurs.* 10:575–81.

Hinton, J. (1981). Sharing or withholding awareness of dying between husband and wife. *J. Psychosom. Res.* 25:337–43.

Imber-Coppersmith, E. (1985). Families and multiple helpers. In D. Campbell and R. Draper (eds.), *Applications of Systemic Family Therapy: The Milan Approach.* London: Grune & Stratton, pp. 203–12.

Kaplan, D.M., R. Grobstein, and A. Smith (1976). Predicting the impact of severe illness in families. *Health Soc. Work* 1(3):71–82.

Kartha, M. and I. Ertel (1976). Short-term group therapy for mothers of leukemic children. *Clin. Pediatr.* 15:803–6.

Knapp, V.S. and H. Hansen (1975). Helping the parents of children with leukemia. *Soc. Work* 18:70–75.

Koocher, G.P. (1986a). Coping with a death from cancer. *J. Consult. Clin. Psychol.* 54:623–31.

Koocher, G.P. (1986b). Psychosocial issues during the acute treatment of pediatric cancer. *Cancer* 58:468–72.

Koocher, G. and J. O'Malley (1981). *The Damocles Syndrome: Psychological Consequences of Surviving Childhood Cancer.* New York: McGraw-Hill.

Lansky, S.B., N. Cairns, G. Clark, J.T. Lowman, L. Miller, and R.C. Trueworthy (1979). Childhood cancer: Nonmedical costs of the illness. *Cancer* 43:403–8.

Lansky, S.B., N.U. Cairns, R. Hassanein, J. Wehr, and J.T. Lowman (1978). Childhood cancer: Parental discord and divorce. *Pediatrics* 62(2):184–88.

Litman, T.J. (1974). The family as the basic unit in health and medical care. *Soc. Sci. Med.* 8:495–519.

Lons, S.B. and B.D. Lois (1982). Curable cancers and fatal ulcers: Attitudes toward cancer in Japan. *Soc. Sci. Med.* 16:2101–8.

McCubbin, H.I. (1979). Integrating coping behavior in family stress theory. *J. Marriage Fam.* 41:237–44.

McCubbin, H. and C. Figley (eds.). (1983a). *Stress and the Family.* Vol. 1, *Coping with Normative Transitions.* New York: Brunner/Mazel.

McCubbin, H. and C. Figley (eds.). (1983b). *Stress and the Family.* Vol. 2, *Coping with Catastrophe.* New York: Brunner/Mazel.

McKeever, P. (1983). Siblings of chronically ill children: A literature review with implications for treatment and practice. *Am. J. Orthopsychiatry* 53:209–17.

Michielutte, R., R.B. Patterson, and A. Herndon (1981). Evaluation of a home visitation program for families of children with cancer. *Am. J. Pediatr. Hematol. Oncol.* 3:239–45.

Miller, M., H. Bernstein, and H. Sharkey (1973). Denial of parental illness and maintenance of familial homeostasis. *J. Am. Geriatr. Soc.* 21:278–85.

Minuchin, S. (1974). *Families and Family Therapy.* Cambridge, Mass.: Harvard University Press.

Minuchin, P. and S. Minuchin (1987). Family as the context for patient care. In L.H. Bernstein, A.J. Grieco, and M. Dete (eds.), *Primary Care in the Home.* Philadelphia: Lippincott, pp. 83–94.

Monaco, G. (1986). Resources available to the family of the child with cancer. *Cancer* 58:516–21.

Mulhern, R.K., M.E. Lauer, and R.G. Hoffman (1983). Death of a child at home or in the hospital: Subsequent psychological adjustment of the family. *Pediatrics* 71:743–47.

Munson, S. (1978). Family structure and the family's general adaptation to loss: Helping families deal with the death of a child. In O.J.Z. Sahler (ed.), *The Child and Death.* St. Louis: C.V. Mosby, pp. 29–42.

Murinen, J.M. (1986). The economics of informal care: Labor market effects in the national hospice study. *Med. Care* 24:1007–17.

Nir, Y., R. Pynoos, and J.C. Holland (1981). Cancer in a parent: The impact on mother and child. *Gen. Hosp. Psychiatry* 3:331–42.

Northouse, L. (1984). The impact of cancer on the family: An overview. *Int. J. Psychiatry Med.* 14:215–42.

Penn, P. (1983). Coalitions and binding interactions in families with chronic illness. *Fam. Systems Med.* 1:16–25.

Perl, M. (1987). Home parenteral nutrition and the family. *Psychiatr. Clin. North Am.* 10:121–27.

Pettle Michael, S.A. and R.G. Lansdown (1986). Adjustment to the death of a sibling. *Arch. Dis. Child.* 61:278–83.

Ringler, K.E., H.H. Whitman, J.P. Gustafson, and F.W. Coleman (1981). Technical advances in leading a cancer patient group. *Int. J. Group Psychother.* 31:329–44.

Rosenfeld, A., G. Caplon, A. Yaroslavsky, J. Jacobowitz, V. Yuval, and H. LeBow (1983). Adaptation of children of parents suffering from cancer: A preliminary study of a new field for primary prevention research. *J. Primary Prevention* 3(4):244–50.

Rosenheim, E. and R. Reicher (1985). Informing children about a parent's terminal illness. *J. Child Psychol. Psychiatry* 26:995–98.

Rudolph, L.A., T.W. Pendergrass, J. Clark, M. Kjosness, and J.R. Hartmann (1981). Development of an education program for parents of children with cancer. *Soc. Work Health Care* 6:43–54.

Sabo, D., J. Brown, and C. Smith (1986). The male role and mastectomy: Support groups and men's adjustment. *J. Psychosoc. Oncol.* 4(1/2):19–31.

Sargent, J. (1985). Physician–family therapist collaboration: Children with medical problems. *Fam. Systems Med.* 3:454–65.

Schuler, D., M. Bakos, C. Zsambor, A. Polcz, R. Koos, G. Kardos, and T. Revesz (1985). Psychosocial problems in families of a child with cancer. *Med. Pediatr. Oncol.* 13:173–79.

Shanfield, S.B., A.H. Benjamin, and B.J. Swain (1984). Parents' reactions to the death of an adult child from cancer. *Am J. Psychiatry* 141:1092–94.

Smith, K.A. (1986). Teaching family members intrathecal morphine administration. *J. Neurosci. Nurs.* 18:95–97.

Sourkes, B. (1977). Facilitating family coping with childhood cancer. *J. Pediatr. Cancer* 2:65–67.

Sourkes, B. (1980). Siblings of the pediatric cancer patient. In J. Kellerman (ed.), *Psychological Aspects of Childhood Cancer*. Springfield, Ill.: Charles C Thomas.

Spinetta, J.J. (1981). The sibling of the child with cancer. In J.J. Spinetta and P. Deasy-Spinetta (eds.), *Living with Childhood Cancer*. St. Louis: C.V. Mosby, pp. 133–42.

Spinetta, J.J. (1984a). Development of psychometric assessment methods by life cycle stages. *Cancer* 53(Suppl.): 2222–27.

Spinetta, J.J. (1984b). Measurement of family function, communication, and cultural effects. *Cancer* 53(Suppl.): 2330–60.

Spinetta, J. and P. Deasy-Spinetta (eds.). (1981). *Living with Childhood Cancer*. St. Louis: C.V. Mosby.

Stam, H.J., B.D. Bultz, and C.A. Pittman (1986). Psychosocial problems and interventions in a referred sample of cancer patients. *Psychosom. Med.* 48:539–48.

Tebbi, C.K., M. Stern, M. Boyle, C.J. Mettlin, and E.R. Mindell (1985). The role of social support systems in adolescent cancer amputees. *Cancer* 56:965–71.

Turk, D.C. and R.D. Kerns (1985). The family in health and illness. In D.C. Turk and R.D. Kerns (eds.), *Health, Illness and Families: A Life-Span Perspective*. New York: Wiley, pp. 1–22.

Vachon, M.L., K. Freedman, A. Formo, J. Rogers, W. Lyall, and S. Freeman (1977). The final illness in cancer: The widow's perspective. *Can. Med. Assoc. J.* 117:1151–53.

Walker, G. (1983). The pact: The caretaker/ill-child coalition in families with chronic illness. *Fam. Systems Med.* 1:6–29.

Walsh, F. (ed.). (1983). *Normal Family Processes*. New York: Guilford Press.

Wellisch, D. (1979). Adolescent acting out when a parent has cancer. *Int. J. Fam. Ther.* 1:230–41.

Wellisch, D.K., K.R. Jamison, and R.D. Pasnau (1978). Psychosocial aspects of mastectomy: II. The man's perspective. *Am. J. Psychiatry* 135:543–46.

Wellisch, D.K., M.B. Mosher, and C. Van Scoy (1978). Management of family emotion stress: Family group therapy in a private oncology practice. *Int. J. Group Psychother.* 28:225–31.

Worby, C. and R. Babineau (1974). The family interview: Helping patients and families cope with metastatic disease. *Geriatrics* 29:83–94.

Zarit, S.H. and J.M. Zarit (1984). Psychological approaches to families of the elderly. In M.G. Eisenberg, L.C. Sutkin, and M.A. Jansen (eds.), *Chronic Illness and Disability through the Life Span: Effects on Self and Family*. Vol. 4. In T.E. Backer (ed.), *Springer Series on Rehabilitation*. New York: Springer, pp. 269–88.

# 48

# Supportive Home Care for the Advanced Cancer Patient and Family

Nessa Coyle, Matthew Loscalzo, and Lucanne Bailey

Meeting the needs of the advanced-cancer patient in the home requires a multidisciplinary approach. Although this is widely accepted, the approach may result in fragmentation of care. As the patient passes through different phases of disease, many specialists may be introduced. In addition, the setting for care may change from community hospital to cancer center, back to the community hospital, to hospice, and/or to home. Continuity of care is difficult to achieve within this multispecialist and multisetting background, and the potential for disjointed care is real (Fig. 48-1). In order to work effectively with the advanced cancer patient at home, both a multidisciplinary approach and continuity of care are important. These may be achieved using the following model.

## A MODEL

A patient-oriented, family-centered, nurse-coordinated model, with a collaboration among nurse, physician, and social worker, is proposed (Coyle et al., 1985) (see Fig. 48-2). A psychiatrist, music therapist, and chaplain are also useful members of the team. The team is based in the hospital or cancer center but is community-oriented. When a cancer patient is first referred to the supportive care program, either as an inpatient or outpatient, the nurse, physician, and social worker establish a plan of care. The nurse and social worker then continue to work with the patient and family in their home environment. This is done through telephone calls, home visits, and clinic visits. Once a patient is accepted into the program, the nurse-clinician contacts the patient's community physician before the patient's discharge home, identifying his or her role, and discussing pain management and other symptom control techniques. He or she will also contact the community nurses and make appropriate referrals as needed. The nurse-clinician will contact the patient's local pharmacy to make sure the prescribed analgesics are available, and if not, will locate a more suitable pharmacy for the family.

If a patient is admitted to a community hospital, the nurse-clinician will contact the hospital physician and head nurse, and again review pain management and other symptom control approaches that have been effective. He or she will keep in touch with the patient and the family throughout their various care settings, in this way facilitating continuity of care and providing a liaison-coordinating role.

This system is effective. It emphasizes the use of community health professionals, with the team's hospital-based nurse clinician and social worker available to the patient, family, and community health workers on a 24-hour basis. In order for the system to work, however, there must be close communication between team physician and nurse-clinician. Just as the nurse is available to the patient and family on a 24-hour basis, so too should the physician be available to the nurse for consultation if needed. It has to be a team effort if the system is to meet the many needs of the patient and family on the one hand, and to ensure optimal coordination of efforts on the other.

A variety of specialists may contribute important types of support within this system. The social worker addresses the psychosocial dynamics of the patient and family in the face of a changing medical status. Approaches include counseling and cognitive-behavioral methods aimed at promoting a greater sense of control in the patient and family. Also, the social worker attends to the practical needs of the patients and family by helping with transportation, acquisition of medical equipment, emergency financial assistance, and engagement of community resources.

The music therapist has been found to be a valuable adjunct member of the team in working with certain patients and families (Bailey, 1986). In the model out-

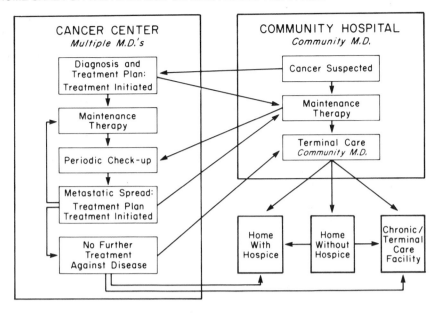

**Figure 48-1.**   Flow diagram showing potential for fragmentation of care in a community hospital and a cancer center.

lined here, referral to the music therapist is made to promote relaxation, reduce anxiety, to supplement other pain control methods, and to enhance communication between patient and family. At times, music becomes a critical way to express affection and to share the sense of impending separation that cannot be otherwise discussed. Because of the unique quality music has of engaging and distracting individuals, music therapy provides a special source of support for many individuals in their efforts to cope with the stresses of terminal illness.

The supportive care team must meet formally on a

weekly basis to discuss patient and family issues, and to maintain a clinical management plan. Guidelines are developed for drug therapy and for all other approaches to patient and family care so that the nurse-clinician and team members have a common framework within which to work.

We have found this model to be an effective way of meeting the multiple needs of patients and families, and of sharing the expertise of a cancer center with the community (Coyle and Loscalzo, 1985). The critical issues in maintaining the advanced cancer patient at home can thus be addressed, namely, continuity of

**Figure 48-2.**   A patient- and family-centered, nurse-coordinated model. PT/OT, Physiotherapy and occupational therapy. *Source:* From N. Coyle, E. Monzillo, M. Loscalzo, C. Farkas, M.J. Massie, and K.M. Foley (1985). A model of

continuity of care for cancer patients with pain and neuro-oncologic complications. *Cancer Nurs.* 8:113. Reprinted by permission.

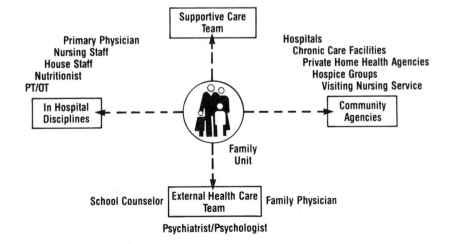

care by the team (which includes coordination with community physicians and public health nurses), 24-hour availability of a team member with physician backup, attention to symptom control (especially pain), help in understanding treatment options, and assistance in decision making within the context of emotional and psychological support to the patient and family.

## CHARACTERISTICS OF PATIENTS AND FAMILIES REFERRED FOR SUPPORTIVE HOME CARE

Our experience suggests that advanced cancer patients and their families referred for supportive home care fall into three major groups (see Table 48-1), ranging from the most stable to the most vulnerable to developing psychosocial problems (Coyle et al., 1985). This framework is helpful in identifying and planning for some of the necessary components of home care.

## Group I

Individuals in this group have good support systems, good coping mechanisms, and good insurance coverage. Usually referred to a supportive home care team at a time of crisis, these patients and families restabilize after appropriate intervention and support. The team's involvement is intense but brief, requiring little maintenance between crises.

### CASE REPORT

Mr. R. was a 34-year-old man with advanced melanoma, metastatic to colon and brain. He was married to a schoolteacher and had two children under 5 years of age. The family was referred in the hospital to the Supportive Home Care Program at a time of crisis when he developed poorly controlled seizures, back pain, and impending paraplegia. The patient and family were overwhelmed by the rapidity of onset of serious neurological complications, as well as by the implications of the changes. They could not visualize how Mr. R. could be cared for at home, although this was their wish.

Our team provided the patient and family with specific information on how to deal with each situation as it arose. This gave the family a sense of control and ability to anticipate problems. Appropriate local medical resources were engaged, and a liaison was established with them. Excellent insurance coverage was utilized to provide the necessary nursing care. Friends and relatives were organized for scheduled visits with assigned tasks; the priest made daily home visits.

These interventions enabled the household to adapt and function adequately around the patient's changing medical circumstances. The wife continued to work; the children continued to interact with their father. Mr. R. remained an involved member of the family.

**Table 48-1** Characteristics of patients and families referred for supportive home care

| Group | Characteristics | Intervention |
|---|---|---|
| I | • Good support systems<br>• Good coping mechanisms<br>• Good insurance<br>• Referred at time of crisis<br>• May regress to group II with prolonged debilitating illness | • Intense and brief<br>• Appropriate symptom management<br>• Community resources mobilized<br>• Family system restabilizes<br>• Team remains available |
| II | • Wavering support systems<br>• Borderline coping mechanisms<br>• May or may not have good insurance | • Ongoing support; liaison and advocacy work<br>• Appropriate symptom management<br>• Community resources mobilized |
| III | • Major psychopathological symptoms<br>• Habitually seek multiple other avenues of treatment and support<br>• Grossly distort reality<br>• Tenaciously maintain unrealistic goals<br>• May or may not have good insurance | • Appropriate symptom management<br>• Community resources mobilized<br>• Attempt to maintain some stability in the system<br>• Accept less than optimal outcome |

## Group II

This group is characterized by individuals who are borderline copers with wavering support systems. Continued support, liaison, and advocacy is required to maintain an intact patient and family system. Patients and families in this group require a treatment plan that incorporates a system of continuous and supportive interventions; the plan must be monitored regularly to determine if it is working. Families originally seen as falling within group I may move into this category when confronted with prolonged, progressively debilitating, painful disease in the patient.

### CASE REPORT

Mrs. G., a 40-year-old married woman with advanced colon cancer, was referred to our program on an inpatient basis, as a major discharge planning problem. The patient and staff concerns revolved around nutrition, pain management, probable escalation of symptoms at home, and an overwhelming fear of the responsibility for the patient's care on the part of the husband and daughter. Mrs. G. was a bright, engaging, anxious, and fearful woman who was accustomed to being in control of situations through meticulous organization. She had always assumed the primary responsibility for paying the bills and running the household. Her husband was withdrawn, rather passive, and appeared overwhelmed, not only by the thought of having to assume responsibility for the household, but also by the actual prospect of his wife coming home. This man did not know how to ask for help; he had become immobilized. The medical bills had accumulated and there were fighting and signs of increased stress among family members.

The 20-year-old daughter was explosive and antagonistic, but eager to learn and assist in her mother's care. Her boyfriend had died of cancer 2 years earlier. This daughter's wish was for her mother to be at home and to be comfortable. The family had several strengths, including a caring commitment to each other and the ability and willingness to tolerate structure and to accept and utilize professional intervention. They also had excellent medical insurance.

The supportive care team established with the family and the staff the viability of home care. They engaged an agency to supply nurses with an expertise in high technology, to give total parenteral nutrition and continuous subcutaneous morphine infusion. The team nurse and social worker worked closely with the patient, family, and private duty nurse in an ongoing way to monitor and manage symptoms and psychosocial stresses. Despite significant medical and psychosocial problems, the family was able, with team help, to manage Mrs. G. successfully at home.

## Group III

In this group, major psychopathological symptoms are present in either the patient or family or both. Such a complication, when it occurs, has a major impact on pain management, symptom control, and supportive care; it also compromises the effectiveness of interventions. Members of this group represent a small minority who, regardless of the intensity of support or intervention, repeatedly seek other avenues for treatment and support, distort reality, and tenaciously maintain unrealistic goals and expectations. As a consequence, the treatment goal is to maintain stability within the system. The team frequently feels ineffectual and frustrated. Team members must set realistic limits on the time devoted to the family and accept a less than optimal outcome. Such families tend to create conflict and divisiveness among staff members by devaluing and praising different members. In these cases, communication between team members becomes critical.

### CASE REPORT

Mr. F. was a 54-year-old married executive with advanced lung cancer metastatic to the spinal cord, who had a history of chronic alcohol abuse. He was a passive-aggressive, guilt-ridden man who had become alienated from his family of origin and his religion, which was a prior source of strength. Mr. F.'s wife was an angry, paranoid, emotionally labile woman with obsessive-compulsive characteristics who was under ongoing psychiatric care. Mr. F. had confidence in conventional medical treatment. His wife tolerated conven-

tional treatment when her husband was doing well, but as the disease progressed, she sought out and engaged multiple unorthodox and fringe health practitioners.

Despite intensive intervention by the supportive care team, this frantic searching by the wife and her inability to come to terms with the progression of the disease continued until the patient's death. In bereavement follow-up, Mr. F.'s wife continued to be quite ambivalent toward the supportive care team, fluctuating between virulent verbal outbursts and sending hand-delivered boxes of expensive chocolates.

Patients and families in groups I and II usually do well throughout the process of maintaining an advanced cancer patient at home and are able to make the necessary adaptations in response to the fluctuating needs. However, those who fall within group III have a great deal of difficulty in dealing with these changing states; the ability to maintain the patient successfully at home becomes tenuous. These latter families need to be carefully assessed, as described later. After careful review, some should be advised against the choice of home care; in other cases a psychiatric nurse-clinician may assume coordination of care of patients–families in this group as discussed in detail in the next section.

## PATIENT, FAMILY, AND COMMUNITY ASSESSMENT

In order to plan for appropriate home care for the advanced cancer patient, and adequate support for the family, it is essential to have not only a medical, psychological, social, and financial assessment, but also a community assessment. It has been shown that in order for home care to be successfully managed, the complexity of the patient's needs must be matched with the ability of the family and supportive network to meet those needs (Baird, 1980). The areas that need to be evaluated as part of this initial assessment process includes *medical variables* in the patient, family, and available community medical system, *psychological variables* in the patient, family, and psychosocial community supports, and *social and financial variables* in the patient and family. Each will be reviewed here.

### Medical Variables

As outlined in Table 48-2, medical variables are evaluated in relation to the patient, the family, and the community. Variables that must be assessed in the patient include the disease status, expected disease progression, present functional level, symptoms, and current management approach. Of particular importance is the patient's functional level, reflecting his or her mobility (e.g., fully bedbound or fully mobile without aids), ability to communicate (from severe as with brain tu-

**Table 48-2** Medical variables in the assessment process of patient, family, and community

| Social level | Medical variables |
|---|---|
| Patient | Present functional level |
| | Level of need in activities of daily living |
| | Disease status and expected progression |
| | Symptoms and management approaches |
| Family | Concurrent medical problems |
| Supports in community | Community physicians' willingness to make home visits and to assume responsibility for home care |
| | Community hospice availability: hospital-based; community-based; none |
| | Community hospital: distance from patient; local doctors affiliated |
| | Community nurses—type of nursing available: visiting-nurse services; private duty nursing agencies; ability to handle complexity of patient needs |
| | Community supports: American Cancer Society, Cancer Care, support groups, Red Cross, I Can Cope, Can Surmount, social service agencies, etc.; religious groups; hospital-based outpatient support and/or education programs; volunteer escort services; volunteer ambulance services, etc. |
| | Community pharmacy: whether it carries or will obtain necessary medications, especially narcotics |

mors to minimal impairment), ability to perform activities of daily living, bowel and bladder function (from incontinence to full self-care), and level of alertness (from coma to full alertness). Concurrent medical problems in a family member, particularly the primary caregiver, also need to be known because the family member's ability to participate may be pivotal to the ability to carry out the home care plan.

In assessing the community medical support network, essential features to assess are the availability of a local physician who assumes responsibility for home care, availability of that physician to make home visits, his or her ability to admit the patient to the community hospital, presence of a hospice in the community (and if so, what level of care it offers), familiarity of the community nurses with pain and symptom control needed in the care of advanced cancer patients, and whether the community pharmacy will obtain necessary medications for the patient (especially narcotic

analgesics). All of this information must be gathered and assessed before the patient accepted for supportive home care is discharged from the hospital. The assessment establishes both the specific care needs for the patient and the level of support available in the community. In this way the nurse-clinician will have the needed data to match patient needs to available resources.

## Psychosocial Variables

The key psychosocial variables relevant to patient and family function are outlined in Table 48-3. Assessment must be an ongoing process that allows a continuous evaluation of response to the rapid changes caused by advanced disease. The process of assessment is designed to lead the health care practitioner to an understanding of the medical and psychosocial situation of the patient and family system, so that effective interventions can be developed (Freidenbergs et al., 1980; Wellisch et al., 1983). It is essential that the perceptions of the patient and family be explored and understood prior to any intervention. Not only does this quickly support the development of rapport, but it also increases the probability that interventions will be acceptable to the patient and family.

It is first necessary to gain from the family an adequate understanding of their major concerns, individually, and as a system. This enables the practitioner to engage the patient and family as active participants in the team and to create an environment of effective problem solving. It is at this time that not only conflicts among the patient, family, and friends surface, but also their goals and expectations, which may be found to differ dramatically from those of the medical staff. Recognition of these differing expectations is the first step in this problem-solving approach.

The issue of control is of major importance in working with the patient and family. For many patients, having a sense of control may lessen the impact of not being able to slow down the disease process in any meaningful way.

The assessment of psychological adjustment to prior traumatic events (e.g., deaths) gives the team a good predictor of likely behavior of the patient and family members in the crises of terminal illness (see Chapters 5 and 49). Prior coping strategies used, and their effectiveness, are important to know. In general, coping strategies ordinarily used by the patient should be supported. Efforts to change someone in time of crisis will only be frustrating to the patient and to the team. In time of crisis, individual family members also revert to previously used strategies that worked. However, such strategies may be inappropriate or ineffective in the current situation.

**Table 48-3** Psychosocial variables in the assessment of patient, family, and community

| | Psychosocial variables |
|---|---|
| Patient | Major concerns at this moment: ability to cope; control issues (perception of loss of control, life–death issues, environment, etc.); expectations of disease process (experience with illness and cancer); work; self-image; independence–dependency issues; significant losses (activities, role change, social supports, etc.); goals and desires |
| | Ability to communicate effectively: feelings, concerns, fears, needs, fantasies (life–death issues, causality, pain, etc.) |
| | Developmental process: age-appropriate behavior (relationships, work, hobbies, aspirations, etc.); life experience (as it influences how one sees things and acts) |
| | Mood (calm, anxious, depressed, etc.): trait (consistent behavioral pattern); state (reaction to recent events) |
| | Preexisting psychopathology: psychiatric illness; psychiatric hospitalizations; substance abuse (use of drugs and/or alcohol causing significant impairment in social functioning); mental illness in family; inadequate coping skills |
| | Coping strategy: tackling, rationalizing, avoiding |
| Family | Same variables as for patient |
| | Preexisting family structure and functioning |
| | Present family structure and functioning |
| | Presence of children at home (age-related ability to comprehend changes caused by the illness process) |
| | Ability to reconcile differences (belief systems, coping styles, treatment decisions, etc.) |
| Supports in community | Clubs; friend network; volunteer group; church; hospice team; counselors |

The coping strategies of the family as a unit are also assessed. A family with a rigid, inflexible coping style is apt to be troubled by episodes of emotional crisis, as compared to one with more flexibility in coping. The potential for alienation of a family member is high in a family known already to be vulnerable to psychological disturbance. The team must be wary of unwittingly being drawn into a collusion with one family member against the other, which represents a part of their disturbed function as a family.

Advanced disease causes greater likelihood of delirium from metabolic encephalopathy, narcotic analgesics, and CNS complications (these are described in Part V). Information concerning prior psychiatric illness (especially alcohol or drug abuse) and prior psychiatric hospitalization is necessary for developing an effective treatment plan. Though difficult for some health care professionals to explore, these are particularly relevant variables for symptom management.

Home care of the advanced-cancer patient, especially if prolonged over a period of months, places enormous stress on the family and community health care providers. If this time period extends into a year or longer, there is a danger that the significance of the cumulative losses on the part of the patient, and mounting strain on the part of the family, may be missed. A type of "status quo" in responses and interventions may occur. All home care patients require a careful reevaluation of their medical, psychological, social, and financial status by the supportive care team at a minimum of every 2 weeks. This lessens the likelihood of the "status quo" phenomenon.

## Social and Financial Variables

Outlined in Table 48-4, a number of social and financial variables must be considered from the point of view of both the patient and family. Essential features include whether the patient lives alone or with others, whether substantial assistance is required in tasks of daily living and whether such help is available, the number of actual hours the primary care provider is unable to spend with the patient and for which coverage must be planned, and whether there is active, consistent, and reliable help from family members and/or friends for the patient's care. Accurate initial assessment of the potential contribution of the proposed caretakers to the patient's care avoids problems later with the family, whose members genuinely want to care for their relative but who overestimated their ability to meet the required investment of time and energy.

The financial impact of advanced disease is widely accepted to be of catastrophic proportions to patient and family members alike (Baird, 1981; Bayer et al., 1983; Bloom and Kissick, 1980; McNaul, 1981; McNaul and Wheeler, 1978). Although most patients have medical insurance, certain essential services are seldom covered by medical insurance, including transportation, medications, and homemakers. It is important that the health care team understand the financial situation of the patient and family so that appropriate interventions and planning can be developed. The psychological, medical, and financial concerns are so in-

**Table 48-4**  Social and/or financial variables in the assessment of patient and family

| | Social and/or financial variables |
|---|---|
| Patient | Living arrangements (lives alone or with others) |
| | Work status |
| | Finances (income, savings, debts, etc.) |
| | Insurance coverage for hospital care (partial or total) |
| | Insurance coverage for home care (partial or total, private duty nurses, community nurses, equipment, medications, etc.) |
| | Medicare or Medicaid eligibility |
| Family | Availability of primary care provider (family, friend, etc.) |
| | Consistency, reliability of family or friend commitment of time |
| | Actively involved friend network |
| | Income other than patient (none, spouse, other) |
| | Structural setup of home (steps, elevator, number of rooms, bathroom, space for equipment, wheelchair accessibility, telephone, etc.) |

**Table 48-5**  Variables in response to the prospect of death

| Pattern | Characteristics |
|---|---|
| I | • Similar to group I (Table 48-1) |
| | • Patient and family openly discuss death |
| | • Attempt to gain control through knowledge; want to know what to expect |
| | • Prepared for death but involved in life |
| | • May or may not continue in active treatment against the disease |
| | • Patient makes a living will |
| | • Patient participates in funeral arrangements |
| | • Patient plans for family's well-being after death |
| | • Patient may achieve some fixed goal after great effort |
| II | • Similar to group II (Table 48-1) |
| | • Possibility of death acknowledged |
| | • Patient attempts to gain control through knowledge; reads about disease, watches for new research, clips out articles on new treatments |
| | • Patient participates in experimental chemotherapy protocols |
| | • Patient values being productive member of society |
| | • Periods of uncertainty and despair with exacerbation of symptoms |
| | • Patient adapts or modifies life-style as functional losses occur |
| III | • Similar to group III (Table 48-1) |
| | • Family may discuss prospect of death with care provider, but not with patient |
| | • If patient broaches subject, family neutralizes it by false assurances |
| | • Patient/family refuse to countenance possibility of death |
| | • Anger frequent as condition deteriorates |
| | • Multiple specialists consulted |
| | • Unorthodox methods of care sought |
| | • Despair and/or rage directed against medical profession |

terrelated that they can become indistinguishable as families perceive these three distressing aspects as one overwhelming dimension.

The purpose of this initial assessment is to identify strengths and weaknesses in the ability of the family, friends, and community to maintain a patient at home. However, the most critical ingredient is a genuine desire on the part of the patient and family to manage the situation at home, coupled with a commitment to face and solve whatever difficulties arise, recognizing that death is the likely outcome. The most painful aspect is often that of dealing with the impending death. Patterns by which the task is approached by families are outlined in the following paragraphs.

## RESPONSES TO THE PROSPECT OF DEATH

Patients and families deal with the prospect of death in different ways (Parkes, 1973, 1978; Tartaglia and Tecala, 1985). Just as assessment of the patient, family, and community resources is the initial step in home care planning, so is a similar assessment needed with regard to the issue of death and dying to provide important information for the care plan (Mount, 1985). We have identified three patterns of dealing with these issues in our families that are frequently encountered. Outlined in Table 48-5, these are discussed briefly in the following paragraphs.

### Pattern I

This response is seen in those situations where the patient and family talk openly about death and may have read books on death and dying. They attempt to gain control of the situation through knowledge. They prepare for the anticipated death, but simultaneously manage to be involved fully in living. The patient may choose to continue in active treatment or to receive supportive care alone. The focus is on dying "well" and remaining in control. Frequently, patients within this group write living wills and seek reassurance that no tubes and machines will be used if they stop breathing. Participation in making funeral arrangements, selecting a burial plot, and writing a eulogy are not uncommon. The patient is involved in planning for the well-being of the family after his or her death; the remaining time is used to put things "in order." The family asks questions about what to expect and how to deal with each situation. One last trip, one last task, or one last family celebration is set as an immediate goal for which survival is attempted. However, even with this preparation and "desensitization" of approaching death, the reality of actual death when it does occur is still experienced as unexpected and ''too soon.'' Shock is expressed by members who may say ''It happened too quickly without enough time to prepare.''

## Pattern II

Here the patient acknowledges the possibility of death but focuses on living. He or she tends to be involved in seeking information from libraries, reading about the disease, looking for new research reports, clipping out articles from newspapers and magazines on new cancer treatments, and seeking to participate in experimental treatment protocols. Interpretation of a new symptom allows it to be seen as more manageable and less threatening. Working and remaining a productive member of society are very important. After each bout or exacerbation of symptoms, and restabilization at a lower level of functioning, modifications in life-style are made and ''pressing on'' with living resumes. ''Roller coaster'' emotions and periods of uncertainty and despair accompany each exacerbation of symptoms. The family is able to support the patient through these periods and remain actively involved as death approaches.

## Pattern III

The pattern here is one of facing approaching death with little open communication between patient and family. In this situation, the family may discuss the prospect of death with the health care provider. However, the family may or may not initiate the conversation, and frequently they do not know what the patient knows about the seriousness of the disease. The patient often does not discuss this with the family, or if he or she does, the subject may be changed or neutralized by reassurances from them. The family may explicitly state that they do not want the subject broached with the patient, or are ambivalent about this, or have been closed off by the patient when attempting to start such a conversation. One also sees the patient and/or family who refuse to countenance the possibility of death. Anger is frequent as the patient's condition deteriorates, and multiple specialists may be consulted and unorthodox methods of care sought. A despairing cry may be heard: ''I want someone to tell me it is not so, that he is cured, that what the original surgeon told me is true, that they got it all out.'' In working with these patients and families, the focus is on confronting their avoidance, redefining the problems in manageable terms, and opening up options and choices. Encouragement of communication between patient and family is critically important. It can be done by having a team member present to initiate discussion of painful facts (Weisman, 1979). This may open up the way to a close bond that can be a great solace to the dying patient and to the survivor during bereavement.

## THE PRIMARY CARE PROVIDER'S EXPERIENCE OF A DEATH AT HOME

During the final stage of a person's illness, the primary care provider, usually the spouse or parent, may be overwhelmed with the feeling of responsibility; ''what if's'' are frequent: ''What if I miss something? What if an emergency occurs? What do I do if he stops breathing? Hemorrhages? Stops eating? Goes into a coma?'' Each of these ''what if's'' must be dealt with, usually repeatedly, in a concrete way. Although it is reassuring to such a relative to have private duty nurses in the home to lessen responsibility, the loss of privacy and sense of intrusion may become an issue.

Intense emotional involvement by the primary care provider is frequent, with the constant anticipation of something monumental and dramatic about to happen. Just before the person dies, his or her final words are given special meaning. If these words are not heard, or the primary care provider is not there at the moment of death, a sense of being cheated is felt. The actual moment of death, so long anticipated and feared, is sometimes anticlimactic, with the relative feeling ''Is that all there is?''

After the family member's death, the primary care provider frequently feels an intense void and loneliness. This may be expressed as a sense of loss of purpose; the most important work they have ever done has been taken from them. Work and everyday life pale in comparison. The ''what if's'' become ''if I had only's'' as normal guilt begins to surface. ''What if I had called the doctor sooner?'' ''What if I lacked sensitivity?'' ''Maybe I thought too much about myself,'' ''Did I do everything I could have done?'' ''Did I give up too soon?'' ''Should I have gone to Mexico or to the Bahamas for further treatment?'' Guilt may also be expressed in relation to the feeling of relief and freedom after death has occurred. ''I didn't think I could live without him and yet here I am doing so.'' Another fear expressed may be that of forgetting the dead one, or fear that the survivor will be able to remember only the last days of illness, and not the earlier, happier times.

Grief leads to recall of prior losses, and to realization of the survivor's own mortality. A reevaluation of self and goals may occur. A medical checkup may be requested. Generalized anger at the ugliness of the death may be expressed, with rage toward the medical profession for not having ''saved'' the relative. Distortion of time occurs: ''It seems so long ago, and yet only a few days have passed.'' The survivor may momentarily forget the patient is gone and, at times, wake up to ''check on'' the patient.

Bereavement counseling is a natural continuation of the activity of the supportive care team. Anticipation of the bereavement with discussions about it prior to death is helpful, contributing to a sense of control and mastery.

## SUMMARY

A model of supportive care at home for patients with advanced or terminal disease is presented that emphasizes several important aspects, including a nurse coordinated multidisciplinary team to assure continuity of care, 24-hour availability, and integration of hospital resources with community care. The team must be able to assess a patient and family for suitability for management at home. This is done by examining medical, psychological, social, and financial variables. The assessment allows classification of the patients and families into groups that predict vulnerability to problems in symptom control, general management, and confronting the approaching death. Involvement of the team at the time of death provides the opportunity for continued support and bereavement counseling.

## REFERENCES

Bailey, L. (1986). Music therapy in pain management. *J. Pain Symptom Management* 1:25–27.

Baird, S.B. (1980). Nursing roles in continuing care: Home care and hospice. *Semin. Oncol.* 7:28–38.

Baird, S.B. (1981). Economic realities in the treatment and care of the cancer patient. In J.W. Rogers and J.H. Fergusson (eds.). *Topics in Clinical Nursing*, 2nd ed. Rockville, Md.: Aspens Systems, pp. 67–80.

Bayer, R., D. Callahan, J. Fletcher, T. Hodgson, B. Jennings, D. Monsees, S. Sieverts, and R. Veatch (1983). The care of the terminally ill: Morality and economics. *N. Engl. J. Med.* 309:1490–94.

Bloom, B.S. and P.D. Kissick (1980). Home and hospital cost of terminal illness. *Med. Care* 18:560–64.

Coyle, N. and M. Loscalzo (1985). For the chronic pain of cancer: A model of comprehensive care. *Pain Analgesia* 1:31–35.

Coyle, N., E. Monzillo, M. Loscalzo, C. Farkas, M.J. Massie, and K.M. Foley (1985). A model of continuity of care for cancer patients with pain and neuro-oncologic complications. *Cancer Nurs.* 8:111–19.

Freidenbergs, I., W. Gordon, M. Ruckdeschel, and L. Diller (1980). Assessment and treatment of psychosocial problems of the cancer patient: A case study. *Cancer Nurs.* 3:111–19.

McNaul, F. (1981). The cost of cancer: A challenge to health care providers. *Cancer Nurs.* 4:307.

McNaul, F. and K. Wheeler (1978). The cancer patient's financial concerns: An element in assessing nursing interventions. *Oncol. Nurs. Forum* 5:1–4.

Mount, B. (1985). Psychological and social aspects of cancer pain. In P. Wall and R. Melzack (eds.), *Textbook of Pain*, 2nd ed. London: Churchill-Livingstone, pp. 462–64.

Parkes, C.M. (1973). Attachment and autonomy at the end of life. In R. Gosling (ed.), *Support, Innovation, and Autonomy*, 2nd ed. London: Tavistock Publications, pp. 151–66.

Parkes, C.M. (1978). Home or hospital? Terminal care as seen by surviving spouses. *J. R. Coll. Gen. Pract.* 28:19–30.

Tartaglia, C. and M. Tecala (1985). Psychosocial aspects of terminal care. In P. Calabresi, P. Schein, and S. Rosenberg (eds.), *Medical Oncology: Basic Principles and Clinical Management of Cancer*, 2nd ed. New York: Macmillan, pp. 1480–84.

Weisman, A. (1979). *Coping with Cancer.* New York: McGraw-Hill.

Wellisch, D., J. Landsverk, K. Guidera, R. Pasnau, and F. Fawzy (1983). Evaluation of psychosocial problems of the homebound cancer patient: 1. Methodology and problem frequencies. *Psychosom. Med.* 45:11–21.

# 49

# Management of Special Psychiatric Problems in Terminal Care: Role for a Psychiatric Nurse-Clinician

Carol Farkas

The ability to provide support for a patient with terminal illness at home is apt to hinge in large measure on the emotional stability of the patient and family members. The presence of serious psychological problems or actual psychiatric illness in either patient or family can compromise care. A home care team must be able to recognize and diagnose these problems and be able to treat them. Families that cope well often require minimal intervention, whereas those with poor coping, poor support, or psychiatric illness require much more help; even that help is often poorly utilized (see Chapter 48). These families with preexisting psychological vulnerability might have compensated during the normal stresses of life, but the presence of one member with advanced cancer being managed in the home is apt to exacerbate old conflicts or prior psychiatric disorders in patient or family, contributing to the risk of psychological decompensation. Since hospitalizations are becoming shorter and home care is being imposed for sicker patients for longer periods, the problems of the "problem" family become significant in home health care.

Because of the special attention these patients and families require, it is helpful to have one member of the home care team who has a background in mental health and expertise in management of the common psychological problems encountered in cancer patients. It is also important that the team have a psychiatric consultant as backup for the management of severe problems. This model has been used at Memorial Sloan-Kettering Cancer Center over the past 8 years (Fig. 49-1).

## THE MODEL

The observations described in the following paragraphs are those of the psychiatric nurse-clinician who functions within the psychiatry service and on the home supportive care team. The nurse provides care for those special patients and families referred because of psychiatric problems that complicate home care, and provides liaison between patient, family, and physicians involved in care.

The psychiatric nurse-clinician works with families referred from several sources, including physicians who recognize special psychological problems and who ask assistance in managing those problems anticipated in home care, the psychiatrist who has seen the patient in the hospital and who recognizes that home care will require special expertise in managing a psychiatric problem, other members of the home care team, as well as social workers, nurses, and other staff.

The nurse-clinician has several functions in these situations:

1. Introduce the service (preferably in the hospital prior to discharge), meeting with the patient and the primary family member and obtaining needed information from the primary physician, psychiatrist (if consultation has been done), and the primary nurse responsible for care.
2. Make a home visit as soon as the patient is discharged to assess the psychological state of the patient in the home setting and review adjustment of family members, the home situation, financial and social resources (see Chapter 48).
3. Assess the other physical problems and symptoms the patient is experiencing and whether symptom control is adequate.
4. Implement measures to ameliorate other symptoms (especially pain, nausea, vomiting, and shortness of breath), on the theory that mental complications in the patient may remit or be reduced by control of other symptoms.
5. Implement a system and schedule of care that structures the time and energy use of the primary caregiver to avoid exhaustion. When appropriate,

**PSYCHIATRIC UNIT**                                    **HOME CARE TEAM**

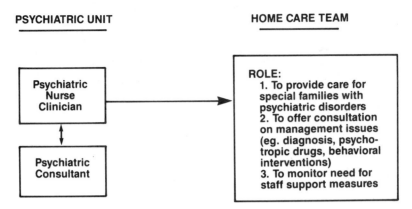

**Figure 49-1.** Psychiatric input to a home care team.

this may include utilizing the services of a home-maker or other relative/friend to give part of the care.

6. Assure patient and family that the nurse-clinician is available at all times by telephone and to make home visits for emergencies. Patient and family are also assured that the nurse-clinician is accessible any time during normal work hours for questions, can be contacted daily to discuss current condition, and will continue to make regular home visits as needed (reducing anxiety associated with feeling "all alone with the problem").

7. Institute counseling that includes clarification of the services, reducing the sense of fragmentation of care, providing information about symptoms and their control, listening to fears, preparing the family about what to do when death occurs, anticipating and planning what is to be done in any of the possible situations that might occur, talking with patient and family separately and together, assuring them of full consideration of their wishes and views, and the availability of medication necessary to relieve symptoms of distress.

8. Assist the family in utilizing other resources to reduce stress, such as home health aide, clergy, extended-family involvement, and community agencies.

9. Implement psychopharmacological symptom control, when indicated, by consultation with the attending physician and psychiatrist who assess the patient for use of an antidepressant, antianxiety, sedative, or antipsychotic medication, or for a family member who is experiencing psychiatric symptoms. The nurse also is able to observe drug effectiveness and report side effects.

10. Teach the patient behavioral techniques as an adjunct to pharmacological efforts to control pain and anxiety, supporting a sense of self-control.

11. Provide continuity of care by assuring availability throughout the illness and by providing bereavement counseling for family members after the death.

The situations that we have successfully managed with this model cover the common problems seen in cancer patients and the range of common psychiatric disorders. An important issue in home care with these families is that there is rarely a single isolated problem but usually multiple problems that make the situation complex to manage. For example, the patient may have mild delirium and major depression. The relative may abuse alcohol, which complicates anticipatory grief and bereavement. There is always the interplay of psychological issues and medical variables that accompanies advancing disease and palliative care, requiring careful consideration of both.

Our clinical experience has identified several frequently occurring problems, some involving patients and others family members (Table 49-1). An early study done by Plumb and Holland (1977) showed that levels of depression in the next of kin were frequently as high as that of the patient. Cassileth and colleagues (1985) have observed increasing distress in patient and relatives as a function of level of illness and treatment, likely reflecting decreasing ability to cope with mounting medical problems, the greatest being those in palliative end-stage care. They found that patients and their next of kin often had similar levels of distress, indicating that one can have an impact on the other, and suggested that intervention with either, especially during terminal care when distress is highest, could enhance the well-being of both. Conversely, exhaustion in a family member can affect the patient's willingness to receive treatment or to continue care at home.

The common problems seen in patients during ter-

**Table 49-1** Common psychiatric diagnosis encountered in home care

| Patient | Family member and/or primary care provider |
| --- | --- |
| Reactive anxiety and depression (about illness, death) | Reactive anxiety and depression (about illness, death) |
| Anticipatory grief | Anticipatory grief |
| Major depression | "Out of sync" with patient |
| Anxiety and/or depression associated with pain or uncontrolled physical symptoms, death | Guilt; "overwhelmed," exhausted |
| | Concerns about moment of death, final symptoms and coping with them |
| Delirium with hallucinations, confusion | Conflicts with patient or other family members |
| Prior psychiatric disorder | Major depression |
| | Prior psychiatric disorder |
| | Bereavement following death |

minal stages of illness at home are reactive anxiety and depression about illness, losses, and death; anticipatory grief associated with advancing illness; anxiety and depression associated with distressing physical symptoms that are not controlled, especially pain, shortness of breath, and nausea and vomiting; major depression; delirium secondary to medication and CNS complications; and prior psychiatric disorder with exacerbation (see Table 49-1).

It is difficult to assess any mental symptoms until pain and other distressing physical symptoms are controlled. Often the panicky, irritable patient becomes calm and pleasant when adequate pain control is instituted. Patients need reassurance about taking narcotics and are helped by discussion of concerns about addiction. Many associate prescribed narcotics with street drugs and will use drugs too sparingly to be effective. The existential distress of illness is expressed by a spectrum of depressive symptoms from sadness to grief, sometimes accompanied by anxiety or major depression, characterized by withdrawal or agitation. Despite its reactive aspects, major depressive symptoms respond to antidepressants that potentiate analgesia and sedation.

Delirium, in one study of patients during terminal illness, was found to be present in 85% of patients prior to death (Massie et al., 1983). These investigators found the causes of this dysfunction were usually multiple, resulting from narcotics, infection, and vital organ failure producing metabolic encephalopathy. Home care must deal with this common complication by explaining the disturbed behavior to relatives—particularly the frightening symptoms of hallucinations and agitation—and by providing sedation and reassurance for the patient. Some patients develop

panic, severe anxiety, or agitation with confusion as death approaches. This terminal anxiety is painful for patient and relatives alike. Its control requires reassurance and sedation with an antianxiety agent, increased analgesic, or addition of low-dosage major tranquilizer (see "Psychopharmacological Management," Chapter 39).

Personality disorders and major psychiatric illness, when they are present, must be managed. Control of physical symptoms may be impossible without attention to those psychiatric issues (see Part IV).

The family member with the key role in care and the closest relationship to the patient has all the existential concerns seen in the patient, including anxiety, depression, and anticipatory grief. In addition, however, he or she must carry on normal activities. These individuals report feeling overwhelmed; they experience guilt about inadequacies in meeting the patient's needs and transient wishes to get on with their lives. Conflicts with others, overriding concern about ability to manage the dying moments, and the sense of exhaustion, hopelessness, and helplessness are difficult to tolerate. Major depression can ensue; prior psychiatric problems recur. Bereavement after the death may call for counseling and monitoring for its severity and resolution.

The extent of the family's fatigue can have a profound effect on the patient. The patient's suicidal ideation, associated with being "a burden," are common, yet suicide is uncommon. Monitoring this is important, especially as a family begins to recognize the futility of treatment as a measure to slow progress of disease. The patient, without support, may sense this as abandonment. Communication between patient and the closest relative, however, may increase as the reality of the situation becomes apparent. As time together becomes shorter the relationship is likely to intensify. This may add to the burden during bereavement.

## CASE HISTORIES

The two case histories that follow demonstrate the multiple problems presented by patients and their families managed at home. One case demonstrates the primary problem in the patient, the other, in a family member.

### CASE REPORT

Mr. L., a 63-year-old married architect who had been treated for colon cancer by surgical resection and placement of a permanent colostomy, developed metastatic disease in the liver and lung within a year, with marked physical impairment.

He had been treated in the past for major depression and

was noted to have an obsessive-compulsive personality. Everything in his home was organized exactly as he wished it to be, including his wife's activities at home and work. He had found learning to manage the colostomy to be a difficult and upsetting task, especially because of his concerns about smells and "accidents." When hospitalized, he was intolerant of waiting for medication or transport to tests. He would become panicky and angry. Evaluation in the hospital by the psychiatrist revealed a profoundly depressed mood, moderate pain, despair about the progressing illness, and thoughts of suicide. He was unable to sleep and had had anorexia over the past 3 months with a 25-pound weight loss. His wife had found the marriage difficult for many years and had increasingly relied on her work to compensate for an unsatisfactory marriage.

Placed on amitriptyline (75 mg hs) and acetominophen/oxycodone (q4h) for pain, Mr. L. became calmer but was felt to constitute a difficult case for home care during advanced illness without assistance for the wife. Referral was made to the psychiatric nurse-clinician for follow-up at home.

An initial home visit identified the need for the wife to continue her work and to have a homemaker for 4 hours per day. Increasing disease and debilitation resulted in a mild encephalopathy with episodes of confusion managed by haloperidol (2 mg bid). Mr. L. received a telephone call every day and was told that he could call the nurse any time in an emergency. Weekly visits were made.

His response to consistent attention and medication proved successful. With control of pain and distress, his appetite and sleep improved and he gained 30 pounds. Depression decreased and he became more able to tolerate his frustrations. He was able to return to work for 12 months.

He was readmitted to the hospital for reconstruction of the bowel and removal of the colostomy at the end of the 12 months. Surgical exploration, however, revealed extensive disease including liver metastases. A debulking procedure was done. A partial obstruction of the small bowel developed shortly afterward and Mr. L.'s depression returned. He did not wish to return home because he felt too weak to direct his own care and he believed that his wife was not capable of managing his care. His attitude reinforced Mrs. L.'s feelings of inadequacy; she did not attempt to transfer care to home. Over 2 weeks, he became lethargic, developed hallucinations and confusion related to hepatic failure, and died in a coma 5 days later.

This case is an example of the frequent presence of depression, delirium, and pain in patients with advanced disease who respond well to symptom control and who may, with good management, have a considerable period of time with good quality of life. In this case, underlying marital problems and the patient's personality were too severe to support final illness and actual death at home.

## CASE REPORT

Mrs. P., a 40-year-old divorced woman, was found at the time of diagnosis of cervical cancer to have infiltration into the retroperitoneal space and lumbar spine. Unable to work,

she gave up her apartment and moved in with her sister, brother-in-law, and their 3-year-old child, as well as her mother. Her own two children had lived with her former husband since the divorce 10 years earlier. Contact with the teenage son was minimal, but the 20-year-old daughter visited her mother once a week at the sister's apartment. Pain, the primary problem, was controlled by 60 mg of liquid morphine q2h. With help, she was able to get out of bed for short periods and to participate in family life. The family resisted all suggestions of additional help in the home until referral to the supportive care program.

The initial home visit disclosed that the patient was comfortable but able to do almost nothing for herself; even eating required some assistance. The sister worked full time for her husband, and was arising at 5 A.M. in order to wash Mrs. P.'s hair, get her bathed and into a clean nightgown, prepare and feed her breakfast. At night, hours were consumed with Mrs. P.'s evening care. Mrs. P.'s brother-in-law was becoming angry at the attention his wife was giving her sister, which he felt was at his expense. He wanted her to go on vacation with him, and was hurt at her refusal to leave her sister. He also was afraid of Mrs. P. dying in his home. He had never witnessed a death and as a child could remember members of his family dying and his father refusing to allow him to attend the funerals, sending him away from home. He felt it would be wrong to expose his young son to death. Mrs. P.'s 69-year-old mother was responsible for the care of her grandson and her ill daughter during the day; she also prepared the meals. She was convinced that a priest in Massachusetts could cure her daughter and refused to listen to anything negative about her daughter's condition. She stated that "voices" told her daily what would happen to her daughter. She had had them in the past with a psychiatric hospitalization but had been well since. A visual hallucination revealed a priest who accused her of failing to cure her daughter, permitting a devil to interfere. At night, she sat by her daughter's bed to protect her from the "devil."

The intervention began with the sister taking a week off from work to care for her son. Mrs. P.'s daughter was given the responsibility of her mother's evening care. Through the visiting nurse service, an aide was arranged for 4 hours a day, to take over the morning care of the patient and prepare meals for the day. A folding bed was set up in Mrs. P.'s room so her mother could sleep beside her. Under the psychiatrist's direction, the mother was started on thioridazine. She was calmer 4 days later, was free of hallucinations, and was sleeping through the night.

As the family situation became calmer, the family accepted 24-hour nursing care. Mrs. P.'s sister went on a 1-week vacation with her husband. The nurse spent a significant amount of time with the brother-in-law. Several home visits were planned solely to see him. He was slowly able to allow his sister-in-law to remain in his home. With 24-hour nursing, he and his wife did not have to assume responsibility for Mrs. P.'s terminal care and he could therefore tolerate her dying in his home, although he anticipated the actual dying with trepidation. He constantly sought information about what to expect.

Mrs. P.'s mother began to accept the reality of her daughter's condition and the painful loss she anticipated.

Mrs. P. became comatose and the family made a joint decision to transfer her to an inpatient hospice program that allowed her mother to remain by her side. She died quietly 2 days later. Her mother tolerated the loss well, continuing to be followed for 6 months by the team, until she could be transferred to a local psychiatrist.

The unusual stressfulness of this situation exacerbated a prior schizoaffective illness in the mother, which responded to environmental manipulation and medication. The terminal care at home hinged on management of the total situation, including working with each individual in the family around their particular problems.

## MENTAL HEALTH OF THE TEAM

Home care exacts a great emotional toll on the team members. The mental health team member and the psychiatric backup should provide a monitoring function in this regard to assess how individual members are managing. Is their caseload realistic? Are they showing signs of stress and fatigue? Regular team meetings to discuss the caseload, deaths, and personal responses to the losses are invaluable. The stresses are offset, however, for most who work in this area by the rewards of assisting patients and families during this time of extreme crisis.

## SUMMARY

Most families who are committed to managing a dying member at home manage well with appropriate home care team support. Occasionally, however, preexisting mental illness in the patient and/or family member calls for more intensive intervention from psychiatric specialists. Using the same structure and approach outlined by Coyle and colleagues in the preceding chapter, a psychiatric nurse-clinician can serve to coordinate and implement successful care in these special cases.

## REFERENCES

Cassileth, B.R., E.J. Lusk, T.B. Strouse, D.S. Miller, L.L. Brown, and P.A. Cross (1985). A psychological analysis of cancer patients and their next-of-kin. *Cancer* 55:72–76.

Farkas, C. and M. Loscalzo (1987). An ultimate ideal in the care of dying patients should be that of death without indignity. In A.H. Kutscher and A.C. Carr (eds.), *Principles of Thanatology*. New York: Columbia University Press, 133–52.

Massie, M.J., J.C. Holland, and E. Glass (1983). Delirium in terminally ill cancer patients. *Am. J. Psychiatry* 140:8–9.

Plumb, M. and J.C. Holland (1977). Comparative study of psychological function in patients with advanced cancer. *Psychosom. Med.* 39:264–75.

# 50

## Bereavement: A Special Issue in Oncology

Harvey Chochinov and Jimmie C. Holland

The experience of the loss of loved ones by death is an inevitable part of adult life; the frequency of such losses increases as an individual grows older. In fact, the annual incidence of bereavement in the population is estimated between 5 and 9% (Imboden et al., 1963; Frost and Clayton, 1977). This large bereaved group is composed annually of those who have lost a parent (most often an older parent), a spouse, a child, or a sibling. While grief has certain universal characteristics, irrespective of the cause of death, it is still true that the circumstances of an illness or accident color the experience of the bereavement.

The likelihood of cancer being the cause of death is quite high, because 20% of all deaths are the result of some form of cancer (American Cancer Society, 1986). This means that one to two percent of the newly bereaved annually in the country are experiencing it as a result of cancer. A substantial part of these newly bereaved individuals will have been intimately involved for a period, sometimes lengthy, as next of kin or family member of the deceased during treatment for cancer. It is a salient aspect of grief resulting from cancer that there is usually a period of anticipatory grieving preceding the death. This fact presents both an opportunity and an obligation for oncologic specialists and their teams, because they are in a unique position to combine care and comfort of the patient with guidance of the family through the phases of terminal illness and death (Koocher, 1986). Done with concern and sensitivity, this can substantially affect the subsequent grieving in a positive way. In particular, the survivor remembers the details of the last days and how the painful issues were handled, how the grave prognosis was conveyed, how sensitive the staff were to family wishes to be present at the bedside, and how the news of death was conveyed. The survivor also has intense but mixed feelings about the oncologist and support staff because of this special role

they have had, and the memories that seeing them evoke. Because they knew the deceased and appreciated him or her as an individual during the fatal illness, they are the recipient of grateful feelings; yet also they are the sole source for answers to the nagging questions that accompany normal grief: ''Was everything done?'' ''What happened?'' ''Could it have been prevented?'' ''Were mistakes made?'' (Pasnau et al., 1987).

Thus, for the several reasons just outlined, those who work with cancer patients are in a unique position to evaluate and manage grief. Vachon (1987) points out that many patients who develop cancer have difficulty adjusting to it because of unresolved grief related to a prior loss. The oncologist also uniquely can assist the relative through anticipatory grieving and through bereavement after the patient's death. It is important that they be able to identify the patterns of normal grief, to expedite its expression, and to guide the individual toward return to normal activities. They should also be able to identify abnormal patterns of grieving for which professional help is indicated. The differentiation is not always easy. This chapter outlines some explanatory models of grief, including phases of grieving, types of abnormal grief reactions, the common psychological symptoms, and the physical morbidity and mortality associated with grief. Like cancer, many myths exist about grief and the frequency of individuals ''dying of a broken heart.'' The actual mortality, based on better controlled studies, appears to be less than previously assumed. The aspects that are special or different when bereavement follows death by cancer are discussed, as well as interventions that have been found effective.

While this chapter deals with bereavement from a medical viewpoint, one must put into perspective that religion is the spiritual and social institution that has been and remains the paramount source of solace and understanding of the meaning of loss by death for the majority of people. Each culture has its own religious practices and rituals that bring comfort. It is important that they also give meaning to a state after death that mitigates its finality. For many individuals, therefore, it is the solace given by the clergy that provides the most important support through painful grieving. The chaplain's role and consultation are critically important in assessing this aspect of a relative's needs in relation to impending or actual bereavement (see Chapter 57) (Rome, 1986).

For clarity of communication in an area where the terms grief, mourning, and bereavement have been used interchangeably, our use of these terms is consistent with the definitions of Osterweis and colleagues (1984) in the excellent monograph on bereavement, which is highly recommended for further reading.

*Bereavement* refers to the loss of someone through death. Bereavement reactions are the psychological, physiological, or behavioral responses to bereavement.

*Grief* is the feeling (affect) resulting from the loss and the associated behaviors such as crying; the grieving process is the changing affect over time.

*Mourning* is used, in the social science sense, to refer to the social expressions in response to loss and grief, including mourning rituals and behaviors that are specific to each culture and religion.

## MODELS FOR UNDERSTANDING BEREAVEMENT

Attempts to explain the phenomenology of normal bereavement and abnormal reactions has resulted in the development of several different models that provide a conceptual framework for understanding symptoms and interventions. The theoretical models are largely empirically derived; they overlap with one another at times in describing the same phenomena from different perspectives, and clinicians often find it easiest to use an eclectic approach in applying them (Osterweis et al., 1984). The models also suggest an increasing convergence of concepts between the psychodynamic and cognitive-behavioral, again supporting a conceptual approach to bereavement that does not adhere to a single rigid viewpoint.

The most thoroughly developed model is the psychodynamic one, based on psychoanalytical theory, which focuses on the intrapsychic processes of grief. According to this theory, the grieving process is accomplished by gradual withdrawal of emotional energy (libido) from the lost love object (Freud, 1976). Because relinquishing the tie is emotionally painful, symptoms of grief can be understood as an initial de-

nial of the loss followed by a period of preoccupation with thoughts of the deceased person during which memories are recalled and reviewed that permits ties to the deceased to be gradually withdrawn. The grief work is completed when the individual has emotional energy released to engage in new relationships.

The interpersonal model of bereavement is based on Bowlby's attachment theory (1977). He viewed the formation of attachment bonds to be instinctual and the psychosocial consequences of breaking them resulting in grieving symptoms. After observing children who were separated from parents in institutional settings, he viewed grieving symptoms as a reflection, initially of protest, followed by search in an attempt to recover the lost object, then despair and disorganization from the unsuccessful attempts, and, finally, resolution and reorganization through forming new ties (Bowlby, 1961, 1980). Parkes (1972) used attachment theory to describe similar phases of initial numbness followed by yearning for the person and efforts to achieve reunion through fruitless searching, resulting in motor restlessness, irritability, and tension. The repeated failures lead to disorganization, depression, disinterest, and despair, which signals the acceptance of the loss as permanent. Reorganization occurs as attachment to the deceased diminishes and new ties to others are established.

Studies of separation in animals has produced a psychobiological model of grief, which builds on attachment theory and has relevance for understanding the psychological and physiological symptoms of bereavement (Lewis et al., 1976). Hofer (1984) viewed attachment bonds as resulting in social interactions that serve as important regulators of internal biological systems throughout life. The behavioral and physiological symptoms of grief, especially the chronic ones, as opposed to the acute waves of distress, represent the withdrawal of the internal regulators that were the result of the emotionally meaningful and constant interactions with an individual to whom there was significant attachment.

Bereavement has also been examined in light of crisis theory in which it is recognized as one of the major stresses of life with both psychological and physiological consequences (Elliot and Eisdorfer, 1982; Osterweis et al., 1984). In fact, loss of spouse is regarded as the event resulting in most change in adult life (Holmes and Rahe, 1967). As such, it represents an acute stressful experience that places demands on coping; ineffective coping can result in major and prolonged disorganization, whereas effective coping may result in emotional growth.

These models provide explanations for the clinical features of normal grief. They are helpful in now exploring the clinical picture of uncomplicated (normal) bereavement and the range of abnormal reactions (American Psychiatric Association, 1987).

## CLINICAL FEATURES OF BEREAVEMENT

Most considerations of the clinical picture of grief begin with the actual loss. However, it is important in discussing the bereavement of those in whom the loss is the result of cancer, to give particular attention to the anticipatory period of grieving and the actual immediate responses to the death. This is important because terminal care in a hospice, hospital, nursing home, or at home allows an opportunity for interventions with family members, which can have a long-lasting impact on the survivor's grief when they are given by staff members who understand bereavement and its management. Thus, clinical features of normal and abnormal responses are described in the following paragraphs with relevance to the phases in which they appear in survivors of a relative's death by cancer, that is, anticipatory grief, responses to news of death, acute grief, and grieving reactions over time.

### Anticipatory Grief

The period of time when death is expected or appears highly likely is clearly a time of intellectual preparation for loss by the next of kin and for attempts at resolution of conflicts. While some observers feel the emotional responses of actual bereavement begin then (Bowlby, 1980; Brown and Stoudemier, 1983), others report observations that confirm our own experience that the true grieving for the loss does not begin until the death has occurred (Vachon et al., 1982a). The attachment is actually transiently enhanced by threat of loss by death. Many of us who work in oncology frequently see the strong efforts made by a relative to avoid facing the impending loss. Some simply refuse to believe it may happen and become angry when efforts to inform are made; many more hear the message but cannot encompass "What it will be like without him." They are emotionally unable to anticipate the loss. This period is often marked by defiant optimism, interspersed with periods of fear and despair that the death will actually occur.

Circumstances also alter the extent of anticipatory response. Relatives who keep their ill family member at home during terminal illness may experience the reality of impending death most intimately because they participate in physical care of the person and see the progressive changes in the body. Care at home and in a hospice also permits early bereavement counseling by the home care nurse or hospice staff (see Chapters 48 and 49). Irrespective of circumstances, advanced

stage of cancer is the time when relatives are told about the grave prognosis (Cassem, 1978). Increasingly today, they and the patient participate in discussions of their wishes about the use of heroic measures (see Chapter 6). Such discussions make impending death more real. In some cases of prolonged illness or pain, the death is seen rationally as a relief for the deceased from intolerable distress. Death is a "blessing," and a religious perspective helps in accepting the outcome as God's will.

Whether or not individuals experience anticipatory grief, the outcome of grief in which the loss is or is not anticipated is of interest here. There is agreement that sudden death, with little or no warning, has greater impact and produces longer lasting disorganization in the survivor than does death that follows warning and longer terminal illness. Parkes (1975) compared a group of survivors who had had less than 2 weeks warning of the seriousness of their spouse's condition and a terminal illness of less than 3 days, with another group who had had 2 weeks or more advance warning of impending death and longer than 3 days of terminal illness. He found much more intense psychological disturbance in those who had had little time to prepare; they remained more socially withdrawn and self-reproachful throughout the first year of bereavement. At 2–4 years later, the majority were still "trapped in a vicious circle of emotional disturbance and withdrawal." Nearly three-fourths or 72% had a moderate to severe level of anxiety and difficulties coping. Only 28% had a positive view of the future. By contrast, those who had anticipated the loss were more likely to have seen the death as a relief from a painful or prolonged illness, and they found less cause of self-reproach during bereavement. By 4 years, 90% were ready to date, and several had remarried. It is of interest that in a study of 30 young widows, of the 5 women who had considered suicide, none had had a chance for anticipatory grieving (Blanchard et al., 1976).

### Responses to News of Death

Ideally, a family should be present at the time of death if they wish to be (Engel, 1964). However, when they are not present, they should be notified as soon as possible. Informing them by telephone is not desirable and usually leaves strong negative feelings. There is no easy way to give news of death, and physicians and nurses receive little instruction in how to handle such sensitive communications. It is usually learned by on-the-job training. There are some caveats in handling the situation that make the bad news easier to hear. It is important because the details of the encounter will be remembered and recounted in great detail for years to come by the bereaved relative, expressing gratitude for a caring manner or anger at perceived insensitivity.

Ideally, the news should be conveyed by the physician who took care of the patient during the illness and who knows the surviving relatives well enough to be able to frame the news in a manner that anticipates the likely responses. Because it is not always possible for the responsible physician to be present, another person, preferably one who is also known to the family, should convey the information. Taking the family member to a quiet place where expression of emotion will not be embarrassing is helpful. Having a relative present is also desirable, so that the person has someone to turn to for comfort. The immediate reaction is usually one of shock and disbelief, even when the death was expected, reflecting the initial phase of bereavement. The range of emotions elicited vary from the stoic and unemotional to hysteria. After the initial response has subsided, it is important that the relative or family be offered time alone with the body of the deceased. This may be comforting and also reinforces the reality. Further discussion should answer medical questions. A full and clear explanation of medical circumstances surrounding death should be given by the responsible doctor present. Open responsiveness to questions and discussion allow the bereaved to understand intellectually the circumstances that led to death and may alleviate misconceptions of personal responsibility ("If I had only not agreed to the surgery"). These facts may need to be stated again later when the family is calmer, can absorb the facts, and wish another discussion of the circumstances around the death.

One of the most controversial and sensitive issues when death occurs in the hospital is the request for autopsy. This task has traditionally been assigned to the house officer, although it should ideally be done by the responsible physician, with great sensitivity for the feelings of the grieving family. While autopsy rates have declined alarmingly because far fewer efforts are made to obtain permission, it is still important with respect to cancer when the cause of death, extent of disease, or response to treatment may be unclear. The information obtained will be of value to the doctor and may clarify the facts leading to death for the family. Neoplasms that have hereditary patterns may be of interest for autopsy study to inform a family better about familial risk. These positive aspects should be emphasized, but the families' decision should be emphatically accepted, irrespective of their choice (Reynolds, 1978).

It is important that the physician follow through by meeting with the family to discuss the results of the autopsy and to provide an opportunity for further questions when the full pathology report is available. Relatives sometimes are tormented by questions that can only be answered with these data. This discussion also allows a follow-up visit with the bereaved in which normal grieving feelings can be explored (Green, 1984).

Pathological responses occur infrequently at the time of learning of the death of a relative. They are usually transient, but some extreme reactions occur that require immediate intervention to assure comfort and safety. The poignancy of the moment complicates the ability to manage the situation expeditiously at times. However, prior psychiatric problems may be exacerbated at this time and result in threat of harm to self or others. Several case reports demonstrate pathological responses that occur.

### CASE REPORTS

*Inability to separate.* Following the death of her 10-year-old boy in the intensive care unit after lengthy treatment for osteogenic sarcoma, the mother clutched her son's body, appearing in a reverie state that responded little to attempts by the staff to encourage her to leave. After half an hour, the staff found it difficult to continue with other routine care. It was clear that attempts to insist that she leave were not heard. She was told she could remain and family members sat with her for another hour. She slowly emerged from her dazed state as family gradually persuaded her to return home with them.

*Homicidal intent.* A 45-year-old father with a history of emotional instability and erratic behavior appeared more and more disturbed during the vigil in his child's room as the child's condition worsened. He began to make menacing overtures toward the doctor, whom he blamed for the downward turn of the illness. When he was told that the child was dead, he became angry, found the doctor, verbally threatened his life, and attempted to hit him. Relatives forcibly held him and took him home. Over the following days, the father recovered and recognized that his anger was at the death itself, not the doctor who had done his best for the child. He later returned to the hospital and apologized for his behavior. Until then, however, the young doctor traveled to and from the hospital with an escort, because the history of prior violent episodes in the father was cause for concern for impulsive violent behavior.

*Suicidal intent.* The wife of a 35-year-old painter had indicated her strong wish to die with her husband. As his illness from cancer progressed and death was near, she took an overdose of diazepam (Valium) in his room. She was found lethargic, the bottle of pills empty. She received emergency treatment for drug intoxication and was hospitalized. Several days later, she recovered and said that she was glad the attempt had failed because she had failed her husband. With relatives accompanying her, she maintained her place at her husband's bedside. She accepted the news of his death with distress, but expressed that she felt the need to carry out several projects that her husband had been unable to complete.

## Acute Grief

The first systematic study of acute grief was reported in 1944 by Lindemann based on his observations of the grief of those who lost relatives in the Boston Coconut Grove nightclub disaster. He described the clinical course of grief and major symptoms of somatic distress, preoccupation with the image of the deceased, guilt, hostility, loss of usual patterns of conduct, and assumption of symptoms or traits of the deceased. The behavioral and physiological symptoms described by Lindemann were used by Hofer (1984) to present his psychobiological perspective on bereavement (Table 50-1). The waves of acute distress coming on several times a day and lasting minutes, are typical of the first few days of acute grief. Although the initial numbness may be continuously present, waves of distress triggered by reminders of the deceased are characterized by agitation, crying, aimless activity, preoccupation with images of the deceased, tears, sighing respirations, choking, and a sense of muscular weakness. In fact, the bereaved person begins to try desperately to avoid stimuli that will precipitate a wave of acute distress.

The constant background disturbance, with the superimposed acute-distress episodes, is characterized by behavioral changes of social withdrawal, decreased concentration, restlessness, anxiety, altered appetite, sad appearance, depressed mood, illusions of the presence of the deceased, dreams, and even hallucinations of hearing or seeing the deceased. Physiologically, weight loss, sleep disturbance, weakness, and cardiovascular, endocrine, and immunological changes develop concurrently with the behavioral changes. Preoccupation with events around death, searching for mistakes, or feeling guilt for not doing enough, are typical. The bereaved feels distant from others, lacking in emotional response to them, and may express anger and envy at seeing others together. This period of acute disorganization is often structured for the individual by the mourning rituals of receiving friends, preparing for the funeral and burial. The individual is seldom left alone, and the sense of numbness may persist as the person goes mechanically through the funeral and expected activities. Families who choose to forego any rituals sometimes suffer more because normal activity is emotionally impossible, and absence of social rituals, such as the funeral, can add to the sense of unreality and disbelief that it has happened. The rituals serve to reinforce the reality of the loss and

**Table 50-1** Bereavement in the human adult

| Behavior | Physiology |
| --- | --- |
| *Acute: Waves of distress, lasting minutes* | |
| Agitation | Tears |
| Crying | Sighing respiration |
| Aimless activity–inactivity | Muscular weakness |
| Preoccupation with image of deceased | |
| *Chronic: Background disturbance, lasting weeks to months* | |
| Social withdrawal | Decreased body weight |
| Decreased concentration, attention | Sleep disturbance |
| Restlessness, anxiety | Muscular weakness |
| Decreased or variable food intake | Cardiovascular changes |
| Postures and facial expressions of sadness | Endocrine changes |
| | Immunological changes |
| Illusions, hallucinations | |
| Depressed mood | |

*Source*: Reprinted with permission from M.A. Hofer (1984). Relationships as regulators: A psychobiologic perspective on bereavement. *Psychosom. Med.* 46:184.

reduce the unreality, which encourages hope of return of the deceased (Averill, 1968).

Acute grief, with its characteristic waves, difficulty concentrating and functioning, was noted by Lindemann (1944) to last for about 6 weeks. This is generally true because most individuals begin to return to some level of function by that time, but the variability is great. Acute grief may be extended in widows who were extremely dependent on their husbands and in whom steps to function independently require an entirely new and unfamiliar set of activities. It may be prolonged, continuing with acute symptoms unabated, in a parent who loses a child. A birthday or holiday will result in marked exacerbation of the first days of grief; in fact "special days" come to be dreaded for the pain they cause (Barton, 1977).

Concerned relatives will usually seek help for the bereaved person in the first 6 weeks of acute grief if an abnormal response appears. Reasons for consultation may be due to a troubled psychological response, psychiatric symptoms or adverse physical sequelae. When the deceased died of cancer, it is not uncommon for the bereaved to fear that they have also developed it. A transient cancerophobia may ensue, confirming the observations of Zisook and colleagues (1982) on the bereaved person's identification with the deceased's disease and symptoms (see Chapter 2). Physiological symptoms may become cause for alarm; if weight loss is extreme, agitation precludes rest, or sleeplessness produces chronic fatigue. Medication to reestablish patterns of sleep each night may be important. If the daytime is experienced with high anxiety, irritability, and agitation, a low dose of a benzodiazepine may allow rest. While medication should be given judiciously, our experience is that a low dose to control particularly distressing symptoms actually expedites the bereavement process rather than inhibiting its expression (see the following intervention).

## CASE REPORT

Julia, a 35-year-old married Italian woman, appeared for psychiatric consultation following her younger sister's death from disseminated lung cancer. She had appeared to cope very well. She arranged the funeral, settled outstanding financial and legal matters, and became guardian of her sister's two preschool children. Within 2 weeks, however, she could not cope with daily routines. Everything was a reminder of her sister, which elicited waves of overwhelming grief. Irritability, anxiety, restlessness, and insomnia also made carrying on daily tasks more difficult. She reluctantly spoke of an occasional feeling that she could hear her sister's voice calling her name; fear that she might be losing her mind resulted in her seeking psychiatric consultation. Over 3 months, she expressed her great sense of loss, came to understand that her responses were normal, and slowly regained full activity.

## Grieving Reactions Over Time

The initial phase of denial of the loss, followed by intense distress, is finally followed by the phase of coming to terms with the loss over the succeeding months as the reality of the death is gradually accepted. It is during these first 12 months that symptoms of grief most resemble depression, and, indeed, it may be impossible immediately to differentiate them. Clayton and colleagues (1974) found crying, depressed mood, and sleep disturbance as the cardinal symptoms during the first year of bereavement. Depression was a problem for 45% of the survivors at some time during the first year, and 13% were still depressed at a year. Clayton (1974) found that when the symptoms in 34 bereaved individuals were matched with those of an equal number of depressed patients, they could not be differentiated on objective criteria for depression. Eventually the bereaved enters a phase of reorganization in which symptoms diminish, old roles are given up, and memories of the deceased can be recalled without sadness. The resolution and readiness for reinvestment in new relationships marks the recovery. The term, however, should not imply full return to the prior emotional state.

These symptoms fall within what is called normal or uncomplicated bereavement. However, within the context of normality there are a range of reactions observed in psychologically healthy individuals. Some require interventions to assure recovery. Several types of reactions are illustrated by case reports.

## CASE REPORTS

*Guilt complicating grief.* A father came to the psychologist at the request of his wife and the oncologist of his deceased son. His 5-year-old son had died 4 months earlier of acute leukemia. He had held himself responsible for the death by not responding to a mild temperature elevation at home, which was the onset of an opportunistic infection from which the boy died in 24 hours. The father vowed never to forget and made daily visits to the cemetery, ignoring the grief and needs of his wife and two older sons. Insight gained over six sessions with the psychologist led to his understanding that this outcome could not have been changed; recognition of his family's needs led to reinvestment in them.

*Survivor guilt.* A childless 50-year-old wife of a devoted husband experienced his death from lung cancer as the end of her life as well. She wished for death, although she would not attempt suicide. She attempted to respond to friend's social gestures, but felt that laughing or experiencing pleasure indicated a lack of dedication to her dead husband. She felt acutely guilty that she could still enjoy life when he could not. She progressively isolated herself, and only the assistance of psychotherapy sessions over several months permitted her to reinvest in activities and friends.

Grief, for all its negative emotions, may be a time of emotional growth, as new responsibilities must be assumed.

## CASE REPORT

*Grief as a stimulus for maturation.* A 40-year-old woman had experienced lifelong dependence on her mother for making decisions for her. Daily phone calls set the pattern of closeness, despite marriage and teenage children. The mother's short illness and death from pancreatic cancer was initially devastating, and acute grief was painful as she missed the source of direction. However, as her family supported her independence, she became more decisive and made an unusually good adjustment, beginning to become a less passive member of the family in activities and planning.

Seeking a fitting memorial to a dear one who has died is another way of handling grief. Many valuable organizations and groups have been developed in response to efforts to help others or memorialize the deceased. The Widow-to-Widow Program grew out of an apparent need of such a group for other women. Candlelighters and Compassionate Friends developed to help parents of ill and deceased children. Many gifts for patient care and cancer research are made in memory of an individual with the intent of improving care for others with the same disease or to support research to prevent others from dying of the same disease. Sometimes the contribution is one of becoming a dedicated volunteer, as the following case illustrates.

## CASE REPORT

*Volunteer for patients.* A single 35-year-old woman came regularly to comfort her mother during a protracted course in the hospital with advanced pelvic cancer. She and her mother were pleasant, cheerful, and loved by the staff. The loss of the mother was shared by the staff. After the daughter recovered from the acute grief, she returned and became a volunteer, assisting patients in obtaining things needed for their comfort. She enjoyed visits to the staff who could reminisce about her mother.

How long normal grieving should continue is a frequent question. There is a common assumption that grief should be resolved by 1 year. For example, the unveiling of the grave headstone on the first anniversary of the death may, like the funeral, be a mourning ritual that points to the end of the formal mourning period. Whereas most individuals are functioning and returning to normal by that time, many are not. Often relatives and friends become annoyed and diminish their support for the bereaved person who continues to grieve actively, sometimes for much longer than a year (Barton, 1977). This is seen often in parents who do not recover fully from loss of a child, and in some spouses.

A 4-year follow-up of widows and widowers by Zisook and Schuchter (1985) provided useful information by pointing out that individual variability is great and chronicity of bereavement is not uncommon. In fact, the time course for grief in their observations was much more prolonged than is generally expected. Affective distress reduced over time, but several widows were still tearful and depressed at 4 years. Guilt diminished, but anger toward those held responsible for the loss persisted in almost 10% of survivors. A continued relationship to the deceased through thoughts and visual images was found; the deceased remained with them indefinitely, so often it was considered part of the norm. Despite this, 23% were remarried by 4 years and 40% were living with someone of the opposite sex. At 4 years, 44% rated an excellent adjustment, but 20% saw their adjustment as fair to poor. Their physical health was unimpaired, except for aging. Most saw themselves and the world in positive terms. These findings suggest that normal grief may often be an ongoing lifelong process, bringing into question the concept that normal grief is a process in which resolution by loss of attachment to the deceased occurs in a circumscribed time period. These observations of the spouse's slow recovery are evidence that our concepts of normal grief need to be reexamined and extended.

## PATHOLOGICAL BEREAVEMENT REACTIONS

Distinguishing between normal and morbid forms of grief is difficult because the abnormal responses largely reflect a greater intensity, a prolongation, or an aberration of normal grief (Volkan, 1966; Worden,

1982). The common forms seen in relation to cancer are chronic grief, cumulative losses and grief, and grief preceding major depression.

### Chronic Grief

This common grief reaction, also called unresolved grief, is marked by continuous symptoms of grief typical of early stages of loss that continue unchanged as grief fails to resolve (Parkes and Weiss, 1983; DeVaul and Zisook, 1976). It is seen often in older women who have lived as the dependent partner in a long marriage. The failure to work through the grief maintains a relationship with the lost spouse and precludes resolution. As a result, the surviving spouse cannot permit resolution despite efforts of those around him or her to assist.

These bereavement reactions often have poor outcome. Clayton and Darvish (1979) found that 12–15% of widowed had unremitting symptoms consistent with clinical depression at 1 year. The connection between clinical depression and bereavement is still unclear. Paykel and co-workers (1969) studied life events in 185 depressed hospitalized and ambulatory psychiatric patients and compared them to a matched community control group. In this sample, 16 of the depressed and 4 of the control group reported death of an immediate family member in the 6 months prior to the onset of the illness. They concluded that losses and events viewed as undesirable distinguished the depressed patients from the control group.

### Cumulative Losses and Grief

Particularly in older individuals, one may see loss of a spouse by cancer followed by loss of independent living because of debts or physical inability to manage alone. The multiple losses of the several aspects of prior life patterns may lead to a difficult and slow recovery. Grief may fail to abate. If depressive symptoms increase, this can be a difficult diagnostic problem requiring judgment about when treatment should be directed toward resolution of normal grief or toward treatment of major depression.

CASE REPORT

A 65-year-old man was seen during the impending death of his wife from colon cancer. He was devoted to her and came for consultation because of his fears that he might become severely depressed because he had had a prior depression 20 years earlier that required hospitalization. He tolerated the death, but 4 months later he became more depressed, agitated, and distraught, and made a suicide attempt. He was hospitalized and improved over 3 weeks to the point that he was able to express his grief more directly. After 6 months he began to seek social contacts and improved despite continuing periods when he acutely missed his wife.

Although studies of treatment of these depressive states emerging from grief are few, our clinical experience and that of others suggest that antidepressants are useful to reduce the dysfunction or dysphoria which are symptoms of major depression. The reduction of symptoms actually facilitates grieving and does not inhibit it (Zisook and Schuchter, 1985; Jacobs, Nelson and Zisook, 1987).

## Grief Preceding Major Depression

Studies of predictors of poor bereavement outcome vary with regard to both the prevalence of mental disorders complicating bereavement outcome and the specific predictors. An association between bereavement and psychiatric hospitalization and care has been shown (Parkes, 1964, 1965; Stein and Susser, 1969). However, it appears overall that about 20% of bereaved individuals (estimates vary from 10 to 36% in individual studies) will develop a psychiatric disorder, primarily depression. Most of those can be expected when one or more of the known predictors of poor outcome are present. These include poor social support, prior psychiatric history, unanticipated death, other significant stresses or losses, high level of initial distress with depressive symptoms, and death of a child (Table 50-2). The first perception that there is no one to talk to or lean on, with the environment failing to meet emotional needs, appears to be a reliable predictor of poor outcome by several investigators (Vachon et al., 1982b; Maddison and Walker, 1967).

Not unexpectedly, prior mental health problems predict poor outcome. A history of alcoholism increases the suicide risk and likelihood of psychiatric hospitalization shortly after bereavement (Murphy and Robins, 1967; Robins et al., 1977). Prior dependence on alcohol, drugs (especially tranquilizers or hypnotic medication), and tobacco predicts increased consumption during bereavement. Mortality data confirm the adverse effects of abuse of these substances on physical health by the increased risk of death by suicide, cirrhosis, and cardiovascular disease.

High initial distress with many depressive symptoms is a predictor of depression at a year (Bornstein et al., 1973; Vachon et al., 1982b). Unanticipated loss, especially in younger widows, or a lengthy period devoted to care of a spouse prior to death, are associated with poorer outcome. The presence of other losses or stresses also complicate recovery. The history of a turbulent marital relationship has not been well confirmed as a risk factor, but it may be assumed that the bereavement is more difficult. Grief is often difficult and outcome is poor in the older woman whose married life spanned the era when homemaking was primary and the husband's role was central in her life. These

**Table 50-2** Predictors of poor bereavement outcome

- Perception of poor social supports
- Prior psychiatric history
- High initial distress with depressive symptoms
- Unanticipated death
- Other significant life stresses and losses
- Prior high dependency on the deceased who provided key support
- Death of a child

widows, uncommonly dependent, often never recover from the loss of the husband.

While few systematic comparisons have been made between the bereavement following the loss of a spouse and a child, Sanders (1979–1980) noted that those who had lost a child had more intense grief reactions with more somatic symptoms, greater depression, anger, guilt, and a loss of meaning and purpose in life. Such a loss is tragic at any age, but the sense of unfairness of a life unfulfilled enhances the sense of anger. A longer and slower recovery period should be expected as well; in fact, grief sometimes intensifies over time. Even so, in a study of 263 bereaved parents, mothers grieved more than fathers, healthy children were grieved for more than ill children, and boys more than girls (Littlefield and Rushton, 1986).

Because death by leukemia and childhood tumors, especially brain tumors, account for 18% of childhood deaths, understanding the bereavement of a parent, irrespective of the age of the child, is important.

### CASE REPORT

*Protracted but normal grief.* A mother of a 17-year-old daughter who died of Hodgkin's disease experienced the loss as painful to the point of inability over the first year to share the loss or any pleasures with her husband. He also grieved quietly, but attempted to hide it from his wife. He felt abandoned and unable to reach her. Psychotherapy with this couple diminished the wife's withdrawal, as she realized her husband's pain. She improved but did not return to her prior outgoing manner. Resigning herself to a loss that she would always feel, she put her grief aside to allow her to give emotionally to her husband. At 3 years she was functioning, with the exception of anniversaries, birthdays, and holidays, which were dreaded and spent away from home when possible.

Participation in the care of a terminally ill child appears to help parents cope, as well as a sense that they communicated closely with the child about the reality of the situation. Rando (1983) found that, as shown with the loss of a spouse, parents who lost a child fared better when the loss was not sudden and death from cancer followed 6–18 months of illness. Deciding about home versus hospital care is an important task for parents (Martinson et al., 1980). The place chosen is less important than their commitment to the choice, because good and poor outcomes occur with both. The impact on siblings at home, though largely positive, has not been fully assessed and, as noted in Chapter 2, the prevalence of overprotection of surviving siblings by the anxious parents, with later hypochondriacal fears of illness and death, is high.

Spinetta and colleagues (1981) found that parents who coped better with their child's death had a philosophy of life (religious or not) and could find some meaning for their loss. Divorce does not appear to be more prevalent but the differential rate of recovery of the parents (with the grief of fathers being briefer than mothers) can reduce the expected supportive communication and sharing of the loss. Replacement children are never a true replacement of the lost child, and advice about postponing a pregnancy until grieving for the child is diminished, if not resolved, should be part of counseling.

The age at which a child dies has an impact on the bereavement, whether as a young child, adolescent, or young adult. The loss appears equally severe at all ages, and bereavement is different but not less painful. Much less studied is the response to the loss of an adult child by middle-aged or older parents. However, clinical experience indicates that they feel vulnerable, unprotected by their child's absence, and severed from their hope for the future through their child. Grief may be similarly intense and protracted.

## HEALTH CONSEQUENCES OF BEREAVEMENT

It has long been widely assumed that bereavement predisposes individuals to exacerbation of existing disease and places them at increased risk of death. The psychosomatic diseases were particularly considered to be exacerbated by threat or actual loss. Anecdotal reports of onset of a range of diseases, including cancer, have readily identified a recent loss in the individual's history. However, the few large studies that have prospectively examined health consequences of bereavement have found a much less clear relationship, for both increased mortality and exacerbation of an existing disease. This discrepancy in retrospective and prospective studies of adverse health consequences of bereavement is well reviewed in the monograph of Osterweis, Solomon, and Green (1984), which concludes that some individuals, though fewer than assumed, are at increased risk of mortality. Whether this comes about by altered behaviors and loss of normal life-style patterns that occur with grieving, such as altered diet, drinking, and smoking, or whether some psychophysiological changes occur that enhance risk is unclear and remains of great research interest. The question whether grief might serve as an initiator or promoter of a malignant process has been asked repeatedly.

The psychobiological model of bereavement proposed by Hofer (1984) is of interest in considering the effects on health. Table 50-1 outlines the physiological consequences, which include effects on the cardiovascular, endocrine, and immunological systems. The concept of interruption of an ongoing relationship causing disruption of biological homeostasis and, thereby, vulnerability to disease—particularly through the endocrine and immune systems—is intriguing in light of the morbidity associated with bereavement.

The seminal psychoendocrine studies by Hofer and colleagues (1972) of parents during the fatal illness and death of their child from leukemia provided the first information on psychological and pituitary-adrenocortical system response to a stressful life event and bereavement. They found that the effectiveness of the psychological defenses modulated the level of cortisol. At 6 months and 2 years after death, cortisol levels generally related to the extent of active grieving, although not all parents fit this pattern.

Two studies have examined immunological function during bereavement. Bartrop and colleagues (1977) in Australia studied the stimulation responses of phytohemagglutinin and concanavalin A on the lymphocytes of widows and widowers, as well as age-matched nonbereaved individuals. Lymphocyte response to the mitogens was significantly lower at 2 months after the loss. Schleifer and co-workers (1983) examined mitogen responses in men before and after the death of their wives from breast cancer. The depressed lymphocyte response was seen only in the bereavement period and was apparent within 1 month. It is of interest, however, that in neither study did perturbations reach levels consistent with clinical immunosuppression.

Irwin, Daniels, and Weiner (1987) extended these studies to examine bereavement, depressive symptoms, NK activity, and T cell subpopulations in three groups of women: those who anticipated their husbands' death from lung cancer, women who were bereaved, and a control group. NK activity was significantly lower in the group anticipating the loss and those studied after the death. Severity of depressive symptoms correlated with reduced NK activity and changes in the ratio of T helper to T suppressor cells, suggesting that the role of depressive symptoms may be more important than the loss per se. Cortisol, elevated only during bereavement, could not be solely responsible for the changes.

Questions still exist as to the clinical significance of the changes in immune function in relation to altering vulnerability to disease. For example, despite the

**Table 50-3**  Summary of major morbidity and mortality associated with bereavement

| Morbidity | Mortality |
|---|---|
| ↑ Psychological distress | ↑ Mortality, largely in older |
| ↑ Physical symptoms | men |
| ↑ Use of health services | Causes of death nonspecific |
| ↑ Self-medication for distress (alcohol, smoking, drugs) | except for infectious diseases, cirrhosis, suicide, and accidents |
| Poor outcome in 20% of bereaved; most predictable by high-risk factors | |

**Table 50-4**  Mortality after widowhood, 1963–1975*

| Sex | Mortality influences |
|---|---|
| Men | Higher for widowed (age 55–74) Lower after remarriage |
| Women | Same for widowed and married Same after remarriage |
| Both | Higher living alone Higher moving to nursing home Not elevated in first year |

*$n = 4032$.
*Source*: From Helsing and Szklo (1981).

stress of their child's illness and death, parents do not develop new illnesses nor do they develop frequent colds or minor illnesses (Martinson et al., 1980). Our observations support this also, even though they smoke and use alcohol and drugs excessively to reduce tension.

Levav and colleagues (1988) have reported a 9-year follow-up study of Israeli parents who lost a son either in the Yom Kippur War or by an accident, to determine their mortality. Neither group of parents had a greater mortality when compared to that of the Israeli general population. There was a subset of parents, those who were widowed or divorced, who had an increased mortality; however, significance was reached only in mothers. Another large and well-designed study by Jones and co-workers (1984) did not find greater mortality among the surviving spouses of those whose partners' death was due to cancer. More studies are needed to clarify the concurrent physiological changes with bereavement and their clinical implications.

The actual health consequences of bereavement that are known are interesting in light of the associated endocrine and immune changes. They can be summarized in the major areas of increased psychological distress, increased physical symptoms, increased use of health services, increased reliance on self-medication for distress (by evidence of increased smoking, drinking, and use of drugs—each contributing to the adverse health consequences), and poor bereavement outcome in 20%, most identifiable by known predictors (Table 50-3). Increased mortality associated with bereavement is not of the magnitude previously assumed. It is discussed later.

The epidemiological studies of mortality following bereavement are based largely on 10 major studies that are described in the review by Osterweis, Solomon, and Green (1984). The most definitive studies on mortality after bereavement were reported by Helsing and colleagues in 1981 and 1982. The 1963 health census of 91,909 persons was followed for 12 years, with the widowed population during that period matched to a

married demographically similar population at the time; both were followed prospectively for mortality. Table 50-4 outlines the findings for both sexes, which showed no elevated mortality in the first year (suggesting failure to confirm increased mortality from existing disease), but greater mortality in both sexes among those living alone or having moved to a nursing home. Women had no greater mortality, irrespective of being widowed or remarrying. Men, however, had an increased mortality that was confined to older ages 55–74, unless remarriage occurred, which returned them to the same risk as their married counterparts (Helsing and Szklo, 1981). Figure 50-1 shows the sex and age differences. Table 50-5 outlines their findings on

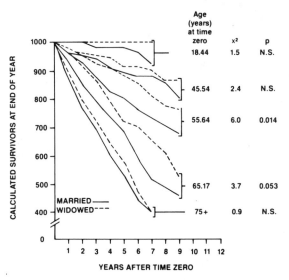

**Figure 50-1.**  Calculated survivorship of widowed (broken lines) and married (solid lines) by years after time zero, for white males of ages indicated: Washington County, Maryland, 1963–1975. Note that $\chi^2$ (1 *df*) calculations are for entire 12 years of study by procedure suggested by Peto et al. (28). N.S., Not significant. *Source:* Reprinted with permission from K.J. Helsing and M. Szklo (1981). Mortality after bereavement. *Am. J. Epidemiol.* 114:49–50.

**Table 50-5** Causes of death (777 widowed, 604 married)

- More deaths occurred among widowed than among married subjects.
- Significant causes of disease-related death, though representing only a small portion of overall excess: men—infectious diseases, accidents, suicide; women—dirrhosis
- "Greater mortality is remarkable nonspecific as to its causes."
- Widowed with chronic disease did not show earlier mortality after bereavement.

*Source*: From Helsing et al. (1982).

causes of death among 777 widowed and 604 married individuals. There was greater mortality among the widowed, but the greater mortality was remarkably nonspecific as to its cause. Several diseases were individually significant in cause of death, but they represented only a small portion of the overall excess: infectious diseases, accidents, and suicide in men; and, cirrhosis in women. The absence of any overrepresentation of cancer is important to note in this large prospective study.

Immune changes during grief must be interpreted with particular caution about their clinical relevance in light of these prospective data, which revealed no increased risk of cancer of any site among widowed individuals. In fact, immunosuppressed individuals, with AIDS or chemically induced immunosuppression (to reduce rejection of organ and bone marrow transplants), experience increased risk of only specific malignancies that include lymphomas and Kaposi's sarcoma. They do not develop other neoplasms with greater frequency.

## BEREAVEMENT FOLLOWING SPECIFIC LOSSES

Other specific losses that warrant particular attention are loss of a parent or sibling during adulthood and loss of a parent or sibling during childhood.

### Loss of Parent in Adulthood

The loss of a parent, particularly an older parent, is a loss that is expected in adult life. In one study 5% of the population had lost one parent in the prior year (Pearlin and Lieberman, 1979). Although it has been studied less than other losses of adulthood, it appears that adults have usually made other attachments and have busy lives that may make the bereavement brief. However, bereavement can be more pronounced and the death more traumatic than what is usually assumed, especially for the daughter or son who has been physically and emotionally close to the deceased. Loss of the mother may be particularly difficult. A lengthy illness of the parent from cancer, requiring extensive

care by a son or particularly a daughter, may result in a more severe bereavement because of the loss of the nurturing role and that the parent had been an integral part of daily life. The death may mean the loss of security, loss of the child role, and assumption of the role of oldest and most responsible family member. It may therefore result in a new level of maturation for the adult child (see earlier case report, *Grief as a stimulus for maturation*).

### Loss of Sibling in Adulthood

Attachment to siblings usually continues into adulthood, which means that death may result in severe bereavement. It often forces an examination of the relationship to other members of the family, resulting in increased sensitivity and concern for surviving members. In neoplasms with high familial incidence, such as in familial polyposis, colon cancer, and breast cancer, the meaning of death of a sibling may carry guilt that another sibling carried the trait and died, but also anxiety about the vulnerability of the survivor to the same disease.

### Bereavement during Childhood

The most painful losses for a child are those of a parent or sibling during childhood. The immediate and long-term consequences have been studied more for parental loss. The age of the child at the time of the loss is of primary importance, because age determines the understanding of death. (See Chapter 43 for review of developmental issues and children's concept of death.) Briefly, it is believed that prior to age 3, death is seen as reversible. From ages 5 to 9, the child comprehends a finality but views it more in terms of a separation. After ages 9–10, a more mature understanding of death and its biological finality develops (Nagy, 1948). It may be, however, that just as observed with children with severe illness who seem to mature more rapidly in the understanding of death, presence of an ill parent or sibling during a lengthy illness with obvious physical deterioration may hasten awareness of death as a cessation of life.

As described with adult bereavement, the anticipation of death from cancer sometimes allows an opportunity for the preparation of a child for the parent's death. Many parents request advice at this time about how much to tell and when they should tell their children about their impending death. Intervention with a family at this time is helpful to monitor reactions and assure that the family is dealing with all members in a constructive way.

A program at Memorial Sloan-Kettering Cancer Center (MSKCC) has provided support for children of terminally ill parents to help them and the family face the impending loss. Especially helpful for the parents is guidance in handling information with the child by a social worker experienced in grief counseling, and counseling about decisions that bear long-term consequences on the child's adjustment after the death (Adams-Greenly and Moynihan, 1983).

Bereavement symptoms in children are variable, but usually include sadness, a sense of vulnerability and insecurity, anxiety, and may include behavioral and disciplinary problems. Anger, guilt, and disorganization occur as well. Longitudinal observations indicate that a significant number of children have maladaptive symptoms, which continue for several years and interfere with academic and social performance (Kaffman and Elizar, 1979).

The long-term effects of childhood bereavement are not clearly known because many studies have focused retrospectively on patient samples rather than community samples. However, the risk of adult depressive disorders of a reactive type appears to increase in those who had an early parental loss. There is no link established to manic-depressive illness. Tennant, Bebbington, and Hurry (1980), on reviewing childhood parental death studies, felt that other considerations, such as quality of relationship to subsequent caretakers, may be more significant in determining the outcome than the loss itself. Because the surviving parent is bereaved, the care may be less consistent, interspersed with irritation and annoyance with the children, which contributes to a sense of insecurity. Extended family may play a critical stabilizing role.

For adults with cancer, having lost a parent to the same disease is a powerful early experience that complicates their adjustment to illness and often predisposes them to greater depression. Sometimes identification is seen by the assumption that they had always known they would also develop cancer.

## Loss of Sibling during Childhood

Cancer is the major cause of death in childhood, after accidents. Because children are kept at home more during illness today, even during terminal stages, the impact on siblings is greater; however, the outcome of grieving appears better when families share in terminal care, including siblings (Rando, 1983; Spinetta et al., 1981). The long-term effect of this more intimate association is not clear as yet. The parents are focused on the ill child, and after the death they may grieve to the point that surviving children continue to receive little attention (Pollack, 1985). The efforts of the surviving child to try to replace the dead child and diminish the parent's pain are often seen. The surviving child may also feel intense secret guilt because he or she harbored wishes for the sibling's death or imagines that he or she contributed to the death. Parents often become hyper-

vigilant about the health of surviving children. As described in Chapter 2, hypochondriases and anxiety disorders in adulthood may result from the emphasis on physical symptoms and fears of cancer.

Interventions for bereaved children have several important aspects that need to address the child, the parents, and the family generally. The child has three common questions, even if not articulated: Did I cause it? Will it happen to me? Who will take care of me? Interventions must deal with these questions (Osterweis et al., 1984). In anticipation of death, visits with the ill parent or sibling are helpful as long as meaningful interaction can occur. They help to reduce the potential for irrational guilt. However, a child should not be forced to visit.

Preventive intervention by counseling with the surviving child, alone or with other family members, may result in a better outcome (Rosenheim and Ichilou, 1979). Counseling with parents about the child's impressions and questions expedites communication and guides management (Pasnau et al., 1987).

Decisions about informing the child of the death should be consistent with the family's culture, religion, and beliefs. The most important caveat is to avoid keeping the death a secret while the child senses the altered mood and behavior in the home. An explanation of the death with regard to the illness and reassurance about his or her own security are adequate, with the offer of answers to questions as they arise. Sharing grief and memories with family members confirms the child's worth and role in the family.

The decision about the child's attending the funeral should be made after explaining what will happen there, again giving permission but not forcing the child to attend. If he or she attends, it may serve positively to make the death more real. Children as well as adults experience the loss again on special days. Sharing the occasion with family support marks it as an expected normal sadness.

In a review of present understanding of childhood bereavement, it is clear that children should be kept informed of illness and death. They should be told in a way that is consistent with their age and understanding. They should be encouraged to participate in events as they are able to tolerate them. Grieving has expected symptoms of sadness, restlessness, and behavioral changes that benefit from counseling for unusual distress; counseling for all children may be helpful to encourage a healthy response (Osterweis et al., 1984).

## INTERVENTIONS FOR ADULT BEREAVEMENT

It is important to recognize first that most bereaved individuals recover from their loss without any professional assistance. When efforts are made to offer counseling and support to a large group of recently bereaved individuals, many do not want it and indeed, likely do not need it. Adequate support is gleaned from family, friends, and spiritual resources. When intervention is attempted, it should be directed toward those who are at known high risk of poor bereavement outcome (Table 50-2). When added support is needed, the two models that are beneficial are the professional interventions (consisting of psychotherapeutic and psychopharmacological approaches) and mutual support through nonprofessional sources.

## Psychotherapy

While most bereaved do well, individuals with persistent anxiety or depression, which is the most common form of pathological grief, should be referred for evaluation and treatment (Raphael, 1983). The individual often responds to six or eight psychotherapeutic visits to assist expression of grief and confrontation with the loss. Sometimes family therapy is the best approach, which includes all the survivors in the family who may be receptive to this approach that enhances their communication with one another. Individuals at high risk, however, may require much more protracted psychotherapeutic intervention, which is not always successful (Rynearson, 1987). Hospitalization is sometimes needed for treatment of severe depression or suicidal intent.

Marmar and colleagues (1988) reviewed the few controlled interventions studies of spouse bereavement and noted that studies that targeted patients with high distress showed benefit to both physical and psychological health. Those that studied unselected subjects, however, showed less benefit. They conducted a trial that compared 12 brief dynamic psychotherapy sessions to a mutual-help group treatment in widows with unresolved grief. While there was a greater attrition rate in the group treatment, the two treatments both caused significant reduction in symptoms to an equal degree. Both had less effect on work and interpersonal relations. These interesting findings suggest that the more cost-effective treatment by mutual-support should be considered further, with efforts to train the leaders to deal with the more distressed individuals who might be most prone to drop out.

Bereavement counseling requires that the therapist know the clinical features of normal and abnormal bereavement, and that the therapist has skills in dealing with the problems of loss, which are so much a part of work with cancer patients and their loved ones. As in dealing with terminal illness, the therapist must be empathic to an individual experiencing great pain; exploring it in repeated sessions can be draining. It requires that the therapist have a good understanding of personal limitations and awareness of personal responses to prior losses that might affect care (see Chapter 38 on psychotherapy). Zisook and Schuchter (1985) offered several key tasks in bereavement counseling: giving permission for expression of feelings and recounting of details of the experience, assessing defenses for dealing with the painful affect, integrating the continuing relationship with the deceased spouse with the present, encouraging healthy functioning, handling altered relationships, and achieving a new view of the personal world and the self in it, with a willingness to try new experiences.

## Psychopharmacology

Medication is best used in combination with psychotherapy and for a limited time (Hollister, 1972). Anxiolytics, most commonly the benzodiazepines, are used frequently during the early weeks of grief for insomnia. Daytime use reduces the feeling of tension, anxiety, and irritability. Although the use of medications in the bereaved has been controversial in the past—based on excessive use of barbiturates to sedate the bereaved during the early period of grief (Morgan, 1980)—cautious use of mild sedation to reduce intolerable anxiety symptoms make it easier to deal with working through the grief. Similarly, the depressive symptoms associated with late-occurring depressions of bereavement are relieved by an antidepressant, especially the vegetative signs of insomnia and agitation. A pilot study of a 4-week open trial of desipramine by Jacobs, Nelson and Zisock (1987) showed moderate to marked improvement of depressive symptoms in 7 of 10 bereaved, depressed spouses. Despite the absence of controlled trials with grieving persons, clinical experience is positive (Zisook and Schuchter, 1985).

## Mutual Help

There is no greater immediate alliance than that which is felt between two individuals who have shared the same stressful experience (see Chapter 41). This is particularly true for the sharing of grief with another who has experienced it. In fact, the Widow-to-Widow program was developed on the premise that the person best qualified to understand and help with the problems of a bereaved person is another bereaved person (Silverman, 1972; Parkes and Weiss, 1983). To help widows through the critical transitions precipitated by bereavement, the multifaceted program offers one-to-one emotional support by an individual who herself presents a positive model of coping. Fundamental information about practical concerns and about bereavement are discussed. Groups promote the personal examination of coping and offer alternative ways that may be more effective. As an advocacy group, they become a source of identification with a group of individuals facing similar problems. And, importantly, the widow who resolves her own grief reinforces the gain by in turn helping others.

Such programs are located throughout the United States, Canada, and the United Kingdom. In a study examining the efficacy of the widow-to-widow model, Vachon and colleagues (1980) randomly assigned widows to the program. Follow-up assessment at 1, 6, 12, and 24 months showed better psychological adaptation in the women using the Widow-to-Widow program. By 24 months, they were better on all measures assessed. Women in the treatment group who were at high risk for poor outcome were significantly better than those at high risk who got no help.

The Candlelighters and Compassionate Friends are two outstanding organizations that have developed mutual help programs for parents who have a child with cancer and for those who have lost a child from any cause. Chapters in many cities and in other countries have been formed. They have become sources of information, referrals, and advocacy for parents with these experiences. The Candlelighters particularly have had an impact on both the medical and humane aspects of pediatric cancer care. Compassionate Friends offer support to many bereaved parents through their chapters.

## Hospice

Hospice care is unique in that it offers both professional and mutual support for the bereaved. Geared to maximal attention to the emotional, social, and spiritual needs of patients, the hospice offers support to many families of cancer patients who constitute the majority of those served (Gaetz, 1981). Most programs assign a bereavement counselor to the families when the patient enters the program. They offer assistance through the terminal phase of the illness and into the bereavement period with home visits, phone calls, letters, support groups, counseling, and referrals to other needed support services.

## SUMMARY

Management of the bereaved family is a common clinical problem faced by the oncology staff. Knowing the symptoms of normal grief and its stages allows support for normal grief and identification of abnormal reactions. Most individuals will recover from acute grief within 1–2 months, and it will be largely resolved within a year, usually without professional help. The anticipatory grieving period that is common with cancer may make the bereavement easier. However, about 20% of individuals will have trouble and will need help. Individuals likely to have trouble include those who have a history of emotional problems, are dependent, have experienced sudden death of the deceased, have poor support, are beset by other stresses and losses besides the death, have high initial distress, or have lost a child. Professional and mutual support are helpful in those who are at high risk or who have unusually intense initial symptoms. Medication may be efficacious if used cautiously for a limited time as an adjunct to psychotherapy. Assumptions about the risk of exacerbation of physical illness and mortality have likely been exaggerated, based on data from more carefully controlled studies. However, in the most extensive study, mortality was increased among older widowers who had increased mortality from suicide, accidents, and infectious diseases. However, there was no overrepresentation of other diseases. It is of interest that, in this epidemiological study, there was not an increased risk of death by cancer. The clinical significance of the perturbations of the endocrine and immune system function demonstrated in psychoimmune studies of bereavement remain unclear.

## REFERENCES

Adams-Greenly, M. and R.T. Moynihan (1983). Helping the children of fatally ill parents. *Am. J. Orthopsychiatry* 53:219–29.

American Cancer Society (1986). *Cancer Facts and Figures.* New York: American Cancer Society.

American Psychiatric Association (1987). *Diagnostic and Statistical Manual of Mental Disorders,* 3rd rev. ed. Washington, D.C.: American Psychiatric Association.

Averill, J.R. (1968). Grief: Its nature and significance. *Psychol. Bull.* 70:721–48.

Barton, D. (1977). *Dying and Death: A Clinical Guide for Caregivers.* Baltimore: Williams & Wilkins.

Bartrop, R., L. Lazarus, E. Luckhurst, L.G. Kiloh, and R. Penny (1977). Depressed lymphocyte function after bereavement. *Lancet* 1:834–36.

Blanchard, C.G., E.B. Blanchard, and J.V. Beeker (1976). The young: Depressive symptomatology throughout the grief process. *Psychiatry* 39:394–99.

Bornstein, P.E., P.J. Clayton, J.A. Halikas, W.L. Maurice, and E. Robins (1973). The depression of widowhood after thirteen months. *Br. J. Psychiatry* 122:561–66.

Bowlby, J. (1961). Process of mourning. *Int. J. Psychoanal.* 42:317–40.

Bowlby, J. (1977). The making and breaking of affectional bonds: I and II. *Br. J. Psychiatry* 130:201–10; 421–31.

Bowlby, J. (1980). *Attachment and Loss.* Vol. 3, *Loss: Sadness and Depression.* New York: Basic Books.

Brown, J.T. and G.A. Stoudemier (1983). Normal and pathological grief. *J.A.M.A.* 250:378–82.

Cassem, N.H. (1978). The dying patient. In T.P. Hackett and N.H. Cassem (eds.), *Massachusetts General Hospi-*

tal: *Handbook of General Hospital Psychiatry*. St. Louis: C.V. Mosby, pp. 300–18.

Clayton, P. (1974). Mourning and depression: Their similarities and differences. *Can. J. Psychiatry* 1:309–12.

Clayton, P.J. and H.S. Darvish (1979). Course of depressive symptoms following the stress of bereavement. In J.E. Barrett (ed.), *Stress and Mental Disorders*. New York: Raven Press, pp. 121–36.

DeVaul, R. and S. Zisook (1976). Unresolved grief: Clinical considerations. *Postgrad. Med.* 59(5):267–71.

Elliott, G.R. and C. Eisdorfer (eds.). (1982). *Stress and Human Health: Analysis and Implications of Research: A Study by the Institute of Medicine/National Academy of Sciences*. New York: Springer.

Engel, G.L. (1964). Grief and grieving. *Am. J. Nurs.* 64:93–98.

Freud, S. (1976). Mourning and melancholia. In J. Strachey (ed. and trans.), *The Complete Psychological Works*, std. ed., Vol. 14. New York: Norton, pp. 243–58 (original work published, 1923).

Frost, N.R. and P.J. Clayton (1977). Bereavement and psychiatric hospitalization. *Arch. Gen. Psychiatry* 34:1172–75.

Gaetz, D. (1981). The case for hospice from a hospital perspective. *Am. Protestant Hosp. Assoc. Bull.* 45:33–40.

Green, M. (1984). Roles of health professionals and institutions. In M. Osterweis, F. Solomon, and M. Green (eds.), *Bereavement: Reactions, Consequences, and Care*. Washington, D.C.: National Academy Press, pp. 215–36.

Helsing, K.J. and M. Szklo (1981). Mortality after bereavement. *Am. J. Epidemiol.* 114:41–52.

Helsing, K.J., G. Comstock, and M. Szklo (1982). Causes of death in a widowed population. *Am. J. Epidemiol.* 116:524–32.

Hofer, M.A. (1984). Relationships as regulators: A psychobiologic perspective on bereavement. *Psychosom. Med.* 46:183–97.

Hofer, M., C. Wolff, S. Freedman, and J. Mason (1972). A psychoendocrine study of bereavement: Parts 1 and 2. *Psychosom. Med.* 34:481–507.

Hollister, L. (1972). Psychotherapeutic drugs in the dying and bereaved. *J. Thanatol.* 2:623–29.

Holmes, T.H. and R.H. Rahe (1967). The social readjustment rating scale. *J. Psychosom. Res.* 11:213–18.

Horowitz, M.J. (1982). Psychological processes induced by illness, injury and loss. In T. Millon, C. Green, and R. Meogher (eds.), *Handbook of Clinical Health Psychology*. New York: Plenum, pp. 53–67.

Imboden, J.B., A. Canter, and L. Cluff (1963). Separation experiences and health records in a group of normal adults. *Psychosom. Med.* 25:433–40.

Irwin, M., M. Daniels, and H. Weiner (1987). Immune and neuroendocrine changes during bereavement. *Psychiatric Clin. N. Am.* 10:449–65.

Jacobs, S.C., J.C. Nelson, and S. Zisook (1987). Treating depressions of bereavement with antidepressants: a pilot study. *Psychiatric Clin. N. Am.* 10:501–11.

Jones, D.R., P.O. Goldblatt, and D.A. Leon (1984). Bereavement and cancer: some data on death of spouses from the longitudinal study of Office of Population Censuses and Surveys. *Br. Med. J.* 289:461–64.

Kaffman, M. and E. Elizar (1979). Children's bereavement reactions following death of father: The early months of bereavement. *Int. J. Ther.* 1:203–29.

Koocher, G.P. (1986). Coping with a death from cancer. *J. Consult. Clin. Psychol.* 54:623–31.

Lazare, A. (1979). Unresolved grief. In A. Lazare (ed.), *Outpatient Psychiatry: Diagnosis and Treatment*. Baltimore: Williams & Wilkins, pp. 498–512.

Levav, I., Y. Friedlander, J. Kark, and E. Peritz (1988). An epidemiologic study of mortality among bereaved parents. *N. Engl. J. Med.* 319:457–61.

Lewis, J.K., W.T. McKinney, L.D. Young, and G.W. Kraemer (1976). Mother–infant separation in rhesus monkeys as a model of human depression—a reconsideration. *Arch. Gen. Psychiatry* 33:699–705.

Lindemann, E. (1944). Symptomatology and management of acute grief. *Am. J. Psychiatry* 101:141–48.

Littlefield, C.H. and J.P. Rushton (1986). When a child dies: The sociobiology of bereavement. *J. Pers. Soc. Psychol.* 51:792–802.

Maddison, D.C. and A. Viola (1968). The health of widows in the year following bereavement. *J. Psychosom. Res.* 12:297–306.

Maddison, D.C. and W. Walker (1967). Factors affecting the outcome of conjugal bereavement. *Br. J. Med. Psychol.* 113:1057–67.

Marmar, C.R., M.J. Horowitz, D.S. Weiss, N.R. Wilner, and N.B. Kaltreider (1988). A controlled trial of brief psychotherapy and mutual-help group treatment of conjugal bereavement. *Am. J. Psychiatry* 145:203–9.

Martinson, I.M., D.G. Moldow, and W.F. Henry (1980). *Home Care for the Child with Cancer*. Final report, Grant CA19490, HHS, National Cancer Institute. Minneapolis: University of Minnesota School of Nursing.

Morgan, D. (1980). Not all sadness can be treated with antidepressants. *W. Va. Med. J.* 76(6):136–37.

Murphy, G.E. and E. Robins (1967). Social factors in suicide. *J.A.M.A.* 199:303–8.

Nagy, M. (1948). The child's theories concerning death. *J. Genet. Psychol.* 73:3–12.

Osterweis, M., F. Solomon, and M. Green (eds.). (1984). *Bereavement: Reactions, consequences, and care*. Washington, D.C.: National Academy Press.

Parkes, C.M. (1964). Effects of bereavement on physical and mental health: A study of the case records of widows. *Br. Med. J.* 2:274–79.

Parkes, C.M. (1965). Bereavement and mental illness: 1. A clinical study of the grief of bereaved psychiatric patients. *Br. J. Med. Psychol.* 38:1–12.

Parkes, C.M. (1970). Seeking and finding a lost object: Evidence from recent studies of the reaction to bereavement. *Soc. Sci. Med.* 4:181–201.

Parkes, C.M. (1972). *Bereavement: Studies of grief in adult life*. Madison, Conn.: International Universities Press.

Parkes, C.M. (1975). Determinants of outcome following bereavement. *Omega—J. Death Dying* 6:303–23.

Parkes, C.M. and R. Brown (1972). Health after bereavement: A controlled study of young Boston widows and widowers. *Psychosom. Med.* 34:449–61.

Parkes, C.M. and R. Weiss (1983). *Recovery from Bereavement*. New York: Basic Books.

Pasnau, R.O., F.I. Fawzy, and N. Fawzy (1987). Role of the physician in bereavement. *Psychiatr. Clin. North Am.* 10:109–20.

Paykel, E.S., J.K. Myers, M.N. Dienelt, G.L. Klerman, J.L. Lindenthal and M.P. Pepper (1969). Life events and depression: A controlled study. *Arch. Gen. Psychiatry* 21:753–60.

Pearlin, L. and M. Lieberman (1979). Social sources of distress. In R.G. Simmons (ed.), *Research in Community and Mental Health: An Annual Compilation of Research*, Vol. 1. Greenwich, Conn.: JAI Press, pp. 217–49.

Pollack, G.H. (1985). Childhood sibling loss: A family tragedy. *Psychiatr. Ann.* 16:309–14.

Rando, T.A. (1983). An investigation of grief and adaptation in parents whose children have died of cancer. *J. Pediatr. Psychol.* 8:3–20.

Raphael, B. (1983). *The Anatomy of Bereavement*. New York: Basic Books.

Reynolds, R. (1978). Autopsies: Benefits to the family. *Am. J. Clin. Pathol.* 69(Suppl. 25):220–22.

Robins, L.N., P.A. West, and G.E. Murphy (1977). The high rate of suicide in older white men: A study testing ten hypotheses. *Soc. Psychiatry* 12:1–20.

Rome, H.P. (1986). Personal reflections: Those who remain. *Psychiatr. Ann.* 16:268–71.

Rosenheim, D. and Y. Ichilou (1979). Short-term preventive therapy with children of fatally ill parents. *Israel: Ann. Psychiatr. Rel. Disc.* 17:67–73.

Rynearson, E.K. (1987). Psychotherapy of pathologic grief. *Psychiatr. Clin. N. Am.* 10:487–99.

Sanders, C. (1979–1980). A comparison of adult bereavement in the death of spouse, child, and parent. *Omega—J. Death Dying* 10:303–22.

Schleifer, S.J., S.E. Keller, M. Camerino, J.C. Thornton, and M. Stein (1983). Suppression of lymphocyte stimulation following bereavement. *J.A.M.A.* 250:374–77.

Silverman, P.R. (1972). Widowhood and preventive intervention. *Fam. Coord.* 21:95–102.

Spinetta, J.J. (1981). The sibling of the child with cancer. In J.J. Spinetta and P.D. Spinetta (eds.), *Living with Childhood Cancer*. St. Louis: C.V. Mosby, pp. 56–82.

Spinetta, J., J. Swarner, and J. Sheposh (1981). Effective parental coping following death of a child from cancer. *J. Pediatr. Psychol.* 6:251–63.

Stein, Z. and M.W. Susser (1969). Widowhood and mental illness. *Br. J. Prevent. Soc. Med.* 23:106–10.

Tennant, C., P. Bebbington, and J. Hurry (1980). Parental death in childhood and risk of adult depressive disorders: A review. *Psychol. Med.* 10:289–99.

Vachon, M.L.S. (1976). Grief and bereavement following the death of a spouse. *Can. Psychiatr. J.* 21:35–44.

Vachon, M.L.S., J. Rogers, W.A. Lyall, W.J. Lance, A.R. Sheldon, and S.J. Freeman (1982a). Predictors and correlates of high distress in adaptation to conjugal bereavement. *Am. J. Psychiatry* 139:998–1002.

Vachon, M.L.S., A.R. Sheldon, W.J. Lance, W.A. Lyall, J. Rogers, and S.J. Freeman (1980). A controlled study of self-help: Intervention for widows. *Am. J. Psychiatry* 137:1380–84.

Vachon, M., A.R. Sheldon, W. J. Lance, W.A. Lyall, J. Rogers, and S.J. Freeman (1982b). Correlates of enduring distress patterns following bereavement: Social network, life situation and personality. *Psychol. Med.* 12:783–88.

Vachon, M.L.S. (1987). Unresolved grief in persons with cancer referred for psychotherapy. *Psychiatr. Clin. N. Am.* 10:467–86.

Volkan, V. (1966). Normal and pathological grief reactions: A guide for the family physician. *Va. Med. Monthly* 93:651–56.

Worden, W. (1982). *Grief Counseling and Grief Therapy: A Handbook for the Mental Health Practitioner*. New York: Springer.

Zisook, S. and S.R. Schuchter (1985). The first four years of widowhood. *Psychiatr. Ann.* 16:188–294.

Zisook, S., R.A. Devaul, and M.A. Click (1982). Measuring symptoms of grief and bereavement. *Am. J. Psychiatry* 139:1590–93.

# PART X

# Oncology Staff: Psychological and Ethical Issues

# 51

# Psychological Problems of Staff and their Management

Marguerite Lederberg

Interest in the psychology of medical staff is a relatively recent phenomenon. In the past, the very ill were cared for at home. The few hospitals were run by religious orders, where faith and obedience sustained the staff. Today these roles are replaced by the secular hospital where staff motivation is more varied and idiosyncratic. The technological revolution in medicine has also meant longer, more stressful encounters under increasingly ambiguous circumstances. It is not surprising that the first studies of staff stress came from high-pressure, high-technology areas such as coronary and intensive care units (Cassem and Hackett, 1975, 1979), dialysis units (DeNour and Czaczkes, 1968), and cancer wards (Vachon, 1978; Vachon et al., 1978). The study of staff psychology also gained impetus from the growing interest in the dying patient, heralded by Kubler-Ross' book "On Death and Dying" (1969). It became apparent that to alter what was happening to the patient, one needed to understand what was happening to the caretakers.

At first, this inquiry took a somewhat critical tone as medicine came under societal reexamination from the consumer movement of the 1970s. There was more scrutiny of the staff's negative behaviors, less empathy and compassion for staff obligations and the associated uncertainties and anxieties. Meanwhile, the entire medical profession came under attack by a more demanding and disillusioned public.

Regardless of the pain for beleaguered medical staff, this has had its bright side. The staff member is now recognized as a fallible human being, whose valid needs and limitations must be considered in designing and evaluating medical care delivery systems (Fox, 1980). The burnout literature (Freudenburger, 1974, 1980; Maslach, 1976, 1979; Cherniss, 1980) has been instrumental in developing the concept and in suggest-

ing remedies (see later section on burnout). There has also been a steady interest in staff support groups, with many positive, albeit anecdotal reports.[1] Increasing attention is being paid to the mental health of medical staff, aimed at effective and timely interventions (Borenstein, 1985; McCue, 1982; Reuben et al., 1984). Today's state of knowledge, while far from complete, should allow us to balance the great demands on and needs of cancer staff, and to offer built-in supports to minimize staff stress and maximize the quality of patient care.

## STRESSES ON CANCER STAFF

Working with cancer patients brings special concerns, because the idea of cancer still conjures up special fears in almost everyone. Some staff members may have had cancer themselves; others fear they may develop it. Almost everyone has experienced cancer in a close family member, and they are also influenced by society's attitudes toward cancer.

### Stresses Common to Other Areas of Medical Care

This section delineates the stresses that are comparable to those experienced by staff in other areas of medicine on specialized high-technology wards such as intensive care, dialysis, and burn units, from which we can

---

1. Nurses: Cassem and Hackett (1979), Eisendrath (1981), Mohl (1980a,b), Moynihan and Outlaw (1984), Simon and Whiteley (1977); medical students: Dashef et al., (1974); house staff: Rosini et al. (1974), Siegel and Donnelly (1978); oncology fellows: Artiss and Levine (1973), Richards and Schmale (1974), Wise (1977).

draw on large bodies of reported experience. Also discussed are death and dying, burnout, and bioethics.

## HIGH-TECHNOLOGY SPECIALIZED WARDS

A number of common themes emerge from the literature on staff response to high-technology settings that share with cancer wards the emotional problems generated by high morbidity, complex technology, and the associated multiple demands and intense pressure on staff (Cassem and Hackett, 1974, 1979):

1. High morbidity, high mortality
2. Complex technology, high pressure
3. High frequency of life–death decisions
4. Terminal care issues
5. Third-party conflicts
6. Interstaff conflicts
7. "Limelight" medicine
8. Response to severe debilitation and disfigurement
9. Response to "difficult" patients (excessive dependency, anger, uncooperativeness)
10. Response to suicidal ideation
11. Issue of inflicting pain as part of treatment

Some studies of nursing staff show that they self-select rather effectively for tolerance of these aspects of intensive medical care (Caldwell and Weiner, 1981). They enjoy the intellectual challenge and the corresponding sense of achievement. However, the pressure may at times be too relentless or the rewards too few, leading to increased turnover and burnout.

The problem is exacerbated by other difficult aspects of cancer care, the consequences of advances in technology (sometimes becoming painfully acute in recent times), which include the need for rapid life-and-death decision making in ambiguous situations; the frequent need for terminal care decisions in the absence of clear-cut guidelines (societal, legal, ethical, or even institutional), and the frequent need for third-party decision making or arbitration involving patient–family groups with strongly held and often divergent views.

Furthermore, these problems occur in a tense, divisive societal setting. Advances in medical care have become big news, and staff must often function in the limelight, answerable to the quixotic demands generated by sometimes exploitative, poorly informed, and easily aroused public scrutiny. The crises and tensions that result are very stressful for staff and can obscure the more respectable and appropriate demands for accountability from the medical profession.

To complicate matters further, conflicts can arise from internal as well as from external sources. Staff members often have strongly divergent feelings in

such controversial situations. At times a covert civil war may develop in a given unit, with some staff members feeling they are being asked to carry out a treatment plan with which they disagree. The resultant emotional corrosion can be significant. In particular, pediatric cases associated with intense disagreements and legal disputes appear in the media with regularity.

Several of the staff stresses listed earlier represent major psychodynamic issues observed in patient–staff relationships on dialysis and burn units (for further details see DeNour and Czaczkes, 1968; Czaczkes and DeNour, 1978; Procci, 1983; Quinbey and Bernstein, 1971; Perry, 1985). Staff psychodynamics in the oncology setting have been described by Spikes and Holland (1975). The extremes of patient dependency and passivity on the one hand and anger and resentment on the other are particularly characteristic of patients in burn and dialysis units, and are also found in cancer patients. Suicidal ideation is also a problem in both settings, especially passive suicide as in the case of the dialysis patient who refuses treatment. Similar problems are seen in cancer patients undergoing a lengthy and arduous course of treatment who experience periods of wondering "Is it worth it?" The impact of disfigurement, a frequent issue in burn patients, is also an aspect of cancer often alluded to by staff and the lay public, expecially in relation to head and neck tumors. The unavoidable necessity of inflicting pain in the course of treatment is a difficult area for burn and oncology units, as suggested by the frequent underestimation of pain and consequent undermedication that can be seen in both areas (Marks and Sachar, 1973; Perry, 1984), despite the lack of evidence to justify it (Kantor and Foley, 1981; Foley, 1985). It has been suggested that pain management should be done by someone other than the treating staff because of their underlying psychological conflicts in dealing with these difficult issues. This solution is an example of the constructive approach recommended by Fox (1980); it attempts to understand the "human condition" of staff members, eliminates the implication of willful disregard for aspects of patient care, and finds ways to assist staff in coping.

All the issues just described arouse painful feelings in staff members, namely, sadness, pity, fear, frustration, and helplessness; at times these uncomfortable emotions can and do give way to transient feelings of irritation and repugnance, anger, and even revulsion. These emotions are surprising and upsetting to the well-intentioned doctor or nurse who may in response experience guilt and institute harsh self-control measures. Another individual may suppress these normal negative feelings and become an overly self-sacrificing and involved caretaker at serious cost to personal adjustment.

## DEATH AND DYING ISSUES

Even though a cancer diagnosis is now viewed more optimistically, death and dying remain important issues for oncology staff. Confrontation with death is a difficult experience for all human beings; this must be acknowledged and dealt with to permit staff members to function effectively over a long period of time. The issues of death and dying are treated in the thanatology literature from several different points of view (Campbell, 1980; Wahl, 1958; Weisman, 1981). Freudian theory has held, with decreasing insistence, that death anxiety was a derivative phenomenon to be translated into more primary components, related to separation and loss. Existential writings view death anxiety itself as primary, with many human behaviors to be understood as manifestations of it. Ultimately, clinical sensitivity should outweigh theoretical bias, and one should strive to stay closely tuned to the factual circumstances. For example, the staff members of a unit who complain of too many deaths may, on closer examination, actually be responding to unsupportive leadership. Then again, on another unit, interpersonal irritability may be a proxy for unacknowledged anguish about the death of several young patients.

Death is a recurring topic of conversation for staff members, which includes the subject of death as premature or long expected and overdue, the ''unfair'' death as in the case of a particularly young, attractive, or deserving individual, and the death that arouses ''gallows'' humor. This last reaction is a fundamental human mechanism used particularly by stressed medical staff. It is difficult for outsiders to understand and is often a source of criticism of staff who are seen as being unfeeling. While it must be restricted to appropriate settings in which only staff are present, it should not be censured (Cassem, 1979; Fox, 1980).

## BURNOUT

The now-extensive burnout literature gives a useful picture of staff stress, with practical interventions to reduce it (Perlman and Hartman, 1982; Savicki and Cooley, 1983; Fullerton, 1983). Cherniss (1980) gives a transactional definition of burnout as a three-stage process. First, the individual experiences stress that occurs because job demands exceed emotional or physical resources. Next, the worker experiences strain with symptoms of tension, fatigue, and irritability. Finally, the worker attempts to cope by becoming emotionally detached, withdrawn, cynical, and inflexible in his or her dealings with patients and colleagues. Subsequent disturbances develop in job performance, personal life, physical and psychological state that become self-perpetuating. Pines and

Aronson (1983) suggest the workshop as a helpful technique to combat burnout. The issues of managing burnout in the patient care setting are reviewed later in this chapter.

## BIOETHICAL ISSUES

There are important ethical dimensions to the problems experienced by staff members, and the impact of these dimensions on staff morale is enormous. These are substantively reviewed in Chapter 59. The emphasis in this section is on the staff's reactions.

The discipline of bioethics, a new branch of applied moral philosophy, reflects a sweeping social change that is far from having run its course. Many of medicine's basic assumptions are brought under critical scrutiny, especially with regard to the ability of high technology to prolong life without a corresponding improvement in quality of life, and to the old doctor–patient relationship and the medical paternalism that characterized it.

These are issues about which public feeling runs high. Critiques have ranged from thoughtful, constructive analyses to angry indictments and harsh accusations. All this takes a toll on the cancer professionals who are working in an area in which the core problems are being addressed daily. Their reactions cover a wide spectrum, but no position anywhere on the spectrum is totally comfortable. At one extreme is the traditionalist, mistrustful of all these changes, practicing medicine in a state of siege. At the other extreme is the covert revolutionary who finds the current system deeply objectionable and works there only out of necessity, while maintaining a negativistic attitude. These individuals are rare, but they can be difficult and disruptive for fellow workers. Most health professionals fall somewhere in the middle, welcoming many of the changes, regretting a few, hoping for more, and making their peace with the current ambiguous and changing situation as best they can. But one should not underestimate the emotional cost to caretakers of the recurrent adversarial tone that informs most of the discussions of these issues. It takes a lot of strength to undergo honest self-scrutiny, tolerate repeated (often uninformed) criticism, and still deliver the level of consistent, disinterested humane care that is demanded.

### Stresses Specific to the Cancer Setting

Many staff stresses are unique to the cancer setting, including the intrinsic nature of the disease, the nature of the treatment and its side effects, the necessity for palliative care, the ambiguity of decision making, dealing with the patient's response to the cancer diagnosis, the staff member's personal reactions to cancer, and the social isolation of staff members. These are discussed in the following paragraphs.

## CHARACTERISTICS OF THE DISEASE

As discussed at length early in this volume (see especially Chapters 1 and 2), cancer's ubiquitous, unpredictable, and often deadly nature makes it as much the source of universal apprehension for professional and ancillary staff as it is for the general public.

A recurrent theme emerges from this situation of uncertainty laced with fear. In facing such a difficult reality, human beings are powerfully motivated to decrease the uncertainty as a way of decreasing the fear. This underlies the growth of popular quasi theories about cancer, with which the public tries to reassure itself; but, in a modified way, it also applies to the oncology staff. They do not adopt quack theories, but as they live through experiences that are unusually bewildering or frightening, they develop a private system of special meanings, associations, and omens that helps them to predict the course of subsequent difficult cases and as such is helpful to them. However, because of its idiosyncratic and irrational nature, this private code can also be a burden. For example, a young female physician had become very involved with a leukemia patient who had died after an unusual symptom presentation and a stormy course. Subsequently, characteristics of this patient's illness remained vividly present for the physician, and colored her emotions and expectations whenever parallel symptoms or responses were present in later cases.

## CHARACTERISTICS OF TREATMENT

Cancer treatment may be difficult to administer for many reasons. Two of the three major treatments used in cancer carry a special fear. The exposure to radiation and powerful chemicals is inescapably associated with major dangers in our society; staff members are not immune to these associations. Realistic fear of these agents (Babich, 1985; Bingham, 1985; Selevan et al., 1985) often plays into irrational reactions and displaced resentments, creating problems even on units with scrupulous safety procedures. These call for a thoughtful response that addresses all aspects of the problem, rational as well as irrational.

## IMPACT OF TREATMENT SIDE EFFECTS

The numerous side effects of treatment are all too familiar to cancer staff members, and tend to reinforce the views just described. Side effects that are not life-threatening (e.g., hair loss and nausea) can be distress-

ing to staff members, involving as they do discomfort and transient altered appearance that is very difficult for some patients to tolerate. However, life-threatening treatment procedures such as bone marrow transplantation or high-dose methotrexate therapy that carry a significant mortality are especially stressful. The emotional tension is high and the potential for anguish ever present during such treatment. As McCue (1982) put it, modern technology can put physicians (and other staff) in "absurdly stressful" situations.

Surgery is ordinarily the least problematic for staff. However, some procedures produce major functional and physical deficits, especially when treatment involves head and neck surgery, hemipelvectomy, or pelvic exenteration. Such extensive postsurgical deficits are difficult to deal with, not only for the patient and family, but for the staff as well. Less obvious long-term side effects, especially infertility, are of great significance, particularly to nurses, many of whom are women in their early childbearing years.

## NATURE OF PALLIATIVE TREATMENT

Much of cancer treatment is still palliative; it is designed to control the spread and the symptoms of the disease, without aspiring to cure. Within the context of this definition, all diabetic, arthritic, and cardiac patients are receiving palliative care; but somehow, palliation with these diseases is viewed as a constructive treatment aimed at sustaining ongoing, future-oriented life. By contrast, palliative treatment in cancer is, for many people, viewed as a "holding action" with the outcome being ultimate defeat. It is interesting to speculate on how much of this attitude is derived from our societal perceptions. At a personal level, it may represent the staff member's personal sense of defeat with patients whose illness is progressing.

## TREATMENT DECISION MAKING

Early in the disease course, when cure or remission are real possibilities, treatment decisions are not ambiguous. Equally, near the end the patient, family, and staff may understand and accept the inevitable. But these are relatively short periods at the two ends of a longer course, most of which is spent in the middle, trying to chart a treatment plan without reliable coordinates. Treatment moves into successive phases. For a great many patients, the shift must be made from curative to palliative intent. That shift may be very difficult to negotiate. It engenders anxiety, confusion, depression, and many negative reactions in patients and families. These reactions are often diverted onto staff, in ways that are widely acknowledged to generate further strain and dissension.

Staff members also vary widely in their degree of comfort with this delicate transition, as well as their philosophy of when and how the transition should occur. This is especially so in complex institutional settings where the medical team is large and the multiple missions of clinical care, teaching, and research coexist uneasily.

Depending on their background, discipline, and specific role on the team, staff members have different ways of reducing stress. Each team may focus on its own facet of care with little sympathy for the other's viewpoint. This can be exacerbated in research settings where ethical and philosophical conflicts between research and clinical care commitments can readily occur, even in objectively well-managed cases. Whether these conflicts are directly acknowledged or not, they may intensify other existing sources of disunity among caregivers.

Some estrangements result from the differing viewpoints of the several disciplines involved in the treatment and care of the cancer patient. The doctor has the most detailed information about the natural history of the disease—its likely course and prognosis in a given patient—from which he or she generates the plan for treatment. This makes it easiest for him or her to assume an intellectual approach (for which he or she is already preselected). In assuming the ultimate responsibility for decisions and outcome, the physician becomes committed to the treatment selected and this enhances his or her ability to accept results that are sometimes less than ideal. In fact, training in oncology and commitment to the field require that the physician be able to accept outcomes that vary from cure in some, to palliation and fatality in others. Many nurses are now trained in oncology to give technologically complex treatments and assume a high level of responsibility, which leads many of them to take "the doctor stance," that is, the same intellectual approach in dealing with the stresses. They are also self-selected for this role. However, a number of nurses do not identify with this approach, because they view themselves more as "nurturers." Although there is no incompatibility between the two stances, nor with good patient care, a primary identification with one or the other dictates a set of emotional responses and sources of professional satisfaction. Failure to acknowledge the existence of these two stances, or valuing one at the expense of the other, can create a schism between staff members that cause tensions on units or within a team.

Besides doctors and nurses, delivery of cancer care today involves a large number of other disciplines, such as medical secretaries, aides, ward clerks, x-ray technologists, laboratory technicians, and transportation, food service, and housekeeping staff. All have varying degrees of patient contact. Many of these interactions have a strong emotional impact on the employee and resonate with their personal feelings about cancer, and about the treatment enterprise in which they play a part. Some feel closely identified with it and derive a sense of pride and security from their association; others feel alienated, yet must continue to work in the institution because they lack job mobility. These emotional conflicts can become chronic and destructive to the quality of life of the staff member and to the quality of care he or she delivers. This situation becomes worse because of the lack of training these workers need to equip them for the troubled patient and family interface they negotiate repeatedly. They may be inappropriately devalued and subject to displaced anxieties and resentments. Self-esteem suffers under these conditions; attempts of the individual to protect it often result in anger toward patients and bitterness toward superiors, with further harm to worker and patient.

In trying to evaluate the reactions of this group, one must keep in mind societal attitudes toward disease and cancer. The highly trained professional can use an intellectualized approach that runs counter to the societal climate. However, ancillary personnel working in a cancer center are more likely to embrace personal beliefs that contradict the center's philosophy and that are strongly molded by their own social milieu.

In summary, reactions to conflicts about cancer treatments affect staff members at all levels, although responses vary with background and specializations. These differences can be, and often are, a source of stress and divisiveness among the members of the staff.

## PATIENT REACTION TO THE DIAGNOSIS OF CANCER

Patient responses to the diagnosis of cancer and to different stages of the disease have been described in Parts III and IV. Some of these responses impinge directly on the staff and include various degrees of regressive behavior that may require great patience from staff, numbness and inappropriate denial that the staff must judiciously confront when it is interfering with needed treatment, panic and grief that the staff must tolerate while continuing to treat the patient, a powerful need to propitiate and bargain that the staff must recognize and gently discourage while understanding it and the magical unrealistic expectations that underlie it, disappointment and anger that the staff must endure without altering their efforts, and a depression that can be the most draining of all. Overall, this is a difficult and often unpleasant set of projections to receive and handle with a professional demeanor. The steadiness of purpose and the steadfastness of personal behavior that is required demands a high level of strength and maturity from each individual.

## STAFF REACTIONS TO CANCER ILLNESS

The staff's personal reactions to cancer consist of conscious and unconscious levels of adaptation.

The conscious adaptation includes having an intellectual grasp of the situation, rejecting superstitions and myths about cancer, feeling proud of problem-solving abilities, feeling proud of the ability to function under pressure and having reliable emotional controls, and feeling proud of the ability to offer constructive interventions in all situations (even those that are hopeless). Much of this is a description of the "medical ego ideal," but the rejection of superstition plays a more important and powerful role here than in other areas of medicine, because fear and superstition play a more powerful role in cancer than in other diseases.

Coexisting with this conscious adaptation are unconscious adaptations that are much more idiosyncratic and often made up of less rational reactions. These responses modify behavior in ways that are difficult to understand or to change voluntarily. They are the sources of these odd little quirks or unexpected reactions that may be found in one's own personality and in co-workers. When queried, the individual will often rationalize the behavior, avoid the issue, or respond with irritation. A good example of this is a capable young nurse who developed a mild cold and became very uncooperative about work assignments, refusing to care for several patients, and finally taking a few days' sick leave. Queried by a sympathetic co-worker upon her return, she stated that she had never forgotten her mother and her aunt suggesting years ago that getting a cold had made her sister "catch leukemia." Although she did not really believe it, her work with leukemia patients when she had a cold made her feel very anxious and frightened.

When the individual becomes aware of these thoughts, as in individual self-reflection, they are often experienced as a sign of weakness or vulnerability, possibly signaling a breakdown of the ego ideal. Such thoughts are seen as incompatible with the professional self-image. These realizations result in embarrassment, shame, guilt, and anger at one's own inadequacy. There is also a sense that these inadequacies must be kept hidden, arising out of the almost universal belief that other people do not feel this way, and that exposure will result in stigmatization.

## ISOLATION OF STAFF OUTSIDE THE WORKPLACE

When the oncology staff leave their workplace, whether hospital or clinic, they enter the world that maintains the "cancer myth." This cancer myth is found in friends and family, and the more staff members share their feelings and experiences, the more they force others to think about a subject that is fundamentally frightening and unpleasant. The oncology staff member who mentions anxiety-provoking subjects or is himself or herself an anxiety-provoking stimulus, elicits from others such varied responses as tense humor, silence, irritation, change of subject, or frank rejection and anger. Another common response is an unrealistic admiration for one's work in oncology. While this is a little easier to accept, in the long term it also creates distancing and isolation.

Thus, the cancer caregiver has the potential for feeling isolated both at work with attempts to hide from other what he or she views as unacceptable weaknesses, and in the outside world when the social environment is unable to tolerate discussions of his or her work. These problems can contribute to a range of stress responses outlined in the following section.

## CLINICAL SPECTRUM OF STAFF STRESS RESPONSES

The spectrum of staff responses can be divided into the categories of normal adaptation and coping, coping accompanied by reactive anxiety and depression, and frank psychiatric syndromes.

### Normal Adaptation and Coping

There is an adaptational process that appears to be universal to all caregivers when they first encounter care of severely ill cancer patients. Dysphoric symptoms of anxiety, sadness, and "numbness" are acute in the beginning, then subside, only to peak again at 3–4 months, to be followed by a more stable resolution over the ensuing 6 months. As discussed in Part I, some new staff members also develop a transient cancerophobia, a fear that their own or a family member's somatic symptoms are due to cancer. Our experience is supported by Vachon's findings. In her research, the stress levels experienced by a group of nurses working on a newly formed palliative care unit initially equaled those of recently widowed women, but had dropped to control levels at the end of 1 year (Vachon, 1978).

The first part of the adaptation process primarily addresses problems of competence. The intellectual and organizational demands on cancer caregivers are significant, and the professional who endures is the one who can control initial emotional reactions sufficiently to focus on mastering the demands of the job. These emotional reactions are powerful, and initially absolute willpower and self-control may have to be exercised. Reassurance about one's ability to endure the stress brings relief, which is mistaken by many for full adaptation. But, in fact, the deeper emotional adaptation takes longer. The personal meaning and impact of this level of exposure to the morbidity and mortality associated with cancer take longer to develop and go beyond the early emotional response engendered by the first personal encounters. Over time the worker's previous experiences with loss are brought into play. Adaptation shapes, and is shaped by, fundamental choices about how to live, to love, and to act in a world in which loss is unavoidable. It may be only during the second phase that the worker acknowledges (to himself or herself and others) the extent of his or her sadness, pain, fear, and guilt, and with it doubt about his or her own personal sense of purpose in the endeavor, the purpose of the endeavor itself, and even doubts about the purpose of life in a broader sense.

The availability of support can be crucial at this time. It need not be psychiatric; its goal is to help the individual recognize his or her feelings as normal, undergo the necessary mourning, and discover his or her inner strengths. If the caregiver is oriented to psychology at this time, there may be an attempt to ascertain a personal meaning in this work and the motivation for doing it. A caregiver who emerges from this period with a continued desire to do oncology work will, given reasonable work conditions, likely have a satisfying career.

Consider the following examples of adaptation reactions.

1. In a staff support group a young male nurse described his heroic efforts in the care of a terminal patient. He was angered by what he experienced as a lack of support from other staff members, who pointed out the futility of his feverish activity. Painful as this was, it opened up a fruitful dialogue with his colleagues, who, upon perceiving his pain, became more explicitly compassionate. A few months later, he was able to look back and see the extent to which he had been denying what was intolerable for him, and how he had been angry at others for not sharing his distortion.

2. In another staff group meeting, several single nurses complained bitterly about their social life. After some general discussion, they made the observation that at least part of their discontent stemmed from anxiety activated by their work with young gynecological cancer patients. This issue was pursued over subsequent meetings with varying outcomes for several nurses. Some nurses stayed on the unit, two transferred out, and one developed a new rehabilitation program for gynecological patients.

3. During his third month of an oncology fellowship, a sensitive, capable physician expressed doubts about his competence and his career choice. Review of his case load revealed a large number of very ill young patients, about whom he felt particularly

hopeless and helpless. He met a few times with the psychooncologist to discuss his perceptions and expectations of himself as a physician. At the same time, a patient's wife sought him out after her husband's death and told him, in moving detail, how much his care and concern had meant to her husband in the preceding months. This unsolicited tribute went a long way in helping this young professional get a clear perspective on both his strengths and limitations, and allowed him to continue his work with greater assurance about his career choice.

## Reactive Anxiety and Depression

A minority of caregivers will develop anxiety and depression greater than that expected from the stresses. Such responses have clear-cut determinants, and they usually resolve spontaneously within weeks or at most a few months. Often they require increased use of resources present in the environment, mainly the informal support of co-workers, or that of an understanding supervisor. Some institutions provide support groups, an employee assistance program, or access to brief counseling and psychotherapy, all of which are helpful. These reactions can occur at any time, even in experienced and senior staff. At worst, the staff member may become temporarily unable to function effectively, and may need a vacation, a short leave, a temporary transfer, or special assignments while still on the job.

The causes include marital or family conflict, and sickness or death of a relative. The cancer caregiver is particularly vulnerable to the stress of having cancer develop in himself or herself, or in a close friend or relative. The problem of cancer in the caregiver is discussed in Chapter 58, but cancer in the family member is discussed here.

During their professional career, half or more staff members will have a family member or intimate friend who develops cancer, and in whose illness they are closely involved. They are often asked to play a supportive and advisory role in treatment decisions. Some staff members welcome this way of dealing with the problem and throw themselves into it, often underestimating the emotional cost to themselves from the ambiguous and potentially conflict-ridden role. Others feel deeply burdened and cheated of the right to react in an untutored, spontaneous way. At work these feelings come to the surface, reactivated by encounters with patients. Workers may reexperience the same acute, nearly uncontrollable dysphoria they felt at the beginning of their career in oncology. Thus, an experienced nurse may come into the lounge in tears, saying "I don't know why, I just can't stop crying." Then again, the person may react with anger at the demands being placed on him or her, and project this anger onto the patient. Or, a usually compassionate physician will say impatiently: ''Oh no, not another depressed breast patient!''

An overinvolved response to the ''special patient'' is a usually milder derivative of this problem. Every cancer caregiver meets patients who are especially significant to them, who engage them intensely, often before they realize it, either because of direct identification or because they remind the caregiver of an important personal figure. In such cases behavioral overinvolvement increases the chance of conflict with other staff. It also involves an intense sense of loss and grief, which comes as a shock to the staff member, because their feelings have seldom been fully acknowledged.

This is one of the staff crises that responds most effectively to support from colleagues. It is reassuring to realize that these occurrences are common and can be tolerated.

The following examples of reactive anxiety and depression are instructive.

1. A male psychologist doing both psychooncology and general psychiatry suffered a deep, personal loss—a noncancer-related death—and took a brief leave. He later resumed his general psychotherapy practice with only a mild sense of effort, but found the resumption of his oncology work much more difficult. Several weeks later when he had better worked through the loss and mastered his reaction, he was able to manage oncology work with his usual enthusiasm.

2. A young nurse's work with leukemia patients brought her into repeated contact with young adults under great stress, often with poor prognoses. She requested counseling because of her overinvolvement with the patients, which had resulted in a self-imposed increase in work load and a sense of guilt about neglecting her personal life. The nurse was seen in counseling at an employee assistance program, with improvement of her depressive symptoms.

3. An oncologist's father was found to have an intraabdominal mass. During the days preceding surgery, while diagnoses of malignancy were under consideration, intrusive images of possible treatment courses made his own work with cancer patients very difficult. At surgery the tumor was found to be benign and the oncologist was able to resume his work with much greater ease, even though his father developed complications and remained quite ill for some time.

## Psychiatric Problems in Staff

Sometimes when a developmental crisis is not negotiated successfully, emotional distress does not respond to the supports available, and job performance suffers

markedly. There may be clear and often multiple causes; however, occasionally none may be obvious. Psychiatric consultation is indicated in such individuals. Evaluation usually reveals preexisting psychological vulnerabilities, and these observed syndromes cover a wide range of diagnoses.

Here are some examples of psychiatric disorders in staff members.

1. A young married aide, father of three, who worked on a bone marrow transplant unit was particularly valued for his capacity to relate well to pediatric patients. His head nurse was therefore surprised when he reacted to the death of a patient with an outburst of sobs and a demand for an immediate transfer. Psychiatric evaluation revealed that this man had always had close supportive relationships to older female relatives, and that two had died in the last 2 years. During this period, he had become increasingly intolerant of patient deaths, feeling that ''everyone dies''; however, he had not shared this feeling with anyone and it had not interfered with the quality of his work. At home, he had become morose and irritable, with uncontrollable episodes of anger and physical abuse toward his own children. Transfer was arranged, pending further psychiatric evaluation and treatment.

2. A young social worker had performed well on an oncological intensive care unit. She went on a 2-week traveling vacation, and upon returning she found that the level of morbidity and suffering, and her conflicted feelings about treatment were so difficult to bear that she requested a temporary rotation to other duties. Her symptoms of anorexia, insomnia, sadness, and work impairment did not improve, and she went on to develop a major depression that responded to antidepressants and psychotherapy. In the course of treatment she recognized preexisting vulnerabilities and a dysfunctional tendency to put herself in overly demanding situations. She requested and was given a permanent transfer to another area, where she performed well.

3. A young male resident rotated to an oncology unit from a demanding general medical floor where he had performed well. During his first 3 months in oncology, he was noted to be hardworking and competent, but unusually anxious and perfectionistic. His anxiety level did not decrease as expected with time. Over the next 6 weeks, he developed a psychosis with paranoid delusions about his co-workers. He required psychiatric admission and responded well to treatment. He resumed his training in another medical subspeciality.

4. A young nurse on a surgical oncology floor went to the psychiatrist at the urging of her co-workers, who were concerned about her inability to function or to work. She was an only child with an intense, am-

bivalent attachment to her parents, although she had lived with peers since college. Despite a history of chronic anxiety, she had never required formal psychiatric treatment. Her mother had, 3 months earlier, received a diagnosis of advanced esophageal cancer and required hospice care. During this period, the nurse had developed increasingly frequent severe panic attacks. She had moved back home with her father and had become almost totally homebound by her anxiety symptoms. She resigned, despite offers of support. Follow-up telephone calls revealed that her symptoms remained severe until after her mother's death. She then slowly improved and started work at a hospital near home.

## REWARDS OF WORKING WITH CANCER PATIENTS

The rewards of working with cancer patients are as important as the stresses, and occur at many levels. The satisfactions of medical practice are very deep, and reflect the opposite of the stresses described.

In their immediate patient encounters, members of the cancer staff are privileged to share powerful, deeply private moments that are seldom shared with others. They often play a significant positive role with patients and families at a critical time. They are in a uniquely strong position to give support to their patients in all stages of their illness, including the later ones. One need only look at ward bulletin boards full of grateful and affectionate messages from patients, to know that there are constantly warm human exchanges going on, from which staff deservedly gain a sense of their own strength and self-worth.

The "cancer myth" has some positive fallout as well, in that it conveys to staff members that they are part of an important, socially valued, and valuable human enterprise. That not everyone can do it makes them feel courageous and "special." On units where interstaff support works well, these feelings are further echoed and reinforced. Some members of the staff feel privileged compared to their friends in other professions whose energies are spent on tasks that appear to them less valuable, or even inconsequential. These values are also reinforced by the esteem received from others outside the profession.

The high-technology environment can also have positive fallout in that it demands alertness and curiosity from staff members who then feel fruitfully challenged. One hears "It's never boring!" said in a half-exasperated, half-delighted tone of voice.

Personal fears of cancer also have a positive aspect. Once the initial cancer fear is resolved, exposure to severe illness can provide a more discriminating outlook on disease in general. Responses to their own and family illnesses show a mature level of concern. This can, however, be carried to an excessive degree as evidenced by the tendency of nurses and physicians to delay in responding to their own symptoms.

Positive effects can extend beyond the hospital to interpersonal relationships. Cancer work can hone many valuable qualities and can give individuals a rich and unusual knowledge base. Staff members take these home and use them to enrich their personal lives in ways that make up for the isolating trends described earlier.

In summary, many of the features that make working with cancer patients special can cut either way, because they can make a staff member feel stressed or they can make him or her feel valuable and worthwhile. For example, one can repress anger or one can feel strong enough to be generous. One can feel numb or one can feel capable of tolerating the human condition. One can flee from overemotional encounters or feel privileged to share extraordinary moments. One can feel guilty or one can feel a special gratitude and refined appreciation for life. One can feel intellectually overwhelmed or intellectually challenged. One can feel useless or proud of one's unique personal contribution. One can feel alienated or anchored in a valuable human enterprise.

What can be done to ensure the latter outcomes? The ways and means of maximizing good staff functioning are outlined in the following section.

## INTERVENTIONS WITH STAFF

### Selection of Staff

Good procedures for choosing staff members are the first consideration in maximizing good staff functioning, but there are few guidelines on what characteristics determine success in oncology. It seems likely that one needs the same positive traits that all leaders desire in their employees, specifically, cognitive skills (namely basic competence plus the will and capacity to keep learning), interpersonal skills, personal attributes such as reliability, dedication, and moral values compatible with the task at hand, and finally a high energy level and an appetite for work. Vachon (1978) discusses the several motivations observed among entering hospice workers and the ways they affect subsequent adaptation. She emphasized the importance of assessing the staff's social network (Vachon, 1978). She also emphasized examining previous experiences with both death and cancer. The latter does appear to be a self-selecting influence for a number of professionals working in oncology; However, its presence does not predict either success or failure. Some staff members go on to committed, satisfying work; others find the reality too difficult and leave.

## Organizational Interventions

There are environmental considerations and personal experiences on the job that do affect staff performance. Organizational interventions addressing such considerations maximize positive outcomes and include the following:

1. Effective leadership
2. Clear lines of authority
3. Unambiguous work assignments
4. Realistic expectations
5. Team approach
6. Open communications about both work issues and burnout issues
7. Respect for time off and vacations
8. Encouragement of group cohesion
9. Good orientation procedures
10. Provision for positive feedback
11. Career enrichment opportunities

There is a growing literature on minimizing the incidence of burnout in the helping professions. Pines and colleagues (1981) described organizational strategies, social support systems, and intrapersonal coping strategies. Pines and Aronson (1983) described a traveling-workshop format. Maslach (1979) has reviewed the special situation of burnout in relation to patient care. Looking to medical settings, Cassem and Hackett (1979) have suggested interventions to improve functioning in intensive care units that have good applicability to cancer units. Gardner and Hall (1981) and Hall and colleagues (1979) have also addressed the problems unique to the medical setting. The problems of cancer nurses have received much attention (McElroy, 1982; Vachon, 1980; Yasko, 1983). Mor and Laliberte (1984) have studied burnout in hospice staff. Finally, interest in the bereaved has spawned a body of work reviewed by Osterweis, Solomon, and Green (1984). The extensive literature on support groups has been described earlier. The information gathered from all these sources is remarkably consistent. The common themes with respect to organizational guidelines, listed earlier are discussed briefly here.

Leadership must be experienced as authoritative yet understanding. To perform well, leaders need good backup and clear lines of authority. They may benefit from special training or support in knowing how to maintain strong leadership and high standards, while showing awareness of human limitations. The latter is perhaps more important than in many other work situations. Examples of this latter problem will appear in the sections to follow.

Work assignments must be unambiguous and expectations realistic. There are two aspects to this. The first

is that the actual work load must remain manageable even if demanding. The second is less tangible; the work goals must remain realistic. It is all too easy for leaders and staff to allow their earnest desire to help to result in an unrealistic drive to achieve ill-defined, unattainable goals in patient care. The role of the leader is particularly crucial, because he or she must monitor this process in himself or herself and in the staff members as well.

In a smoothly functioning unit, experienced staff also play an important role in helping new and young colleagues to develop a practical working stance. Rotating the most thankless tasks or the most difficult patients is a good practical intervention in this respect, because it gives a welcome respite and conveys an important symbolic message of fairness and acceptance of human limitation.

The team approach is another useful technique that increases opportunities for sharing of expertise and constructive staff development, and ensures that no individual feels indispensable. It realistically eases coverage problems and allows time off, with minimal disruption of patient care. It follows from this that staff vacations and time off must be valued and respected.

Keeping open lines of communication is all-important. This includes communication vertically between staff members and leaders, and horizontally among coequals. This should serve to help define problems, work out solutions when possible, ventilate feelings, provide information, clarify misunderstandings, and negotiate partial solutions. The topics of communication are related to the tasks of the team, but they can also address burnout issues.

Because high morale is important to group cohesion, group activities (both work and social) can be encouraged, but the kind and amount must be monitored so that it remains compatible with the setting. If a unit or a team appears to have become overinvolved with itself, the leader must reestablish work discipline while seeking to understand the reasons that led to the problem. A simple laxness of standards can be at fault; but members can also be responding to difficult and unresolved work problems that are not being addressed directly or to unusual neediness in a few members who co-opt the work group to meet personal needs.

Leaders should be able to identify the individuals who cause conflict because of personal problems. They should be able to confront them, work with them, and if necessary, refer them for additional help. Leaders may need help to perform this task. In an unsupportive climate, they may set high standards without seeing the human cost that is being paid. But more often, in a more supportive vein, they may collude with their staff to overlook problems and support a co-worker in distress. Leaders should have readily available to them one or more confidential sources of help. This can be a liaison psychiatrist or other specially trained mental health worker, or an employee assistance program.

It is equally important for leaders to identify and reinforce good performance and to make an ongoing effort to give positive feedback to their staff, both individually and as a unit.

Adequate orientation of new and young staff is very important. Sessions should include a concrete portion with detailed formal teaching, as well as an emotional component that is directed to helping staff recognize and accept the feelings they will experience. An apprenticeship is helpful, be it in a form of a preceptorship or a buddy system, so that the initial weeks of work take place under the aegis of a supportive and experienced colleague.

The issues that almost universally arise are confrontation with death, and encounters with especially meaningful patients. Less evident but always also present are fears about cancer, both reality-based concerns and irrationally based fears. Staff members function better when they are given repeated educational and in-service training programs to organize and allay their anxieties. In the case of irrational fears, ventilation and sharing also bring relief. Staff fears about certain treatments also call for the same management, that is, acknowledgement, ventilation, and education.

Ambivalence about treatments is more complex. Not only does it engender guilt in staff members about administering treatments they are not sure they would want for themselves, but it can also engender anger, divisiveness, and mistrust among staff members of different persuasions about aggressiveness of treatment. It may sometimes be desirable to arrange a lateral transfer without prejudice, to a position that is less emotionally conflicted.

Ongoing support groups may supplement the measures just described to monitor and manage intrastaff tensions of a more pervasive nature. They may help some staff members to come to terms with their conflicted feelings about work. They almost always help to cut down on inappropriate scapegoating of a single individual, emotional confusion, and escalation of negative feelings. Groups are an important modality with which to address staff problems and are reviewed in the following section.

## STAFF SUPPORT GROUPS IN AN ONCOLOGY SETTING

Beneficial effects of group meetings have been reported with both doctors and nurses in several medical settings including oncology. Although there are few research studies on the effectiveness of groups in the oncology setting, there are many descriptive accounts in the literature, and there is wide agreement about their usefulness. The format and content vary widely between the two extremes of a highly structured educational emphasis on the one hand (Collins and Grobman, 1983), and an open, self-expressive one on the other. A position somewhere in between these extremes seems desirable. It has been observed that the work groups that are most effective and that endure the longest are those that meet the members' sentient needs, while recognizing the work task as the fundamental objective of the group. Clear structure and goals make it easier for staff members to participate, because purposes and rewards are apparent, and the threatening aspects of group participation are decreased. At the same time, there should always be flexibility and built-in opportunities for expression of feelings and personal support. Keeping a good balance between these two poles is a leadership task that can be very demanding. Abrams and Sweeney (1982) address the destructive processes that can occur in staff support groups when this balance fails, and outline responses to them. Eisendrath (1981) addresses the more usual problems encountered and speaks of the reactions and needs of the group leader. Qualifications for an effective leader include understanding of both group process and the task at hand.

The ideal general goals of staff support groups can be seen as a flow of accomplishments, each one facilitating the next. Improving communications and decreasing the sense of isolation in a constructive, educational setting decreases staff anxiety and raises staff self-esteem. This, in turn, leads to better morale and better patient care.

The group format depends on the skill of the leader whose role it is to ensure that the group functions as a support and not a therapy group, because participants will initially not know the difference. The leader must establish appropriate boundaries. The content discussed should focus on work-related issues. "Special" cases that have obvious personal meaning for one member require that the leader help the staff member and the group stay within a conservative range of personal disclosure in which the group gains an increased sense of mutual understanding without the individual feeling unduly exposed.

For example, a young nurse began to cry in a group upon saying that a certain patient reminded her of her mother. Several members responded warmly and shared similar experiences. The young woman acknowledged this support and pulled herself together rapidly, showing a desire to remove herself from the emotional center of attention. Although group members wished to pursue the topic, the leader supported the nurse's desire to end her role in the discussion and guided the group away from her and back toward work-related aspects of the issue.

The difference between therapy and support groups in oncology work can be illuminated by comparing the latter to four other modalities, namely, outpatient, inpatient, family, and self-help groups. They are briefly considered here.

The usual group therapy frame of reference is the outpatient psychotherapy group in which patients freely contract to work on psychotherapeutic issues in a setting that is clearly defined, with many rules that must be honored, and with the clear possibility that there will be anxiety-provoking moments that must be endured. Adherence to this model would be counterproductive in cancer staff support groups, in which there is neither a therapeutic contract nor an agreement to tolerate anxiety or accept discipline. The leader must abandon most of the procedures he or she may have been taught in regard to psychotherapy groups. Different ground rules apply here and include open, variable membership, shifting attendance, tolerated lateness and cancellations, subgrouping that goes unconfronted, and limited contracts that are abrogated.

It is also relevant to compare staff support groups to inpatient groups. Articles on inpatient groups (Klein, 1977; Klein and Kugel, 1981; Rice and Rutan, 1981) have emphasized the consequences of the ward setting for inpatient group dynamics; in fact, all events that affect the unit have a major impact on the process of staff groups as well. Major policy issues under discussion, ongoing power struggles, and impending administrative changes are very important for the members, even when they are covert. The group's work is strongly affected by these events, and the leader's effectiveness is diminished by lack of awareness of them. Deciding how much to bring them into overt discussions is a matter of judgment.

It is often said that a cohesive work unit is "like a family." Accordingly, family theory has a lot to say about the dynamics of staff support groups. The group members share a history that excludes the leader. They have preexisting loyalties that may outweigh the potential transference to the leader, and can work effectively at manipulating the leader's role in the group. Powerful mechanisms operate to maintain the status quo. These are often appropriate and must be respected. Patients, staff, and leaders may come and go, but the ward culture must endure because the ward task endures. This gives the long-term support group a cyclical quality reminiscent of inpatient or family groups.

Self-help groups also present some parallels. In particular, members are not patients and would resent being labeled as such. Also, the leader participates by invitation, and his or her expertise is not necessarily viewed as belonging to the process. An honest presentation of one's professional expertise, coupled with more openness, support, and participation is most effective in the staff support group setting.

## Setting Up Groups

Several points must be addressed in setting up a staff support group. These issues are also discussed by Zimberg in Chapter 54 in relation to support groups for nurses.

## TERMINOLOGY

A term must be found for group meetings that is acceptable to the participants. Support groups need not be called groups at all. They can be designated as rounds, workshops, crisis meetings, or ad hoc task forces. The necessary components are several staff members gathered for discussion of work-related issues, with a leader who will encourage discussion along the lines just described.

## LOCATION AND COMPOSITION

Meetings can have a geographic base such as a specific ward or clinic, or a functional one such as a team or a discipline. They can be homogeneous or heterogeneous for discipline and level of training. Heterogeneity, while harder to achieve, has the merit of directly improving communications across professional lines; the desirability of this goal has been discussed earlier.

## DURATION

Duration can vary from regular weekly meetings to recurrent clusters of sessions, ad hoc meetings, or periodic co-option of other scheduled meetings.

## OPENING AGENDAS

When a group session is requested, the overt agenda should be addressed, but it should be borne in mind that the situation is usually more complex than has been stated and that there are always covert agendas that do not relate to the request. It is important for the leader to understand these covert agendas, but it is not always necessary to address them, unless they are directly opposed to the overt agenda.

## ROLE OF DE FACTO LEADERS

Support groups stand or fall with the amount of genuine support they receive from the working leaders of the group—that is, the superiors such as head nurses and service chiefs. One exception is the group in se-rious conflict with its unit leader that may use the group as a forum of opposition, but this is not the usual situation. More often the group will be poorly attended if staff members perceive a lack of interest or respect from the unit leader. Therefore, it is important for group leaders to develop and maintain a good rela-tionship with unit leaders. Some staff group leaders feel that staff groups are most effective if the superior attends regularly.

## STRUCTURE AND CONTENT

When planning to start a group, one should offer struc-ture and content that would be practical and useful (e.g., in-service training or case conferences), but leave the format flexible enough to allow open discus-sion and change of agenda, which almost always oc-curs. For example, a unit may request support in deal-ing with patient-oriented issues, but it may become obvious they are really troubled by interpersonal issues.

## CONFIDENTIALITY

Confidentiality, as usually understood, is impossible because there is no therapeutic contract among the members. One should avoid making hollow statements on the subject, but it may be helpful to explore realistic boundaries and the limits of discretion. This also rein-forces the importance of helping members control their level of personal disclosure.

## IDEAL GROUP CONDITIONS

The ideal conditions for an ongoing group include a regular and convenient meeting time and place, with stable multidisciplinary attendance, genuinely positive input from de facto authorities, and a blend of structure and open discussion.

### Contents and Dynamics of Support Groups

Having outlined the mechanics of starting groups, let us now turn to a consideration of the developmental stages of ongoing support groups in relation to both content and dynamics. Early, middle, and late stages recur in a cyclical fashion and are outlined in the fol-lowing paragraphs.

## EARLY STAGES OF GROUP DYNAMICS

The topics of the early group stage deal with work issues and are outlined here:

1. Overwork; hectic pace
2. Understaffing; sense of exploitation
3. Problems with co-workers: intrashift, intershift
4. Problems with other disciplines
5. Doubts about treatment
6. Confusion and displacement between items 4 and 5
7. Problems with authority
8. Difficult patients and families
9. Confrontations with death

Ventilating these issues in a nonjudgmental atmo-sphere is welcome. An emotionally loaded issue is usually a mix of several issues, and it is helpful to identify and label the components. First, the emo-tionality is defused. Second, one can analyze the com-ponents, discover possible interventions, and help the members concentrate their energy on rationally se-lected achievable goals. Because a sense of passivity and helplessness is common and demoralizing, any-thing that mitigates it is helpful.

The problem of authority requires special discus-sion. Classic psychoanalytical group theory views al-most all early group content as reflecting competing bids for the group leader's attention. This is not neces-sarily the case here, because support groups already have de facto leaders, such as senior attending physi-cians, department chairs, head nurses, or supervisors. These are people with real power and therefore, they are strong transference figures as well. The trans-ference to the group leader is consequently always diluted, displaced, or split. If the transference is dis-placed, the group must be led as if one had an absent coleader. If it is split, one must make strenuous efforts not to be brought into the struggle, and not to allow a real-life split to develop between yourself and the de facto leader.

The issue of difficult patients and families presents problems that are obvious and easy for staff to de-scribe. They make it possible to examine human be-havior under stress, with several helpful conse-quences. First, better understanding decreases nega-tive feelings and increases effectiveness of manage-ment. Second, given the universaly of much human experience, discussing patients is a nonthreatening way of helping staff to better understand their own reactions. Finally, the shared knowledge usually re-sults in better teamwork and better patient care.

Staff confrontations with death deserve special men-tion. The theme recurs at all stages of groups and in all levels of the staff. With young or new staff this is a "rite of passage," but the issue is sufficiently over-whelming that it recurs in all levels of staff associated with feelings of fear, inadequacy, and grief. All staff members benefit from repeated opportunities for ven-tilation, validation, and support of their reactions to death and dying.

## MIDDLE STAGES OF GROUP DYNAMICS

Groups that do not meet regularly usually do not proceed beyond the early stage. In those that do, while the topics may remain the same, the dynamics undergo a change. More trust is developed; the discussion becomes more introspective and revolves around themes of self-definition as a professional and personal vulnerability to special patients and issues in the work setting. At this time, staff are also able to discuss interpersonal problems with a more personal focus on their own style of coping and confrontation, reducing the tendency to respond with anger and blame.

## LATE STAGES OF GROUP DYNAMICS

The concerns of the middle stage are on the boundary between work issues and private concerns, and they demand skill from the leader if a successful balance is to be maintained. When well managed, the discussions are experienced as very meaningful by group members and are associated with positive change. Morale is high, a sense of intimacy is achieved, and members may push further in a direction that blurs the difference between a work and a therapy group. But the push is not well advised, and the attempt must fail because a more therapeutic emphasis brings increased intensity and vulnerability. This, in turn, is associated with increased anxiety and acting out that cannot be managed, because there are no ground rules and there is no therapy contract. This brings a threat of disruption in the workplace, which is an unacceptable outcome to all concerned. Hence, the group must either disband or return to safer levels, thus accounting for the episodic, cyclical quality described in these groups.

### Support for "Nonprofessional" Staff

The ongoing groups described earlier are generally offered to doctors, nurses, social workers, and other staff trained for and deeply involved in patient care. However, ward clerks, secretaries, and technicians also have important responsibilities and interact with patients and families in very stressful circumstances. Ironically, they are often left to manage the desks and telephones while staff groups and conferences are meeting. An effective intervention for these staff members (if they are not participating in heterogeneous support groups) is a time-limited workshop, organized around a core of didactic material on human behavior under stress, which helps to prevent them from personalizing the behavior of patients and families. Opportunities must always be provided for open discussion, during which feelings about cancer and the myths about it emerge, along with strongly held idio-

syncratic beliefs about cancer treatment. Searching questions about quality of care and staff competence are expressed, and conflicted feelings about the group endeavor in which they are playing a role and about their own role in it are shared. Feelings of trust and pride also emerge.

If not well directed and if the goals and limitations are not clear at the outset, these workshops become subject to the hazard of turning into personnel grievance sessions.

### Role For Mental Health Supporting Staff

There are several important staff support roles for a mental health professional on a cancer unit. The first is that of support and backup to unit leaders. This ranges from support from colleagues to help in identifying and dealing with particularly troubled employees. The second role is that of facilitator of communications about difficult issues. Leading groups or conferences is the main route, but smaller meetings and individual sessions may be useful if indicated.

The mental health consultant can be an outsider, but this usually hampers his or her usefulness and effectiveness. Ideally, an active role on the unit makes him or her most likely to identify and understand problems. However, too great an involvement can distort perceptions, especially because the consultant is subject to the same emotional stresses as everyone else. Therefore, he or she should make a point of self-monitoring, seeking an outside source of criticism, support, and validation.

A liaison psychiatrist with experience running support groups and a good knowledge base about psychological issues in cancer is the most highly trained professional available; however, psychologists, social workers, and nurses also function well in this setting, provided they obtain special training in the areas outlined. (See also Chapter 54 on nurse-to-nurse consultation, and the section on support for pediatric oncology staff in Chapter 45.)

## SUMMARY

Working with cancer patients is both challenging and rewarding. The demands are varied and have been outlined in detail. Many are shared by other high-technology, high-stress areas of medicine. A few are specific to cancer, deriving from the special negative aura that cancer still carries in our society, and from the toxic or frightening aspects of cancer treatments.

However, for staff who are able to deal with these problems, the rewards are very profound and represent the quintessence of the satisfactions that have always made medicine so meaningful to generations of dedicated professionals.

The clinical spectrum of staff stress responses includes the following several points. First, a near-universal normal adaptation period lasting several months, during which the staff member makes an early, competence-based adaptation, is followed by one that is emotionally deeper. Second, occasional episodes of reactive anxiety and depression occur that may be briefly incapacitating. These are characterized by having definite causes and being time-limited; moreover, they may benefit from psychiatric intervention but do not usually require it. Third, the rare psychiatric problems that occur with or without obvious causes are typically self-aggravating unless they receive prompt and effective psychiatric care.

An understanding of the stresses faced by cancer staff members enables one to design work conditions that minimize them, and to develop effective interventions to treat them. Organizational guidelines to achieve this goal have been offered. Particular attention was devoted to support groups, including a theoretical discussion and a practical guide on setting up, running, and understanding the dynamics of staff support groups.

Despite the many difficulties just described, the mood for cancer professionals can be cautiously optimistic. Treatment results continue to improve, albeit too slowly, and the sweeping changes in society's outlook and expectations about medical care (though bewildering and inconsistent for now) herald a change that is welcomed by most professionals, who more than anyone are familiar with the problems being addressed and are eager for workable solutions.

Professionals working in oncology settings can be glad that the depth of their contributions is more clearly recognized, and coincidentally, that their needs are acknowledged as well. It is becoming more routine to address issues of staff morale and to build in supports and interventions to maintain them.

These are important developments, ensuring that professionals in cancer care, rather than experiencing their work merely as a drain on their resources, feel privileged above all to share in such a meaningful human endeavor.

## REFERENCES

Abrams, R.C., and J.A. Sweeney (1982). A critique of the process-oriented approach to ward staff meetings. *Am. J. Psychiatry* 139:769–73.

Artiss, K.L. and A.S. Levine (1973). Doctor–patient relation in severe illness. *N. Engl. J. Med.* 288:1210–14.

Babich, H. (1985). Reproductive and carcinogenic health risks to hospital personnel from chemical exposure—a literature review. *J. Environ. Health* 48:52–56.

Bingham, E. (1985). Hazards to health workers from antineoplastic drugs. *N. Engl. J. Med.* 313:1220–21.

Borenstein, D.B. (1985). Should physician training centers offer formal psychiatric assistance to house officers? A report on the major findings of a prototype program. *Am. J. Psychiatry* 142:1053–57.

Borenstein, D.B., and K. Cook (1982). Impairment prevention in the training years. A new mental health program at UCLA. *J.A.M.A.* 247:2700–2703.

Caldwell, T. and M. Weiner (1981). Stresses and coping in ICU nursing. I. A review. *Gen. Hosp. Psychiatry* 3:119–27.

Campbell, T.W. (1980). Death anxiety on a coronary care unit. *Psychosomatics* 21:127–36.

Cassem, N.H. (1979). Internship, liberty, death and other choices. *Harvard Med. Alumni Bull.* 53:46–48.

Cassem, N.H. and T.P. Hackett (1975). Stress in the nurse and therapist in the intensive-care unit and the coronary care unit. *Heart Lung* 4:252–59.

Cassem, N. and T.P. Hackett (1979). Psychiatric medicine in intensive care settings. In T. Manschrek (ed.), *Psychiatry Medicine Update: MGH Reviews for Physicians.* New York: Elsevier, pp. 135–61.

Cherniss, C. (1980). *Staff burnout: Job stress in the human services.* Beverly Hills, Calif.: Sage Publications.

Collins, A.H. and J. Grobman (1983). Group methods in the general hospital setting. In H.I. Kaplan and B.J. Saddock (eds.), *Comprehensive Group Psychotherapy,* 2nd ed. Baltimore: Williams & Wilkins, pp. 289–93.

Czaczkes, J.W. and A.K. DeNour (1978). *Chronic Hemodialysis as a Way of Life.* New York: Brunner/Mazel.

Dashef, S.S., W.M. Espey, and J.A. Lazarus (1974). Time-limited sensitivity groups for medical students. *Am. J. Psychiatry* 13:287–92.

DeNour, A.K. and J.W. Czaczkes (1968). Emotional problems and reactions of the medical team in a chronic haemodialysis unit. *Lancet* 56:987–91.

Eisendrath, S.J. (1981). Psychiatric liaison support groups for general hospital staffs. *Psychosomatics* 22:685–94.

Foley, K.M. (1985). Medical progress. The treatment of cancer pain. *N. Engl. J. Med.* 313:84–95.

Fox, R.C. (1980). *The Human Condition of Health Professionals.* Distinguished lecture series, School of Health Studies, University of New Hampshire. Durham, N.H.: University of New Hampshire, pp. 11–39.

Freudenberger, H.J. (1974). Staff burnout. *J. Soc. Issues* 30:159–65.

Freudenberger, H.J. (1980). *The High Cost of High Achievement.* New York: Anchor Press.

Fullerton, S. (1983). Burnout (Book review). *Child. Youth Services Rev.* 5 (Special issue):301–14.

Fullerton, S. and E. Weeks (1983). Burnout. *Child. Youth Services Rev.* 5 (Special issue):225–313.

Gardner, E.R. and R.C.W. Hall (1981). The professional stress syndrome. *Psychosomatics* 22:672–80.

Hall, R.C.W., E.R. Gardner, M. Perl, S.K. Shickney, and B. Pfefferbaum (1979). The professional burnout syndrome. *Psychiatr. Opinion* 16:12–17.

Kantor, P. and K. Foley (1981). Patterns of narcotic use in a cancer pain clinic. *Ann. N.Y. Acad. Sci.* 362:161.

Klein, R.H. (1977). In-patient group psychotherapy: Practical considerations and special problems. *Int. J. Group Psychother.* 27:201–4.

Klein, R.H. and B. Kugel (1981). In-patient group psychotherapy from a systems perspective: Reflections through a glass darkly. *Int. J. Group Psychother.* 31:311–28.

Kubler-Ross, E. (1969). *On Death and Dying.* New York: Macmillan.

Marks, R.M. and E.J. Sachar (1973). Undertreatment of medical inpatients with narcotic analgesics. *Ann. Intern. Med.* 78:173.

Maslach, C. (1976). Burned out. *Hum. Behav.* 5:16–22.

Maslach, C. (1979). The burn-out syndrome and patient care. In C.A. Garfield (ed.), *Stress and Survival: The Emotional Realities of Life-Threatening Illness.* St. Louis: C.V. Mosby, pp. 111–20.

McCue, J.D. (1982). The effects of stress on physicians and their medical practice. *N. Engl. J. Med.* 306:458–63.

McElroy, A.M. (1982). Burnout—a review of the literature with application to cancer nursing. *Cancer Nurs.* 5:211–17.

Mohl, P.C. (1980a). Group process interpretations in liaison psychiatry nurse groups. *Gen. Hosp. Psychiatry* 2:104–11.

Mohl, P.C. (1980b). A systems approach to liaison psychiatry. *Psychosomatics* 21:457–61.

Mor, V. and L. Laliberte (1984). Burnout among hospice staff. *Health Soc. Work* 9:274–83.

Moynihan, R.T. and E. Outlaw (1984). Nursing support groups in a cancer center. *J. Psychosoc. Oncol.* 2:33–47.

Osterweis, M., F. Solomon, and M. Green (eds.). (1984). *Bereavement Reactions, Consequences, and Care.* Washington, D.C.: National Academy Press.

Perlman, B. and E.A. Hartman (1982). Burnout: Summary and future research. *Hum. Relations* 35:283–305.

Perry, S. (1984). Undermedication for pain. *Psychiatr. Ann.* 14:960.

Perry, S.W. (1985). Irrational attitudes toward addicts and narcotics in iatrogenic addiction: Developing guidelines for the use of sedatives and analgesics in the hospital. *Bull. N.Y. Acad. Med.* 61:706–27.

Pines, A. and E. Aronson (1983). Combatting burnout. Burnout. *Child. Youth Services Rev.* 5 (Special issue):263–76.

Pines, A.M., E. Aronson, and D. Kafry (1981). *Burnout: From Tedium to Personal Growth.* New York: Free Press.

Procci, R. (1983). Psychiatric sequelae of chronic dialysis. In S. Akhtar (ed.), *New Psychiatric Syndromes: DSM-III and Beyond.* New York: Jason Aronson, pp. 219–42.

Quinbey, S. and N.R. Bernstein (1971). Identity problems and the adaptation of nurses to severely burned children. *Am. J.Psychiatry* 128:90–95.

Reuben, D.B., D.H. Novack, T.J. Wachtel, and S.A. Wartman (1984). A comprehensive support system for reducing house staff distress. *Psychosomatics* 25:815–20.

Rice, C.A. and J.S. Rutan (1981). Boundary maintenance in in-patient therapy groups. *Int. J. Group Psychother.* 31:77–93.

Richards, A.I. and A.H. Schmale (1974). Psychosocial conferences in medical oncology: Role in a training program. *Ann. Intern. Med.* 80: 541–45.

Rosini, L.A., M.C. Howell, I.D. Todres, and J. Dorman 1974). Group meetings in a pediatric intensive care unit. *Pediatrics* 53:371–74.

Savicki, V. and E. Cooley (1983). Theoretical and research considerations of burnout. Burnout. *Child. Youth Services Rev.* 5 (Special issue):227–38.

Selevan, S., M.L. Lindbohm, R. Hornung, and K. Hemminki (1985). A study of occupational exposure to antineoplastic drugs and fetal Loss in nurses. *N. Engl. J. Med.* 313:1173–78.

Siegel, B. and J.C. Donnelly (1978). Enriching personal and professional development: The experience of a support group for interns. *J. Med. Educ.* 53:908–14.

Simon, N. and S. Whiteley (1977). Psychiatric consultation with MICU nurses: The consultation conference as a working group. *Heart Lung* 6:497–504.

Spikes, J. and J. Holland (1975). The physician's response to the dying patient. In J.J. Strain and S. Grossman (eds.), *Psychological Care of the Medically Ill.* New York: Appleton-Century-Crofts, pp. 138–48.

Vachon, M.L.S. (1978). Motivation and stress experienced by staff working with terminally ill. *Death Educ.* 2:113–22.

Vachon, M.L.S. (1980). Care for the caregiver. *Can. Nurse* 76:28–33.

Vachon, M.L.S., W.A.L. Lyall, and S.J.J. Freeman (1978). Measurement and management of stress in health professionals working with advanced cancer patients. *Death Educ.* 1:365–75.

Wahl, C.W. (1958). The fear of death. *Bull. Menninger Clin.* 22:214–23.

Weiner, M.F. and T. Caldwell (1981). Stresses and coping in ICU nursing. II. Nurse support groups on intensive care units. *Gen. Hosp. Psychiatry* 3:129–34.

Weisman, A.T. (1981). Understanding the cancer patient: The caregiver's plight. *Psychiatry* 44:161–68.

Wise, T.N. (1977). Training oncology fellows in psychological aspects of their specialty. *Cancer* 39:2584–87.

Yasko, J.M. (1983). Variables which predict burnout experienced by oncology clinical nurse specialists. *Cancer Nurs.* 5:109–16.

# 52

# Special Problems of Physicians and House Staff in Oncology

Kathryn M. Kash and Jimmie C. Holland

During the past decade there has been an increasing recognition of the psychological and physical impact that providing medical care has on physicians. The stresses have increased as medical practice has become more dependent on technology (McCue, 1982). In the modern cancer center, there are particular challenges for the physician who must deal daily with illnesses for which curative treatments are limited and for which progressive disease and death are frequent outcomes. It is important as the field of oncology grows to identify the stresses and their consequences and methods to reduce both, because studies of other health professionals have shown deleterious effects of stress (Cartwright, 1979).

First, the word *stress* is so widely and often uncritically used that one must define the word to understand it in relation to work in cancer. Caplan (1981) defined stress as that state of emotional and physiological arousal that occurs when the demands of work, personal life, or both exceed one's ability to cope or respond effectively. This takes into account the personal stresses of the individual's social environment and his or her ways of coping with it. We have examined these issues at Memorial Sloan-Kettering Cancer Center (MSKCC) for the past 2 years from a slightly different viewpoint: specifically, given the recognized high level of stress in both oncologists and house staff, why do some seem to thrive on stress and others falter under the strain?

To examine stress in the field of oncology, one must call on a relevant body of work from studies of medical students, house staff, and physicians from other specialities. The first section of this chapter reviews the sources of stress. The next looks at the consequences of stress, including physical symptoms, psychological distress, occupational signs of ''burnout,'' and physician impairment caused by substance abuse and psychiatric disorders. The third is concerned with the

ways physicians adapt and cope with stress. The fourth section investigates the intervention strategies that have been used to reduce stress, including one presently being tested as an educational/supportive approach to alter the environment of an oncology unit. These aspects of physician stress and its modification are conceptualized in a model (Figure 52-1) developed by Kobasa and adapted for study in the cancer center. It outlines the personal and hospital stresses that contribute to adverse psychological and physical symptoms and the personal factors (e.g., personality and support from others) that serve to decrease the adverse effects of stress.

## SOURCES OF STRESS

One must begin by examining the personal characteristics that physicians bring to medicine and the impact that medical school and training has on them. Individuals who choose medicine, irrespective of later decisions about specialty, have strong obsessive-compulsive traits that lead them to choose a career in which long hours of study, heavy responsibility, and devotion to work are required. In fact, the more these traits are exaggerated the more outstanding a student may be (Reuben, 1983). Feifel (1959) observed that doctors have greater fear of death than laypersons, a concern that could have preceded or been acquired in training. These personal attitudes about death and overconscientiousness may cause increased distress as the physician agonizes over a decision that he or she sees as a personal failure to save a patient's life (Spikes and Holland, 1975). This compulsiveness, when present in conjunction with other characteristics of overly controlled emotions and low need for relaxation and pleasure, makes the medical student, and later the physician more vulnerable than others to depression, alcoholism, psychiatric disorders, and suicide. Medi-

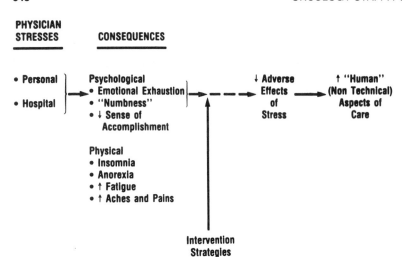

**Figure 52-1.** Intervention strategies, personality, and social supports as a means of reducing stress and decreasing its adverse effects. *Source:* Adapted from Kobasa (1982), Commitment and coping in stress resistance among lawyers. *Journal of Personality and Social Psychology, 42,* pp. 707–717.

cal students relate their sense of being stressed also to financial burdens, an overload of knowledge to be acquired, challenges to their competence (especially in the clinical years), social isolation, fatigue, and discomfort with the early experiences of dealing with death and dying patients (Gaensbauer and Mizner, 1980).

The clinical training that follows for the intern and resident involves spending 80 hours a week at the hospital and staying awake 30–36 hours when on call. Friedman and colleagues (1973) showed the impact of sleep loss and fatigue on interns who read electrocardiograms with less acuity after prolonged periods of work than when they were fresh. New York State has taken recent steps to reduce the time on duty to reduce the hazard of poorer performance. In addition, work affords the house officer very little time with family, friends, and peers. Guilt for not being available to the family, especially children, adds to the stress. Loneliness, social isolation, and work overload combined with an overwhelming sense of responsibility create major stress for the house officer.

Again, as students, the personal qualities that contribute to success as house officers also contribute to the hospital stresses; that is, compulsiveness, a tendency to be overly conscientious and self-doubting, a strong sense of responsibility, a feeling of never having read enough, and choosing to take little time off from work. Coupled with lack of sleep, absence of social life, anger about "scut" work, and overwork, it is not surprising that a "house officer syndrome" has been described with characteristic symptoms, including episodic cognitive impairment due to lack of sleep, chronic anger and resentment about demands on time and energy, family discord (especially marital prob-

lems), and a pervasive cynicism (with an accompanying shift from wanting to help those in distress to wanting to protect limited time and energy available) (Small, 1981). Some house officers become concerned about their unaccustomed callousness and change from their prior personality.

While house officers usually rotate to an oncology unit or cancer center for a limited period of time (usually 5 weeks to 3 months), oncology fellows training for 2 years requires their full time in treating seriously or terminally ill cancer patients or related clinical or basic research. In fact, their training is the result of the decision to devote their career to care of these patients. This makes their adaptation in oncology all the more important, not only for their personal well-being, but for their ability to give sensitive care to patients throughout their careers. Thus, the sources of stress for them must be considered not only for the short term, but also from the perspective of long-term adaptation to the stresses of the work.

The modern cancer center imposes significant stresses on both staff and patients as technology has provided a more complex environment (e.g., Bard, 1984; Holland, 1982). Vachon (1987) described some of these stresses that are regularly encountered by oncologists and oncology nurses, including caring for patients who are extremely ill, dealing with the deaths of patients of all ages, poor staff communications, being intensely involved with patients and their families, conflicts between research and clinical care goals, and the work load imposed by the complicated and taxing work of palliative care. Both the gravity of the illness under treatment and the emphasis on clinical investigation in a cancer center present many similarities of the modern cancer treatment setting and the social environment to the metabolic research ward described elegantly by Renée Fox (1962) more than two decades ago when the initial use of steroids for otherwise fatal diseases was being tried. We see the same problems today in dealing with uncertainty, frustration with failure, and concerns about outcome of often hopeless illness.

However, the contemporary oncologist must also cope with the rapid changes in cancer care, increase in technology, and greater dependence on laboratory data that result in a more impersonal environment and, some say, greater emotional distance between physician and patient. In fact, because of these impediments to the doctor–patient relationship, patients place even greater importance on that bond with the physician. Several deaths in a short period of time, especially when it includes a ''special'' patient with whom identification is closer, such as an ill physician or a patient who resembles a loved one, takes its toll on the physician (see Chapter 58).

Trust and communication between doctor and patient are of the utmost importance for the emotional well-being of the patient. This becomes crucial in advanced stages of cancer when it becomes necessary to discuss the painful reality, including initiation of a do not resuscitate order. Communications with the patient around these issues are particularly stressful. In fact, Mount (1986) has described this difficult conflict in the care of cancer patients when the decision must be made to change from active treatment of disease to palliation and comfort. This transition and the decisions that follow (e.g., the do not resuscitate order) are among the most painful aspects of oncology. These decisions are the most frequent cause of conflict among staff, because the views are so intertwined with personal values and beliefs. Katz (1984), who provides a social history of medicine, notes that physicians must learn to live with failure and the awareness of the uncertainty of clinical judgments yet be able to proceed in any case; finally, the doctor, and especially in relation to managing advanced cancer, must decide which aspects to share with patients.

A different but real and very stressful problem is the demanding and uncooperative patient who, while rejecting most help, also seeks much attention (Holland and Holland, 1985; McCue, 1982). Some of these patients threaten malpractice suits, which adds to the tension in giving care. They create stress in the physician because they are noncompliant with treatment, and many have psychiatric problems that are beyond the scope of the physician's training. Also, communication skills with patients generally, and particularly with problem patients are not taught to physicians, thus their stress is compounded because they are less than well prepared to handle the patient.

The personality of many doctors also leads them to have difficulty denying patient requests, other professional obligations, and scholarly and academic pressures. This results in few avocational outlets and frequent absence from home. Even while at home, the beeper and telephone calls take time away from the family. Emotional distancing and withdrawal from family may occur, which creates conflicts at home and in turn reduces the support of family and increases stress (McCue, 1982). While the divorce rate is not disproportionately high for physicians (Fine, 1981), the impact of taking work home and seeing patients on the weekends are problems. One physician was afraid to retire because he had never spent time with his family and didn't know how he would fare at home with them (Bendix, 1984). When personal grief occurs after the loss of a family member or friend, emotional response to patients' deaths at work are more painful. Oncologists particularly are apt to be brought into the care of relatives with cancer, complicating the family role with one that is quasi-medical. A physician's own health problems are often ignored or denied because physicians often feel guilty asking colleagues for a personal consultation, leading to poor care at times (see Chapter 58). There is some suggestion that they tolerate recognizable symptoms of disease longer than others. Financial worries, especially student loans and expenses of a practice, can be significant. A random sample of 147 physicians approached as members of the American Society of Clinical Oncology found several indications of stress among oncologists whose average age was 43 (Schmale et al., 1987). They felt challenged by oncology. Nevertheless, they felt pressured, suffering from the negative responses of patients and families as well as their emotional problems, dealing with dying patients, ineffective treatments and the negative impact on personal life. They identified a need for more emotional support for themselves as well as for patients.

The cumulative stressors on physicians include the following:

Work load and patient care related stresses
Conflicts at work (e.g., boss, peers, and staff)
Conflicts in personal life (e.g., spouse, patients, and children)
Personal illness
Personal grief (e.g., loss of family members or friends)
Personal financial worry.

It is important to take into account the inevitability of personal losses, illnesses, and conflicts, at times coinciding with work stresses. These salient sources of stress for oncologists have both personal and professional consequences. They are described in the following sections.

## CONSEQUENCES OF STRESS

During their education medical students frequently need help in coping with stress. One-third of students seek professional counseling because they suffer anxiety or depression secondary to academic pressures or because they feel emotional distance from others (Weinstein, 1983). This is likely an underestimate of the numbers who actually need help, because many schools still have inadequate counseling resources and some students still fear the stigma and potential retaliation for seeking a psychiatric consultation. That suicide is the second leading cause of student death speaks for the need (Ross, 1971).

As for house officers, one-third of the interns in one study had experienced significant depression during their internships; approximately 25% stated they had had suicidal ideation (Valko and Clayton, 1975). Another study found that, during the years 1979–1984, 55.5% of the internal medicine programs granted leaves of absence to residents because of emotional problems (Smith et al., 1986). While 79% of these residents ultimately returned, 10% dropped out of medicine and 2% committed suicide. A survey of 1805 interns, residents, and fellows in Ontario, Canada revealed that 23% had some degree of distress or depression on the Center for Epidemiological Studies of Depression Scale (CES-D); women were 1.5 times more likely to be depressed and 3 times more likely to be severely depressed than men. Among the male respondents ($N = 1162$), interns had the highest frequency of depression and distress ranging from mild to severe, and 26% of them had high scores on the CES-D. Among the specialities, male residents in obstetrics and gynecology had the highest mean scores, followed by interns and residents in psychiatry. Among the female respondents ($N = 585$), a pattern similar to the male house staff emerged, with interns receiving the highest scores in the distress and depression ranges; 38% of these women had high scores on the CES-D. Women residents who specialized in psychiatry followed by women in obstetrics and gynecology had the highest average scores on the CES-D. No data were provided on those in oncology (Hsu and Marshall, 1987).

For physicians, there are four categories for the consequences of stress, namely, physical symptoms, psychological symptoms, burnout (combining both personal and organizational), and more serious psychiatric impairment (e.g., alcoholism, drug abuse, and major mental illness). The most frequent physical symptoms of chronic stress include frequent tension headaches, exhaustion, fatigue, insomnia, gastrointestinal disturbances (with increase or decrease in appetite) when no medical explanation can be found, and

**Table 52-1**  Psychological symptoms of stress in physicians

- No enthusiasm for work
- Hard to get up to go to work
- Mood characterized by depression, tension, irritability, easy frustration
- Detachment characterized by cynicism, negativity, "why bother," tuned out, shortening hours, less responsible about obligations
- Overinvolvement characterized by "nobody can do it right but me," "nobody works but me," stretching work hours, but less efficient, taking work home

minor aches and pains (often questioned as signs of leukemia or cancer). For those working close to cancer, there is the fear that minor symptoms in one-self or a family member might be the onset of a neoplastic disease. Attempts at self-medication along with delay in seeking the professional help of another physician are common and may complicate the problem.

Coupled with the physical symptoms are the signs of psychological distress (Table 52-1); loss of enthusiasm for work, depression, irritability and frustration, and a cynical view of medicine and colleagues (Hall et al., 1979; Holland and Holland, 1985; Maslach, 1979; Mount, 1986). Simultaneously, the doctor becomes overinvolved with excessive dedication and commitment, longer hours with less productivity and decreased sensitivity to the emotional needs of patient and others; conversely, he or she may become detached and disinterested in medical practice. These two presentations of burnout in oncologists have been described as the "*I must do everything*" syndrome and the "*I hate medicine*" syndrome. The known potential outcome of both of these two syndromes, if allowed to progress, is alcoholism, substance abuse, mental illness, and suicide (Hall et al., 1979; Holland and Holland, 1985; Mount, 1986).

Many of the signs in health care professionals were described by Maslach (1979) as the "burnout" syndrome, specifically, emotional exhaustion, depersonalization, and lack of a sense of personal accomplishment. Emotional exhaustion is felt as being emotionally overextended and exhausted by work. Depersonalization is a poor term to describe the sense of distance and reduced sympathy that the person usually feels toward patients. Lack of personal accomplishment is experienced as "What do I ever accomplish anyway." In oncology it is expressed often by house officers as a feeling that all treatment is futile in cancer, so why bother at all. Millerd (1977) conceptualized these problems as a form of survivor syndrome in health caregivers who have dealt repeatedly with losses from death; some of the adverse symptoms are the same as those seen in survivors of natural disasters.

**Table 52-2** Degrees and characteristic signs of physician stress

| Stages | Degree of stress | Characteristics |
|--------|------------------|-----------------|
| 1 | Mild | Hard to get up, tired, aches, somatic complaints, fatigue, exhausted |
| 2 | Moderate | Negative outlook, cynical, suspicious, alienated |
| 3 | Severe | Absenteeism, work slowdown, disgust, alcohol and/or drug abuse |
| 4 | Extreme | Withdrawal, collapse, suicidal risk |

Table 52-2 shows the progression in severity of symptoms from mild (Stages 1 and 2) to more severe, when actual inability to function and a psychiatric illness, frequently depression, ensue; alcohol and drugs become a solace. Access to prescription drugs and those available on hospital units leads to easy abuse. The more serious consequences of stress occur when the early signs and symptoms of distress are ignored or denied by the physician (and family and colleagues). Physicians fear knowing that they are ill because with substance abuse they may no longer be regarded as competent; they also fear the stigma of seeing a psychiatrist. The use of alcohol and drugs to reduce distress and symptoms escalates the dysfunction at work.

Far less studied are the physicians who have 10–15 years of practical postacademic experience and who appear most frequently with actual work impairment at an average age of 40. There is ample evidence that impairment among physicians is common, has been underreported, and is now on the rise at least partially because of more active reporting by medical societies and monitoring by hospitals (Scheiber and Doyle, 1983).

Alcoholism is estimated to affect from 7 to 8%, or approximately 40,000 U.S. physicians, at some point during their careers (Steindler, 1975). While this prevalence rate is not greater than that of the general population, the second leading cause of death among physicians is cirrhosis of the liver (Sakinofsky, 1980). The drink or two after work to relieve stress may be innocuous, but dependence and increasing use is the usual onset of alcoholism and, at times, drug addiction. Physician drug addiction rates are 30–100 times greater than the general population (Modlin and Montes, 1964).

A study of alcoholism and drug addiction in physicians found that the predisposing personality (e.g., obsessive-compulsive) traits of the physician with vulnerability to depression and the easy availability of drugs were the primary contributing factors. One interesting finding was that more than 50% of addicted

physicians had had alcoholic fathers. Despite these findings, the physicians themselves reported the causes of their problems to be overwork, fatigue, and physical illnesses (e.g., migraine, colitis, hypertension, and ulcers), suggesting the tendency to deny the psychiatric aspects of illness in themselves (Modlin and Montes, 1964).

The pattern that leads to addictive behavior in physicians is characterized by a history of an inefficient and disorganized work routine, as well as poor eating and sleeping habits. Over time this pattern contributes to chronic anxiety, emotional withdrawal, depression, and symptoms of the burnout syndrome. Alcohol or drugs, or both, are employed to ameliorate symptoms. When this does not work, and the family supports are weak, the physician may engage in acting-out behaviors to reduce distress, such as extramarital affairs or gambling. When these activities fail to reduce distress, then fatigue, irritability, and depression increase, as well as the alcohol or drug abuse. The end stage is actual drug addiction, alcoholism, divorce, depression, and attempted suicide, which may be the precipitant for hospitalization (Scheiber, 1983). Special hospitals for health professionals with drug and alcohol problems have been effective in offering inpatient care to doctors and nurses.

Although the divorce rate for physicians is no higher than in the general population, a controlled study indicated that 47% of physicians had unsatisfactory marital relationships when compared with 32% of controls (Vaillant et al., 1972). A study of physicians' wives revealed that, of those hospitalized for depression, the majority reported feelings of abandonment by their husbands; 82% of these women report unsatisfactory sexual relationships (Evans, 1965). For female physicians, the divorce rate is higher than that of men and higher than the general population (Rosow and Rose, 1972). Among addicted physicians, 75% had difficulties in their sexual relationships (Modlin and Montes, 1964). Thus, it appears that physicians under stress from professional obligations are in marriages that are often troubled and more attention and study should be given to spouses, beginning during medical training.

Suicide, the most tragic consequence of depression, is committed by approximately 100 U.S. physicians each year, the equivalent of one medical school class (Scheiber and Doyle, 1983). Alcohol and drugs are frequent means of suicide in themselves or are used in conjunction with some other lethal methods. There are conflicting reports of suicide rates for male physicians, although it is generally accepted that the rates for men are not greater than their counterparts in other professions (Rich and Pitts, 1979). For female physicians, however, the rate was similar to that of male physicians, but was three to four times greater than women in other professions (Pitts et al., 1979; Steppacher and Mauser, 1974). Others have questioned the comparison groups, and the interpretation of the finding is unclear. Among specialties, psychiatrists commit suicide at twice the expected rate (Rich and Pitts, 1980). The rate among oncologists is not known, but it is of interest in view of the daily proximity to death.

On a more reassuring note about deleterious consequences of practicing medicine, Valliant and colleagues (1972) studied 47 physicians and 79 socioeconomically matched controls not in medicine. Physicians, especially those involved in direct patient care, had more problems and had more often sought psychotherapy. However, the problems of poor marriages and heavy use of alcohol and drugs were clustered among those physicians who had had the least stable childhoods and more troubled adolescence. This may be important in identifying the house staff and physicians who are most vulnerable and emphasizes that work stress alone is usually not the cause. Combined work and personal characteristics, some of which could be predicted by history, appear the more reliable predictors. The need for measures to ameliorate the deleterious effects of stress are clear from the facts just outlined. Exploring personal, social, and professional interventions that could be used to enhance coping has been an important concern in studying stress in oncology.

## ADAPTING AND COPING WITH STRESS

There is an interaction of influences between the physician and the environment that results in a range of ways of adapting and coping. There are actually both personal (personality type and coping style) and interpersonal (social support and support of the work environment) resources available to counter professional stresses.

An effort to reinforce certain personality characteristics that lead to better coping with stressful situations is one approach to reducing stress. Kobasa (1979) described the "hardy" personality that copes well in stressful environments; one that has three characteristics—commitment, control, and challenge. The combination of a sense of commitment to one-self and the various areas in life including work, an attitude that one has influence over what occurs, and a sense of being challenged in the face of a changing environment has been shown, when present, to be associated with fewer mental and physical symptoms of stress. Hardiness is said to lead to a perception, interpretation, and handling of stressful events that prevents excessive activation or arousal and therefore results in fewer symptoms of stress.

Empirical research has found that business execu-

**Table 52-3**  Coping strategies

- Recognize and monitor symptoms.
- Change pace and balance diet.
- Decrease overtime.
- Exercise.
- Maintain sense of humor.
- Seek consultation if symptoms are severe.
- Discuss work-related stresses with others who share the same problems.
- Visit counterpart in other institutions; look for new solutions to problems.
- Note stress symptoms in colleagues and discuss with them; suggest referral, if needed.

tives, lawyers, army officers, and others with a high number of stressors, who had a strong sense of commitment to self and work, a more positive attitude toward change, and a greater belief in control over life, reported fewer physical symptoms than those who did not have this personality style (Kobasa, 1979; Kobasa, 1982; Kobasa et al., 1982; Kobasa and Puccetti, 1983). These were all professional groups that are similar to physicians in socioeconomic status. Preliminary findings from studies of house officers at MSKCC suggests that it likely holds true for coping with the stress of working in a cancer center.

This personality type is useful in influencing effective ways of coping with stress. These coping methods can be introduced on both the personal and organizational levels and are useful in the prevention and management of burnout (Koocher, 1979; Hartl, 1979; Mount, 1986). Some of these are shown in Table 52-3. One of the most important strategies is to be able to recognize the physical and psychological symptoms of stress in oneself. It is additionally important to identify them in colleagues and point out that such symptoms are common, transient, and reversible when dealt with early. Discomfort in pointing out emotional distress in a colleague should not be any greater than suggesting a consultation for a medical symptom.

Oncologists who take a positive attitude toward themselves and their work deal better with it. Daily challenges are less overwhelming. Maintaining self-esteem and self-confidence, often shaken when caring for cancer patients, is helpful and contributes to a doctor patient communication characterized by mutual respect.

Maintaining a sense of humor through the use of black or gallows humor allows laughing at tragedy as a way to lighten it. It is sometimes poorly understood by others who see it as disrespectful. It is actually an important coping device that, when shared with close colleagues, contributes to the esprit de corps. The "MASH" mentality evidenced by the familiar Korean

War film of surgeons in a field hospital portrays its use extremely well.

Exercise and diet are useful. Exercise, particularly if practiced on a regular basis, reduces stress symptoms. Adequate sleep prevents the associated problems of fatigue and irritability.

Change of pace by taking breaks and vacations is important. The fresh look at the work problems that comes after time away confirms its value. The sabbatical is a long-standing academic device to assure a time for self-assessment, too often missing in medical environments.

Attention to an avocation also assures a change of pace. When it entails vigorous physical exercise, it helps relieve frustration and physical symptoms of stress, especially tension. Relaxation is another way to cope with symptoms of stress. Meditation, yoga, biofeedback, and progressive relaxation work well. Consistency in using relaxation is the key to making it work.

In addition to coping strategies that can be used on a personal level, organizational and supportive measures have been undertaken to assist physicians in their adaptation to clinical care in oncology.

## INTERVENTIONS

Consultation–liaison psychiatry has addressed the major attention to this area, studying both the patients' psychological reaction to illness and the physicians' responses to giving clinical care (Strain and Hammerman, 1978). The care of patients with life-threatening and fatal illnesses has long been identified as the most stressful, and those giving these services are in most need of support (Spikes and Holland, 1975). Far more interventions have been studied for nurses (see Chapters 53 and 54). However, the need for support of oncology fellows was noted by Artiss and Levine (1973). The overall ideal support likely comes from having a single individual, usually a liaison psychiatrist, who constitutes a ''psychological presence'' in both inpatient and outpatient settings, and to whom problems can be brought without fear of ridicule or embarrassment.

Most efforts have been directed toward house staff distress, aimed at providing both group and individual assistance, and toward altering the work load. Reduced frequency of night call has slowly changed from several decades ago when on-call availability was 7 days and nights a week to the present every third, or even every fourth night. Shared on-call assignment and better backup have developed. Support groups have been shown to be effective with pediatric house staff in promoting cooperation and reducing isolation (Siegel and Donnelly, 1978). Special mental health

programs, such as a free service at UCLA for psychiatric consultation and brief psychotherapy, has been effective (Borenstein and Cook, 1982). Also, orienting house staff, especially chief residents, about problems that may arise, assures their identification.

At MSKCC, the rotating house staff have received orientation about stresses and resources by a liaison psychiatrist who is also available on rounds for consultation and case discussions. Rotations through oncology are dreaded, and most are ill-prepared for the many seriously ill patients. Transient cancerophobia is also not uncommon because fears about having cancer arise as a variant of the medical student syndrome (see Chapter 2). Personal problems are often taken to the liaison psychiatrist as a known and trusted colleague who has credibility and is seen as one to be trusted. When this visibility on a medical unit is coupled with close coordination with the chief resident, potential problems are identified and often averted early. Separate orientation is given to medical oncology fellows which focuses on the stresses that will occur and the types of reactions that can be expected. This sets up awareness of problems and identifies a resource if help is needed later.

At the National Cancer Institute, a series of seminars have been held by a psychiatrist and an oncologist since the early 1970s and have continued as an annual support for the oncology fellows, usually extending over the first 5–6 months of the training year (Artiss and Levine, 1973). They meet on a weekly basis for 90 minutes and discuss selected articles they have read prior to the seminar. Discussions take place about various aspects of the doctor and patient relationship and the practical application of the reading material. Using small-group dynamics, the seminars focus first on the emotional needs and problems of patients and later on the responses of the fellows to various psychological problems, especially those dealing with the terminally ill. They come to recognize those situations that arouse their anger, depression, denial, and displacement of emotional distress from one situation to another and that affect the quality of care. This model is used in different forms in many oncology programs.

A similar approach was introduced at the University of Rochester in New York, where psychiatric input to medical oncology resulted in a biweekly formal 90-minute conference, which was attended by fellows, nurses, attending physicians, social workers, clergy, and medical students (Richards and Schmale, 1974). It was led by an oncologist who had trained in the psychological medicine program and who discussed a patient presented by a trainee, with discussion geared to specific patient problems and treatment.

Yet another approach, and a more open-ended one, was used at the Johns Hopkins Hospital in Baltimore

(Wise, 1977). In this group, the issues raised revolved around the problems that the oncology staff themselves were experiencing. This group, led by a liaison psychiatrist and a psychiatric nurse-clinician, was composed of nurses, oncology fellows, medical students, house officers, and social workers from the oncology unit. Wise points out the initial responses in discussions; including anxiety about helplessness in the face of terminally ill patients, distress about how to dispel the hospital myth of the oncologist as the "poison peddlar," and dealing with the dying patient. The liaison psychiatrist and a nurse worked with the group and, by looking at responses and identifying where expectations were inappropriate, increased skills developed in working with patients psychologically. It also allayed some dysphoric feelings and promoted a sense of acceptance of role and limits. This ongoing group helped foster a collaborative team spirit among the staff members and increased their ability to deal effectively with their feelings about cancer patients.

In a similar manner, Strain and Hammerman (1978) developed ombudsman rounds on the oncology floor at Montefiore Hospital in the Bronx. These rounds, led by an oncologist and psychiatrist, were attended by all staff members who were related to patient care on the unit, including house officers, nurses, aides, medical students, social workers, the attending physician, secretary, and clergy. These rounds often also brought the patient to the meeting with a family member, to discuss their own reactions. They also, as the only forum that included all staff members provided a place for airing of conflicts and for resolutions through discussions. It was described as the only time other than the Christmas party that all staff met together. Understanding of patient behavior and that of the staff helped improve communication and increased psychological support of staff members for each other.

At MSKCC, a similar weekly meeting has been effective on the neurooncology unit where dealing with patients with brain tumors is particularly stressful. Run by the head nurse and liaison psychiatrist, it serves to identify special problems and patients, and facilitates their management. A similar group run by a liaison psychiatrist has been effective in the intensive care unit. On a medical oncology floor, a supportive intervention model has been studied for effectiveness in reducing stress on house staff members and nurses through enhanced information, communication, sense of cohesiveness and support. It also seeks to examine the impact on patients' perception of that portion of their care that relates to sensitivity of the staff members support and communication. The intervention seeks to increase the staff person's sense of control, commitment, and challenge at work, thereby reducing the physical and psychological symptoms of stress and

avoiding negative impact on care. This model was designed to use existing staff and to meet criteria of simplicity, economic feasibility, and easy implementation and integration in other centers.

The intervention has several components: orientation for new house staff prior to the day of arrival for assignment, when observations repeatedly showed that anticipations of stresses were exaggerated; weekly meeting with house staff members to listen to their "gripes" at "pizza lunch"; a weekly interdisciplinary unit meeting, the collaborative practice meeting, which explores patient and staff issues, and attempts to identify problems and seek resolutions; finally, a weekly attending rounds for house staff members where patients are presented whose problems pose particularly stressful issues for the staff (such as the do not resuscitate order, AIDS dementia, or an angry patient), and the management principles for each.

Baseline measures of stress and coping were initially obtained at the beginning of the year for fellows, interns, residents, and nurses. Figures 52-2 and 52-3 indicate the scores on emotional exhaustion and reduced empathy that are on the burnout inventory. Emotional exhaustion and reduced empathy (depersonalization scale of the burnout measure) were extremely high for interns and residents, and moderately high for fellows and nurses as compared to other health care professionals. While there were no significant differences between the groups on emotional exhaustion, there were differences on diminished empathy. Interns and residents had a significantly greater sense of diminished empathy than did fellows and nurses, although the fellows' scores were significantly greater than the nurses. As for the sense of personal accomplishment scale on the burnout measure, nurses, residents and fellows reported a moderate sense of accomplishment while interns reported a lower sense of accomplishment.

The results of this year-long educational and supportive intervention, as compared to a control unit, indicate that it was significantly effective for the residents. The impact was less obvious for interns and nurses, perhaps because of their great levels of stress for which the intervention was not powerful enough to show an impact. For all studied it was clear that there was less burnout and psychological distress in those who had a hardy personality style. One of the most important findings was that patients expressed greater satisfaction with the "art" of their medical care (e.g., interest, sensitivity, and compassion from the staff) on the intervention unit than did patients on the control floor. Thus, one could conclude that increasing sensitivity, support, and communication for the staff members also increased the patient's positive perception of the "human" side of care.

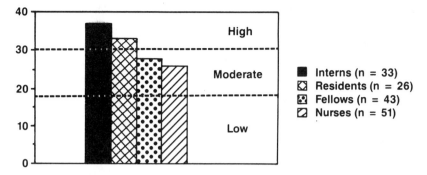

**Figure 52-2.** Baseline emotional exhaustion scores for each group: interns, residents, nurses, fellows.

The intervention strategies were directed to the unit as a single social system, recognizing that any change in a single group's behavior affects the others. By modifying the stresses of patient care, many of which relate to interstaff conflicts, the symptoms of house officer syndrome should be prevented, with their particularly deleterious effect on the ability to feel empathy and compassion for the patient and to prevent the development of cynicism that reduces usual pleasure in patient care and likely affects interaction with patients negatively. These burnout symptoms are often interpreted by patients as signs that the staff places less value on the "human" side of care, which is viewed as highly important by patients especially in the current context of high technology in medical care.

Research in this area lags behind clinical and empirical trial and error methods. Our experience suggests that interventions aimed at one or another professional group are too narrow and do not take into account the full social environment of an oncology unit, where interdisciplinary interactions and stresses are often troublesome. For optimal support to an oncology unit, our experience suggest that the following interventions offer the ideal model. While few units have all components, the presence of one or more is beneficial.

1. The primary intervention model is the liaison psychiatrist as just described, who accompanies house staff on rounds, sees patients in both formal and informal consultation, and is identified as the unit psychiatrist. This model is used with patients with leukemia and lymphoma and is described by Lesko in Chapter 16. This method also allows observation of staff members, particularly house staff, to assess who is vulnerable and who needs an offer of help and support.

2. A weekly staff conference that includes all staff members involved in patient care, which addresses both patient and staff issues; it also serves as a teaching resource for management of special problems. These are often run by the nurse manager, attending physician or resident, and a social worker or psychiatrist. The collaborative practice meeting described earlier is a successful example.

3. A conference meeting every 1–2 weeks for oncology fellows (as described earlier) at which discipline-related issues can be shared in a more confidential setting. Ideally, these are run by a psychiatrist and an oncologist with an interest in psychological problems. Separate nurses support groups are important and are described in Chapters 53 and 54.

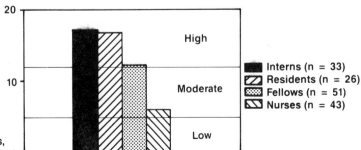

**Figure 52-3.** Baseline diminished empathy scores for each group: interns, residents, fellows, nurses.

4. Conferences for patients' families, held weekly by nurses, social workers, or a mental health professional, identify their problems and promote mutual support.

5. Integration with ambulatory care is more difficult to achieve. However, a model that permits nurses and house staff who work primarily in one setting to be familiar with the other setting where their patients are treated would be helpful. The same liaison psychiatrist who works with the inpatient staff should ideally relate to the ambulatory unit and follow outpatients as well. A pediatric model at MSKCC allows a team of the pediatric oncologist, nurse and social worker to work in the clinic and follow their patients in the hospital unit. This offers excellent continuity.

Finally, it is important to note that for all the stresses recounted and supports recommended, the rewards for most individuals outweigh the risks. In the final analysis, it is a personal satisfaction in the work that keeps doctors working year after year. Peabody (1926) showed the quality required to survive, both personally and professionally, in his superb article written more than 60 years ago about ''caring for the patient.''

What is spoken of as a ''clinical picture'' is not just a photograph of a man sick in bed; it is an impressionistic painting of the patient surrounded by his home, his work, his relations, his friends, his joys, sorrows, hopes and fears. . . . Thus the physician who attempts to take care of a patient while he neglects this [emotional] factor is as unscientific as the investigator who neglects to control all the conditions that may affect his experiment . . . the treatment of disease immediately takes its proper place in the larger problem of the care of the patient. . . . The treatment of a disease may be entirely impersonal; the care of a patient must be completely personal. . . . One of the essential qualities of the clinician is interest in humanity, for the secret of the care of the patient is in caring for the patient.

## SUMMARY

The oncology unit or cancer center carries with it basic stresses on the house staff members who train there, on the fellows who choose oncology as a career, and on the attending physicians. Those who choose medicine are often individuals who are conscientious, feel responsibility heavily, and work long hours. Training reinforces these traits and, because it is physically and psychologically stressful, may result in symptoms of stress that, if unrecognized, can progress to a burnout syndrome and development of a psychiatric disorder in a vulnerable individual. Commonly seen is depression with dependence on alcohol or drugs; suicide is an outcome in some cases. Support for house staff and oncology fellows is important, both as a single group

and as part of a meeting for all staff of a unit. Each has advantages; both are effective. Most physicians who work in oncology find it personally rewarding, outweighing the daily stresses that are readily acknowledged, but tolerated in the context of giving the most sensitive care.

## REFERENCES

Artiss, K.L. and A.S. Levine (1973). Doctor–patient relation in severe illness: A seminar for oncology fellows. *N. Engl. J. Med.* 288:1210–14.

Bard, M. (1984). The cancer center as a social system. In M.J. Massie & L.M. Lesko (eds.), *Current Concepts in Psycho-oncology: Syllabus for a Postgraduate Course.* New York: Robert Gold Associates, pp. 109–11.

Bendix, J. (1984). Physicians and stress: How to cope. *Physician's Management* 24:232–33, 236–37, 240–41, 247, 250–51.

Borenstein, D.B. and K. Cook (1982). Impairment prevention in the training years: A new mental health program at UCLA. *J.A.M.A.* 247:2700–2703.

Caplan, G. (1981). Mastery of stress: Psychosocial aspects. *Am. J. Psychiatry* 138:413–20.

Cartwright, L.K. (1979). Sources and effects of stress in health careers. In G.C. Stone, F. Cohen, and N.E. Adler (eds.), *Health Psychology.* San Francisco: Jossey-Bass.

Evans, J.L. (1965). Psychiatric illness in the physician's wife. *Am. J. Psychiatry* 122:159–163.

Feifel, H. (1959). *The Meaning of Death.* New York: McGraw-Hill.

Fine, C. (1981). *Married to Medicine: An Intimate Portrait of Doctors' Wives.* New York: Atheneum.

Fox, R. (1962). *Experiment Perilous.* Glencoe, Ill.: Free Press.

Friedman, R.C., D.S. Kornfeld, and J.D. Bigger (1973). Psychological problems associated with sleep deprivation in interns. *J. Med. Educ.* 48:436–41.

Gaensbauer, T.J. and G.L. Mizner (1980). Developmental stresses in medical education. *Psychiatry* 43:60–70.

Hall, R.C.W., E.R. Gardner, M. Perl, S.K. Stickney, and B. Pfefferbaum (1979). The professional burnout syndrome. *Psychiatr. Opinion* 16:12–17.

Hartl, D.E. (1979). Stress management and the nurse. In D.C. Sutterley and G.F. Donnelly (eds.), *Stress Management.* Germantown, Md.: Aspen.

Holland, J.C. (1982). Psychological aspects of cancer. In J.F. Holland and E. Frei (eds.), *Cancer Medicine,* 2nd ed. Philadelphia: Lea & Febiger, pp. 991–1021.

Holland, J.C. and J.F. Holland (1985). A neglected problem: The stresses of cancer care on physicians. *Primary Care Cancer (Oncol. Rounds)* 5:16–22.

Hsu, K. and V. Marshall (1987). Prevalence of depression and distress in a large sample of Canadian residents, interns and fellows. *Am. J. Psychiatry* 144:1561–66.

Katz, J. (1984). *The Silent World of Doctor and Patient.* New York: The Free Press.

Kobasa, S.C. (1979). Stressful life events, personality, and health: An inquiry into hardiness. *J. Pers. Soc. Psychol.* 37:1–11.

Kobasa, S.C. (1982). Commitment and coping in stress resistance among lawyers. *J. Pers. Soc. Psychol.* 42:707–17.

Kobasa, S.C. and M.C. Puccetti (1983). Personality and social resources in stress resistance, *J. Pers. Soc. Psychol.* 45:839–50.

Kobasa, S.C., S.R. Maddi, and S. Kahn (1982). Hardiness and health: A prospective study. *J. Pers. Soc. Psychol.* 42:168–77.

Koocher, G.P. (1979). Adjustment and coping strategies among the caretakers of cancer patients. *Soc. Work Health Care* 5:145–50.

Maslach, C. (1979). The burnout syndrome and patient care. In C.A. Garfield (ed.), *Stress and Survival: The Emotional Realities of Life-Threatening Illness.* St. Louis: C.V. Mosby.

Maslach, C. (1982). *Burnout: The Cost of Caring.* Englewood Cliffs, N.J.: Prentice-Hall.

McCue, J.D. (1982). The effects of stress on physicians and their medical practice. *N. Engl. J. Med.* 306:458–63.

Millerd, E.J. (1977). Health professionals as survivors. *J. Psychiatr. Nurs. Ment. Health Services* 15:33–36.

Modlin, H.C. and A. Montes (1964). Narcotic addiction in physicians. *Am. J. Psychiatry* 121:358–63.

Mount, B.M. (1986). Dealing with our losses. *J. Clin. Oncol.* 4:1127–34.

Peabody, F.W. (1926). The care of the patient. *J.A.M.A.* 88:877–82.

Pitts, F.N., A.B. Schuller, and C.L. Rich (1979). Suicide among U.S. women physicians. *Am. J. Psychiatry* 136:694–96.

Reuben, D.B. (1983). Psychologic aspects of residency. *South. Med. J.* 76:380–82.

Rich, C.L. and F.N. Pitts (1979). Suicide by male physicians during a five-year period. *Am. J. Psychiatry* 136:1089–90.

Rich, C.L. and F.N. Pitts (1980). Suicide by psychiatrists: A study of medical specialists among 18,730 consecutive physician deaths during a 5-year period (1967–1972). *J. Clin. Psychiatry* 41:261–63.

Richards, A.I. and A.H. Schmale (1974). Psychosocial conferences in medical oncology. *Ann. Intern. Med.* 80:541–45.

Rosow, J. and K.D. Rose (1972). Divorce among doctors. *J. Marriage Fam.* 34:587–98.

Ross, M. (1971). Suicide among physicians. *Psychiatr. Med.* 2:189–98.

Sakinofsky, I. (1980). Suicide in doctors and wives of doctors. *Br. Med. J.* 281:386–87.

Scheiber, S.C. (1983). Emotional problems of physicians: Nature and extent of problems. In S.C. Scheiber and B.B. Doyle (eds.), *The Impaired Physician.* New York: Plenum.

Scheiber, S.C. and B.B. Doyle (1983). *The Impaired Physician.* New York: Plenum.

Schmale, J., N. Weinberg, and S. Pieper (1987). Satisfactions, stresses, and coping mechanisms of oncologists in clinical practice (Summary). *Proc. Am. Soc. Clin. Oncol.* 6:255.

Siegel, B. and J.C. Donnelly (1978). Enriching personal and professional development: The experience of a support group for interns. *J. Med. Educ.* 53:908–14.

Small, G. (1981). House officer stress syndrome. *Psychosomatics* 22:860–69.

Smith, J.W., W.F. Denny, and D.B. Witzke (1986). Emotional impairment in internal medicine house staff. *J.A.M.A.* 255:1155–58.

Spikes, J. and J.C. Holland (1975). The physician's response to the dying patient. In J.J. Strain and S. Grossman (eds.), *Psychological Care of the Medically Ill.* New York: Appleton-Century-Crofts, pp. 138–48.

Steindler, E.M. (1975). *The Impaired Physician.* Chicago: American Medical Association.

Steppacher, R. and J.S. Mausner (1974). Suicide in male and female physicians. *J.A.M.A.* 228:323–28.

Strain, J.J. and D. Hammerman (1978). Ombudsmen (medical-psychiatric) rounds. *Ann. Intern. Med.* 88:550–55.

Tokarz, J.P., W. Bremer, and K. Peters (1979). *Beyond Survival.* Chicago: American Medical Association.

Vachon, M.L.S. (1987). *Occupational Stress in the Care of the Critically Ill, the Dying, and the Bereaved.* Washington, D.C.: Hemisphere Publishing Co.

Vaillant, G.E., N.C. Sobowale, and C. McArthur (1972). Some psychological vulnerabilities of physicians. *N. Engl. J. Med.* 287:372–75.

Valko, R.J. and P.J. Clayton (1975). Depression in the internship. *Dis. Nerv. System* 36:26–29.

Weinstein, H. (1983). A committee on well-being of medical students and house staff. *J. Med. Educ.* 58:373–81.

Wise, T.N. (1977). Utilization of group process in training oncology fellows. *Int. J. Group Psychother.* 27:105–11.

# 53

## Stress on Nurses in Oncology

Phyllis Shanley Hansell

The practice of nursing, once viewed as little more than a function of motherhood practiced outside a domestic setting, has evolved into a formal health care discipline that is distinct from medicine and in many cases highly specialized. The art and science of contemporary nursing are practiced in high-technology environments and have a rapidly expanding scientific basis. The American Nurses Association, ANA in its *Social Policy Statement* (1980, p. 6), has defined nursing as

a profession committed to the care and nurturing of sick and well people, individually and in groups and [states] that the practice of nursing entails diagnosis and treatment in three areas that together comprise the core of practice: (1) human responses to actual or potential health problems; (2) self-care deficiencies; and (3) adaptive and maturational functions of individuals.

Advances in nursing science, however, have not altered the basic elements of nursing, namely, concern, solicitude, affection, observation, and ministration (Abdellah, 1972). Indeed, one of the distinguishing characteristics of nursing practice is the performance of acts that are nurturing, protective, and therapeutic in nature. This emphasis on caring is at once the great source of stress and strength in the practice of oncology nursing. Regardless of the nurse's area of expertise, to be effective she or he must achieve a comfortable balance between the science and art of patient care.

### ONCOLOGY NURSING: A BRIEF HISTORY

Before discussing cancer nursing stress, it is helpful to glance at the history of oncology nursing and distinguish it from other, older nursing specialty areas. Oncology nursing is a relatively new area of practice concerned with the nursing care of cancer patients. It has developed simultaneously with major scientific ad-

vances in cancer treatment, which require that nurses in oncology receive specialized training to manage the increasingly complex care requirements that arise from sophisticated diagnostic and treatment procedures. Graduate programs in oncology nursing that lead to a master's degree have recently begun to be offered at many universities. Individuals with a nursing license and 3 years of nursing experience including 1 year of oncology experience could, for the first time in 1986, take a certification examination in oncology nursing offered in conjunction with the eleventh annual congress of the Oncology Nursing Society.

The practice of oncology nursing was confined to major cancer centers 25 years ago. Today, however, nurses who specialize in the care of cancer patients can be found in comprehensive cancer centers, university and community hospitals, home health care agencies, hospices, and private practice (Johnson, 1985). The development of oncology nursing as a distinct specialty throughout the world has occurred largely through the efforts of the Oncology Nursing Society.

Although many of the stressors experienced by nurses working with cancer patients are shared by other "front-line" health professionals, the nature of the nurse's role as a primary care provider imposes a unique set of demands on individuals. Personal resources may be depleted by the intensity of the emotions aroused by the constant and close exposure to the distress of cancer patients and their families (Newlin and Wellisch, 1978). This is particularly true in hospital units where the emotional demands are greatest and need even closer monitoring (Klagsbrun, 1970). Thus, stresses associated with oncology nursing arise from individual (personal) as well as situations specific to care of the oncology patient, which often entails managing increasing levels of dysfunction in the patient, the family's response to progressive illness, and the management of terminal illness and death.

Studies of nursing stress conducted in units requiring highly technical care, such as intensive care units (ICUs), and those in oncology units are both relevant to this subject and are discussed here.

## STUDIES OF NURSING STRESS

### High-Technology Settings

Over the past three decades, studies of work stress encountered by nurses have been conducted predominantly in units where patient mortality is high, such as dialysis units (Oskins, 1979; Stehle, 1981). Early studies were largely anecdotal and descriptive involving small groups of nurses. Stress was often poorly defined and measured (Huckabay and Jagla, 1979). Although there was little consensus in this literature regarding the major sources of stress for nurses, an important observation was that an apparent frequent outcome of the stressful work environment for nurses was increased staff turnover (Maloney, 1982; McElroy, 1982). One of the first studies that described the stresses associated with the practice of nursing was by Menzies (1960), who reported his personal observations over a 4-year period. He described stressful situations in which nurses were exposed to patient suffering, frequent deaths, heavy work loads, and disturbing patient relationships. His pioneering work was the stimulus for numerous subsequent studies revealing nurses' stress. In fact, in 1974 the U.S. Department of Labor identified nursing as a highly stressful occupation (McLean, 1974).

A study by Huckabay and Jagla (1979) identified several variables as significant predictors of high stress in ICUs, including problems in interpersonal communication, need for an extensive amount of readily available knowledge, the demands of highly technical equipment, and the complexity of patient care. Another study by Oskins (1979) found that the presence of inexperienced or inadequate staff on a unit, conflict with a patient's family, or a personal crisis were associated with more stress.

Norbeck (1985a,b) found that higher levels of perceived stress were related to lower levels of job satisfaction. In her research, the top-ranked stressors were the number of rapid decisions required, heavy work load, frequency of cardiac arrests, and extent of knowledge needed to function effectively. One study compared ICU nurses to those on other units for presence of burnout (Keane et al., 1985). It was interesting that levels of burnout were not different; however, nurses who scored higher on the personality variable of "hardiness," characterized by qualities of commitment, control, and challenge in relation to work, experienced less burnout.

**Table 53-1** Sources of stress in nursing

| Source | Characteristics |
|---|---|
| Organizational | Low status of nurses |
| | Lack of opportunity for advancement or enrichment |
| | Multiple educational entry points to nursing practice |
| | Poor staff support services |
| Situational (Unit or clinic level) | General: |
| |   Complex technology and treatments |
| |   Need for a broad knowledge base |
| |   Critically ill patients |
| |   Multiple ethical issues |
| |   Absent or weak psychological support services |
| | Specific: |
| |   Inexperienced staff |
| |   Inadequate staff |
| |   Heavy work load |
| |   Communication problems among staff |
| |   Communication problems with patient and/or family units |
| |   Multiple deaths, treatment crises |
| Personal | General: |
| |   Poor coping capacity |
| |   Few social supports or activities |
| |   Low socioeconomic status |
| |   Psychiatric history, substance abuse |
| | Specific: |
| |   Family or personal crises |
| |   Conflict with staff or patient |
| |   Death of a "favorite" patient |
| |   Beginning on a new unit |
| |   Lack of adequate "time off" |

These studies and others support the idea that stress in nurses needs to be approached from a multidimensional perspective (Gentry et al, 1972; Claus and Bailey, 1980; Caldwell and Weiner, 1981). Table 53-1 shows that stress can result from problems occurring at several different levels, including organizational, situational, and personal. Some are more amenable to alleviation than others. At times, one source of stress depends on another for change. For example, it might be highly desirable to institute a staff support group on a unit to help members deal with the stresses of critically ill patient care. Such an effort would be impossible without institutional support. Similarly, whereas it is impossible to alter the complexity of care, the critical nature of illness, or exposure to death on a unit, it is possible to recognize need for time off and to monitor work assignments carefully at such a time. The personal dimension is clearly equally important, determined by the emotional maturity and experience of the nurse, as well as stresses in his or her personal

**Table 53-2** Summary of studies on nursing stress

| References | Personal stressors | Situational stressors | Organizational stressors |
|---|---|---|---|
| *Specialty unit studies* | | | |
| Menzies (1960) | | Patient suffering and deaths Disturbing patient relation- ships | Heavy work load |
| Huckabay and Vagla (1979) | Interpersonal communication problems | — | High-technology care Patient care complexity |
| Oskins (1979) | Personal crisis | Patient and/or family conflicts and threats | Inadequate staffing Inexperienced staff |
| Keane et al. (1985) | Personality variables | — | — |
| Norbeck (1985a,b) | Low level of job satisfaction | Knowledge required Cardiac arrests | Heavy work load |
| *Oncology unit studies* | | | |
| Stewart et al. (1982) | Decision making Patient relationship reservations Disruption of interpersonal relationships | Length of patient relationships Administration of debilitating chemotherapeutic regimens | — |
| Chiriboga et al. (1983) | Negotiation style Poor coping | Perceptions of disease by pa- tient, physician, family Problems of patients' families Patient care requirements Terminal illness | — |
| Yasko (1983) | Youth Inexperience Lower educational level | High-stress setting | Inadequate psychological support |

life at the time. Specific situational stressors on units are the negotiation required by the nurse to reconcile differing patient–family or patient–physician percep- tions of the disease and treatment, dealing with family members, providing care for terminal illness, and in- terpersonal communications (Chiriboga et al., 1983; Moynihan and Outlaw, 1984; Gentry and Parkes, 1982). In most of the studies reviewed, the lists of problems cited as being major determinants of stress for nurses include individual as well as environmental characteristics (see Table 53-2).

## Oncology Settings

Nurses who specialize in the care of cancer patients are often viewed as particularly vulnerable to stress. Re- search in this area suggests that it is the nature of the patient care demands that is the most pervasive stressor for oncology nurses. While heir also to the personal and contextual sources of stress faced by other high- technology specialists, oncology nurses may be partic- ularly susceptible to the more chronic situational stressors associated with the nature of their respon- sibilities and patients' needs.

As cancer progresses and the prospect of cure dimin- ishes, patient care demands become significantly more

stressful. This is particularly true if the nurse has come to know the patient and family well. The loss becomes more personal. The nurse who spends day after day caring for the patient not only is keenly aware of the signs of disease progression, but must also respond to the increasing level of care required by a patient who may previously have been wholly self-sufficient (Moynihan and Outlaw, 1984; Yasko, 1983). Equally distressed families react to what they see and may blame the nurse for the change. This added inappropri- ate burden of blame requires maturity to accept without personal discomfort.

In one study outpatient oncology nurses were com- pared to nurses in similarly stressful inpatient settings (e.g., CCU, ICU, and operating room units) to deter- mine if they experienced greater stress as a function of their job (Stewart et al., 1982). The four groups of nurses did not differ on their daily stress leading to physical and emotional exhaustion. However, cancer nurses reported significantly more daily mood swings and greater difficulty in discussing the patient's condi- tion with him or her than the other nursing specialty groups. The perceived long-term stress of their work also appeared to increase over time and was signifi- cantly greater in the cancer nursing group. This dif- ference was attributed to the greater contact of these

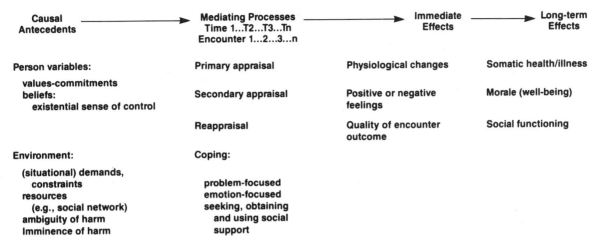

| Causal Antecedents | Mediating Processes Time 1...T2...T3...Tn Encounter 1...2...3...n | Immediate Effects | Long-term Effects |
|---|---|---|---|
| **Person variables:** | Primary appraisal | Physiological changes | Somatic health/illness |
| values-commitments beliefs: existential sense of control | Secondary appraisal | Positive or negative feelings | Morale (well-being) |
| | Reappraisal | Quality of encounter outcome | Social functioning |
| **Environment:** | **Coping:** | | |
| (situational) demands, constraints resources (e.g., social network) ambiguity of harm Imminence of harm | problem-focused emotion-focused seeking, obtaining and using social support | | |

**Resolutions of each stressful encounter**

**Figure 53-1.** A theoretical schematization of stress, coping, and adaptation. *Source:* Reprinted with permission from R.S. Lazarus (1981). The stress and coping paradigm. In C. Eisdorfer, D. Cohen, A. Kleinman, and P. Maxim (eds.), *Models for Clinical Psychopathology*. New York: Spectrum, pp. 117–214.

nurses with patients who showed progressive dysfunction and who had more side effects of chemotherapy to be managed by nurses. Influences identified by the authors as contributing to long-term stress were reservations about forming relationships with patients and the effect of the job on other interpersonal relationships.

Yasko (1983) explored characteristics that predicted burnout in oncology nurse specialists using a multidimensional perspective focusing on personal resources, personal perceptions, and role-related variables. Findings from this study indicated that these clinical specialists had significantly lower burnout scores on the Jones Staff Burnout Scale for Health Professionals than other groups of nurses previously tested with the scale. However, staff characteristics that were correlated with significantly higher levels of burnout included being younger with fewer children, receiving inadequate psychological support at work, having a high level of stress at work, expressing dissatisfaction with the nursing role, and experiencing feelings of apathy and withdrawal.

The complexity of the sources of stress in oncology nursing is reflected in the theoretical model of stress, coping, and adaptation developed by Lazarus (1981; Lazarus and Launier, 1978). The Lazarus and Folkman (1984) model conceptualizes stress as multidimensional and incorporates influences that have an impact on health, morale, and social functioning (Fig. 53-1). The dimensions of the model include characteristics predisposing an individual to stress that relate to values and beliefs, situational constraints and resources, appraisal of stress, coping strategies, ability to use available social resources, and adaptive status. This conceptual model was used in a study of stress in hospice nurses (Chiriboga et al., 1983). The findings from this study suggest that the nature of coping strategies used and the individual's appraisal of the stress of work were the most significant features in adaptive status.

Thus stress experienced by oncology nurses seems to be the result of a dynamic interplay of internal and external influences that determine how well an individual nurse manages stress. Bruhn and Cordova (1982) have developed a model that illustrates the process and outcome of coping (Fig. 53-2), which is applicable to the practice of oncology nursing. It suggests that personal aspects of prior experience and personal attributes lead to perception of a work situation in a particular way, which then engenders a coping behavior that, if successful, leads to personal growth and maintenance of personal and professional stability.

Attention to stress on oncology nurses should be a priority for nursing administrators and educators. How to handle stress needs to be included in basic education, in in-service programs, and in planning of staff support (see Chapters 51 and 54). If oncology nurses are to provide high-quality, sensitive patient care that meets their own standards of care and compassion, they must not feel so hassled; in these contexts they cannot be adequately caring for the patient. Certainly more studies of this dimension of patient care are needed. Our own studies show nurses at Memorial Sloan-Kettering Cancer Center to be high on emotional exhaustion, but relatively lower than house staff members on the dimension of diminished empathy—a find-

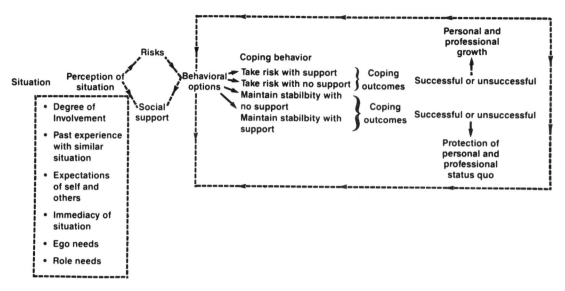

**Figure 53-2.** The process and outcomes of coping.
*Source:* Reprinted with permission from J.G. Bruhn and F.D. Cordova (1982). Coping with change professionally and personally. In J. Lancaster and W. Lancaster (eds.), *Concepts for Advanced Nursing Practice: The Nurse as a Change Agent.* St. Louis: C.V. Mosby, p. 438.

ing in this latter group that we hypothesize may have a particularly adverse effect on sensitivity and compassion in patient care.

## SUMMARY

The studies of stresses on nurses in oncology indicate that the sources of stress can be viewed as arising from personal, organizational, and situational areas. Personal features important in dealing with stress are personality, maturity, experience, and absence of personal crises. Organizational characteristics encompass the need for attention to distribution of work load and recognition of emotional concerns of nurses working with cancer patients by provision of adequate supervision, staffing, and support. Situational stressors are associated with the care of patients through progressive and terminal illness with whom personal ties have developed, maintaining supportive interpersonal communications, negotiating family–physician conflicts, and simultaneously carrying out complex treatment procedures. At times strengths in one area help buffer stresses in another. In all cases, being able to draw effectively on available personal and institutional resources is critical to optimal patient care and to individual growth and well-being of oncology nurses.

## REFERENCES

Abdellah, F. (1972). Evolution of nursing as a profession. *Int. Nurs. Rev.* 19:319–27.

American Nurses Association (1980). *Social Policy Statement.* Kansas City, Mo.: American Nurses Association.

Bruhn, J.G. and F.D. Cordova (1982). Coping with change professionally and personally. In J. Lancaster and W. Lancaster (eds.), *Concepts for Advanced Nursing Practice: The Nurse as a Change Agent.* St. Louis: C.V. Mosby, pp. 429–41.

Caldwell, T. and M.F. Weiner (1981). Stresses and coping in ICU nursing: A review. *Gen. Hosp. Psychiatry* 3:119–27.

Chiriboga, D., G. Jenkins, and J. Bailey (1983). Stress and coping among hospice nurses: Test of analytical model. *Nurs. Res.* 32:294–99.

Claus, K. and J. Bailey (eds.). (1980). *Living with Stress and Promoting Well Being.* St. Louis: C.V. Mosby.

Gentry, W.D. and K.R. Parkes (1982). Psychologic stress in intensive care unit and nonintensive care unit nursing: A review of the past decade. *Heart Lung* 11:43–47.

Gentry, W.D., S.B. Foster, and F. Froehling (1972). Psychologic responses to situational stress in intensive and nonintensive nursing. *Heart Lung* 72:793–96.

Huckabay, L. and B. Jagla (1979). Nurses' stress factors in the intensive care unit. *J. Nurs. Admin.* 9:21–26.

Johnson, J.L. (1985). Building on the past planning for the future. *Cancer Nurs.* 8:1–4.

Keane, A., J. Ducette, and D.C. Adler (1985). Stress in ICU and non ICU nurses. *Nurs. Res.* 34:231–36.

Klagsburn, D.C. (1970). Cancer emotion and nurses. *Am. J. Psychiatry* 126:1237–44.

Lazarus, R.S. (1981). The stress and coping paradigm. In C. Eisdorfer, D. Cohen, A. Kleinman, and P. Maxim (eds.), *Models for Clinical Psychopathology.* New York: Spectrum, pp. 117–214.

Lazarus, R.S. and R. Launier (1978). Stress-related transactions between person and environment. In L.A. Pervin and M. Lewis (eds.), *Perspectives in Interactional Psychology.* New York: Plenum, pp. 287–322.

Lazarus, R.S. and S. Folkman (1984). *Stress, Appraisal, and Coping.* New York: Springer.

Maloney, J.P. (1982). Job stress and its consequences on a group of intensive care and nonintensive care nurses. *Adv. Nurs. Sci.* 1:31–42.

McElroy, A.M. (1982). Burnout. A review of the literature with application to cancer nursing. *Cancer Nurs.* 5:211–17.

McLean, A. (1984). *Occupational Stress*. Springfield, Ill.: Charles C Thomas.

Menzies, I. (1960). Nurses under stress. *Int. Nurs. Rev.* 12(7):9–16.

Moynihan, R. and E. Outlaw (1984). Nursing support groups in a cancer center. *J. Psychosoc. Oncol.* 2:33–48.

Newlin, N.J. and D.K. Wellisch (1978). The oncology nurse: Life on an emotional roller coaster. *Cancer Nurs.* 1:447–49.

Norbeck, J.S. (1985a). Perceived job stress, job satisfaction and psychological symptoms in critical care nursing. *Res. Nurs. Health Care* 8:253–59.

Norbeck, J.S. (1985b). Types and sources of social support for managing job stress in critical care nursing. *Nurs. Res.* 34:225–30.

Oskins, S. (1979). Identification of situational stressors and coping methods by intensive care nurses. *Heart Long* 8:933–60.

Stehle, J.L. (1981). Critical care nursing stress: The findings revisited. *Nurs. Res.* 30:182–86.

Stewart, B.E., B.E. Meyerowitz, L.E. Jackson, K.L. Yarkin, and J.H. Harvey (1982). Psychological stress associated with outpatient oncology nursing. *Cancer Nurs.* 5:383–87.

Yasko, J.M. (1983). Variables which predict burnout experienced by oncology clinical nurse specialists. *Cancer Nurs.* 5:109–16.

# 54

## The Psychiatric Nurse Clinician in Oncology

Marianne Zimberg

Over the past 20 years, nurses with expertise in psychiatry have increasingly provided consultation to their peers about psychological care of medical patients (Nelson and Schilke, 1976; Hackett and Cassem, 1978). Such consultation was initially provided on an ad hoc basis by nurses with full-time responsibility on a psychiatric unit, who often lacked practical or "hands-on" experience with medical and surgical patients. As special care units evolved, each with its own types of psychological problems, this informal service soon proved to be inadequate. It became clear that the nurse-consultant needed expertise in medical, surgical, and psychiatric nursing. Out of this need came the development of the psychiatric nurse-clinician (PNC), a Master's degree prepared nurse educated to provide assistance in psychological management, particularly in high-stress units of the intensive (ICU), neonatal, and dialysis units (Robinson, 1982). The mandate of these individuals is to provide consultation in psychological problems of patients, and to serve as liaison to administration, and as an educator and supporter for nurses in the general hospital (Fife, 1983).

Formal psychiatric nurse consultation in oncology developed somewhat later, growing out of the expertise acquired in consultation to cancer patients scattered among other patients and, most recently, from work with oncology. Psychiatric expertise has emerged in oncology, however, in the context of a strong tradition of nursing's concerns about quality of psychological care of patients with cancer. Nursing has had a long important commitment to giving emotional support to cancer patients with advanced disease. The initial psychosocial concerns that nurses addressed centered around revealing (or concealing) the cancer diagnosis and issues of death and dying. Nurses were strongly influenced by Kubler-Ross' work (1969) on psychological stages of dying, which supported their position on the desirability of increased communication about diagnosis and prognosis. The encouragement to talk more openly with dying patients was an important emphasis through the 1960s and 1970s. Some of the seminal contributions to psychosocial oncology were made by nurses, particularly Jean Quint-Benoliel, who was an early pioneer in this area (1967).

The current need for the PCN in an oncology unit has expanded as the functions of staff nurses have broadened (MacNeil-Zimberg, 1984; Zimberg, 1986). Today, the oncology nurse is responsible for giving complex chemotherapy regimens, overseeing management of side effects, caring for patients with severe levels of illness due to both disease and treatment, making acute care a central issue in his or her work (Asadorian et al., 1984). The nurse must also be sensitive to those patients on a ward whose condition is deteriorating, and who require palliative and comfort care. Thus, the oncology nurse is caught in the dilemma created by the competing needs of patients for both the best psychological and medical care. Because the nurse also sees the same patients and their families over many admissions, she or he develops a close relationship with these patients and the families. Because patients have anxiety, depression, and anger associated with lengthy treatment and life-threatening complications, the nurse is also at greater risk of experiencing these same emotions, either in response to a particular patient's problems, or as a consequence of repeated exposure to losses. Finally, there is the potential for conflict with doctors and other staff members about level of aggressive medical care, use of investigative treatments, and selective reduction of life supports, stresses that are repetitive on units giving acute care.

In this current context of oncology nursing, the PCN is a valuable consultant, educated as he or she is to recognize the psychological problems in the nurse, the conflicts on the unit, and those of the patient and family (Rankin, 1986). The ability to intervene and to reduce tensions is most important on the oncology unit where high stress, when combined with nurses' personal reactions, may contribute to staff turnover and "burnout" (Vachon, 1981; Maslach, 1976).

## THE ROLE OF AN EXPERT

### Creating the Position

The PNC has a unique role in the institution; it is important that he or she be based firmly in nursing, yet also be autonomous enough to function in a liaison role with the psychiatric consultant, or department (if present) in the institution. She or he must often point out the need for a psychiatric consultation, educating staff to recognize symptoms and behaviors, such as suicidal ideation, that need evaluation. Toward this end, educating the staff nurse to observe and document accurate psychiatric symptoms and behavioral changes can be invaluable. Helping the nurse to recognize that a psychiatric consultation "doesn't mean the patient is crazy" can be important, as well as encouraging his or her role in pointing out the need for a consultation by observations gained from an interview with the patient. The PNC also consults with social workers, clergy, physiotherapists, and other support personnel on special patient problems. It is crucial that he or she be able to work well in an interdisciplinary role (Barbiasz et al., 1982; Berarducci et al., 1979).

### Selecting the Individual

To carry out this unique role, the PNC must have two areas of competence: first, adequate education in oncology and psychiatry, and second, personal attributes of maturity. In terms of education the individual must have credibility as an oncology nurse in the eyes of the floor and clinic nurses. The individual should ideally have had experience as a staff nurse caring for cancer patients. In cases where this is not possible, and as an adjunct to such experience, the PNC should organize an initial period of orientation to the units to which he or she will consult, becoming familiar with the responsibilities of the nurses. To function most effectively, nurses must feel that the PNC understands their problems from "having been there." The PNC must also have adequate psychiatric nursing expertise and, ideally, some experience with psychiatric care of medical, surgical, or oncology patients. Interviewing skills, psychiatric syndromes (especially those common in cancer), personality theory, knowledge of psychodynamics, individual or group psychotherapeutic techniques, psychopharmacology, and pertinent issues of consultation–liaison psychiatry must be part of the repertoire of the PNC.

The second area of necessary competence is in the realm of personal attributes. The PNC must have an emotional maturity that commands respect from other nurses. She or he must be seen as sensitive to emotional problems, a good listener, and reflect an integrity which assures respect for confidential communications and exposure of feelings. This person must be able to assess systems issues and be able to avoid or recognize when she or he is being drawn into conflicting alliances. A supervisor from outside the nursing department, with whom these complex systems issues can be explored and the PNC's own reactions examined and discussed in a confidential relationship is helpful to the functioning of the PNC.

### What the PNC Does

The PNC who works in oncology provides four major services. First, and central, is clinical consultation to nursing staff on the nursing management of psychological problems involving patient or family distress and conflicts with staff (particularly those that compromise optimal medical care). Second, staff education in psychosocial problems through teaching is carried out in conjunction with the consultation and through the provision of inservice courses on special problems (e.g., common psychological problems and recognizing depression). Third, the PNC provides for nursing support groups concerning specific patient problems and problems arising from the work environment. The final important service of the PNC is that of monitoring the quality of psychological care given to patients by nurses, and raising awareness of the emotional as well as physical aspects of care. Figure 54-1 provides a diagram of these overlapping yet discrete functions. Each is described in more detail in the following paragraphs.

### CLINICAL CONSULTATION

The PNC takes several steps in performing a consultation. First, he or she must discern the reason that the consultation was requested—both the overt and covert reasons, because they are often different. A referral may be called because of distress in the patient or family, because the nurse is distressed by some aspect of the situation, or because of a "systems" problem, arising out of conflicts either among nurses or between staff members of different specializations involved in the patient's care. This latter category of referrals is frequent in teaching hospitals and tertiary care centers, where it is common to have staff from several different specialties involved in a patient's management.

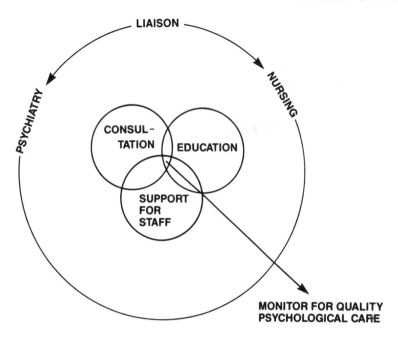

**Figure 54-1.** Diagram of the overlapping functions of the psychiatric nurse-clinician.

The PNC begins by obtaining a history from the nurse, chart, and others involved. She or he may also choose to interview the patient, preferably with the referring nurse present. This should be sufficient to determine the problem and develop a nursing care plan. The plan takes into account the nature of the problem and the psychological nursing care appropriate to managing the patient. For example, if the patient were depressed, the plan would include monitoring for signs of suicidal thoughts or behavior, conducting frequent checks, and encouraging activity and visitors. If the problem derives from the nurse's distress, the PNC explores the nature of the problem, specifically the nurse's anger, guilt, sense of inadequate support, or unrealistic expectations of himself or herself. It may be that some quality of the patient, such as age or similar background, elicited overidentification or personal anxiety about the illness, which will require further exploration and support to correct the problems in giving care. A "systems" problem calls for further exploration of the staff conflicts that may result in distress in the patient, a task that requires sensitivity and diplomacy. Such problems often arise with very ill patients in whom adequacy of pain control, resuscitation, and continuation of life supports produce highly emotional responses and sharp disagreements that can be difficult to resolve. These situations may be resolved through meetings to review the issues, through individual discussions, or through referral to ethics committees, which in many institutions serve to provide review and suggestions.

The astute clinician also assesses the "emotional climate" of a ward or unit when providing a consultation. Have they had many deaths? Experienced staff turnover, nursing shortage? Do they function cohesively? Support one another? Is it a unit that lacks stable leadership? Lacks support for staff nurses? The PNC takes into account the nurse, the staff, the unit, and the supervisor in assessing what was presented at the outset as "the patient's problem."

As information is gathered from the patient, family, and staff members, the clinical assessment of the PNC takes the following aspects into account in evaluating the patient/family problem.

- Present level of the illness and treatment of the patient and the implications for nursing care
- History of mental illness and prior personality or coping ability
- Family and social supports
- Patient's reaction to present illness and treatment; stresses associated with these responses, and his or her reaction to nurses and physicians involved (conflicts, relationship) as well as their duration

Assessment of the nurse who is giving primary care to the patient about whom the consultation is called includes the following:

- Level of nursing care required by the patient
- Nature of the nurse's relationship to and interaction with the patient (overly close, negative, or distant)
- Level of the nurse's education and prior experience (e.g., young and inexperienced versus mature and experienced in cancer nursing)

- Level and nature of the nurse's personal distress and its origin (e.g., personal life, conflicts at work)

When all the information is evaluated, the care plan is formulated. The plan may need to be presented to all shifts, particularly if the problem centers around a patient with delirium resulting in violent behavior, a suicidal patient who must be managed on the unit, or one who is manipulative. A conference format also allows the underlying feelings of frustration, fatigue, grief, or anger to be presented, an opportunity that makes it possible for staff members to recognize or discover that others may have felt the same but had not expressed it. Of course, the clinician must have a prior relationship with the staff in order to be able to facilitate a productive meeting where "raw" feelings may be expressed. It is expected that he or she will protect participants from undue exposure.

The nursing care plan that evolves from the conference will have addressed key areas for the staff nurse and provided some concrete suggestions. These should include the following:

1. Communication of the underlying psychological problems and why the patient behaved as he or she did (e.g., the patient who is panicky in anticipation of surgery)
2. Help for the patient in assessing the situation, with reassurance that distressed feelings are normal
3. Identification of a patient's prior ways of coping with a crisis that have been effective
4. Identification of available supports (e.g., family member or friend) who can be called on to offer additional assistance as needed
5. Organization of a consistent plan that will include all shifts
6. Written nursing care plans and nursing notes to inform others of the patient's problem
7. Instruction of the staff to minimize conflicting information (only one person to give information about procedures and plans)
8. Notation that it may be necessary to ask the physician to call for a psychiatric consultation if reassurance is not adequate to reduce anxiety

Persistent significant distress indicates the need for further evaluation to determine the underlying cause that may be, in cancer patients, a metabolic disorder or abnormality resulting in mental symptoms (e.g., cerebral hypoxia due to lung cancer or pneumonia, encephalopathy with liver failure, renal failure, and hypercalcemia). Other common problems in cancer patients that cause delirium are the effects of narcotics and steroids. The alert nurse, through consultation with the nurse-clinician, can be important in identifying an early treatable delirium.

## STAFF EDUCATION

The PNC bears responsibility for developing content and organizing the nursing curriculum with respect to its psychological teaching content. The areas can be divided into three, namely, orientation and teaching of new staff, inservice educational programs, continuing education for community based nurses.

When nurses begin work on an oncology ward, they need to review or become familiar with the special psychological problems of cancer patients, as well as to be given information about their management and the reactions they themselves may experience in response to the care of cancer patients. Several major topics that should be covered are listed here.

1. Stages of illness and how patients adapt to them (e.g., diagnosis, during treatment, recurrence, and advanced disease)
2. Characteristics of patients who are at high risk for poor coping (e.g., those with prior mental illness and poor supports)
3. How to evaluate and manage common problems (e.g., anxiety, depression, and delirium)
4. How to recognize psychological problems that require psychotropic drugs for management
5. Symptoms and behaviors for which a psychiatric consultation should be requested by the doctor, and appropriate referrals to social workers and chaplain
6. Guidelines for nurses in how to assess their own reactions to stress, which include attention to common responses to starting to work in oncology (e.g., increased fears of having cancer, and fears of minor symptoms in oneself or family), the need to recognize signs of overidentification with patients, the importance of balancing work with recreation, how to recognize symptoms of fatigue and stress, and sensitivity to potential interaction between personal and work problems that can create distress; encouragement for nurses to obtain professional help when needed

Inservice and continuing education on psychological care is done by informal teaching on individual units and by formal seminars. A series can be developed that meets weekly and focuses on different management problems, including the patient who is angry, or depressed, or emotionally regressed, or anxious, or isolated. For supervisors and clinical specialists, nursing leadership skills can be taught to emphasize group dynamics, communication skills, how to resolve conflicts, and theories of motivation and how to encourage it. Nurses also need further teaching in communications skills if they are to lead patient and family support groups, and present educational information to patients. The training of nurses responsible for the supervision of the licensed practical nurses, in particular in their use of role modeling and group discussion as teaching tools, is an important and often-overlooked task in which the PNC can offer helpful consultation.

## STAFF SUPPORT

Staff support for nurses is conducted largely through groups. It is a highly effective way to deal with psychological problems encountered by nurses in oncology clinics and wards (Lederberg, 1982; Mohl, 1981; Fawzy, Wellisch and Pasnau, 1983). The focus of the group is generally on emotional problems related to the work environment with a direct effort at problem solving (Eisendrath, 1981). The personal issues of nurses are examined within the context of the work issues. Several major themes come up repeatedly in the support group setting, that is, dealing with dying patients, death itself, "special" or difficult patients, and conflicts with doctors, peers, and supervisors. (Lipowski, 1979).

Staff support groups can be led by a member (or members) of any discipline (e.g., nurse, social worker, psychiatrist, or psychologist), provided the individual(s) has been educated and has had experience in group work. There is an advantage in having the PNC as leader or coleader because the shared nursing background fosters the sense that the leader "understands" the feelings, the conflicts, and the circumstances as viewed by the nurse. In this capacity, the PNC readily serves as a role model in the handling of problems, reflecting mature judgment about behavior with regard especially to conflict resolution (Lewis and Levy, 1982).

The decision to develop or take responsibility for the leadership of a staff support group must be thoughtfully considered; the restraint necessary to elucidate hazards can be applied by insisting on developing a contract in which the expectations and goals are clearly defined (see Lederberg, Chapter 51). The stated goals may not be the actual ones (and often they are not). Primary issues to be covered in the contract and resolved before beginning any sessions are who is to lead the group, who are the participants (e.g., supervisor, staff members), are meetings to be closed or open, how often and for how long will meetings be held, what is the time course for the group—time-limited (e.g., 6–10 sessions) versus open-ended, and what will be the format and agenda for meetings.

Once these issues are resolved, the sessions are often devoted to discussion of a number of common topics. Work-related issues that nurses report as the most frequent sources of problems include the hectic pace of work and unrealistic expectations of others, problems concerning management of dying patients and families, or difficult patients, feelings of exploitation (e.g., by doctors, by the "system"), lack of respect from other professional disciplines (particularly doctors), complaints about supervisors (authority) and peers (interpersonal), and strain in maintaining personal and professional roles.

These oft-mentioned topics quickly arouse an array of personal responses and raise issues about how to handle them. The major feelings evoked and those that are considered most troublesome include dealing with negative emotions (e.g., anger, conflict, and frustration) toward others (patient, family, and staff), handling grief and loss about patients or from personal life, and concerns about professional adequacy (sometimes responses to guilt about aspects of patient care or unrealistic expectations of oneself or others).

These central themes require sensitivity to assure the nurse that his or her feelings are valid and that the problems may be a result of the situation and that the ways to handle them constructively must be tried.

## MONITORING QUALITY OF CARE

The last area of involvement for the PNC consists of monitoring the quality of psychological care given by the entire nursing service in the institution. The PNC may point out weaknesses in the system and advise the director about changes needed to improve quality. This may also require suggestions for the creation of task forces to examine a particular problem or issue. At times a particular issue may be addressed by a survey or by a clinical research study in a large institution. The development and implementation of a quality assurance program is a primary role for the PNC.

Irrespective of the size of the institution or the resources, special attention within nursing must be given to the psychosocial needs of cancer patients and their families. Employing a psychiatric nurse-clinician, even on a part-time basis, makes available a consultant who can not only assess the needs but also institute, if necessary, basic support programs. By using existing staff, providing educational programs, and having a PNC available on an "on-call" basis, such programs can meet an institution's needs and be maintained at a low cost. (Robinson, 1986).

## SUMMARY

The psychiatric nurse-clinician assumes a unique role in an institution. Visible to patients, families, nurses on floors and in clinics, administration, other disciplines, and departments, she or he must have a broad knowledge of the fundamentals of nursing oncology, psychiatry, combined with personal skills that encompass diplomacy, leadership, empathy, sensitivity, and personal integrity. She or he must monitor psychological care given by nurses, units, the nursing divisions, and indeed the institution. She or he must be a staunch advocate, along with those staff members from psychiatry and other support disciplines, in encouraging within the institution and its members a firm commitment of quality psychosocial care.

## REFERENCES

Asadorian, M., M.H. Brown, A. Powers, M. Sheehan, K. Studva, K. Sullivan, and L. Wollnik (eds.). (1984). *A Century of Oncology Nursing 1884–1984*. New York: Memorial Sloan-Kettering Cancer Center.

Barbiasz, J., K. Blandford, K. Byrne, K. Horvath, J. Levy, A. Lewis, S.P. Matarezzo, K. O'Meara, L. Palmateer, and M. Rossier (1982). Establishing the psychiatric liaison nurse role: Collaboration with the nurse administrator. *J. Nurs. Admin.* 12:14–18.

Berarducci, M., K. Blandford, and C.A. Garant (1979). The psychiatric liaison nurse in the general hospital, three models of practice. *Gen. Hosp. Psychiatry* 1:66–72.

Eisendrath, S.J. (1981). Psychiatric liaison support groups for general hospital staffs. *Psychosomatics* 22:685–94.

Fawzy, F.I., D.K. Wellisch, R.O. Pasnau, and B. Leibowitz (1983). Preventing nursing burnout: A challenge for liaison psychiatry. *Gen. Hosp. Psychiatry* 5:141–49.

Fife, B. (1983). The challenge of the medical setting for the clinical specialist in psychiatric nursing. *J. Psychiatr. Nurs. Ment. Health Services* 21:8–13.

Hackett, T.P., and N.H. Cassem (eds.). (1978). *Massachusetts General Hospital Handbook of General Hospital Psychiatry*. St. Louis: C.V. Mosby.

Kubler-Ross, E. (1969). *On Death and Dying*. New York: Macmillan.

Lederberg, M.S. (1982). Support groups to prevent burnout. In J.C. Holland (ed.), *Current Concepts in Psychosocial Oncology: Effects of Cancer and Its Treatment on Patient, Family, and Staff*. New York: Memorial Sloan-Kettering Cancer Center, pp. 89–91.

Lewis, A. and J. Levy (1982). *Psychiatric Liaison Nursing: The Theory and Clinical Practice*. Reston, Va.: Reston Publishing.

Lipowski, Z.J. (1979). Consultation liaison psychiatry: Past failures and new opportunities. *Gen. Hosp. Psychiatry* 1:3–10.

MacNeil-Zimberg, M. (1984). The liaison nurse clinician: Support for patient and staff. In J.C. Holland (ed.), *Current Concepts in Psycho-oncology*. New York: Memorial Sloan-Kettering Cancer Center, pp. 113–17.

Maslach, C. (1976). Burned-out. *Hum. Behav.* 5:16–20.

Mohl, P.C. (1981). A review of systems approaches to consultation–liaison psychiatry, a need for synthesis. *Gen. Hosp. Psychiatry* 3:103–10.

Nelson, J.K.N. and D.A. Schilke (1976). The evolution of psychiatric liaison nursing. *Perspect. Psych. Care* 14:61–65.

Quint-Benoliel, J.C. (1967). *The Nurse and the Dying Patient*. New York: Macmillan.

Rankin, E.A.D. (1986). Psychiatric/mental health nursing. *Nurse Clin. N. Am.* 21(3):381–86.

Robinson, L. (1982). Psychiatric liaison nursing 1962–1982: A review and update of the literature. *Gen. Hosp. Psychiatry* 4:139–45.

Robinson, L. (1986). The future of psychiatric/mental health nursing. *Nurse Clin. N. Am.* 21(3):537–43.

Vachon, M.L.S. (1981). Losses and gains: Some comments on staff stress in oncology. In G. Hongladarom and R. McCorkle (eds.), *Grief, Loss and Support in Cancer Care, Proceedings of Third Annual Cancer Nursing Symposium*. Seattle: Fred Hutchinson Cancer Research Center, pp. 1–28.

Zimberg, M. (1986). Psychosocial care. In M.H. Brown, M.E. Kiss, E.M. Outlaw, and C.M. Viemontes (eds.). *Standards of Oncology Nursing Practice*. New York: Wiley, pp. 37–58.

# 55

# Social Work in Oncology

Grace H. Christ

Some of the professional issues confronting oncology social workers are outlined in this chapter; these include the diversity built into the social work role, expanded social work functions and treatments, and the challenge of maintaining good staff morale.

The social work role in oncology has become much more complex in recent years. First, the increased use of high technology in the treatment of cancer challenges social workers to find ways to bridge the gap between complex technology and the human experience of the patient. New interventions are required to limit the negative impact of such treatments on the quality of patients' lives. Patients now require help in integrating new information and in making informed decisions about undergoing innovative treatments. Such treatments offer advantages over traditional treatments in some areas, but more compromised functioning in others.

A second issue is the prolonged survival of cancer patients and the evolution of chronic debilitating diseases from what were previously rapidly fatal illnesses, which has increased the numbers of patients who need social work services. The social worker must also develop a broader range of interventions that include supporting patients not only during acute crises, but during long periods of chronic illness as well (Christ and Adams-Greenly, 1984; Christ et al., 1987).

Third, massive changes in the health care delivery system have led to a dramatic increase in outpatient care. This is complicated by inadequate resources in many communities to support patients in their homes or inadequate insurance coverage to obtain existing resources. Therefore, the social worker must often coordinate services from a number of different agencies for a single patient, which creates a complex and at times fragile home care plan. Extensive outpatient treatment also requires the development of new strat-

egies for monitoring patients' condition outside of the institution. Social workers devote increasing amounts of time to developing new resources in the community for their patients and advocating for better insurance coverage and less expensive services.

Fourth, increased specialization in cancer treatment has placed new demands on social workers as well as other health care professionals to find ways to prevent fragmentation and discontinuity in patient care. For example, outpatient and inpatient care are often not provided by the same social worker. Developing effective strategies for communication and collaboration among team members is vital when many different professionals are involved in the patient's treatment.

Fifth, in order to meet the broadening range of patient needs, social workers have had to learn new methods of intervention. Such new methods and techniques include the use of relaxation, hypnosis, visual imagery, social skills training, health education, sex therapy, and network therapy (Loscalzo, 1985).

A sixth major focus for social work interventions is supporting the caretakers of cancer patients. The prolonged survival of the cancer patient and the movement to outpatient care have placed an ever-increasing burden on the patients and their caretakers.

## DIVERSITY IN THE SOCIAL WORK ROLE

An ongoing challenge for the oncology social worker is to clarify his or her role in the minds of other health professionals who tend to differentiate medical social work from psychiatric social work. Unfortunately, this dichotomy is often reinforced because these professionals do not understand its negative implications for social work practice or its historical significance in the social worker's professional education and training. As a result of this lack of understanding, many tend to view medical social workers as discharge planning technicians and psychiatric social workers as non-disease-related therapists. For example, medical social workers are not expected to understand psychiatric issues, while psychiatric social workers are not expected to appreciate medical issues or the need for discharge planning (Goldberg et al., 1984).

This dichotomy also tends to reinforce the notion that the two social work specialties require different skills rather than that they represent different emphases within the general framework of social work practice. In fact, misperceptions about the social work role occur in part because of the enormous diversity and multidimensionality of the role, which is required by the complexity of patients' needs.

In actual practice, the oncology social worker must assess both the psychosocial and medical situations to plan adequately for a patient's care after discharge. Similarly, the worker often must deal with the patient's emotional state so that the patient will be able to follow through on treatment and participate actively in recovery or rehabilitation. In other words, patients' thoughts and plans regarding the practical aspects of their care and their emotional reactions constantly interact. Many patients are unable to separate their need for help in planning for their posthospital care, their need for an accurate understanding of the stage of their disease, and their emotional reactions to these facts. Another example occurs when patients learn that they will need special equipment and nursing care after discharge, which may be the first time they have confronted the disease-related changes that have occurred in their bodies or the reality that they will be forced to rely on others for personal care, transportation, and other tasks that they formerly handled themselves. Having to rely regularly on another person for these activities can be demoralizing for patients, who may then delay seeking care until a medical or family crisis develops.

Similarly, social workers cannot provide effective psychological treatment unless they are knowledgeable about the disease process and have a clear idea of how to help patients adapt to the disease and its treatment. Knowledge of the disease process includes thorough understanding of the biological aspects of cancer, the continuum of the disease experience, and the differences in how patients and family members react to each stage of the disease and each aspect of treatment.

Oncology social work reflects an ecological systems perspective, in that the worker's focus is to change the environment and the context in which patients experience stress as well as to help them cope with that stress more effectively (Germain, 1977). Because of this perspective, the worker must be involved in all aspects of a patient's treatment and care, and carry out a broad range of functions.

## SOCIAL WORK FUNCTIONS IN ONCOLOGY

The functions of oncology social workers fall into three broad categories, namely, clinical practice, education, and research. The first two functions are already well developed within the field of oncology, whereas psychosocial research is still in the evolutionary stage.

### Clinical Practice

In their clinical role, oncology social workers counsel patients and families and help them with task management, the complex plans and decisions that often must be made during times of extraordinary stress, and financial and other practical problems.

### COUNSELING

As a counselor, the worker's primary goal is to help patients and family members adapt to the stresses of diagnosis and treatment within today's complex health care system, whether these individuals are psychologically healthy, disturbed, or from a different culture. Social workers can and do treat psychopathology, but their major focus is to support the optimal adaptation of all patients to the disease and its treatment. To achieve the goal, they rely on a broad range of counseling modalities and therapeutic techniques, including individual, group, and family therapy, education, behavior modification, crisis intervention, supportive techniques, and insight-oriented interventions. The counseling role clearly includes the role of therapist. However, workers also may have to assume the more active roles of broker and patient advocate.

### TASK MANAGEMENT

Another clinical function of the oncology social worker is to help patients deal effectively with the social and psychological tasks confronting them at each stage of the illness. With improved technology and medical treatment, prospective payment systems, an increasing number of cancer patients are either cured or living with cancer as a chronic disease. Because the preterminal and terminal phases of cancer also have become prolonged, new demands on both caregivers and patients have developed. The worker monitors the adaptive challenges facing patients and families at each stage of illness and attempts to develop educational and supportive interventions that will help them master those challenges. In other words, oncology social workers must be truly "Janus-faced," maintaining their perspective while helping patients solve problems related to the progression of the disease, terminal illness, and death, and at the same time preparing other patients to live with long-term chronicity and cure.

## STRESS MANAGEMENT

Stress management involves helping patients develop ways of handling specific stresses related to diagnosis, treatment, the side effects of treatment, and the impact of treatment on body image, emotional state, and personal and social relationships. As an increasing number of patients have been cured, health professionals—especially mental health professionals—have had to shift from focusing exclusively on survival to improving quality of life by identifying and minimizing the effect of impairments, enhancing the ability to function independently, and mitigating the impact of social barriers (Christ, 1987). This shift has led to a broad range of new rehabilitative interventions such as sex therapy, social skills training, hypnosis, relaxation, behavior modification, and social and political advocacy.

## PLANNING AND DECISION MAKING

Helping patients with the complex planning and decision making that confront them during periods of extreme stress (at diagnosis, or when the disease recurs, metastasizes, or becomes chronic or terminal) is a relatively new clinical function in oncology social work. For example, more than one treatment for breast cancer can lead to excellent results. Although each treatment has an equal effect on the patient's chances for survival, it can affect the quality of life differently, namely, to better functioning in some areas and to compromised functioning in others. Thus, patients must make complex treatment decisions at diagnosis, a time when their ability to make decisions is severely compromised.

The social worker also develops strategies for helping patients make complex decisions throughout the course of the illness. For example, after a mastectomy, the patient must decide whether she wants cosmetic repair procedures such as breast reconstruction, which necessitates weighing the value of an improved appearance against the cost of additional surgery. A patient with osteosarcoma often must decide between amputation and a limb-sparing procedure that retains a body part and potentially improves body image, but may limit mobility. Another difficult decision is whether to participate in an experimental treatment program. As the disease progresses, patients must weigh the impact of the effects and side effects of research treatment against the possibility of longer survival. Frequently patients and families are left wondering whether they fought hard enough to live or compro-

mised too much functioning for an increase in survival time. Patients also can choose where they will be treated and by whom, and they often must decide what kind of care they need at home and whether they can afford it. Finally, if their treatment is unsuccessful, they must choose how they wish to die and where—in a hospital, in a hospice, or at home.

The social worker helps patients make these decisions by informing them about options, clarifying their misconceptions and misunderstandings, encouraging them to evaluate the outcomes of different choices, identifying and mitigating the barriers to decision making, facilitating family communication about the patient's decisions, and helping patients understand, accept, and adapt to the outcomes of their choices.

## ACCESS TO PRACTICAL RESOURCES

When the federal government imposed limits on institutional care to reduce costs, oncology social workers increased their emphasis on another important function, that is, helping patients gain access to financial and other practical resources they need after discharge from the hospital and during recuperation. Since the advent of prospective payment systems, an increasing number of patients have been treated in ambulatory care settings, where reimbursement is inadequate and requires more payments out of pocket. Because community services have not been expanded (and in some cases not even developed) in response to the demand for more home care, social workers must spend more time trying to develop new resources and to use existing agencies and foundations creatively.

In this role the worker must identify a large network of services that are specific to cancer. The more services in the network, the more likely the worker will be able to meet the diverse needs of cancer patients effectively throughout the course of the illness. Some of these services, such as transportation and home care, are well known. Others—such as the Make-a-Wish program, which attempts to gratify the wishes of dying children—are not.

One important new resource involves advocacy on behalf of patients who have survived cancer and need help in finding employment and insurance. The increasing numbers of cured and chronic patients have highlighted the need to remove the social barriers that hinder patients from living productive lives.

Finally, because patients tend to focus on their immediate needs rather than on those that may arise in the future, the worker needs to enhance their awareness of services that will meet future needs in a timely way. Unfortunately, it is becoming increasingly difficult to obtain services in the community because of bureaucratic complexities. Thus, even the most sophisticated patients and families often require professional help in gaining access to those services.

## Education

Oncology social workers have developed expertise in the education and training of both patients and professionals. Educating and training patients has become an increasingly important method of helping patients and families cope with complex medical treatments and new methods of service delivery. As more patients are treated and cared for at home, they and their families must become active partners in care to ensure that the treatment is carried out safely and effectively. Furthermore, the longer periods of chronic disease and cure have created a demand for less expensive services after treatment has ended and the support services of acute care institutions are less likely to be available. Developing education and assessment strategies for monitoring the changing needs of large numbers of ambulatory patients is a new challenge in oncology.

Because anxiety often interferes with the patient's retention of information, patient education requires a multimodality approach that accommodates a broad range of individual preferences and supportive methods. For example, social workers direct and participate in multidisciplinary workshops such as ''I Can Cope,'' integrate discussions with physicians into existing patient support groups, and develop printed and audiovisual educational materials for distribution to patients.

Finally, education is a vital method of helping patients gain a sense of control during overwhelming medical and psychological crises. Thus, it has been integrated increasingly into social work counseling and psychosocial treatment (e.g., for patients treated on research protocols, groups facilitate ongoing understanding of effects and give feedback).

Oncology social workers also have developed innovative programs for educating other professionals as well as social work students about psychosocial oncology. For example, in 1973 the social work department of Memorial Sloan-Kettering Cancer Center (MSKCC) in New York, assisted by a grant from the American Cancer Society (ACS), developed a postgraduate training program for social workers and has conducted the weeklong program 10 times a year for the past 15 years. Approximately 100 social workers from cancer centers and other institutions throughout the country participate in the program each year, and the program was recently expanded to include other mental health professionals and more specialized content.

This program was followed by the Social Work Oncology Group, developed at the Sidney Farber Cancer Center with the support of the National Cancer Institute (NCI), which reaches out to practitioners in rural and metropolitan areas of New England. Similar programs were subsequently developed at the Fox Chase Cancer Center in Philadelphia, the California Division of the ACS, and, most recently, the M.D. Anderson Cancer Center in Texas. Many social work oncology support groups have also been developed in rural and urban areas throughout the United States.

In 1985 oncology social workers from postgraduate training programs, cancer centers, and treatment institutions and agencies throughout the country formed the National Association of Oncology Social Workers with support from the ACS. The purpose of this organization is to (1) promote the members' clinical, educational, and research development, (2) devise and maintain professional standards for oncology social workers, and (3) serve as an advocate for the right of patients and their families to obtain necessary services.

## Research

The primary objective of social work research in oncology is to contribute to the existing knowledge base and enhance the understanding of processes such as adaptation and the provision of support in a way that will improve clinical practice and delivery of services to patients and families. Areas include the full range of research in psychosocial oncology. Ideas for the research frequently grow out of issues that have emerged in the staff's work with patients and families. Typically, some clinical issue presents itself and captures a worker's interest. A researcher then helps shape that issue into a question that can be studied systematically. Other staff members often cooperate in implementing the research and in collecting data. When the research is completed, the results are usually discussed with clinical staff, who help interpret the findings and use those findings to develop new interventions which will improve their practice. Research findings also may suggest new avenues for investigation.

Psychosocial research is supported by organizations such as the ACS, the NCI, the National Institute of Mental Health (NIMH), and philanthropic agencies. It has its roots in studies of quality assurance and service delivery that have been conducted since the late 1970s in social work and health care. Social workers participate as investigators in a wide range of biomedical and psychosocial studies on service delivery, patient-related matters, and family and other support systems.

Because service delivery has changed dramatically in recent years, research in this area focuses increasingly on the practical and administrative needs of patients and families, and on identifying patients who are most likely to have difficulty having their needs met. For example, Berkman and colleagues (1983) investigated the characteristics of elderly cancer patients who require institutional care.

Evaluating new methods of monitoring patients who live at home while receiving treatment is a current focus of psychosocial research (Siegel et al., 1987). A major thrust of research on concrete needs is the development of replicable interventions that will improve the quality of service delivery. For example, the social work department at MSKCC tested the feasibility and acceptability of utilizing a computer-automated telephone outreach system to assess the needs of chemotherapy outpatients for a range of practical services (Siegel et al., 1987). The fully automated system was programmed to (1) place telephone calls to 79 patients, (2) conduct a 12-question survey in a high-quality, digitally stored voice, (3) interpret, confirm, and record the patients' answers, and (4) flag patients who identified one or more unmet needs, so these patients could receive prompt, direct professional attention.

The results of the pilot study indicated that computer-automated surveys are likely to have broad-based acceptance among cancer outpatients and that outpatients are able to comply with instructions for completing the interview. This method could provide a cost-effective, universal, and ongoing assessment of patients' needs that would facilitate timely intervention and the efficient use of professional staff.

Patient-related research focuses on the impact of diagnosis and treatment on quality of life at all stages of illness. Examples of such research include the studies of Fobair and colleagues (1986) and Siegel and Christ (1988), who examined the consequences of long-term treatment on survivors of cancer. In the past few years, social workers have undertaken research on the psychosocial impact of acquired immune deficiency syndrome (AIDS) (Christ et al., 1986; Christ and Wiener, 1985). The AIDS epidemic also has provided a unique opportunity for interdisciplinary studies of a major public health problem, as it develops, and with a special emphasis on prevention.

There are also examples of research on family and other support systems. For example, Adams-Greenly and colleagues (1985) and Adams-Greenly and Moynihan (1983) studied the children who had a parent dying of cancer to identify the process of childhood grief and develop interventions that could be used during the course of the parent's illness to prevent long-term adjustment problems in the children. In another study, Bauman, Gervey, and Siegel (1988) asked questions such as the following about patients who participate in self-help groups: How do participants differ from nonparticipants? Do participants generally cope better than nonparticipants with the stresses of cancer and its treatment? What, according to partici-

pants, are their motives for taking part in these groups? Finally, a critical new area for research is the stress and burden experienced by the caretakers of patients with cancer.

## MAINTAINING GOOD STAFF MORALE

Maintaining good staff morale in the midst of such emotional intensity, system change, and increasing complexity and diversity of treatments requires the development of a conceptual framework and specific strategies to address these issues and to support optimal staff functioning. Most studies of morale among health care staff members working with the seriously ill and dying patients have found that administrative and management problems have a greater negative impact on staff members than the stress associated with direct work with patients and families (Yancik, 1984). "The stress of the job has as much to do with the working conditions, the administration, and the co-workers as it does in any similar job situation" (Yancik, 1984, p. 31). These findings match our own clinical experience in providing support to other health care workers (Moynihan and Outlaw, 1984) as well as to mental health professionals including social workers. The components we have found useful in maintaining good staff morale include a focus on the development of professional competence, specific efforts to create a supportive work environment, and the continuous development of effective multidisciplinary team functioning.

### Focusing on the Development of Competence

We have found that a focus on the development of competence and mastery of the complexities and demands of the job is a more useful approach to maintaining staff morale than an excessive concentration on the enormity of the patient-related stresses confronting staff members. The latter approach can inadvertently increase a sense of being overwhelmed and helpless rather than instilling confidence in the individual's ability to master job demands. New workers need adequate orientation to the job and both formal and informal opportunities to learn, whereas more experienced staff need opportunities for continuing education and teaching experiences with students and newer workers. Individual social work supervision and staff support groups are examples of formal on-the-job teaching frequently used by social workers. Peer support and education also provide both formal and informal training. As individual social workers gain expertise in new interventive techniques, they can be most effective teachers of these techniques to their peers.

Such formal and informal teaching structures will not occur by chance; they need to be planned, organized, and systematically implemented. It is useful for each department to develop a formal written strategy for on-the-job training with periodic monitoring of its effectiveness in meeting workers' training needs. A survey of staff education needs can identify emerging areas of interest. The costs of such training can be reduced by the liberal use of peer and group education and support.

The development of special areas of interest and expertise within the generic role is another means of enhancing competence and mastery. Individual social workers and multidisciplinary units of professionals can gain recognition for their specialized expertise by their demonstration of competence in the daily management of patients.

## Creating a Supportive Environment

Facilitating the development of an environment in which emotional intensity can be experienced, shared, and integrated is effective in increasing staff morale. For example, social workers are encouraged to express their strong emotional reactions to specific patient situations to each other and to provide mutual support. The expression of these emotional responses is not viewed as pathological, but as a normal and expected reaction to being involved with patients in such emotionally intense and personally meaningful situations.

Social workers also provide emotional support and training to medical, nursing, and other health care staff with whom they work, but who may find emotional expression more difficult. Social workers' special skills in stress management and in moderating intense affects are frequently used by other disciplines (Moynihan and Outlaw, 1984). This support may be organized and provided in formal group sessions, especially for newer staff members, or it may be provided informally.

When a group of social workers or members of an interdisciplinary unit are able to communicate effectively with each other about emotional issues and provide mutual support, they develop a sense of cohesion and community that buffers them against the stresses of poignant, emotionally wrenching situations. Staff morale can remain high even with significant system change and new job demands.

Open communication between administrative and patient care personnel is also an important dimension of a supportive environment that enhances good morale. Such communication addresses and seeks to im-

prove the conditions of the work situation (i.e., personnel conflicts, administrative problems, work overload, as well as emotional overload).

## Maintaining Effective Team Functioning

Because a sense of group cohesion is such an important source of staff morale, social workers and other health professionals are often especially affected by conflicts and difficulties in team functioning. Today, a well-functioning multidisciplinary team is viewed as essential for the survival of the health care system; it is expected to be efficient, cost-effective, and able to respond quickly to constantly changing demands. The team is regarded as a vital means of sharing resources, expertise, and knowledge, and of developing systems for effective communication among diverse but interdependent professionals. Thus, the roles and functions of each team member must be clearly defined so that he or she can carry out those functions efficiently with a minimum amount of discussion. This type of efficiency is viewed as necessary to avoid discontinuity in patient care and wasteful duplication of services.

To reduce confusion, avoid duplication or overlap of services, and enhance the coordination and continuity of the services provided, the interdisciplinary team must make continuous efforts not only to define the role and tasks of each member but to manage conflict constructively as well.

## DEFINITION OF ROLES

Defining one's role is an ongoing process, not a one-time event, and involves at least three processes, namely, describing the role, demonstrating competence, and developing programs that increase the team's awareness of the role.

When the role and function of each member of the multidisciplinary team are clearly defined, the team can rely on each member to provide specific services with a minimum amount of discussion. This presents a major challenge to social workers and other mental health professionals, who have more difficulty articulating their role and function than other specialists whose procedures are discrete and easily described.

Social work often involves procedures that physicians, nurses, and administrators do not automatically accept as such and do not necessarily regard as part of an overall dynamic process. For example, they may view counseling as little more than talking to the patient or "hand-holding." Social workers also often work in private with patients and families or during phone calls to community agencies. If their roles are not clearly defined, health care members of the team tend to rely on their previous experiences with social workers or on stereotypes of the role. The increasing diversity and complexity of the role makes it even more difficult to convey its dimensions to other disciplines.

## TASK FOCUS

The most important organizing concept for effective team functioning is that of task. What is the task to be accomplished? Who has the knowledge, expertise, time, and resources required to accomplish it? Who should lead the effort? This more collaborative approach replaces the traditional hierarchical structure in which team membership and leadership depended on the institutional hierarchy. It is a more effective strategy when many different disciplines are involved in the care and treatment of patients.

## CONFLICT MANAGEMENT

Because the team members represent a variety of disciplines, a certain amount of conflict is inevitable. In fact, the absence of conflict may reflect incompetence, demoralization, or discouragement. Although conflict is not inherently negative, how it is handled will determine whether it is constructive or destructive.

In a team that handles conflict destructively, members harbor resentment, try to assign blame, feel put upon, build negative coalitions, and, in extreme cases, form alliances with patients against other team members or detach themselves from the team. In a team that handles conflict constructively, all team members are willing to collaborate, compromise, reduce the amount of conflict (or even increase it when necessary), and use it proactively and creatively to demonstrate a member's role or clarify a patient's need. The team that focuses on the patient's needs and how those needs are best addressed is a team that achieves the maximum degree of consensus. In other words, a patient focus is a vital element in an effective team.

## SUMMARY

Oncology social work is one of a growing number of mental health professions that constitute the newly emerging field of psychosocial oncology. The many changes in the health care delivery system and in the treatment of patients have placed new demands on these professions to develop innovative approaches to the current health care system that are both effective and efficient. In social work this has meant that an already multidimensional role has become even more diverse and complex. As social workers and other mental health professionals have responded proactively to this challenge, they have grown professionally, become more vital and productive, and thus experienced a greater sense of effectiveness in the care and treatment of cancer patients.

## REFERENCES

Adams-Greenly, M., and R.T. Moynihan (1983). Helping children of fatally ill parents. *Am. J. Orthopsychiatry* 53:219–29.

Adams-Greenly, M., R.T. Moynihan, and N. Beldoch (1986). Helping adolescents whose parents have cancer. *Semin. Oncol. Nurs.* 2:133–38.

Adams-Greenly, M., R.T. Moynihan, G. Christ, and H. Slivka (1985). Helping the children when a parent is dying. In J.A. Billings (ed.), *Outpatient Management of Advanced Cancer*. Philadelphia: Lippincott, pp. 269–81.

Bauman, L.J., R. Gervey and K. Siegel (1988). Factors Associated with Cancer Patients' Participation in Self-Help Groups (Final report). New York: Ittleson Foundation. In press.

Berkman, B., C. Stolberg, J. Calhoun, E. Parker, and N. Stearns (1983). Elderly cancer patients: Factors predictive of risk for institutionalization. *J. Psychosoc. Oncol.* 1(1):85–100.

Christ, G.H. (1987). Social consequences of the cancer experience. *Am. J. Pediatr. Hematol. Oncol.* 9:84–88.

Christ, G.H. and M. Adams-Greenly (1984). Therapeutic strategies at psychosocial crisis points in the treatment of childhood cancer. In A.E. Christ and K. Flomenhaft (eds.), *Childhood Cancer: Impact on the Family*. New York: Plenum, pp. 109–28.

Christ, G.H. and L.S. Wiener (1985). Psychosocial issues in AIDS. In V. DeVita, Jr., S. Hellman, and S. Rosenberg (eds.), *AIDS: Etiology, Diagnosis, Treatment, and Prevention*. Philadelphia: Lippincott, pp. 275–97.

Christ, G.H., M.E. Bowles, and L.J. Bauman (1987). Educational and support groups for breast cancer patients and their families. In J. Harris, S. Hellman, I.G. Henderson, and D.W. Kinne (eds.), *Breast Diseases*. Philadelphia: Lippincott, pp. 648–56.

Christ, G.H., L. Wiener, and R. Moynihan (1986). Psychosocial issues in AIDS. *Psychiatr. Ann.* 16:173–79.

Fobair, P., R.T. Hoppe, J. Bloom, R. Cox, A. Varghese, and D. Spiegel (1986). Psychosocial problems among survivors of Hodgkin's disease. *J. Clin. Oncol.* 4:805–14.

Germain, C.B. (1977). An ecological perspective on social work practice in health care. *Soc. Work Health Care* 3:67–76.

Goldberg, R.J., R. Tull, N. Sullivan, S. Wallace, and M. Wool (1984). Defining discipline role in consultation psychiatry: The multidisciplinary team approach to psychosocial oncology. *Gen. Hosp. Psychiatry* 6:17–23.

Loscalzo, M. (1985). Behavioral approaches: Applications. In *Management of cancer pain* (Syllabus of the Postgraduate Course, Memorial Sloan-Kettering Cancer Center, November 14–16, 1985). New York: Memorial Sloan-Kettering Cancer Center, pp. 261–73.

Moynihan, R. and E. Outlaw (1984). Nursing support

groups in a cancer center. *J. Psychosoc. Oncol.* 2(1):33–48.

Siegel, K. and G. Christ (1990). Psychosocial consequences of long-term survival of Hodgkin's disease. In M. Lacher and J. Redman (eds.), *Hodgkin's Disease: The Consequences of Survival.* Philadelphia: Lea & Febiger.

Siegel, K., G. Christ, and L. Weinstein (1987). Concrete needs of cancer outpatients. *Proc. Am. Soc. Clin. Oncol.* 6:254 (Abstract No. 998).

Yancik, R. (1984). Sources of work stress for hospice staff. *J. Psychosoc. Oncol.* 2(1):21–31.

# 56

## Stresses on Mental Health Professionals

Jimmie C. Holland

The treatment of patients with cancer was originally the exclusive domain of surgeons. Radiotherapists joined them early in this century, and by midcentury medical oncologists began providing chemotherapy. There was traditionally little role for any other professional in patient care, except for the nurse who assisted the doctor and gave psychosocial support. It was social workers who in the early 1950s, with their feet firmly planted in both medicine and mental health, began to function admirably as providers of psychosocial support. They also began to contribute to the understanding of the emotional problems of patients. Ruth Abrams at the Massachusetts General Hospital described the changing pattern of communication of cancer patients during illness (Shands et al., 1951). At about the same time, Sutherland, a psychiatrist at the Memorial Sloan-Kettering Hospital in New York headed the first psychological clinical and research group in cancer, which counted a psychologist, Morton Bard, and social worker, Ruth Dyk, among its members (see Chapter 1).

As consultation–liaison psychiatry emerged in the 1960s, the psychological problems of both cancer patients and staff began to be recognized. Most attention was given to the psychological difficulties caused by not revealing the diagnosis of cancer and to assisting patients in facing a poor prognosis, within the constraints of revealing little information. The development of a role for mental health professionals in oncology units and clinics has been a relatively late development, especially in light of the significant stresses faced by cancer patients, and their doctors, and nurses (Holland, 1982). However, the past decade has seen a marked increase in assignment of psychiatrists, psychologists, and psychiatrically trained nurses to oncology divisions. They have joined social workers as members of increasingly multidisciplinary treatment teams to give psychological support.

Not surprisingly, far less attention has been given to the stresses mental health professionals experience in relation to their work in cancer, because they do not represent the ''front-line'' staff. Much of the work on professional burnout has addressed health professionals in general, although Wise (1981) described the burnout syndrome in psychiatrists working in consultation–liaison psychiatry on general medical and surgical units. Many of the stresses they outlined apply to the mental health professional working in oncology, with some unique additions created by the special problems of cancer (Reiser and Rosen, 1984). These problems are outlined later, and some strategies are proposed for combating the stress experienced by this increasingly visible and important group of mental health professionals working in oncology. Most of the observations are based on our 10 years' experience at the Memorial Sloan-Kettering Cancer Center (MSKCC), and the application of observations from other health care areas that has provided a base for more meaningful interpretation of our observations (Holland, 1982; Vachon et al., 1978; Tull, 1975).

## MAJOR STRESSES ON MENTAL HEALTH PROFESSIONALS AND ONCOLOGY SOCIAL WORKERS

### Attitudes of Others

One of the ways that ''problems I had at work today'' are made more tolerable is by discussing them with family and friends. There are few cocktail party conversations or family dinners at which mention of the emotional problems confronted in a day's work with cancer patients and their families is welcome. Even revealing that one works in a cancer hospital is met with ''Isn't it depressing?'' Comments to the contrary are scarcely heard. The image of a cancer ward as a depressing place is hard to dispel for one who has not visited. Thus, work in oncology sets one apart and diminishes some usual sources of social support away from work.

## Isolation from Collegial Peers

Training in mental health is usually given in settings in which patients are physically healthy and have psychological problems; the focus is on mental health and the mental health professional has the central role in care. A problem, particularly for young clinicians who come to train in the psychological problems of oncology, is the sudden loss of a supportive group of psychologically oriented peers. It is combined with the feeling that one is an outsider working in "someone else's specialty." This is true, and it constitutes a major entry problem. Becoming familiar with cancer and its problems to the point that the field is at least partially "one's own," mitigates the sense of "being in another's shop." The evolution of the oncology subspecialty of psychooncology has helped because it identifies an area of oncology with its own body of literature, training and identified skills.

## Ambiguity of Role

Unlike the oncologic specialists who accept jobs with discrete functions and roles, there are far fewer guidelines and expectations of what the mental health professional in oncology will do, in part because the role has not yet been defined in most oncology units, and is therefore subject to more idiosyncratic definition, based on the personality and wishes of the individuals involved. The person new to a setting feels the absence of a defined role and must search to develop one. This usually occurs over a period of months in which seeing consultations, doing rounds with staff members, and bringing mental health concepts to unit meetings begin to define the job. This very ambiguity, and that several mental health professionals are attempting to work in the same area, leads at times to conflicts that stem largely from this poor definition and the absence of a source from which the definition can be made. Some have solved this by developing a human services division in which all those who give psychosocial services constitute a unit. Other places have a psychosocial or mental health team, which also divides the labor and assures cooperation.

## Absence of a "Tool"

The sense of helplessness that every health professional experiences when caring for a patient with advancing illness is felt even more keenly by the mental health professional, whose only "tool" is the psychological support for the painful events that he or she cannot prevent. The experience of multiple losses is felt particularly by the mental health practitioner who repeatedly offers empathy and involvement with many patients over time. Professional distance and an appropriate level of involvement become difficult to judge in oneself. It is essential that the mental health practitioner monitor his or her responses and those of colleagues. The necessity to be more personally active and involved in working with cancer patients, as compared to working with physically healthy patients, makes it even more important to be aware of oneself and one's "loss history," which may heighten the vulnerability to stress in this role (Sourkes, 1982). The issues are reviewed more extensively under psychotherapy and in the chapters on psychosocial interventions (Chapters 38, 51–56).

## Response of Medical Colleagues

The medical staff members are also unclear about the role of the mental health professional and what he or she can offer. The common ambivalence toward psychology and psychiatry becomes greater in a setting in which the urgency of life and death is so much the mode. The usual way out of this dilemma is the establishment of a professional credibility and a relationship to the staff members that assumes mutual respect. When this is accomplished, the stage is also set for the informal support to be given to staff members as they experience work-related stresses.

## Stresses of Patients

The patients who are requested to be seen in consultation by the mental health professional are frequently those who pose difficult adjustment and personality problems that lead to demanding or inappropriate behavior. The role of interpreting the behavior of the patient that is causing the staff to be angry can be difficult and stressful as the mental health professional tries to identify the problems and resolve them. Sometimes the anger is displaced onto the mental health practitioners. Consultations are often requested only when the situation has become dire, which adds to the emotional tension. Such patients often manipulatively create conflicts among the staff members which can result in great stress in the individual who tries to explain the cause of the conflicts and mediate to reach a solution.

## Work Conditions

In liaison work, contact with one's own peers is limited and the nature of the way patients are referred (by informal or formal consultation) precludes careful scheduling of hours and distribution of the work load. In both the hospital and clinic, the consultations are apt to be done in less than ideal conditions of privacy and comfort, and because of this, there is a risk of confirming a sense of less importance attached to the work.

## Low Status of Psychosocial Issues

With a busy staff, far more excitement will be created by a lecture on interleukin 2 than on the management of psychologically difficult cases. Psychological problems are usually appreciated only after house staff members and fellows enter practice on their own and realize that the absence of psychological management is indeed a major deficit (Schmale et al., 1987). The need to try to "sell" the importance of these issues to some staff members who are not interested creates a sense of devaluation of the work that can be felt personally.

## Dealing With The Sense of Urgency

The issues of life and death are often so pervasive that the consultation–liaison staff member feels compelled to seek answers and make recommendations quickly, even prematurely. These problems are discussed in Chapter 38 on psychotherapy in crisis situations.

## Fears of Cancer and Phases of Emotional Reactions

Transient cancerophobia, a typical medical student syndrome, occurs in mental health professionals as well as staff members who are confronted with initial contact and work in oncology (see Chapter 2). The awareness of this phobia and a familiarization with the actual facts about cancer become part of the initiation rites and adaptation. Not only anxiety but also depressed feelings are felt after the initial period of numbness. After about 3 months, one feels a sense of depression about the difficulties of the work and the burden of frequent patient deaths. After that, a sense of resolution allows for the weighing of rewards from the work against its stresses. Individuals who remain beyond a year usually become engrossed and satisfied in the field.

## Systems Problems

The mental health professional must be able to think of the whole system and to identify the nature of the problem that is presented, which may be the patient, or a member of the health care team, or the social system

itself. Interventions that are based on this more comprehensive perspective are complex and far less amenable to solution, because they may require action of administrators in several different disciplines (Strain and Grossman, 1975).

## Solving Insolvable Problems

The consultation–liaison staff member may be called to "fix" a situation that is not correctable. The failure to resolve the problem increases the sense of helplessness unless the problem is viewed in the realistic light of being insolvable. Several interventions have proved useful from the experiences and teaching of consultation–liaison psychiatry (Strain and Grossman, 1975).

## TECHNIQUES FOR ADJUSTING TO WORK IN ONCOLOGY

Recognizing the problems just outlined, there are some guidelines and techniques for assisting doctors and nurses in the ability to understand psychosocial issues and to reduce personal stresses. They are covered in Chapters 52 and 53 on the stresses of doctors and nurses. Many apply to the mental health professional as well. Several important measures that enable adjustment in working in oncology are outlined in the following paragraphs.

## Orientation

Mental health professionals beginning to work in an oncology setting must be oriented to the succession of emotions they may feel, including transiently increased fears of cancer, anxiety, some depression, and finally adaptation to its stresses. They must also receive some formal instruction about the types of neoplasms and their treatment, as well as the prognosis associated with each.

## Critical Mass and Mutual Support

The work of consultation–liaison in oncology results in professional isolation from peers of the same specialty, and therefore it is important not to attempt the work unless there is a source of peer and mutual support. Consultation–liaison psychiatrists recognize the need for peer groups and for senior staff members who offer leadership and who can place problems and goals in a larger context. The psychiatry service at MSKCC finds it essential to have weekly support sessions for fellows in which patients are presented and personal reactions discussed; additionally there are private conferences with a supervisor in which personal issues can be more comfortably raised. The individual also achieves a sense of being part of a group that takes on difficult tasks and carries them out well. Elitism can have its positive aspects in creating a high level of esprit de corps often seen in these groups.

## Awareness of Stresses

The mental health professional should know burnout symptoms and be aware of their development. Vacations, and reducing the load of very ill patients, when several have died in a short period, may be necessary.

## Integration in a Medical Unit

The sense of "belonging somewhere" is enhanced by allocating time to a single group, which promotes a sense of being part of one unit although work may have to be done elsewhere as well. This also allows more personal interaction with staff members who utilize the mental health professional better in this liaison model.

## Organize a Body of Information

Organization of teaching materials, lectures, and information based on research studies to teach about psychological problems to medical staff creates the scientific credibility for the field and gives the mental health practitioner a sense of a professional identity.

## Research Orientation

The emotional issues in care of cancer patients and the interaction of biological and psychological aspects of illness, when viewed from a research perspective, allow painful problems to be seen in a different way; a research question can be posed and an investigation of the problem undertaken. It is best within a mental health team to have some member or members of the group working primarily with research issues that promotes this different way of looking at clinical problems. They can also teach research skills to clinicians, and the clinicians in turn can assist them in identifying key questions to address in a research design, and by identifying the personal issues that arise in doing clinical research with patients with cancer and AIDS. The research mode is also a route to enhanced collegiality and collaboration with those doing biomedical research. Particularly valuable contributions can be made by the mental health professional to collaborative efforts in methods of monitoring and quantifying subjective data, including pain, psychological symptoms, and quality of life. They also contribute to

the awareness of psychological issues in research, such as investigator bias and compliance (see Part XII on research). The potential for collaborative research in areas such as psychoneuroimmunology is also great in institutions geared to clinical care and research.

## Recognizing the Need for Time and Patience

It is tempting to assume that one will overturn long-ingrained patterns in oncology house staff members or nurses by some "new" approach. The review of efforts with peers and senior staff members helps to reduce the disappointment when the novice liaison professional recognizes that the only change is that all participants are 1 year older. The counsel of others helps to achieve the patience and tolerance that such work requires.

## Refer a Problem

It is clear at times that a particular patient kindles some emotion in the mental health professional that makes that patient's care more stressful than that of others. Self-reflection and referral to another, if needed, is useful, particularly when doing psychotherapy.

## SUMMARY

Stresses are significant on those who choose to work as mental health professionals in cancer care. However, some of the stresses have an opposing positive side, in that there is little opportunity for boredom, little repetition in daily activities, and constant exposure to new information from other fields. New cases frequently present novel areas for clinical investigation. There is the sense of being a part of a group capable of doing a difficult job; one meets bright, dedicated colleagues who stimulate new ideas. The sense of challenge and excitement in exploring new areas in which psychiatry and psychology overlap with oncology make the stress for most worth the effort.

## REFERENCES

Holland, J.C. (1982). Selected new developments: Psychologic aspects. In J.F. Holland and E. Frel III (eds.), *Cancer Medicine*, 2nd ed. Philadelphia: Lea & Febiger, pp. 2325–31.

Reiser, D.E. and D.H. Rosen (1984). *Medicine as a Human Experience*. Baltimore: University Park Press.

Schmale, J., N. Weinberg, and S. Pieper (1987). Satisfaction, stresses and coping mechanisms of oncologists in clinical practice. *Proc. Twenty-Third Annu. Mt. Am. Soc. Clin. Oncol.* 6:255 (Abstract No. 1003).

Shands, H.C., J.E. Finesinger, S. Cobb, and R.D. Abrams

(1951). Psychological mechanisms in patients with cancer. *Cancer* 4:1159–70.

Sourkes, B.M. (1982). The deepening shade: Psychological aspects of life-threatening illness. Pittsburgh: University of Pittsburgh.

Strain, J.J. and S. Grossman (1975). *Psychological Care of the Medically Ill: A Primer in Liaison Psychiatry.* East Norwalk, Conn.: Appleton-Century-Crofts.

Tull, A. (1975). The stresses of clinical special work with the terminally ill. *Smith Coll. Studies Soc. Work* 45:137–58.

Vachon, M.L., W. Lyall, and S.J. Freeman (1978). Measurement and management of stress in health professionals working with advanced cancer patients. *Death Educ.* 1:365–75.

Wise, T.N. (1981). Burnout: Stresses in consultation–liaison psychiatry. *Psychosomatics* 22:744–51.

# 57

# Psychological Stress on Clergy

## Rev. George Handzo

In recent years the chaplain has become an increasingly important member of the health care team in oncology. Chaplains fulfill some of the basic needs of patients, family members, and staff members that might not otherwise be met. The role of the chaplain has broadened from one that was purely sacramental (e.g., prayer, communion, anointing) to one that encompasses much wider areas of support. The chaplain also represents an extension of the patient's personal life into the hospital, and thus offers some continuity in the life of the patient.

## SPECIAL ROLE OF THE CLERGY

It is generally agreed that all patients have spiritual needs and therefore need spiritual care. The spiritual realm is broadly defined as that which is beyond human knowledge (Berryman, 1983). The special role of the clergy on health care teams is based on this need for spiritual care. Everyone, at some time, and especially in times of crisis, deals with insurmountable questions, such as "Why is this happening to me?" or, "What sense does this all make?" These are questions for which science and medicine have no answer. These questions have a unique language often involving symbol, story, and ritual. The chaplain has the unique expertise to deal in this language and therefore with the questions of this realm.

Some of these questions and concerns might be stated in the language of faith. God might be invoked and statements of faith used to deal with some of these questions. However, other questions, such as the attempt to make sense out of one's life, might be dealt with in more existential terms. The diagnosis of cancer invokes in an individual the need suddenly to make sense of life on an existential and spiritual level (Mudd, 1981; Sontag, 1977). The chaplain deals with this issue in terms of how the world works, how God

works, and what we consider the essence of "life" to be.

Clergy implicitly represent the presence of God in the hospital. Even when employed by the hospital, they are the official representatives of the religious community by virtue of their ordination or commission. They are responsible to a "higher authority." The chaplain's relationship to the patient is centered in the formation of an emotional bond. The main goal for a chaplain is to support the patient and to be present for him or her emotionally. The chaplain has to accept the patient as a worthy and respected fellow human being (Mundhenke, 1982). Chaplains do describe their own faith, but only when that is requested of them. This ministry of presence is centered around acceptance, caring, a nonjudgmental stance, consistency of care, and physical and emotional availability. The patient is given complete autonomy in the relationship. Cancer patients have a disease that is beyond their control. Therefore, enabling them to have control in the relationship is especially important.

## PRACTICE OF CHAPLAINCY IN THE ONCOLOGY ENVIRONMENT

There are two major models by which chaplaincy services are delivered, namely, the denominational and the "one for all." In the denominational model, the chaplain serves all patients of his or her denomination (e.g., Catholic, Protestant, or Jewish). This model is more traditional and has the advantage of giving all patients a chaplain from their own religion. Its disadvantage is that the chaplain cannot be integrated into any one unit or treatment team, reducing integration with the staff. In the "one for all" model, one chaplain is designated to one or more specific nursing units. This latter model emerged to address the disadvantage of the denominational model and coincided with the general evolution of team care. Many institutions provide a mixture of these two systems, trying both to offer intensive presence and to serve specific denominational needs.

This lack of definition is both the central strength and the central frustration in the practice of chaplaincy. There is no objective scientific task, such as giving chemotherapy or curing an illness. There is not even a standard form of practice. The unstructured nature of the work is necessitated by the centrality of the personal relationship in the pastoral process (Holst, 1984). However, one way to deal with the lack of role definition is to improve on and broaden the old model of the chaplain as the person who deals with ''God talk.'' Chaplains do have unique training and expertise to talk about God. However, this training also gives them the much broader ability to deal in the realm of indirect language as described by Berryman (1983). This expertise can be called religious counseling and defined as the explicit interaction between the chaplain and the faith system of the patient or family member. In doing religious counseling, the chaplain would seem to have four major tasks, specifically, assessment, emotional faith support, intellectual faith support, and interpretation.

## Assessment

The first task, assessment, involves finding out what people really believe. The assumption has often been made that a person's belief system is described by their denominational affiliation or lack of one. While there is some truth to this statement, the range of belief systems within any denomination is quite broad. A Jew can be Reform or Orthodox. A Roman Catholic can be strongly charismatic or traditional. A person who claims no religious affiliation may still have a highly developed theology. For example, within some ethnic groups, the beliefs of Roman Catholics with respect to disease and death may be virtually identical to those of their Pentacostal neighbors. Also, a simple faith statement can have several possible meanings. For example, the statement, ''God will take care of me,'' could mean that God will cure me without help from doctors, or God will cure me through doctors, or God may or may not cure me but will support me through illness and even possibly through death. The chaplain needs to be able to assess and interpret faith statements such as these and place them within the context of the person's total faith system as is done with physical and psychological issues (Pruyser, 1976). To be most effective with a cancer patient or family member, a chaplain must have an understanding of the individual's faith system.

One aspect of this task is assessing the person's belief of how God works in the world. For many people, God seems to be primarily either a doer or a supporter. The doer is a God of action: creating, destroying, healing, inflicting, and so on. This God is omnipotent and omnipresent, more distant or transcendent, and capable of coldness. The person with this belief wants to understand and know the reasons for God's actions. The important thing is to understand. This person agonizes over ''why'' questions. The person seeks to know God. He or she is more likely to suspect that he or she is being punished by God, because God causes everything and must have some reason for causing this disease.

On the other hand, the supportive God may also be a doer but is primarily a God who makes sure we get by. This God tends to be closer or more imminent and loving, and will not abandon us in time of need. The supporter God seems the more helpful for cancer patients because they feel loved, accepted, and cared for no matter what the outcome of their illness. These patients who feel supported are also those who may seem overly optimistic, until one discovers that their hope is not in cure but in God's continued presence. They are the people who often insist that God will take care of them. An example is a mother whose child was dying with neuroblastoma. Although she knew the medical realities, she was in a generally good mood because she believed that God was not the source of her troubles, that God would give her the support she needed, and that God would give her son eternal life. Harold Kushner's *When Bad Things Happen to Good People* and John Claypool's *Tracks of a Fellow Struggler* represent these two positions. Both authors are reflecting on the death of one of their children. Kushner is primarily interested in why God would do this or allow it. Claypool is concerned, almost exclusively, with how the support and love he felt from God helped him survive. Knowing where a patient is on this supporter–doer continuum is helpful to the chaplain in his or her dealings with the patient. The chaplain can then know whether to reinforce God's basic supportiveness or whether to help deal with the ''why'' questions and the feelings behind them.

As exemplified by Kushner's title, it is also important to know how the cancer patient views good and evil operating in the world. Where do suffering and death come from, and who or what causes them? Do they come from God, is there a devil or other evil force, or are they created by humans themselves? However, Kushner's title points to what may be the most difficult and persistent issue with which chaplains deal. The issue is, in psychological terms, ''low self-esteem.'' While many people profess to believe that their God is forgiving and loving, most really believe that they have to earn their way into God's favor. Stated simply, this belief says "be good and God will love you." This need for acceptance and forgiveness is acted out in myriad ways. Many patients believe their disease is a punishment for some real or imagined past sin. For them, this is the only logical reason why an omnipotent God allows cancer. Some maintain an outwardly flawless faith because they secretly believe that God will surely not help a doubter. Mothers of pediatric patients have fasted until they fainted, hoping to demonstrate to God their love for their child as King David tried to do in the biblical story.

The last assessment issue is not essentially faith-related but comes up in a chaplain's normal conversations and has to do with whether or not the patient has a supportive religious community. Some religious communities are tremendously supportive, and sometimes this support can be transferred to a local group if the patient is far from home. This information can be added to that gathered by other staff to form an overall picture of the patient's supports. In this assessment, the chaplain is trying to determine how the patient views disease, suffering, and death from a religious or existential perspective. The chaplain identifies which parts of this faith system are supportive, and which parts may hinder the patient's coping. It should also be pointed out that, as in any other kind of assessment, the process itself may help clarify the patient's thinking and thereby help him or her use a faith system more effectively.

## Emotional Faith Support

The second part of religious counseling, emotional faith support, is part of the general emotional support mentioned earlier. The task for the chaplain is to support the patient's faith system as it is, to help the patient strengthen it, and to deal with the emotions related to faith issues. The chaplain tries to reinforce the positive aspects of the faith system by accepting and affirming them, thereby strengthening the faith system's overall usefulness to the patient. The patient often needs to hear that doubts intruding on a previously solid faith are normal and not to be feared. He or she may need to hear from someone else what they already believe and find helpful. For example, a 50-year-old woman with metastatic colon cancer who was resisting further treatment was feeling separated from God and simply wanted someone to confirm her basic belief that God was there for her.

The most prevalent emotion the chaplain deals with is hope. This hope is not for physical healing, although that can be included when appropriate. It is hope that the patient will not be abandoned, will not have more than he or she can bear, and will always be cared for

and loved. It is one of the central goals of chaplaincy to continue to support hopefulness. The chaplain can often help the patient deal with anger at God by acting as the lightning rod that draws the anger to it. Many patients need permission to be angry at God and need to hear that their anger is symptomatic of a close relationship rather than one that is broken. Lastly, the chaplain is the agent of forgiveness and grace that can help relieve anxiety and elevate self-worth. Given the lack of self-worth noted earlier, many patients feel separated from God. Late one night, a dying teenager asked to see the chaplain who had been working with him throughout his illness. The young man was quite agitated and wanted to be assured that he would go to heaven. His parents had tried to reassure him, but he wanted to hear it from the chaplain. The thrust of emotional faith support is not to change the patient's faith system, but to help the patient maximize the support that it provides.

## Intellectual Faith Support

However, the third task in religious counseling, intellectual faith support, involves the chaplain in changing the patient's faith system or refocusing on its positive aspects rather than simply supporting it. In practice, the separation of emotional and intellectual faith support is not always sharp. However, changing the patient's faith system is primarily a cognitive process, whereas supporting it as it is is primarily an emotional process. The chaplain and the patient work together to change parts of the patient's faith system that both agree are not helpful. The difference between intellectual faith support and proselytizing is the need for agreement between the chaplain and the patient on the parts of the system to be changed. The most common issues in this area revolve around the belief that God causes cancer as a punishment. Most people include punishment as one of the functions of an authority figure. However, most people also want to believe that God is not vengeful. They need help to restructure their theology in the direction of a beneficent God.

Another role of the chaplain is to help patients see their God as a supporter and focus less on the "why" questions. For many people, the "why" questions are rhetorical and a way of expressing their emotional pain. Most people find only frustration in searching for answers. No answer can justify why they as an individual should have cancer. Even if they find answers, they are left only with understanding, which provides no support. They may need the understanding in order to feel some control over the situation, but it is normally not sufficient to enable them to feel connected to and supported by God. Many patients are also helped by thinking about the nature of evil. Ever since the concept of Satan went out of fashion in many religious groups, little thought has been given to the possible nature of evil. Especially helpful to some cancer patients is the idea that, regardless of how we think about evil, part of its nature is randomness. In other words, many of the bad things that happen to good people are so terrible exactly because there is no reason why that specific person should be chosen. Other areas of concern can include how God works in the world, the nature of God's plan if there is one, and how we can feel more supported by God. Generally, this area of support calls for the chaplain to share his or her faith rather than simply affirming the patient's.

## Interpretation

The final part of religious counseling is the interpretive function of the chaplain, which involves representing faith issues and faith systems to the staff. Some of these issues are relatively minor points of information such as what kinds of condolences or other gestures are appropriate for families of a specific faith. The medical staff may want information on certain religious beliefs and customs that are foreign to them, such as the beliefs of Jehovah's Witnesses about receiving blood. The chaplain should be a resource for the medical staff in understanding patients from religious groups not commonly found in the area or whose beliefs are very pronounced. For example, some patients from fundamentalist Christian groups may seek to impose their beliefs on others. The hospital staff may need help in accepting these patients and limiting them at the same time. Orthodox Jews have many needs and customs that can be provided for if the staff has adequate information and planning is done. The chaplain can also serve to mediate between patients and doctors when misunderstandings occur about faith questions. Medical staff are often uneasy with patients who say God will take care of them. The doctors assume that the patient is about to sign out. The same thing happens with patients who are visited by a faith healer. In the vast majority of cases, these statements and visits do not indicate any loss of confidence in doctors. They are often attempts by patients to cope with times of uncertainty and crisis. They tend to vanish when the patient feels in control. Patients who might refuse medical treatment on religious grounds generally do so well before they arrive at a cancer center. This interpretive function can be seen as part of a larger advocacy role that the chaplain fulfills. Finally, it is helpful in this interpretation if the chaplain can speak both in the language of religion and in the language of psychology.

## STRESSES ON CLERGY

Like other staff, chaplains are subject to burnout, the intrusion of outside personal issues into their work, hopelessness and despair, the need to work with patients they do not like, and their own fears concerning illness and death. However, these issues are exacerbated in clergy by the need for chaplains to be constantly available on an emotional level. The chaplain is constantly breaking and forming relationships. Unlike many other professionals in the medical setting, there is almost no part of a chaplain's job that does not require emotional input. A chaplain who cannot give of himself or herself cannot function.

Allowing the patient autonomy in the relationship may be a source of stress. It can be frustrating to have to conform to the patient's agenda and not to one's own. The chaplain risks personal rejection, a special problem for women in chaplaincy. All chaplains can be rejected, but some patients or family members of every denominational group will be resentful or simply will not accept ministry from a woman, even though that ministry is officially recognized by their denomination.

Because the chaplain is expected to care genuinely for every patient, the problems of working with disagreeable patients can be particularly stressful. The chaplain is sometimes put in the position of having to support a faith system that is helpful to the patient but antithetical to his or her own faith. A common example is the patient who resolutely believes that God will perform a miracle even though he or she seems to be dying and knows the medical realities. This belief is clearly helpful to the patient's coping. The chaplain is caught between being supportive of the patient and true to the chaplain's belief that God's miracles are not predictable. In a profession in which being true to one's belief is central, this predicament is not insignificant. This is one area in which the emphasis on acceptance over evangelism is clear.

While it is important for the chaplain to discover the patient's faith system, this may at times be difficult. Many chaplains are not trained to interview patients or family members with respect to their religious beliefs and practice. Assessment is not a widely accepted part of the practice of chaplaincy. From the other side of the relationship, the patients do not expect the chaplain to question their faith system and may see any attempt at assessment as a challenge. Until a chaplain gains enough experience in being able to maintain a supportive position while gaining sufficient information to know what it is they are supporting, undertaking such assessment can be stressful.

Chaplains have no concrete way to evaluate their

work or their style of relating to patients. They do not do psychotherapy, diagnose illness, or give physical care. Knowing the number of visits they make only means that the chaplain has been there but says nothing about effectiveness. There is no change in blood cell counts or physical markers against which to chart the impact of his or her therapy. This openness and lack of direction fostered in the ideal chaplain–patient relationship, while beneficial to the patient, may be frustrating for the chaplain precisely because of its lack of goals. The need to be responsive to patient concerns also means that the limits of the chaplain's relationship to the patients are, at best, unclear.

Finally, the chaplain often feels peripheral to the work of both the hospital and organized religion. Chaplains have little to do with the main business of the hospital, which is treating disease. The health care system creates all other roles in the hospital. However, the religious community creates and empowers the chaplain. The hospital can only give permission and support for the acting out of this role. However, chaplains are also generally not engaged in the main work of organized religion, which takes place in local churches and synagogues. The chaplains are in, but not of, the hospital, and of, but not in, the religious community. They are able to stand uniquely with the patient because they do not belong primarily to the traditional health care system. However, they do have some lack of role definition because they do not stand fully within either the religious or the health care community. Living on the boundary makes it difficult to have a sense of belonging.

Dealing in the spiritual rather than the scientific realm and having authority from outside the medical community also sets the chaplain apart from the rest of the staff and makes it difficult to feel part of the team. The basic problem is one of definition, namely, is the chaplain a representative of organized religion, a health care professional, or both? Clearly, chaplains are primarily representatives of religion, although they also function as health care professionals. However, maintaining that stance can be difficult in the face of the frequent temptation to become more of a member of the health care team by dealing in the language and processes of science.

## MANAGING STRESS

Managing stress for clergy understandably has some of the same components as it has for other staff members. There is a need for emotional outlets both inside and outside the hospital, for the ability to process feelings well so that they do not lead to "burnout," and for direct support from the staff and from other chaplains.

The sharing of verbatim reports has become common as a form of continuing education among chaplains. This ongoing mutual support should include encouragement to grow in areas of weakness, such as assessment of patients' faith systems.

Working with cancer patients exacerbates virtually every chaplaincy issue and stress. The uncertainties associated with the cause, treatment, and prognosis of cancer lead patients to look more often to their faith systems for explanation and support. Especially tragic cases such as cancer in young parents and children strain even the strongest faith systems. It is often necessary to monitor stress on an individual patient basis to allow full involvement with each. Chaplains must be especially disciplined about maintaining their faith systems as well as using their support systems.

Chaplains do have one special strength intrinsic to their profession: they have well-developed faith systems that, in most cases, have been fine-tuned to deal especially well with disease and death. Although this system often cannot be used to the patient's advantage, it is the chaplain's major support against his or her own stress. One particular strength of this faith system normally is that physical health and even avoidance of physical death are not the highest values. Although the death of a patient is experienced as a loss, it does not carry the same sense of failure as it does for many other health professionals.

## SUMMARY

Chaplaincy with cancer patients and their families requires that curious mix of understanding, training, creativity, and intuition present in the practice of any art form. The chaplain needs to be emotionally present to patients and family members as well as having thorough understanding of spiritual issues involved in sickness and death. The chaplain needs to deal with each person as a unique individual, while knowing what general issues and questions might be important to him or her. Lastly, the chaplain must be continuously aware of living at the interface between the spiritual and the scientific, be able and willing to work in both worlds, and be ready to interpret one realm to the other.

## REFERENCES

Berryman, J. (1983). *The Chaplain's Strange Language: A Unique Contribution to the Health Care Team.* Paper presented at the Eighth Mental Health Conference of the Department of Pediatrics, M.D. Anderson Hospital and Tumor Institute, Houston.

Claypool, J. (1974). *Tracks of a Fellow Struggler.* Waco, Texas: Word Books.

Holst, L. (1984). The hospital chaplain—a ministry of paradox in a place of paradox. *Care Giver—J. Coll. Chaplains* 1(2):7–13.

Kushner, H. (1981). *When Bad Things Happen to Good People*. New York: Avon Books.

Mudd, R. (1981). Spiritual needs of terminally ill patients. *Bull. Am. Protestant Hosp. Assoc. (Spec. Ed. on Pastoral Care)* 45(3):1–5.

Mundhenke, C. (1982). Living with cancer. *Bull. Am. Protestant Hosp. Assoc. (Spec. Ed. on Pastoral Care)* 46(3):86–89.

Pruyser, P. (1976). *The Minister as Diagnostician.* Philadelphia: Westminster.

Sontag, S. (1977). *Illness as Metaphor.* New York: Farrar, Straus & Giroux.

# 58

## Caring for the Physician with Cancer

Kenneth Cohn and Jimmie C. Holland

With the estimated annual incidence of cancer approaching 870,000 cases in the United States, it is likely that a physician who takes care of patients with cancer will eventually treat a fellow physician. Although the physician as patient shares a common medical knowledge with the treating physician, this creates unique problems and can lead to misunderstanding and unnecessary stress. Feelings of isolation and distance between doctor and patient may develop if these problems are not addressed. Similar principles apply to other health care professionals, such as nurses (Johnson, 1982) and social workers (Harker, 1972). This chapter addresses these unique issues, using as a model the physician who requires treatment for cancer.

## PROBLEMS FACED BY THE PHYSICIAN AS PATIENT

The physician as patient faces several problems that are rather unique.

- Abrupt change in status; loss of independence and self-esteem; transition from care taker to patient
- Inside knowledge of complications of therapy and limits of oncology
- Helplessness due to dependence on others, loss of privacy especially in one's own hospital, treatment-related side effects, and inability to plan
- Fear of the stereotypes of physician as patient; difficulty asking questions and expressing anger

One of the most overwhelming initial problems for the physician as patient is the often abrupt transition from the role of independent health care provider to dependent recipient-patient. According to White and Lindt (1963), accepting the role of patient was the most common obstacle to care for the physician-patients they studied. F. Mullan, a physician treated for a primary seminoma in the mediastinum in 1983, wrote, "No amount of medical training could prepare me for so sudden and drastic an alteration in self-perception." The strong feelings that accompany such a rapid change in status are exacerbated by the loss of self-esteem associated with inability to work. The physician as patient also feels embarrassed and ashamed to be "abandoning" his or her patients because of this illness. Thus, it is not surprising that, despite their medical knowledge, physicians frequently delay seeking medical consultation for a symptom suspicious of cancer and continue working after the onset of significant symptoms (Robbins et al., 1953; Stoudemire and Rhoads, 1983). A study of delay in seeking consultation among women with breast lumps found that health professionals, especially nurses, appeared later with larger lesions (Buttlar and Templeton, 1983). The adverse effect of medical training on personal health should be examined further.

Prior medical knowledge may lead to two problems not commonly found in patients from nonmedical backgrounds, namely, enhanced understanding of illnesses and the complications of therapy, and recognition of the limitations of many cancer treatments. After treatment for lymphoma, Cohn wrote in 1982 that "After taking care of patients with a variety of illnesses, I was unable to dismiss the threat of a side-effect as an abstract concept. Many potential complications about which I was informed before consenting to chemotherapy triggered memories of patients who had the worst imaginable complications of their disease." Second, physicians recognize that oncology is a relatively young field and that many treatment protocols are empirical. The insecurity of knowing that the duration and even the type of therapy are still uncertain in a number of malignancies arouses feelings of anxiety and mistrust when one's own life is on the line.

For physicians accustomed to successful mastery of most challenges from elementary school through residency training, helplessness is sometimes a new personal emotion. The helplessness associated with life-threatening illness has previously largely been observed in patients and not personally experienced. The abrupt change in status renders physician-patients helpless in a number of ways. For those who choose to be treated where they work, there is the unaccustomed feeling of loss of privacy; the ill doctor becomes the topic of hospital gossip. Some physicians choose not to be treated in their own hospital for this reason, and because colleagues and members of the staff rarely observe the "No Visitors" sign when a friend is ill.

Accustomed to maintaining a tight schedule, the physician as patient feels particularly helpless when illness and the side effects of treatment make it impossible to make short-term or long-term plans. Finally, treatment, especially chemotherapy, may result in temporary body changes that cause feelings of deformity, embarrassment, and lowered self-esteem. Weakness, fatigue, weight loss, and susceptibility to infection are unexpected complications of daily existence, which lead to greater dependence on others and enhanced feelings of helplessness. Cohn summarized these feelings in a 1982 statement:

Surprise spits in the eye. Any event that occurs unpredictably, regardless of the cause, should be expected to produce feelings of helplessness and outrage. The most difficult situations for me to deal with were not the diagnosis of lymphoma or the initial hair loss, because they were events for which I was prepared. The most challenging events were a drug-induced grand mal seizure, a toxic reaction to phenytoin, and the stresses of terminating chemotherapy, because they were events for which I had not been prepared. The only times I considered terminating chemotherapy prematurely were during these "surprises." each one made me feel as though the light at the end of the tunnel was not daylight but an oncoming train. Intermittent desire to stop chemotherapy represented my inability to cope with these unpredictable side-effects of treatment rather than an objective calculation of the amount of medicine necessary for cure.

The implications regarding therapy are clearly significant. Education of the doctor as patient regarding possible side effects and the development of realistic expectations for therapy are as important as with any other patient.

Frequent mild physical activity is also helpful for the physician as patient. Cohn (1982) nicknamed swimming "hydrotherapy" because it renewed feelings of control over his body, promoted his self-esteem, and helped dissipate tension and anger. Wigs and prostheses are important for physician-patients, who are especially sensitive to the need to maintain appearance in interpersonal and professional roles.

In addition to helplessness, other troubling emotions may surface. Those who have placed their trust in reason may find themselves at a loss to control their emotions, much as they feel at a loss to control their lives after diagnoses of cancer. Anger is ubiquitous and sometimes irrational in its direction (Romm, 1983). It is often directed at those providing treatment, or at the family and friends who provide the most crucial support. However, as impatient as physician-patients seem toward others, they are equally critical of their own behavior. Sanes (1979) frequently demanded "Why can't I adjust?" However, toward the end of his illness he concluded that in addition to reason and determination, it also takes time to adjust.

Like other patients, physician-patients may hesitate to ask a question of the treating physician because they might appear ignorant. It is even more difficult for the physician as patient to complain or to express anger because of fear of being labeled by the stereotype "Doctors make the worst patients." Fear of being refused treatment if too "difficult," or of being abandoned by those supervising their treatment are other common emotions. Physician-patients need to be reassured that their situations and responses are not unique; moreover, they need to be told repeatedly that it is acceptable to show emotions. Even anger is a positive emotion, associated with spirit and determination when directed at the disease rather than at the health care team (Sanes, 1983). However, a stable relationship between the doctor as patient and his or her colleague who has become the treating physician should be able to tolerate expression of the patient's occasional anger and frustration.

In most ways, responses of physicians facing major illnesses in themselves are identical to those reactions observed in other patients who do not have medical training, including initial shock, denial, numbness, and emotional turmoil in attempting to adapt to diagnosis and treatment (Holland, 1982). The physician as patient may also unexpectedly experience a feeling of purposelessness:

I became increasingly self-preoccupied. My fears were not so much for my life but for the loss of all that had made life worthwhile and enjoyable—useful work, multiple interests, professional and personal relations. . . . One must combat a host of fearful thoughts and feelings. These include uncertainty, inadequacy, isolation, morality, guilt, anxiety, depression, withdrawal, and even, for some, the temptation of suicide. . . . A college student covered in three words the whole struggle. . . . Mope, hope, cope. (Sanes, 1979)

In coping with the demands of chronic illness, Cohn (1982) found parallels between the stresses of chronic illness and those of surgical residency, in which he had learned to deal with unpleasant situations by thinking of only one day at a time and accepting the fact of functioning at less than peak efficiency on some days.

In addition to preparing the physician as patient for the negative aspects of treatment, it is also important for the treating physician to stress the gains resulting from treatment:

- Recognition of opportunity for personal growth
- Increased appreciation of health, life, and family
- Improved bedside manner; enhanced sensitivity to patients' emotional needs

The treating physician should emphasize that, in addition to improved survival, individuals often sense a greater enjoyment and appreciation of life. The personal growth and sense of accomplishment that result from successfully completing a course of arduous treatment heighten self-esteem and confidence. During treatment and convalescence, nonmedical avocational interests should be encouraged by the physician. The broadening of horizons enhances self-esteem and gives new interests to pursue when morale is poor.

At the end of treatment, physician-patients often feel a heightened awareness and appreciation of good health (Stoudemire and Rhoads, 1983). Moreover, most physicians find that spending some time on the receiving end of the health care system makes them far more compassionate toward patients. As Thomas wrote in 1983,

I know a lot more than I used to know about hospitals, medicine, nurses, and doctors. . . . But I wish that there were some easier way to come by this level of comprehension for medical students and interns. . . . Every young doctor should know exactly what it is like to have things go catastrophically wrong, and to be personally mortal. It makes for a better practice.

Cancer has been called a social disease because it inevitably involves family and friends as well as the patient. Colleagues especially may feel uncomfortable and, in their discomfort about what to say, will shun the friend who is now a patient (Rabin, 1982). Illness can be a time, however, when a loyal friends become clearly separated from those who drop away. Most physician-patients report becoming closer to supportive friends and family in the course of undergoing the challenging experience together. There is often also the sense of guilt for "putting the family through this," and especially concern for the effects on one's spouse and young children.

Finally, those who believe in God ultimately find their faith strengthened rather than weakened by their illness. The emotional acceptance of the helpless state results in enhanced inner strength and a diminished sense of isolation:

[A]nger and despair may initially lead a person to deny his religious beliefs, but the rejection is seldom more than temporary. The people who have turned to God at other times for lesser reasons will turn to Him again. . . . Unable to control their situation themselves, they are led to rely more and more on the spiritual. (Sanes, 1979)

## INTERPERSONAL DILEMMAS FACED BY THE TREATING PHYSICIAN

Although it is clear that becoming a patient creates a unique situation for a physician, the interpersonal dilemmas confronting the treating physician are also considerable:

- Providing adequate information without feeling condescending
- Abdicating responsibility in advising the physician as patient
- Finances: limits of professional courtesy
- Preparing patient for stresses of terminating therapy

The initial problem often involves how to relate to a colleague who has become a patient. Faced with the abrupt change in status of a colleague who is now a patient, the treating physician may feel uncomfortable that he or she will talk down to the physician as patient about medical facts. These apprehensions may result in inadequate explanations of diagnostic procedures, therapy, and possible side effects (Stoudemire and Rhoads, 1983). It is important to remember that a physician as patient *is above all, a patient* (Sanes, 1979). Specialization in medicine makes it likely that most physician-patients will know little more about a disease outside their specialty than a patient who is not medically trained. If one is concerned about being patronizing to a colleague, it is easy to preface information with, "As you know, . . .." Probably, the physician as patient will not have known, or will have forgotten, and will be grateful for the information.

It is important for physicians to beware of causal personal consultations in the hallway with a colleague about personal symptoms, which may reflect the colleague's difficulty in seeking a formal consultation. They should insist on an appointment in the office, where an adequate history and physical examination can be taken, or refer the colleague to a mutually respected physician (Stoudemire and Rhoads, 1983). Despite the reticence that a doctor may have about asking personal questions of a colleague, he or she must realize that information not sought or revealed at the initial examination may lead to delays or errors in diagnosis or treatment. If the relationship impairs the taking of an adequate history, it may be wise not to treat the colleague but refer him or her to a less closely associated physician. A physician should generally *not* tackle the burden of treating a close friend for cancer if decisions that will need to be made may be too emotionally difficult for the friend to maintain needed objectivity.

The treating physician must always be mindful of how easy it is to hide behind medical jargon, especially when discussing a sensitive issue. One cannot expect physician-patients to respond to a bedside discussion of their own health in the same way they would respond to a discussion of another patient's case:

[P]hysicians seemed to find difficulty in talking to me as a patient rather than as a medical colleague. Nearly four weeks after the end of chemotherapy, I became dyspneic with a $Po_2$ of 41 mm Hg. Yet, as breathing became easier, I became increasingly anxious, listening to the residents discuss the contingencies of my care as though they were chatting with a fellow physician in the cafeteria rather than with a patient at the bedside. (Cohn, 1982)

It is important for the treating physician to encourage the physician as patient to direct questions about the illness and its treatment to him or her. Reading the medical literature on the disease in question should be discouraged. The objectivity of the medical literature will sound callous and disheartening when read, but the same facts can be made to seem more encouraging when presented by the physician. It is also important to advise the physician as patient about the recommended treatment in the same manner as a patient without medical training. The tendency to allow a physician as patient to choose his or her own treatment or to feel that he or she is directing the care should be avoided. Stoudemire and Rhoads (1983) suggested that being allowed to give up the burden of self-care and total decision making can be of considerable relief to the physician as patient.

Financial issues should also be discussed early in the course of the illness. Professional courtesy may create a sense of obligation on the part of the physician as patient, making it difficult to receive adequate care without feeling bothersome (Stoudemire and Rhoads, 1983).

Even more vexing are the issues that arise near the end of therapy on how to provide reassurance and hope in the face of uncertainty about recurrence and death. Despite the difficulties that the physician as patient encounters during therapy, the months following the end of treatment may be the most stressful, because of awareness of the possibility of recurrence and fear of delayed complications of therapy (Cohn, 1982). The physician as patient may feel vulnerable that the lifeline of treatment has been taken away, similar to the feelings of other cancer patients (Holland et al., 1979). Also, the patient may feel a moral responsibility to resume work soon after the last treatment, when physical and psychological resources are still limited. Family resentment and anger, not expressed during the course of the illness, may surface once therapy has

ended. Discrimination regarding employment and insurability may make the patient feel insecure or trapped by the present situation (Mullan, 1983).

The best way to deal with the termination stresses is to begin discussing them with the patient well before the end of therapy, preferably at the time when approximately 75% of the therapy has been given. It should be stressed that fear of recurrence and death is an inevitable part of the recovery process and that coping with this fear takes time and patience. Patients should be urged to set concrete goals for the next day, week, and year with the understanding that each day builds hope (Sanes, 1979). The progress that has been made in treating certain types of malignancies should be stressed. Perhaps the word "cancer" should be replaced by "cancers" to denote a diverse group of diseases with different prognoses, contrary to the public expectation of a uniformly fatal outcome.

Mullan (1985) describes the ambivalence toward "extended survival," as it blends slowly into "permanent survival." "No matter how long we live, cancer patients are survivors—at once wary and relieved, bashful and proud." Regardless of the outcome as perceived by the treating physician, the physician as patient will require repeated reassurance after treatment ends, and over some time of "extended survival." This chapter should trigger a mental alarm against the concept that "because my doctor-patient is cured he does not need me any longer."

## INTRAPERSONAL DILEMMAS FACED BY THE TREATING PHYSICIAN

Intrapersonal difficulties often arise in the treating physician:

- Unwelcome reminders of personal mortality
- Anger
- Identification with physician as patient
- Helplessness

Having a physician for a patient may challenge the treating physician's usual sense of invulnerability to illness and raise disturbing questions about his or her own health, serving as an unwelcome reminder of mortality. This phenomenon, which occurs with the care of any seriously ill patient, is heightened when the patient is a physician (Spikes and Holland, 1975). These questions are usually overlooked and avoided, because of time pressure and healthy denial that "patients" are different from "us." It is a startling revelation that "they" are in fact "us," a revelation made more painful by identification with another physician of similar age or background, or with one who reminds the treating physician of a beloved family member. Overidentitification with the physician as patient can be a difficult burden for the treating physician, requiring an awareness to avoid mistakes in treatment due to these associations. Anger toward the physician-patient may be felt for forcing questions of personal mortality to the surface and for producing a sense of helplessness, when, despite optimum care, the ill physician experiences advancing disease and death. A treating physician may perceive the death of a colleague as a true mark of failure and may experience considerable grieving following the death, akin to that seen with loss of a family member. Depression may also ensue in a physician already burdened by other troubling personal issues.

The major intrapersonal issues just described cannot be ignored for long without resulting in avoidance of the patient (Rabin, 1982) and/or unnecessary occupational or domestic conflicts.

## SUMMARY

The treatment of a physician creates a challenging but rewarding situation that involves unique responsibilities for the treating physician and for the physician receiving treatment. Some of the usual problems experienced by all patients are accentuated in the doctor as patient and in other health care professionals (especially nurses), including unaccustomed helplessness, dependence on a prior colleague for care, and loss of privacy and self-esteem. Coupled with these general problems are the inside knowledge of the limitations of oncology, fears of complications of therapy, and anxiety about being a "difficult patient."

The treating physician also faces special dilemmas in providing information without seeming condescending. The experience may awaken unwelcome thoughts of personal mortality, identification with the ill doctor, and anger and helplessness, if treatment fails. It is essential that the physician as patient and the treating physician be alert to unique issues that can create challenging problems for both but that, if properly addressed, can contribute to a rewarding human as well as medical experience. During the "inadvertent fellowship in oncology," the physician as patient requires gentle but firm guidance from the treating physician.

## REFERENCES

Buttlar, C.H. and A.C. Templeton (1983). The size of breast masses at presentation: The impact of prior medical training. *Cancer* 51:1750–53.

Cohn, K. (1982). Chemotherapy from an insider's perspective. *Lancet* 1:1006–9.

Harker, B. (1972). Cancer and communication problems: A personal experience. *Psychiatry Med.* 3:163–71.

Holland, J.C. (1982). Psychiatric aspects of cancer. In J.F. Holland and E. Frei (eds.), *Cancer Medicine,* 2nd ed. Philadelphia: Lea & Febiger, pp. 1175–1203; 2325–31.

Holland, J.C., J. Rowland, A. Lebovits, and R. Rusalem (1979). Reactions to cancer treatment: Assessment of emotional response to adjuvant radiotherapy as a guide to planned intervention. *Psychiatr. Clin. North Am.* 2:347–58.

Johnson, J. (1982). Call me healthy. *Oncol. Nurs. Forum* 9:73–76.

Mullan, F. (1983). *Vital Signs: A Young Doctor's Struggle with Cancer.* New York: Farrar, Strauss & Giroux.

Mullan, F. (1985). Seasons of survival: Reflections of a physician with cancer. *N. Engl. J. Med.* 313:270–73.

Rabin, D. (1982). Compounding the ordeal of ALS: Isolation from my fellow physician. *N. Engl. J. Med.* 303:506–9.

Robbins, G., M. MacDonald, and G. Pack (1953). Delay in the diagnosis and treatment of physicians with cancer. *Cancer* 6:624–26.

Romm, S. (1983). *The Unwelcome Intruder: Freud's Struggle with Cancer.* New York: Praeger.

Sanes, S. (1979). *A Physician Faces Cancer in Himself.* Albany: State University of New York Press.

Spikes, J. and J.C. Holland (1975). The physician's response to the dying patient. In J. Strain and S. Glassman (eds.), *Psychological Care of the Medically Ill.* New York: Appleton-Century-Crofts, pp. 138–48.

Stoudemire, A. and J. Rhoads (1983). When the doctor needs a doctor: Special considerations for the physician-patient. *Ann. Intern. Med.* 98:654–59.

Thomas, L. (1983). *The Youngest Science.* New York: Viking Press.

White, R.B. and H. Lindt (1963). Psychological hazards in treating physical disorders of medical colleagues. *Disorders Nerv. Syst.* 24:304–9.

# 59

## The Confluence of Psychiatry, the Law, and Ethics

### Marguerite Lederberg

The current practice of medicine has been profoundly altered by deep changes in our social climate. An expression of this is the increasing importance of bioethical and legal issues in case management. Several controversial concerns often converge in the care of cancer patients. These include informed consent (in ordinary clinical situations as well as in research settings), terminal care issues (e.g., the institution of cardiopulmonary resuscitation orders, the termination of life supports, and the allocation of intensive care beds), and proxy consent (especially in the case of children with tumors). (These and other problems are discussed in Chapters 6 and 48).

Although these issues are being actively explored and defined in many arenas (e.g., hospital ethics committees, philosophy journals, and courts of law), any given case in medicine still tends to be surrounded by legal and ethical uncertainty. There may be no laws or regulations to cover a given situation. Where regulations do exist, they vary by jurisdiction. The vigor with which they are enforced—or ignored—also varies from community to community. The whole area arouses much general interest and strong feelings. Unfortunately the tone of debate is often adversarial, which is especially unconstructive when pursued by people who lack an intimate understanding of the situation.

Increasingly inflexible demands for cost containment and the growing intrusion of third-party payers into case management represent another major complication of medical care. These processes have only begun. In the long run, they may simplify ambiguous situations by making certain options unavailable; in the near future, they are likely to complicate them by restricting expenditures before society has formally acknowledged and accepted the moral implications of these restrictions. Institutions with heavy research and teaching obligations, among which cancer centers figure prominently, are particularly hard-hit by these constraints.

The conditions just described add a large element of stress to the already stressful situation of the cancer patient, the family, and the treatment team. Not surprisingly, this is often translated into increased interpersonal tensions, conflicts, and dysfunctional reactions, which may become severe enough to result in psychiatric consultation. While these troubled responses actually reflect societal pressures affecting behavior, psychiatric labeling can occur in such situations, and, indeed, reactive psychopathology may develop as well. In both situations psychiatric consultation is often requested. To be effective, the evaluation must take these contributing considerations into account.

The converse situation may also occur in which psychological problems in the patient or family members complicate clinical care; such cases may result in a consultation for what appears to be a legal or ethical controversy. This represents another situation in which there is an overlap of psychiatric, bioethical, and legal issues. The just-cited examples reflect the uneasy confluence of the three areas. This relationship takes on added importance and poignancy in the context of the life-and-death issues that come up so frequently in the care of cancer patients.

Thus, psychiatry is very frequently involved in legal and ethical problems. There is some argument as to the credentials of psychiatrists to play this special role. Stone (1984) has explored the special relationship between psychiatry, ethics, and law in a broad philosophical framework. Perl and Shelp (1982) have explored it more briefly in a clinical setting. Whatever one's ultimate philosophical and ethical conclusions, one guideline remains all-important, that is, the need to distinguish between psychiatric, ethical, and legal dimensions of a case. When a psychiatric problem is present, it calls for accurate assessment and active treatment recommendations. Legal and ethical issues should be explicitly defined and a broadly based decision-making process set in motion, in which the psychiatry consultant may be one of several participants.

Several areas of knowledge are necessary to make a solid contribution to this process, including a clear understanding and delineation of exactly what issues are under scrutiny, a current and precise understanding of local, state, and federal laws and regulations that apply in the case, and knowledge of—and access to—skilled local referral resources that include psychiatrists familiar with the psychiatric issues in medically ill patients, bioethics committees, or bioethicists and/or lawyers.

In many cases psychiatric treatment as needed, plus clarification of the legal and ethical problems, reduces tensions sufficiently so that the patient, family, and treatment team can reach decisions in a spirit of mutual cooperation. Occasionally this does not happen, and a more formal consultation process must be instituted, calling on the resources just mentioned. In institutional settings bioethics committees are becoming increasingly common. Where they do not exist, legal counsel is usually available and can at least establish the boundaries of the problem. In private practice, or in more isolated settings, the professional can call on his or her professional organization and ask to be referred to the ethics committees, which have become *de rigueur* in all such organizations.

When all is said and done, it cannot be overemphasized that the mainstay of management is the implementation of unhurried friendly discussions conducted in a spirit of open inquiry and genuine respect to encourage better communication between the principal parties. psychiatrists and other mental health professionals with good communication skills and experience in conflict reduction can and do play a valuable role. However, they may confuse their special contribution with ethical expertise. They must recognize that it is their psychiatric training, not their moral insight—excellent as the latter may be—which is being utilized.

Elucidation of these complex issues and clarifying the three overlapping and contributing considerations is often best demonstrated by case studies. For this reason the rest of the chapter is devoted to annotated case examples, illustrating a few facets of these complex issues. The major problems to be addressed are the psychological problems of decision making, the problems of when and how the "truth" is told, ethical problems that appear as psychological problems, psychological problems that appear as ethical dilemmas,

ethical problems created by third parties, ethical problems in the case of children with cancer, and the need for psychiatric vigilance, even in the apparent absence of ethical and psychiatric problems.

## THE PERILS OF BEING A MODERN PATIENT

### CASE REPORTS

*Case 1:* O.C. was a 35-year-old white housewife with a 2-cm mass in the left breast, who, after extensive research and multiple consultations, had elected to undergo lumpectomy with radiation therapy. The night before surgery her anxiety level rose so high that an emergency psychiatric consultation was requested. The patient was found to have an adjustment reaction with anxiety, overlying a personality with moderately severe obsessive-compulsive traits, but without any previous psychiatric history. Surgery was delayed 2 days while she again reviewed her options. Following this, she agreed to the surgery without difficulty. In the 3 months after surgery, despite negative axillary nodes and an uneventful course of radiation therapy, she remained very anxious, requiring minor tranquilizers, relaxation techniques, and supportive psychotherapy. The focus of her overt concerns continued to be the treatment decision.

*Case 2:* L.S. was a 32-year-old white, single business professional, who had been diagnosed with breast cancer and was scheduled for mastectomy the following day. Emergency psychiatric consultation was requested because the patient was manifesting an unusual and rising level of anxiety. At interview the patient described and demonstrated severe symptoms of distress, including psychophysiological ones (palpitations and hyperpnea), cognitive ones, (racing, repetitive thoughts and inability to concentrate), and periods of depersonalization. She gave a history of obsessive character traits. Consistent with her personality, she had consulted several doctors and had learned a great deal about all the treatments available to her. However, as the moment for surgery approached, all her knowledge seemed meaningless and she felt overwhelmed with terror. She was treated with oxazepam (30 mg po q8h), and her surgeon was advised of her feelings. He postponed the surgery and had several more discussions with her. She was able to undergo surgery 3 days later without complication. No follow-up information is available.

### Commentary

As medical paternalism has become increasingly unacceptable, greater demands have been placed on patients to play a responsible decision-making role in their treatment. This change is welcomed by some and tolerated by others, but there is a minority of patients who cannot emotionally tolerate this new requirement for full participation. The enormous and controversial publicity surrounding the treatment of early breast cancer, particularly when it emphasized medical shortcomings and inadequacies, has added to the woman's burden of anxiety by unnecessarily lowering her sense of trust, without giving her enough knowledge to feel truly confident about her own decisions.

In this climate, even the most sensitive physicians, who provide extensive opportunity for discussion of treatment options, will see an increased number of severe anxiety reactions and occasional frank psychiatric decompensations. As Marzuk (1985) has outlined, there is, more than ever, a place for "the right kind of paternalism" as doctors try to help their patients reach increasingly complicated treatment decisions.

## ON THE VICISSITUDES OF TRUTH-TELLING

### CASE REPORTS

*Case 3:* R.G. was a 46-year-old, single, white woman executive with advanced metastatic breast cancer of 10 years duration who was admitted with symptoms of cord compression. A CT scan showed widespread disease in the thoracic spine and upper mediastinum. In the previous 3 years, as her disease had worsened, the patient had returned home to be cared for by her elderly, diabetic mother. The patient requested psychiatric consultation in the hospital to help her deal with the enforced dependency on her mother, an issue that had only recently become very irritating. She was a woman with a warm personality who related well to the interviewer. Her coping abilities had been admired throughout her illness. She always had a clear understanding of her disease, yet she now denied the implications of the newest findings, and behaved as if she believed that the disease would continue indolently, as it had in the past. Her mother also requested an interview and revealed that her daughter's attitude caused her enormous pain because it deprived her of the opportunity to speak frankly to her, making their daily dealings flounder in irritating trivia. This was worsened by the ritualized optimism that her daughter's attitude induced in the treatment team, an attitude that left the mother feeling isolated and angry. The patient's sister had left her husband and children in another town to come and help their mother. She was pressing for the patient to be forced to "confront reality," so as to move to her home town where the sister could more conveniently fulfill her responsibilities to both her nuclear family and her mother and sister. The physician refused, saying the patient had always coped well, and deserved to face things at her own pace. The psychiatric consultant held several meetings with the patient and her mother. They worked effectively on long-standing relationship issues between them. However, the key issue of the patient's immediate prognosis could not be confronted. The patient would act increasingly confused, perplexed, and uncomprehending when the subject was approached. Her mother would signal a halt with a reassuring embrace and a change of subject. The psychiatrist followed the physician and the mother's lead, and did not push matters. She held supportive meetings with the patient's sister. As the course of palliative irradiation drew to an end, the

attending physician evaluated the patient's condition in relation to discharge planning. Home care was beyond the mother's physical and emotional capacity. He decided that the time had come for the patient to participate in a frank discussion of available options. In the presence of family, primary nurse, and psychiatric consultant, he patiently and skillfully led her to an overt realization of her terminal condition. She responded with appropriate sadness and thanked him for having "done such a good job." Over the next few days she and her mother enjoyed a new level of closeness and did a great deal of reminiscing. She focused primarily on saying goodbye, and died suddenly, while still in the hospital, 4 days later.

*Case 4:* S.B. was a 50-year-old married white electrician with advanced carcinoma of the colon, who had flown in from a distant state over the last 3 years to receive treatments in a research center. He was admitted to the hospital as complications developed from abdominal disease. Psychiatric consultation was requested because of a toxic psychosis due to steroids that responded to a brief course of neuroleptics. It was noted that the patient and his wife were deeply religious, and very involved in a supportive church community, which they missed very much while in a strange city. They stated they understood the nature of his illness, and added confidently that their faith would give them strength to accept whatever God chose to bring upon them. As his condition worsened, the treatment team felt that they should be given the option of returning to their home community for palliative care. The attending physician met with the patient, family, and psychiatric consultant, and explained the situation in a kind, supportive way, making it clear that he wished to give them the choice of returning home because active therapy was no longer feasible. Nevertheless, the couple responded poorly, feeling betrayed by the onslaught of bad news for which they felt they were unprepared. They experienced the doctor's suggestion that they might prefer to be home as a callous rejection of the patient. They made plans to return home, all the while complaining of having been deprived of hope in a cruel and inhumane way. Follow-up calls 3 weeks later revealed that they were still very angry and were having some difficulty reintegrating into their home community because their faith had been so seriously shaken by the experience.

*Case 5:* G.W. was a 12-year-old white boy with acute lymphocytic leukemia whose parents had, throughout his course, asked the doctor to use all treatments, including experimental ones, in his care. His attending physician placed the child on an institutionally approved investigational treatment protocol, but he was scrupulous in alerting them to their son's poor prognosis. Upon admission for his third relapse, psychiatric consultation was requested for his mother, who was found to have a major depression. She showed a partial response to psychological support and to imipramine (150 mg po, hs). After his death her depression took on a paranoid cast. She stated that she had been lied to, "experiments" had been done on her son against her will, and that he had been kept alive only to be "used as a guinea pig." She pointed to his cushingoid appearance as evidence of the doctor's evil intent, and for the several months she was known to follow-up, kept his room untouched while neglecting her other children.

## Commentary

Case 3 illustrates many intertwined problems. First, there is the question of differential rates of information processing. R.G. had maintained a lucid view of her disease until the end when it became too much to bear, and she retreated into denial. This created no problems for the staff, who responded with the optimism that comes easily to them, but it created serious family problems that resulted in the request for a psychiatric consultation.

The second issue is that of the purpose of information processing. Each participant had a different reason for wanting the patient to face the truth. Both mother and sister would resolve severe emotional conflicts, and would cope with reality issues more effectively, once the patient faced the truth. On the other hand, they and the physician acknowledged that the patient needed her denial and they agreed to protect her as long as possible. The consultant supported this and worked with the patient and family in ways that brought them closer and paved the way for a later confrontation. When the confrontation finally came, it was because of external necessity at the end of active treatment. The patient had to be discharged or transferred, and responsible planning required her participation. For better or for worse, many ethical dilemmas come to practical, not ethical, solutions!

Case 4 illustrates the difference between religiousness and "religiosity," or between the kind of faith that gives courage and hope in adversity and that which is a mask for dependent needs and magical expectations and provides no strength in extremity. The author has observed many cases in which the participants' faith served them reliably and enabled them to endure a terminal period with admirable serenity. Psychiatric intervention is rarely needed in such cases; when called for, it is usually because of a specific problem such as delirium, and not because of complicated problems with ethical and social implications. In the case of "religiosity," however, psychiatric complications are more likely to occur, as they did in case 4. Therefore, it behooves the consultant to examine religious manifestations closely and not take them automatically at face value. Case 12, described later, further illustrates this point.

Case 5 might be called a case of retroactive "untruth" telling. This bereaved mother recast her son's course in the light of her grief and felt that people had "lied" and that her son had been "used," even though she had been kept clearly informed and had agreed to the use of an investigational protocol. While one sees a great deal of "micro-optimism" on the wards—namely, a determined focusing on small goals and small gains—it is unlikely the mother was not aware of the truth about her son's illness. The gloomy larger picture is always fully discussed at major junctions, although it may be taken for granted at other times. Staff members do this in order to make their work tolerable, and they cannot easily behave otherwise. But potential problems must be recognized. It is possible for this approach to create a false sense of hope in patients and families who are eager to deny the other aspects of reality. It can also be misleading, if the base of knowledge on which patients and families are operating is too incomplete. Finally, it plays into the potential distortions of people who have strong magical beliefs, as was seen in case 4 and the mother in case 5.

Some patients and families are so wedded to irrational hope as their main way of coping that they always experience truth-telling as an assault. If it is given to them fairly early, they feel attacked and rejected as in case 4. If it is left for them to discover slowly, they feel betrayed and lied to as in case 5. In any case they will always be angry. This is worsened in cases in which families have elected aggressive or investigational treatment. When such treatment fails, the families feel overwhelming guilt for having prolonged suffering and become angry at the staff for having "pushed" these treatments.

## ETHICAL DILEMMAS LURKING BEHIND PSYCHIATRIC SYMPTOMS

### CASE REPORTS

*Case 6:* G.C. was a 54-year-old white male, married physician with advanced gastric carcinoma, who was admitted for treatment of pneumonitis. He had been getting worse and was currently receiving vasopressors as well as antibiotics. Psychiatric consultation was recommended because the patient was intermittently confused and consistently irritable, angry, and difficult to deal with for both staff and family. Review of the chart confirmed the episodes of confusion, but during the psychiatric interview, the patient showed only minimal cognitive impairment on formal testing. He also revealed a deep desire to stop all treatment, which he felt unable to convey to his wife and daughter. As a result, he felt isolated, frustrated, and angry. Family meetings were arranged and his attending physician was alerted. During the 2 days that the treatment discontinuation was being discussed, the patient became quiet, relaxed, and pleasant. He elected to stop all treatment, including vasopressors, and died 1 day later, after a peaceful interval.

*Case 7:* C.B. was a 48-year-old white female, married teacher who had been maintained on total parenteral nutrition at home for 3 years because of a "cement-block abdomen" following radiation therapy for a lymphoma. The patient had multiple fistulas and was admitted because of sepsis, thought to originate in the gallbladder. Her surgeon recommended cholecystostomy, explaining the advantage of clearing up the source of infection, but he also advised her that she was a poor surgical risk. The patient alternated between agreeing to the operation and refusing it. Her husband and daughter appeared at the bedside politely, but were emotionally distant and reluctant to play any role in her decision. Psychiatric consultation was requested to help her make up her mind. At the first visit the patient demonstrated mild reactive depression, anxiety, and a mild fluctuating delirium. After 2 days of receiving low-dose haloperidol and supportive psychotherapy, she was calmer, had a longer attention span, less cognitive impairment, and much less anxiety. Despite continuing depressive symptoms, she elected to undergo the surgical procedure, saying that to die in surgery held no fear for her, but that she would welcome any improvement in her current condition. She had no suicidal ideation, and no self-denigration. She was able to speak cogently and consistently to the surgeon, who then agreed to perform the procedure.

## Commentary

Both of these cases required making decisions with ethical implications, but psychological issues interfered in both of them. In case 6, the patient's frustration at feeling unable to express—much less carry out—his decision to discontinue treatment, led to his developing a stress syndrome that functioned effectively as a signal. To resolve the situation, someone had to recognize the signal for what it was, and to respond appropriately to it. In case 7, the patient's unwillingness to make a decision created an ethical dilemma for her surgeon. Her family refused to play a role in the decision, and because she was indecisive (not incompetent), one could not name a proxy. Medications and supportive psychotherapy helped her reconstitute enough to reassure her surgeon that she wanted him to proceed. However, in the intimacy of the psychotherapeutic relationship, she remained disconcertingly passive and continued to offer decisions that in fact represented acts of gratitude for the care and concern she was receiving. The psychiatric consultant earnestly suggested that she must do what she "really wanted," but this was a hollow request because the only thing she really wanted was care and concern. In its absence, the decision really did not matter to her. What is the ethical meaning of informed consent in such a case?

It has been suggested (Perl and Shelp, 1982) that psychiatric consultations masking a moral dilemma are often associated with attempts at therapeutic coercion. This may have been more frequent in the past and the potential still exists; but it has not been true in our experience. Consultations are usually called on the

basis of well-documented observations as demonstrated in case 6, or because the physician is in a true quandary as in case 7.

## PSYCHOLOGICAL DISTRESS MASQUERADING AS ETHICAL DILEMMAS

### CASE REPORTS

*Case 8:* C.U. was a 46-year-old single black secretary with carcinoma of the uterus for whom psychiatric consultation was requested to evaluate whether she was competent to refuse treatment. The patient had been scheduled for surgery 2 days before but it had been cancelled because of operating room scheduling problems. By the time it was rescheduled, the patient angrily changed her mind and refused. At the interview she was loud, irritable, and uncooperative, and was incensed at being asked to speak to a psychiatrist. She showed no cognitive impairment. It became clear that she was extremely upset and disappointed because her family had not come to see her during the preoperative delay. She was sad, angry, and very frightened that no one would take care of her if she went ahead with the surgery. Meetings with her family and surgeon reassured her of support and she proceeded with treatment.

*Case 9:* M.M. was a 55-year-old male Hispanic mechanic with recurrent malignant melanoma, who had just undergone exploratory laparotomy to establish the extent of the current disease. Psychiatric consultation was requested to help the family with terminal care issues that the staff felt they were handling inappropriately. Interviews revealed a divisive situation in which the brother of the patient (a health professional who prided himself on his understanding of the ethics of medical care) was pushing insistently for "facing the inevitable," stopping treatment, and starting anticipatory mourning. The patient's wife wished to "hope as long as possible" and was waging an ineffective battle for her point of view. The patient had become withdrawn and morose during this period, and his children were grieving about his withdrawal from them. A family meeting was held at which the wife was given overt support for her denial, which was felt to be an important coping resource at this time, and had the added advantage of reinforcing the nuclear family. The brother was given a separate channel for expressing his grief in his own way. Subsequently, despite receiving bad news about the extent of disease, the family reconstituted, and the patient returned to his previous friendly, emotionally reactive manner.

## Commentary

These two cases represent situations that the staff and/or family initially perceived as ethical problems, but that essentially dissolved when the psychological stresses that had led to their development were defused. In case 8, the surgeon correctly questioned his patient's sudden refusal of surgery as being unexplained, and requiring further scrutiny. In case 9, the brother's need to force anticipatory grieving propelled the family prematurely into explicit terminal care issues. The consultant made a choice (one with ethical implications) and elected to support temporarily the denial helpful to the nuclear family, while still trying to respect the brother's different needs.

## ETHICAL DILEMMAS ROOTED IN THE FAMILY

### CASE REPORTS

*Case 10:* F.S. was a 77-year-old white widower with renal cell carcinoma who had recently been started on dialysis. Psychiatric consultation was requested because of episodes of agitation and depression. At the interview the patient was found to have no acute or chronic psychiatric disorder. He was sad to be dying, but because of pain and the discomfort of repeated dialyses, he wanted to stop treatment. However, his 32-year-old only son was still living at home and was so dependent on his father that he demanded that his father continue treatment because he could not tolerate his death. The crises observed by the staff members occurred when the patient would talk of stopping dialysis and his son would then become overtly angry, pressuring him in highly guilt-provoking and verbally aggressive ways. The consultant evaluated father and son separately, then held a joint interview at which many current and old issues were frankly confronted. The thrust was to affirm the father's feeling that his son's demands, though understandable, were inappropriate. It also demonstrated to the patient that his son was stronger than he realized. Finally, the son was offered an empathic relationship through which to begin anticipatory grieving. The consultant also suggested improvements in comfort measures for the patient, who then agreed to continue dialysis. He received three more treatments, at which time he stated firmly that he wished to stop. His son did not place any undue pressure on him, and he died 3 days later.

*Case 11:* C.H. was a 52-year-old white woman with breast cancer that had metastasized to the central nervous system. She was cachectic and had considerable cognitive impairment, but normal affect, cooperative behavior, and no evidence of distress. Psychiatric consultation was requested because of the staff's uneasiness with her husband, who had refused to leave the ward for many days, and because the patient was being upset by an increasing number of acrimonious scenes taking place at her bedside between her husband and their three young adult children. The psychiatric consultant briefly evaluated the patient to verify that she was indeed not part of the problem, and ascertained that the correctly identified psychiatric patient was the husband, who was totally dependent on his wife, and by history was known to become periodically violent. He was afraid to be at home alone both currently and after his wife's death, and was demanding that his children return home to take care of him. The psychiatric consultant interviewed the children and found that the youngest child, a daughter, showed signs of atypical depression. She was offered a referral to a psychiatrist and said she would think it over. Psychiatric referral was

also offered to the father, but he refused. At the time of his wife's death, the consultant participated in discussions to negotiate the husband's departure from the hospital, and supported the youngest daughter's faltering attempts to avoid becoming her mother's substitute in the care of her father. All family members were advised about the father's great need for psychiatric treatment and were given instructions on how to help him obtain it. A phone call 2 weeks later revealed that he had moved in temporarily with his older cousin and the daughter had gone to live with an aunt.

## Commentary

Consultations are often called for in cases in which the patient does not demonstrate any psychopathological symptoms, but the family is so troubled, and troubling that they upset patient and staff, and interfere with the delivery of care. It has been suggested that some of these patient care problems are an outgrowth of the staff's own attitudes. The pros and cons of this are discussed by Hengeveld and Rooymans (1983). In our experience, inappropriate staff projections are rare. Treatment teams usually make earnest persistent efforts to deal with these difficult cases, and call for a psychiatric consultation in a spirit of honest perplexity. The main criticism one can make is that they often call too late, because they have not recognized the problem or have been trying to solve the problem themselves.

The treatment team's primary responsibility is to the patient, but it can be difficult to discharge this duty when it is in direct conflict with family members. This is even more difficult when patients are in conflict about their loyalty to themselves versus their family. Thus, in case 10, the patient was experiencing an ethical conflict between his desire to die without further treatment, and his paternal responsibility for his dependent son. The psychiatric consultant clarified the issues, labeled them clearly for both father and son, and took some of the pressure off the father by confronting the son and offering him support. Given this help, the patient was better able to go on a few more days, during which time his son slowly accepted the inevitable and began to behave more appropriately. This in turn set the stage for the patient to feel finally able to make a firm decision to discontinue treatment and die.

Case 11 presented more difficult problems. In this case, the ethical conflict lay entirely with the staff, who had to decide how much to become involved in an acute crisis involving only family members. In the narrowest definition of their responsibility to the patient, the staff could have protected her by enforcing strict visiting rules that allowed only one person in the room at a time. However, this would have instigated arguments over who should go in, and would have resulted only in intensifying the conflict and moving it from the bedside into the hallway. The consultant chose to attempt a cautious exploration of the family situation, to diagnose treatable psychopathology, to identify strengths and weaknesses, to offer referral and treatment where needed, and to support emotional health where it existed. The consultant was quite clear that while she functioned in a psychiatric capacity in evaluating the family members, there were strong ethical components in the intervention decisions, such as how much to intervene, and whom to support, in this highly conflicted family whose long-standing problems erupted acutely around the issue of the mother's death.

The practice of any profession is value-laden, psychiatry perhaps more than most. It has even been said that psychotherapy is applied ethics (Breggin, 1971). Although that is probably an overstatement, it is true that the practice of clinical psychiatry constantly thrusts the practitioner into situations where complex ethical decision making is required. Given the inevitability of this, it is especially important to keep in mind the difference between making objective observations with resulting clinical decisions, and making value judgments. Psychiatrists should be skillful and confident about the former function, but humble and open-minded about the latter one.

## ETHICAL ISSUES IN CHILDREN WITH CANCER

### CASE REPORTS

*Case 12:* P.N. was an 11-year-old white, only child of divorced parents, who had acute lymphocytic leukemia in a second relapse. Her mother was deeply involved with a religious group and had elected to refuse all further treatment to allow ''God's will to take its course.'' The father's whereabouts were unknown. The staff was upset by this decision, in part because the nurses who knew the child well felt that she wished to continue treatment, but she had agreed with her mother to avoid conflict. They also described the mother's unwillingness and inability to discuss the child's illness with any staff members. Any attempt to talk about prognosis and treatment was greeted with an immediate change of subject. A psychiatric consultant evaluated the mother, finding that she was overcome with anxiety and that the ''no-treatment'' course, far from being a religious decision, was a desperate move to escape from an overwhelming situation. The staff were advised to stop all attempts to discuss the child's illness in any substantive way with the mother and to focus on giving her warmth, support, and simple concrete suggestions. Within a week she felt more secure, could hear reasons for treatment, and could acknowledge her daughter's desire for it. She agreed to it, and the child readily followed.

*Case 13:* O.S. was a 16-year-old white adolescent with a diagnosis of osteogenic sarcoma without metastases. He had a long history of delinquency and truancy, and his chemo-

therapy had fallen far behind schedule because his parents could not make him keep regular appointments. As time passed, his family became discouraged and their efforts all but ceased. During a brief hospitalization, psychiatric consultation was called and, despite an inconclusive clinical picture, a diagnosis of possible depression was made. The patient was given doxepin (150 mg hs), which he was said to have received at home for 3 weeks, with no obvious response. At this time the patient announced his determination to stop all treatment. The issue of a psychiatric hospitalization was entertained, but it received no support from the family or patient. The several residential treatment centers approached declared themselves unable to handle the complex medical problems associated with his chemotherapy. Work was done to engage his family, but they would not come for any appointments and further exploration revealed a deep alienation from the patient. In the light of his poor scholastic history, an extensive mental status examination was performed by an outside consultant; it showed no significant cognitive impairment. A meeting was held for all staff involved in his care to make sure all avenues had been explored. Following this, the case was referred to the bureau of child welfare; however, they declared themselves unable to intervene. At this time the staff acquiesced to the patient's wishes, his Broviac catheter was removed, and he was allowed to leave.

### Commentary

These two cases involving minors are more complex, because they require assent of both parents and child. Nevertheless, case 12 was managed easily, once it was clear that the mother's refusal of treatment was not an ethical decision but an act of panic. Once her panic abated she accepted treatment readily. It would have been enormously more difficult to resolve had her refusal been on ethical grounds and the staff had had to decide whether to confront the discrepancy between the wishes of the mother and the child. In that case, management would have hinged on the correct assessment of that discrepancy and might well have been scuttled by the child's desire to spare her mother further suffering, even at the cost of her own survival. This may seem like a dramatic assessment, but in fact it is not uncommon for very sick and dying children to sacrifice themselves covertly for the sake of their families.

Unlike the first case, which resolved itself with simplicity, case 13 was one in which everything that could go wrong, did. The patient was a mature minor, close to his majority. But, from school and other sources, he was felt to be functioning at less than his chronological age. Extensive interviewing and testing, research into school, family, and social sources, plus collected staff observations were all used to determine his level of functioning. Second, the patient had irrevocably lost family support, which was not revived by the staff's repeated multipronged efforts. Third, external limitations played an important role. There could be found no facility, psychiatric or medical, to hold this unwilling 16-year-old delinquent for a course of high-dose methotrexate treatment, requiring complex medical support and patient cooperation, over a period of 1 year. This limitation was difficult for the staff to accept. One psychiatric consultant emphasized the patient's behavior as a depressive gesture, to the neglect of its manipulative, adolescent characteristics, and wanted a psychiatric commitment for suicidality. Even when the bureau of child welfare refused the case, a legal expert suggested that the case be taken to court, even though a court order would not carry any means of enforcement. The treatment team put in many hours, but finally, and sadly, abandoned efforts to force a potentially curative treatment.

## THE "NO PROBLEM" CASE

### CASE REPORT

*Case 14:* M.M. was a 66-year-old white widower of 1 year, with a diagnosis of multiple myeloma, whose recent course showed severe weight loss, weakness, and fatigue. His physician felt that his medical condition was poor and that it was time to ascertain his wishes about resuscitation and life supports. A psychiatric consultant was asked to sit in, to provide backup and advice if needed. The doctor and patient knew each other well and the discussion proceeded smoothly. The patient affirmed his long-standing desire not to have any extraordinary measures. His son was consulted and agreed that these were indeed his father's wishes and that he too wanted them honored. The patient made it clear, however, that he wanted all other treatment to continue aggressively. He had a cooperative and warm manner, and he spoke philosophically about accepting death "when your time comes"; he showed no evidence of suicidal ideation guilt, low self-esteem, or ruminatory thinking, but did show continuing active bereavement. On formal cognitive testing he showed mild impairment of short-term memory and concentration. He denied any previous psychiatric history.

The consultant was concerned by the continuing grief response and the mild cognitive impairment, and wondered if the current physical decline could be partly due to vegetative signs of depression. She suggested a trial of amitriptyline (50 mg hs), to which the patient responded in 1 week with increased vigor, appetite, and weight gain. On reevaluation his cognitive testing was slightly improved; however, his mental state was unchanged and he reaffirmed his decision about resuscitation.

## Commentary

This last case presented itself as a nonproblem, both psychiatrically or ethically. The resuscitation decision was being made rationally, with no special pressure, in a stable historical context with a supportive relationship between patient, physician, and family. A careful psychiatric assessment revealed a few depressive symptoms, certainly not enough for a diagnosis of major depression if one assumed that the physical symptoms were due to the disease. But a high index of suspicion, and the readiness to treat promptly, unearthed the presence of a treatable depression, to the patient's obvious benefit. It was appropriate to reopen the question of resuscitation once his depression had responded, on the outside chance that he would react differently, but in fact he did not. It has been our experience that when these discussions are well conducted as this one was, they are quite reliable; but patients must still be given repeated chances to express their wishes.

This case leads one to reiterate again the importance of making a careful psychiatric assessment, taking abnormal findings seriously, and always erring on the side of aggressive treatment, even in what seem like terminal circumstances.

## SUMMARY

It is apparent from the cases just discussed that psychiatry in oncology is intrinsically involved in situations that go far beyond the medical or psychiatric dimension. Ethical issues are absolutely pervasive; legal issues must always be kept in mind and religious issues come up frequently.

It seems that the initial task of the psychiatric consultant is not to diagnose the psychiatric problem, but to discover the broader issues imbedded in the psychological phenomena for which they have been called. These phenomena often act as a signal, but just as often they act as camouflage. What are the ethical issues driving the psychiatric symptoms? Conversely, are the ethical issues outgrowths of underlying psychiatric problems? Are the religious issues masking psychiatric problems? What legal constraints must be considered? Are family issues the true driving force behind all that is being observed?

This could be called making a situational diagnosis, and only once it has been made, is it possible to address the narrower task of psychiatric diagnosis and treatment, if any is indicated. That task must be addressed with firmness and an activist stance. This exhortation would be superfluous in a standard psychiatric setting, but the oncology setting with its high level of morbidity and mortality has, in the past, at times induced passivity and defeatism in the psychiatric profession. Happily, this stance is changing, but the process still needs encouragement.

The nonpsychiatric issues must also be dealt with,

but it is extremely important for the psychiatric consultant to remain clear that, in these areas, he or she is only one of many participants and must remain flexible, open-minded, and humble. It is obvious that psychiatric, ethical, legal, and religious issues are so intertwined that one cannot stay rigidly in one's own area. There are cases in which one's mere presence on the scene forces one to make so-called "ethical decisions," to weigh legal requirements, or to evaluate religious declarations. Eventually there is no escaping it: one must act. But first, one must consult other participants carefully, and in detail (including staff, patient, family, outside sources as needed), and one must give the principals the maximum amount of decision-making power they can tolerate.

There are no easy guidelines here; one must walk a line between two poles. The first abandons patients to decisions that are beyond their endurance, a form of moral evasion that has been given philosophical respectability under the rubric of respecting patient autonomy. The second underestimates the patient's capacity and slips into overprotection and manipulation, the old kind of unnecessary "paternalism" that has been justly criticized. Walking the proverbial tightrope sometimes looks easy by comparison.

In many situations, one's intervention can so dramatically relieve human suffering as to allay any personal doubts. But in the frequent situations in which one cannot help so easily, one must conscientiously review the situation and analyze one's management. Then one must accept helplessness without guilt if helplessness was indeed inevitable, or one must try to learn from one's errors without defensiveness.

This process is immeasurably helped by the use of consultation or extensive review and sharing with one's peers. Indeed, adequate support can make the difference between this work being very draining or uniquely rewarding.

The cases just described all illustrate issues and problems that the author has experienced. However, the case material has been rewritten and invented to prevent any resemblance to real cases. (Some cases are so universal and the problems so common that some feeling of recognition is unavoidable even if inaccurate. Others appear sufficiently unusual that one should be reminded that the facts and details are indeed fictitious.)

## REFERENCES

Breggin, P.R. (1971). Psychotherapy as applied ethics. *Psychiatry* 34:59–74.

Hengeveld, M.W. and H.G.M. Rooymans (1983). The relevance of a staff-oriented approach in consultation psychiatry: A preliminary study. *Gen. Hosp. Psychiatry* 5:256–64.

Marzuk, P.M. (1985). The right kind of paternalism. *N. Engl. J. Med.* 313:1474–75.

Perl, M. and E.E. Shelp (1982). Psychiatric consultations masking moral dilemmas in medicine. *N. Engl. J. Med.* 307:618–21.

Stone, A.A. (1984). *Law, Psychiatry and Morality*. Washington, D.C. City: American Psychiatric Press, Inc.

# PART XI

# Psychosocial Considerations in Cancer Cause and Survival

# 60

# Behavioral and Psychosocial Risk Factors in Cancer: Human Studies

## Jimmie C. Holland

The possible role of psychological, social, and behavioral influences in cancer risk and in survival, after it develops, has intrigued researchers for centuries. Cancer was one of several diseases explored in the 1950s when there was a surge of interest in psychosomatic research in this country. The research over the past three decades has been influenced by work in several areas, including epidemiological studies linking cancer to environmental exposure (especially smoking), animal and human studies on the physiological consequences of stress, and studies of the impact of emotional states on cancer risk and survival through links between the brain and the immune and endocrine system (Table 60-1). This has led to investigations along two lines: exploration of the *indirect* effects on cancer risk of behavior that exposes the individual to carcinogens or alters survival, as with delay in seeking treatment or noncompliance (the "external loop"), and the *direct,* or "internal loop," whereby psychological, social, and behavioral factors affect the internal milieu and tumor growth (Table 60-2). The biopsychosocial model in cancer has been explored in recent years with the far more sophisticated techniques of psychoneuroimmunology (see Chapter 61). Far more is known about the transformation from a normal cell to a malignant one (initiation of neoplastic growth) and about promoter factors that affect tumor progression (Weinstein, 1982). Collaborative research by psychobiological investigators and those working in tumor biology offers new potential to explore the possible role of psychosocial and behavioral factors in cancer.

To examine psychosocial and behavioral risk factors in human cancer, one must consider two large domains, namely, those factors that influence vulnerability to cancer and those that may affect length of survival, once a particular tumor has developed (Cullen, 1982). Both domains, but particularly the lat-

ter, are frequently the subject of questions posed to cancer staff by patients who attempt to assess the "why" of getting cancer, and as they attempt to review the options open to them to assure the most positive outcome of cancer treatment. Common questions asked are, "Did I bring the cancer on myself?" What can I do to improve my outlook?" "Am I making my cancer worse when I cry and get down in the dumps?" "Should I have a mental health checkup before beginning chemotherapy?" Many questions are based on reports of research in the media that imply positive answers to these questions. Thus, it is important for clinicians to be aware of the actual research studies and the status of their findings. Current information about the human studies is summarized in this review (further reading in the specific areas can be found in Ader, 1981; Levy, 1985; Fox and Newberry, 1984). The animal studies that contribute to psychoneuroimmunology and its relevance to cancer are explored in Chapter 61.

## PSYCHOSOCIAL AND BEHAVIORAL FACTORS IN THE BROADER CONTEXT

There are several important, well-established causes of tumor initiation and promotion: viruses, chemicals, radiation, hormones, chronic trauma, parasites, and genetic and physical characteristics of the host. Fox (1981) cautioned that, with the exception of environmental exposures, psychosocial factors (by an internal loop) likely contribute a small fraction to total risk in relation to these other powerful carcinogens. Also, given our current knowledge, psychosocial or behavioral variables may also act either to reduce or to enhance risk, albeit contributing a small amount in either direction.

Another important caveat to keep in mind is that just as psychological variables represent a wide range of

**Table 60-1** Overview of research in psychosocial variables in cancer risk and survival

| Decade | Study objectives |
| --- | --- |
| 1950s | Retrospective studies of premorbid personality in patients with cancer of breast, cervix, and lung<br>Smoking and lung cancer association found |
| 1960s | Animal studies on cancer vulnerability and survival by environmental manipulations (e.g., housing conditions, shock, cold)<br>Human stress studies (started by H. Selye)<br>Environmental carcinogens identified |
| 1970s | Psychoendocrine studies of response to surgery and grief<br>Studies of psychosocial and biobehavioral variables in cancer risk and adaptation |
| 1980s | Psychoneuroimmunology identified as a field that integrates biopsychosocial variables in health, cancer risk, and cancer survival |

responses, cancer also represents a range of neoplasms that may be sensitive to different potentiating influences. However, the carcinogenic process, irrespective of site, proceeds in multiple steps from initiation to promotion and progression (Weinstein, 1982). Synergistic effects of many factors likely occur in the multiple-step progression of carcinogenic transformation. Progression is influenced by age, sex, and nutritional status of the host. Psychological or social factors could potentially act as co-factors in promotion and progression of malignant change in a cell that had already undergone initiation of the carcinogenic change. In humans, most interest in a potential role for psychological and social factors has generally been in the endocrine-sensitive tumors, especially breast, where hormonal influences are thought to play a prominent role in development. Tumor sites that are in part hormone-dependent offer one of the fruitful areas for further study of psychological variables.

**Table 60-2** Two proposed routes whereby psychosocial and behavioral factors may alter cancer risk and survival

| Route | Factors |
| --- | --- |
| External loop (indirect effect) | Behaviors that alter risk (e.g., tobacco, alcohol, diet, delay and noncompliance) |
| Internal loop (direct effect) | Effect of psychological and social factors on internal milieu, altering cancer risk and survival through effect on tumor growth (research in psychoneuroimmunology) |

**Table 60-3** Major influences that may alter cancer risk and survival

| Major influences | Personal characteristics |
| --- | --- |
| Life-style and behaviors | Social habits (tobacco and alcohol)<br>Diet<br>Sexual habits<br>Environmental exposures |
| Social environment | Socioeconomic status<br>Social ties |
| Personality and coping style | |
| Emotional states | "Stress," loss, and grief |

## AN ASSESSMENT OF PSYCHOSOCIAL AND BEHAVIORAL RISK FACTORS

The psychosocial and behavioral factors that may alter cancer risk and length of survival are best considered in the following four areas explored in this section (see Table 60-3): life-style and behaviors, social environment and social ties, personality and coping style, and emotional states ("stress," loss, and grief).

### Life-style and Behaviors

Life-style is a concept that has not been firmly defined by cancer epidemiologists. It is used here in a broad sense, as suggested by Higginson and Muir (1979) to mean the exogenous and endogenous factors that may modify cancer risk, including social habits (tobacco and alcohol), diet, sexual habits, and environmental exposures, especially those in the workplace. Doll and Peto (1981) estimated the proportion of cancer deaths attributed to the several known factors or classes of factors (Table 60-4). The contribution of exogenous carcinogens to cancer risk is great and contributes a fruitful area for cancer prevention.

### TOBACCO USE

In 1950 the single most important epidemiological finding in cancer research was reported when lung cancer was linked to cigarette smoking. More than 30 retrospective studies have confirmed the association and a dose-dependent relationship (Doll and Peto, 1978). The epidemic of lung cancer in American men in the twentieth century appeared about 20 years after cigarette smoking became fashionable in the 1890s. It has continued to rise over the ensuing 50 years and has only begun to level off, because there has been less smoking among men and lower tar cigarettes have become popular. Nevertheless, smoking remains the largest preventable cause of premature death and dis-

**Table 60-4** Proportions of cancer deaths attributed to different factors

| Variable or class of variables | Percentage of all cancer deaths | |
|---|---|---|
| | Best estimate | Range of acceptable estimates |
| Tobacco | 30 | 25–40 |
| Alcohol | 3 | 2–4 |
| Diet | 35 | 10–70 |
| Food additives | <1 | −5–2 |
| Reproductive and sexual behavior | 7 | 1–13 |
| Occupation | 4 | 2–8 |
| Pollution | 2 | <1–5 |
| Industrial products | <1 | <1–2 |
| Medicines and medical procedures | 1 | 0.5–3 |
| Geophysical variables | 3 | 2–4 |
| Infection | 10? | 1–? |
| Unknown | ? | ? |

*Source*: Reprinted with permission from R. Doll and R. Peto (1981). *The Causes of Cancer*. New York: Oxford University Press, p. 1256.

ability, and accounts for 30% of cancer deaths annually (USDHHS, 1982). Prevalence figures show that 30.5% of adults and 11.7% of adolescents (12–18 years) were current smokers in 1985 (USDHHS, 1986b). The rates in women are regrettably rising precipitously as the result of cigarette smoking, which became popular in the 1920s and has continued. The mortality from lung cancer in women is presently equal and will exceed that of breast cancer by 1990. Control of cigarette smoking would eliminate 90% of all lung cancer and would significantly improve health and prolong life in developed countries. Incidence is rising in underdeveloped countries as well, because high-tar cigarettes (no longer permitted for sale in Western countries) are being advertised and widely sold there. An epidemic of lung cancer like that in the United states is anticipated in Africa within 20–30 years.

While smoking is declining among some groups of men, particularly physicians, it is not diminishing among women, and has actually increased among some groups of women, surprisingly including nurses. The effective application of social and psychological information to this area has been difficult, but a major effort launched by the National Cancer Institute as part of its year 2000 goal of 50% reduction in cancer mortality includes reducing smoking rates by more than half (Greenwald and Sondik, 1986).

This effort has already begun by encouraging physicians to become better informed about known effective methods of smoking cessation, which can be recommended to patients, to become models for nonsmok-

ing, and to offer counseling more aggressively, suggesting the use of nicotine-containing chewing gum and referring patients who still smoke to programs that will aid in breaking the addiction. This approach is particularly relevant to pediatricians who may be able to influence the teenager who will usually start to smoke before the senior year of high school. Obstetricians, who have access to families through the pregnant mother, and family physicians, who can inform parents about the risks of parental smoking on children, are other potentially effective antismoking counselors. Oncologists have an opportunity to intervene with patients at the time of workup for cancer, and with the patient's children and families. Also, physicians need to be advocates for legislation to limit cigarette advertising and to encourage institutions, public transportation, and workplaces to become smoke-free environments. This movement has gained momentum as passive or sidestream smoking has been shown to increase the risk of lung cancer by the surgeon general, particularly among nonsmoking wives of husbands who smoke (Hirayama, 1981; USDHHS, 1986a).

The behavioral sciences have contributed to knowledge about factors that are barriers to smoking cessation: withdrawal symptoms, stressful situations, anxiety, depression, social situations associated with smoking, and likely weight gain. All of these are addressed by the use of cognitive and behavioral approaches in most cessation programs.

Multiple influences have been found in the development of smoking addiction among adolescents: parental smoking habits, peer acceptance, low achievement, "sophistication," symbolic rebellion, anxiety reduction, and the adolescent's inability to consider a health hazard 30 years hence. No helpful consistent characteristics separate those who become habitual smokers from those who remain nonsmokers. Efforts in education have been directed at increasingly earlier ages and most recently toward the preadolescents in whom health education may still outweigh the influences that favor smoking. Sweden's experiment with the antismoking education of young couples in order to develop a generation of nonsmokers by influencing family and national attitudes of a generation of unborn children offers a thoughtful long-term effective approach. Cooperation of physicians with public health efforts at all levels, national Smoke Out Days, nicotine chewing gum, and behavioral interventions are all worthwhile efforts that work best when physicians and staff are committed to and involved in prevention.

Supportive techniques and counseling for smoking cessation have been investigated. No single technique, whether it be hypnosis, group therapy or pharmacotherapy, has emerged as ideal. Many programs sponsored by the American Cancer Society and the

National Cancer Institute use a range of methods. Several factors are known to contribute to success: motivation, expected benefits, specific coping methods used consistently during the immediate quitting period, good social support, and even prior successful cessation attempts for half a year or more (Orleans, 1985). A growing characterization of smoking as a socially and physically undesirable habit may begin to dispel the effect of years of advertising that portrayed the smoker as more attractive, desirable, and sophisticated than others.

However, not only cigarette smoking but also smokeless tobacco is hazardous. Tobacco, in one form or another, is the most important worldwide cause of oral cancer. This has been demonstrated in many studies of tobacco chewing, snuff dipping, betal nut chewing mixed with tobacco and lime, beedi smoking in India, and cigar and pipe smoking. The association of tobacco use with increased risk of cancer of the lip, oral cavity, tongue, hypopharynx, larynx, lung, esophagus, bladder, kidney, and pancreas has also been demonstrated. The rise of smokeless tobacco use among young adults and teenagers, who have begun to use chewing tobacco and snuff, has already resulted in increased buccal tumors in these young people.

Interaction of smoking with other risk factors must be kept in mind in terms of the special risk of certain individuals. Asbestos workers who continue to smoke after knowledge of prior exposure have a greatly increased risk of mesothelioma and lung cancer. Women who use oral contraceptives and who smoke have a greater risk of stroke. Smoking increases risk of cervical cancer as well.

## EXCESSIVE ALCOHOL INTAKE

Little public attention has been given to the data that strongly associate excessive alcohol consumption with cancer of the mouth, pharynx, larynx, esophagus, and possibly pancreas (USDHEW, 1974). Head and neck cancer in the United States is strongly associated with a history of alcoholism; it contributes not only to cause but often complicates management and rehabilitation (Chapter 17). Primary cancer of the liver is almost nonexistent in developed countries, except in the presence of preexisting alcoholic cirrhosis. Because heavy smoking is an almost invariable accompaniment of heavy drinking, the risk of cancer rises sharply in individuals who use both. The relative contribution of one versus the other is often hard to assess in these individuals. Data suggest that heavy intake of both has a synergistic (not simply additive) effect on risk, perhaps by exerting a cocarcinogenic effect in the esophagus, mouth, pharynx, and larynx. Figure 60-1 indicates the relative risk of increasing the number of

drinks consumed and cigarettes smoked per day in oral cancer, demonstrating the synergistic effect of up to 15 times the relative risk in heavy drinkers who also smoke (Rothman and Keller, 1972). The mechanism hypothesized is that alcohol may act as a promoter or co-factor with tobacco acting as the initiator, accounting for the synergistic effect. Ethanol may act as an irritant to membranes, making them vulnerable to other carcinogens, to the adverse effects of vitamin deficiency and malnutrition, or to immune suppression. Whether alcohol acts as an irritant, as an augmenter of other carcinogens, or indirectly through associated malnutrition is unknown, but the data are persuasive concerning increased risk with distilled spirits, primarily whiskey. While less risk exists with wine and beer, heavy beer drinking is associated with increased risk of colon and bladder cancer. The absence of a public health campaign about the carcinogenic effects of alcohol is remarkable, given the recent attention to tobacco. While the relative number of cases of cancer annually attributed to alcohol is 2–4% (considerably below those attributed to cigarette smoking), the incidence of head and neck cancer among heavy drinkers, most of whom smoke, is high. Encouraging national efforts have appeared recommending warnings on alcohol bottles and limiting of alcohol advertising.

Malnutrition and anemia, often present in patients with alcoholism, are also associated with increased risk of oral, hypopharyngeal, and esophageal cancer. Women with oral cancer often have a history of Plummer–Vinson syndrome with brittle nails, glossitis, and loss of teeth, related to dietary deficiencies.

A history of alcoholism is found in both men and women with esophageal cancer, although other factors clearly play a role as well. There is an extremely high incidence in the eastern provinces of Iran where no drinking of alcohol occurs. The steady rise of esophageal cancer in black men has leveled off some in the United States. Although a relationship between alcohol and pancreatic cancer is not clear, some studies have suggested a relationship.

## DIET

Diet has become increasingly important in understanding cancer risk, particularly as it relates to high-fat diet and obesity (see Table 60-4). A weight significantly above the ideal increases the risk of several tumors, including cancer of the endometrium, breast, gallbladder, ovary, prostate, and colon. Doll and Peto (1981) attributed 35% of cancer deaths to increased risk from dietary factors that included both overnutrition and high-fat diet. A 1979 American Cancer Society survey of deaths confirmed the risk for women (Lew and Gar-

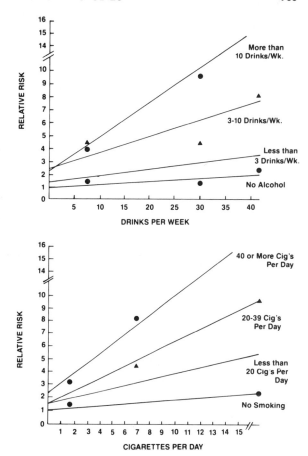

**Figure 60-1.** Relative risk of oral cancer according to level of exposure to alcohol and smoking. Plotted with conversion of drinking scale from ounces of alcohol per day to "drinks per week." Regression lines fitted by eye. Risk is expressed relative to a risk of 1.00 for persons who neither smoked nor drank. *Source:* Reprinted with permission from K. Rothman and A. Keller (1972). The effect of joint exposure to alcohol and tobacco on risk of cancer of the mouth and pharynx. *J. Chron. Dis.* 25:711–16.

finkel, 1979). However, a recent review of several studies at the National Cancer Institute noted less risk of prostate and premenopausal breast cancer, but increased risk of endometrial and postmenopausal breast cancer (Editorial, 1987). The cause appears to be prolonged exposure to higher levels of estrogen stored in fat tissues, adding to postmenopausal breast and endometrial cancer risk. Trials of reduced dietary fat content, both as a means of reducing cancer in those with genetic high risk, and as a means of reducing risk of recurrence in women with stage I breast cancer are under way. Evidence appears particularly strong in relation to breast and endometrial cancer, suggesting an appropriate basis for large clinical trials of reduced-fat diets, from the usual 40% to less than 20% fat. The level to which fat must be reduced is regarded by some as almost incompatible with compliance. The association of obesity with shorter survival in breast cancer, and as the second most significant factor after nodal status, suggests the importance here as well (see Chapter 14).

Both epidemiological and animal data suggest that colon cancer is positively correlated with total dietary fat intake. The mechanism proposed is that fat in the diet enhances cholesterol and bile acid synthesis by the liver, leading to increased amounts of sterols and their metabolites in the colon that act as promoters in colon carcinogenesis. Lipkin and Newmark (1985) have found in several studies that increased proliferation of colonic epithelial cells is associated with higher cancer risk; oral calcium reversed this proliferation and the mitogenic effects of fatty and free bile acids by conversion to insoluble cancer compounds.

Fiber is also a recommended ingredient in the diet, because it may help reduce the risk of colorectal cancer. Increased bran cereals and whole wheat are recommended because they may shorten the time that the stool is in the colon, or alter possible carcinogens or bacteria in the stool. Combining reduced fat intake with increased fiber is therefore recommended. Table 60-5 outlines a food guide to assure attention to dietary aspects of cancer prevention (Greenwald, 1985).

## SEXUAL BEHAVIOR

Sexual mores vary with the culture as do the circumstances and age of the initiation of sexual activity and circumcision for boys. They affect cancer risk in

**Table 60-5**  Cancer prevention food guide at a glance

| Type of food | Choose | Limit | Avoid |
|---|---|---|---|
| Fats and oils | Fats within daily allowance: low-fat salad dressings, low-fat mayonnaise, vegetable oils, butter, margarine | | All other fats, including regular salad dressings, cooking fats, mayonnaise, fried nuts, and olives |
| Dairy foods | Skim milk: fluid, evaporated, and powdered<br>Buttermilk (skim)<br>Fat-free yogurt<br>Cottage cheese (1% fat, rinsed)<br>Skim farmer cheese<br>Sapsago cheese | Low-fat and part skim (1% and 2%) milk and milk products, including yogurt, cottage cheese, frozen yogurt, farmer cheese, and ricotta cheese<br>Sherbert<br>Ice milk | Whole (homogenized) milk and whole-milk products including yogurt, cottage cheese, and ricotta cheese<br>Cream, nondairy creamers<br>Sour cream<br>Cream cheese<br>Hard cheeses |
| Meat and protein | Lean veal, fish, poultry<br>Legumes (beans, lentils, and peas)<br>Tofu and tempe<br>Egg whites | Red meat<br>Duck<br>Lamb<br>Egg yolks<br>Nuts<br>Peanut butter | Sausage, bacon, luncheon meat, hot dogs, fried meat, and fried fish |
| Bread, cereals, and other starches | Whole-grain breads, rolls, bagels, cereals, pasta, brown rice, and potatoes with skins | Muffins, tea biscuits, crackers | Doughnuts, croissants, commercial baked goods, fried potatoes, fried rice, potato chips, and corn chips |
| Fruit and vegetables | All fresh and frozen fruit and vegetables | Canned fruit<br>Avocado | Coconut |
| Sugar, alcohol | | Honey, molasses, maple syrup, jams, and hard candy<br>Alcoholic beverages | Sugar, chocolate, caramel, toffee, and nougat |
| Beverages | Juice<br>Herbal tea<br>Club soda, seltzer, and water | Beverages containing caffeine (e.g., coffee, tea, hot chocolate, cola)<br>Sweetened beverages (naturally and artificially carbonated beverages not containing caffeine) | Drinks made with ice cream or cream |

*Source*: Courtesy of Mahoney Institute for Health Maintenance, American Health Foundation. Reprinted with permission from P. Greenwald (1985). Prevention of cancer. In V.T. DeVita, Jr., S. Hellman, and S.A. Rosenberg (eds.), *Cancer: Principles and Practice of Oncology*. Philadelphia: Lippincott, p. 202.

positive and negative ways. For example, an early full-term pregnancy reduces the risk of breast cancer, an apparent result of the pregnancy's reduction of prolactin levels—in comparison with nulliparous women or those who have a late first full-term pregnancy (Musey et al., 1987). A high relative risk of anal cancer in men has been reported in those who have a history of receptive anal intercourse in homosexual sexual relations (Darling et al., 1987). The association of genital warts, caused by papillomavirus, may be the cause of anal cancer in such situations.

The clearest association of sexual behavior and cancer relates to cervical cancer, which is most common among women with a history of early sexual intercourse with multiple partners. The incidence is much greater in lower socioeconomic groups, especially among black and Hispanic women. There is a strong suggestion that cervical cancer results from sexual transmission of the herpesvirus to the woman which is carried by the man who has wider exposure (Graham et al., 1982). The number of sexual partners during and following adolescence appears to be the most important period of increased risk, perhaps reflecting the period of most vulnerability of cervical cells to sexually transmitted cancer-causing agents (USC Cancer Center, 1987). The mortality from cervical cancer has been decreasing steadily in North America for 50 years, probably because of increased detection of precancerous cervical lesions by virtue of more cervical smears, earlier diagnosis, and better feminine hygiene.

The current campaign to increase the use of condoms as a means of preventing the spread of AIDS is also the best potential preventive for invasive cervical cancer.

## SUNLIGHT EXPOSURE

The exposure to sunlight, especially among fair-skinned individuals is a risk factor for skin cancers, which appear largely on the exposed face, arms, and hands. Older individuals, especially men who have worked outside for many years, develop basal-cell and squamous-cell carcinomas. The ultraviolet radiation in sunlight increases the melanin content in the cells and hence encourages the development of deeper color, tan, and freckles. Chronic exposure encourages the formation of keratosis, premalignant lesions, and finally carcinoma.

The role of solar exposure in formation of melanoma is less clear, but it is a risk factor in susceptible individuals. While exposure related to outdoor work can be minimized by wearing sleeves, gloves, and a head covering, the exposure to sunlight as part of the "healthy tanned look" cult is a needless risk. Education is needed about the risk of excessive exposure, especially in southern climates, and of fair-skinned, vulnerable individuals. Sunscreens have become highly effective, and their use should be encouraged (Levy, 1985).

## OCCUPATIONAL EXPOSURES

Awareness of the association between environmental exposures and increased incidence of a particular cancer is not new—nor is procrastination in eliminating the risk. Sir Percivall Potts observed scrotal cancer in chimney sweeps in London, England and suggested that it was the result of a constant exposure to soot-laden clothes. It was 200 years before efforts were successful in protecting these young men. Table 60-6 shows occupational exposures associated neoplasms, and evidence for carcinogenicity (Pitot, 1985). Chromates and aniline dyes have long been known to in-

**Table 60-6** Occupations and chemical agents presenting carcinogenic risk to humans on the basis of epidemiological studies

| Chemicals, process, or industry | Associated neoplasm | Evidence for carcinogenicity |
|---|---|---|
| Acrylonitrite | Lung, colon, prostate | Limited |
| Arsenic | Lung | Sufficient |
| Asbestos | Lung, mesothelioma, gastrointestinal tract(?) | Sufficient |
| Manufacture of auramine | Bladder | Limited |
| Aromatic amines (aminobiphenyl, benzidine, 2-naphthylamine, 4-nitrobiphenyl) | Bladder | Sufficient |
| Benzene | Leukemia | Sufficient |
| Beryllium and its compounds | Lung | Limited |
| Bis(chloromethyl)ether | Lung | Sufficient |
| Boot and shoe manufacture and repair | Nasal carcinoma | Sufficient |
| Cadmium and its compounds | Lung, prostate (?) | Limited |
| Chromium and some of its compounds | Lung | Sufficient |
| Furniture manufacture (hardwood) | Nasal carcinoma | Sufficient |
| Hematite mining (underground) | Lung | Sufficient |
| Isopropyl alcohol manufacture | Cancer of paranasal sinuses | Sufficient |
| Nickel refining | Lung, nasal sinuses | Sufficient |
| Occupational exposure to phenoxyacetic acids and herbicides | Soft tissue sarcoma | Limited |
| Rubber industry (certain occupations) | Leukemia, bladder | Sufficient |
| Soots, tars, and oils | Skin, lung, bladder, gastrointestinal tract | Sufficient |
| Vinyl chloride | Liver (angiosarcoma) | Sufficient |

*Source:* Reprinted with permission from H. Pitot (1985). Principles of cancer biology: Chemical carcinogenesis. In V.T. DeVita, Jr., S. Hellman, and S.A. Rosenberg (eds.), *Cancer: Principles and Practice of Oncology.* Philadelphia: Lippincott, 2nd ed., p. 92.

**Table 60-7**  Classes of preventive action for intermediate and proximal environmental causes of cancer

| Class | Preventive action |
|---|---|
| In the physical environment | Change in laws or government regulations |
| | Product regulation |
| | Work situation (substance enclosure, shielding, smoking, etc.) |
| | Industry regulation (pollution, manufacturing methods) |
| | Local environments (movies, office, government premises, homes) |
| | Medical regulations (screening controls, use of x rays, carcinogens) |
| | Institutional regulations |
| | Self-regulation by industry |
| | Role by medical associations or hospitals |
| | Insurance requirements |
| | Union contract requirements |
| In the individual's behavior (by informing, changing attitudes) | Personal lay communication or behavior |
| | Mass media |
| | Formal education |
| | Orienting local cultures to prevention |
| | Changing doctors' attitudes |
| | Physician effects on the patient's behavior |
| | Specific incentives: insurance premiums reduced for not smoking; damage suits |

*Source*: Reprinted with permission from B.H. Fox (1984). Remote life-style causes of cancer. *Cancer Detect. Prev.* 7(1):21–29.

crease frequency of certain tumors. Asbestos, used as insulation on pipes in ships, homes, and schools, was found to be a substance whose fibers remain in the body and produce mesothelioma of the peritoneum and pleura, as well as lung cancer. Previously an uncommon tumor, it has become more common. It appears following a lag of 20–30 years in individuals and their families who were exposed from the workman-father's clothes containing the fiber. Selikoff and Hammond (1979) estimated that the risk of exposed asbestos workers increased eightfold if the worker was also a heavy smoker. Vinyl chloride has been shown to cause hepatoma, a primary liver tumor, which otherwise is rarely seen.

Particular responsibility for dealing with occupationally related carcinogens lies with labor, management, and regulatory agencies. Table 60-7 gives the classes of preventive actions outlined by Fox (1984). Chemical carcinogens in industrial plants and particu-

larly radioactive materials emerge as major problems for the future where accidents may expose the adjacent community as well as plant employees. Storage and containment of radioactive waste is an increasing issue as safe disposal sites become more difficult to find.

## COMBINED EFFECTS

Many cultural, social, religious, and psychological influences contribute to the daily pattern of the life of an individual. The life-style of Seventh-Day Adventists who maintain strict observance of religious tenets is of considerable interest. While otherwise full participants in urbanized American society, they strictly abstain from tea, coffee, alcohol, soft drinks, and tobacco, maintaining a simple and nutritious diet and living as close-knit large families with strong ties. Although the reduced exogenous exposures likely reduce their cancer mortality, their close family ties and philosophy of life are interesting subjects for study of life-style and cancer mortality.

### Social Environment and Social Ties

The two components of the social environment that affect both cancer risk and cancer survival are socioeconomic status and social support.

Socioeconomic status was studied by the American Cancer Society in 1986 to examine cancer among the economically disadvantaged. The ACS noted that 34 million of the 238.8 million inhabitants of the United States live below the poverty line. The report indicated that in studies that have considered cancer mortality in terms of socioeconomic status and ethnic differences, the differences assumed to be ethnic were found to be largely based on socioeconomic variables affecting both nonwhites and whites equally at low income levels.

There are consistent excesses of cancer mortality among the economically disadvantaged, both overall and by several specific sites. It is estimated that the survival differential is due to later diagnosis, largely reflecting poor access to medical care. In a study commissioned by the ACS Committee on Cancer in the Economically Disadvantaged, Lerner (1986) examined cancer mortality in Baltimore from 1949 to 1981 by comparing high- and low-income groups. As with other diseases, cancer mortality in the lower income groups exceeded the rates of those with high income, often substantially. Income exerted a significant effect independent of race for all sites. Second, race had a significant effect independent of income, *but only* among low-income individuals, suggesting that race may have been a proxy for adverse environmental and social conditions.

Jenkins (1983) examined additional social variables in cancer mortality that extended beyond simple sociodemographic risk factors. He assessed cancer deaths in 39 mental health catchment areas in Boston, in which detailed demographic, economic, social, household structure, and educational data were available. Cancer mortality in men, but not women, was higher than expected in several clusters: where a high proportion of families and children lived in poverty and where high proportions of men were unemployed or underemployed (Tables 60-8 and 60-9). Housing units located in large buildings were overcrowded; there were few family units with children under 18, few husband–wife households, and many households with only one person, of whom many were aged. The neighborhoods had a high percentage of divorced and separated men and women, disabled individuals, single women, and households headed by a woman. The two cancer types with highest correlations were stomach and colon.

Jenkins drew conservative conclusions, but these findings support Lerner's study of low socioeconomic status and high cancer mortality, because the highest excess cancer mortality (37% and 32% above Massachusetts state averages) was in the two catchment areas in Boston that were most economically deprived, had lowest educational level, highest unemployment, and highest death rates from all causes. The issues for

**Table 60-8** Correlation of economic status, housing, and neighborhood composition with mortality from cancer in male residents of Massachusetts, 1971–1973

| Parameters | Tau value* |
|---|---|
| Economic status | |
| Families in poverty (%) | 0.361 |
| Children in poverty (%) | 0.329 |
| Median income | −0.295 |
| High occupational status, men | −0.258 |
| Unemployed persons (%) | 0.273 |
| Underemployed men (%) | 0.308 |
| Type of housing | |
| Housing units single, detached (%) | −0.390 |
| High-rise apartments (>7 stories) | 0.313 |
| Apartments with >20 units | 0.286 |
| Units renter-occupied (%) | 0.370 |
| Households in over-crowded units (>1.51 persons per room) (%) | 0.293 |
| Neighborhood composition | |
| Male residents per 100 female residents | −0.442 |
| Youth dependency ratio (children under 18/persons 18–64 years) | −0.291 |
| Population disabled and unable to work (%) | 0.403 |

*Tau >0.30 significant at $p = 0.01$.
*Source*: Reprinted with permission from C.D. Jenkins (1983). Social environment and cancer mortality in men. *N. Engl. J. Med.* 308:395–98.

**Table 60-9** Correlation of household composition, marital status, and household size with mortality from cancer in male residents of Massachusetts in 1972–1973

| Parameters | Tau value* |
|---|---|
| Household composition | |
| Households with husband–wife (%) | −0.381 |
| Children living with both parents (%) | −0.384 |
| Families with children <18 years (%) | −0.289 |
| Households (%) | |
| Having female head | 0.437 |
| Having female head and including children | 0.426 |
| Having female head, including children, and in poverty | 0.364 |
| Marital status | |
| Men divorced or separated (%) | 0.311 |
| Women divorced or separated (%) | 0.417 |
| Men (>25 years) never married (%) | 0.245 |
| Women (>25 years) never married (%) | 0.333 |
| Women who are widows (%) | 0.411 |
| Household size | |
| Median household size | −0.371 |
| One-person households (%) | 0.392 |
| Aged persons living alone | 0.378 |
| Households with >6 persons (%) | −0.295 |

*Tau >0.30 significant at $p = 0.01$.
*Source*: Reprinted with permission from C.D. Jenkins (1983). Social environment and cancer mortality in men. *N. Engl. J. Med.* 308:395–98.

research are challenging because many of the findings suggest absence of integrated families, in which lifestyle would include adherence to reasonable health and dietary practices, regular eating and sleeping, and access to health care as needed in a timely fashion. The stresses of living in such an environment lead to speculation about its added role in individuals who are vulnerable for other reasons.

The effects of marital status on the diagnosis, treatment, and survival of patients with cancer were examined in population-based data on 27,779 cancer cases. Unmarried persons with cancer (single, divorced, or widowed) had decreased overall survival. Unmarried persons were more apt to be diagnosed with a more advanced stage of cancer and they were more apt to be untreated for cancer. And, even after adjustment for stage and treatment, unmarried persons still had poorer survival (Goodwin et al., 1987). These data support the importance of psychological and social support in diagnosis, treatment, and survival.

A study by Marshall and Funch (1983) used crude indicators of social stress and support in 283 women who had died after diagnosis of breast cancer between 1958 and 1960. Because it is limited to a single tumor site, the study is of interest. Stage of disease was the most powerful predictor, as expected; however, 9% of the variance could be explained by social indicators of stress and support, in younger women. Limited psychosocial data were available for study, but it is interesting that the findings point in the same direction as those of Jenkins just cited.

The links among life-style, nutritional deficiency, and chronic stress, all of which can contribute to impaired immune function and poor cancer outcome, offer challenging directions for more extensive epidemiological studies. There is little question that these data, even now, suggest that this part of the population is in greatest need of education and access to health care.

There is considerable evidence that social ties within the social environment serve to modulate stress in such a way that they have an impact on illness and mortality. The study of Berkman and Syme (1979) found, among 87,000 individuals studied over a 10-year period, that those who lacked social and community ties were more apt to die from a range of diseases than those with more ties. Blazer (1982) studied 331 persons 65 years of age and older, and found that relative mortality was significantly increased among those elderly who perceived poor social support and felt fewer attachments were available. There was, however, no excess of deaths from cancer. A review by House, Landis, and Umberson (1988) on social relationships and health indicates that several prospective studies, which were controlled for baseline health status, consistently show increased mortality among individuals who have few or poor social ties. While the mechanisms through which this is mediated remain elusive, studies in humans and animals show that social isolation increases mortality from a range of causes.

## Personality and Coping Style

Personality, incorporating early childhood experiences, enduring traits, styles of coping, and defense mechanisms usually employed by an individual, has been suggested for centuries as a factor in both risk of cancer and length of survival. Human and animal studies have explored both risk and survival. The simplistic view of a ''mind–cancer'' link is giving way to testable models and hypotheses that place the aspect of psychoneuroimmunology which relates to cancer on a more scientifically sound basis (Temoshok and Heller, 1984; Lippman, 1985). Present information about personality in risk and survival is outlined in the following paragraphs.

## PERSONALITY AND CANCER RISK

### Retrospective Studies

The first studies were retrospective case comparison studies of cancer patients who were queried about their

**Table 60-10**   Design of clinical studies assessing cancer risk and personality

| Study design | Assessment |
|---|---|
| Retrospective | Assessment of patients after cancer diagnosis for premorbid personality and events |
| Quasi-prospective | Assessment of patients after seeking medical consultation but prior to definite cancer diagnosis |
| Retroprospective | Examination of cancer incidence and mortality among a cohort studied psychologically for some other reason (e.g., job evaluation) |
| Prospective | Baseline psychological assessment of a cohort who are followed for cancer morbidity and mortality |

*Source*: Adapted from Temoshok and Heller (1984).

personality and psychological responses before having cancer (Table 60-10). These investigations supported the observation by some clinicians of a role of emotions in cancer risk. The findings described a personality in which there was a tendency to repress and deny emotions (LeShan, 1959; Bahnson and Bahnson, 1966), and to have poor expression of emotions, especially negative ones (Greer and Morris, 1975; Kissen, 1967; Cox and Mackay, 1982; Todd and Magarey, 1978). Many clinicians have felt that the picture of a repressed, cooperative, uncomplaining person was typical of many cancer patients in general, particularly in earlier decades when physicians were viewed as authoritarian figures who had to be pleased. Fear of abandonment was great when few active treatments were available and supportive care for advanced disease was poor. However, these early findings of a repressed expression of emotions in cancer contributed to the construct developed by Temoshok of a type C personality bearing these characteristics (Temoshok and Heller, 1984). A retrospective study by Kneier and Temoshok (1984) supported the idea of this personality type when they found that patients with malignant melanoma, in comparison to patients with cardiovascular disease, showed greater psychophysiological arousal to electrical skin stimulation but reported less emotional perturbation in response to the potentially upsetting stimuli. From a series of studies, Temoshok has proposed the type C personality, using concepts from types A and B in cardiovascular disease. Type C maintains emotional control and pleasant interpersonal relations despite internal unexposed distress (Temoshok and Fox, 1984).

The other dimension, which has continued to be actively pursued, is that the cancer-prone person copes with stressful life changes and loss by depressive symptoms and hopelessness (Greene et al., 1956; Jacobs and Charles, 1980; Becker, 1979). These two characteristics, a personality style with repressive attributes and chronic depressive affect, appear to persist as the two major distinct and separate lines of study.

The observations from the retrospective studies have been criticized because an individual's view of the past is altered by a cancer diagnosis, leading Fox (1978) to say that all retrospective data are suspect. Temoshok and Heller (1984) have pointed out, however, that traits, as opposed to state, should be less affected by retrospective account and that the findings should be considered in that light. Certainly some types of factual information, such as demography, should be unbiased by illness, whereas recall of prior relationships and emotional events might be recalled differently, particularly when the individual is depressed.

It is surprising that these constructs hold despite the major limitations in study design posed by the absence of control for site (in some studies), stage, and treatment of cancer, as well as demographic variables such as age, which is important in identifying control or comparison groups. The ideal retrospective study should clearly also control for such known risk factors as family history and smoking. Critiques of the retrospective studies have pointed out the methodological problems and the evolution of increasingly better designed studies (Perrin and Pearce, 1959; Fox, 1978; Wellisch and Yager, 1983; Bielianskas and Garron, 1982; Fox and Newberry, 1984).

## Quasi-prospective Studies

Another method of study designed to improve on the retrospective model is the quasi-prospective, a term used by Temoshok to denote those studies in which patients are assessed before diagnosis of cancer is known from biopsy but after the person has developed sufficient symptoms to seek medical attention. This window between health and illness offers some advantages over the retrospective studies (Table 60-10). Schmale and Iker (1966) used this method to study women with suspicious cervical lesions, showing more hopeless affect among those with cervical cancer. Effects of anxiety about cancer, subtle cues from the physician, and disease effects on mood also limit this method. Goodkin and colleagues (1986) studied women prior to definitive diagnosis but with known abnormal Pap smears. The more severe stages of dysplasia were associated with low levels of cooperative coping style and high premorbid pessimism, sense of future despair, somatic anxiety, and reaction to life threat. The hypothetical mechanisms suggested were possible elevated corticosteroid production with decreased T-cell growth factor or elevated epinephrine

levels and stimulation of cyclic adenosine monophophate with a similar consequence of immunosuppression and promotion.

Katz and co-workers (1970) showed that women who coped poorly at the time of biopsy for breast cancer showed arousal of the hypothalamic-pituitary-adrenal axis, as compared to women whose defenses allowed them to maintain emotional equilibrium. The effect of such arousal has not been examined for its immunological consequences.

Greer and Morris studied women before breast biopsy (1975), as did Muslin, Gyarfas, and Pieper (1966) obtaining information from a quasi-prospective method. Horne and Picard (1979) used a similar method studying patients with lung lesions but prior to diagnosis of malignant or benign origin. They found that composite psychosocial data about childhood and losses significantly predicted malignant versus benign disease. Abse and colleagues (1974) showed that those young patients who were studied before the biopsy, and who were later diagnosed with lung cancer, were more rigid and controlled.

A large study by Cooper and colleagues (1986) of 2,163 women in England compared those with breast cancer to those with cysts, benign disease, and no illness on type A behavior, coping, and social support. Women were queried at the time of breast examination and before diagnosis was known: repressed emotions and passivity were initially found in the breast cancer and cyst groups, but this correlation was not supported when the variable of age, an important variable in breast cancer, was controlled.

## Retroprospective Studies

Using Temoshok's classification of studies, the retroprospective studies have made significant contributions (Table 60-10). These studies have taken large cohorts of individuals who were assessed psychologically at some earlier point in time and examined their subsequent morbidity and mortality from cancer and other diseases over 20 years or more. The major limitations have been the use of assessment tools that were unsophisticated or inappropriate, and the absence of accurate medical records for cancer diagnosis and cause of death.

Dattore and colleagues (1980), using the retroprospective design, found more repression and less self-reported depression among those who developed cancer of multiple sites, in a cohort observed for medical outcome over 10 years.

Shekelle and co-workers (1981) designed a retroprospective study using data obtained from the MMPI which had been routinely given to 2020 Western Electric employees at the time of being hired 17 years earlier. They identified these individuals and reviewed the cause of death 17 and 20 years later among those who had died. Controlled for other known risk factors, an elevated depression score on the MMPI (but not at the level associated with clinical depression) was associated with a twofold increase in the odds of death from cancer, combining all sites. Persky, Kempthorne-Rawson, and Shekelle (1987) have confirmed the association of mortality from cancer and depression as measured by the D Scale on the MMPI at 20 years as well. The relationship to incidence was only evident at 10 years, but the association with mortality was observed for the full 20 years. Subjects were examined for other known risk factors and the findings were adjusted for age, smoking, alcohol, occupation, family history of cancer, body mass, and serum cholesterol. Repression, using the Welsh R scale in the MMPI, was not associated with cancer risk in this cohort. The question of a possible role of depression as an initiator or promoter of cancer, based on these unbiased prospective data, requires further study.

A similar prospective study has examined data from the cohort of 3,154 men on which the identification of type A behavior was based. Psychological data have been analyzed in relation to their cancer mortality over 22 years. Type A individuals had a 1.5 relative risk of cancer mortality, as compared to Type B. When controlled for age, smoking, and education, the association held for Type A in relation to cancer mortality from sites other than lung. Although the meaning is not clear and may represent chance alone, the findings are nevertheless of interest and serve as a stimulus for further study (Ragland et al., 1987).

## Prospective Studies

The fourth type of studies are prospective; they have obtained baseline psychological data and followed the individuals for subsequent development of disease and mortality. Vaillant's longitudinal study (1979) of a class of Harvard graduates from the 1940s is an example in which it was shown that poor mental health predicted poor physical health, even when controlled for the obvious influences of smoking, drinking, and overweight. An even earlier study was reported by Hagnell (1966), in which those who developed cancer were compared to healthy controls. Using a Swedish personality scale, Hagnell found that women who were low on emotional control and who tended to inhibit emotions when depressed tended to be in the cancer group.

Grossarth-Maticek and co-workers (1983, 1985) have reported two prospective studies, the first of 1,353 inhabitants of Cverenka, a Yugoslavian village, and another in Heidelberg, Germany, in an attempt to

replicate the first and to improve the design. In the Heidelberg study, 872 individuals were randomly accessed and asked to identify a person whom they knew was stressed. Those who were followed 10 years in the Yugoslavian study and who developed cancer showed chronic hopelessness resulting from painful life events, or they showed low emotionality. In the initial study and the Heidelberg replication, four personality type descriptions were given to the subject and relatives to determine which was closest to being representative of the subject. Type I personality (cancer-prone) was highly correlated (46%) with cancer death (Eysenck, 1987). The personality is described as dealing with loss by hopelessness, helplessness, and retention of closeness to withdrawing objects that are idealized, while also repressing emotions. Type II was defined in terms similar to type A personality. Types III and IV were described as intermediates between the two extremes posed by types I and II. The data were remarkably consistent with the hypothesized personality and mortality from cancer (type I) and cardiovascular disease (type II). The data are being scrutinized for accuracy, however, there has been much interest generated by these studies.

The extensive studies by Caroline Thomas and colleagues of Johns Hopkins medical students who graduated between 1948 and 1964 have provided helpful information on the psychological characteristics of the medical students who later developed cancer, as compared to those who developed other diseases (Thomas and Duszynski, 1974). No actual traumatic events correlated with later development of cancer, but reported emotional distance from parents during childhood was noted in the physician-subjects who later developed cancer (Duszynski et al., 1981). Questionnaires available at that time limit the interpretation of findings to some degree. A study was reported in 1986 of the Rorschach findings of these students in relation to subsequent development of cancer (Graves et al., 1986). Using the Rorschach Interaction Scale based on cards showing two related figures, they identified six patterns of relatedness to others, ranging from flexible and empathic to ambivalent and avoidant. The relative risk of developing cancer over the 19–35 years of follow-up was 3.02 and 4.10 among those with greatest trouble in relating to others, as compared to the normal relative risk of 1.0, even when controlled for other variables including smoking. These long-term patterns of social behavior and impact on cancer vulnerability are of interest. The information gleaned from the prospective data on Johns Hopkins medical students is a rich source of information available because of the foresight of Dr. Thomas in the late 1940s. The annual data obtained on their morbidity and mortality continue to yield provocative findings. Unfortunately, the low incidence of cancer from multiple sites limits the possible interpretations of the findings.

An important series of prospective studies by Reynolds and Kaplan (1988; Kaplan and Reynolds, 1986), using the Alameda County (California) study of healthy individuals followed from 1965 to 1982 for cancer incidence and mortality, offer provocative leads that poor psychological well-being, lower level of satisfaction with life, and feeling socially isolated enhance risk of cancer. However, a meta-analysis of reported studies explored the support for existence of a "disease-prone" personality. They found the evidence present, but weak, except for heart disease (Friedman and Booth-Kewley, 1987). Studies of this kind suggest the need for research strategies that use a general, not cancer-specific perspective.

The effect of stress on disease vulnerability has also been examined to find characteristics that buffer stress and prevent stress-associated symptoms and illnesses (Maddi and Kobasa, 1984). The investigators found that the "hardy" personality (characterized by viewing stress as a challenge, by attempting to control stressful situations and by exercising a strong sense of commitment), had fewer physical illnesses, complaints, and psychological distress than those who lacked these qualities.

## CANCER RISK IN INDIVIDUALS WITH PSYCHIATRIC ILLNESS

There has been a long-standing interest in whether mental illness protects against development of physical illness, particularly cancer. The effect of schizophrenia and its treatment with phenothiazines was examined in the 1960s for impact on cancer mortality. A review by Fox and Howell (1974) of the studies concluded that the differences observed in mortality related to length of hospitalization. Increased cancer mortality was found among the psychiatric patients who died shortly after admission, which was likely related to selective variables, such as age and physical disability. Significant decrease in mortality was found from cancer of the lung, bronchi, gastrointestinal system, and all other sites combined in the patients hospitalized for more than 10 years. It was hypothesized that the hospital environment led to less exposure, not only to environmental carcinogens, but also to cigarette smoking, high-fat, and a high-calorie diet.

A 1986 report by Black and Winokur used the Iowa Record-Linkage data bank to correlate psychiatric diagnoses of patients admitted to state hospitals and their subsequent medical illnesses and mortality. Information on 5,412 psychiatric patients showed that the number who died had no overall excess of deaths from cancer. However, significant excess mortality from cancer was seen among those who died within 2 years of admission, and particularly among women and those with organic brain disorders. Their interpretation of the findings was that underlying physical illness likely contributed to the psychiatric admission and subsequent diagnosis of cancer in the psychiatric hospital.

Two other studies found no relationship between having a psychiatric disorder and cancer mortality. Mortality among subjects in a large population who had received psychiatric treatment, either as ambulatory or hospitalized patients, was found to be no greater from cancer than that seen in the general population (Babigian and Odoroff, 1969). Additional negative data were found in the studies of cancer mortality among World War II veterans who were discharged with a psychoneurotic diagnosis. They had experienced no excess in cancer mortality at follow-up (Keehn et al., 1974).

That reserpine elevates prolactin became a concern in the 1970s in relation to whether its chronic administration in psychiatric patients in the 1960s had increased the risk of breast cancer in women. A panel reviewing data on the association confirmed that while elevated prolactin is associated with mammary tumor growth in mice, the association does not appear to hold in humans. Even women who received chronically high-dose reserpine treatment for psychiatric illness did not show a later increased incidence of breast cancer (Hoover, 1977). Concern about giving psychotropic drugs that elevate prolactin to women at high risk of breast cancer, or to those who are being treated for it, does not appear warranted.

## PERSONALITY FACTORS CONTRIBUTING TO CANCER SURVIVAL

The ability of individuals to will themselves to die or to live, in the face of overwhelming odds, is a common literary theme. The possible contribution of elusive psychological factors that might contribute to the length of survival with cancer has been a topic of major interest over the past decade, although the contribution of such factors is likely small, if it exists at all, as suggested by Fox (1978). The role of psychological factors in influencing tumor growth has also been reexamined as links between the brain and the immune and endocrine systems have been identified in the emerging field of psychoneuroimmunology (Ader, 1981; Riley et al., 1981; Sklar and Anisman, 1981; see also Chapter 61). Animal studies of stress and immune modulation, provocative human studies, and patients' testimonials that describe the importance of their own "will to live" in surviving cancer have stimulated interest in possible ways to enhance the immune sys-

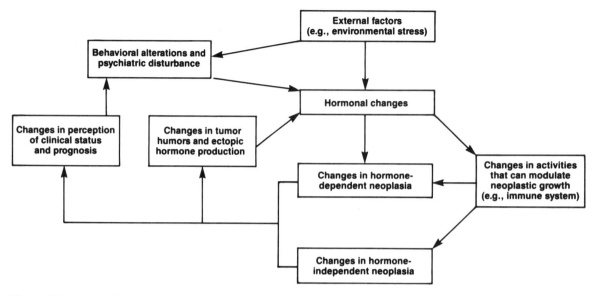

**Figure 60-2.** Interaction of psychic and endocrine factors with progression of neoplastic disease. *Source:* Reprinted by permission from M.E. Lippman (1985). Psychosocial factors and the hormonal regulation of tumor growth. In S.M. Levy (ed.), *Behavior and Cancer.* San Francisco: Jossey-Bass, pp. 134–47.

tem's effectiveness and thereby the body's ability to control tumor growth. For these reasons, emotional factors that may contribute to length of survival from cancer by a direct route have taken on more clinical relevance than has the search for psychological factors that may directly affect cancer risk.

The same psychosocial factors that are hypothesized to alter risk have also been examined for their effect on survival. It has generally seemed more logical to assume that a psychosocial variable might act as a promoter of malignant cell division in a tumor cell that had already been affected by an initiator of a malignant cell process. With this concept, impact on tumor progression becomes a more reasonable pursuit for research study. However, the time lag between initiation of a neoplastic process and tumor growth to a level of clinical recognition is known to be long, therefore discouraging a simplistic explanation of a stressful event being followed by development of cancer. However, rate of tumor progression is affected by many hormonal influences that might be perturbed by strong emotional states through the psychoneuroendocrine axis (Lippman, 1985). The converse is also true, because ectopic hormones produced by tumors affect psychological state. Knowledge of tumor regression or progression affect the patients' mood and emotional state from enhanced well-being to demoralization. Lippman (1985) proposed a model that outlines the potential for psychic and hormonal interaction in tumor progression (Fig. 60-2).

Longitudinal studies that have assessed personality variables and survival are outlined in Table 60-11. They have relied on the patients' view of their personality after presence of symptoms of illness. They have also not usually had the advantage of stratification for known factors impacting on length of survival (e.g., performance status, stage, nodal status in breast cancer, and treatment). However, several studies are of interest. Weisman and Worden (1975) studied 35 patients' survival time with one of five tumor sites: breast, cervix, colon, lung, lymphoma, and stomach. Psychosocial studies were obtained by open-ended interviews and standardized tests. They applied a survival quotient that compared observed versus expected survival for the site and examined antemortem and postmortem information, using the method developed from the psychological autopsy. Applying multiple-regression analyses to the identified variables, they found longer survival in patients who had good relationships, who asked for and received medical and psychological support, and who recognized the nature of their serious illness, but were not depressed or angry. Shorter survivals were seen in individuals who reported long-term poor social relationships (especially evident in the terminal period), more psychiatric disorders, depression, and pessimism, even stating a wish to die.

In 1979 two studies of psychological variables and survival appeared; one examined patients with stage II malignant melanoma, and the other studied women with stage II breast cancer (Table 60-11). The latter study of Derogatis, Abeloff, and Melisaratos (1979)

**Table 60-11**  Psychosocial variable and cancer survival in human studies

| Reference | Psychological variable | Biological condition |
|---|---|---|
| Weisman and Worden (1975) | Poor social relationships, depression, psychiatric disorders in short-term survivors | Observed versus expected survival by tumor site |
| Derogatis et al. (1979) | Long-term survivors—more distress; short-term survivors—well adjusted | Survival ($<1$ year or $>1$ year) with advanced breast cancer |
| Rogentine et al. (1979); reanalyzed by Temoshok and Fox (1984) | "Little adjustment to disease required" among those with early recurrence | Increased frequency of recurrence found at 1 year; reanalysis at 3 years failed to confirm |
| British group (1975–1985); Pettingale et al. (1985) | Stoic, resigned, helpless, hopeless: shorter survival time; fighting spirit or denial: long survival time | Survival at 5 and 10 years with breast cancer |
| Temoshok (1985); Temoshok and Fox (1984); Temoshok et al. (1985) | Type C personality: lower self-report of dysphoric emotions, passive responses | Increased recurrence in melanoma |
| Levy et al. (1985) | Adjusted, undistressed, apathetic, decreased family support | Lower NK* activity and greater number of positive nodes at surgery |
| Levy et al. (1987) | Depressive, fatigued, decreased family support | At 3 months, decreased NK persisted |
| Cassileth et al. (1985) | No correlation of psychosocial variables with time to recurrence or length of survival | Survival of patients with stage IV disease; patients with stage II breast cancer or melanoma |
| Holland et al. (1986) | No correlation of psychosocial scales of SCL-90 with time to relapse or death | Stage II breast cancer disease-free interval and mortality |
| Jamison et al. (1987) | Controlled for time since diagnosis, no psychosocial variable predicted short-term or long-term survival | Metastatic breast cancer |

*Natural killer cells.

showed that 35 women with stage III and IV breast cancer who were studied with the Symptom Checklist-90 (SCL-90) and separated into long ($>1$ year) and short ($<1$ year) survival varied on psychological characteristics. The long-term survivors both experienced and expressed more negative emotions—especially anger—whereas the short-term survivors were uncomplaining and cooperative. In actuality, however, scores were elevated less than one standard deviation on 11 of the 12 subscales (Cella, 1985). The confounding of treatment variables is also important in analyzing the results, because 85% of short-term survivors versus 55% of long-term survivors had had prior chemotherapy, and as a group, short-term survivors had also been on chemotherapy longer (mean of 407 versus 181 days), suggesting that more advanced disease in the short-term survivors could have accounted for the results. The critical variable of number of positive nodes at surgery was not reported, although it is the most reliable predictor of time to recurrence and death.

Rogentine and colleagues (1979) studied patients who had had wide excision of a malignant melanoma and lymph node dissection. Using data from a self-rated scale obtained at the time of surgery, recurrence at 12 months was related to number of positive nodes and, via a self-report rating, that the disease had not required major adjustment in their life. However,

when patients were reexamined at 3 years, the psychological predictor was no longer significant, indicating the need for lengthy time interval of study (Temoshok and Fox, 1984).

The series of studies by the London, England, research group under S. Greer have been important for over a decade. Beginning in 1975, they have critically examined psychological variables in survival from breast cancer, developing hypotheses and assessment instruments based on their earlier work. The notion of a "fighting spirit" being associated with better survival came from their systematic clinical observations. They have reported 5- and 10-year survival among women with breast cancer who had simple mastectomy without axillary node dissection. A randomly selected proportion had radiotherapy to the axillary nodes (Pettingale et al., 1985). The women were controlled for stage of disease and other key medical variables with the exception of number of positive axillary nodes. Data from structured interviews done at 3 months after the mastectomy placed women into three defined psychological categories, namely, those who showed either fighting spirit or denial, those with stoic acceptance of illness, and those showing helplessness and hopelessness. At 5 years, and again at 10, those women who showed fighting spirit or denial at 3 months after their mastectomy were more apt to be alive and

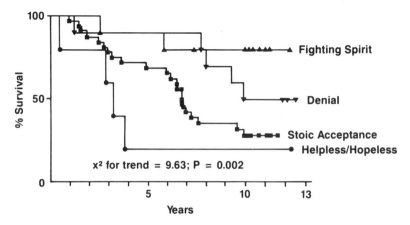

**Figure 60-3.** Psychological response and survival from breast cancer. $\chi^2$ for trend = 9.63; $p$ = 0.002. *Source:* Reprinted with permission from K.W. Pettingale, T. Morris, S. Greer, and J.L. Haybittle (1985). Mental attitudes to cancer: An additional prognostic factor. *Lancet* 1:750.

disease-free; those with stoic acceptance or helplessness–hopelessness were more apt to have poor outcome (Fig. 60-3). Absence of information about number of axillary nodes, and the small sample size, suggest the data should be interpreted with caution. It would also be important to know whether their initial coping style following mastectomy had actually persisted over the 10-year time interval of study.

Temoshok has carried out a series of studies in psychosocial variables and prognosis in melanoma patients (Temoshok and Fox, 1984). Known prognostic characteristics are size of lesion and depth of invasion at the time of excision. Outcome therefore depends on early diagnosis. Because the course of melanoma is highly variable, markers to predict progression are absent, but it is known to be sensitive to hormonal and immunological influences. Melanoma lends itself well to the exploration of possible psychosocial or behavioral variables. From her studies, Temoshok identified two variables relative to prognosis, namely, delay in consultation and a hypothesized type C behavior pattern. The personality of these individuals appears patient and pleasant with others, rarely expressing anger. The key feature of type C described was nonexpression of dysphoric emotions—found at 18 months follow-up to predict those who had died or relapsed. Interviewers had rated these patients as more depressed, although the individual did not report a dysphoric affect. The studies supported less expression of negative emotions as a prognostic characteristic in this group. Using a videotaped structured interview and self-report instruments, Temoshok found that the two groups who were identified by personality type did not differ significantly on thickness of the primary lesion and level of invasion. However, both variables (delay and personality) contributed, even though each was independent of the other.

Temoshok (1985) reported a series of seven studies that investigated different biopsychosocial aspects of cutaneous malignant melanoma. In addition to the study of delay, she identified a type of repressive coping in patients with melanoma as compared to patients with cardiovascular disease. Repression was measured by the discrepancy between reported anxiety in response to an electrodermal stimulation. Melanoma patients were more repressive in responding to it, suggesting that self-reported and observer-reported data may be quite different in these individuals. This could contribute to some of the contradictory findings across studies that use observer versus self-report approaches. She also found that emotional expression was associated positively with host response, whereas it was negatively correlated with metastatic configuration of the melanoma that was predictive of rapidity of tumor growth and spread. Temoshok's continuing work with one tumor is an important model for study of psychosocial survival variables.

The studies by Levy and colleagues (1985, 1987) have provided a useful model of concurrent examination of psychological and biological variables, particularly immunological status, in women with breast cancer. Measuring psychosocial state and immunological characteristics at time of mastectomy and at 3 months, Natural Killer (NK)-cell activity was an important predictor of axillary nodal status. Using multiple-regression analysis, 51% of the NK variance was accounted for by three distress indicators: adjustment, lack of social support, and fatigue and depressive symptoms. At 3 months, NK activity had not been affected by administration of chemotherapy and/or radiotherapy. However, NK-activity levels remained markedly lower in patients with positive nodes. Of the NK-activity variance at 3 months, 30% was consistently accounted for by fatigue and depression, and by the lack of social support identified at baseline. They concluded that, while tumor burden was associated with NK-activity level, a significant amount of baseline and 3-month NK activity could be predicted on the basis of CNS-mediated effects. These studies address the complexity of medical and psychological variables, and they serve as a model for consideration of psychological and biological status. Levy has also provided helpful reviews of this intriguing area (1982, 1985).

The Levy studies are of particular interest because of the findings from studies of Kiecolt-Glaser and colleagues that NK activity is negatively perturbed in physically healthy individuals under stresses of examinations (1984), and loneliness (1986) in medical students. Similar findings were identified in college students (Heisel et al., 1986). These psychoneuroimmunological studies,, are important parallel areas of research that show the psychoimmune linkages (see Chapter 61). Their reports are also important in that NK-cell activity is important in response to tumors of viral origin, such as herpesvirus and cervical cancer (Herberman, 1982).

The affective state described as helplessness–hopelessness as an outcome predictor in human cancer has received considerable attention, in part because of the animal studies (Sklar and Anisman, 1981). Animals that lacked control over environmental stress (such as inescapable shock) had shorter survival from tumors than animals that could control it. Cox and Mackay (1982) have used these studies to hypothesize that helplessness is associated with depletion of catecholamines; in turn, adrenocorticotrophic hormone (ACTH) release stimulates the release of corticosteroids, which suppresses immune function. The intense need to regain control of events in patients with cancer has led to extrapolation of these concepts to the clinical arena. Regaining a sense of control has been seen as not only promoting coping but also enhancing host resistance to tumor growth. Clearly, it is an intriguing hypothesis that needs further testing.

## STUDIES OF SURVIVAL WITH NEGATIVE PREDICTION

Cassileth and colleagues (1985) prospectively examined 204 patients with Stage IV pancreatic, gastric, lung, and colorectal cancers, and glioma. They sought to determine the relationship of seven psychosocial characteristics to survival. Given by a self-report method, the variables used were chosen because they had been reported to influence survival: social ties, marital status, job satisfaction, use of psychotropic drugs, life satisfaction, health, and hopelessness–helplessness. They also similarly studied a group of 155 patients with Stage I and II melanoma and Stage II breast cancer to evaluate the effect of these variables

on time to recurrence. They found that the most powerful predictors were the known medical prognostic variables. When these were taken into account first, no single or combined psychosocial variables appeared to influence survival. The strength of the biology of the disease appeared to outweigh any psychosocial variables that might have been present. The study is straightforward, although Temoshok (1985) has noted that self-report instruments might obtain different results because of the tendency of patients with type C personality to underreport dysphoric affect.

The cooperative clinical trial group, the Cancer and Leukemia Group B (CALGB), was used to conduct a study that attempted to replicate in women with stage II disease the Derogatis, Abeloff, and Melisaratos (1979) findings of personality variables in survival with metastatic breast cancer. The clinical-trials setting provided an opportunity to study a large number of women, stratified carefully for disease stage, number of axillary nodes at surgery, estrogen receptor status, and treatment by a standard protocol. Using the self-reported SCL-90 given at the time of entry to the study between 1980 and 1984, women receiving adjuvant chemotherapy for stage II breast cancer were followed 3 or more years to 1986 (Holland et al., 1986). Of the 346 women studied, 106 had died or relapsed at the time. Axillary nodal status was the most powerful predictor of time to relapse; psychological scale scores, when examined alone or combined with medical variables, did not predict survival. Further analysis of these patients in 1988 has found similar negative results.

Jamison, Burish, and Wallston (1987) replicated the Derogatis and colleagues (1979) study exactly, examining women with metastatic breast cancer. Controlling for time since diagnosis, and using eight psychological instruments to measure well-being, anxiety, depression, and anger, no scale identified those who died in the group with a mean of 10 months versus those termed long-term survivors who lived a mean of 30 months.

These studies generally suggest that while psychosocial variables may contribute to survival, the biological contribution to prognosis overshadows the ability to identify a strong psychosocial determinant. The issue is not an argument about whether psychosocial variables may play a role at all, but the relative strength of such variables, confronted by tumor biology. Data from the related fields of immunology and endocrinology suggest that the exploration is important, especially as patients seek to bring every possible self-generated support they can to their struggle with cancer. Eysenck (1987) and others suggest to patients that psychological interventions alter risk of cancer and tumor growth, and should be actively pursued. It is important that information be given by investigators in a way that neither negates nor overstates (thereby making false promises) the importance of these findings. The complex interactions of brain, neuroendocrine and immune systems, especially showing CNS modulation of the immune system through neuropeptides and hormones, make these issues highly relevant and challenging to researchers in psychoneuroimmunology (Stein et al., 1976; Besedovsky et al., 1986). It is premature to apply them at the clinical level.

### Emotional States: "Stress," Loss, and Grief

Distress in the form of emotional response to stressful life events and losses has been explored for its impact on survival with cancer. Most data are available on grief. Studies of the morbidity and mortality associated with grief are described in Chapter 50. Grief results in predictable distress in response to loss and, as such, constitutes one of the major stressful events in life. Bereavement has been assumed to be a risk factor for development of cancer from anecdotal accounts of clinicians who have observed development of cancer following a major loss. The affect of hopelessness, helplessness, depression, and traumatic life events resulting in chronic depression is one of the lines of research in both cancer risk and survival, as described earlier. Greene and colleagues (1956) showed the onset of a hematological malignancy in the context of a major loss in children and young adults. Jacobs and Charles (1980) found that losses in children antedated cancer onset. These observations have been pointed out as likely not having a relationship to the initiation of a neoplasm that would have to have occurred from months to years earlier. Whether the distressed emotional state of bereavement might serve as a promoter of tumor growth, after initiation, has been the subject of conjecture, especially as psychoimmune studies have shown perturbations of immune function during bereavement.

The concept of bereavement as a psychobiological response to loss of a relationship has been of interest (Hofer, 1984). New interest in grief has arisen since the two studies of Bartrop and colleagues (1977) and Schleifer and co-workers (1983), showed diminished immunocompetence during the first two months of bereavement; the latter study found no changes during anticipation of the loss. Phytohemaglutinin (PHA) and pokeweed mitogen (PWM) levels were perturbed during the 4- to 8-week period of grief. Although both studies suggested perturbation of immune function during the acute grief period, levels of immune function tested did not, however, reach pathologically low levels in either study. Studies by Irwin, Daniels, and Weiner (1987) examined NK activity and T-cell subpopulations in three groups of women: those who were bereaved, those anticipating their husbands' death from lung cancer, and a control group. NK activity was significantly lower in women anticipating loss and after husbands' death, as compared to controls. Those with most depressive symptoms, however, had the most reduced NK activity and changes in the ratio of T helper to T suppressor cells. Since cortisol levels were elevated only during the bereaved period, they could not be solely responsible for the changes.

Despite these findings, the most carefully controlled studies of mortality among spouses, while showing increased deaths from suicide, alcoholism, and infectious diseases, have not shown an excess of deaths from cancer (Helsing and Szklo, 1981). Although mortality was increased, it was limited largely to older men. The most important observation is that cancer does not appear to be responsible for any excess mortality among bereaved spouses (see Chapter 50).

### AN INTEGRATIVE MODEL AND FUTURE RESEARCH

Temoshok (1987) has noted the absence of theoretical constructs in psychosocial studies. She has proposed a model that attempts to reconcile contradictory findings and identify a type C personality in which the individual has little expression of chronic dysphoria from life stressors. The type C person develops blocked expression of emotions and chronic but masked hopelessness. This enduring pattern could contribute to adverse cancer outcome through immune and hormonal pathways. Figure 6-4 shows her proposed process model.

Recommendations for research are based on Temoshok and Heller's 1984 review:

1. Terms used are poorly defined, both theoretically or operationally, and need to be clearly defined for future clarity of findings, especially in those clustered around repressive emotions and depressive affect.
2. Studies should control for independent variables related to disease and environment.
3. Hypotheses tested should be specified.
4. Instruments used should be standardized.
5. Researchers should try to replicate previous findings and also attempt to extend those findings from one site or stage to another.

### SUMMARY

That psychosocial factors play a role in cancer risk and progression is documented primarily as it relates to behaviors that lead to exposure to environmental carcinogens, including smoking, sunlight, diet, personal

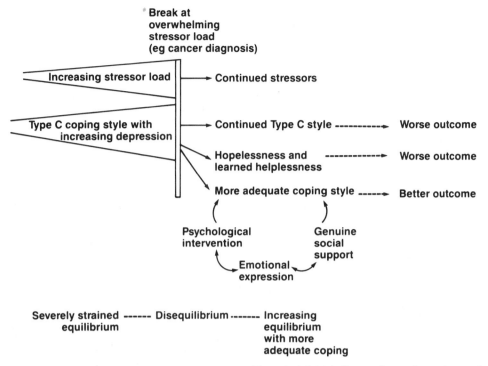

**Figure 60-4.** Proposed model for process by which type C personality pattern may contribute to adverse cancer outcome. *Source:* Reprinted by permission from L. Temoshok (1987). Personality, coping style, emotion, and cancer: Towards an integrative model. *Cancer Surv.* 6:545–67.

habits, and occupational exposures. Thus, life-style and risk behaviors are areas for active intervention at the level of both individuals and communities. The second area of social environment and social ties suggests that poverty is a risk factor for increased cancer mortality, along with other diseases. The association of absent or poor social ties with increased mortality from all diseases, including cancer, though not disproportionately, suggests their importance especially in older individuals.

Personality as a risk factor for developing cancer via a cancer-prone personality remains debatable. The concept of a type C personality with decreased expression of dysphoric emotions is being explored as a possible influence in cancer risk and progression. Here, too, conflicting data exist with regard to the possible contribution of psychosocial factors to tumor progression, beyond ways in which it relates to behavior. Most studies that have controlled carefully for the biological contribution have found the magnitude of psychosocial influences to be small. However, the increasing focus in our society on a potential personal contribution to disease and its control makes this an area of great research interest, particularly in light of the emerging evidence of perturbation of the immune system by psychological states, and the modulation of immune function through hormonal and CNS-mediated neuropeptides.

## REFERENCES

Abse, D.W., M.M. Wilkins, R.L. Van DeCastel, W.D. Buxton, J.P. Demars, R.S. Brown, and L.G. Kirschner (1974). Personality and behavioral characteristics of lung cancer patients. *J. Psychosom. Res.* 18:101–13.

Ader, R. (1981). *Psychoneuroimmunology.* New York: Academic Press.

American Cancer Society (1986). *Cancer in the Economically Disadvantaged: A Special Report.* New York American Cancer Society.

Babligian, H.M. and C.L. Odoroff (1969). The mortality experience of a population with psychiatric illness. *Am. J. Psychiatry* 126:470–74.

Bahnson, C.B. and M.B. Bahnson (1966). Role of the ego defenses: Denial and repression in the etiology of malignant neoplasm. *Ann. N.Y. Acad. Sci.* 125:846–55.

Bartrop, R., L. Lazarus, E. Luckhurst, L.G. Kiloh, and R. Penny (1977). Depressed lymphocyte function after bereavement. *Lancet* 1:834–36.

Becker, H. (1979). Psychodynamic aspects of breast cancer; younger and older patients. *Psychother. Psychosom.* 32:287–96.

Berkman, L.F. and S.L. Syme (1979). Social networks, host resistance, and mortality: A nine-year follow-up study of

Alameda County residents. *Am. J. Epidemiol.* 109:186–204.

Besedovsky, H., A. Del Rey, E. Sorkin, and C. Dinarello (1986). Immunoregulatory feedback between Interleukin-1 and glucocorticord hormones. *Science* 233:652–54.

Bieliauskas, L.A. and D.C. Garron (1982). Psychological depression and cancer. *Gen. Hosp. Psychiatry* 4:187–95.

Black, D.W. and G. Winokur (1986–1987). Cancer mortality in psychiatric patients: The Iowa Record-Linkage study. *Int. J. Psychiatr. Med.* 16:189–97.

Blazer, D. (1982). Social support and mortality in an elderly community population. *Am. J. Epidemiol.* 115:684–94.

Cassileth, B.R., E.J. Lusk, D.S. Miller, L.L. Brown, and C. Miller (1985). Psychosocial correlates of survival in advanced malignant disease. *N. Engl. J. Med.* 312:1551–55.

Cella, D.F. (1985). Psychological adjustment and cancer outcome: Levy versus Taylor. *Am. Psychologist* 40:1275–76.

Cooper, C.L., R.F. Davies-Cooper, and E.B. Faragher (1986). A prospective study of the relationship between breast cancer and life events. Type A behavior, social support and coping skills. *Stress Med.* 2:271–78.

Cox, T. and C. Mackay (1982). Psychosocial factors and psychophysiological mechanisms in the aetiology and development of cancers. *Soc. Sci. Med.* 16:381–96.

Cullen, J.W. (1982). Behavioral, psychological, and social influences on risk factors, prevention and early detection. *Cancer* 50(Suppl., November 1):1946–53.

Darling, J.R., N.S. Weiss, T.G. Hislop, C.M. Maden, R.J. Coates, K.J. Sherman, R.L. Ashley, M. Beagrie, J.A. Ryan, and L. Corey (1987). Sexual practices, sexually transmitted diseases, the incidence of anal cancer. *N. Engl. J. Med.* 317:973–77.

Dattore, P.J., F.C. Shantz, and L. Coyne (1980). Premorbid personality differentiation of cancer and non-cancer groups. A test of the hypothesis of cancer proneness. *J. Consult. Clin. Psychol.* 48:388–94.

Derogatis, L., M. Abeloff, and N. Melisaratos (1979). Psychological coping mechanism and survival time in metastatic breast cancer. *J.A.M.A.* 242:1504–8.

Doll, R. and R. Peto (1978). Cigarette smoking and bronchial carcinoma: Dose and time relationships among regular smokers and lifelong non-smokers. *J. Epidemiol. Community Health* 32:303–13.

Doll, R. and R. Peto (1981). *The Causes of Cancer.* New York: Oxford University Press.

Duszynski, K.R., J.W. Schaffer, and C.B. Thomas (1981). Neoplasms and traumatic events in childhood: Are they related? *Arch. Gen. Psychiatry* 38:327–31.

Editorial (1987). Hope for fatties: Avoirdupois may not increase risk after all. *Cancer Lett.* 13:7–9.

Eysenck, H.J. (1987). Personality as a predictor of cancer and cardiovascular disease and the application of behavior therapy in prophylaxis. *Eur. J. Psychiatry* 1:29–41.

Fox, B.H. (1978). Premorbid psychological factors as related to cancer incidence. *J. Behav. Med.* 1:45–133.

Fox, B.H. (1981). Psychosocial factors and the immune system in human cancer. In R. Ader (ed.), *Psychoneuroimmunology.* New York: Academic Press, pp. 103–57.

Fox, B.H. (1984). Remote life-style causes of cancer. *Cancer Detect. Prev.* 7(1):21–29.

Fox, B.H. and M.A. Howell (1974). Cancer risk among psychiatric patients: A hypothesis. *Int. J. Epidemiol.* 3:207–8.

Fox, B.H. and B.H. Newberry (eds.). (1984). *Impact of Psychoendocrine Systems in Cancer and Immunity.* Lewiston, N.Y.: C.J. Hogrefe.

Friedman, H.S. and S. Booth-Kewley (1987). The "disease-prone personality": A meta-analytic view of the construct. *Am. Psychologist* 42:539–55.

Goodkin, K., M.H. Antoni, and P.H. Blaney (1986). Stress and hopelessness in the promotion of cervical intra-epithelial neoplasia to invasive squamous cell carcinoma of the cervix. *J. Psychosom. Res.* 30:67–76.

Goodwin, J.S., W.C. Hunt, C.R. Key, and J.M. Samet (1987). The effect of marital status on stage treatment and survival of cancer patients. *J.A.M.A.* 258:3125–30.

Graham, S., W. Rawls, M. Swanson, and J. McCurtis (1982). Sex partners and herpes simplex type Z in the epidemiology of cancer of the cervix. *Am. J. Epidemiol.* 115:729–35.

Graves, P.L., LA. Mead, and T.A. Pearson (1986). The Rorschach Interaction Scale as a potential predictor of cancer. *Psychosom. Med.* 48:549–63.

Greene, W.A., L.E. Young, and S.N. Swisher (1956). Psychological factors and reticuloenthelial disease. *Psychosom. Med.* 18:284–303.

Greenwald, P. (1985). Prevention of cancer. V.T. De Vita, Jr., S. Hellman, and S.A. Rosenberg (eds.), *Cancer: Principles and Practice of Oncology.* Philadelphia: Lippincott, p. 202.

Greenwald, P. and E.J. Sondik (1986). Cancer control objectives for the nation: 1985–2000. *National Cancer Institute Monographs,* No. 2. U.S. Department of Health and Human Services, Public Health Service, National Institutes of Health.

Greer, S. and T. Morris (1975). Psychological attributes of women who develop breast cancer: A controlled study. *J. Psychosom. Res.* 19:147–53.

Greer, S. and M. Watson (1985). Towards a psycho-biological model of cancer: Psychological considerations. *Soc. Sci. Med.* 20:773–77.

Grossarth-Maticek, R., D.T. Kanazir, H. Vetter, and P. Schmidt (1983). Psychosomatic factors involved in the process of cancerogenesis. *Psychother. Psychosom.* 40:191–210.

Grossarth-Maticek, R., D.T. Kanazir, P. Schmidt, and H. Vetter (1985). Psychosocial and organic variables as predictors of lung cancer, cardiac infarct and apoplexy: Some differential predictors. *Pers. Indiv. Diff.* 6:313–21.

Hagnell, D. (1966). The premorbid personality of persons who developed cancer in a total population investigated in 1947 and 1957. *Ann. N.Y. Acad. Sci.* 125:846–55.

Heisel, J.S., S.E. Locke, L.J. Kraus, and R.M. Williams (1986). Natural killer cell activity and MMPI scores of a cohort of college students. *Am. J. Psychiatry* 143:1382–86.

Helsing, K.J. and M. Szklo (1981). Mortality after bereavement. *Am. J. Epidemiol.* 114:41–52.

Herberman, R.B. (1982). Possible effects of central nervous

system on natural killer cell activity. In S.M. Levy (ed.), *Biological Mediators of Behavior and Disease: Neoplasia*. New York Elsevier, pp. 235–48.

Higginson, J. and C.S. Muir (1979). Environmental carcinogenesis: Misconceptions and limitations to cancer control. *J.N.C.I.* 63:1291–98.

Hirayama, T. (1981). Nonsmoking wives of heavy smokers have a higher risk of lung cancer: A study from Japan. *Br. Med. J.* 282:183–85.

Hofer, M.A. (1984). Relationships as regulators: A psychobiologic perspective on bereavement. *Psychosom. Med.* 46:183–97.

Holland, J.C., A.H. Korzun, S. Tross, D.F. Cella, L. Norton, and W. Wood (1986). Psychosocial factors and disease-free survival in Stage II breast cancer. *Proc. Am. Soc. Clin. Oncol.* 5:237 (Abstract No. 928).

Hoover, R. (1977). Breast cancer: Epidemiologic considerations. Reserpine and Breast Cancer Task Force, Department of Health, Education and Welfare. Washington, D.C.: U.S. Government Printing Office.

Horne, R.L. and R.S. Picard (1979). Psychosocial risk factors for lung cancer. *Psychosom. Med.* 41:503–14.

House, J.S., K.R., Landis, and D. Umberson (1988). Social relationships and health. *Science* 241:540–45.

Irwin, M., M., Daniels, and H. Weiner (1987). Immune and Neuroendocrine changes during bereavement. *Psychiatric Clin. N. Am.* 10:449–65.

Jacobs, R.J. and E. Charles (1980). Life events and the occurrences of cancer in children. *Psychosom. Med.* 42:11–24.

Jamison, R.N., T.G. Burish, and K.A. Wallston (1987). Psychogenic factors in predicting survival of breast cancer patients. *J. Clin. Oncol.* 5:768–72.

Jenkins, C.D. (1983). Social environment and cancer mortality in men. *N. Engl. J. Med.* 308:395–98.

Kaplan, G.A. and P. Reynolds (1988). Depression and cancer mortality and morbidity: Prospective evidence from the Alameda County study. *J. Behav. Med.* 11:1–13.

Katz, J.L., P. Ackman, Y. Rothwax, E. Sachar, H. Weiner, L. Hellman, and T.F. Gallagher (1970). Psychoendocrine aspects of cancer of the breast. *Psychosom. Med.* 32:1–18.

Keehn, R.J., L.D. Goldberg, and G.W. Beebe (1974). Twenty-four year mortality followup of army veterans with disability separations for psychoneurosis in 1944. *Psychosomatic Medicine*, 36:27–46.

Kiecolt-Glaser, J.K., W. Garner, C. Speicher, G.M. Penn, J. Holliday, and R. Glaser (1984). Psychosocial modifiers of immunocompetence in medical students. *Psychosom. Med.* 46:7–14.

Kiecolt-Glaser, J.K., R. Glaser, E.C. Strain, J.C. Stout, K.L. Tarr, J.E. Holliday, and C.E. Speicher (1986). Modulation of cellular immunity in medical students. *J. Behav. Med.* 9:5–21.

Kissen, D.M. (1967). Psychosocial factors, personality and lung cancer in men aged 55–64. *Br. J. Med. Psychol.* 40:29–43.

Kneier, A.W. and L. Temoshok (1984). Repressive coping reactions in patients with malignant melanoma as compared to cardiovascular patients. *J. Psychosom. Res.* 28:145–55.

Lerner, M. (1986). Cancer mortality differentials by income, Baltimore 1949–51 to 1979–81. In *Cancer in the Economically Disadvantaged: A Special Report*. New York: American Cancer society. Appendix B.

LeShan, L. (1959). Psychological states as factors in the development of malignant disease: A critical review. *J.N.C.I.* 22:1–18.

Levy, S.M. (ed.). (1982). *Biological Mediators of Behavior and Disease: Neoplasia*. New York: Elsevier.

Levy, S.M. (1985). *Behavior and Cancer*. San Francisco: Jossey-Bass.

Levy, S., R. Herberman, M. Lippman, and T. d'Angelo (1987). Correlation of stress factors with sustained depression of natural killer activity and predicted prognosis in patients with breast cancer. *J. Clin. Oncol.* 5:348–53.

Levy, S., R. Herberman, A. Maluish, B. Schliew, and M. Lippman (1985). Prognostic risk assessment in primary breast cancer by behavioral and immunological parameters. *Health Psychol.* 4:99–113.

Lew, E. and L. Garfinkel (1979). Variations in mortality by weight among 750,000 men and women. *J. Chron. Dis.* 32:563–76.

Lipkin, M. and H. Newmark (1985). Effect of added dietary calcium on colonic epithelial-cell proliferation in subjects at high risk for familial colonic cancer. *N. Engl. J. Med.* 313:1381–84.

Lippman, M.E. (1985). Psychosocial factors and the hormonal regulation of tumor growth. In S.M. Levy (ed.), *Behavioral and Cancer*. San Francisco: Jossey-Bass, pp. 134–47.

Maddi, S.R. and S.C. Kobasa (1984). *The Hardy Executive: Health under Stress*. Homewood, Ill.: Dow Jones-Irwin.

Marshall, J.R. and D.P. Funch (1983). Social environment and breast cancer: A cohort analysis of patient survival. *Cancer* 52:1546–50.

Musey, V.C., D.C. Collins, I.P. Musey, D. Martino-Saltzman, and J.R.K. Preedy (1987). Long-term effect of a first pregnancy on the secretion of prolactin. *N. Engl. J. Med.* 316:229–34.

Muslin, H.L., K. Gyarfas, and W.J. Pieper (1966). Separation experience and cancer of the breast. *Ann. N.Y. Acad. Sci.* 125:802–6.

Orleans, C.T. (1985). Understanding and promoting smoking cessation: Overview and guidelines for physician intervention. *Ann. Rev. Med.* 36:51–61.

Osterweis, M., F. Solomon, and M. Green (eds.). (1984). *Bereavement: Reactions, Consequences, and Care*. Washington, D.C.: National Academy Press.

Perrin, G.M. and I.R. Pierce (1959). Psychosomatic aspects of cancer. *Psychosom. Med.* 21:397–415.

Persky, V.W., J. Kempthorne-Rawson, and R.B. Shekelle (1987). Personality and risk of cancer: 20-year follow-up of the Western Electric Study. *Psychosom. Med.* 49:435–49.

Pettingale, K.W., T. Morris, S. Greer, and J.L. Haybittle (1985). Mental attitudes to cancer: An additional prognostic factor. *Lancet* 1:750.

Pitot, H. (1985). Principles of cancer biology: Chemical carcinogenesis. In V.T. DeVita, Jr., S. Hellman, and S.A. Rosenberg (eds.), *Cancer: Principles and Practice of Oncology*. Philadelphia: Lippincott, 2nd ed., p. 92.

Ragland, D.R., R.J. Brand, and B.H. Fox (1987). Type A behavior and cancer mortality in the Western Collaborative Group Study (Abstract). *Psychosom. Med.* 49:209.

Reynolds, P. and G. Kaplan (1986). Psychological well being and cancer: Prospective evidence from the Alameda County study. *Am. J. Epidem.* 124:503–504.

Riley, V., M.A. Fitzmaurice, and D.H. Spackman (1981). Psychoneuroimmunologic factors in neoplasia: Studies in animals. In R. Ader (ed.), *Psychoneuroimmunology*. New York: Academic Press, pp. 31–102.

Rogentine, N., D. van Karnmen, B. Fox, J. Docherty, J. Rosenblatt, S. Boyd, and W. Bunney (1979). Psychological factors in the prognosis of malignant melanoma: A prospective study. *Psychosom. Med.* 41:647–55.

Rothman, K. and A. Keller (1972). The effect of joint exposure to alcohol and tobacco on risk of cancer of the mouth and pharynx. *J. Chron. Dis.* 25:711–16.

Schleifer, S.J., S.E. Keller, M. Camerino, J.C. Thornton, and M. Stein (1983). Suppression of lymphocyte stimulation following bereavement. *J.A.M.A.* 250:374–77.

Schmale, A. and H. Iker (1966). The psychological setting of uterine cervical cancer. *Ann. N.Y. Acad. Sci.* 125:807–13.

Selikoff, I.J. and E.C. Hammond (1979). Asbestos and smoking (Editorial). *J.A.M.A.* 242:458–59.

Shekelle, R.B., W.J. Raynor, Jr., A.M. Ostfeld, D.C. Garron, L.A. Bieliauskas, S.C. Liu, C. Maliza, and O. Paul (1981). Psychological depression and seventeen-year risk of death from cancer. *Psychosom. Med.* 43:117–25.

Sklar, L. and H. Anisman (1981). Stress and cancer. *Psychol. Bull.* 89:369–406.

Stein, M., R. Schiavi, and M. Camerino (1976). Influence of brain and behavior on the immune system. *Science* 191:435–40.

Subcommittee on Cancer on the Economically Disadvantaged (1986). *Cancer in the Economically Disadvantaged. A Special Report.* New York: American Cancer Society, pp. 1–20.

Temoshok, L. (1985). Biopsychosocial studies on cutaneous malignant melanoma: Psychosocial factors associated with prognostic indicators, progression, psychophysiology and tumor–host response. *Soc. Sci. Med.* 20:833–40.

Temoshok, L. (1987). Personality, coping style, emotion, and cancer: Towards an integrative model. *Cancer Surv.* 6:545–567.

Temoshok, L. and B.H. Fox (1984). Coping styles and other psychosocial factors related to medical status and to prognosis in patients with cutaneous malignant melanoma. In B.H. Fox and B.H. Newberry (eds.), *Impact of Psychoendocrine Systems on Cancer and Immunity*. Lewiston, N.Y.: C.J. Hogrefe, pp. 258–87.

Temoshok, L. and B.W. Heller (1984). Chapter 10. On comparing apples, oranges and fruit salad: A methodological overview of medical outcome studies in psychosocial oncology. In C.L. Cooper (ed.), *Psychosocial Stress and Cancer*. London: Wiley, pp. 231–60.

Temoshok, L., B.W. Heller, R.W. Sagebiel, M.S. Blois, D.M. Sweet, R.J. DiClemente, and M.L. Gold (1985). The relationship of psychosocial factors to prognostic indicators in cutaneous malignant melanoma. *J. Psychosom. Res.* 29:139–53.

Thomas, C.B. and K.R. Duszynski (1974). Closeness to parents and the family constellation in a prospective study of five disease states: Suicide, mental illness, malignant tumor, hypertension, and coronary heart disease. *Johns Hopkins Med. J.* 134:251–70.

Todd, P.B. and C.J. Magarey (1978). Ego defenses and affects in women with breast symptoms: A preliminary measurement paradigm. *Br. J. Med. Psychol.* 51:177–89.

U.S. Department of Health, Education and Welfare (1974). Alcohol and cancer. In *Alcohol and Health*. Second special report to the U.S. Congress. U.S. Department of Health, Education and Welfare, Public Health Service, pp. 53–67.

U.S. Department of Health and Human Services (1982). *The Health Consequences of Smoking: Cancer. A Report of the Surgeon General*. USDHHS, Public Health Service, Office on Smoking and Health. DHHS Publ. No. DHHS (PHS) 82-50179. Washington, D.C.: U.S. Government Printing Office.

U.S. Department of Health and Human Services (1986a). *The Health Consequences of Involuntary Smoking. A Report of the Surgeon General*. USDHHS, Public Health Service, Centers for Disease Control, Office on Smoking and Health, DHHS Publ. No. DHHS (CDC) 87-8398. Washington, D.C.: U.S. Government Printing Office.

U.S. Department of Health and Human Services (1986b). *Advances Data from Vital and Health Statistics*. No. 126 DHHS Publ. No. (PHS) 86-1250. Public Health Service, Hyattsville, Md, September 9.

University of Southern California Cancer Center (1987). Barrier contraceptives prevent cervical cancer. *Cancer Center Rep.* 11:1–11.

Vaillant, G.E. (1979). Natural history of male psychologic health: Effects of mental health on physical health. *N. Engl. J. Med.* 301:1249–54.

Weinstein, I.B. (1982). The scientific basis for carcinogen detection: Primary cancer prevention. *CA* 32:348–62.

Weisman, A. and J. Worden (1975). Psychological analysis of cancer deaths. *Omega: J. Death Dying* 6:61–75.

Weiss, S.M., J.A. Herd, and B.H. Fox (eds.). (1981). *Perspectives on Behavioral Medicine*. New York: Academic Press.

Wellisch, D. and J. Yager (1983). Is there a cancer-prone personality? *CA* 33:145–53.

# 61

# Psychoneuroimmunology and Cancer

Dana Bovbjerg

The possibility that psychological and social factors may contribute to the development and progression of cancer by their effects on the immune system will be explored in this chapter. The impact that the diagnosis and treatment of cancer can have on a patient's psychological health has been underscored in other sections of this book. The converse may also be true. As reviewed in the previous chapter, some researchers have reported that psychosocial factors can modify the risk of developing cancer, the progression of the disease, and the response to treatment. The relative importance of psychosocial factors compared to other known risks for cancer is not yet clear. It may be small. The important implication of the research is not that one should "blame the victim" for bringing the cancer on himself (Sontag, 1978), but rather that there may be as yet poorly understood natural mechanisms for the control of cancer. Greater understanding of the mechanisms by which the brain can influence cancer could potentially lead to the development of novel treatment strategies, including new drugs as well as behavioral interventions.

The study of interactions between the central nervous system (CNS) and the immune system, psychoneuroimmunology (or behavioral immunology), has received increasing attention in the last decade. This emerging interdisciplinary field of research has been the subject of several international meetings, a number of books, and a new journal, *Brain Behavior and Immunity*. Clearly, an exhaustive review is well beyond the scope of this chapter; the reader should refer to several recent books (Ader, 1981; Berczi, 1986; Cotman et al., 1987) and review articles for a more comprehensive examination of this topic (Fauman, 1982; Ader and Cohen, 1985; Blalock and Smith, 1985; Hall and Goldstein, 1986; Cohen, 1987).

In lieu of a comprehensive review, the following discussion of some of the key findings in psycho-neuroimmunology is intended as a background for the subsequent discussion of research relevant to cancer. The central research finding is that neural activities can influence the immune system. Psychosocial factors (presumably reflecting as yet unknown neural processes) have been shown to influence a number of different immune responses in humans as well as experimental animals. More direct manipulation of neuroendocrine activity (e.g., experimental lesions of the brain or manipulation of the neuroendocrine axis) has also been shown to influence the immune system (Roszman and Brooks, 1985). These findings suggest that there are neuroendocrine efferent pathways between the brain and the immune system. The existence of such pathways has received further support from studies of neuroanatomy. The organs of the immune system (the lymphoid organs such as the thymus, spleen, and lymph nodes) have been found to be richly innervated by neurons of the autonomic nervous system (Felten et al., 1985). The ability of the cells of the immune system, the leukocytes, to respond to neuroendocrine signals is suggested by the presence of specific receptors for both classical hormones and neurotransmitters (Plaut, 1987). Experimental treatment with these substances either by injection (in vivo) or by direct addition to cultures of cells (in vitro) has been shown to alter a variety of immune functions (Comsa et al., 1982).

Other experiments have revealed that communication between the brain and immune system also flows *from* the immune system to the brain. Induction of an immune response has been shown to alter neural activity in experimental animals (Besedovsky et al., 1983). Although these findings must be viewed as preliminary, they imply that there is an afferent pathway between the immune system and the CNS (Blalock, 1984). The physical basis of this pathway has not yet been well characterized (and is likely to include multiple mechanisms). One example of communication from the immune system to the brain is the induction of a fever. Infectious agents induce leukocytes, in the monocyte family, to secrete interleukin 1 (IL-1, formerly known as endogenous pyrogen) into the bloodstream. The temperature-regulatory areas of the brain respond to this IL-1 and increase the set point for body temperature. The higher temperature is then sustained by peripheral mechanisms. Febrile temperatures can kill some pathogens directly, and have also been shown to augment a number of protective immune responses (Dinarello, 1984). Thus, a signal from the immune system induces the brain to increase body temperature, which in turn enhances the activities of the immune system.

The existence of both afferent and efferent pathways for communication between the CNS and the immune system provides the essential elements of a regulatory loop (Blalock and Smith, 1985). The functional significance of this loop is suggested by evidence for both feedback (Besedovsky et al., 1986) and feedforward (Bovbjerg and Ader, 1986) regulation of the immune system by the CNS. Feedforward regulation has been supported by a series of studies that immune responses in experimental animals can be modified by classical conditioning procedures (Ader and Cohen, 1985; Bovbjerg and Ader, 1986). In one particularly apposite study, tumor growth in mice was increased by classical conditioning; the apparent mechanism was a conditioned suppression of immune defenses (Gorczynski et al., 1985).

The extent and specificity of neural regulation of the immune system have yet to be determined (Melnechuk, 1985). Neural influences may be limited to generalized augmentation and suppression, or may be capable of more specific modulation of immune responses to particular challenges. Whatever the capacities of neural regulation are found to be, it is clear that the immune system has an extensive capacity to regulate itself (Asherson et al., 1986). The autonomous regulatory mechanisms within the immune system involve both specific and nonspecific components in a complex cellular circuitry that is only beginning to be understood. Immune-regulatory mechanisms include both cell–cell contact and the secretion of regulatory factors. How the neural-regulatory influences interface with these immune-regulatory mechanisms is not yet known, but could well prove to be complex. For example, neural influences could increase an immune response by direct communication with effector cells or indirectly by communication with regulatory cells that would otherwise suppress the effector cells. Further complexity is introduced by regulatory signals with more than one target. It is already known that IL-1 released from monocytes not only reaches the brain

where it induces fever, but also has a direct effect on T lymphocytes, causing augmented proliferation (Dinarello, 1984).

Can psychoneuroimmunology provide the mechanism(s) by which psychosocial factors influence the development or progression of cancer? Although there has been considerable speculation to that effect, and a few researchers in the field have begun to put the question to experimental test, not enough work has been done to provide a definitive answer (see Fox and Newberry, 1984). Before considering the relatively few studies that have concurrently investigated psychosocial factors, immunologic mediators, and the development of cancer, we should first consider the evidence that led investigators to propose a connection.

The plausibility of psychoimmune involvement in cancer is based on three largely independent research literatures that have explored the following critical hypotheses:

1. Cancer incidence and progression are affected by psychosocial variables.
2. Cancer incidence and progression are influenced by the activities of the immune system.
3. The kinds of immune responses that influence cancer incidence and progression are themselves affected by psychosocial variables.

Let us briefly examine the evidence for each of these.

## EVIDENCE OF A ROLE FOR PSYCHOSOCIAL VARIABLES IN CANCER

A large number of studies have investigated the possible involvement of psychosocial factors in the etiology of cancer in humans. This literature will only be touched on here, because it has been extensively reviewed elsewhere (Fox, 1978, 1981, 1983; Levy, 1982; Levy et al., 1985) as well as in this volume (see Chapter 60). Studies in humans have been of three basic types: retrospective, semiprospective, and prospective.

### Retrospective Studies

Retrospective studies have been the most common. In these studies, psychosocial factors have been assessed in patients who already have cancer in an attempt to find differences that distinguish them from control subjects without cancer. Three general categories of psychological variables associated with cancer have been proposed: a history of psychological stress, personality attributes, and social contact. For instance, cancer patients have been reported to have a history of life stress that preceded their illness. These studies have included both self-reported measures of past stress as well as documentation of the loss of an important emotional relationship (e.g., loss of a spouse through divorce or death). One or another study has proposed a considerable number of personality attributes to be associated with cancer. The wide variety of psychosocial variables with claims for an association with cancer may reflect a weakness of the field. As Fox (1983) has pointed out, researchers often do not mention negative findings, which makes it difficult to assess the replicability of the significant correlations that are reported in the literature.

The difficulties in interpreting such retrospective results have been discussed at length, notably by Fox (1978, 1981, 1983). The critical problem is that the reported correlations do not allow one to distinguish cause from effect. The patient's knowledge of the diagnosis is likely to influence not only measures of current psychological attributes and social support, but also the interpretation of past experience (e.g., searching after meaning). Moreover, even if patients are not aware of their diagnosis, the cancer itself may induce psychological changes as a result of brain metastases or as a result of various physiological responses to the tumor.

## Semiprospective Studies

The confounding effects of a patient's knowledge of diagnosis are eliminated in semiprospective studies. In such studies, the investigator either attempts to predict the diagnosis of cancer based on an assessment of psychosocial factors prior to the patient's diagnosis, or the investigator attempts to predict the subsequent course of the disease based on an assessment of psychosocial factors just after the patient learns of a positive diagnosis. The possibility that the presence of cancer itself may influence psychosocial measures is obviously not eliminated. It is important to consider the possible effects of the stage or severity of the disease at the time the study begins and to assess the possible contributions of the response to treatment.

## Prospective Studies

Prospective studies would provide the strongest evidence for psychosocial influences on cancer. Although a number of studies have reported such influences, interpretation of the results has been challenged for a number of reasons (see Fox, 1983). For example, because the interval between the initiation of malignancy and the clinical discovery of cancer can be many years, prospective studies have been challenged on the grounds of possible influence of the developing cancer on psychological variables.

## Human Versus Animal Studies

Other difficulties in interpretation of positive findings are common to most studies in humans. It is important that the contribution of psychosocial factors to behaviors known to increase the risk of cancer (e.g., psychosocial connections with smoking) be assessed. The demonstrated relationship between some types of cancer and genetics raises another difficulty for the interpretation of prospective studies of psychosocial factors. Because genetic influences also appear to contribute to personality, the apparent causal relationship between certain psychological factors and cancer may actually represent an underlying genetic predisposition with two manifestations.

Most of the variables that confound human studies of psychosocial influences on cancer could, in principle, be brought under experimental control in studies of animals. The contribution of genetic variability can be eliminated (or explored) by the use of inbred strains. Psychosocial effects on the incidence of tumors can be studied in animals known to have a high genetic risk or by application of well-characterized carcinogens at specific doses. Psychosocial effects on the growth of tumors can be explored by experimental challenge with well-characterized tumor cell lines transplanted in known quantities at a specified time. Various types of psychosocial factors can be imposed at specified times in relation to the tumor challenge. In short, the use of animal models allows the experimental manipulation of variables that may influence the development of tumors; such interventions allow one to infer causal relationships. In humans, ethical considerations (as well as cost) largely preclude any experimental manipulations.

Despite such potential advantages, the research in experimental animals has yet to fulfill its promise. As reviewed in more detail elsewhere (LaBarba, 1970; Sklar and Anisman, 1981; Riley, 1981; Borysenko and Borysenko, 1982; Newberry et al., 1984), psychosocial influences have been variously reported to enhance or to suppress tumor induction, growth, and metastasis. This literature includes a large number of isolated studies that demonstrate that some psychosocial factor (usually the imposition of a ''stressor'') can influence the development of some tumor model. Unfortunately, there have been few systematic attempts to clarify which of the wide variety of variables in these studies is responsible for the divergent results in the literature. Many different stressors have been applied to different strains or species of animals, of different ages, at different times relative to challenge with different types of tumors (to note just a few of the possibly relevant variables). There is evidence that some of the variability in these studies is the result of exposure to uncontrolled stressors associated with conventional animal housing facilities (Riley, 1981). Differences between the effects of acute and chronic exposure to stressors have also been reported (Sklar and Anisman, 1981; Teshima and Kubo, 1984). Interpretation of a number of studies is problematic because some experimental manipulations, characterized as stressors (e.g., irradiation), clearly have direct physical consequences that might account for their effects on cancer quite independently of putative psychological influences.

Two research designs that have used electrical shock as a stressor are particularly noteworthy. Experimental animals allowed to "cope" with electrical shock (by escape) show reduced growth of transplanted tumors (mouse P815 mastocytoma or rat Walker 256 sarcoma) compared to "yoked" control animals receiving the same amount of shock but unable to cope (Sklar and Anisman, 1979; Visintainer et al., 1982). Because the experimental animals and the yoked controls differ only in their ability to control the shock, the studies underscore the possible psychological effects on tumor growth. The second design involves a regimen of electrical foot shock that has been found to provoke temporary analgesia in rats, apparently by inducing endogenous opioid mechanisms (Shavit et al., 1985). Pretreatment with the opioid, but not a nonopioid shock regimen (with identical shock intensity and total duration), was found to reduce the mean survival time of rats implanted with a mammary adenocarcinoma (MAT 13762B); this effect was blocked by the opiate antagonist naltrexone, and was mimicked by morphine treatment (Shavit and Martin, 1987).

## EVIDENCE OF A ROLE FOR THE IMMUNE SYSTEM IN CANCER

A thorough review of the huge body of literature addressed to the question of a possible association between the immune system and cancer is well beyond the scope of this chapter; however, a number of books are available (e.g., Herberman, 1983; Hancock and Ward, 1985). A brief analysis of some key points may serve to highlight the difficulties of this complex topic. Cancer is thought to develop from the unchecked proliferation of a single cell after several sequential induction and tumor promotion events at the nuclear level (Klein and Klein, 1985). Tumors can be induced by DNA tumor viruses, retrovirus insertion near a cellular oncogene, or cellular oncogene activation that occurs spontaneously or following carcinogen exposure. One possible role for the immune system in the defense against cancer is to recognize cells in which such changes have occurred and to eliminate them before a tumor can develop, as hypothesized by "immune-

surveillance" theories (Thomas, 1982). Additional immune defenses might come into play to block the subsequent growth or metastasis of tumors that escaped surveillance (Rees and Ali, 1985). The capability of the immune system to perform any of these tasks remains controversial (Stutman, 1985).

## The Search for Tumor-Specific Antigens

In order for the immune system to recognize malignant cells, there must be some cell surface markers (antigens) that are unique to the malignant state. Tumors induced by oncogenic DNA viruses might be expected to bear viral proteins that could be recognized as nonself by lymphocytes and targeted for destruction. In fact, specific immune defenses against such tumors are well documented, particularly in experimental animals (Klein and Klein, 1985). The possible surface markers on cells that have undergone spontaneous activation of cellular oncogenes are less obvious (but could include reexpression of developmental antigens). Attempts to demonstrate such tumor-related antigens have met with mixed results, particularly in humans (Doherty et al., 1984). In experimental animals the existence of such antigens has been inferred from the finding that preexposure to some spontaneous tumors results in increased resistance to subsequent challenges with the same tumor. Demonstrating tumor-specific antigens in humans has proved to be more difficult. Differences between the results of human and animal research underscore the importance of keeping species dissimilarities in mind when attempting to assess the generalizability of research findings. For example, many spontaneous rodent tumors are viral (and therefore tend to express viral antigens that can be recognized by specific immune defenses), whereas relatively few human tumors are known to have a viral etiology (Fox, 1983). Also, much of the research in animals has involved transplantation of tumor cells that were originally induced in other hosts (by viral or chemical challenge). This technique has allowed the study of responses to established tumors, but cannot be used to study immune defenses against the early (induction) phases of malignancy. The animal studies of transplantable tumors are thus analogous to studies of disease progression in humans with established tumors.

## Tumor-Induced Immune Suppression

Although one possible explanation for the lack of strong specific immune defenses against cancer is the absence of recognizable cell surface markers of the malignant state, tumors have also been reported to induce immune suppression (Hancock, 1985; Naor, 1979; North, 1985). Humans and experimental animals with tumors have increased activity of a number of different types of suppressor cells that can suppress responses to the tumor by both specific and nonspecific mechanisms (Naor, 1979; North, 1985). Because the consequences of inappropriate (i.e., false positives) immune defense can be severe (e.g., autoimmune disease), the existence of such suppressor mechanisms is perhaps not surprising. Although the clinical significance of immune suppression in cancer patients is still controversial, the possible influence of suppressor mechanisms adds another layer of complexity to attempts to investigate antitumor immune responses. Further complexity may be introduced by dynamic changes in the normal balance between effector and suppressor mechanisms. For example, during the first 2 weeks after animals receive a tumor graft, the ratio of suppressor T cells to effector T cells has been reported to increase gradually, until suppressor mechanisms become completely dominant (North, 1985).

### Nonspecific Immune Defenses

Specific immune responses to cancer may prove to be limited to tumors with a viral etiology (which therefore express viral proteins): however, nonspecific immune defenses including macrophages and killer cells may play a wider role (Herberman, 1984). Recent clinical studies of the effects of interleukin 2 (IL-2) treatment for cancer have provoked considerable interest in lymphokine-activated killer (LAK) cells (Rosenberg and Lotze, 1986). The antitumor activity of LAK cells, as with natural killer (NK) cells, does not appear to depend on recognition of tumor-specific antigens (Herberman, 1984; Uchida, 1986). NK cells have been shown to kill a variety of different tumor types in culture, although not all tumors are equally sensitive. This subset of large granular lymphocytes has been shown in both experimental animals and humans to be active in the elimination of metastatic tumor cells. In addition, both in vitro and in vivo studies of NK cells have recently provided some evidence for immune surveillance against primary tumors. Low NK activity has been reported to be associated with increased tumor incidence (mostly lymphomas) in both patients and mice (Herberman, 1984), although this evidence has been challenged (Stutman, 1985).

In summary, the possibility that the immune system plays a major role in defense against cancer remains controversial. Specific immune responses (e.g., as provided by T and B cells) do not appear to be important in defense against most human cancers. Recent research has emphasized that nonspecific immune defenses such as NK-cell activity may play a larger part in protection against at least some types of cancer. Both specific and nonspecific defenses are thought to be subject to immune-regulatory influences (e.g., suppressor cells). It should also be noted that immune mechanisms have been reported to augment tumor development in some instances.

## EVIDENCE OF A ROLE FOR PSYCHOSOCIAL VARIABLES IN IMMUNE RESPONSES THAT DEFEND AGAINST CANCER

As discussed earlier, both the overall importance and the specific immune mechanisms that may be critical to the defense against various types of cancer remain controversial. Nonspecific immune defenses have received increasing attention.

Kiecolt-Glaser and Glaser (1986) have reported a relationship between psychosocial influences and NK activity in studies of three different populations, namely, medical students, geriatric residents of independent-living facilities, and nonpsychotic psychiatric inpatients. NK activity in blood samples collected from medical students during their final-examination period was compared to a baseline sample collected 1 month earlier. NK activity was found to be lower during exam week and lower in students with scores above the median on the UCLA Loneliness Scale (Kiecolt-Glaser et al., 1984a). A subsequent study of another medical school class confirmed that self-reported distress was higher during exam week and that potential confounding variables such as nutrition, concurrent illness, or sleep did not appear to be responsible for the effects on NK activity (Glaser et al., 1986). Enhancement of NK activity as an apparent result of psychosocial influence was reported in a study of 45 geriatric residents of independent-living facilities (Kiecolt-Glaser et al., 1985a). Relaxation training was found to decrease self-rated distress and increase NK activity compared to control groups given social contact or no intervention. In a group of newly admitted nonpsychotic psychiatric inpatients, subjects with loneliness scores below the median were found to have significantly lower NK activity (Kiecolt-Glaser et al., 1984b). Responses to several scales of the Minnesota Multiphasic Personality Inventory (MMPI) differed in the low- and high-loneliness subgroups, but correlations with NK activity were not reported. Other investigators have reported a correlation between reduced NK activity and psychopathology as assessed by the MMPI in a sample of college students (Heisel et al., 1986).

In experimental animals, NK activity has been shown to be altered by environmental stressors. In a series of studies with rats, Shavit and his colleagues (Shavit et al., 1985; 1987) have reported that exposure to prolonged, intermittent foot shock that induces opioid-mediated analgesia also induces suppression of NK activity. On the other hand, brief continuous shock (of the same intensity and equated for the total duration of shock) induces nonopioid analgesia with no changes in NK activity. These investigators have also reported preliminary data that NK activity is suppressed by inescapable but not escapable shock (Shavit et al., 1985). Although these findings suggest a potential neuroendocrine pathway by which neural activity may influence the activity of NK cells, the path may be indirect because adrenalectomy apparently blocks these opioid effects (Shavit and Martin 1987).

The evidence for an influence of psychosocial variables on any immune defenses (e.g., NK-cell activity) thought to play a role in the development of cancer is all relatively recent and has yet to be widely replicated by independent research groups.

## SUMMARY

In this chapter we have briefly considered the research support for the three hypotheses underlying an interest in possible psychoneuroimmunological processes in cancer, and have found that the development and progression of some cancers may be affected by psychosocial influences, and that some cancers are influenced by the activities of the immune system. Furthermore, it appears that at least one immune response (NK activity), thought to influence cancer, appears to be affected by psychosocial factors. Although the evidence for each is not incontrovertible, together they do suggest that alterations in immune defenses should be explored as a possible mechanism by which psychosocial variables could influence the development of cancer.

Other possible mechanisms must also be considered, however. Immune responses are only one among a number of potential body defense mechanisms against cancer that may be influenced by psychosocial variables (Greenberg et al., 1984). The first line of defense against chemically induced cancer may be provided by carcinogen-transforming enzymes. Another line of defense is provided by nuclear DNA repair mechanisms. Such mechanisms have been shown to be suppressed in experimental animals (Glaser et al., 1985b) following exposure to a stressor and in humans (Kiecolt-Glaser et al., 1985b) who evidence high levels of distress on the MMPI. Stress has also been reported to alter a wide variety of neuroendocrine hormone levels (Irwin and Anisman, 1984), including endogenous opiates. Because many tumors are sensitive to endocrine levels, endocrine changes induced by psychosocial factors could have a direct effect. Also, hormonally driven changes in metabolic activity (e.g., by altering body temperature or the availability of nutrients) may result in altered tumor growth.

The investigation of the role of psychoneuroimmunology in cancer will require carefully designed studies linking psychosocial variables, immune media-

ators, and altered incidence or progression of cancer in the same subjects. To date, almost no such studies have been reported. One exception has been provided by a semiprospective study of breast cancer patients in which psychological factors, NK activity, and prognostic indicator of disease (the number of axillary lymph nodes positive for cancer) have been assessed (Levy et al., 1985, 1987). Levy and associates (1985) have reported that 51% of the baseline NK-activity variance in patients with breast cancer could be accounted for by three "distress" indicators. Three months later following chemotherapy 30% of the variance in NK activity was accounted for by psychosocial factors included in the original three. Psychosocial factors were not found to be significantly related to the prognosis indicator of positive nodes, although NK activity was found to be lower in women with positive nodes. This report has been criticized on a number of methodological grounds (Talmadge and Alvord, 1987); obviously, it is correlational, but it does at least attempt to provide direct evidence of a linkage among psychosocial factors, an immune mediator, and the progression of cancer.

Animal models allow the types of experimental interventions that are necessary for the direct assessment of causal relationships among psychosocial factors, immune defenses, and cancer. Further studies in psychoneuroimmunology may begin to uncover the physiological mechanisms that are responsible for these interactions. We can hope that some of the old questions will soon be put to rest, and look forward to the new ones that will undoubtedly arise.

## REFERENCES

Ader, R. (ed.). (1981). *Psychoneuroimmunology*. New York: Academic Press.

Ader, R. and N. Cohen (1985). CNS–Immune system interactions: Conditioning phenomena. *Behav. Brain Sci.* 8:379–425.

Asherson, G.L., V. Colizzi, and M. Zembala (1986). An overview of T-suppressor cell circuits. *Ann. Rev. Immunol.* 4:37–68.

Berczi, I. (ed.). (1986). *Pituitary Function and Immunity*. Boca Raton, Fla.: CRC Press.

Besedovsky, H., A. Del Ray, and E. Sorkin (1983). What do the immune system and the brain know about each other? *Immunol. Today* 4:342–46.

Besedsovsky, H., A. Del Ray, and E. Sorkin (1986). Regulatory immune-neuro-endocrine feedback signals. In I. Berczi (ed.), *Pituitary Function and Immunity*. Boca Raton, Fla.: CRC Press, pp. 241–49.

Blalock, J. (1984). The immune system as a sensory organ. *J. Immunol.* 132:1067–70.

Blalock, J. and E. Smith (1985). A complete regulatory loop between the immune and neuroendocrine systems. *Fed. Proc.* 44:108–11.

Borysenko, M. and J. Borysenko (1982). Stress, behavior,

and immunity: Animal models and mediating mechanisms. *Gen. Hosp. Psychiatry* 4:59–67.

Bovbjerg, D. and R. Ader (1986). The central nervous system and learning: Feedforward regulation of immune responses. In I. Berczi (ed.), *Pituitary Function and Immunity* Boca Raton, Fla.: CRC Press, pp. 252–57.

Cohen, J.J. (1987). Immunity and behavior. *J. Allergy Clin. Immunol.* 79:2–5.

Comsa, J., H. Leonhardt, and H. Wekerle (1982). Hormonal coordination of the immune response. *Rev. Phsyiol. Biochem. Pharmacol.* 2:116–88.

Cotman, C., R. Brinton, A. Galaburda, B. McEwan, and D. Schneider (eds.). (1987). *The Neuro-Immune-Endocrine Connection.* New York: Raven Press.

Dinarello, C. (1984). Interleukin-1. *Rev. Infect. Dis.* 6:51–95.

Doherty, P., B. Knowles, and P. Wettstein (1984). Immunological surveillance of tumors in the context of major histocompatibility complex restriction of T cell function. *Adv. Cancer Res.* 42:1–65.

Fauman, M. (1982). The central nervous system and the immune system. *Biol. Psychiatry* 17:1459–82.

Felten, D., S. Felten, S. Carlson, J. Olschowka, and S. Livnat (1985). Noradrenergic and peptidergic innervation of lymphoid tissue. *J. Immunol.* 135:755s–65s.

Fox, B. (1978). Premorbid psychological factors are related to cancer incidence. *J. Behav. Med.* 1:45–133.

Fox, B. (1981). Psychosocial factors and the immune system in human cancer. In R. Ader (ed.), *Psychoneuroimmunology.* New York: Academic Press, pp. 103–57.

Fox, B. (1983). Current theory of psychogenic effects on cancer incidence and prognosis. *J. Psychosoc. Oncol.* 1:17–31.

Fox, B.H. and B.H. Newberry (eds.). (1984). *Impact of Psychoendocrine Systems in Cancer and Immunity.* Lewiston, N.Y.: C.J. Hogrefe.

Glaser, R., J. Kiecolt-Glaser, C. Speicher, and J. Holliday (1985a). Stress, loneliness, and changes in herpesvirus latency. *J. Behav. Med.* 8:249–60.

Glaser, R., J. Rice, C. Speicher, J. Stout, and J. Kiecolt-Glaser (1986). Stress depresses interferon production by leukocytes concomitant with a decrease in natural killer cell activity. *Behav. Neurosci.* 100:675–78.

Glaser, R., B. Thorn, K. Tarr, J. Kiecolt-Glaser, and S. D'Ambrosio (1985b). Effects of stress on methyltransferase synthesis: An important DNA repair enzyme. *Health Psychol.* 4:403–12.

Gorczynski, R., M. Kennedy, and A. Ciampi (1985). Cimetidine reverses tumor growth enhancement of plasmacytoma tumors in mice demonstrating conditioned immunosuppression. *J. Immunol.* 134:4261–66.

Greenberg, A.H., D.G. Dyck, and L.S. Sandler (1984). Opponent processes, neurohormones and natural resistance. In B.H. Fox and B.H. Newberry (eds.), *Impact of Psychoendocrine Systems in Cancer and Immunity.* Lewiston, N.Y.: C.J. Hogrefe, pp. 225–57.

Hall, N. and A. Goldstein (1986). Thinking well. *Sciences* 86:34–40.

Hancock, B. (1985). Immunosuppression in cancer. In B.W. Hancock and A.M. Ward (eds.), *Immunological Aspects of Cancer.* Boston: Martinus Nijhoff, pp. 147–61.

Hancock, B.W. and A.M. Ward (eds.). (1985). *Immunological Aspects of Cancer.* Boston: Martinus Nijhoff.

Heisel, J., S. Locke, L. Kraus, and R. Williams (1986). Natural killer cell activity and MMPI scores of a cohort of college students. *Am. J. Psychiatry* 143:1382–86.

Herberman, R. (ed.). (1983). *Basic and Clinical Immunology.* Boston: Martinus Nijhoff.

Herberman, R. (1984). Possible role of natural killer cells and other effector cells in immune surveillance against cancer. *J. Invest. Dermatol.* 83:137s–40s.

Irwin, J. and H. Anisman (1984). Stress and pathology: Immunological and central nervous system interactions. In C.L. Cooper (ed.), *Psychosocial Stress and Cancer.* London: Wiley, pp. 93–147.

Kiecolt-Glaser, J. and R. Glaser (1986). Psychological influences on immunity. *Psychosomatics* 27:621–24.

Kiecolt-Glaser, J., W. Garner, C. Speicher, G. Penn, J. Holliday, and R. Glaser (1984a). Psychosocial modifiers of immunocompetence in medical students. *Psychosom. Med.* 46:7–14.

Kiecolt-Glaser, J., R. Glaser, D. Williger, J. Stout, G. Messick, S. Sheppard, D. Ricker, S. Romisher, W. Briner, G. Bonnell, and R. Donnerberg (1985a). Psychosocial enhancement of immunocompetence in a geriatric population. *Health Psychol.* 4:25–41.

Kiecolt-Glaser, J., D. Ricker, G. Messick, C. Speicher, W. Garner, and R. Glaser (1984b). Urinary cortisol, cellular immunocompetency, and loneliness in psychiatric inpatients. *Psychosom. Med.* 46:15–24.

Kiecolt-Glaser, J., R. Stephens, P. Lipetz, C. Speicher, and R. Glaser (1985b). Distress and DNA repair in human lymphocytes. *J. Behav. Med.* 8:311–20.

Klein, G. and E. Klein (1985). Evolution of tumours and the impact of molecular oncology. *Nature* 315:190–95.

LaBarba, R. (1970). Experimental and enviornmental factors in cancer: A review of research with animals. *Psychosom. Med.* 32:259–76.

Levy, S. (ed.). (1982). *Biological Mediators of Behavior and Disease: Neoplasia.* New York: Elsevier.

Levy, S., R. Herberman, M. Lippman, and T. D'Angelo (1987). Correlation of stress factors with sustained depression of natural killer cell activity and predicted prognosis in patients with breast cancer. *J. Clin. Oncol.* 5:348–53.

Levy, S., R. Herberman, A. Maluish, B. Schlien, and M. Lippman (1985). Prognostic risk assessment in primary breast cancer by behavioral and immunological parameters. *Health Psychol.* 4:99–113.

Melnechuk, T. (1985). Why has psychoneuroimmunology been controversial? *Advances* 2:22–38.

Naor, D. (1979). Suppressor cells: Permitters and promoters of malignancy? *Adv. Cancer Res.* 29:45–125.

Newberry, B.H., A.G. Liebelt, and D.A. Boyle (1984). Variables in behavioral oncology: Overview and assessment of current issues. In B.H. Fox and B.H. Newberry (eds.), *Impact of Psychoendocrine Systems in Cancer and Immunity.* Lewiston, N.Y.: C.J. Hogrefe, pp. 225–57.

North, R. (1985). Down-regulation of the antitumor immune response. *Adv. Cancer Res.* 45:1–43.

Plaut, M. (1987). Lymphocyte hormone receptors. *Ann. Rev. Immunol.* 5:621–69.

Rees, R. and S. Ali (1985). Antitumor lymphocyte responses. In B.W. Hancock and A.M. Ward (eds.), *Immunological Aspects of Cancer*. Boston: Martinus Nijhoff, pp. 11–50.

Riley, V. (1981). Psychoneuroendocrine influences on immunocompetence and neoplasia. *Science* 212:1100–1109.

Rosenberg, S. and M. Lotze (1986). Cancer immunotherapy using interleukin-2 and interleukin-2-activated lymphocytes. *Ann. Rev. Immunol.* 4:681–709.

Roszman, T. and W. Brooks (1985). Neural modulation of immune function. *J. Neuroimmunol.* 10:59–69.

Shavit, Y. and F. Martin (1987). Opiates, stress, and immunity: Animal studies. *Ann. Behav. Med.* 9:11–15.

Shavit, Y., G. Terman, F. Martin, J. Lewis, J. Liebeskind, and R. Gale (1985). Stress, opioid peptides, the immune system, and cancer. *J. Immunol.* 135:834s–37s.

Sklar, L. and H. Anisman (1979). Stress and coping factors influence tumor growth. *Science* 205:513–15.

Sklar, L. and H. Anisman (1981). Stress and cancer. *Psychol. Bull.* 89:369–406.

Sontag, S. (1978). *Illness as Metaphor*. New York: Farrar, Straus & Giroux.

Stutman, O. (1985). Immunological surveillance revisited. In A.E. Reif and M.S. Mitchell (eds.), *Immunity to Cancer*. New York: Academic Press, pp. 323–45.

Talmadge, J. and W. Alvord (1987). Editorial: Stress factors and breast cancer outcome. *J. Clin. Oncol.* 5:333–34.

Teshoma, H. and C. Kubo (1984). Changes in immune response and tumor growth in mice depend on the duration of stress. In B.H. Fox and B.H. Newberry (eds.), *Impact of Psychoendocrine Systems in Cancer and Immunity*. Lewiston, N.Y.: C.J. Hogrefe, pp. 208–24.

Thomas, L. (1982). On immunosurveillance in human cancer. *Yale J. Biol. Med.* 55:329–33.

Uchida, A. (1986). The cytolytic and regulatory role of natural killer cells in human neoplasia. *Biochim. Biophys. Acta* 865:329–40.

Visintainer, M., J. Volpicelli, and M. Seligman (1982). Tumor rejection in rats after inescapable or escapable shock. *Science* 216:437–39.

# PART XII

# Research Methods in Psychooncology

# 62

# Research Methods in Psychooncology

David F. Cella, Paul B. Jacobsen, and Lynna M. Lesko

Having reviewed the many psychosocial aspects of cancer treatment and survival as they relate to patients, family, and staff, this book closes with a perspective on research. Some of the key methodological considerations in planning and conducting studies in this field are outlined in this chapter. It also provides a historical background, identifies potential funding sources, and offers practical guidelines for approaching some of the perils and pitfalls identified by others (Yates and Edwards, 1984). We encourage beginning investigators to be creative, flexible, and adaptive in their efforts to overcome these potential obstacles. This chapter provides a departure point for further reading and a review of methods and measures that can be applied to clinical research in psychooncology.

## HISTORY AND RESEARCH PRIORITIES

Systematic research in psychooncology is a recent endeavor. Before 1970 research on psychosocial issues in cancer was noticeably absent. There was no formal governmental support for such research until the cancer control effort that began with the National Cancer Plan in 1972 (Holland, 1984). Most philanthropic support and individual efforts were previously directed toward patient education and service, with the task of research left only to a few highly motivated individuals. Consequently, the field of psychooncology is quite young in relation to its parent disciplines. Before 1972, research in psychooncology suffered from the limitation that most investigators were either social scientists with little knowledge of oncology or oncologists with insufficient knowledge of social science or psychology. Notable exceptions were Sutherland's group in the 1950s and Weisman's Project Omega in the 1970s (see Chapter 1).

Until the Division of Cancer Control and Rehabilitation was established by the National Cancer Program

within the National Cancer Institute (NCI) in 1972, there was no U.S. governmental unit systematically addressing problems of prevention, treatment, rehabilitation, and palliative care in cancer patients. In 1975 the first conference was held to review the research directions in these areas (Cullen et al., 1976). Participants from the disciplines of rehabilitation, oncology, psychiatry, psychology, social work, and nursing convened to discuss common interests and patient needs. Support was generated for demonstration studies and investigator-initiated research. Later reorganization led to the present Division of Cancer Prevention and Control (DCPC), which reviews the psychooncological studies submitted to the NCI.

A review of research opportunities in 1982 led DCPC to increase its emphasis on prevention and intervention strategies. At that time the division put forth a formal definition of its purpose: "Cancer control is the reduction of cancer incidence, morbidity, and mortality through an orderly sequence from research on interventions and their impact in defined populations to the broad, systematic application of the research results" (Greenwald and Cullen, 1985). Accompanying this broad definition is the concept of phased research in cancer, which maintains a connection on one end to basic research and on the other end to large-scale demonstration programs. The five research phases follow a logical progression from hypothesis development to demonstration and implementation in the community at large (see Fig. 62-1). Because most research in psychooncology fits this broad definition, it is advisable to consider these phases when conceptualizing research studies, particularly those that will be submitted for governmental funding.

*Phase I studies* (hypothesis development) seek to identify and define clinically relevant problems in cancer and develop hypotheses about possible intervention strategies that are testable in later phases of re-

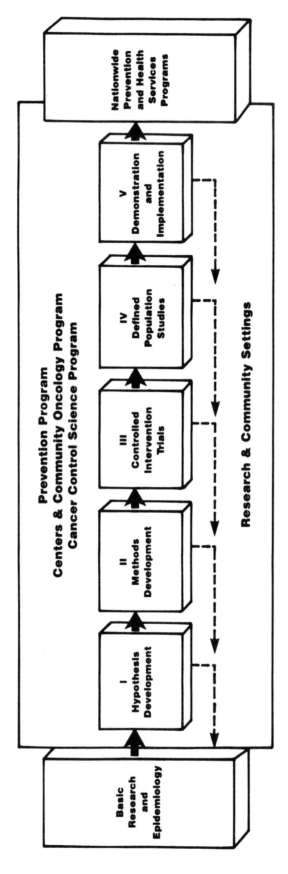

**Figure 62-1.** Phases in cancer control research.

search. Many studies to date have necessarily been hypothesis-gathering, clinical Phase I studies. *Phase II studies* (methods development) address development and testing of assessment instruments and procedures to conduct pilot studies. These have figured prominently in early psychooncology studies in which instrument development has been central to the ability to proceed to Phase III and IV studies (testing proposed interventions). Phase II studies are exceedingly important and yet undervalued by investigators. It is only after successful methods development that a large-scale intervention study can be considered feasible and its conclusions valid. Phase III and IV studies are intervention trials. *Phase III studies* (controlled-intervention trials) focus on successful research management; *Phase IV studies* require sampling of specific (defined) populations. *Phase V studies* (demonstration and implementation) are those that apply effective interventions in large community trials and test their effectiveness on a public health basis. Nationwide cancer education programs and public screening clinics are good examples of such large-scale implementation research.

In the early 1980s, concurrent with the establishment of DCPC by NCI, the American Cancer Society (ACS) began actively assembling acknowledged experts in the field of psychooncology as part of their effort to encourage research in psychological and behavioral areas. In 1981, 60 clinical investigators in the medical, behavioral, and social sciences held a working conference to identify and establish priorities for research and education concerning psychosocial and behavioral problems in cancer. As a result of this conference, six major areas of research were identified: (1) adaptation to cancer and psychosocial interventions to improve general adjustment, (2) biobehavioral interventions in behavioral medicine and their application to cancer, (3) behavioral and psychosocial research in childhood cancer, (4) behavioral, psychological, and social determinants of cancer risk, prevention, and early detection, (5) psychopharmacological applications to cancer, and (6) attitudes, communication, and teaching models (ACS, 1982).

The primary outcome of this 1981 conference was the recognition of the critical need for improved assessment methodology in psychosocial and behavioral cancer research. The investigators proposed several steps to address the need: critique available measuring instruments, explore necessary modifications of those instruments, and design new measures where none existed. A second ACS conference, convened in 1983, outlined the core issues in psychometric assessment of cancer patients (ACS, 1984). The major problem identified was that most available measures were inappropriate because they were designed for assessment

**Table 62-1**  Important areas in psychooncology

| Areas | Specific components |
|---|---|
| Patient characteristics | Physical performance |
| | Somatic functioning: pain, nausea, vomiting |
| | Psychological functioning: distress, anxiety, depression |
| | Cognitive functioning |
| | Quality of life: work, social, leisure, sexual |
| Social environment of the patient | Family |
| | Social support |
| | Cultural influences |
| Treatment environment of the patient | Satisfaction with treatment |
| | Perceptions of health care |
| | Physician–patient communication |

of either physicially healthy individuals or those who were psychiatrically impaired. Such instruments were poorly applicable to assessment of psychologically healthy individuals with cancer.

A useful tripartite framework for research in psychooncology emerged from this 1983 ACS conference. Research issues were broken down into three conceptual areas: characteristics of the patients being treated, characteristics of the social environment of the patient, and characteristics of the treatment environment. Table 62-1 outlines these three general areas and details the specific components of these areas that were thought to be influential. Patient research areas included subjective experience (anxiety, depression, hypochondriasis, demoralization, hopelessness, and cognitive function), somatic function (pain, nausea, vomiting, and sexual functioning), and quality of life (work, family relations, social functioning, leisure activities, physical status, and disease and treatment impacts). Social environment issues included general family functioning during illness, family and social communication, cultural influences, and social support as a buffer against distress of illness. The treatment environment was also seen to have had an important bearing on patients' adaptation to illness, adherence to treatment, and quality of life. The major issues in this domain included patient satisfaction, perceptions of health care, and communication between the patient and the health care provider.

These three broad domains clearly overlap and interact with each other, suggesting that comprehensive multidisciplinary research programs are valuable when addressing the range of research questions in the field. To facilitate multidisciplinary research, the NCI supported the formation of the Psychosocial Collaborative Oncology Group (PSYCOG) in 1977 under the chairmanship of Arthur Schmale. For a decade, this multi-center group (University of Rochester, Johns Hopkins, and Memorial Sloan-Kettering Cancer Center) carried out studies addressing the prevalence of psychiatric disorders and cognitive dysfunction in cancer patients, the development of brief assessment tools to measure adjustment to illness, and the use of psychotropic drugs in cancer patients.

In 1976 the Cancer and Leukemia Group B (CAL-GB) became the first NCI-supported clinical trials group to add psychiatry to its multimodal constituency. This permitted the first collection of sociodemographic and quality-of-life data on patients receiving treatment on national protocols. Many psychological and social questions can only be answered with such large samples in which disease and treatment variables are controlled. Even with minimal funding support, "companion" studies that add a psychosocial component to an existing experimental design can address many important research questions that are only possible with large multicenter samples. For example, difference in quality of life across treatment arms can be assessed in protocols that randomize patients after they have been stratified according to important clinical and prognostic variables.

Since 1980, the European Organization for Research and Treatment of Cancer (EORTC) has made major strides in including quality-of-life questions in EORTC treatment protocols (Aaronson, 1986). Their recent collaboration with the World Health Organization (WHO) is aimed at developing and testing a quality-of-life instrument that can be used across diverse cultures. When appropriate norms are developed for this instrument, it may have broad research and clinical applications.

## SEEKING FUNDING SOURCES

Undertaking any large study without the cooperation of a multidisciplinary team is virtually impossible today. This team should include an individual or small group of individuals whose specified job or jobs is the actual execution of the study, management of data entry, and use of statistical software. Consultation from a biostatistician is usually mandatory for initial study design and later data analysis. Support for such teams is expensive. After a research question has been identified and pilot data obtained, most investigators begin to seek outside funding sources. In the past decade the number of funding sources for psychooncology studies has grown tremendously.

There has also been a recognition of a shortage of trained social scientists who are willing to make a major commitment to oncology. The DCPC at NCI has developed initiatives that offer support for research

done in pursuit of the doctoral degree when the work relates to cancer. The NCI also supports career development awards encouraging social scientists to become active in cancer prevention and control research. Likewise, the DCPC often targets specific areas for research. These areas are listed in the NIH *Guide to Grants and Contracts* (Distribution Center, National Institute of Health, Bethesda, Maryland 20892), in the form of Requests for Proposals (RFPs), and Requests for Applications (RFAs).

A new investigator in the psychological, social, and behavioral aspects of cancer should also be aware of other organizations such as the American Cancer Society and the Leukemia Society of America that encourage psychological research. Recognizing the dearth of accomplished investigators in this field, they too have initiatives to encourage and train new investigators. Support via the ACS is provided by means of Research and Clinical Investigation grants and through grants in Support of Personnel for Research. Descriptive brochures are available on request from the American Cancer Society (ACS, 3340 Peachtree Road, NE, Atlanta, GA 30026). The Leukemia Society of America (733 Third Avenue, New York, New York 10021) has developed a funding track for new and young investigators at different levels of their research careers. Fellows, special fellows, and scholars' grants are available that provide salary support for researchers for 2, 3, and 5 years, respectively. To meet other financial needs of researchers, the society has developed two additional grants: short-term scientific exchange and travel grants to promote the exchange of research information, and the President's Research Development Award to cover expenses for critical research projects when funding is not immediately available.

## DESIGNING A RESEARCH STUDY

With this historical background in psychooncology research in place, we will proceed to more general considerations in research design. Examples are presented from psychological and behavioral aspects of cancer as they relate to the general issues of research methodology in this field.

Research design refers to the plan, structure, and organization of data collection—In other words, the selection of the patients to be studied, time of the study, and the method for collecting and measuring the information. While principles of research design are generally straightforward, their application to research in psychooncology is often complex. Difficulties arise for several reasons, including limitations in access to patients, imprecise research questions, and inadequate measuring instruments. To help readers avoid these and other problems in conducting psychooncology research, we review in the remainder of this chapter the major stages in designing a study, specifically, formulating the research question, reviewing the literature, determining which patients to study, selecting the appropriate variables and measuring instruments, and evaluating the design's validity or "soundness."

## Formulating the Question

Research questions usually arise out of clinical experience or from the suggestions of oncologists caring for patients. Interest in a particular problem leads to a review of the literature about clinical issues and prior research in the area. This in turn serves to refine the question. It is useful to ask whether the research question is one that will have some application to clinical care, or to the advancement of theoretical understanding. A research question must also be examined in terms of whether it can be answered in a particular context, given the number of available patients, existing instrumentation, and uncontrollable confounding variables. This is why pilot studies to determine study feasibility is important.

## Reviewing the Literature

An extensive review of the clinical and research literature is important because it provides information about who has already examined the question, about how thoroughly the question has been studied, about the adequacy of previous designs and available instruments, and about the relevance of the question. The advent of computer-assisted literature searches provides, at a very low cost, extensive information about past studies. Unfortunately there is no single abstracting service that searches all the relevant journals, because psychooncology crosses several disciplines. For example, *Index Medicus* does not include many social science journals, whereas *Psychological Abstracts* is weak in its coverage of medical journals. It is best not to rely on computer searches at the exclusion of recent review articles that permit working backward from the reference list. Proceedings of recent scientific meetings at which psychosocial and behavioral aspects of cancer have been presented are also useful. Psychooncology research is frequently presented at meetings of the American Cancer Society, the American Society of Clinical Oncology, the Society of Behavioral Medicine, and the American Psychological Association.

## Determining Feasibility

The feasibility of a study must be considered in the context of collaboration with medical oncology per-

sonnel. The first issue faced by the researcher is that the access to patients is determined by both the physician responsible for the patient and the oncology treatment team. The most useful approach is to become a part of that team, learning the clinical problems of patients, families, and staff, and then to introduce a social science perspective to those problems. The result of this approach is that collaborative research follows naturally and the research questions asked are assured of being both appropriate and relevant. Many elaborate studies are planned without giving due consideration to developing collaborative ties with the physicians, nurses, social workers, and clerical staff responsible for patient care and hospital administration. Although there may initially appear to be adequate numbers of patients or families in a particular setting, actual accrual may identify far fewer subjects than anticipated. Very often, this is due to insufficient motivation on the part of the treatment staff to collaborate or even support a study. Studies in which all participants feel a commitment and a sense of participation are far more likely to be successful.

Time and effort must be devoted not only to developing working relationships with staff, but also to the needs of patients and families. Psychosocial questions are often viewed as gratuitously intrusive, and they must therefore be carefully and parsimoniously drafted. Refusal rates as high as 53% have been reported due to physician, patient, and family resistance arising from their perception of psychological research as irrelevant if not intrusive (McCorkle et al., 1985). Pilot testing of instruments helps to determine acceptability to physicians, patients, and families; furthermore, a well-written consent form can prepare patients for the measures to be administered by advising them of the nature and purpose of the inquiries.

## Patient Selection

### SAMPLING

Sampling is the process of accruing research participants from the target population. For example, if one is interested in studying patients' quality of life or psychological response to treatments for lung cancer, the most representative sample would be randomly selected from among all patients receiving those treatments. With the participation of many hospitals throughout the country utilizing identical treatment protocols in carefully defined patient groups, the national clinical trials groups come closest to providing this opportunity. Conclusions from a well-designed study using patients from numerous hospitals have a great deal more generalizability, or external validity, than conclusions drawn from a study done at one hospital. However, very few investigators have access to multihospital clinical trials groups. A more common strategy is to study a representative or random sample of lung cancer patients at a given hospital. One might study every eligible patient or, if resources do not permit, every third patient who comes to an outpatient clinic. Without such a strategy, the cohort of participants will likely be reduced to a "sample of convenience," in which people are studied according to the availability of the researchers or participant accessibility. This approach is less desirable than random sampling, because study conclusions may be biased by variables that are related to the selection method. For example, a researcher might have more time for interviewing patients during a holiday period, and therefore draw a disproportionate number of patients into the study at that time. Because it is also true that certain types of patients might be more willing to come to the clinic during the holiday period (e.g., those in full-time employment or students away at college), the resulting sample could be biased in its representation of the population. Similarly, a telephone study that relies on reaching people at home may end up over-representing homebound or nonworking patients.

## INCLUSION AND EXCLUSION CRITERIA

The knowledge that many studies are limited by the number of available participants is very important when establishing criteria for including or excluding potential study participants. It is in the interest of study feasibility to set minimal exclusion criteria so as not to turn away any potential participants. However, most research in psychooncology requires consideration of the patient's disease and treatment as well as personality and cognitive functioning. All these considerations may in themselves alter psychological responses and therefore dilute study results. The answer to how much or how little control should be exercised over inclusion and exclusion criteria depends on the question being asked in the study. For example, if one were seeking to determine the psychological impact of receiving a diagnosis of breast cancer, it would be important to control for the stage of disease. Stage I disease, which is known to be largely curable, and stage IV disease, which is far less responsive to available treatments, would be likely to evoke different psychological responses. Unless the study's purpose was to examine differences across stage of disease, it would be inadvisable to include all stages in the eligibility requirements.

Issues related to psychosocial development often arise in determining subject eligibility. Consider a study seeking to examine the adjustment of men to testicular cancer. The meaning of such a tumor may be very different for a single 20-year-old who is trying to develop an intimate relationship, compared to a 30-year-old who is married with two children. Age and developmental phase of life are variables that deserve careful consideration in setting eligibility requirements. There are other cases, however, in which it may not be known, or may be open to debate, whether age or developmental phase are important variables with which to determine inclusion or exclusion. For example, the development of anticipatory nausea or other treatment side effects may not be strikingly different across age groups, so exclusion on that basis would deprive the investigators of potential individuals for study.

In general, when no known relationship exists between entry characteristics and the responses of interest, the investigator ought not to exclude patients simply on the basis of being different on some variable at entry. It is important to keep in mind that even though two sites of cancer may be treated by different means, the psychological issues being studied may not be so different. The work of Jessop and Stein (1984), and that of Cassileth and colleagues (1984), has suggested that there is probably not as much specificity in the psychological responses and coping of patients to different illnesses as we might imagine. If an investigator is skeptical about including different disease sites or different treatment regimens in a protocol looking at responses to illness, there is always the possibility of recording these variables when the data are collected and looking at subgroup differences in a post hoc analysis. If inclusion criteria were strictly set, these differences could never be examined because all participants would be equivalent on these questionable entry characteristics.

## SAMPLE SIZE

A question frequently asked of methodological consultants is, "How many patients do I need to conduct this study?" Very often the question should be rephrased to, "Do I have a sufficient number of available patients to answer the study question, and will I be able to enlist these participants in my study?" This rephrasing is given as an example of the reality considerations that confront the investigator. Without prior knowledge of the available number of patients, and without prior support of the medical personnel to help enroll and study these patients, the finest design will simply remain an idea.

Sample size is important because it can affect power, or the likelihood of a study to yield accurately significant results. Another influence affecting power is effect size, which refers to the extent or degree to which the phenomenon under study varies across groups. (Cohen, 1977). Power analysis is a statistical technique that can be used to examine the relationships between sample size, effect size, and power. For example, power analysis may indicate that, for a given effect size, the likelihood of obtaining significant ($p < .05$) results would be only 20% with 30 subjects but would be 80% if the sample size were increased to 100 subjects. In other words, a larger sample size would increase the sensitivity of the research design to detect the true effect. Differences in effect size also have to be considered in determining sample size, with larger samples being needed to detect smaller or more subtle effects. Thus, a small sample size may be all that is necessary to establish that relaxation training reduces anticipatory nausea in chemotherapy patients; however, dozens of people may be required to demonstrate that quality of life is better on one treatment arm than in another, and hundreds may be needed to test whether psychological distress or depression present at the outset of therapy is associated with length of survival.

## Variables

### INDEPENDENT AND DEPENDENT VARIABLES

The terms independent variable and dependent variable are derived from the classic experimental design in which the setting (laboratory) is controlled, the independent variable is manipulated along certain dimensions, and the dependent variable is measured for changes caused by the manipulation of the independent variable. Most research in psychooncology does not take place in a laboratory and precludes the ability to control the setting to this degree.

Because of the relative lack of experimental control in clinical situations, the issue of confounding variables presents itself in practically every clinical study. A confounding variable is one that may systematically affect results and thereby account for the findings assumed by the investigator to be attributable to the independent variables. For example, in a study examining the impact of delirium on the development of depression one must consider other variables that could cause depression (e.g., current medications, type of disease, extent of disease, personal history or family history of depression, and social support). After considering all the possible confounding variables, the task is to control them. One strategy is to enter them as independent variables into the design, but this quickly becomes a problem because more variables require more subjects. Another strategy is to measure these potentially confounding variables and then to analyze them after the study is completed to see if they are significantly associated with the dependent variables. Those that are associated with the dependent variables can be entered into the analysis as covariates. This technique allows one to control statistically for the effects of other variables before examining the independent–dependent variable relationship of interest. This strategy is recommended when the potentially confounding variables are more of a "nuisance" to the investigator than a subject of interest. If these confounding variables are of interest themselves, then they should be included as independent variables in their own right.

### Selection of Measures

One of the most difficult tasks in doing research in psychooncology is to select measures and develop questions that obtain sufficient information, are sensitive to the physical condition of patients who are ill and tire easily, are perceived as nonintrusive, and have a clearly explained potential contribution to future patient care. Table 62-2 lists measures that have been used to assess variables of interest in psychooncology research.

Although many areas of psychooncology are still in need of adequate measuring instruments, there have been a number of notable developments in the assessment area. For example, in the area of patient adjustment, Derogatis and colleagues have put forth a number of self-report, structured interview, and observer-rated measures that assess disease-specific adjustments to illness. The Psychosocial Adjustment to Illness Scale (PAIS) and its self-report version (PAIS-SR) measure seven areas of adjustment: health care orientation, vocational environment, domestic environment, sexual relationships, extended-family relationships, social environment, and psychological distress (Derogatis and Lopez, 1983). The PAIS and PAIS-SR can be applied to medical patients other than those with cancer, facilitating questions about cancer-specific impact. Similarly, it can be used across disease sites and treatments. Another advantage of the instrument is that, with the exception of health care orientation, the subtests can be administered to cancer survivors who have completed treatment, permitting the collection of longitudinal data.

For many areas of psychooncology research there are no assessment instruments that have been developed specifically for use with cancer patients. In such instances an investigator must choose between two less desirable options. The first is to construct one's own instrument based on clinical knowledge of the problem. Test construction is itself a science, and putting a new instrument through all the necessary steps to demonstrate its psychometric properties may take years. For those who wish to undertake this task, consultation

**Table 62-2** Commonly used measures in psychooncology research

| Variable | Measure | Reference |
|---|---|---|
| Physical status | Karnofsky Performance Status Scale | Karnofsky and Burchenal (1949) |
| | ECOG Performance Status Scale | Zubrod et al. (1960) |
| | WHO Drug Toxicity Scale | Miller et al. (1981) |
| Pain | McGill Pain Questionnaire | Melzack (1975) |
| | Visual Analog Pain Scale | Scott and Huskisson (1976) |
| Nausea and vomiting | Morrow Assessment of Nausea and Emesis | G.R. Morrow (1984) |
| | Visual Analog Nausea Scale | Redd et al. (1982) |
| Sexual functioning | Derogatis Sexual Functioning Inventory | Derogatis (1975c) |
| Cognitive functioning | Mini-Mental State Examination | Folstein et al. (1975) |
| | Cognitive Capacity Screening Examination | Jacobs et al. (1977) |
| Psychological distress | Symptom Check List-90 | Derogatis (1975b) |
| | Brief Symptom Inventory | Derogatis and Spencer (1982) |
| | Profile of Mood States | McNair et al. (1971) |
| | Multiple Affect Adjective Checklist | Zuckerman et al. (1965) |
| Psychopathology | Minnesota Multiphasic Personality Inventory | Hathaway and McKinley (1967) |
| Depression | Beck Depression Inventory | Beck et al. (1961) |
| | Hamilton Depression Scale | Hamilton (1960) |
| Anxiety | Hamilton Anxiety Scale | Hamilton (1959) |
| | State–Trait Anxiety Inventory | Spielberger (1983) |
| Coping and adjustment | Impact of Event Scale | Horowitz et al. (1979) |
| | Ways of Coping Checklist | Lazarus and Folkman (1984) |
| | Psychosocial Adjustment to Illness Scale | Derogatis and Lopez (1983) |
| Staff stress | Maslach Burnout Inventory | Maslach and Jackson (1981) |
| Quality of life | Global Adjustment to Illness Scale | Derogatis (1975a) |
| | Psychosocial Adjustment to Illness Scale | Derogatis and Lopez (1983) |
| | QL-Index | Spitzer et al. (1981) |
| | Functional Living Index-Cancer | Schipper et al. (1984) |
| Social adjustment | Social Adjustment Scale | Weissman and Bothwell (1976) |
| Family functioning | Family Environment Scale | Moos and Moos (1981) |
| Stressful life events | PERI Life-Events Scale | Dohrenwend et al. (1978) |
| | Recent Life Changes Questionnaire | Rahe (1975) |
| Psychiatric symptoms | Schedule for Affective Disorders and Schizophrenia | Endicott and Spitzer (1978) |
| | Structured Clinical Interview for DSM-III-R | Spitzer et al. (1986) |
| Social support | Interpersonal Support Evaluation List | Cohen et al. (1985) |

with a statistical expert and familiarization with textbooks on scale construction (e.g., Nunnally, 1978) are recommended.

The second and more frequently exercised option is to select an established instrument that was developed for use with populations other than patients with cancer. This places the investigator in the uncomfortable position of worrying that the really important information may be untapped by an insensitive measure. Consequently, the tendency is to burden the patient with several measures and hope that one or more of them will be sensitive. For many reasons (e.g. responder

burden; experiment-wide error), this practice is inadvisable. It is useful to remember that as patient burden rises, accrual rate drops and attrition rate increases. Investigators are advised to keep the number of measures to a minimum. It is better to administer one well-aimed measure than to shoot haphazardly with many, hoping for the best.

Careful and parsimonious selection of measures should not be confused with the importance of assessing all the relevant variables. Particularly with treatment studies, multiple measures are preferred over single measures for two very distinct reasons. First, most outcomes being measured tend to have several dimensions and/or different vantage points along which they can be measured. For example, if one is trying to examine and seek methods to improve self-care and general well-being in patients who have been discharged home from the hospital, it may be necessary to obtain information from the patient, a family member, and an objective interviewer. Each of these sources of information provides different and potentially disparate data, so the omission of one or two of them would diminish the validity of the claim that ''self-care'' was assessed. Thus, in many instances the use of both self-report and observer-rated measures is needed.

The second reason for preference of multiple measures over a single measure is breadth of coverage. It may be worthwhile to examine dependent variables that are peripheral to the central medical study because they may provide useful information when the study itself yields negative results. A very good example of this is the assessment of quality of life in clinical trials that compare two or more treatment regimens. Often, a large-scale clinical trial will contrast treatment regimens that possess different potentials for toxicity. The advantage of adding quality-of-life measurement in such studies is that differences in quality of life become part of the test of efficacy of treatment. When differences in response rate and survival are similar, quality-of-life differences become important, especially in choosing among palliative treatments. This was demonstrated in the comparison of two chemotherapy protocols for treatment of lung carcinoma, for example, within the cooperative clinical trials setting (Silberfarb et al., 1983). Companion psychosocial assessment can also add information about treatment effects that can be included in later treatment considerations. For example, neuropsychological studies have shown that cranial irradiation as CNS prophylaxis in childhood acute lymphocytic leukemia is associated with long-term deficits in attention and overall intellectual function (Rowland et al., 1984). This has led to the limiting of prophylactic cranial irradiation to those children considered to be at high risk for CNS recurrence. It is interesting that despite these and other demonstrations of the value of assessing nonmedical sequelae of cancer treatment, fewer than 5% of clinical trials reviewed as of 1982 by the Department of Health and Human Services (DHHS) were using any form of psychosocial measure, and the majority of those were simply physician ratings of performance status.

Given the difficulties in constructing new tests, it is likely that most investigators will continue to select a measure from among existing measures and supplement it with some study-specific interview questions. Therefore, it is useful to review some basic issues about reliability and validity of measurement that can be applied when searching for an appropriate measure.

Table 62-2 lists many frequently used measures in psychooncology research and includes references describing the measures' psychometric properties.

## Reliability of Measurement

Reliability refers to the dependability of a measure and its ability to yield the same score with repeated use (Cronbach et al., 1972). Generally speaking, a test cannot be considered valid until it can be demonstrated that it possesses satisfactory reliability. Depending on the measure being used, there are up to four different kinds of reliability, although not all four are necessarily important for a given test.

*Test–retest reliability* refers to the stability of measurements over time. Will a measure of family adjustment to illness give the same score if readministered 1 month later?

*Alternate-form reliability* deals with the question of whether two versions of a test measure the same thing. These two versions are usually administered at different times, so that alternate form reliability is limited by the test–retest reliability of either form. Only a few measures (e.g., Spielberger's State–Trait Anxiety Inventory) actually have alternate forms; however, they can be very useful when one is doing a study involving repeated measurements over a short period of time.

*Internal consistency* examines whether certain items within a test contribute as expected to the total score obtained. If a test is made up of 20 items that purport to measure one construct (e.g., coping style or demoralization), then all responses to each of the 20 items should correlate positively with the overall score.

*Interrater reliability* is generally the only form of reliability that an investigator will need to report when using an existing instrument. Any time the unit of measurement is an observer rating, it is important to demonstrate that this rating is consistent across different observers. The usual way to do this is to use two or more raters who are unbiased by knowledge of the study hypotheses or status of the patient on the critical variables. The two raters then independently assess and quantify the patient's behavior on the rating scale, and these independent ratings are then correlated with each other to determine the extent of concordance or agreement.

## Measurement Validity

Validity addresses the extent to which a test really measures what it claims to measure. Does a score on a depression scale really measure depression when the patient is physically ill, or does it mistakenly identify symptoms of disease as somatic symptoms of depression? Test items designed to assess vegetative symptoms of depression often have compromised validity when administered to patients with cancer (Bukberg et al., 1984; Endicott, 1984).

Validity can be elusive and complex, and may never be fully obtained. Three central components of validity are content validity, criterion-related validity, and construct validity.

## CONTENT VALIDITY

Face validity (does a measure appear to measure what it claims to measure?) and true content validity (does a measure successfully sample all the domains typically associated with the variable?) constitute content validity. A scale measuring compliance with treatment regimens has face validity if it asks about things like keeping appointments. However, the measure may lack content validity if it fails to ask patients about other aspects of compliance such as missed doses of oral medication. Pill taking is generally viewed as a necessary component of compliance with a treatment regimen, so a measure that does not include this domain may be considered to have insufficient content validity.

Content validity is not a great concern when a test has been constructed on an empirical basis. The Minnesota Multiphasic Personality Inventory (MMPI, Hathaway and McKinley, 1983) is a good example of an empirically derived test in that its subscales were drawn from the responses of specified groups. With such a test, it is less important to know whether all domains of the construct have been sampled, because a criterion group was used to establish the items of the scale.

## CRITERION-RELATED VALIDITY

This refers to the ability of a measure to correlate with the score on another more widely accepted measure or indicator of the same thing (*concurrent validity*), or to predict a relevant future behavior (*predictive validity*). A measure of quality of life during treatment has concurrent validity if it correlates significantly with measures of life satisfaction, pain, distress, or treatment toxicity given at the same time. It also has predictive validity if it is correlated with measures of life satisfaction and adjustment administered after treatment has been completed.

## CONSTRUCT VALIDITY

The most elusive and the most important of all forms of validity (Cronbach and Meehl, 1955), construct valid-

ity must be conceived within a theoretical framework and is central to the measurement of any abstract construct. In social science research, construct validity is a concern when measuring any theoretical construct, such as depression, anxiety, hopelessness, family enmeshment, adaptation, coping style, fighting spirit, or quality of life. Construct validation of any measure involves three steps. First, the theoretical relationships between related concepts must be clarified. Second, the statistical relationships between the measures of these concepts must be examined. Third, the empirical data must be analyzed and interpreted in terms of how they clarify the construct validity of the measure in question. Campbell and Fiske (1959) have discussed the terms convergent validity and divergent validity in this regard. To demonstrate *convergent validity,* one must show that a test correlates with other measures of the same thing. To demonstrate *divergent validity,* one must show the reverse, that the test does not correlate with measures of other constructs. Construct validity becomes particularly relevant in psychooncology when, as described earlier, constructs such as depression are contaminated by the concurrent presence of physical symptoms that may not reflect true depression in the physically ill. Standardized depression scales may require revision to account for the overlap of symptoms when measuring depression or other psychological conditions that have physiological correlates in healthy individuals (Bukberg et al., 1984; Plumb and Holland, 1977).

## Design Validity

An important consideration in conducting any study is to evaluate the soundness or validity of one's research design. Are there any variables extraneous to the phenomenon under study that are influencing or could serve to explain the results? Threats to the soundness or internal validity of a research design can include the passage of time, the measurement process, and the sampling process.

Two threats are commonly present in any study that involves the passage of time: history and maturation. The threat of *history* is that some unplanned or uncontrolled event may occur between pretest and posttest. Imagine a study examining the impact of a patient education program on compliance with treatment. Unless there is a randomly assigned control group that does not receive the program, or that receives some placebo program, one can never be sure that measured changes were due to treatment. It is possible that there was a major campaign to improve cancer awareness and treatment compliance, which was launched between pretest and posttest. Differences over time could just as likely be due to this campaign as to the educational program. In cases in which random assignment is not possible, historical effects can often be dealt with by staggering pretest and posttest times in a way that amounts to a series of replications at different time points.

*Maturation* of the participants can also explain differences over time. An example might be the effort to study the impact of cancer longitudinally on the sense of identity in adolescents with cancer over an extended period. Without an appropriate control or comparison group, one could not be certain whether the identity changes over time were due to the cancer experience or to maturation in general. One way to handle the problem of maturation is by including a pretest measure that tests the developmental trend and establishes its nature.

Threats that occur in the measurement process are testing and instrumentation. Asking a set of questions can itself induce change and therefore alter later responses to the same or similar questions. This phenomenon is reminiscent of the Hawthorne effect; that is, the knowledge of being studied is itself enough to induce change. Consider a lung cancer prevention program that includes an effort to reduce the number of cigarettes smoked per day. If the study begins by assessing in detail the average number of cigarettes, participants are likely to try to reduce their cigarette intake simply because they know they are being evaluated.

Threats related to *instrumentation* occur because a measure can lose its reliability or validity between pretest and posttest ("instrument decay"). This is one reason why the test–retest reliability of a measure is so important. Observational measures are particularly vulnerable to this threat. If one is measuring depression on a rating scale or assessing DSM-III diagnosis with observer ratings, it is very easy for raters to lose their reliability over time. This can result in the appearance of significant results when in fact only the measure has changed. For this reason, the reliability of raters over the course of a study period should be checked. Similarly, it is inadvisable to administer different instruments to test the same construct at pretest and posttest points, because the differences found could obviously be attributed to differences in the measure and not to true differences between groups.

Two other common threats to internal validity that result from imperfect sampling procedures are statistical regression and selection. *Statistical regression* refers to the probability that someone selected on the basis of a high pretest score will show a lower score at posttest. A study looking at the ability of relaxation training to reduce anxiety in patients before getting treatment is likely to yield significant results due to statistical regression alone if the participants are selected on the basis of high anxiety scores. This is one reason a randomly selected control group is important. The problem of *selection* refers to differences between

treatment and control groups that might have existed before the study itself began. In studying differences in adjustment between women who choose mastectomy over lumpectomy, or between women who choose breast reconstruction versus those who do not, how can the investigator be certain that these differences do not predate the treatment decision? In other words, would differences found between women be due to the personality characteristics that also entered into the decision about treatment, or due to the differential stressors that present themselves after receiving the selected treatment, or perhaps even to some unknown third confounding variable? The investigator must examine these potential biases by concurrent measurement of confounding variables and by ex post facto statistical control.

Most threats to internal validity can be effectively ruled out by the use of random assignment to treatment and control groups. However, in many contexts in which psychooncology research is conducted, random assignment is not possible. West (1986) has identified five strategies for reducing threats to internal validity. Listed in decreasing order of preference, these are: 1) random assignment to treatment groups whenever possible; 2) patchwork design improvements to address specific threats to internal validity; 3) ex post facto measurement and statistical adjustment (covariate analysis); 4) discussion of the current results in the context of a pattern that makes alternate explanations unlikely; and 5) reference to previous research that has effectively ruled out the alternate interpretations to which the current design is vulnerable. With each strategy adopted, the investigator is increasing the likelihood that extraneous variables are not responsible for the study results.

## SUMMARY

Psychooncology is an exciting and vibrant new discipline that examines the common ground between oncology, consultation–liaison psychiatry, health psychology, and social science. Opportunities for the study of adjustment to illness, psychopharmacology, neuropsychology, psychoneuroimmunology, quality of life, and the social environment of the cancer patient, family members, and medical staff are among the many new avenues currently being pursued. Improvements in methodology, measurement, and theoretical sophistication have recently elevated the discipline to one that allows the investigator to make valuable contributions to patient care, family adjustment, the health care delivery system, and cancer control.

## REFERENCES

Aaronson, N.K. (1986). Methodological issues in psychosocial oncology with special reference to clinical trials. In

V. Ventafridda, F.S.A.M. van Dam, R. Yancik, and M. Tamburini (eds.), *Assessment of Quality of Life and Cancer Treatment.* Amsterdam: Elsevier, pp. 19–28.

American Cancer Society (1982). Proceedings of the working conference on the psychological, social and behavioral medicine aspects of cancer: Research and professional education needs and directions for the 1980's. *Cancer* 50(Suppl):1919–78.

American Cancer Society (1984). Proceedings of the working conference on methodology in behavioral and psychosocial cancer research—1983. *Cancer* 53(Suppl.):2217–84.

Beck, A., C. Ward, M. Mendelson, J. Mock, and J. Erbaugh (1961). An inventory for measuring depression. *Arch. Gen. Psychiatry* 4:561–71.

Bukberg, J., D. Penman, and J.C. Holland (1984). Depression in hospitalized cancer patients. *Psychosom. Med.* 46:199–212.

Campbell, D.T. and D.W. Fiske (1959). Convergent and discriminant validation by the multitrait–multimethod matrix. *Psychol. Bull.* 56:85–105.

Cassileth, B.R., E.J. Lusk, T.B. Strouse, D.S. Miller, L.L. Brown, P.A. Cross, and A.N. Tenaglia (1984). Psychosocial status in chronic illness: A comparative analysis of six diagnostic groups. *N. Engl. J. Med.* 311:506–11.

Cohen, J. (1977). Statistical power analysis for the behavioral sciences. Orlando, Fla.: Academic Press.

Cohen, S., R.J. Mermelstein, T. Kamarck, and H. Hoberman (1985). Measuring the functional component of social support. In I.G. Sarason and B. Sarason (eds.), *Social Support: Theory, Research and Applications.* The Hague: Martinus Nijhoff.

Cronbach, L.J. and P.E. Meehl (1955). Construct validity in psychological tests. *Psychol. Bull.* 52:281–302.

Cronbach, L.J., G.C. Gleser, N. Rajaratnam, and H. Nanda, (1972). *The Dependability of Behavioral Measures: Theory of Generalizability for Scores and Profiles.* New York: Wiley.

Cullen, J.W., B.H. Fox, and R.N. Isom (1976). *Cancer: The Behavioral Dimensions.* U.S. Department of Health, Education and Welfare, National Cancer Institute.

Department of Health and Human Services (1982). *Compilation of Experimental Cancer Therapy Protocol Summaries,* 6th ed. Washington, D.C.: U.S. Government Printing Office.

Derogatis, L.R. (1975a). *Global Adjustment to Illness Scale.* Baltimore: Clinical Psychometric Research.

Derogatis, L.R. (1975b). *The SCL-90-R.* Baltimore: Clinical Psychometrics Research.

Derogatis, L.R. (1975c). *Derogatis Sexual Functioning Inventory (DSFI).* Baltimore: Clinical Psychometrics Research.

Derogatis, L.R. and P.M. Spencer (1982). *The Brief Symptom Inventory (BSI): Administration, Scoring and Procedures Manual—I.* Baltimore: Authors.

Derogatis, L.R. and M. Lopez (1983). *PAIS & PAIS-SR: Administration, Scoring and Procedures Manual—I.* Baltimore: Clinical Psychometric Research.

Dohrenwend, B.S., L. Krasnoff, and A.R. Askenasy (1978). Exemplification of a method of scaling life events: The PERI Life-Events Scale. *J. Health Soc. Behav.* 19:205–29.

Endicott, J. (1984). Measurement of depression in patients with cancer. *Cancer* 53(Suppl.):2243–48.

Endicott, J. and R. Spitzer (1978). A diagnostic interview: The schedule for affective disorders and schizophrenia. *Arch. Gen. Psychiatry* 35:837–44.

Folstein, M.F., S.E. Folstein, and P.R. McHugh (1975). "Mini-Mental State." *J. Psychiatr. Res.* 12:189–98.

Greenwald, P. and J.W. Cullen (1985). The new emphasis in cancer control. *J.N.C.I.* 74(3):543–51.

Hamilton, M. (1959). The assessment of anxiety states by rating. *Br. J. Med. Psychol.* 32:50–55.

Hamilton, M. (1960). Rating scale for depression. *J. Neurol. Neurosurg. Psychiatry* 23:56–62.

Hathaway, S.R. and J.C. McKinley (1967). *The Minnesota Multiphasic Personality Inventory: Manual for administration and scoring,* rev. ed. Minneapolis: University of Minnesota Press.

Hathaway, S.R. and J.C. McKinley (1951). *Minnesota Multiphasic Personality Inventory: Manual (rev.).* New York: Psychological Corp.

Holland, J.C.B. (1984). Need for improved psychosocial research methodology: Goals and potentials. *Cancer* 53(10)(Suppl.):2218–20.

Horowitz, M.J., N. Wilner, and W. Alvarez (1979). Impact of Event Scale: A measure of subjective stress. *Psychosom. Med.* 41:209.

Jacobs, J.W., M.R. Bernhard, A. Delgado, and J.J. Strain (1977). Screening for organic mental syndromes in the mentally ill. *Ann. Intern. Med.* 86:40–46.

Jessop, D.J. and R.E.K. Stein (1984). A non-categorical approach to psychosocial research. *J. Psychosoc. Oncol.* 1:61–64.

Karnofsky, D.A. and J.H. Burchenal (1949). The clinical evaluation of chemotherapeutic agents in cancer. In C.M. Macleod (ed.), *Evaluation of Chemotherapeutic Agents.* New York: Columbia University Press.

Lazarus, R.S. and S. Folkman (1984). *Stress, Appraisal, and Coping.* New York: Springer.

Maslach, C. and S.E. Jackson (1981). *Maslach Burnout Inventory: Research edition manual.* Palo Alto, Calif.: Consulting Psychologists Press.

McCorkle, R., N. Packard, and Landenburger, K. (1985). Subject accrual and attrition: Problems and solutions. *J. Psychosoc. Oncol.* 2(3/4):137–46.

McNair, D.M., M. Lorr, and L.F. Droppleman (1971). *EITS Manual for the Profile of Mood States.* San Diego, Calif.: Educational and Industrial Testing Service.

Melzack, R. (1975). The McGill Questionnaire: Major properties and scoring methods. *Pain* 1:277–99.

Miller, A., B. Hoogstraten, M. Staquet, and A. Winkler (1981). Reporting results of cancer treatment. *Cancer* 47:207–14.

Moos, R. and B. Moos (1981). *Family Environmental Scale Manual.* Palo Alto, Calif.: Consulting Psychologists Press.

Morrow, G.M., M. Feldstein, L.M. Adler, L.R. Derogatis, A.J. Enelow, C. Gates, J. Holland, N. Melisaratos, B. Murawski, D. Penman, A. Schmale, M. Schmitt, and I.

Morse (1981). Development of brief measures of psychosocial adjustment to medical illness applied to cancer patients. *Gen. Hosp. Psychiatry* 3:79–81.

Morrow, G.R. (1984). The assessment of nausea and vomiting: Past problems, current issues, and suggestions for future research. *Cancer* 53(Suppl.):2267–78.

Nunnally, J.C. (1978). *Psychometric theory,* 2nd ed. New York: McGraw-Hill.

Plumb, M.M. and J.C. Holland (1977). Comparative studies of psychological function in patients with advanced cancer—1. Self-reported depressive symptoms. *Psychosom. Med.* 39:264–76.

Rahe, R.H. (1975). Epidemiological studies of life change and illness. *Int. J. Psychiatr. Med.* 6:133–46.

Redd, W.H. and M.A. Andrykowski (1982). Behavioral interventions in cancer treatment: Controlling aversion reactions to chemotherapy. *J. Consult. Clin. Psychol.* 50:1018–29.

Redd, W.H., G.V. Andresen, and R.Y. Minagawa (1982). Hypnotic control of anticipatory emesis in patients receiving cancer chemotherapy. *J. Consult. Clin. Psychol.* 50:14–19.

Rowland, J.H., O.J. Glidewell, R.F. Sibley, J.C. Holland, R. Tull, A. Berman, M.L. Brecher, M. Harris, A.S. Glicksman, E. Forman, B. Jones, M.E. Cohen, P.K. Duffner, and A.I. Freeman (1984). Effects of different forms of central nervous system prophylaxis on neuropsychologic function in childhood leukemia. *J. Clin. Oncol.* 2:1327–35.

Schipper, H., J. Clinch, A. McMurray, and M. Levitt (1984). Measuring the quality of life of cancer patients: The Functional Living Index–Cancer: Development and validation. *J. Clin. Oncol.* 2:472–83.

Scott, P.J. and E.C. Huskisson (1976). Graphic representation of pain. *Pain* 2:175–87.

Silberfarb, P.M., J.C.B. Holland, D. Anbar, G. Bahna, L.H. Maurer, A.P. Chahinian, and R. Comis (1983). Psychological response of patients receiving two drug regimens for lung carcinoma. *Am. J. Psychiatry* 140:110–11.

Spielberger, C.D. (1983). *Manual for the State–Trait Anxiety Inventory.* Palo Alto, Calif.: Consulting Psychologists Press.

Spitzer, R.L., J.B.W. Williams, and M. Gibbon (1986). *Structured Clinical Interview for DSM-III-R Personality Disorders.* New York: Authors.

Spitzer, W., A. Dobson, J. Hall, E. Chesterman, J. Levi, R. Shepherd, R. Battista and B. Catchlove (1981). Measuring the quality of life of cancer patients: A concise QL index for use by physicians. *J. Chron. Dis.* 34:585–97.

Weissman, M.M. and S. Bothwell (1976). Assessment of social adjustment by patient self-report. *Arch. Gen. Psychiatry* 33:1111–15.

West, S.G. (1986). Beyond the laboratory experiment: Experimental and quasi-experimental designs for interventions in naturalistic settings. In P. Karoly (ed.), *Measurements Strategies in Health Psychology.* New York: Wiley.

Williams, A.W., J.R. Ware, and J.E. Donald (1981). A model of mental health, life events, and social circumstances applicable to general populations. *J. Health Soc. Behav.* 22:324–36.

Worden, J.W. (1984). Response. *Cancer* 53(10)(Suppl.): 2241–42.

Yates, J.W. and B. Edwards (1984). Practical concerns and pitfalls in measurement methodology. *Cancer* 53(10) (Suppl.): 2376–79.

Zubrod, C.G., M. Schneiderman, E. Frei, C. Brindley, G.L. Gold, B. Shnider, C. Orieto, J. Gorman, R. Jones, G. Jonsson, J. Colsky, T. Chalmers, B. Ferguson, M. Dederick, J. Holland, O. Selawry, W. Regelson, L. Lasagna, and P.H. Owens (1960). Appraisal of methods for the study of chemotherapy of cancer in man: Comparative therapeutic trial of nitrogen mustard and triethylene thiophosphoramide. *J. Chron. Dis.* 11:7–33.

Zuckerman, M., B. Lubin, and T. Robins (1965). *Manual for the Multiple Affect Adjective Checklist.* San Diego, Calif.: Educational and Industrial Testing Service.

# PART XIII

## Appendices

**Appendix A.** Childhood development

| Age stage | Physical | Cognitive |
|---|---|---|
| *Birth–2 years: Infancy to toddler* | Rapid growth and development; maturation of CNS with motor system, facilitating progression from coordinated sucking to directed vision, eye–hand coordination, grasping, object tracking, sitting with support, standing, and finally walking unaided; acquisition of deciduous teeth; refinement of grasping and releasing maneuvers such that by the end of the period most children can feed themselves, and put on and take off some clothes; acquisition of bladder and bowel control | *Sensorimotor Period:* Infant develops from dependency on reflex activity, to purposive, goal-oriented interaction with environment. Infant learns to differentiate between self and external world; child comes to see objects as separate from self (object concept) and develops capacity to represent objects and persons mentally in their absence (object permanency and representational ability; preconceptual). |
| *3–5 Years: Early childhood* | Development of gross motor coordination (manipulation of scissors, buttons, utensils) Early drawing Alteration in body proportions Hemispheric dominance established Early writing and printing | *Preoperational Period:* Transition to symbolic thought occurs paralleling developing language. Using words, child can talk about and imagine objects not present or events and feelings. Thinking is, however, egocentric; child is unable to take another's viewpoint and exerts little effort to adapt communication to listener's needs. Thinking is also limited by inability to take into account two aspects of observation or object simultaneously (nonconservation). Child also cannot differentiate between a symbol and the object it represents (Intuitive thinking; prelogical). |
| *6–11 Years: Middle childhood and latency* | Eruption of permanent teeth Elaboration of fine motor coordination Increase in athletic prowess<br><br>Onset of puberty (girls) | *Concrete Operational Period:* Stage characterized by acquisition of elemental logic about concrete events, perceptions, representations. Child demonstrates ability to understand relationships among observations and to show experience independent of thought. Principles of reversibility and conservation are learned: child realizes steps in problem solving can be reversed or retraced as can actions performed on objects. Egocentricism in this period limits child's ability to distinguish between what he or she thinks and what is. |

**Appendix A.** *continued*

| Age stage | Physical | Cognitive |
|---|---|---|
| *12–18 Years: Adolescence* | *Puberty*: Development of secondary sexual characteristics: menarche, breast development, axillary and pubic hair growth, chest expansion, change of voice, muscular development<br><br>Growth spurts with stature attaining full adult size by end of this age period | *Period of Formal Operations*: Mastery of ability to apply logical rules and reasoning to abstract problems and propositions—even to extent of including counterfactual thinking; adolescent is able to generate hypotheses, juggle many variables at a time and even to think about thinking. Preoccupation with own thinking at this stage, often leads to adolescent's assumption that everyone sees things in a like manner (See also Appendix E, young adult.) |

| Linguistic | Affective and social | Psychosexual | Concepts of life and death |
|---|---|---|---|
| Bubble-blowing, babbling<br><br>First words<br><br>Understanding of sentences<br><br>Says simple sentences<br><br>Uses 40 words and understands 250<br><br>Uses plurals | Mother–infant bonding: initially infant does not experience self as separate from others, especially mother (normal autism). With smiling and play, infant begins to separate though mother seen as extension of self (provides care or frustrates—symbiotic stage). Father–infant bonding; stranger anxiety (strongest at 8 mos.); early sibling relations. Finally, with decreasing separation—individuation, child gains a sense of entirely separate being; increased independence from mother though vacillating between independent functioning and reattachment; separation anxiety. | Establishment of a primary gender identity as boy or girl dependent on assignment at birth (phenotype) and social response of family | Studies indicate perception of differences between sleeping and waking may represent early development of appreciation of being and nonbeing.<br><br>Death is thought to be understood as separation from parents; loss of parents' comfort. |
| Says full sentences with primitive verb forms<br><br>Demonstrates ability to communicate by language out- | "True socialization"—interaction with close and extended family; continued dependency on parents, but begins striving toward autonomy; bathes self; helps a little at household tasks; nursery school involvement (separation issues); control of anger; active | Acquisition of primary sex role identity (masculine or feminine behaviors) through adoption of same or opposite-sex parent as | Expansion of death concept to include loss of loving and protective object.<br><br>Death is seen as temporary departure, hence reversible; child sometimes ex- |

| | | | |
|---|---|---|---|
| side family (decrease in idiosyncratic expressions); early reading and writing | fantasy play, imitation, and role modeling<br>Beginning to play competitive games | a role model in play<br>Preoccupation with adequacy of body for role<br>Foundations laid for sense of sexual body image<br>Masturbation | hibits thoughts that indicate that he or she believes it is possible to come back to life (magical thinking).<br>Appreciation of removal from one kind of physical existence to another (e.g., angels in heaven) is gained by latter part of period. |
| Enriched vocabulary and sophisticated grammatical manipulations; reading; pleasure in word games and verbal skills, spoken as well as written (acquisition of second language difficult after age 10) | Formal school and separation from mother and home; begins to tell time to quarter hour<br>Growing peer relationships with same and opposite-sex friends<br>Sharing games at home and school<br>Conformity to social rules: competition, groundwork for self-esteem and self-acceptance | Latency (see Freud and Erikson)<br><br>Response to beginning development of secondary sexual characteristics—physical (girls) | Latency-age child begins to understand death as permanent, nonreversible, contributing to fears of mutilation and physical injury.<br>Death is personified (e.g., "bogey man").<br>Death is associated with grief for anticipated separation from loved ones; and fear when seen as punishment for wrong acts. |
| (Damage to language centers after age 12 commonly results in communication deficits.) Acquisition of complex propositional grammar constructions; enjoyment of books, magazines, newspapers; writes lengthy papers | Capable of full self-care; peer group conformity; increasing independence from parents; growth toward autonomous self; peak athletic and growing academic achievement; involvement with chores and jobs; consolidation of self-image and reevaluation of societal norms and values; formulation of love concepts and search for intimacy; sexual experimentation and establishment of sexual orientation; establishment of control over emotions. | Adjustment to adult sexual role: pubertal development of internal and external genitalia results in reevaluation of sexual self-concept and image; masturbation, heterosexual experimentation and homosexual experiences occur.<br>Conflicts with resolution of sexual orientation | Death comes to be recognized as a final and irrevocable act, yet is accompanied by disbelief in the possibility of one's personal death(adolescent egocentricity). |

**Appendix B.** Childhood development: Life stage models

| Age stage | Erikson | S. Freud | A. Freud |
|---|---|---|---|
| *Birth–2 Years: Infancy to toddler* | *Basic Trust versus Mistrust (birth–1)*: Dependent on the quality of care he or she receives, the child comes to recognize the level of consistency of response to outer providers as well as internal stimuli leading him or her to feel trust (or mistrust) and to have a sense of rudimentary ego identity, an early appreciation that people will come to respond to him or her in a certain fashion and he or she will be able to meet their expectations. Trust enables a child to let mother go (or not) because her return is reliable.<br><br>The key word for this period is hope. | *Oral*: Child is entirely dependent on mother; primary gratification is oral (feeding, sucking).<br><br>Attitudes of basic trust in the environment are developed. | *Separation to Individuation* |
| | *Autonomy versus Shame and Doubt (1–3)*: Characteristic of this period is the child's struggle to master and control his or her internal and external environment; degree of success here leads to depth of autonomy. Effort is to attain independence without loss of self-esteem; need for protectors to be firm to guard against potential anarchy of child's inability in his or her exuberance to discriminate or to discern when to hold on or to let go. Failure at mastering these tasks leads to shame and doubt.<br><br>The key words for this period are self-control and willpower. | *Anal*: Child's attention turns to excretion, which is also a source of pleasure. This corresponds to an age at which environmental demands are beginning to be made on the child, particularly toilet training. Attitudes toward authority figures begin to be formed. Attitudes of ambivalence and stubbornness are predominant. | |
| *3–5 Years: Early childhood* | *Initiative versus Guilt*: Child at this stage is involved in undertaking, planning, and attacking tasks. Primitive morality is manifested in struggle with sense of | *Phallic* (Oedipal): Child is increasingly interested in sex differences; opposite-sex attachment is pronounced with | *Dependency to Independence* |

anxiety about disruption of relationship with same-sex parent (castration anxiety in boys, penis envy in girls)

guilt (superego) over impulsive goals or acts initiated in exuberance. Growth is initiated by facility for getting around (nursery school). This is a time of sibling rivalries and castration complexes.

The key words for this period are purpose and direction.

*Autonomous Play to Work Role*

*6–11 Years: Middle childhood latency*

*Latency:* Successful positive identification with same-sex parent and internalization of parental values to form conscience achieved in prior stage enable child to relegate sexual impulses to lesser emphasis and increase concern with mastery of external environment: school, hobbies, sports, peers.

*Industry versus Inferiority:* Mastery of school life and harnessing exuberance of earlier period to fit laws of impersonal realm (3 *R*'s) are goals of this stage. Recognition is gained by producing things. Cultural and social identity is acquired. Mastery of this stage can be hindered if child despairs of adequacy of personal skills, tools or status among peers.

The key word for this period is competence.

*12–18 Years: Adolescence*

*Genital:* Individual's sexuality reawakens and is directed toward heterosexual union and reproduction; procreative functions are emphasis of this and later ages.

*Identity versus Role Confusion:* Fruition of ego identity; identity formation or development of self; discovery of self as having continuity between how one views oneself and one's personal meaning for others from past to present; growth of sexual identity; search for young love; creation of occupational identity. Doubts or sense of differentness can lead to role confusion sexually, socially, and culturally.

The key words for this period are devotion and fidelity to principle(s) and persons.

Levinson

*Early Adult Transition (17–22):* Questioning of the nature of adult world and one's place in it; key relationships are reappraised, modified, terminated and self is reevaluated in context of these changes; consolidation of initial adult identity and testing of some choices for adult living.

757

**Appendix C.** Childhood development: Age stage-related disruption of illness

| Age stage | 1. Altered interpersonal relationships | 2. Dependence–independence issues | 3. Achievement disruptions | 4. Body–sexual image and integrity | 5. Existential issues |
|---|---|---|---|---|---|
| *Birth–2 Years: Infant to toddler* | Separation from family; altered family interactions leading infant to become withdrawn, apathetic, helpless<br><br>Inconsistent caregiving and caregivers<br><br>Exaggeration of stranger anxiety; parental sense of helplessness and guilt; toddler may experience acute separation anxiety | Unexpected handling (e.g., forced feedings, painful procedures) causing helpless feelings, fears, inconsistent daily routines<br><br>Sense of mistrust | Potential for disruption, regression, and/or retardation in psychomotor, emotional, and social growth; setbacks in maintenance or achievement of age-specific milestones (e.g., coordination, locomotion, speech) | Failure to develop sense of separateness from "external" happenings<br><br>Lack of body image apart from that of environment | Parental and sibling confrontation with uncertainty and possible death of infant; inability to let go of dying child<br><br>↔<br><br>↔ |
| *3–5 Years: Early childhood* | Parental conflict about caretaking; other children at home demand attention; sibling anger or depression in face of brother's or sister's illness and diverted focus of attention; exacerbation of preexisting parental marital discord; abandonment or withdrawal of one or both parents from ill child and/or each other | Constraints on independence and first efforts at autonomy precipitating anger, depression, withdrawal | Occasional loss of recently acquired skills and motor functions (e.g., bowel control) and/or apparent precocious maturity (e.g., accelerated speech development and apparent emotional "supermaturity") | Alterations through disease or treatment of nascent body image; threat to fragile self-esteem and early sex role identity; fear of physical harm | Death perceived as separation from parents; may precipitate acute anxiety and withdrawal in ill child; frequent fears of abandonment |

758

| | | | | |
|---|---|---|---|---|
| *6–11 Years: Middle childhood and latency* | Isolation from peers; (see also problems in younger age groups above); fear of being rejected by parents, especially during hospitalization periods; problems of "reentry" upon discharge | Parental overprotection and/or child fearful of actions (overdependency); fear of inability to cope; loss of a sense of mastery that may lead to ego and self-image-threatening regression | School disruption (absence, poor performance); loss of sense of competence; academic and social position compromised; increased fears of inadequacy leading to behavior problems (e.g., acting out, overdependency, school phobias); threat to "reputation," "stigmatization" | Mutilation anxiety; fears of painful procedures (esp. surgery and anesthesia); increased shyness and embarrassment; concerns regarding physical inadequacy; fantasies in response to intrusive procedures, of being punished, attacked, disfigured, mutilated (e.g., EEG will turn me into Frankenstein) | Concerns with illness as a punishment for misdeed or "bad" thoughts; fear of own actions causing disease or recurrence or death; nightmares of "monster" taking one away from family; concrete fears of death (being buried alive); disquiet about family circle in his or her absence |
| Threatened loss of or alteration in role in family or peer group and school | | | | |
| *12–18 Years: Adolescence* | Isolation from supportive peer group; concern for social isolation <br><br> Disruption in ability for an intimate relationship with sexual object | Increased dependency on parents and feelings of helplessness; loss of control (castration anxiety) often leading to alienation, distrust, and uncooperativeness; overprotection of parents; anger, acting out, uncooperative; loss of privacy; concerns about body disintegration and "insanity" | Perception of self as diminished in value and worth; fears of inability to fulfill ambitions; shame; sports and academic status jeopardized or lost | Shyness and embarrassment about body exposure; deviation from crucial peer conformity; delay of physical growth and sexual maturation; fears of being somehow "dirty"; threat to nascent sexuality (masturbation associated with weakness, guilt or shame); loss of adolescent sense of physical invulnerability | Fears of recurrence seen as punishment of self (masturbation guilt) or punishing others (form of noncompliance) or punishment by God; search for life meaning; survival associated with guilt and/or special purpose in life; faltering belief in immortality; anguish at not living to "grow up"; anxiety |

**Appendix D.**  Childhood development: Illness-related interventions by age stage

| Age stage | Theme and Intervention |
|---|---|
| *Birth–2 Years: Infancy to toddler* | *Parents* |
| | 1. Support maximal family contact: encourage participation in infant's hospital care with flexible visiting privileges; sleep-in and home-like housing arrangements (e.g., Ronald McDonald); maintain consistent caretakers. Evaluate resources of family unit (emotional, social, financial). Monitor parental and sibling reactions: provide counseling for family members who exhibit disturbed responses in relation to ill infant or toddler (irrational guilt, inappropriate anger). |
| | 2. Maintain consistent caretaking. |
| | 3. Provide social, physical, and play stimulation (holding, cuddling, talking, playing); special focus on using motor and sensory skills. |
| | 4. Keep procedures to a minimum; facilitate play and manipulation of environment by the child and his or her body. |
| | 5. Mobilize supports from religious affiliation; encourage emotional "working through" of threatened or actual loss; visit with parents and siblings in bereavement period. |
| *3–5 Years: Early childhood* | *Play* |
| | 1. (See item 1 above); group meetings for education and support with staff (doctors, nurses, mental health professionals). Facilitate interaction with parents of other ill children, and use of "veteran parents." Medical and psychological support for families who maintain a critically ill child at home. |
| | 2. Establish trusting relationship with child *before* arduous procedures; rehearsal of medical procedures through play (injections, anesthesia). Encourage parents to maintain as normal as possible a growing experience (limit need to overindulge); encourage social autonomy appropriate for age. |
| | 3. Attention to child's "real" level of understanding and capabilities or limitations. Maintain motor development and skills; foster peer play groups. |
| | 4. Discuss body changes with child and family (cushingoid face, baldness, increased appetite, fatigability) and possible responses of others (esp. peers and family, siblings). Minimize sense of looking or feeling "different" from peers. |
| | 5. Reassure child he or she will not be abandoned. Work with parents' own fears, anger, guilt, sadness regarding possible death and loss (see item 5 above). |

*Milieu*

6–11 Years: Middle childhood and latency

1. (See item 1 above for both younger age groups). Foster peer interaction in and out of hospital, play groups, therapeutic play sessions. Maintain role in family in hospital (visits, pets, telephone calls, videotapes, cassettes) and at home (give former chores, responsibilities).

2. Help parents to support child while still setting limits and boundaries. Describe and rehearse with child anticipated procedures and consequences; establish trust. Understand meaning of illness for individual child. Enlist child's cooperation through understanding reasons for treatment. Prehospitalization–treatment teaching valuable especially with this age group. Enlist parents' aid in assessing child's coping level.

3. Minimize absenteeism, provide tutoring as necessary; discuss with teacher and classmates special needs of student. Provide tasks that can be mastered. Facilitate peer interaction on ward and appropriate competitive games and/or hobbies.

4. Respect child's need for privacy (see also item 4 above for both younger age groups).

5. Minimize fantasies about cause of illness; talk about fears and nightmares. Discuss child's concepts about life after death. Open discussion of peer patient's death, no secrets. Respond to child's concern about family life without him or her.

*Peers*

12–18 Years: Adolescence

1. Use peer support groups and "veteran patient" to model effective coping strategies. Family counseling regarding overpassivity and regression issues.

2. Respect need for privacy both physically and emotionally. Avoid any signs of secrecy or dishonesty. Encourage self-care and as much autonomy as possible. Decisions made *with* adolescent *not* parents alone (mutual respect, confidence, honesty).

3. Encourage gradual return to prior activities or when not possible, explore new areas of expertise or mastery (e.g., intellectual pursuits). Emphasis in this age on physician as "ego-idea" and role model. Strive for fullest return to premorbid abilities with as near normal school attendance as possible (include extracurricular activities). Reinforce self-esteem through review of prior accomplishments (vs. emphasis on future and present limitations).

4. Provide explanations regarding meaning of delays in maturation and explore ways of looking normal. Counseling about self and sexual image, especially with veteran peers.

5. "Dose" anxiety. Foster expression of fears and means of coping with them. Airing of concerns regarding illness as shameful or a weakness. Reassurance about ability to take control of their lives and find meaning. Open communications between staff and parents regarding outcomes of illness. Counseling regarding irrational fears of punishment, conflicts of childhood, reasonable expectations of self, positive realistic appraisal of achievements.

**Appendix E.** Adult development

| Age stage | Physical | Cognitive |
|---|---|---|
| *19–30 Years: Young adult* | Peak cardiovascular work performance; physically and sexually mature adult body<br><br>Peak sexual and reproductive activity<br><br>Pregnancy changes in female | (see also appendix A, adolescence.)<br>Because reflexive thinking constitutes a new and unique experience, the person is apt to think that he or she is the first to experience ideas of this nature despite historical evolution of thought.<br><br>One of the tasks of the adult is to overcome the ego-centristic thinking experienced in adolescence and in early adulthood. Ability to deal with more and more subjects on the formal operational level (logical reasoning) is extended. |
| *31–45 Years: Mature adult* | Decrease in bone density<br><br>Limited regeneration of cartilage in joints leading to increases in arthritic complaints<br><br>Acquired obesity<br><br>Linear decrease in functioning capacity of organs<br><br>Presbyopia | Peak of intellectual ability |
| *46–65 Years: Mature adult* | Redistribution of fatty deposits; skin changes; beginning loss of musculoskeletal integrity; decrements in bone density and mass<br><br>Changing hormonal patterns; menopause or climacteric<br><br>Trend toward weight increase despite decrease in body mass; gradual vertebral compression | Slow decrease in intellectual acumen, being more pronounced on tasks involving sensorimotor and visual perception skills, which are more susceptible to interference by normal aging processes (e.g., poorer eyesight, slower reflex times) |
| *66+ Years: Aging adult* | Decrease in functional capacity of organ systems: basal metabolic rate, cardiac index, respiratory capacity, renal filtration rate<br><br>Less energy reserve; decrease in activity; decline in capacity for physical work<br><br>Sharp increase in prevalence of chronic diseases and metabolic dysfunctions<br><br>Senescence (varying in deficit) | Occasionally progressive memory loss |

*continued*

**Appendix E.** *continued*

| Linguistic | Affective and social | Psychosexual | Concepts of life and death |
|---|---|---|---|
| Perfection of speaking and writing skills for more formal settings | Formalization of personal values and goals: work, marriage, family, avocations<br><br>Completing educational goals (advanced degrees); striving for career and work goals<br><br>Commitment to another person in marriage and movement toward parental roles<br><br>Adjustment to parenthood and role with small children | Establishment of a relationship with appropriate sexual partner with potential for parenthood and/or nurturing<br><br>Reconciliation of sexual identity with work and career goals<br><br>Response to changes in psychosexual image resulting from parenthood<br><br>Assumption of family and childrearing roles | Death viewed as universal and natural end point of physical life |
| | (Establishment of family—late)<br><br>Childrearing<br><br>Readjustment of ties to growing children and older parents<br><br>Definition of work roles; maintenance of home; striving toward job recognition and upward mobility<br><br>Stabilization of personal identity | Optimal sexual life | (Anticipation of and preparation for parental death) |
| | Adjustment to growing children and children as adults: "empty nest" | Redefinition of sexual role: response to | Change in time perspective leads to individu- |

al's awareness of being on the upper half of the age curve: time perceived as "years left" versus "years since birth"; personalization and mental rehearsing for death: men with heart attacks; women with widowhood

Realistic assessment of life expectancy

Concerns for dying more than for death itself

menopause and male climacteric—male moves from active to more passive mode of mastery, becomes more nurturant, while women increase their instrumental and assertive roles (role-reversal shift)

More global, androgynous perspective on sex role adopted

Normal "unisex" of later life

Four-generational perspective

New family roles and reclaimed intimacy with readjustment of relationships between spouses; nurturance of grandchildren; responsibility as a guide and mentor to young associates; assumption of "parent-caring"; heightened introspection and reflection; "stock taking"; increased sense of physical vulnerability—"body monitoring"

Retirement: yielding of authority or status; life review of successes and failures; focus on legacy rituals

Adaptation to aging process; preoccupation with fears of dependency and physical and mental deterioration

Limitations on abilities, income, and mobility; restriction of habitual contacts and potentially of sense of purpose; accommodation to loss of spouse, siblings, family, and peers

Shift from sense of controlling, to yielding to environment's demands; sense of wisdom, "knowing it all"; affectional love dominant over physical love

Beginning disengagement? "Adaptational paranoia" or combative quality seen sometimes as a survival asset

(Occasionally inability to remember common words or referents)

**Appendix F.** Adult development: Life stage models

| Age stage | Erikson | Levinson |
|---|---|---|
| *19–30 Years:*<br>*Young adult* | *Intimacy versus Isolation*: Emotional and physical commitment to social, educational, career affiliations, and partnerships and the willingness to abide by the constraints of these relationships despite some sacrifices and compromises<br><br>Excessive fear of loss of personal identity or rejection can lead to avoidance of the above relationships and result in isolation and self-absorption<br><br>Attainment of mature sexual relationships<br><br>Key word for this period is love.<br><br>(Vaillant: career consolidation vs. self-absorption) | *Youth*: Quest for comfortable fit between self and society and preparation of script for one's life (see also Appendix B, early adult transition)<br><br>*Entering the Adult World* (22–28): First adult life structure: exploration of adult life possibilities and alternatives in context of trying to create a stable life structure; growing new roots while striving for achievement; investing in others yet achieving individuation<br><br>*Age 30 Transition* (28–30): Changing first life structure: life goals, structure, become more "for real"; time to work with flaws and limitations of first adult structure and create basis for more satisfactory structure (reform vs. revolution) |
| *31–45 Years:*<br>*Mature adult* | *Generativity versus Stagnation* (>40): Concern in establishing and guiding the next generation (productivity, creativity); may be in terms of one's own family and/or the younger generation of the culture at large<br><br>Key words for the period are production and care.<br><br>(Vaillant: keepers of meaning vs. rigidity) | *Settling Down* (33–40): Second adult life structure: efforts toward establishing a niche in society and working at "making it"; striving toward sense of a future, "becoming one's own person"; investment in major life aspects as they are important (work, family, friendship, etc.); making self heard, becoming more senior in one's world<br><br>*Midlife Transition* (40–45): Termination of early adulthood and initiation of middle adulthood |

Questioning every aspect of life: searching for optimum expression of desires, aspirations, talents, values; neglected parts of self seeking expression; intentionality

*Entering Middle Adulthood* (45–50): Changes in certain crucial aspects of life, either dramatic (divorce, change of profession) or subtle (increase or decrease in satisfaction and creativity);

Shift from outer-world to inner-world of orientation, "interiority"

Provides an initial basis for life in a new era

*Age 50 Transition* (50–55): Mid-era period for modifying, perhaps improving middle-adult structure; "senior" members of one's own world; responsibility for one's own and work of others—new generation; culmination of middle adulthood (55–60)

*Late Adult Transition* (60–65): Boundary period between middle and late adulthood; preparing for next life era; putting store of memories in order: dramatizing some, seeking consistency in others; reworking of past by life review; (creation of late, third-fourth, adult life structure?)

| | |
|---|---|
| *46–65 Years: Older adult* | Failure to attain a sense of producing and creating can lead to personal impoverishment, pseudointimacy, and premature disengagement and excessive dependence. |
| | *Ego Integrity versus Despair* (>60): This stage is characterized by one who "has taken care of things and people and has adapted himself to the triumphs and disappointments adherent to being the originator of or the generator of products and ideas." |
| *66+ Years: Aging adult* | There is a sense of dignity of life-style and a genuine feeling of the meaningfulness of one's life; emotional integration is apparent as well as a new and different love of parents |
| | Others at this stage may feel despair about accomplishments or meaningfulness, leading to a fear of death |
| | Key word for this era is wisdom. |

Vaillant, G.E. and E. Milofsky (1980). Natural history of male psychological health. IX. Empirical evidence for Erikson's model of the life cycle. *Am. J. Psychiatry* 137:1348–1359.

**Appendix G.   Adult development: age stage-related disruptions of illness**

| Age stage | 1. Altered interpersonal relationships | 2. Dependence–independence issues | 3. Achievement disruptions | 4. Body-sexual image and integrity | 5. Existential issues |
|---|---|---|---|---|---|
| *19–30 Years:*<br>*Young adult* | Fear and guilt about close personal ties; tendency toward isolation and self-absorption; previously established relationships strained by illness. Patient and family feel stigmatized by illness; rejection of patient by family, friends, and society due to illness, disruption of daily routines and usual role; concern for children growing up without one parent | Concern about increased dependency on others (family, friends, co-workers; new and unexpected dependency on health care system (anger: non-compliance); over-protection by family or excessive dependency by patient | Uncertainty in planning future; concern for performance of and ability to meet achievement goals; confrontation with delay in achieving milestones or giving up hoped-for level of performance for physical, social, or emotional reasons | Decreased sense of attractiveness to others and in particular to sexual partners due to site of cancer and/or treatment effects (e.g., hair loss, scarring); lowered libido; impaired self-esteem regarding sexuality (sterility, infertility, impotence); any physical symptom feared as possible metastases | Finality of death; threat to personal identity and continuity of generations (especially if patient is an only child or unmarried) |
| *31–45 Years:*<br>*Mature adult* | Absence from family circle (partners, children); fears of abandonment in patient or partner; crisis of illness strains faltering relations; what to tell aging parents; fears of or real social isolation related to "communicability" of cancer; regrets about leaving partner or children with concern for survivors (social, financial, educational) | Dilemma of role reversals caused by illness (esp. increased male dependency); overdependency giving in to illness; overcompensation (counterphobic behavior)—too excessive and/or early return to physical or work activity | Job interruption; anxiety about ability to maintain or achieve promotion and confrontation with unfulfillable life goals; worry about long-term financial commitments (child education, business, mortgages, loans) | (See above regarding lack of libido, impotence); extant sexual problems exacerbated by illness; premature loss of reproductive ability. Illness accentuates body vulnerability experienced with aging: minor physical symptoms of aging interpreted as return or progression of disease; fears about contagion | Disruption of developed identity<br><br>Religious concerns: questioning about God's purpose; concerns about afterlife; concern about doubts and faltering faith |
| *46–65 Years:*<br>*Older adult* | Concern for welfare of surviving parents; regret for possible loss | Excessive bad feelings about having to be "cared for"; concerns | Anger, frustration with possible enforced early retirement: sense of | Acceleration (real or imagined) of aging due to effects of disease or | Depression associated with less denial of death as outcome of |

| | 66+ Years: *Aging adult* |
|---|---|
| illness; heightening of introspection and reflection characteristic of age period leading to potential despair about one's accomplishments and hence meaningfulness of one's life | Concerns for "how one will die" (pain, disability); additive effect of illness to multiple life losses—grief (bereavement overload); sudden acceleration of need for constructive life review; remorse, sense of inability to "contribute"—loss of personal dignity; despair; urgency to settle relationship to religion |
| treatment; threat to sense of physical vulnerability; concern about sexual image already threatened by physical changes of aging; acute embarrassment and demoralization with alopecia, seen esp. in women; distress concerning feminization effects of female hormones in men (prostate cancer—female habitus, loss of libido, breast development), masculinizing effect of hormonal treatment in women (breast cancer—hirsute face, deep voice, altered libido) | Inability to carry out personal hygiene; compounding of common diseases of aging by cancer (e.g., blindness, deafness, heart disease); greater difficulty perceiving and assimilating complex information (e.g., pill schedules); increased susceptibility to complications of illness: lower tolerance to lung side effects, greater risk of CNS dysfunction related to treatment. |
| being cheated out of "healthy" retirement; disappointment about curtailment of potential achievements (esp. second career); concerns about loss of emotionally significant enterprise(s)—inability to maintain business and home | Anxiety about dissolution of planned financial security for self and survivors; anger for loss of enjoyment in later life (pursuit of avocations, relaxing, traveling) |
| about becoming an invalid, dependent on others for physical care (esp. one's children); threat to ability to live alone and sustain independence; financial burden on others; concerns about ability to meet illness costs on fixed income | Fears of being an invalid and a burden to others particularly children; or opposite, unnecessary dependency and giving up to illness; shame about having to ask for help (esp. about incontinence) |
| of opportunity to know and nurture grandchildren; inability to maintain adequate level of social life; confrontation with chronically unhappy marriage or social relations; conflict about changing nature of interactions | Isolation increased; fewer physical, social, and emotional resources; less adaptability to stresses of unfamiliar environments and treatments; suspiciousness about treatment and staff; fears of abandonment by staff, family, friends, and healthy spouse; diminished ability to nurture (work, cook, sew) |

**Appendix H.** Adult development: Illness-related interventions by age stage*

| Age stage | Theme and intervention |
|---|---|
| *19–30 Years:* Young adult | *Counseling* |
| | 1. Hospital and home family visits; encourage role functions that can be maintained (e.g., decision making). Guidance and support in what information about illness should or needs to be given to children, parents, friends, and colleagues. Assess key relationships with person sharing illness. Counseling regarding attitudes, beliefs, and feelings about cancer; planning for family security (wills, substitute caregivers). |
| | 2. Early assessment of rehabilitative potentials to prevent the fixation of maladaptive responses (e.g., overdependency, poor motivation, unrealistic expectations and efforts). |
| | 3. Help in redefining life goals after illness; encourage clarification of job security (e.g., amount of sick leave entitlement, absence, disability); review and refinancing of liabilities and obligations. |
| | 4. Appendix D, item 4, Adolescence. Explore meaning of illness to individual's sense of self-worth and future. Adapt sex counseling therapies to special problems and needs (e.g., inability to have usual form of intercourse due to surgical ablations). |
| | 5. Offer pastoral counseling. |
| *31–45 Years:* Mature adult | *Interpersonal Relations* |
| | 1. Maintain normal patterns of home life and ADL; foster visits by family, friends, and peers; counsel about interpersonal relations. Provide groups for patients and/or significant others to deal with shared feelings about illness and goals, and negative information, attitudes about cancer. Financial planning for illness and decreased income; homemaker as necessary. Communicate with children about parental illness with monitoring of their response and opportunity to visit parent. |
| | 2. Maximal self-care. Concrete rehabilitation goals involving the patient in his or her own care and striving for as normal as possible living and working conditions. Patient encouraged to feel a partner in care with physician. "Veteran patient" counseling. |
| | 3. Facilitate return to home, school, job as quickly as possible with rehabilitation and retraining as necessary. Counseling to adjust to goal limitations. |
| | 4. Support normal appearance and function (e.g., wigs, prostheses, clothes, physical retraining such as esophageal speech); sex counseling for patient and/or couple (address special needs: sperm banking, penile prostheses, adoption advice); use of veteran patient models (esp. with breast, GI, GU, GYN patients). Reassurance for anxiety about recurrent disease through physical examinations. |
| | 5. Guide search for meaning to past and remaining life, death, and after death. |

## Personal Integrity

**46–65 Years:**
**Older adult**

1. Social work consultation regarding welfare of family and patient; evaluate social support systems and develop alternative resources where lacking. Consider conjoint or personal therapy to deal with conflicts in context of disease and death.

2. Institute rehabilitative measures necessary to achieve maximal independence: provide mechanical aids for ADL. Encourage patient to tolerate dependency on others when required. Explore available financial benefits and alternatives for nursing care.

3. Counseling focuses on grief associated with loss of hoped-for life-style and goals; realistic financial planning.

4. *Special* attention to well-fitted and functional prostheses. Counseling must deal with practical management of alterations in physical appearance and body functions (e.g., baldness, colostomy); focus on good and regular personal hygiene. Refer for psychiatric evaluation: severe depressive symptoms. Explanation about nature of side effects of treatment and reassurance about sexual identity despite cross-sexualizing changes.

5. Self-esteem building life review. Reinforce adaptive coping mechanisms and behaviors. Philosophical and religious meaning of life and death explored.

## Social Support

**66+ Years:**
**Aging adult**

1. Maintain and reestablish or develop social support network (religious, social, familial). Stress orientation to new environments and treatments. Stress continuity of care by trusted and familiar staff. Support shared activities and affectional ties with family and friends.

2. Strive for level of care that does not exceed need. Explore home or alternative care options (home visits, "Meals-on-Wheels," nursing home, hospice). Discuss feelings about dependency and helplessness.

3. (see also item 3 in older adult category). Plan best use of available financial assets. Tap community financial aid resources (e.g., Medicare, ACS). Explore meaningful hobbies and recreation.

4. Plan daily routine with help as needed (bathing, etc.). Obtain aids for sensory losses (hearing aid, glasses, large-print news, talking books). Aid time-and-place orientation (large clocks, calendars, night-lights). Encourage consistent caregivers and support of family members for sense of security. Close monitoring for complications of illness and treatment.

5. Allow discussion if desired, and plans about death, funeral, and burial. Arrange visit with clergy or chaplain. Foster positive review of past life and achievements. Supportive understanding of personal and physical losses.

---

*Abbreviations: ADL, activities of daily living; GI, gastrointestinal; GU, genitourinary; GYN, gynecological.

# Index